Textbook of Community Medicine

Preventive and Social Medicine

Fifth Edition

Key Features of the Fifth Edition

Unique features: The fifth edition updates all the chapters and incorporates recent developments in public health such as Mother and child tracking system, death review, India Newborn Action Plan (INAP), operational guidelines for injection vitamin K prophylaxis at birth, kangaroo mother care, use of gentamicin by ANMs for management of sepsis under specific conditions, use of antenatal corticosteroids in pre-term labour (under specific conditions by ANMs), reproductive maternal, newborn, child and adolescent health (RMNCH + A), Rashtriya Bal Swasthya Karyakram, Rashtriya Kishor Swasthya Karyakram (National Adolescent Health Programme), adverse events following immunization, National Urban Health Mission, Multi-year Strategic Plan 2013–17 for universal immunization programme, National Drug Policy on Malaria 2013, National Policy on Mental Health 2014, Integrated Biological and Behavioural Surveillance in HIV, Ebola and Zika virus disease, epidemiological basis of National Health Programmes, National Health Policy 2015 (draft). National Oral Health Programme, National Programme for Prevention and Management of Burn Injuries, National Iron + Initiative, WHO Global Action Plan and Monitoring Framework for Prevention and Control of Non-communicable Diseases, besides account of premature deaths in India, and national deworming day, human resources (workforce) in health care delivery, strategies to be followed in polio-free India, Introduction of IPV and switch from tOPV to bOPV and rotavirus vaccine besides sustainable development goals NFHS-4 and HMIS version 1.1.6. International Conference on Population and Development (IPCD) and Beti Bachao Beti Padhao.

Core domains of community medicine (social and preventive medicine/public health) are epidemiology and biostatistics, health management, health policies, national health programmes and legislations, behavioural and management sciences including health communication and applied nutrition.

Teaching and training programmes of undergraduates/postgraduates and orientation of public health managers/practitioners must primarily focus on these core domains with specific learning objectives. In Indian context human behaviour, environments, organized health services and nutrition are the key determinants of 'health', to achieve "Health in All" remain a cherished goal. Accordingly this textbook on community medicine purposely focuses on behavioural and managerial sciences—community organization and participation, leadership and motivation, health communication/behaviour change communication in first four chapters, which in fact are the basis/foundations of epidemiology and health management and biostatistics, environments and applied nutrition. Case studies in social and behavioural sciences (clinical-social case review), reproductive maternal and child health, environmental health, applied nutrition, and national health programmes enriches the learning of bio-behavioural and health managerial sciences. health education/behaviour change communication, community participation, and environmental sanitation (environment modification/manipulation) which form an integral part of all national health programmes and policies, on communicable, non-communicable, diseases, reproductive, maternal and child health, have been presented in an integrated manner rather than focussing on individual isolated disease entity, to reinforce the learning of community medicine.

Besides the chapter on applied epidemiology, the science of epidemiology has been given its rightful place/slot in all the national health programmes to reinforce the learning of epidemiology and biostatistics. health management chapter focuses on managerial function which are to be read in combination with behavioural and managerial sciences (first four chapters) for better comprehension and application. Human resources in health system consume over 70% of the budget, their role in health care delivery system is critical. Involvement of NGOs/Private practitioners and specialists is essential to fill the gap in human resources. This component has been dealt to a desirable extent. System approach in health care delivery system has been highlighted. Public health practitioners working at district, state, CHC, PHC as also health volunteers, PRIs must be involved in training/teaching programmes to make it more vibrant, viable and sustainable, going beyond the prescription of MCI. This textbook gives this message very clearly, and forcefully says that over 80% teaching/training should be based in the community setting. Sequential and integrated presentation of comprehensive text material enhances the learning of community medicine, which no other textbook could do so in such a comprehensive manner.

Feedback and comments received from learned and experienced teachers like Director Professor Dr DK Taneja, Late Prof AK Sharma, Late Prof RK Sachar, Director Prof Suneela Garg, Prof Lahiri, Prof Dominic Misquich, Prof Dara S Amar, Prof MK Sudershan, Prof Rajesh Kumar, Prof Sandeep Kumar Ray, Prof SC Mohapatra, have been included in appropriate chapters to make the book more comprehensive and learner-friendly.

Part I

Part I of this comprehensive textbook on community medicine covers basic sciences related to the discipline of community medicine—application of social and behavioural sciences, clinicosocial case review, pedagogy, organization behaviour, leadership, motivation, group dynamics, behaviour change communication, counseling in health and disease, health economics, concept of health and disease, health policy and goals, demography and population problem, applied nutrition, environmental health, epidemiology and its application, and applied biostatistics, medical entomology and medical genetics. The subject of epidemiology is covered in chapters on epidemiology and its application in epidemiology of CCD and NCD and research methodology, applied statistics and national health programmes, sub-centre action plan, planning, monitoring and evaluation of health systems. The reproductive and child health, policy and programmes in India has been intentionally linked with demography and population problem and included in this part for the purpose of continuity and sequential learning. Generally, Part I conforms to the Paper 1 in theory, excluding maternal and child health. The demarcation of theory papers to Paper 1 and Paper 2 varies from university to university but generally it covers the above mentioned areas.

Part II

Part II of the text covers epidemiology of communicable and non-communicable diseases, national health programmes, health management—health care delivery system, health management functions—planning, monitoring and evaluation of services/programmes, health care financing and hospital statistics. It also incorporates occupational health, geriatrics, disaster management, hospital waste management, research and medical ethics and international health regulations apart from international statistical classification of diseases and related health problems (ICD-10). These areas generally form the contents of theory Paper 2 of community medicine which also includes maternal and child health but may differ from university to university.

Textbook of Community Medicine

Preventive and Social Medicine

Fifth Edition

Dr (Brig) Sunder Lal MBBS, DPH, MD

Former

Professor and Head, Department of Social and Preventive Medicine
Pt BD Sharma Postgraduate Institute of Medical Sciences
Rohtak and AIMSR, Bathinda (Punjab)
Professor, Community Medicine at MM University—Mullana (Ambala)
Deputy Director-General, TA (Medical)
Chairman, Board of Studies of Medicine and Allied Sciences, MDU, Rohtak
Member, National Commission on Population, GoI; Consultant, ICDS
Member, National Technical Advisory Group on Immunization and Child Health
Member, Technical Resource Group on Women, Children and ICDS
NSS Programme Officer
Honorary Professor, IMACGP and
President of IAPSM

Adarsh MBBS

Former

Senior Medical Officer, HCMS (I)
Medical Officer-incharge, Postpartum Centre, PGIMS, Rohtak
Medical Officer-incharge, Urban Family Welfare Centre, Rohtak
Urban Health Centre attached with PGIMS, Rohtak

Pankaj MDS

Associate Professor, Department of Public Health Dentistry
Rajasthan Dental College, Jaipur
(Rajasthan)

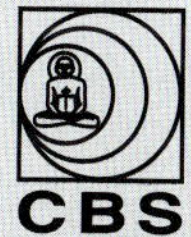

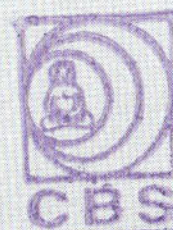

CBS Publishers & Distributors Pvt Ltd

New Delhi • Bengaluru • Chennai • Kochi • Kolkata • Mumbai
Hyderabad • Nagpur • Patna • Pune • Vijayawada

Disclaimer

Science and technology are constantly changing fields. New research and experience broaden the scope of information and knowledge. The authors have tried their best in giving information available to them while preparing the material for this book. Although, all efforts have been made to ensure optimum accuracy of the material, yet it is quite possible some errors might have been left uncorrected. The publisher, printer and the authors will not be held responsible for any inadvertent errors, omissions or inaccuracies.

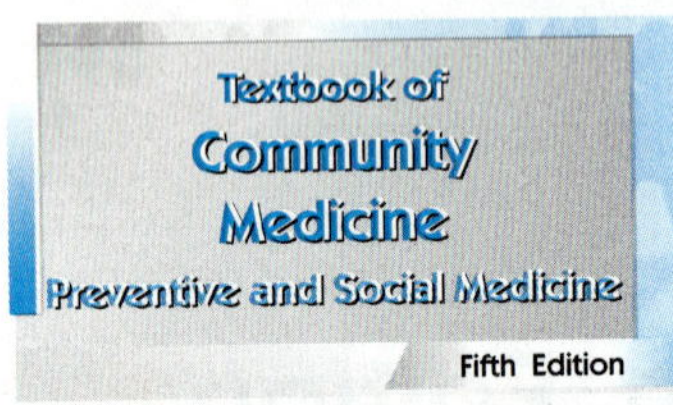

ISBN: 978-93-86217-55-4

Fifth Edition 2017

First Edition 2007
Second Edition 2009
Third Edition 2011
Fourth Edition 2014

Published by Satish Kumar Jain and Produced by Varun Jain for
CBS Publishers & Distributors Pvt Ltd
4819/XI Prahlad Street, 24 Ansari Road, Daryaganj, New Delhi 110 002, India.
Ph: 23289259, 23266861, 23266867 Website: www.cbspd.com
Fax: 011-23243014 e-mail: delhi@cbspd.com; cbspubs@airtelmail.in.
Corporate Office: 204 FIE, Industrial Area, Patparganj, Delhi 110 092
Ph: 4934 4934 Fax: 4934 4935 e-mail: publishing@cbspd.com; publicity@cbspd.com

Branches

- **Bengaluru:** Seema House 2975, 17th Cross, K.R. Road, Banasankari 2nd Stage, Bengaluru 560 070, Karnataka, India
  Ph: +91-80-26771678/79 Fax: +91-80-26771680 e-mail: bangalore@cbspd.com
- **Chennai:** 7, Subbaraya Street, Shenoy Nagar, Chennai 600 030, Tamil Nadu, India
  Ph: +91-44-26680620, 26681266 Fax: +91-44-42032115 e-mail: chennai@cbspd.com
- **Kochi:** Ashana House, No. 39/1904, AM Thomas Road, Valanjambalam, Ernakulam 682 016, Kochi, Kerala, India
  Ph: +91-484-4059061-65 Fax: +91-484-4059065 e-mail: kochi@cbspd.com
- **Kolkata:** 6/B, Ground Floor, Rameswar Shaw Road, Kolkata-700 014, West Bengal, India
  Ph: +91-33-22891126, 22891127, 22891128 e-mail: kolkata@cbspd.com
- **Mumbai:** 83-C, Dr E Moses Road, Worli, Mumbai-400018, Maharashtra, India
  Ph: +91-22-24902340/41 Fax: +91-22-24902342 e-mail: mumbai@cbspd.com

Representatives

- **Hyderabad** 0-9885175004
- **Nagpur** 0-9021734563
- **Patna** 0-9334159340
- **Pune** 0-9623451994
- **Vijayawada** 0-9000660880

Printed at Rashtriya Printers, Dilshad Garden, Delhi, India

Foreword

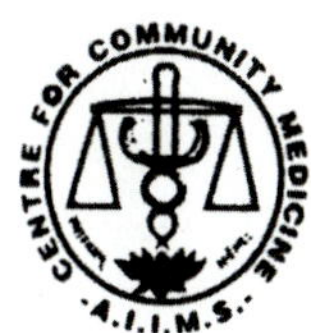

अखिल भारतीय आयुर्विज्ञान संस्थान

ALL INDIA INSTITUTE OF MEDICAL SCIENCES

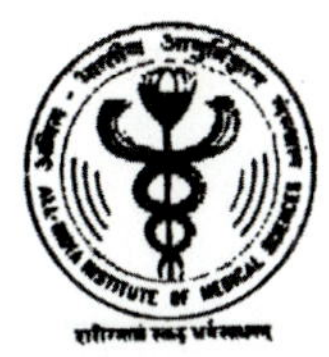

डॉ चन्द्रकान्त एस पांडव
एम बी बी एस, एम डी (एम्स)
एम एम सी (मैक्मास्टर युनिवर्सिटी, कनाडा) एफ ए एम एस
आचार्य एवं विभागाध्यक्ष
सामुदायिक चिकित्सा केन्द्र
अंसारी नगर, नई दिल्ली 110029, भारत
फोन : 91-11-26588522, 26593553
फैक्स : 91-11-26588522

Dr. Chandrakant S. Pandav
MBBS, MD (AIIMS)
M.Sc. (McMaster Univ. Canada), FAMS
Professor and Head
Center for Community Medicine
Ansari Nagar, New Delhi-110029, India
Phone: 91-11-26588522, 26593553 Fax: 91-11-26588522
E-mail : cpandav@iqplusin.org.cpandav@indiatimes.com

It is a matter of great privilege for me to write the Foreword of the Fifth Edition of *Textbook of Community Medicine* by Prof (Dr) Sunder Lal and coauthors (Dr Adarsh and Dr Pankaj). It is a unique book that not only imparts theoretical concepts but also lays emphasis on the applied and practical aspects of the preventive, promotive and curative health. This book fulfils the tenets of Miller's Triangle in developing competence in community medicine in terms of knows, knows how, shows how and does. While being precise, the book has not compromised with essential information.

Immense popularity of earlier editions, especially among students of community medicine, and the everchanging public health scenario in the country, have made it necessary to revise and update the earlier edition to suit the present day requirement. Authors have incorporated all the recent developments in the field of community medicine and have been successful in presenting the information in lucid manner. Authors have also adhered to the current global trend in medical education of integration of clinical disciplines with preventive medicine with the focus of the integrated information on primary health care. This will provide proper perspective to the readers of the book.

I hope that this book will be of a great interest and use equally to students as well as professionals of Community Medicine and Public Health. I am quite confident that this book will be widely referred to and will be put into practice. I hope that like previous editions, this edition will also be a great success.

I congratulate the authors for bringing out the fifth edition of *Textbook of Community Medicine*.

Chandrakant S Pandav

Book Review

There has been a rapid progress in the field of community medicine in the last few years which compel the authors to continuously revise their book. After going through the *Textbook of Community Medicine* written by Dr Sunder Lal, Dr Adarsh and Dr Pankaj, I am happy to note that almost all the chapters have been thoroughly revised, especially the demography, national health programmes, HIV, RCH, communicable and non-communicable diseases and the concepts of health apart.

Also the health management, hospital statistics, HIV, medical ethics and research have been very well written and presented in a lucid manner.

However, the topics like telemedicine, GIS, e-waste management, medical tourism, recent update on immunization are the need of the hour and to be covered in the next edition.

This edition of the book will be definitely useful to undergraduate/postgraduate medical students/faculty of community medicine, family medicine as well as program implementers of public health services.

Muralidhar Tambe

Professor of Community Medicine
BJ Government Medical College
Pune 411001, Maharashtra

Phone: 9423007898/02026128000 Fax: 02026126868
Email: muralidhartambe@rediffmail.com

Preface to the Fifth Edition

The text on communicable and non-communicable diseases and related National Health Programmes has been integrated to avoid fragmentation and to enhance the learning of subject of epidemiology and management of National Health Programmes. Health financing in India and chapter on health management, besides health economics, organization behavior, gender issues, adolescent reproductive and sexual health (ARSH), hospital statistics, health management and information system, national authority on disaster management, Infection Management and Environmental Plan (IMEP), HIV and AIDS Programme, HIV sentinel surveillance and integrated biological and behavioural surveillance surveys and case studies are the unique features of fifth edition which no other book has been able to cover in its entirety. Chapters on applied biostatistics and epidemiology cover the examples of national health programmes/problems reinforcing the learning of specific programme. Building clear concept of community medicine starting with historical aspects, elucidating community structure and functions, community diagnosis leading to family health and home-based records facilitating the learning of community medicine—a stepwise approach-based on real practice of public health in the community/life situation leading to thinking epidemiologically and acting socially.

Sunder Lal
Adarsh
Pankaj

Preface to the First Edition

To write quality textbook on community medicine (preventive and social medicine) is a challenging task, however, this challenge was accepted by the authors. Departure has been made from conventional textbooks to accommodate the requirements of Medical Council of India as also to incorporate newer challenges, hitherto not attempted by most textbooks available in the market. The author has incorporated the most recent advances in the field of community medicine besides the practical field experiences in the form of case studies. Field experiences/observations cannot be substituted by any textbook material; the authors have made a bold and conscious attempt to bring back live situations and field experiences into the textbook, which is the unique feature of this book. Another unique feature is to restrict to the specific areas of concern to public health (epidemiology, application of biostatistics, health management, communication and biosocial and sciences of humanity) to avoid duplication of areas/concerns of other specialities. The sequencing of chapters is purposeful to highlight the priority health problems and concerns of community medicine (preventive and social medicine). Hopefully the textbook will meet the needs of health managers and decision-makers at various levels besides, the teachers of community medicine, postgraduate students and predominantly the undergraduates (MBBS and BDS students), and teachers of community medicine, graduate nurses, general nursing students in the discipline of community medicine. It would indeed be a pleasure to get positive as well as negative feedback from the readers to effect improvement in future editions of the book.

Sunder Lal
Adarsh
Pankaj

Acknowledgements

The support, guidance, encouragement and material help received from learned colleagues and friends like Late Prof AK Sharma of LHMC, New Delhi; Prof Rajesh Kumar, PGI, Chandigarh; Dr DK Taneja, Professor at MAMC, New Delhi; Late Prof RK Sachar, DMC, Ludhiana; Prof AS Sekhon, Head, Department of Community Medicine, Govt. Medical College, Patiala; Prof AS Wantamutte, Head, Department of Community Medicine, JLNMC, Belgaum (Karnataka); Prof Sandip Kumar Ray, KPC Medical College and Hospital, Jadavpur, Kolkata; and Dr SC Mohapatra, Professor, Community Medicine, Institute of Medical Sciences, Banaras Hindu University, Varanasi (UP), are sincerely acknowledged. The authors owe deep sense of gratitude to World Health Organization which has kindly permitted us to use the valuable published material, and to UNICEF, NICD-DGHS, MOH and FW, New Delhi, whose published material was used extensively to enrich the contents of the book for dissemination of scientific information to the teachers and the students.

Help received from Dr Kuldip, Dr Manish Goyal and Dr Shankar Prinja is sincerely acknowledged.

Sunder Lal
Adarsh
Pankaj

Contents

Part II

Abbreviations

AIDS	Acquired Immunodeficiency Syndrome
AKD	Acetone Killed and Dried Typhoid Vaccine
ANC	Antenatal Care/Clinic
ANM	Auxiliary Nurse Midwife
APL	Above Poverty Line
ARSH	Adolescent Reproductive and Sexual Health
AWW	Anganwadi Worker
BCC	Behaviour Change Communication
BObC	Basic Obstetric Care
BPL	Below Poverty Line
CBHI	Central Bureau of Health Intelligence
CCDs	Communicable Diseases
CHC	Community Health Centre
CRS	Congenital Rubella Syndrome
CNAA	Community Need Assessment Approach
DGHS	Director-General of Health Services
DOTS	Directly Observed Treatment Short-course
EAG	Empowered Action Group
EHP	Essential Health Package
EObC	Essential Obstetric Care
FOGSI	Federation of Obstetric and Gynaecological Societies of India
FP	Family Planning
FSWs	Female Sex Workers
GDP	General Domestic Product
GNI	Gross National Income
GOI	Government of India
HDI	Human Development Index
HIV	Human Immunodeficiency Virus
IAP	Indian Association of Paediatrics
HLEP	High Level Expert Group
IAPH	Indian Association of Public Health
IAPPD	Integrated Action Plan for Pneumonia and Diarrhoea
IAPSM	Indian Association of Preventive and Social Medicine
ICDs	International Classification of Diseases
ICDS Scheme	Integrated Child Development Services Scheme

ICMR	Indian Council of Medical Research
ICTC	Integrated Counselling and Testing Centre
IDSP	Integrated Disease Surveillance Programme
IDU	Injecting Drug Users
IEC	Information Education and Communication
IPV	Injectable Polio Vaccine
IEAG	India Expert Advisory Group
IHR	International Health Regulations
ILO	International Labour Organization
IMA	Indian Medical Association
IMNCI	Integrated Management of Newborn and Childhood Illness
IMR	Infant Mortality Rate
IPHS	Indian Public Health Standards
IRS	Indoor Residual Spray
IUCD	Intrauterine Contraceptive Device
JSY	*Janani Surakshya Yojna*
LBW	Low Birth Weight
MCH	Maternal and Child Health
MB	Multi-bacillary Leprosy
MCI	Medical Council of India
MDG	Millennium Development Goals
MGNREGA	Mahatma Gandhi National Rural Employment Guarantee Act
MMR	Maternal Mortality Ratio
MOHFW	Ministry of Health and Family Welfare
MCTS	Mother and Child Tracking System
MPHW	Multipurpose Health Worker
MSM	Men Having Sex with Men
MTPA	Medical Termination of Pregnancy Act
NCD	Non-communicable Diseases
NGO	Non-Governmental Organization
PNMR	Postneonatal mortality Rate
NMR	Neonatal Mortality Rate
NHM	National Health Mission
NIDs	National Immunization Days
NIPCCD	National Institute of Public Cooperation and Child Development
NRHM	National Rural Health Mission
NSSK	*Navjat Shishu Swasthya Karyakram*

NVDCP	National Vector-borne Disease Control Programme
NTAGI	National Technical Advisory Group on Immunization
NSP	New Sputum Smear Positive
NUHM	National Urban Health Mission
OOP Expenditure	Out of Pocket Expenditure
ORS	Oral Rehydration Salt
PB	Pauci-bacillary Leprosy
PC–PNDT	The Pre-conception and Prenatal Diagnostic Technique Act
NMR	Neonatal Mortality Rate
PNMR	Perinatal Mortality Rate
PNMR	Post-neonatal Mortality Rate
ORT	Oral Rehydration Therapy
PHC	Primary Health Centre
PPTCT	Prevention of Parent to Child Transmission
PPP	Public–Private Partnership
PRIs	Panchayati Raj Institutions
RCH	Reproductive and Child Health
RDA	Recommended Dietary Allowances
RDT	Rapid Diagnostic Test
RTI	Reproductive Tract Infection
SBR	Still Birth Rate
SC	Sub-centre
SES	Socioeconomic Status
SRS	Sample Registration System
SSA	*Sarava Shikshya Abhiyan*
STD	Sexually Transmitted Diseases
STI	Sexually Transmitted Infections
TAS	Transmission Assessment Surveys
TSC	Total Sanitation Campaign
TGR	Total Goitre Rate
UIP	Universal Immunization Programme
UNS	United Nations
UHC	Urban Health Centre
UnHC	Universal Health Coverage
VHSC	Village Health and Sanitation Committee
VHND	Village Health and Nutrition Day
WHO	World Health Organization

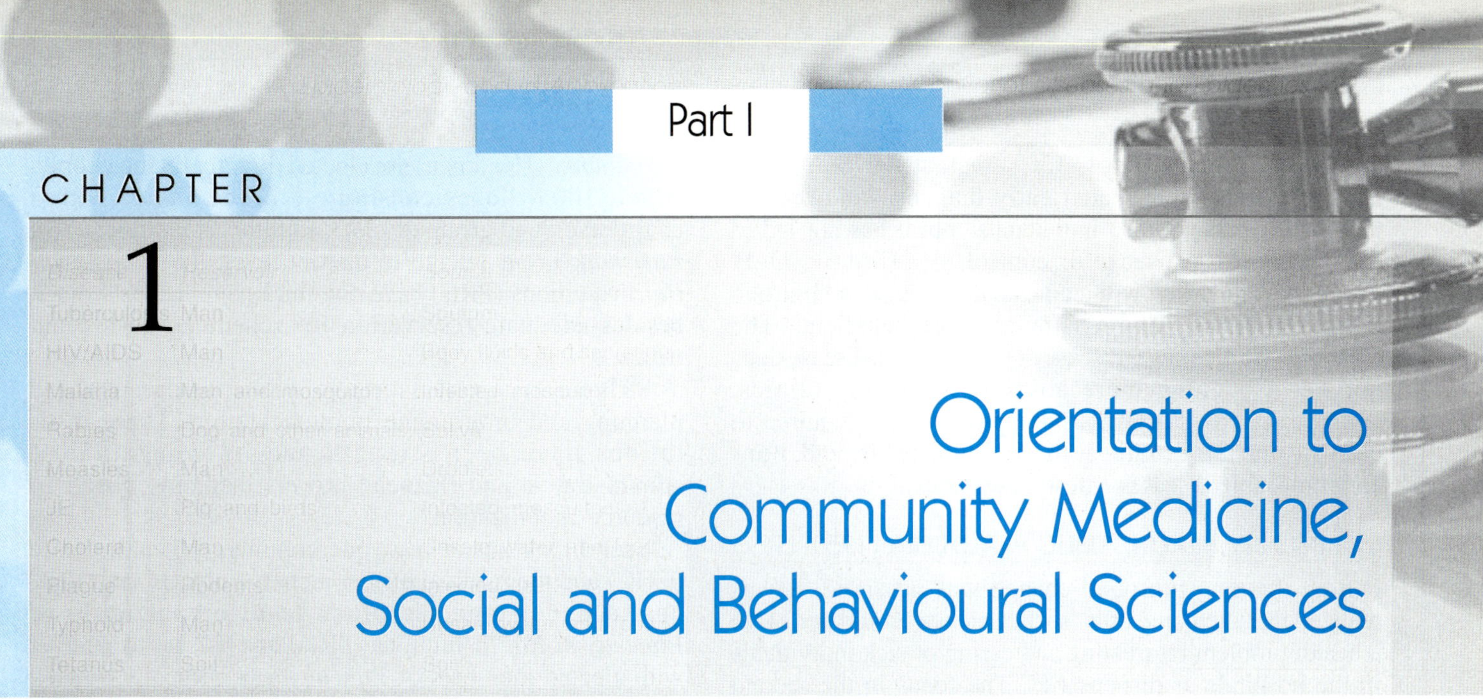

Part I

CHAPTER

1

Orientation to Community Medicine, Social and Behavioural Sciences

HISTORICAL ASPECTS OF COMMUNITY MEDICINE
From Symptoms to Science to Universal Coverage

Evolution of medicine has passed through various stages. These can be segmented into various eras.

EMPIRICAL ERA (Until 1850)

During this period, the medicine and health science belonged to empirical era. The focus was on *symptoms*. The art of medicine revolved around the diagnosis and treatment of symptoms by all kinds of available home-medicaments considered appropriate at that time, which had no basis of science or scientific evidence. People put the blame on witches or evil spirits and treated the sickness or symptoms with magic cures, cupping and application of leaches to draw bad blood out of the body and administered a variety of purgatives. People held several kinds of wrong beliefs like evil eyes, past sins, curse of god, and being possessed by an evil or evil spirits (ghost/bhoot-pret intrusion into body) in case of all mental illnesses. Yet like the three monkeys of Mahatma's talisman, we do not see, hear or speak about mental illness because of stigma attached to it. Accordingly, people resorted to treatment through various magic centres, religious centres, wearing charms, amulets, and talisman, exorcism and faith healers. Some of these beliefs and practices are still prevalent in urban, rural, and tribal areas.[1]

BACTERIOLOGICAL ERA (1850–1900)

During this era, medicine became a science. Micro-organisms of various diseases were discovered or isolated and grown on cultures. The focus shifted from *symptoms* to *disease*. Much more emphasis was laid on diagnosis and treatment of disease. This era was also called basic science era and there was a profound change in the focus (Table 1.1).

PREVENTIVE MEDICINE AND CLINICAL SCIENCE ERA (1900–1950)

Hospitals, dispensaries and health centres were developed and focus shifted from diagnosis and treatment of disease to diagnosis and treatment of *patient*. This was an era of preventive medicine, treating/curing the sick in hospitals/health centres by using the advanced knowledge of clinical sciences, laboratory tests and other advances. The whole approach was *patient-centred*. Subsequently, it was realised that an individual needs to be treated as a whole in totality, including family. The concept of family physicians

Table 1.1: Historical development of medicine

Period ⟶	*Before 1850*	*1850–1900*	*1900–1950*	*1950–1977*	*1977–2017 and beyond*
Eras ⟶	Empirical health era	Bacteriological or basic science era	Preventive medicine and clinical science era	Community health or public health era	Health for/in all era 'Universal coverage'
Focus ⟶	**Symptoms** ⟶	**Bacteria or disease** ⟶	**Individual** ⟶	**Community** ⟶	**Community**
Sciences ⟶	Unknown	Basic sciences	Social sciences and clinical sciences	Community health sciences (social and managerial sciences)	Community health sciences, behavioural sciences, and management sciences

developed. But we know for sure that the *individual approach* or for that matter early diagnosis and prompt treatment has benefited "individuals" but it has not led to eradication of a disease or control of a disease. Only *community approach* will eradicate the disease or control a disease ultimately and it is much more beneficial. The answer to eliminating a disease or controlling a disease does not lie in opening more hospitals and more clinics. Community-based actions and approaches are required to control and eliminate both communicable and non-communicable diseases (lifestyle diseases).

COMMUNITY HEALTH/PUBLIC HEALTH ERA (1950–1977)

During this era, profound change was observed. It was realized that medicine as a "social science" could not solve a health problem by treating and caring of sick individuals in the hospitals or dispensaries. The focus in the second half of the 20th century shifted to *community* and *community diagnosis and treatment*. The whole *community* should be the focus of health. Ensure health to total community and meet the health needs of the "community".

Accordingly, the approach to medicine shifted from treatment to care, coverage, reduction of incidence of disease burden and disability and "development of community" to achieve positive health.

During the year 1952, India adopted a strategy and National Policy of all round community development through "Community Development Block". This was a unique approach and unique movement wherein "health" was considered as a part and parcel of all round development. "Health" became an integral part of agriculture, industrial, social and human development. One Community Development Block (CDB) with population of 1,00,000 was considered as the smallest development unit for all round development.

COMMUNITY DEVELOPMENT BLOCK (CDB)

Block or the Community Development Block is the smallest administrative unit for organizing integrated development activities in rural areas in India. On an average, one block consists of about 100 or more villages, with an average total population of 1,00,000 and 400–500 sq km area.[2] Each village has about 1000 population on an average. There are 5,50,000 habitated villages in India. There are 5652 community development blocks in India.[3] Each village has *Gram Panchayat* in the form of local self-government. *Village Panchayat* represents the democratic decentralized local self-government and it has been made responsible for decentralized planning for health, family welfare, and education and many other areas of village development under the 73rd and 74th Constitutional Amendment Act.[4]

Each village or a group of villages elects village *Panchayat*. All adult members (persons above the age of 18) constitute *Gram Sabha*, who have the right to vote and elect village *Panchayat*. Village *Panches* and *Sarpanches* (Headmen) are elected directly by the people. About 100 villages constitute a *Block Samiti* with a chairperson and group of block samities constitute a *Zila Parishad*. From village to district level, the *Panchayati Raj* Institutions (PRIs) have one-third members as women besides adequate reservation for scheduled castes and tribes.

PRIs are an important means of furthering decentralized planning and programme implementation. These institutions have been strengthened by delegation of administrative and financial powers including power of resource mobilization.

Each block has at least one community health centre (CHC) and the medical officer incharge of CHC and PHC has to understand the block level organization of *Panchayati Raj* Institutions (PRIs) and as also to interact with elected members of *Panchayat* periodically to seek their support and participation in all the health programmes and activities. As a health team leader, the medical officer has to interact with development functionaries and other sectors at the block and village level. Each block has chief executive officer known as block development and panchayat officer (BDPO) who is a government officer made responsible to execute the development works.

In essence, the mapping up of all villages of the block, the location of facilities, drinking water sources, educational institutions, road communication and number of villages, and their population has to be known thoroughly to manage the health functions in a block area. Without the support of people and PRIs of the block, the health activities and programmes cannot succeed. They are more than equal partners in health activities; hence all planning and especially village health plan and subcentre action plans should be developed with their consultation.

"Health for All Era" 1977 Onwards—Global Strategy

During the year 1977, WHO adopted the strategy of "Health for All by 2000". The emphasis was clearly focused on *community* to achieve a level of health which would permit all individuals to lead a socially useful and economically productive life through primary health care approach (Table 1.1).

Thus it can be summed up that during various eras profound changes were taking place and focus was shifting from 'Symptoms' to 'bacteria or disease' to 'individual' to 'community'. As of now, the 'Community' is the focus or concern of all health sciences or medicine. The community concern or focus means that whole population (urban, rural, tribal, desert areas and slum dwellers) need to be ensured "health" and their "health needs" must be responded through community diagnosis and need assessment.

As a follow-up measure of International Conference on Population and Development held at Cairo in 1994, the Government of India made a paradigm shift by launching "Community Needs Assessment Approach (CNAA)" in 1997 wherein the total community is covered and its reproductive and health needs are assessed and care is provided with as much coverage as possible. Our concern is to achieve "health" for total "community".

Community health centre for 100,000 population, primary health centre for 30,000 population and subcentre for 5000 have been set up to look after the "health" of assigned "community". A primary health centre has been given the responsibility of 30,000 population or "defined community" spread over in many villages and the health team at primary health centre level is to ensure "health" of total community (30,000 population) under its jurisdiction. Thus in "community health/medicine", focus is total community and not an individual. It does not mean that the sickness of a person is not given importance, it is duly treated, but the goal remains to ensure "health" to prevent occurrence of diseases by treating environments, or modifying environments, by raising community immunity by mass vaccination and ensuring 100% coverage, by disease surveillance, and national health programmes by involving community and many other sectors related to health (like agriculture, education, ICDS, development), etc.

EVOLUTION OF HEALTH SERVICES REFORMS AND POLICY DEVELOPMENT IN INDEPENDENT INDIA

Health services and policy development in independent India can be divided into following phases of development.[5,6]

Phase I (1947–1972)

1 Health was considered a development function and a part of community development programme. Community development programme started in 1952.

2 One primary health centre was established in each community development block.

3 Expansion of primary health care infrastructure occurred in this phase.

4 Family planning needs and services were recognized as priority problem and National Family Planning Programme commenced on voluntary basis in 1952.

5 A separate department of family planning was set-up in the Ministry of Health and Family Welfare (MOH and FW).

6 Many national health/disease control/eradication programmes were launched as vertical programmes.

Phase II (1972–1977)

During this phase, India launched:

1 Minimum needs programme.

2 Multipurpose health workers scheme.

3 Health guides were introduced.

4 Dais training programme was stepped up.

5 Integrated child development services (ICDS).

Phase III (1977–1996)

Important policy developments during this phase were:

1 Alma Ata Declaration of "Health for all" 1978.

2 Reorientation of medical education 1978

3 National Health Policy was formulated in 1983.

4 National Education Policy was adopted in 1986.

5 Universal Immunisation Programme was initiated in 1985.

6 Child Survival and Safe Motherhood Programme (CSSM) started in 1992.[7]

7 73rd and 74th Constitutional Amendments Act, 1992.

Phase IV (1997–2012)

1 A paradigm shift in policy: Reproductive and Child Health (RCH) Programme was launched.

2 National Population Policy of 2000 was adopted.

3 Millennium Development Goals were adopted in 2000.

4 Revised National Health Policy of 2002 was launched.

5 National Rural Health Mission was launched in 2005.

6 National Urban Health Mission Launched.

Phase V (2012–17)

- Rolling out a system of 'Universal Health Coverage'.
- NRHM transformed to National Health Mission.
- Phase IV of national AIDS control programme started.
- National health policy 2015 drafted.

First Generation Reforms

First generation reforms in India commenced way back in 1946, based on outstanding recommendations of "Health survey and development committee" (Bhore committee). Through successive five years plans efforts were made "to establish and develop health care delivery systems in India" to cover its vast population.

The major recommendations of this committee were:

- No individual should fail to secure adequate medical care because of inability to pay for it.
- Health services should provide all, consultant, laboratory and institutional facilities for proper diagnosis and treatment.
- The health services should be placed as close as possible to the people in order to ensure maximum benefit to the communities to be served.
- Health consciousness should be stimulated by providing health education on a universal basis as well as by providing opportunities for individual participation in local health programmes.
- Medical services should be free to all without distinction.
- Three-tier system—subcentre, PHC, subdistrict and district level health care model, be set up.
- The establishment of one primary health centre for 10,000 to 20,000 population in the long-term perspective and one centre for 40,000 population in the short-term perspective.

- One bed for 175 persons, one doctor for 1600 and one nurse for 600 persons. One 650-bedded hospital at *Taluka* (3 lakh population) and one district hospital of 2500 beds. It recommended 15% of Government expenditure on health care.

2 ***Mudaliar Committee 1961 (health survey and planning committee):*** The major policy recommendations were:
- Integration of curative and preventive services.
- Establishment of one primary health centre for 40,000 population.
- One bed for 1000 population and one doctor for 3000 population.
- One 50-bedded hospital with specialist services for each *Taluka* and 500 beds hospital at district level.
- One medical college for 5 million population.

3 ***Chadha Committee 1963***
- Integration of maintenance phase of malaria with general health services in the country consisting of subcentres, primary health centres and district level organisations.
- Designating the malaria surveillance workers as basic health workers at the scale of 1 per 10,000 population.
- One sanitary inspector/health inspector at the rate of one per 20–25,000 population.
- One laboratory technician at the level of PHC.
- One family planning field worker at the rate of 1 per 30,000 population for intensification of family planning measures.
- Utilisation of extension educators for all national health programmes.

4 ***Mukherjee Committee 1966 Recommendations***
- One family planning field worker (FPFW) for every two subcentres or 20,000 population.
- One lady health visitor for 40,000 population.
- One part-time worker for motivating population for acceptance of IUD be appointed with honorarium.
- Campaign for opinion leader (opinion leaders training camps) for intensification of motivation campaign for acceptance of family planning services.
- Incentives to Government doctors and practitioners.

5 ***Jain Committee 1966 Recommendations***
- One bed per 1000 population.
- One 50 beds hospital at *Taluka* level.
- Enhancing maternity facilities at each level.
- Health insurance for larger population coverage.

6 ***Kartar Singh Committee 1974 Recommendations***
- Change of uni-purpose workers to multipurpose health workers.
- Integration of health services and programmes.
- One male and one female multipurpose health workers for each subcentre.
- One supervisor for 4 ANMs or four health workers.
- One PHC for 50,000 population.

7 ***Srivastava Committee 1975 (group on medical education and support manpower)***
- Health guides at the community level one for 1000 population.
- One male and one female health worker per 5000 population.
- One additional doctor and nurse at PHC for MCH services.
- Increase in PHC drug budget.
- Compulsory national service of two years at PHC by every doctor.
- Establish medical and health education commission
- Integration of various health systems.

8 ***ICMR-ICSSR joint panel 1980 (Ramalingaswami committee)***[8]

i Formulation of comprehensive national health policy.

ii The basic objectives of this policy should be:
- Development of health system should be integrated with overall plans of socioeconomic development.
- To ensure access to adequate food, provide environment conducive to health and adequate immunisation where necessary.
- Devise an educational programme for health.
- To replace the existing model of health care services by an alternative new model of health care which will be:
  - Village or community health volunteer/health guide for 1000, subcentre for 5000 population, community health centre for 100,000 population, district health centre for one million population.
  - The specialist centre for 5 million population.

SECOND GENERATION REFORMS: NATIONAL HEALTH POLICY (NHP)-1983 "HEALTH FOR ALL"

The second generation reforms in India led to formulation of "National Health Policy" in 1983 to achieve "Health for all" through "Primary Health Care". Policy focused on:
- Provision of universal, comprehensive primary health care services.
- Involvement of private practitioners and NGOs to expand coverage of services.
- Transfer of knowledge and simple skills to village-based workers.
- Evolving a decentralised system of health care and establishment of a referral system
- Establish nationwide chain of epidemiological stations.
- Encourage private investment in health sector to reduce Government burden.
- Specification of health and demographic outcomes targets to be achieved by the year 2000.

NATIONAL POPULATION POLICY (NPP)-2000

a Immediate goal is to meet the unmet needs of contraception, health care infrastructure, personnel and provide basic RCH services.

b Medium-term goal was to achieve total fertility rate of 2.1 by 2010.

c Long-term goal was to have stable population by 2050.

- Decentralised planning and programme implementation with involvement of Panchayati Raj institutions (PRIs).
- Promote intersectoral approach between a number of key Government departments.[9]

REVISED NATIONAL HEALTH POLICY-2002

The objectives of NHP-2002 were to:

- Achieve an acceptable standard of good health in general population.
- To ensure more equitable access to health services.[10]

Approach

- To increase access to the decentralised public health system by establishing new infrastructure in deficient areas and by upgrading the existing institutions.
- To increase public health investment through substantially increased contribution by the central Government.
- To enhance participation of non-governmental organizations.
- To increase public private partnership (PPP).
- To invest 55% of public health investment in primary health care, 35% for secondary and 10% for tertiary care to achieve equity.
- To provide *essential drugs* and equipment at primary health centre by the central Government.

National Rural Health Mission (NRHM) 2005–2012

The objectives of NRHM were:

- To raise public spending on health from 0.9% of GDP to 2–3% of GDP.
- To strengthen Subcentres, PHCs, CHCs and Districts health services.
- To achieve convergence of services of various sectors like health, nutrition, water supply and sanitation at various levels.
- To enhance community participation by enhancing capacity of PRIs.
- To promote access to health care through accredited social health activist (ASHA).[11, 12]

The Third generation reforms were on account of development of market oriented economies and globalisation and these reforms respond more to demand ushering in an era of competition within stakeholders of private sector focusing on health. Insurance mechanism including privately financed insurance. "Rashtriya Bima Swasthya Yojna" has been launched by government of India to cover BPL families and several other weaker sections of community.

National Urban Health Mission (NUHM)-2008

To address the health needs of the urban poor, mission document on National Urban Health Mission (NUHM) was approved in 2008.

Nation Health Mission 2012–17 and Health Reforms

National Health Mission (NHM) envisages universal access to equitable, affordable and quality health care services that are accountable and responsive to people's needs. NHM has two Sub-missions, the National Rural Health Mission and the National Urban Health Mission. The Pogramme components include Health System Strengthening in rural and urban areas, Reproductive Maternal, newborn, Child and Adolescent Health and control of communicable and non-communicable diseases.

12th five-year plan (2012–17): Raising public spending on health from 1.04 to 1.87% of GDP" and cashless OPD health care in government hospitals as also accelerating **universal health coverage** (UnHC).[13]

REFERENCES

1 McGavaran EG. Community as patient. JAMA 1956 Oct. 20; 162(8): 724–7.

2 Dhillon H, Dasgupta S, Menon K, Shah PM. Delivery of care to mothers and children in a community development block. Miller FJW (editor). Geneva: World Health Organization; 1983.

3 GOI. Provisional population totals. Census of India. Paper I of 2001and 2011. New Delhi: GOI; 2001 and 2011.

4 Planning Commission (GOI). Tenth Five-Year Plan 2002–07 (II). New Delhi: GOI; 2002.

5 NIHFW. Management Training Modules for Medical Officer, PHC. New Delhi: NIHFW; 1987.

6 GOI: Health manpower, planning, production management. Report of expert committee. New Delhi: MOH and FW GOI; 1987.

7 MOH and FW. National Child Survival and Safe Motherhood Programme—Module for health workers. New Delhi: GOI; 1992.

8 ICSSR and ICMR. "Health for all" an alternative strategy—report of a study group. Pune, India: Indian Institute of Education; 1981.

9 GOI; 2000: National Population Policy 2000. New Delhi.

10 GOI; National Health Policy 2002. New Delhi; GOI; 2002.

11 GOI; National Rural Health Mission—New Delhi; GOI; 2005.

12 GOI; Towards Faster and More Inclusive Growth. An Approach Paper to 11th Five-Year Plan; Govt. of India, Planning Commission, Yojna Bhawan, New Delhi, Dec 2006.

13 GOI; 12th Five Year Plan 2012–17 Health Sector. High level expert group on universal health coverage.

COMMUNITY ORGANISATION AND COMMUNITY DIAGNOSIS

COMMUNITY

"*Nation's Greatest Asset is its People*"

The community is the "heart" of the system of health care or for that matter of any development programme. The "community" is the essential laboratory for practice of teaching, training and research in the subject of community medicine. Community medicine without "community" means no community medicine. The concern and focus of community medicine is total community.

What is a Community?

It is difficult to define a community because of its diversity and complexity. No universal definition should be attempted. "Community is a group of people who occupy a well-defined territorial area, have common interests, heritage, shared assets and needs and have common pattern of socioeconomic relationship, derive a common bond of solidarity from the conditions of its abode, have a constellation of social institutions and are subject to some degree of group control."[1]

Each community is different from other. The community may be rural or urban or tribal. Community can be small (a few families) or one village or group of villages or as large as district, state or nation.

Understanding of community is not only essential but also is imperative for the practice of community medicine. Take a good look at your community, respect your people, their traditions, ideas and culture and help them build on the knowledge and skills they already have.

It is common proverb:

Go in search of your people
Love them, learn from them
Plan with them, serve them
Begin with what they know
Build on what they have
But of the best leaders
When their task is accomplished
Their work is done
The people all remark
"We have done it ourselves"

The first requirement is to understand the community you serve. Go to your people, visit their homes, fields, gathering places, schools and market places, understand how they have organized themselves, their attitudes, beliefs and practices and their health needs and resources they have to meet their felt needs.[2]

Take a Good Look at Your Community

Those who have grown up in the community and locally resident know their people well. You may be already familiar with many of their problems and may have inside view. But in order to see the whole picture, you will need to look carefully at your community from many points of view.

Since community medicine practitioners are concerned with the well-being of all the people—not just those, who come to them or are known to them. They must go to people, visit their homes, fields, gathering places and schools, understand their joys and concerns. Examine them or observe their habits, lifestyles—the things in their daily lives that bring about good health and those that may lead to sickness and injury.

Know Community Structure and Organization (Community Anatomy)

Geographical area, terrains, roads and accessibility and means of access to community, total number of villages and hamlets in your area. How many people (size of community) live in the community? How many are infants, children in age group 1–5, 5–14 years, 10–19 years, persons in age group 15–49 years (eligible couples) and elderly people above the age of 60 years? How many houses, households and families are there in each village and number of subcentres in the area manned by multipurpose health workers? How many can read and write? What good is schooling? How many schools are there? Are these accessible to girls? What are the major occupations of your people? Life of economically weaker sections, below poverty line families, land holding pattern, (landless and land-owners) caste structure, and religious institutions. What are common "customs, beliefs and practices" in relation to health and disease, health seeking and "reproductive health behaviour"? What are their "lifestyles"?

What is Leadership Pattern? Who are Elected Representatives?

Any organised groups, such as women (*Mahila Swasthya Sangh* or *Mahila Mandal*) or men group or youth groups. How the people have organised themselves? The power structure, local self-government (at village, block and district level), village *Panchayat*, leadership pattern, influential persons, opinion makers, system of collection of revenue, economic structure and caste groups.

Housing and Sanitation (Community Physiology)

Know the sources of drinking water, system or practice of garbage and excreta disposal, i.e. where do the people go for defecation, how the animal excreta and garbage is disposed off? Is the source of drinking water safe? What common animals or pets are kept? Is there menace of dogs, rats, flies, mosquitoes, and pigs? What are different houses made of?

Community Pathology—Health Status

Community Nutrition

What are the "breastfeeding practices" in the area? What are the main staple foods grown and eaten in the area? What foods are preferred for children? Do people give enough food to young children, additional food to pregnant women? Do people continue feeding during illness? How many children are *underweight* in the village or in the community particularly in families below poverty line? What are supplementary nutrition programmes which operate in the area? What are the important green leafy vegetables grown in the area or in their kitchen gardens? What are the cooking and food storage practices in the area? What is the incidence of low birth weight in the area?

Deliveries

Who conducted deliveries in the area? What proportions of deliveries are conducted in the *home* and *institution*? How many trained birth attendants are available in each village? Do they have enough material in their kit? Are disposable Dai kits available? Are mothers and neonates being provided care after delivery?

Service Coverage and Disease Burden

What is the coverage level of *immunisation* in young children, pregnant women and school children? How many pregnant women have been provided full essential obstetrical care? How many births and deaths are registered in the area? What are the important *diseases prevalent* in the area and what are most important *killer diseases* in the area? This can be gauged from the records of subcentre or primary health centre.

Reproduction

What are the contraceptive practices in the area? How many *eligible couples* have been *protected* with what method? What is the crude birth rate of the area? How many families have more than 2 children?

Assess Felt Need

What things in your people's daily lives (living conditions, lifestyles, ways of doing things, beliefs, etc.) do they feel help them to be healthy? What do people feel to be their major problems, concerns and needs—not only those related to health, but also in general?

1. *Felt needs:* Means what people feel are their biggest problems?
2. *Real needs:* As determined by experts and steps people can take to meet these problems in lasting way.
3. Willingness or readiness of people to plan and take the needed steps.
4. *Resources:* "People" themselves are the biggest resource.

People count first in resources, their skills, materials, and/or money needed to carry out the activities decided upon.

Example: Let us suppose that a man who smokes a lot comes to you complaining of cough that has been steadily getting worse:

1. His felt need is to get rid of cough.
2. His real need is (to correct the problem) to give up smoking.
3. To get rid of his cough will require his willingness to give up smoking. For this he must understand how much it really matters.
4. One resource that may help him to give up smoking is information about the harm it can do to him and his family. Another is the support and encouragement of his family, his friends and you.[2,3]

Self-help

For how many of their problems, can people care for themselves? How much outside help is required? Are people ready to generate resources and cooperative to solve their problems? Do people work together to meet common needs? Do they share or help each other when needs are great. What are their opinions to make the village better and healthier place to live? Where might you and your people begin?

Describing India as Community—Case Study

India is a land of diversities. It has 29 states and seven union territories and 671 districts. India's most important resource is its people-1210 million as on 1st March 2011. Nearly 69% of population lives in 6,40,000 villages (rural areas) and urban population is 31% and it is growing fast due to rapid urbanisation. Major proportion, i.e. 62% of population depends upon agriculture. The sex ratio of 940 females per 1000 men is unfavourable for females. Similarly falling child sex ratio of 914 is also not very encouraging sign and many of the states which are progressive: like Punjab have child sex ratio of 846 and Haryana with 830 is a bad news and most probable explanation is foeticide practice (sex selective abortions). Overall literacy rate is 74%; males have better level of literacy (82.5%) against female literacy (65.46%). The total fertility rate is 2.4 (2012), infant mortality rate of 40/1000 live births (2013); maternal mortality rate 167 per lakh (in 2011 to 2013) and human development index ranking was 130 in year 2015. About 350 million people are living below poverty line (38% in the year 2009), life expectancy was 68 years in 2013. Population having access to proper sanitation was 36% in 2012, and population having access to improved water supply was over 90% in year 2009. Health expenditure public (% of GDP) was 1.10 in 2009 and health expenditure private (% of GDP) was 4.13 in 2009. Allopathic doctor population ratio is 1: 1319. Of the total amount spent on health in general, Government expenditure accounts for 26% while private spending amounts to 74%.

The crude birth rate is 21.4/1000 and death rate is around 7 per 1000.

Rural Community—Case Study

India lives in 640,000 villages, of these 550,000 are inhabited. Nearly 69% of Indian population lives in rural areas spread over to more than 10 lakh habitations of which 60% have population of less than 1000. Density of population is low. The rural community is scattered in small villages, hamlets which may be difficult to reach. The characteristic of rural community are: the people are engaged predominantly in agriculture work or farm work, 40% are landless and work as manual casual labourers, their relationships are intimate, kinship is very strong, most families lead a joint family life, whole village is just one family in a way, the system of governance is by local self-government, each village has a common land (Shamlat) for pasture, animal grazing and forestry or it may be leased out for cultivation and income generated is used for village development, pond is a universal phenomenon and is life for village. On the bank of pond are shallow wells to provide drinking water. Each village or a group of villages has/have a village *Panchayat* and headman (*Sarpanch*) and one-third of seats are reserved for women members by an Act. Village community gives land for schools, subcentre and primary health centre or community health centre and place for *Anganwadi* to run. The caste system is very strong in rural community. Each village has dominant caste (landholders), occupational caste and subservient weaker sections or schedule castes and backward castes. Each caste has its own "community centre" used for social activities, such as social meetings, marriages, day care leisure centre for men. Community centre in each village is a hub of activities for aged people who gossip, play cards and smoke in groups and discuss and share the news. Village community has **organised women groups** in the form of *Mahila Mandals*, *Mahila Swasthya Sanghs* (MSS) and self help groups (SHG) who work for women development and women empowerment. Daughters-in-law have to put a veil or cover her face as a mark of respect to men, she is considered to be "daughter-in-law" of total village. Daughters-in-law have to work for family, farm, fetch fuel, fodder and water, take care of animals, kitchen besides bearing and rearing of children and all this consumes lot of her energy or calories. The child rearing practices are traditional and 25–40% of deliveries are home deliveries. Women are confined to home, outward mobility and interaction with outside world is minimal. Interaction and socialisation of women occur at the source of water or group defecation in the field. School is a universal feature of every village. If the high school is at a distance, the girls are not sent to school because of insecurity.

Village *Panchayat* is a democratic decentralised system of local self-government. Village *Panchayat* has a responsibility to register births and deaths and it is responsible for village development, including health and holds its meetings regularly. All adult members of the village constitute *Gram Sabha* (who have voting right) and *Gram Sabha* keeps watch over village *Panchayat's* activities.

Cattle wealth: Rearing cattle is almost universal in villages. Cattle sheds are located in dwellings or very close by. Dietary needs and fuel needs are met by cattle rearing. Disposal of animal excreta is not very far from dwellings. Unprocessed biomass fuel (dung of animals) is the most common fuel used by the families (over 80%) and is cause of indoor air pollution. Cow-dung cakes are stored in beautiful pyramidal structures near dwelling or on the outskirts of village.

The health and development parameters, such as infant mortality, maternal mortality, under-five mortality are much higher in rural areas as compared to urban community. Similarly, literacy rates are much lower in rural community. Birth and death rate tends to be much higher in rural community only 3.45% of eligible people being graduates. In rural community, over 70% of population have no toilets and practice of open field defecation is rampant, leading to soil pollution and worm infestation.

Rural community profile must be known to doctor for practice of community medicine. All characters explained above have implications and have bearing on planning, organisation, implementation and evaluation of health services. System of health services for rural community of necessity has to be based on their culture, and health needs. Accessibility of community health services is the prime need in rural areas. Government alone may not be able to afford the cost and it has to depend on the village people, local health volunteers, traditional birth attendants besides non-governmental organizations and private sector.

Urban Community—Case Study

31% of people in India live in urban areas. Census of India defines urban areas as "(a) all areas with municipality, corporation, cantonement board or notified area committee, etc., (b) place satisfying the following three criteria simultaneously: a minimum population of 5000, at least 75% male working population engaged in non agricultural vocation and density of population of at least 400 per sq km".

In the urban community, the pattern is different. One-third of urban people or even more may be living in urban slums with deplorable or subhuman conditions. (Congested locality, unhygienic environment usually with inadequate infrastructure and lacking in proper sanitary and drinking water facility.) Slums are notified by state/local Govt and UT administration.

Urban dwellers have less interaction with each other and live in isolation. The occupation is business, service or industrial work. The class system predominates not the caste. The system of governance is by local self-government in the form of Municipal Corporation/Committee (Nagarpalika). The facilities or amenities like piped water supply, electricity, roads, developed markets, hospitals, nursing homes and private practitioners are well established. The economic condition of most of urban dwellers is much sound and health services are easily accessible. Over 80% of hospitals and 80% of doctors are available in urban areas, yet the urban slum dwellers are deprived of health services. Some of the urban slums are worst of rural areas as living conditions may be delporable with poor basic amenities. There is overcrowding and space available is less, land prices are very high.

Urbanization is inevitable, people migrate from rural areas to urban areas to improve their quality of life and access to education of their children and search of jobs and get a livelihood in industry. Industrialization and urbanization are inseparable. Life in an industrial town and work place is quite different. Air pollution is a problem in most cities due to increased population of vehicles and human population besides industrial activities. Density of population is much more in towns/cities.

Most health parameters in urban areas are much better as compared to rural areas. Infant mortality rate, maternal mortality rate, under five mortality rate and disease rates are much lower as compared to rural areas. Similarly birth rates are lower and literacy rates much higher in urban set-up. Health facilities are much more and paying capacity much better.[4]

Urban community of necessity has to have a different community health service set-up in view of the structure and function of urban community and much more so for urban slum community, industrial community and well to do urban community. Using private practitioners and philanthropists and religious and voluntary organisations for community health is a necessity as the governmental health services alone cannot meet the entire needs of preventive—promotive, curative and rehabilitation services. Hence, there is imperative need of people-public-private participation (PPPP) model of health services.

Since community medicine is deeply entrenched in the community. The community must be thoroughly studied and intimate relations and interactions have to be developed. Public Health practitioner and teacher has to know the structure of community, community organisation, target service groups (infants, children, pregnant women, lactating mothers, women between 15 and 45 or 15 and 49 years, adolescents), resources available with the community, functions of the community for development including health, willingness to help themselves and eagerness to seek outside support.

Tribal community is explained in Chapters 5 and 15.

Essential Skills for Community Medicine Practice

The most essential skills/competence include:

1 Positive attitude of mind to work for community.
2 Ability to organize community or groups in the community.
3 Ability to generate resources from community.
4 Ability to elicit community participation.
5 Give responsibility to community (sanitation, birth and death registration, report outbreaks, maintenance of wells—chlorination of water—disposal of human excreta and animal excreta, etc.).
6 Ability to assess community health needs.
7 Ability to meet community health needs.
8 Ability to share the health information with community.
9 Ability of training of community volunteers (birth attendants, health guides, *Anganwadi* workers, ASHAs, school teachers, *Mahila Swasthya Sanghs* and others).

The pivotal responsibility of 305 dental and 404 (189 Govt. and 215 private) medical colleges in the country is to develop positive attitudes towards community health and develop above-mentioned competence through curricular and extracurricular activities.

COMMUNITY DIAGNOSIS AND TREATMENT

Objectives of community diagnosis are:

i To determine the major health problems and needs and to identify resources to deal with these problems.
ii To ensure community participation.

The whole community is our patient and concern should develop for whole community. The focus of community medicine is "community". Community diagnosis is essential step. Steps involved in community diagnosis are similar to patient diagnosis but tools of diagnosis differ and basically involve *epidemiological*, *statistical* and "*social sciences*" tools.

Steps in community diagnosis:[4]

1 Listening to people.
2 Observations on community.
3 Examination of community.
4 Survey and investigation in community.
5 Tentative diagnosis.
6 Treatment of community (community therapy).
7 Follow-up of community.
8 Evaluation of therapy.
9 Re-planning of services.

1. Listen to People—Their Chief Complaints

The public health approach puts people first. Their chief complaint: Community expresses its needs through demands. Listen to community leaders, women groups, youth groups, *Panchayat* members, Urban local body members and note down their health demands. People usually want hospitals, subcentres, primary health centres, drugs and doctors, safe water, roads, schools and other developments in their area or they raise their voice by way of lodging complaints/dissatisfaction. Regular contacts and dialogue with people are most essential to get their feelings and demands and assess their health needs.

People's opinion matters most. Consultation of community is a must or essential before launching any programme hence, it is first and foremost step in community diagnosis.

People identify their own needs, priorities and work hard to achieve these needs. The expert determines the *real needs* based on scientific evidence. People express their *felt needs* in the form of demands. It is better to begin with areas where there is overlap of demands expressed by people and needs identified by the expert. In the second step, take those areas which are significantly determined by expert and left out by people.

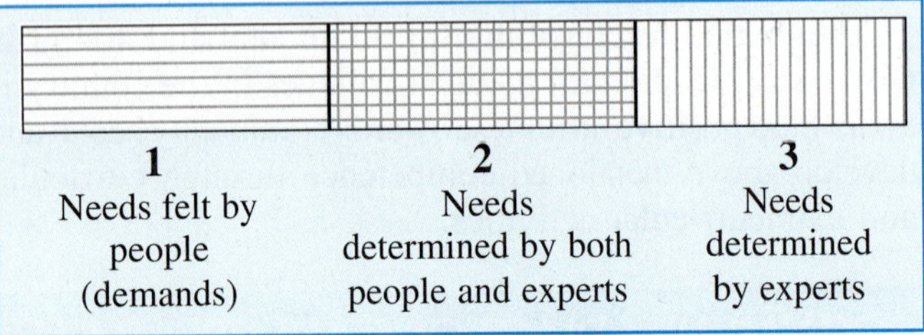

Begin with second segment as the chances of success are much more. Needs determined conjointly by people and the expert together will enhance community participation.

2. Observation on Community (Descriptive Epidemiology)

Go in search of your people, love them, learn from them, plan with them and serve them. Begin with what they know and build on what they have.

Epidemiological observations of community involve: geographical area, the size (total population), distribution of population; number of villages, wards in municipal area, their accessibility and terrain, resources available in terms of subcentres, schools, *Panchayats*, *Mahila Swasthya Sangh*, traditional birth attendants, health guides and indigenous practitioners. Rapidly assess the sanitary conditions, sources of drinking water, excreta disposal practices, water storage practices, major occupations, community leadership, community organization, economically weaker sections, power structure, age and sex composition of population, religious institutions, cropping pattern, "health customs and practices" as also health seeking behaviour. The other significant observations include, work sampling observations, i.e. when the health workers are working their quality of work can be observed, their "acceptability" in the community as also their problems. Always involve health workers and their supervisors in diagnosis of community.

Observations provide direct evidence of the extent of health problem/needs of the area, these can be interpreted and analysed with chief complaint and community examination to arrive at community diagnosis.

3. Examination of Community (Analytical Epidemiology)

It is essentially examination and review of available service data, its *analysis* and *interpretation* to draw information. Health records examination provides valuable clues, look through immunisation register to know the coverage level, number of antenatals registered in each village, birth records, nutritional status of 0–6 years children from *Anganwadi* workers, how many deliveries were done by health staff, institutional and home deliveries, number of pregnant women given tetanus toxoid, iron and folic acid, etc. number of eligible couples protected, number of traditional birth attendants trained, availability of drugs, equipment and material at subcentre, PHC, immunisation sessions held, birth rate of the area, infant mortality and common diseases as revealed through PHC morbidity-outdoor attendance register or subcentre clinic register, surveillance data, and health programmes reports and records. Surveillance data and monthly reports of health workers and *Anganwadi* workers when analysed and interpreted provide important lead/information on health needs of the community.

Analysis of data will give you the information on *health status of the community*: nutritional status of 0–6 years children, level of fertility, morbidity pattern, immunisation status and proportion of safe deliveries and "acceptance of maternal and child health services". These records are available routinely at the level of subcentre and primary health centre. These may be incomplete, or inaccurate, never mind—these provide useful clue of health status of the community and community needs in your area at no cost or at very low cost.

4. Survey and Investigations in Community

Eligible Couple Surveys—Household Surveys

These are carried out routinely once in a year and health workers generate information on couples protected by different methods of contraception, parity-wise acceptance of contraception, age-wise distribution of eligible couples and contraceptive acceptance. You can determine the approximate level of contraception acceptance rates method-wise and can come to conclusion as to which method needs to be promoted, besides availability and accessibility of various contraceptives at various levels. Household survey data provides information on age and sex of all members, their marital status, literacy level, economic status, source of drinking water, excreta disposal and "health practices" which forms the basis of health needs assessment. Mother and child Tracking system provides information on coverage of services and outcomes.

Investigations

The investigation in community diagnosis consists of monitoring of samples of drinking water for coliform counts, investigation of an outbreak, disease surveys and surveillance, screening of diseases by health check-ups, mass screening, stool examination, haemoglobin estimation, dietary survey, identification of mosquitoes, mass blood smears for malaria parasite, sputum examination for tuberculosis and screening for cataract and disability as also screening for sexually transmitted disease/ infections besides testing of salt samples for iodine.

Facility Surveys in Rural and Urban Areas

Health supervisors and medical officers carry out facility survey by visits to health facilities and supervise availability of manpower, drugs, functional status of equipment, training status of workers. This provides useful information on essential inputs available for services.

Monthly Meetings and Sector Meetings

These are fora where health workers and *Anganwadi* workers meet once a month. These workers bring wealth of information with them in the form of monthly reports and rich experiences of observations and community contacts. The health problems or needs can be quickly or rapidly ascertained in these meetings. These are no cost methods of getting information on health needs or health status.

5. Tentative Diagnosis and Final Diagnosis

From information derived by listening to people, epidemiological observations, and examination of service data/records you can come to conclusion of community diagnosis or health needs of your community. The tentative diagnosis can be changed to final diagnosis by having supplementary information from investigations, monthly meetings, facility surveys and supervisory visits. The extent and nature of needs can be thus worked out by going through these steps. It can lead to information on most important killer diseases, major disease problems and environmental problems.

Examples:

- Need of infant is survival and protection by feeding, immunisation, supplementary nutrition, prevention and control of diarrhoeal diseases and acute respiratory infections.
- Needs of pregnant woman are care and check-ups, adequate nutrition, iron and folic acid supplementation, tetanus toxoid (essential obstetrical care) and safe delivery, as also emergency obstetrical care as and when required.
- Need of eligible couple (sexually active persons) is contraception, safe sex and prevention of STD and HIV.
- School children and adolescents need to be provided information on STD/HIV and population, nutrition and environmental sanitation and promotion of healthy lifestyles.
- Need of village is sanitation, safe water, safe disposal of human excreta and prevention of fly and mosquito breeding, better roads, electricity and schools.

After assessing the needs, you have to meet these needs through interventions/package of services. Periodic surveys, such as village household survey, district rapid household surveys, national family health survey also provide clue for community diagnosis but it can never substitute your own observation on community to assess local problem by use of local service data, "local health beliefs, practices and utilisation of services".

6. Community Therapy (Treatment of Community) (Intervention-Epidemiology)

It may include:

1 *Treatment of environment or modification* and manipulation *of environment:* Chlorination of water at source or home, proper storage of water at home, prevention of contamination of water at source, safe disposal of human excreta, prevention of fly and mosquito breeding, animal birth control (ABC) for stray dogs, vaccination of dogs, rodent control, prevention and control of air pollution, and pasteurisation of milk and improving macro-environments—better housing, better drainage, and safe water.

2 Enhance community immunity by immunisation of young children and pregnant women.

3 Salt iodation, iron and folic acid supplementation.

4 Adolescent health in school and out of school, providing them information on prevention of STD/HIV, adequate nutrition, population problem, age of marriage and clean environments, promotion of sanitary latrines, mass deworming and personal hygiene.

5 Training of birth attendants for safe home delivery.

6 Promotion of institutional and safe deliveries.

7 Contraception services.

8 Safe abortion at PHC level.

9 Services for chronic non-communicable diseases like early detection of cancer, cataract and prevention of accidents in home, at school and on road.

10 Improving registration of births and deaths, marriages and pregnancy.

11 Enrolment of girls in schools.

12 Educating people on health/disease and "Behaviour change communication" and healthy lifestyles.

13 Improving dietary practices, prevention of food adulteration and other legislative measures (Acts).

14 Surveillance of diseases for prevention and control.

The interventions include not only treatment of illnesses but go far beyond that, i.e. legislation, environmental control and surveillance of diseases, besides "education and communication on health" for behaviour change.

7. Follow-up of Community

The follow-up of clients in their home at regular interval is essential to motivate the clients to continue the treatment or prophylaxis to complete the immunisation, to limit and space their children and report marriages, pregnancy, births and deaths to subcentre, apart from encouraging them for initiating early breastfeeding and exclusive breastfeeding, start supplementary feeding at right age, give enough semisolid food to child and observe rules of hygiene. Follow-up ensures regular contacts, development of trust as also increased utilisation of service.

Follow-up also ensures the progress of antenatal period and weight gain or development of any complication or danger signs, growth of children and reinforcing the messages for appropriate action.

8. Evaluation of Therapy

The impact of interventions can be assessed by monitoring of activities through annual reports or annual surveys and rapid methods of assessment, by eliciting "client satisfaction", improvement of malnutrition, increased levels of coverage of immunization and maternal and child health services. Regular monitoring of drinking water supply by orthotoluidine test and coliform count provides useful information on quality of water supply. The results of evaluation can be generated at each level, i.e. Subcentre, PHC, CHC and District level.

9. Replanning of Services

The results of evaluation should be fed back to the system for improving the services/programmes and replanning of services. Community diagnosis is thus a scientific and epidemiological approach for identification of community problems/needs step by step. It involves essentially a team work and requires help from other sectors as well like ICDS, education and village *Panchayat*.

Community involvement is essential. Community diagnosis and need assessment is a dynamic process. Some of the parameters are collected once a while say once a year, but most of the information on needs assessments are continuous like marriages, pregnancy, childbirth, death and occurrence of disease, etc. hence surveillance programme is built into the system of health for continuous assessment. Doctor provides leadership in community needs assessment or diagnosis.

Distinction between Clinical and Community Medicine

The approaches in clinical medicine and community medicine are distinct. The purpose of this elucidation is not to undermine the discipline of clinical medicine or hospitals, but to emphasize that the "medicine as a social science" has much wider scope and bigger responsibility. The preventive and social medicine/community medicine specialists have to be best physician first to accomplish the tasks in the community. The areas and skills of two disciplines are clear cut and distinction has been drawn between the two to enhance the understanding of students of community medicine. Clinical medicine and preventive and social medicine (community medicine) need each other and interdepend and interrelate in many of the critical areas; however, the approach differs (Table 1.2).

The prevention is not the monopoly of preventive and social medicine alone the "preventive outlook and attitude of mind" applies equally to all branches of medicine and its specialities. All branches of clinical medicine—surgery, obstetrics and gynaecology, paediatrics or any of their sub-specialities, aim at early diagnosis and prompt treatment and application of preventive aspects in their respective speciality.

India's Share in Global Health Problems

- 17% of the population
- 21% of Global disease burden
- 17% of total deaths
- 23% of child deaths
- 20% of maternal deaths
- Lymphatic filariasis 40%
- 58% of leprosy cases
- 23% of tuberculosis cases
- 10% of HIV infected persons

(*Source:* 10th and 11th Five-Year-Plan document)

Major Health Problems in India 2015

Population in 2014	**1295 million**
Sex ratio:	**940**
Female illiteracy:	**65.46%**
People below poverty line: 2012	**21.8%**
Population without sanitary conditions:	**60%**
Human development index rank 2015	**130**
DISEASE BURDEN	
India's global disease burden	**21%**
Tuberculosis: Incidence per year	**2.2 million**
HIV/AIDS: Burden	**2.16 million**
STIs/Reproductive tract infections:	**30 million**
Malaria incidence per year:	**1.50 to 2.0 million**
Filariasis-endemic districts:	**250 districts**
People suffering from goiter and other Iodine deficiency disorders	**71 million**
Polio-since 2014 India is polio free	
Anaemia in pregnancy:	**58.8%**
Safe deliveries:	**76%**
High maternal mortality rate	**167**
High infant mortality rate	**40**
High total fertility rate	**2.4**
Low birth weight babies:	**28%**
Underweight children below five years:	**47%**
Proportion of deaths due to non-communicable diseases:	**42%**
Deaths due to accidents and injuries:	**10%**
Proportion of deaths due to communicable diseases:	**38%**
Emerging and re-emerging infectious diseases:	**Epidemics**
Allopathic doctor population ratio	**1:1319**

Table 1.2: Distinction between clinical medicine and community medicine (PSM)

Areas/outlook	*Clinical medicine*	*Community medicine/preventive and social medicine/public health*
Focus	Treats individual	Treats community
Concern	Sick persons	Sick persons and healthy people both
Responsibility	Of those who come to seek help	Whole community
Goal	To relieve symptoms, signs and to cure patient	• To eliminate and eradicate disease. • To reduce incidence and prevalence of diseases
Skills/competence	Clinical skills	Epidemiological-biostatistic and managerial skills
Treatment/prescription	Treats patients with pills-drugs-injections and therapeutics	• Treats causes through National Health Programmes • Treats environments—safe water—safe excreta disposal. • Raises community immunity by mass immunization • Mass treatment like MDA for filaria vitamin A prophylaxis • Iodized salt • DOTS (directly observed treatment short course chemotherapy) • Health legislation and behaviour change communication.
Work station	Hospitals and special clinics	Health centres, community/institutions
Teaching training	Bedside—patient side	In community
Diagnostic and evaluation tools	Uses clinical parameters	• Uses epidemiological tools: – Surveys, surveillance and outbreak investigations – Health records and epidemiological studies – Reduction of disease, death, and disability rates
Requirement	Patient compliance and cooperation	Community participation
Intersectoral Coordination	Mainly health sector	Intersectoral coordination is essential between health, ICDS, education, development and agriculture.
Results	Quickly achieved and visible	Takes longer time to see the results
Laboratory	Hospital-wards	Community

FAMILY

Family is a universal institution in all the cultures. In India, family occupies a pivotal position and is a significant system in the social fabric. The family thus is a biological unit, or a social unit and a universal institution in every society.

Several definitions of family have been given from time to time; some of these are being reproduced:

- McLver defines family as a group defined by a sex relationship, sufficiently precise and enduring to provide for the procreation and upbringing of children.
- According to Burgess and Locke, a family is "A group of persons united by ties of marriage, blood or adoption, constituting a single household, interacting and intercommunicating with each other in their respective social roles of husband and wife, mother and father, son and daughter, brother and sister, creating a common culture".[5]
- Ninkoff defines a family "As a more or less a durable association of husband and wife with or without children or a man or woman along with children".
- Elliot and Merrill define family as "The biological social unit composed of husband, wife and children."
- The definition given by Bureau of Census (USA) is easier. According to Bureau, the family is "A group of two or more persons related by blood, marriage or adoption and residing together."

Household

The term family differs from household, in that, all members of household may not be blood related, e.g. servants.

House and Household

The term "house" means a structure with a single roof, where one or more than one family may be residing during the enumeration of population.

The number of households in a house is determined according to number of kitchens (chulahs) in a house. For examples, if there are four families living in a house and their food is being cooked in three kitchens, the total numbers of households will be three. In a house, there may be more than one household and each should be assigned a separate identity number.

Characteristics of Family

Out of these definitions, the following characteristic can be summed up:

- ***A mating relationship:*** The family comes into existence when a man and woman establish mating relationship between them. The relation may be of shorter duration or lifelong. When a marital relation breaks down, the family disintegrates.
- ***A form of marriage:*** Mating relationship is established through the institution of marriage, it may take one of the several forms, monogamous or polygamous, partners may be selected by the parents or elderly persons in the family in arranged marriages or an individual himself/herself may select the partner.
- ***A common habitation:*** Family lives in home or household for child bearing and rearing.
- ***System of nomenclature:*** Every family is known by name and it has its own system of reckoning and descent. The descent may be reckoned through the male line or through the female line. Usually the wife goes and joins her husband's relatives but sometimes husband also may go and join his wife's relatives (in North-East India).
- ***An economic provision:*** There is some source of income to sustain economic needs of the family. Head of the family performs certain vocation to earn money.

Types or Forms of Families

The families can be classified on the basis of authority or else on the basis of structure.

On the basis of authority vested the families can be either:

- *Patriarchal:* Where male member as head of family is authority in decision-making and controlling the family affairs and the female is subordinate. Patriarchy defines life patterns and culture and even way men and women think about one another. The descent is recokned through the male line.
- *Matriarchal:* The authority is vested in female head of the family. In rural areas 12.8% of households are headed by women.

On the basis of marriage pattern, the family may be classified as:

- *Monogamous* in which one man marries one woman. Only such a marriage where there is only one regular trusted sexual partner and both are free from HIV infection have no chance of acquiring sexually transmitted infections like HIV and other STDs.
- *Polygamous family:* Husband has more than one wife or multiple sexual partners, such a marriage relationship in these families involves the greater risk of transmission of STDs and HIV infections.
- *Polyandrous family:* In this kind of family, one woman marries many men and lives with all of them or with each of them alternatively. This also involves the risk of multiple sexual partnerships. If it is regular partnership the risk of HIV transmission is somewhat less but certainly it carries more risk if the partnership is irregular and involves multiple sexual partnership behaviour is prevalent in men.

Similarly the family could belong to various groups as per sanctions of marriage.

An endogamous family is one which sanctions marriage only within members of in-groups. Consanguineous marriages, i.e. marriages amongst cousins have more risk of transmission of genetic disorders.

An exogamous family is one which sanctions or allows marriages of in-groups with members of an out-group. Such a marriage carries low risk of transmission of genetic disorders.

On the basis of the structure, the family has been classified as nuclear, joint or extended family.

Nuclear Family

Nuclear family is one which consists of the husband, wife and their children who stay together. These types of families are common in urban settings when the male adult members get married, they leave their parental home and start their life as an independent unit. Compelling reasons for development of nuclear family are—the male member getting an employment in urban settings far away from parental house or the newly married couples wish to stay away from their parental house. Industrialization, urbanization and employment pattern are some of the compelling reasons for development of nuclear family. In a nuclear family, both the parents may be employed for the job or work for wages, children are left under the care of some agency or at home under the care of servant.

The strain and stress of bringing up children (feeding and care) is real in nuclear family. If the wife is housewife, the worry of care of child gets reduced. The development of children in such families is a challenge. The extra-familial institutions, such as creches, child care centres, balwadi centres or nurseries are utilised for the care and development of young children by most nuclear families. These institutions charge heavy money which may be beyond the earning capacity of parents. Sometimes the agency like Red Cross or women and child welfare department provides these creches in urban settings.

Joint or Extended Family

The culture of joint family is widely prevalent in rural India and even in urban areas. Married couple/couples live with their parents. The children of these couples are looked after by the grandparents as the men and women are away for field work or are in the job. The joint family shares the common kitchen. All the property is held in common; including land. To save the land from division or fragmentation, joint families played their pivotal role. The authority is vested in the eldest member who is the head of the family/household. Joint family is characterised by large size, common residence, common purse, common kitchen and common land and there is great degree of interdependency.

The merits of joint family are—that it provides social and economic security to all its members—working, non-working, old age people and young children, sick people, widows and handicapped/disabled. The widow's re-marriage is common and it is a kind of rehabilitation to save the property in the name of joint family.

Apart from merits, there are several demerits of joint family, such as it hinders the development of personality, privacy to couple is least, and it leads to uncontrolled births. Merits overweigh demerits.

Three Generation Family

It is also a joint family but it denotes that three generations stay together and share common house and kitchen. Grandparents, their married sons and their offsprings are an example of three generation family.

Functions of Family

Biological Function

The basic/essential function of family is to bear children and propagate its progeny. Bearing and rearing children is to preserve its species. In the process of bearing children, there may be too many children, which add to the size of family and in some states like Bihar, Rajasthan, Uttar Pradesh and Madhya Pradesh, the family size tends to be large and acceptance of contraception may be low. Biological function should have emphasis on quality of life. Though the total fertility rate has declined from 6.0 (1951) to 2.4 in 2012, we have a long way to go to achieve replacement level of fertility of 2.1. Interruption of biological function by contraception adds on, the essential responsibility of ensuring the survival of the children born as also adequate quality of life.

Rear Children

Rearing children is another essential or obligatory function. Rearing children means nurturing; transmitting values and culture till such period the children attain adulthood and become independent. Rearing practices vary from culture to culture and family to family. Child learns moral values and develops "lifestyle" within the family as family and parents are eternal and first school of learning for a young child. The basic values and practices are transmitted from parents and family members to their children/offsprings. In this process, the parents and other family members have to be good role models for their children.

Child may acquire the habit of smoking from parents or grandparents, habit of use of toilet, brushing teeth, washing hands and personal hygiene is acquired in the family. Family needs to be supported in this function by all other social institutions like *Anganwadi* centres, creches, balwadis and formal system of schools. The total child development and growth is family-based but conditioned by the environments.

Culture Transmission

The family is an institution that transmits traditional values, ideals, beliefs, practices and traditions. The child who is born in the family is a "clean slate" and he imbibes and learns the values, beliefs, practices from his family. Some of the things which cannot be taught by any other institution are best learnt within the family.

Security

Family provides social and income security to its members. It provides shelter, food, clothing and other necessities of life to dependent members. Similarly, family provides security to old age person, to sick and disabled person. Mentally retarded and other disabled are best cared for in the family. Old age homes are homes away from home and do not provide family environments hence family in Indian set-up is the best institution for care of the elderly people. All efforts should be directed to sustain and maintain the institution of family.

Shaping Personality and Lifestyles of an Individual

Family takes pride in shaping of personality of an individual. Behaviour pattern of a person, obedience, respectfulness, cooperativeness, truthfulness, discipline, self-reliance, ability to stand against stress, gender respect, develops in the milieu of family. Children learn by imitation and this learning can be further enhanced by extra-familial institutions like non-formal education imparted through ICDS *Anganwadi* workers and continued through the formal education system of school.

Thus, family is sheet anchor for sustaining and providing social and economic security, developing personality traits and transmission of values and culture to its members. The family would be referred and quoted in all "lifestyle diseases", "chronic non-communicable diseases" and "behavioural problems" because all have their origin at the place of living and in the family and the natural history of disease can be traced to the setting of family. The first response to illness of young children or any other falling ill comes from family. It is the family response which matters most in child survival may it be initiation of breastfeeding, exclusive breastfeeding, administration of home available fluids (HAF) in diarrhoea, continuing feeding during diarrhoea, smokeless kitchen, supplementary feeding, spacing and limitation of births, home delivery/institutional delivery, seeking antenatal care, immunisation services and treatment of tuberculosis, the decisions of family are critical. Therefore, the families need to be empowered and well informed and supported by all the primary health centres, subcentres, ICDS system, education and development department. How this support comes is a matter of national, state, district and local policy of village *Panchayat*. Disparity between boys and girls and adverse sex ratio (gender discrimination) is ultimately family or at the most a community choice.

Food availability at the household level is seldom a problem for children between the ages of 6 and 24 months, the amounts required are small, the issue is proper care and attention to child's need and attitudes of the family which deliberately denies food (cereals) to children, due to wrong beliefs.

Social attitudes at the family level are at heart of environmental concerns. Much of the hygiene and sanitation is in the mind, rooted in conceptions of purity, pollution, and dignity of labour. Family level storage of drinking water and its use, protection from contamination by use of clean hands are decisions of the family. Safe disposal of garbage, refuse, waste water and excreta disposal are ultimately the decisions of the family. Sanitation costs nothing when people cooperate and take it by themselves. People's programme on sanitation succeed but Government programmes on sanitation quite often fail. Sanitation and hygiene is essentially a way of life deep rooted in the cultural practices and only determined efforts of families can make it successful.

Family and Health

What people do with their lives and those of their children affect their health far more than anything that Governments do but what they can do is determined, to a great extent, by their income and knowledge—factors that are not completely within their control.

Poverty reduction programmes and universal elementary education and education for all especially for girls (*Sarva Shikhsha Abhiyan*) by the Government if pursued and implemented vigorously can change the scenario. Similarly, primary health care for all can make the differences.

Reaching Families

The primary health care is reaching families through network of subcentres, PHCs, CHCs and *Anganwadis*. This appears to be the major means of reaching families. It is mandatory for health workers female and *Anganwadi* worker to maintain family records of each household. This household register (family register) connects families to the system of subcentres and *Anganwadis* under ICDS. Family register is updated once every year and it forms the basis of formulation of village and subcentre action plan and community needs assessment. The needs of each family are assessed by the health workers by establishing contacts with each family. The family register provides wealth of information relevant to the health and action to be initiated/undertaken by the worker.[6–8] The objectives of this register are:

To assess the health status of each individual in the household and its environment and for identifying eligibles for initiating relevant health care activities.

The information of household register consists of—household information and individual information.

The household information consists of:

House No........... Household No........... Single couple or Joint Family........... Religion/Caste........... Source of drinking water........... Type of latrine...........Above/below Poverty line.

The information on individual is given in Table 1.3.

Armed with this information the health workers, Anganwadi workers and ASHAs are required to visit 10 families per day and to cover the entire area within 3 months period. The priority houses where visit is required are chosen and priority includes:

- Eligible couple
- Pregnant women—unregistered.
- Registered pregnancy with any complications or not turning up for 2nd dose of tetanus toxoid/or IFA tablets.
- Postnatal case not seen after delivery.
- A low birth weight neonate.
- A new acceptor of oral pill/IUD.
- Child with suspected pneumonia.
- Child with diarrhoea with some dehydration.
- Child with vitamin A deficiency not turning up for second therapeutic dose.
- An infant not turning up for immunisation.
- Follow-up after tubectomy and follow-up of referred to PHC/CHC/hospital by you.
- A person acutely and seriously ill.
- A child who has had an adverse reaction to any immunisation.
- Maternal, neonate or child death.
- A recent case of acute flaccid paralysis.
- Severely malnourished child.

In summary, it includes priority houses of "scheduled caste, below poverty line families or landless families", and families having either infant or pregnant woman.

Table 1.3: Individual information (Household survey)

1 Eligible couple and child register no.	2 Name	3 Age	4 Sex	5 Relation to head of household	6 Marital status			7 Immunization status	8 Morbidity status	9 Disability if any	10 Significant events (births-deaths-marriages-migration)	11 Remarks or any other information (below poverty line family occupation and literacy)
					Unmarried	Married (date and year)	Widowed/ divorced					

1

Before making home visits, the workers are required to look into the relevant individual health card, immunisation card, or family record and note the urgency of the health needs. The workers review any procedures to be carried out, specific advice to be given or demonstration to be done. Workers carry the required articles and records with them and visit the priority houses/families.

This example indicates that the primary health care services are family-based. Family health services have been further reinforced by community need assessment approach; similarly the National Active Surveillance Programme for malaria (now named as National Vector-borne Disease Control Programme) is family-based wherein beat programme to cover all households/families is ensured. Family health awareness campaign is yet another example to reach all families to target persons between 15 and 49 years of age.

Family Size

In general, the family size means total number of persons in family, however demographically it means the number of children a woman has born at a point in time. The total fertility rate (TFR) means the average number of children born to a woman during her lifetime or else the number of children that would be born per woman if she was to live to the end of her child-bearing years (15–49 years) and bear children at each age in accordance with prevailing age specific fertility rate (see measures of fertility).

$$\text{TFR} = \frac{5\sum_{15\ 19}^{15\ 49} \text{Age specific fertility rate}}{1000}$$

During the year 1951, the TFR was 6.0. The current level of TFR is 2.4 (2012). We want to bring it down to the level of 2.1 by 2017 this in other words means two child norm. In states like Uttar Pradesh, TFR is 3.3, Bihar 3.5, Rajasthan 2.9 and Madhya Pradesh 2.9.

The large size of the families in these states is attributable to early marriages, lack of practice of contraception due to illiteracy, ignorance and poverty, unfavourable attitudes and disbelief in contraception. These states are very high focus states for Family Planning Programme.

Large-sized family means where the number of children are more than average of the nation, these families are at risk families.

Broken Family

These are those families where the parents have separated or divorced due to disharmony or else one or both parents have died and the children become orphans. Such a situation profoundly affects the physical, social and mental development of children since the family support is lost or it is partial. Children of such families may drift to abnormal development and likely to develop behavioural problems. *Orphanages* provide support to such children.

Broken homes are due to inter- and intra-family quarrels and is the bed rock on which personality and psychological breakdown starts in children.

Problem Families or High-risk Families

Such families like large-sized families, families below poverty line, broken families, addiction in husband, and long illness of child or in any other member are called problem families and these families need to be targeted as priority families for health care, social development and poverty alleviation. Children in these families run the risk of poor health, development problems and social problems.

Socioeconomic Status (SES) of Family

The socioeconomic status of family can be determined on the basis of *education*, *occupation* and *income* level. Based on these variables, socioeconomic status has been measured by following methods.

Kuppuswami's Method (for Urban Area)

Kuppuswami's method takes into consideration the education, occupation and monthly income of respondent to classify or determine socioeconomic status. Each component is given a weighted score and then the total score is summed up and the individual/family can be classified into a socioeconomic class I, II, III, IV and V. The level of income is generally updated on the basis of consumer price index (CPI) (Table 1.4).

Udai Pareek's Method (For Rural Areas)

Pareek has evolved to determine socioeconomic scale and class for rural area.[7] It takes into consideration–caste, occupation, education, land holding, social participation, family size, housing and farm power and material possession. Each of these components is given weighted score and by summing up all the components the SES can be determined and categorised into several classes, as given in Table 1.5.

This way individual and families can be classified into a socioeconomic class. Income may be concealed and it may not be easy to determine. To determine the level of poverty, these criteria can be adopted to classify the family as below poverty line (BPL) or above poverty line (APL).

Prasad's Method (1961)[8]

Socioeconomic status of family can also be known by criteria proposed by BG Prasad in 1961, which includes per capita monthly income of an individual as given in Table 1.6.

Standard of living index (SLI)[9] based on household amenities and possession of some selected household items, the SLI can be developed by allocating scores to

Table 1.4: Kuppuswami's method of social classification of an individual (urban areas)

Component	Weighted score	Component	Weighted score
(A) Completed educational qualification		**(C) Monthly income (2003)**	
• Professional degree	7	• Above ₹ 20000	12
• Graduate	6	• 10000–19999	10
• Intermediate/diploma	5	• 7500–9999	6
• High school	4	• 5000–7499	4
• Middle school	3	• 3000–4999	3
• Primary school	2	• 1001–2999	2
• Illiterate	1	• Below ₹ 1000	1
(B) Occupation		**Calculation**	
• Professional	10	***Total score = A+B+C***	***Social class****
• Semiprofessional	6	• 26–29	I
• Clerical/shop/farm	5	• 16–25	II
• Skilled worker	3	• 11–15	III
• Semiskilled worker	3	• 5–10	IV
• Unskilled worker	2	• Below 5	V
• Unemployed	1		

*Class I is highest socioeconomic class; while class V is lowest economic class.

Table 1.5: Pareek's method of socioeconomic classification (rural areas)

Components	Weighted score	Components	Weighted score
(A) Caste		**(F) Family members**	
• Scheduled caste	1	• Up to 5	1
• Lower caste	2	• Above 5	2
• Artisan caste	3	**(G) House**	
• Agriculture caste	4	• No house	1
• Prestige caste	5	• Kutcha house	2
• Dominant caste	6	• Mixed house	3
(B) Occupation		• Pucca house	4
• None	0	• Mansion	6
• Labourer	1	**(H) Farm power**	
• Caste occupation	2	• No. draught* (buffalow/cows) animal	1
• Business	3	• 1–2 draught animals	2
• Independent profession	4	• 3–4 draught animals	3
• Cultivation	5	• 5–6 draught animals or tractor	6
• Service	6	**(I) Material possession**	
(C) Education		• Bullock cart	1
• Illiterate	0	• Cycle	1
• Can read only	1	• Radio	1
• Can read and write	2	• Chairs	1
• Primary	3	• Improved agriculture equipment	2
• Middle	4	• None	0
• High school	5	**Socioeconomic class**	
• Graduate and above	6	***Total score***	***Grading***
(D) Land		Score more than 43	I
• No land	0	Score 33–42	II
• Less than 1 acre	1	Score 24–32	III
• 1–5 acre	2	Score 13–23	IV
• 5–10 acre	3	Score less than 13	V
• 10–15 acre	4		
• 15–20 acre	5		
• 20 and above	6		
(E) Social participation			
• None	0		
• Member of one organization (like *Panchayat* member, *Nambardar*, etc.)	1		
• Member of more than one organisation	2		
• Office holder in such organisation	3		
• Wider public leader	6		

*Draught animal—animal used for pulling heavy load.

Table 1.6: Prasad's social classification

Social class	*Per capita monthly income limits (₹)*	
	Prasad's classification 1961	*Modified (proposed in March 1991*)*
I	100 and above	1000 and above
II	50–99	500–999
III	30–49	300–499
IV	15–29	150–299
V	Below 15	Below 150

*Proposed by Kumar P., IJCM 1993; XVIII (2): 60–61.

items. The total of scores may vary from lowest of 0 to maximum of 40. On the basis of total score households are divided into three categories as:

a Low—if total score is less than or equal to 9.

b Medium—if total score is greater than 9 but less than or equal to 19.

c High—if the score is greater than 19.

These three categories of SLI have been used in district level household surveys and NFHS in India (Table 1.7).

Socioeconomic criteria determine the level of "well-being", lifestyles, and utilisation of services apart from social status and recognition and position in the society. Wealth does not ensure or guarantee good health as wealthy may adopt unhealthy lifestyles. Poor may spend money on alcohol or tobacco and wealthy persons may smoke, drink and consume unhealthy diets (more saturated animal fats, animal food, etc.). Income level or socio-economic status of families can be assessed by rapid observation methods and family can be described as economically well-off or economically weaker or middle class family. Middle class income families in India are under transition and obesity, hypertension, coronary heart disease and diabetes (all lifestyle diseases) are emerging in this socioeconomic class, while poor families bear the burnt of malnutrition, repeated infections due to diarrhoeal diseases, acute respiratory infections, and worm infestation, etc.

Social Mobility

The socioeconomic status of an individual/family can change or advance over a time period with attainment of literacy, better occupation and enhanced income. Person/family of low socioeconomic status may move to upward scale (higher socioeconomic status) or from higher status to poor economic status. This phenomenon is known as social mobility. Stories of rags to riches are most common.

Table 1.7: Standard of living index (SLI)

Sr. No.	*Variables*	*Categories*	*Scores*
1	Source of drinking water	i Tap (own)	3
		ii Tap shared	2
		iii Hand pump+well	1
		iv Others	0
2	Type of house	i Pucca	4
		ii Semi-pucca	2
		iii Katcha	0
3	Source of lighting	i Electricity	2
		ii Kerosene	1
		iii Others	0
4	Fuel for cooking	i LPG	2
		ii Kerosene	1
		iii Others	0
5	Toilet facility	i Own flush toilet	4
		ii Own pit toilet	2
		iii Shared toilet	2
		iv No toilet	0
6	Ownership of items	i Fan	2
		ii Radio/transistor	2
		iii Sewing machine	2
		iv Television	3
		v Telephone	3
		vi Bicycle	2
		vii Motor cycle/scooter	3
		viii Car	4
		ix Tractor	4

1

Below Poverty Line (BPL) Families

Poverty itself is a disease which cripples access to and success in school/college. Ill health comes in the way of working harder and longer and reduce productivity and income and thus sets a vicious cycle.

a According to World Bank criteria of new poverty line of $ 1.25 per day at 2011 Purchasing Power Parity (PPP) 33% of Population of India is now living below poverty line. This is much above the earlier estimates based on $ 1 per day. If Asian Development Bank Criteria of $ 1.35 per day per person is applied 54.8 percent of India's population is living below poverty line which is almost double the poverty estimates of 28.5 per cent (Planning Commission of Government of India, 2004).[10] The Planning Commission's latest poverty estimates (year 2009) of 38 per cent is a 10 per cent jump from its last estimates in 2004–05 which was 28.5 per cent. The new estimate is based on monthly expenses of a household on health, food, education, sanitation and income indicators. A family of five with total income of less than ₹ 3000 a month in urban areas and ₹ 2250 in rural areas, should be considered poor. Until now, using standards laid down in 1998, an urban family of five earning ₹ 2200 per month and rural family earning ₹ 1650 were considered poor.[11]

b Planning Commission (Govt. of India) defines poverty line as a total household per capita expenditure sufficient to provide in addition to basic non-food items-clothing, transport—a daily intake of 2400 calories per person in rural areas and 2100 in urban area. Govt. of India defines poverty line as expenditure class-wise distribution of persons less than ₹ 560 per person per month in urban area and below ₹ 368 in rural area (at 2004–2005 prices). According to these criteria, 28.5% of population is below poverty line in India.

c However, income and expenditure approach to determine BPL was adopted in 10th plan by 13 indicators, by giving a weighted score to each indicator, ranging from 0 to 4. The sum of score of all indicators obtained ranges from 0 to 52. The list of BPL so prepared should be approved by *Gram Sabha*. The indicators included land holding, type of house, average availability of normal wear clothing (per person in pieces), food security, sanitation, ownership of consumer durables, literacy status of highest literate adult, status of household, labour force, means of livelihood, status of children (5–14 years), type of indebtness, reasons for migration from household and preference for assistance. Below poverty line families are at risk families. Over 47% of population in Odisha, 42.60% in Bihar, 37.43% in Madhya Pradesh, 31.15% in Uttar Pradesh, was below poverty line against the national figure of 28%.

The Government of India (2008) has decided to redefine poverty as deprivation by including seven indicators of deprivation to arrive at deprivation index:

1 Average income
2 Out of school kids
3 Accessibility to basic health services
4 Access to clean drinking water and sanitation
5 Whether children work
6 Electric connection
7 Link with all weather road.

In 75% of 179 million rural households monthly income of the highest earning member is less than ₹ 5000 per month. About 106 million households (60%) being deprived household (socio-economic and caste census 2011).

Sustainable Development Goal 1 states: "End poverty in all its forms eveywhere" Target is to halve between 2015 and 2030, the proportion of people whose income is less than $ 1.25 per day. Latest estimate of poverty in India (2011) is 29.8%. At the current rate of progress it may take 41 years to eradicate poverty in India. For inclusive development the centre and states focus more on handouts to the poor than spending on water, nutrition, affordable houses, education, health and employment generation. In the year 2012 GOI estimated poverty at the level of 21.8%, based on per capita monthly consumption expenditure of less than ₹ 1640 in rural and ₹ 2500 in urban areas at current prices (2014). Population below international/ poverty line-living on less than US$ 1.90 per day in India (2009–2013) was 21% (UNICEF 2016).

Family-based Household Records

Home based pregnant mother and infant immunization card is powerful tool to educate family as also to motivate them to complete all the health actions up to 3 years of age. (Mother and child protection card prepared by Ministry of Women and Child Development GOI and Ministry of Health of Family Welfare). This is a ready-made tool to evaluate the services and outcome thereof by the family itself. Simplified records (with pictorial and action photographs) of this kind are quite valuable and helpful to both the family and the health care system to evaluate their performance and to quickly know, what remains to be done. Apart from this, it generates demand for maternal and child health services and is a useful tool for referral centres, as well as to monitor the progress of these services (Fig. 1.1).

Family Medicine

"Family Medicine" is an academic discipline and a speciality recognised by National Board of Examination and the Medical Council of India leading to degree awarded called Diplomat of National Board (DNB), on par with other postgraduate degrees. However, the universities and medical colleges have not set-up the departments of family medicine so far. Only a few MBBS doctors in practice or Government service have acquired DNB.[12]

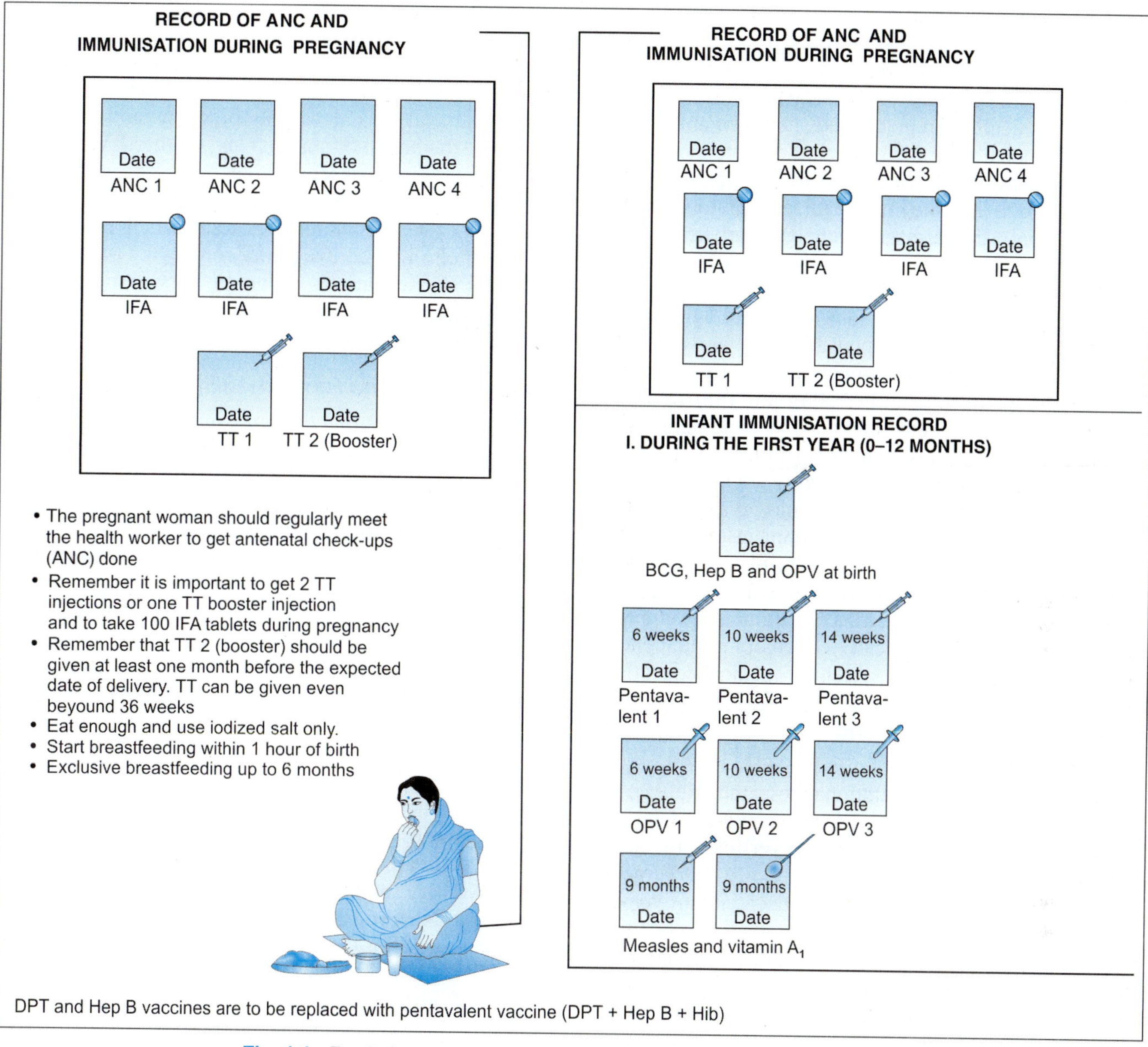

Fig. 1.1: Family/home-based records (Mother and Child Protection card)

There is need for creating awareness in the public about family medicine as an independent speciality. Family physician is the first level contact for the patient and his family. In a country with large population spread over to vast rural and urban areas, the need for adequately trained, properly qualified, competent general practitioners is acutely felt. National Board is a unique body which conducts postgraduate degree examinations in family medicine to the award of Diplomat of National Board (family medicine).

"Family" being the basic unit of community is a well-defined entity and fundamental unit of clinico-epidemiology. "Family" being a recognized unit of both development and social growth, it is a unit of living as well as unit of illness. Individual reacts on the family and the family reacts on the individual and as such illness is a family event.

The practitioner of "family medicine" is a basic doctor or physician who has to concern himself with the promotive, preventive, curative and rehabilitative family oriented approach in health and disease. Thus, the concept of family medicine endeavours comprehensive and continuity of care covering the total life cycle (all phases of life). In essence, "family medicine" is total medicine, for total family in its total environment and it goes far beyond the concept of general practice. Family medicine emphasizes attention to responsibility for total health care for sick and healthy both. Family doctor who combines preventive with curative medicine, with the full background of total environment is able to see persons in the *prepathogenic period*, as well as *pathogenic period* of disease and he is able to study all the elements that produce disease or make the family healthy.

After obtaining DNB such a doctor should be able to render health services to the community by providing primary health care to all members irrespective of age, sex, culture and socioeconomic background. He should be able to decide for appropriate referral in order to provide secondary/tertiary health services when necessary. He should be clinically competent and should be able to take personal responsibility for rendering comprehensive and continuing care of his patients in their own setting. He should be able to institute immediate resuscitatory and first aid measures in different emergencies apart from taking administrative responsibility of health centre and training of medical and paramedical staff.

Family physician should think epidemiologically and act socially. Accepting the responsibility of family in health and disease becomes the cardinal skill. Ability to assess the health problems in the assigned families in a geographical area and ensuring adequate and appropriate response is the major task which is similar to community diagnosis and treatment of community (families).

Practice of family medicine has almost disappeared due to advances in medicine and development of specialities and super-specialities but we certainly need general practitioners. MG Institute of Medical Sciences and Research at Sewagram (Wardha) is a unique example in the country which took a lead in developing the concept of 'general practice' in the system of medical education.

Research in Family Medicine

'Family' is a unique biological unit where one can undertake applied and operational research. Research is really attitude of mind. The process consists of making observations which are objective and verifiable by others. The opportunities for research in family medicine lie essentially in the area of primary health care improvement.

There are opportunities for family medicine practitioner to undertake clinical, epidemiological, behavioural and educational researches. Most important method of research available with family practitioners is *clinical* and *observational methods*. He may use simple tests; out of his observations arise a problem and he develops a hypothesis and begins to test it. *Epidemiological research* provides special opportunities in the work of family medicine practitioner. It identifies *risk factors* rather than specific agents, it requires no complex technology except the field data processing and so much has come out of these researches. The diseases can be related to behaviour, lifestyles and maladaptation. The *case study* method is most appropriate for family practitioner. It is a detailed study of a single and well-defined social life or a case in its natural environment. In depth, exploration of case leads on to several evidences which can be verified further. The case study is associated with qualitative approach in particular with ***anthropological*** and ***ethnographic research***. (Scientific description of people and culture with respect to their customs and characteristics).

The information is gathered by interviews, observations, reviews of various records, reports and tests. A notebook and pencil are considered very important instruments. This kind of research provides answer to leading causes of morbidity, death, who dies most often, what is economic burden of ill health, what are feeding habits, outlook of people (attitudes) and various practices and how these influence the health of children and mothers. Many of the answers to big problems have come through simple observations of this kind. John Snow observed deaths occurrence due to contaminated water which provided the basis of cholera control and control of water-borne diseases. Observations serve as very important epidemiological tool to explain *natural history of disease* and build appropriate intervention.

Family Studies and Family Health Services[13,14]

It is a matter of routine that undergraduates and postgraduates in community medicine are given family studies in urban slums or rural areas depending upon the resources. Each medical college has adopted some urban area in their vicinity for the purpose of family studies and some institutions go on changing the area after one or two years. Very few institutions have taken the total responsibility of geographical area for *provision* of *primary health care services* on *continuous basis* especially *maternal* and *child* health *services*, and services for national health programmes. Further very few institutions have established linkages with the urban health authorities and municipal corporations to avoid duplication and to enhance coordination for health services. The essential requirements for meaningful family studies include, having an urban health centre (UHC) or health posts established in urban slum, take responsibility for essential services on continuous basis (at least National Health Programmes) and have adequate staff for urban health centre as per requirement of MCI. Lastly establish linkage and submit a progress report of performance to health authority or municipal corporation every month and attend the review meeting with the authorities and involve them in teaching and training programmes of undergraduates and postgraduates, since they are the real practitioners of Public Health/Community Medicine.

What is the Purpose?

The major purpose of family study is to offer educational experiences with focus on "learning" the natural history of disease, the levels of prevention apart from assessing health needs of family.

Demography, medical sociology, behavioural sciences, art of interview and communication, vital statistic and biostatistics, epidemiology, health care delivery system, health management, health information system and National Health Programmes can be the focus of family studies. In brief, family studies help learning most aspects of community medicine. The art and science of community medicine can be seen, perceived and learnt best in families or in community. There is no exaggeration if we say that the whole subject of community medicine can be best learned and practiced in the families and community, hence most of the teaching and training should be based in the community. Wherever possible the system of ICDS (*Anganwadis*) in urban or rural setting should be used to the maximum as it (ICDS) is community-based and family-linked and it creates positive influence on the minds of over 51979 MBBS students admitted every year.

In our experience, the following aspects can be easily covered in planned manner to achieve the stated objectives:

- Composition of family (structure). Birth interval, age and sex composition. Large-sized and problematic families, and their unmet health needs.
- Most vulnerables in the family.
- Gender issues and practices in the family.
- Socioeconomic profile (literacy, occupation and income). Below poverty line, and above poverty line families.
- Benefits reaching below poverty line families.
- Vital events, disabilitics—agc of marriage and registration of events (pregnancy, birth and deaths).
- Social factors related to health and disease.
- Environments—sources of drinking water, water storage practices, garbage and excreta disposal, problem of over-crowding and Indoor air pollution.
- Health beliefs, attitudes and practices—reproductive health behaviour, gender biases, gender analysis contraception practices and beliefs.
- Infant and young child feeding practices.
- Interaction and interrelation between family members, and Addiction/substance abuse in family.
- Dietary surveys (qualitative and quantitative methods).
- Growth monitoring of young children.
- Health and nutrition education and communication.
- Supplementary nutrition—therapeutic nutrition.
- Health check up of family members for communicable and non-communicable diseases and care of elderly.
- Outreach session on immunisation.
- Motivation exercises.
- Health care seeking behaviour/utilisation.
- Common illnesses and management of these by family. (Tuberculosis, Malaria, Filaria, Addiction).
- Community-based rehabilitation.
- Cost of illness (health economics).
- Mosquito breeding and fly breeding and collection of larvae and adult mosquitoes.
- Existing health care delivery system in these families.
- National health programmes (malaria surveillance, immunisation, control of anaemia, directly observed treatment short course chemotherapy, leprosy, and filaria, elimination, etc.).
- Health records and family-based health records.
- Organised primary health care/reproductive child health care.
- Functioning of NGOs in slums and ICDS in slum areas.
- Working of NGOs their role and positive contribution besides village health and sanitation committee.
- Practitioners in the area and their involvement in health programmes.
- Observe meeting of *Mahila Mandals*/woman groups.

These are indicative areas, much more can be added and these can be enriched by advance preparation. The family exercises done by the students can be compiled and the data thus generated can be pooled and used for teaching of health statistics, behavioural sciences, managerial sciences and epidemiology. Similarly, case studies or caselets, problem-based learning and clinical-social case-review exercises can be generated out of these. Much will depend on the teachers and preceptors of the students and their orientation, attitudes and preparedness. Spot exercises like testing of residual chlorine at home and iodized salt testing or simple test of food adulteration can be quite impressive and effective. Similarly, collection of sample of water, stool, blood smear, blood, throat swabs, etc. can be starting point in surveillance of disease or evaluation of a programme. Practice and art of interview and how to observe and what to observe are essential elements in family studies. *Listening* to people is the hallmark. *Counselling* can be most rewarding. These exercises require a great element of creativity and programming. Each learning exercise must have learning objectives, methods of learning, the observations made and inferences drawn and key health needs of family are to be documented by all students. Mere collection of data from families could be a frustrating experience. Minimum *service* component is essential to develop confidence and sustain the interest. Demonstrations can be organised by the faculty members or postgraduates and return demonstration to be done by students or family members, e.g. preparation of ORS solution, preparation of blood smears, staining and examination. At family level, emphasis is on "action" or "activities" and no time is wasted on theory or lecture. A small act is better than tonnes of advice or lecture, "actions" speak louder than "words".

PROTOCOLS

Most institutions have temptation to introduce family folders containing varieties of household registers, maternal and child health card, immunisation card, growth charts, etc. which are much different from the one's used under the national health programmes and ICDS system. In our experience use of same household survey register and cards being used in NRHM, RCH and ICDS programmes are much more meaningful. That makes more sense as it gives an opportunity to update the local record, identification of beneficiaries as also follow-up services. The observations can be cross-matched with those of health workers and gaps can be discovered for rectification. This mechanism reinforces the system and helps the system.

Clinical-social Case Review (*see* page 32)

REFERENCES

1 Young PV. Scientific Social Surveys and Research. New York: Prentice Hall; 1950.

2 David Warner. Where there is no doctor. A Village Health Care Handbook, 3rd edition, California: The Hesperian Foundation Palo Alto; 1978.

3 NIN. Community action—Family nutrition programmes, Generation of interrelated activities. Guidelines on policies and procedures. Prepared by working group. Conference of the International Union of Nutritional Sciences; 1976 Oct. 17–21; Hyderabad, India.

4 NIHAE. Steps in diagnosis of the community as a patient. Background document. Seventh staff college course; 1970 July 20–Sep. 11; New Delhi.

5 Bhushan V, Sachdeva DR. The family In: Bhushan V, Sachdeva DR (eds). An Introduction to Sociology. 34th ed. Allahabad: Kitab Mahal Publishers; 2002. p. 134–9.

6 GOI. Health management information system (version 2.0) subcentre registers and reporting formats (model). New Delhi: MOH and FW, GOI; 1992.

7 NIHFW. Survey instruments for collection of information from household developed by NIHFW for collaborative activity of the National Consortium of Public Health. New Delhi: NIHFW; 2003.

8 Kumar P. Social classification need for constant upgrading. Ind. J Comm Med; 1993, 18(2): 60–1.

9 IIHMR Jaipur–Rajasthan. Reproductive and Child Health-2. District level Household survey-2004 Haryana–Ambala. 6–7.

10 Asian Development Bank. Comparing poverty across countries. The role of purchasing power parities. Asian Development Bank; Manila; 2008.

11 Chauhan C. Hindustan Times, Thursday, August 20, 2009. "38% of Indians are poor says plan panel report".

12 National Board of Examinations. Guidelines of competency based training in family medicine. New Delhi; NBE; 2003.

13 MCI. Regulation on graduate medical education. New Delhi: MCI; 1997.

14 Lal S. Present and future status of family medicine—a speciality. New Delhi: NIPHC Publication; 1994.

COMMUNITY PARTICIPATION IN HEALTH MANAGEMENT AND DEVELOPMENT

There cannot be "health" without people participation. Goal of health can only be realised by community involvement and participation. The most valuable resources for the health of the people are the people themselves. They are the biggest resource for health and development. If community takes responsibility and becomes self-reliant, it is considered as the biggest achievement.

The community is the "heart" of primary health care system and should no longer be viewed as periphery of the system or passive recipient of services: Consumer or user is 'King' in the health care delivery system.

The existing approaches, instead of improving awareness and building self-reliance, have tended to enhance dependency and weaken the community capacity to cope with its problems.[1, 2] Various health programmes have by and large, failed to involve individuals, and families in establishing a self-reliant community. The ultimate goal of achieving a satisfactory health status for all our people cannot be secured without involving community in identification of their health needs and priorities as well as in the implementation and management of various health and related programmes.

What is Community Participation?

1 "Community participation is a process by which individuals and families assume responsibility for their own health and welfare and for those of community and develop capacity to contribute to their and the community's development" (WHO).[3,4]

2 Community participation is "an educational and empowering process in which people, in partnership with those who are able to assist them, identify the problems and needs and increasingly assume responsibility themselves to plan, manage, control and assess the collective actions that are proved necessary". Ideally true or active participation means people should be knowledgeable about their own health problems/needs, draw out the plans for action according to priority and resources available, organise and implement programme and monitor and control their progress and periodically evaluate for getting the feedback and do the reprogramming. However, under the prevailing conditions, it may be hard to expect spontaneous participation from people. To begin with, the motivational factor may be external force or help and gradually it may transform to self-motivation.[5]

Characteristics of External Stimulus

- The external stimulus or in personal term the "stimulator" has certain characteristics. He or she should aim at eliciting a response from the community in the form of strengthened organization and an increase in the level of awareness of its needs.
- The stimulator should also be able to give some support to projects emanating from the organised community and to act as a link to external, governmental or non-governmental resources.
- The stimulator should be knowledgeable of community structure, capable of communicating not only with formal leaders, but also with community at large and further identifying potential new leaders.

- Should have technical knowledge in specific field: health, nutrition, agriculture and cottage industry, etc.
- He or she should be acceptable to community.

Types of Community Participation

1. The participation in development efforts, not only at all levels, but also in all sectors, including those of food and water and others which have (sometimes barely recognised) bearing on health.
2. Participation at all levels in planning and decisions concerning the structure and functioning of health services.
3. The provision of facilities, materials, funds, labour and other support for health.
4. The provision of health services to others, e.g. elderly people in good health, helping to care for other elderly people who need assistance, or members of the family helping with a patient's physical and social rehabilitation.
5. Attention by individuals to personal hygiene, diet and self-care.

The first type may be considered the ideal form of participation, representing as it does the genuine participation of citizens at all levels in genuine types of decision relating to all aspects of development. Although seldom fully realised, it remains a standard against which other forms of participation must be measured.[5]

Observed Pattern of Community Participation in Development and Health

Community Development

The community development movement initiated way back in 1952 tried in its earnest to lay strong base of people's organizations, however, the highly centralised planning process kept the people out of focus and their involvement in planning was negligible. Someone else planned for them and subsequently the plans were implemented and executed by the executives and the government infrastructure to achieve the targets. Programmes after programmes were pushed to develop infrastructure without "preparing the community" and its active involvement.

Panchayati Raj

Introduced in 1959, is a three tier structure of local self-government at village, block and district levels. On the recommendations of the Balwant Rai Mehta Committee (1957), it was decided to create "an interconnected system of democratic institutions at the village, block and district levels" and provide general transfer of authority and responsibilities to these institutions by way of transferring resources to them for development programmes. This means progressive transfer of power and responsibility to the people through their elected representatives. Panchayati Raj Institutions (PRIs) were established in whole of India by 1964. The three-tier system consists of:

Levels	System of administration	Membership
1 **Village**	Gram Panchayat	Sarpanch and members by direct election from the village; their number varies on the size of population
2 **Block**	Panchayat Samiti	All Sarpanches (village headmen)
3 **District**	Zila Parishad	Presidents of Panchayat Samitis

PRIs are responsible for economic, social and women and child development. Control and management of subcentres, primary health centres, primary schools, water and sanitation, family welfare, animal husbandry, fisheries, adult education, and many other areas have been vested with PRIs. The implementation is, however, very slow. PRIs have been involved in all the national health programmes and in some states their participation in health and development has been marvellous.

73rd and 74th Constitutional Amendment Act, 1992, made health and family welfare and education responsibility of village Panchayats. The Panchayati Raj Institutions (PRIs) are important means of furthering decentralised planning and programme implementation in the context of NPP, 2000. However, Panchayats need further delegations of administrative and financial powers including powers of mobilisation of resources. Control of Subcentres and PHCs has been given to village Panchayats in Kerala. In some states, only control of subcentres has been given to village Panchayats. In this process, the PRIs will plan and administer the activities of subcentres and PHCs. This is power in the hands of people for their self-reliance. The progress of this movement is very slow and variable from state to state. Further one-third of seats in village Panchayats, Block Samitis and Zila Parishads have been reserved for women to empower women and mainstreaming women in development process.

Mahila Mandals

"Mahila Mandals" (women's organizations) programme under the community development movement intended to organise women groups at the village level for social, economic and health development of women (women empowerment). This programme established "core group of women" at the village level to speak for women and bring women at one platform. The activities were primarily confined to registered women group of 25–30 middle-aged women members, who enrolled themselves voluntarily. Other women and particularly women from weaker sections of community were out of reach of *Mahila Mandals* programme. Middle-aged and elderly women dominated the proceedings. However, positive contribution of these groups included—promotion of kitchen gardens, home management, female functional literacy, food preservation, smokeless chullah, sanitary latrines, small savings, craft centres, family planning and feeding of young children, Balwadis and other village-based technologies. In fact, all the Government departments made use of these "Mandals" to involve women groups in their programmes. More or less these mandals acted on the advice of official organs like Gramsevikas and Block Development and Panchayat Officer (BDPO), who were responsible for giving meagre government grant as bait. The initiative of mandals to organise other women in the village was minimal. With the passage of time, these mandals became dormant and subservient to the Government functionaries. Attempt was made to revitalise these organisations by integration with Integrated Child Development Services Scheme (ICDS), but not much could be achieved.

In the early phase of community development movement, primary health centres were integral part of the community development and *health was perceived as development function*. Village Panchayat and Block Samiti controlled these primary health centres and thus, the community had the ownership of health institutions and played pivotal role in the affairs of health care delivery system. Gradually, the Government took over the control of these health centres, process of centralisation started and thereafter this grew to over-centralisation, and people participation were marginalised.

Orientation Training Camps

National Family Welfare Programme initiated country wide programme of "orientation training camps" for men and women leaders at village level to build favourable environment as also to build partnership with people and ultimately involve people to assume responsibility to control fertility and propagate the norms of two-child family. These camps involved elderly men and women and young couples were left out of the purview of these camps. Elderly men and women were too shy to propagate the message on contraception and child bearing to younger people and vice versa young people maintained distance from elderly people because of several cultural taboos. Thus, the programme of family welfare with a stigma of 100% "centrally sponsored programme" remained a government programme, involvement of community and their participation remained marginal. The planning of family welfare programme was highly centralised and targets were set from the top with universal prescription till 8th plan period.

Orientation training camps could not generate enough information, education and communication at the level of community to lead to adoption of contraception practice and prevention of boom of unwanted pregnancies. The issues discussed in these camps related to nation and had little relevance to that community. This incongruity of perception between the people and the providers of services cost the programme dearly.

People's Health in People's Hands

The programme of community health workers/volunteers (village health guides) was adopted as a distinct strategy to universalise primary health care in the year 1977, all over India, to enhance community participation in health programmes. Over 600,000 health guides were recruited and trained to realise the dream of "People's health in people's hands". Health guides were selected by village community and they were accountable to community. During the initial phases, they did contribute in eliciting community involvement in village sanitation, taking responsibility for chlorination of wells and anti-malaria activities. However, majority of health guides overwhelmingly adhered to distribution of medicines for minor ailments. One of the disturbing observation and experience was that the Panchayat leaders and other leaders perceived this scheme essentially as Government scheme. This went against the spirit of new scheme, which sought to increase involvement of people in solving their own problems through self-help. In 1986, the Government of India dispensed with the services of male village health guides and directed the states only to appoint female health guides.[6]

ICDS

ICDS introduced *Anganwadi* workers (AWWs) as honorary workers at the village level chosen by the people themselves with an objective of enhancing women and community participation. Over 13 lakhs AWWs are in position to enhance community participation. This is the strongest base for community involvement. The AWWs have mobilised women of economically weaker sections of the community and their participation in the services of women and child development has increased enormously. ICDS services have inbuilt component of community participation, however, active participation of the community is not forthcoming to the extent desired and community linkages are very weak in spite of voluntary base and great potential of ICDS system. Like any other programme, the major drawback in the system of ICDS has been inadequate "preparation" of the community for effective participation in the programme. Sakhshar Mahila Samooh (literate women groups) have been constituted under ICDS in Haryana, to enhance community participation. The community contributions have been in the form of buildings of Anganwadi centres, fuel for cooking and furniture and selection of AWWs. It was intended that one day the community will take over the responsibility of running Anganwadi centres but that remains a dream till now. ICDS programme is viewed as yet another government programme; like health guides the AWWs have also expressed their strong feelings to become Government servants and this must be resisted to maintain the voluntary/honorary base of the scheme.[7–13]

Mahila Swasthya Sanghs (MSS)

It was yet another attempt to enhance participation of women in reproductive and child health. MSS were established in village having population of 1000 or 200 households, consisting of 5 official members (ANM, AWW and TBA, school teacher and *Gramsevika*) and ten prominent women members from village community. This scheme is operative since 1990–91. The major task entrusted to them was empowering women on health and development through interpersonal communication. These groups have not taken any significant responsibility. The health workers and their supervisors have limited capacity to organise such groups and use their potentials for health and development. Around 79,512 MSS were functioning in the country. A nominal amount of ₹ 1200 per year is allocated to each MSS for organising monthly meetings.[14]

Target Free Approach (Community Needs Assessment Approach)

Under RCH there has been a major *paradigm shift*. Emphasis in RCH is laid on decentralised participatory planning and management at various levels. Health teams were entrusted the task of contacting communities, leaders, men and women apart from various Governmental and Non-Governmental organisations (NGOs) to evolve "action plans" at the level of village, subcentre, primary health centre and community health centres, respectively. The essence of "Action Plan" was to consult and involve people, but "how to involve" people was left to imagination of workers. This is new culture as all along these years, the health staff has worked on the "targets" given from the top and they are not used to this new approach. It will take quite sometime to put the things into operation.

But the approach holds great promise. It needs to be stated that district health teams, primary health centre and subcentre teams have not been trained well in their basic training and during continuing education programme, on the subject of "community participation" and working with community and mobilisation of community resources. All of them have perceived their role as "providers of services" focusing on supplies and services and reporting to higher levels or superior officers. They are not answerable to community and community has no control over these set-ups. Reversal of "top down approach" to "bottom up approach" as envisaged under RCH programme will have to be pursued aggressively to achieve community participation. It requires change of mindset at all the levels and within many sectors related with health and development.[15–17]

Accredited social health activists (ASHAs) have been inducted by National Rural Health Mission in 2005 to enhance community participation in rural areas. Ten lakh ASHAs have been recruited so far.

Village health sanitation and Nutrition committees have been constituted under National Rural Health Mission (NRHM) which will initiate village health plan. Untied fund of ₹ 10,000 per annum has been provided for local action. Hopefully, it would enhance community participation. Village is the first level of convergence of programmes of the Ministry of Health, Education, Social Welfare Development as well as that of others Ministries.

Examples of a few successful Indian experiences of community participation like VADU Rural Health Project (Maharashtra, Comprehensive Rural Health Project, Jamkhed (Maharashtra), Participatory Health Communication and Action (Madhya Pradesh), Cooperative Development, Tilonia (Rajasthan), Sewa rural (Gujarat), Sunderban Project (West Bengal) and many other projects cited in Anubhav series, have been documented. All these models were projects for a shorter duration to demonstrate high degree of success with dedication and commitment of charismatic personality, inspired by funding from a donor agency. These projects could not be reproduced or sustained for long. All these approaches indicated that different models are needed for community participation in a vast country like India where diversities prevail to a great extent. Some of the directions and the lessons learnt could be the guiding force for involving people in health and development. One of the critical and disturbing observation about all these projects stands out clearly, i.e. these operated in isolation of the existing health and development infrastructure. Monetary incentives for project functionaries played the trick in achieving the results in a limited geographical area.[18–22]

Community is endowed with multitude of resources. The institution of village Panchayat is prime mover for village development including health activities. Subcentre buildings and land for subcentre building, maintenance of these centres/payment of rent is borne by village Panchayat. Birth and death registration is an obligatory responsibility of village Panchayats. Village sanitation work has been entrusted to Panchayats. Pavements of streets, construction of drains, manure pits, promotion of sanitary latrines, Gobar gas plants and maintenance of wells by each community have been distinct areas, under sanitation programme. However, the resources with PRIs are limited and work is enormous. Maintenance of water posts, and hand pumps is enormous responsibility. Because of increasing population, the standards of sanitation are going down and environmental diseases continue to show their ugly heads. People are to help themselves and Government has symbolic support.

Village cooperative societies: Cooperative banks and village milk cooperative societies have been quite effective in mobilizing village people for development activities.

The initiative taken by National Rural Health Mission by allocating untied money to village Panchayat for local health and sanitation activities is encouraging indeed, but this is just symbolic, much remains to be done for involvement of PRIs.[21–23]

People themselves are the biggest resource for development.[22] NRHM recognises the value of "Village Health Sanitation and Nutrition committee" to promote community participation[23–25] and establish control over

PHCs and subcentres with PRIs. Community based monitoring of health services is the key strategy of National Rural Health Mission apart from citizen's charter at every level.

The community participation identified as essential supportive component of primary health care remains a weak component.

Now under NHM there have been concerted efforts to make health services accessible and accountable to the people. It strives for people-public-private partnership (PPPP). The NHM tries to ensure that more than 70% of resources are spent through bodies that are managed by people's organizations. Funds, functions and functionaries have been given to local community. National Urban Health Mission has been set up to give primacy to Urban Local Bodies.

REFERENCES

1 GOI. National Health Policy 1983. New Delhi: MOH and FW GOI; 1983.

2 Lal S. Let people operate and government cooperate in health development programmes. Ind J Comm Med 1999; 24(3).

3 WHO. Health system support for primary health care. Proceedings of thirty-fourth world health assembly; 1981. Public Health Paper 80. Geneva: WHO.

4 ICSSR. "Health for All" an alternative strategy. New Delhi: MOH and FW; 1983.

5 Roy S, Sharma BBL. Community Participation in primary health care. Technical paper 6. New Delhi: NIHFW; 1986.

6 MOH and FW. Agenda Notes. Proceedings of 6th Conference of Central Council of Health and Family Welfare; 1999 Feb. 16–18; New Delhi, India.

7 ICDS. A study of some aspects of the system. Nutrition Foundation of India. Scientific Report No. 7. 1988.

8 NIPCCD. National Evaluation of Integrated Child Development Services. New Delhi: NIPCCD; 1992.

9 Nagendra N, Subhash R. Community participation in ICDS–A case study of Garden Reach Calcutta. Technical Bulletin (NIPCCD) No. 8. New Delhi; 1993.

10 Murthy LSN, Kumar K, Nath N. Management of Community Participation in ICDS. Technical Bulletin NIPCCD No. 6, March 1993.

11 UNICEF. Immunizing more children. Towards greater community participation. Lodhi Estate New Delhi: UNICEF; 1984.

12 Rhode JE. Promoting healthy child growth – an occasional publication of NIPHC 1989; 16: 3–15.

13 GOI. Integrated Child Development Services Scheme. New Delhi: Department of Social Welfare Ministry of Education and Social Welfare; 1975.

14 GOI: MOH and FW Annual Report 2006–07 NRHM, New Delhi.

15 GOI. Manual on Target Free Approach in family planning programme. New Delhi: MOH and FW, GOI; 1996.

16 GOI. Annual Report 1993–94. New Delhi: MOH and FW GOI.

17 Measham AR, Heaver RA. Directions in development. India's Family Welfare Programme moving to a Reproductive and Child Health Programme. Washington DC: The World Bank; 1996.

18 Measham AR, Heaver RA. Directions in Development (Supplement) India's Family Welfare Programme moving to a Reproductive and Child Health Programme. Washington DC: The World Bank; 1996.

19 Dubey DC, Trakroo PL. Community Participation in Health and Family Welfare: A situational analysis. New Delhi: NIHFW.

20 Community action—family nutrition programmes (Generation of Interrelated Activities). Guidelines on policies and procedures. Proceedings of Conference of International Union of Nutritional Sciences; 1977 Oct. 17–21; NIN, Hyderabad.

21 Prinja S, Lal S, Singh A and Verma R. Role of PRIs in decentralized village health Planning in North India. SAJOSP ISSN 0972-4613 vol 7: (2) Jan-June 2007, 23–26.

22 UNICEF. Community participation. Current issues and lessons learnt. Assignment Children 59/60: UNICEF; 1982.

23 GOI. National Rural Health Mission (2005–12) MOH and FW, GOI; New Delhi.

24 Warner D. Where there is no doctor – A village health care handbook. 3rd ed. California, USA: Hesperian Foundation; 1978.

25 Prinja S, Lal S, Verma R. Operationalization of the Community needs assessment approach under the Reproductive and Child Health Programme at subcentre level in north India. WHO South-East Asia Region Regional Health Forum November 2, 2007; 11:39–47.

CHAPTER

2

Application of Social and Behavioural Sciences in Health and Disease Management

HUMANITIES AND COMMUNITY MEDICINE

Health has been defined as "State of complete physical, mental and social well-being and not merely the absence of disease or infirmity". Therefore, one of the dimensions of health is "social well-being" or "social health". To understand the social component of health, knowledge of social and behavioural sciences is essential.

Social sciences: It is the study of people in society and how individuals relate to one another and to the group. "A nation's greatest asset is its people." This discipline consists of *sociology*, *psychology*, *economics, political science*, and *history* or *anthropology*. Sociology, social psychology, social and cultural anthropology are known as ***behavioural sciences***.

Sociology is one of the human biosocial or behavioural science. It deals with social relationships of man with his fellow human beings. Sociology means study of society or group of people. The word sociology is derived from Latin, Socio (for society) and Greek, logos (study). The word society is derived from the associated words: Socius (individual) and societas (group). Men around man (groups and individuals) both interact and interrelate and influence each other. The pattern of relationship could be in terms of economic, cultural, political, religious, familial or social groups and caste groups. Medical sociology aims at study of individual, family, groups and their relationships and group dynamics and their behaviour. In essence, the sociology involves study of structure and functions of group life or community life.

Areas of Medical Sociology

Structure and **functions** of society (age and sex composition, caste, class, power structure and size of group), family life, customs, and habits, population movements and trends (birth rate, death rate and growth rate), urbanisation, industrialisation, income structure (economic status), occupations, structure of family and community, leadership in community, community organisation and development, housing conditions, water sources, human and animal waste disposal, what integrates the society and what disintegrates the society, etc.

Medical sociology essentially includes the structure and functions of community, community organization, community power structure, groups, leadership, resources and economics of community, responsibilities of community for health and development, lifestyles, ways of life and practices in relation to health and disease, health care delivery in the community, community participation in health programmes and doctor community relationship. Family is the universal institution in the community and society, family-based services, home visits and interaction with family members are other essential areas of medical sociology.

Social Factors in Health, Disease and Disability

The various social factors, such as age, sex, literacy levels, income, occupation, habits, marital status, and health seeking behaviour, way of life, aggregation and dispersal of population, migration, urbanisation, industrialisation, globalisation and geographical area play an important role in initiating, perpetuating and distribution of a disease in the process of natural history of disease.

The total development of society, its economic and health development, development of women and women groups and organisations, industrial and agriculture development, equity and social justice remain cherished goals. Most of the health problems are as much sociological as biological.

Study and understanding of humanities (behavioural sciences) is essential to understand an individual, group/society or community structure, function, interrelationship of man with his fellow-men and their ways of life. Behavioural sciences enhance the skills and competence of students, to elicit correct history, inculcates the art and skill of interview and communication, to assess the communication needs, and to formulate health education programmes. The knowledge of humanities is also essential to understand the role of socioeconomic factors in the *natural history of disease* as also to enhance client satisfaction and doctor-patient relationship. Integrated Bio-behavioural Survey (IBBS) and behavioural surveillance survey data have been extensively used in National programme on HIV/AIDS epidemic in India.

Social Psychology

Social psychology studies the behaviour of individual and group. Essentially, it provides understanding of processes involved in thinking, perception, motivation, learning, attitudes and opinions among individuals and groups.

Anthropology

It studies the physical, social and cultural history of man. Anthropology is study of human in holistic manner. Anthropology has been divided into three divisions:

1. ***Physical anthropology*** is study of races and evolution of mankind, by physical measurement of skulls and skeleton and inherent racial characteristics.
2. ***Social anthropology*** deals with the institutions and human relationship of the past and present.
3. ***Cultural anthropology*** which studies the 'way of life' or development of social and cultural life of people.

Culture is "way of life" or sum total of customs, beliefs, attitudes, practices, values, goals, laws, traditions and moral codes of people, as also the language they speak, dress they wear, rearing of children, services utilisations and dietary patterns.

Acculturation

It means diffusion of culture between groups and communities. "Way of life" is influenced by contacts. Indian migrants acquire the culture of Western countries and change their "lifestyles" way of eating, smoking and alcohol consumption or Western people may adopt Indian culture and may become vegetarian and adopt Indian diet and Yoga or meditation. The culture diffusion or acculturation occurs, because of migration, urbanisation, industrialisation, and social mobility (education, trade, globalisation, and information technology).

The knowledge of social sciences is essential to assess the community health needs, and community diagnosis. Understanding the culture of people is essential to implement a programme or to get a service or programme accepted by people. Acceptance of family planning programme necessitates thorough understanding of reproductive behaviour of people, their knowledge beliefs, attitudes and practices in relation to reproduction.

Launching a programme of health education or behaviour change communication (BCC) strategies and their implementation requires thorough understanding of community and its 'way of life'. The knowledge of social sciences is also essential in the areas of:

- Strategy of effective communication with patient/client/community on health matters.
- Policy for allowing visits of relatives and near ones in hospitals.
- To develop good interpersonal relationships between staff and team leader or health team and community members.
- Motivating people and identification of priority group.
- Community needs assessment.
- To understand role of social factors in health and disease and diagnosis of social-medical problem.
- Helps to understand the natural history of disease process or epidemiological triad of disease/health.
- To enhance people or community participation in health programmes.
- To enhance the compliance of treatment and follow up of instructions.
- To develop user-friendly health services.
- To tailor the health services according to the felt needs of the people.
- For effective organization and management of health services, especially to understand, to predict and control the behaviour of people in an organisation and to marshal resources of the community.
- To enhance patient or client satisfaction.
- To enhance utilization of services (Health seeking behaviour) and to create demand for services.

Social diagnosis and social therapy: Social diagnosis of an illness needs the application of behavioural sciences to arrive at community diagnosis and accordingly the therapy is social therapy in the form of education, legislations, individual and group counselling and motivation and team building apart from providing services on equity basis without any discrimination with priority focused on economically weaker sections of the society.

Social Health Problems

A disease is called a social problem and its social relevance becomes high:

- When it has predominant behavioural component in its causation.
- When it is widespread over to large geographical area and it affects many people (incidence and prevalence is very high).
- When it is severe and mortality is very high.
- When it leads to permanent disability or crippling.
- When it leads to discrimination and ostracism.
- When it disrupts the trade, and affects the economy of the nation.

- When it affects the economically productive population most and leads to poverty.
- When it threatens the growth and development of young children.
- When the treatment is beyond the reach of many.
- When the disease is incurable.

Examples

Almost all diseases have some or other element of social factors but some of these are major social problems, as shown in Table 2.1.

The social therapy is directed towards removing the cause or changing behaviour through education, individual and group counselling, motivation, involvement of community and by legislation to curb the bad practice or else to provide the missing services.

Specific: Social factors and behavioural components in relation to diseases, reproduction, child rearing, environmental health, health management and health services utilisation, gender related issues have been discussed in relevant chapters and "case studies or caselets" have been cited to enhance learning of behavioural sciences. Case studies have been highlighted in the chapters on community and community diagnosis (Chapter 1), environmental health—safe water and excreta disposal (Chapter 7), epidemiology (Chapter 8), geriatrics (Chapter 16), mental health (Chapters 12 and 13), applied nutrition (Chapter 6), maternal mortality (Chapter 4), and RCH (Chapter 5). These case studies and caselets should be linked to the chapters (Chapters 1 and 2) on behavioural sciences for better comprehension.

Teaching vs Learning

People resent being taught. No body wishes to be taught but everyone wishes to learn and people have strong desire to learn. Emphasis should be on learning. Learning is a lifelong process. Child learning and adult learning differs. There are four ways of learning:

1. **Trial and error** by trying for oneself (trial and error) and learning from each trial (experiential learning).
2. **Being told** by receiving instructions either orally or in writing or by demonstration.
3. **Imitation** by copying the actions of another person usually an instructor or a skilled person.
4. **Thinking** by organizing one's thoughts about a topic or problem to arrive at an explanation or solution.

Best way of learning is learning by doing. Common saying is:

"I hear I forget
I see I remember
I do I know."

Adult learning should be problem-centered and experience-centered.

Table 2.1: Social problems and their behavioural components

	Social problems	Behavioural components
1	(a) Population explosion	High fertility, early marriages, non-acceptance of contraceptive or no belief in contraceptives
	(b) Adverse sex ratio and falling child sex ratio	Female foeticides, infanticide and gender biases/disparity
2	Smoking or tobacco and alcohol use	Habit or smoking in the family and peer groups, socially acceptable practice in the society or status symbol
3	Accidents and suicides	High speed driving and not obeying the traffic rules or driving under the influence of drugs or alcohol and stress
4	Drug abuse (substance use)	Drug trafficking, illicit drug use by adolescents and youths sharing of needles and syringes
5	HIV/AIDS and STDs	Pre-marital, extra-marital sexual relationships, unprotected sex with multiple sex partners
6	Prostitution	Economic compulsions, poverty and exploitation of young girls and women
7	Mental disorders and behavioural problems in children	Broken families, problem families, unable to cope with stress and adjustment problems
8	Insanitary environments, wide-spread filthy conditions	Habit of open field defecation, non-acceptance of latrines and belief that excreta of children is harmless and poor personal hygiene practices
9	Unsafe water	Poor water storage practices and drawing of water from pot or pitcher by dipping hands and non-acceptance of chlorination as also non-use of piped water supply for drinking purposes
10	Leprosy and tuberculosis	Social stigma, hiding disease, fear of loosing job, and non-utilisation of treatment facilities, thought to be incurable and disabiling and fatalistic attitudes
11	Poor utilisation of health services (antenatal care immunisation, vitamin A prophylaxis, etc.	Lack of knowledge, no belief in facility, non-accessibility (because of distance), non-affordability and non-acceptance due to cultural reasons
12	Poor management of health services	Lack of motivation, poor leadership, lack of interaction and involvement of community, lack of coordination
13	Illiteracy, poverty, unemployment and urban slums	Rising population, large sized families, prolonged and recurring illness, addiction in the family, lack of facilities of schooling for girls, migration and industrialisation.
14	Diabetes, hypertension cancer, CVD and strokes	Life styles—physical inactivity, diet, tobacco and excess use of alcohol

Pedagogy

The art and science of learning/teaching is known as pedagogy. It includes different teaching/training methods and technology to change the knowledge, attitude and behaviour of an individual, group and community.

Curriculum: It is "a sum total of all educational experiences which include learning objectives, content areas, a time table, methods of learning and evaluation."

Pedagogic methods: Teaching technology and methods in medical education are—lecture, lecture discussion, demonstration, return demonstration, tutorial, clinical teaching, group discussion, brain storming, buzz session, problem-based learning, panel discussion, symposia, seminar, workshop, conference, convention, institute, completion of project, focus group discussion and case study method.

Teaching aids: Include audiovisual and other aids, such as tape recorder, over-head projector, mike, transparencies, video-tapes/cassettes, pictorials, blackboard, computer, laptop, etc.

Problem-based Learning

Education is a process to bring about change in behaviour of students. Three domains—*cognitive* (knowledge) *affective* (attitudes) and *psychomotor* (practical skills) are the main focus of behaviour change.

Behaviour change can be done by conventional method of *teacher-centred training* in which the knowledge and skills are imparted to students by traditional methods of lectures and demonstrations; it is passive process. The second method is, in which the students participate and take active part in self-directed learning. Here the teacher acts as a facilitator. The learning here is *student-centred*.

At present, undergraduate medical education is subject based *teaching* in various semesters. One course is not related to other. In the traditional subject-based curriculum, it is assumed that the knowledge gained in pre- and paraclinical periods will be remembered and will be transferred to illness situations. Both assumptions are unsupported. Forgetting is massive and rapid. Basic science teachers present material in *cause-effect logic* in which they organise their own knowledge and in which the textbooks are written. The students as clinician has to relearn it in the *effect-cause sequence* within which clinical problems must be worked out.

That is, the clinical problem start with an effect of a disease process. The student must work backwards from *effects* through possible explanation to identify what is likely to *cause*. This can be best achieved by integrated curriculum and integrated teaching. Various techniques have been used to have integrated curriculum, like *system-based learning*, *community-based* and *problem-based learning*.

Problem-based learning is defined as learning that results from the process of working towards the understanding or evalution of a problem. Problems are used as spring board for learning. The problem is encountered first. It serves as a stimulus for the application and development of problem-solving skills and search for knowledge to understand the mechanisms responsible for the problem and its solution. The process involved facilitates self-directed learning. Once the information has been gathered, digested and understood, the knowledge obtained can be used to solve other problems. The key features of problem-based learning are:

1. Analysis of health care problems as main method of acquiring and applying knowledge.
2. Self-directed lifelong learning
3. Use of small tutorial groups.
4. Develop a clinical reasoning process.

The problem-based learning creates an atmosphere which encourages active participation, emphasizes the personal nature of learning, accepts the differences between the learners, recognizes the learner's right to commit mistakes, tolerates imperfection, encourages openness of mind and trust in self, facilitates discovery, puts emphasis on self-evaluation and accepts confrontation of ideas.

The Problem

The problem selected should be major public health problem. The entire subject may be taught on the basis of problems.

a. Problems are presented to the students as written cases or live simulations or actual cases.
b. The students analyse these problems and discuss these problems and generate issues which may be basic or clinical.
c. These issues are framed into objectives of learning by the students.
d. The teacher has a list of learning objectives for that problem with him. He helps the students to identify the objectives of learning by themselves.
e. The students seek the information from library, books, journals and resource persons in the college and wards of the hospitals.
f. In subsequent tutorials, the students appraise the information; share it with other students in the group and discuss all aspects of the problem. They critically evaluate their own performance.
g. Once the students and tutor are satisfied that the pre-determined objectives have been met, the students write down the summary of discussions. Later on other problems are taken up in the same sequence.
h. *Assessment:* The evaluation of students performance is based on their achievement of the programme objectives and their performance in problem-based learning excercises, self-evaluation, peer evaluation and the evaluation by the tutor. Objective-structured clinical examination (OSCE) and objective-structured practical examination (OSPE) and special exercises can be given.

(*Source:* Souvenir-Diamond Jubilee celebration MCI)

Clinical-social Case Review (CSCR)

This is yet another method to learn and comprehend the natural history of disease and effective interventions (levels of prevention).

This approach has two distinct components. One—the clinical review—which consists of standard case management (history taking, examination, clinical diagnosis, confirmative diagnosis, treatment, counselling and follow-up). This is best done by treating physicians and their teams in the outdoor or indoor set up. Objective here is to treat the illness and reduce its prevalence. Second part is social review: Social review essentially consists of identification of specific *social factors* and their analysis in respect of presenting *disease* with the *objective*:

a To *recognize* the *sufficient causes* or risk factors or underlying determinants of presenting disease.

b To *treat* the *cause* by effective intervention in order to prevent the disease, reduce its incidence, prevalence and ultimately elimination of disease.

The social review thus begins with a *disease* and searches for its *causes* which are often *multiple*—host factors, environmental factors and factors relating to causative agent of disease.

Example: **Host factors**—age, sex, habits, personal hygiene marital status, age of marriage, birth interval, migrant worker/labourer, social class (determined by income, education, housing and occupation), immunity and heredity may predispose a person to an illness.

Social and Cultural Factors

Similarly, use of tobacco, excessive alcohol, physical inactivity, high speed driving and not obeying traffic rules, unprotected sex with multiple sex partners (lifestyles), non-utilization of available health services or delay in seeking care, incomplete treatment, faulty choice of food—junk food, fast food, inadequate food, delayed initiation of breastfeeding, and weaning, large sized family, lack of information and knowledge, wrong beliefs and attitudes, are other factors which could initiate a disease, help in its progression or precipitate a disease or an event. Many harmful cultural practices may worsen a disease.

Environmental Factors

- Unsafe environments, such as unsafe water, indiscriminate defecation, soil pollution, air pollution, overcrowding, urban slums, breeding of mosquitoes, flies, rodents, insects, presence of stray dogs, animals and pets, bad working environment/occupational hazards, could be sufficient causes for disease occurrence.
- Economic loss due to an illness to individual, family, community and nation and cost of treatment and care.
- Impacts of illness on individual, family, community and nation or state are other dimensions of CSCR.

In essence, social factors have their significant role in either initiating a disease, its progression, recovery or cure.

Example: Inadequate breastfeeding and delayed weaning initiates malnutrition in young children, and an episode of diarrhoea in malnourished child precipitates malnutrition. Girl child or lesser child is predisposed to malnutrition. *Causative Agent Factors* see Chapter 8 and 12.

CASE STUDY

Clinical Review

A low birth weight (1.8 kg) male baby was born to Maya at first referral unit. Baby could not suck the breast milk and expressed milk was given to this baby by nurses. Baby was kept with mother for 10 days when the breastfeeding got established and baby started thriving on breastfeeds. Thereafter, the mother and baby were sent home. This baby started having episodes of cough and difficult breathing requiring hospitalization on two occasions. At the age of 10 months, the hospital admission was on account of difficult and fast breathing and the child recovered after 7 days time and sent home after counselling. The baby was due for measles vaccine and this opportunity was missed in the hospital. Weight-for-age at the time of discharge was 6 kg.

Social Review

Maya was lesser child and most of her time got spent in care of younger brother and sister and household chores. She could not be enrolled in school and got married around 16 years of age, she looked very weak and pale and got easily tired after household work, became pregnant after two months of marriage. She had to work in farm and family, to bring fodder, fuel and cook meals. Anganwadi worker registered Maya as pregnant women around 5th month and this family was identified as below poverty line family, but Maya could never go to Anganwadi because she was too much occupied. Similarly, antenatal care visits to subcentre located at a distance of 2 km could not happen. At last Maya was brought to subcentre with swollen face and legs with labour pains. Female health worker with the help of ASHA arranged free transport up to first referral unit (FRU). Free medicines and material were provided at FRU for safe delivery and incentive money was given to Maya from funds under *Janani Suraksha Yojna* (JSY) under the umbrella of National Rural Health Mission.

Several issues can be identified out of this clinical-social case review, such as girl child—the lesser child, deprivation of education to girls, undernutrition, age of marriage and teenage pregnancy, workload, anaemia and pregnancy, toxaemia, below poverty line family, health seeking behaviour, incentives for safe delivery, missed opportunities, causes of low birth weight babies, breastfeeding and management of low birth weight babies, weight gain pattern in low birth weight babies, etc. It could be part of problem-based learning and learning of epidemiological methods. Similarly, presenting illness can be linked to total prevalence or occurrence of that illness in the community and national/community efforts to deal with that problem.

These reviews can be an opportunity for *integrated teaching* by the departments of paediatric, obstetric and gynae and community medicine, to identify causes of low birth weight and occurrence of repeated episodes of illness in young children as also integrated management of childhood illness (IMCI) apart from gender disparity.

ORGANIZATIONAL BEHAVIOUR (OB) (LEADERSHIP STYLES, GROUP DYNAMICS AND MOTIVATION)

Organizational Behaviour (OB)

OB means "better understanding and managing people at work". The medical officer incharge of CHC or PHC works with health volunteers and honorary workers (Anganwadi workers, traditional birth attendants, health guides and ASHAs), health workers, health supervisors and above all with Panchayati Raj institutions (elected representatives of people) and village leaders formal and informal both.[1–3] Since manpower for primary health care is of varied background and around 70% of the total budget and sometimes more than that is spent on manpower alone, hence to *understand the behaviour of health teams, predicting their behaviour, and controlling* their behaviour becomes an important task, in the hospital and community setting.

Health Organization

The health organization, which is constituted by above-mentioned group of people who all work towards some common goal. Bringing positive change in their behaviour is an important job function of health manager (or health team leader).[1–3]

Knowing health teams intimately, their personality, aptitudes, attitudes, family responsibility, training background, motivational level and job satisfaction is essential. The leader must analyze after collecting these attributes about each member of the health team and this analysis provides him useful information for **making decision.** In order to influence others' behaviour, the best way is to understand and know each other well.

Leadership—A Health Management Function

The medical officer is a leader of health teams, who by virtue of his position in the health organization influences the behaviour of others. Wherever the leadership is effective, the performance of health team has been much better.

Who is a Leader?

Any person or an individual in **an organization** who **influences** the **behaviour of others** is a health team leader. A medical officer is a leader to health workers and health assistants and other persons in the organization.

A health worker and supervisor is a leader to health guides, Anganwadi workers, ASHAs, and traditional birth attendants. Each individual in health team plays the role of health leader at various levels and influences the behaviour of others who come in contact with him in day-to-day activities. A school teacher is a leader to his class students.

Individuals differ in their degree of leadership. There are two prime concerns:

1. Concern for the "people" (Humanistic approach)
2. Concern for the "task" (Mechanistic approach).

Balanced leadership has equal concern for both "people" and the "task" or "work".

Leadership Styles

The manner in which the leader influences the behaviour of health team is known as leadership styles.

There are four styles of leadership. It all depends upon the development levels of the followers.

Style 1—Directing (Directive Behaviour)

This involves telling people what to do, how to do it, where and when to do it and then supervising their performance closely. The leader in this situation provides specific instructions (written job description and tasks to be done) and closely supervises the task accomplishment. This style is applied to health workers who have *low competence* (newly recruited persons) but *high commitment* (eager to perform or are enthusiastic).

Style 2—Coaching

It involves directing and supporting the workers. The leader continues to direct and closely supervises the task accomplishment, but also explains decisions, solicits suggestions and supports progress.

This style of leadership is observed for workers or supervisors who have *some competence* but *low commitment.*

Style 3—Supporting

Supportive behaviour involves listening to people, providing support and encouragement for their efforts and then facilitating their involvement in problem-solving and decision-making. The leader facilitates and supports subordinate's efforts towards task accomplishment and shares responsibility for decision-making with them.

This style is applicable in a situation where the subordinates have *high competence* but *variable commitment.*

Style 4—Delegating

It means turn over responsibility for day-to-day decision-making. The leader hands over responsibility and authority for decision-making and problem-solving to subordinates. This style is applicable for those subordinates who have *high competence* and *high commitment.*

There is no best way to influence others. The leader needs to assess the situation in the organization and accordingly choose a style of leadership. One has to become situational leader. The most important criterion in deciding the leadership style is the characteristics of the subordinates or health teams.

There is no one best leadership style. You need to adapt your style to fit the needs of each person. Leadership style is how a manager behaves when trying to influence the behaviour of someone else. The appropriate styles will vary for each person but will be a combination of directive and supportive behaviours.

- **Competence** means sound scientific knowledge and skills.
- **Commitment** means highly motivated and confident person.

Medical officer is a leader of health team at primary health centre and he provides day-to-day directions to his subordinates, provides supportive supervision, and conducts continuing education to improve their skills. Maternal and child health activities (antenatal care, deliveries, postnatal care and immunization, etc.) have been delegated to health workers. Untied money of ₹ 10,000 per annum has been given to female health workers for local action: an example of delegation of financial powers—**a best practice.**

How to Lead?

Apply LEAD model. Leaders can use a simple four-step model to ensure their participation and increase productivity.

1. **L**ead with clear purpose.
2. **E**mpower to participate.
3. **A**im for consensus.
4. **D**irect the process.

The LEAD model includes key leadership functions: setting clear goals and objectives, getting people involved, reaching consensus on important items and paying attention to both tasks (the work) and relationship (the team).[1–3]

Best Way to Influence Others: Lead by Examples

Observe high standards and lead by examples. Practice what you teach or who will listen to you. If you smoke yourself and advise others not to smoke that is bad example. Set examples first for yourself and then the followers will follow you. If you set an example of coming in time the others will follow. A good leader does not tell people what to do, he sets examples.

Qualities of a Leader Facilitator[1–3]—Best Practices

1. Sets examples for correct behaviour.
2. Facilitates work.
3. Actively listens and solves problems.
4. Takes responsibility for both his actions and the people he supervises.
5. Knows himself and his limits and constantly seeks to improve himself.
6. Is available
7. Looks after the welfare of his employees.
8. Makes sound and timely decision.
9. Sets goals that are achievable.
10. Knows his job and stays abreast with current events.

Some other attributes of a good leader:

- He makes decision based on: Information and data and his own observations and facts.
- Gives credit to team members for high performance and gives them recognition for high performance.
- Encourages different view points.
- Teaches and coaches others without telling them what to do.
- Organizes information and data so that others can understand and act on it.
- Models the behaviour he or she would like to see in others.
- Knows how to bring the right people together for a task.
- Is aware of his own limitations and knows who is better qualified to make a decision or complete a task.
- Understands that diversity can affect team work in a positive way.
- Understands that different people are motivated by different things and are willing to work hard to address their individual needs.
- Shares powers and authority with others.
- Encourages team members to take responsibility for issues, problems, actions and projects.
- Looks for ways to help the team achieve its goals.
- Finds opportunities to reward appropriate behaviour, minimizes punishment for inappropriate behaviour.
- Is firm about goals, but flexible about the process used to reach those goals.
- Is not afraid to address conflict.
- Understands and acknowledges that people's, individuals' needs (social, personal career, lifestyle, work preferences), may affect team work and accordingly works with and not against these needs.

The health system is adequately designed to provide a comprehensive, high coverage of promotive, preventive and curative services throughout India. A large trained staff of workers and health volunteers and Anganwadi workers, with task appropriately defined to meet the major public health needs of rural poor are in place. There remains a question of motivated leadership of each health team, their continued education, supervision and encouragement, if the potential is to be fulfilled. Wherever the leadership has been good dramatic improvement in the health can be seen in poor Indian rural population. Most medical officers are unwilling or unable to assume the role of effective leadership. They have most probably been not trained well, not prepared or motivated to take this role.

MOTIVATION

The health team leader or manager motivates health team for better efficiency of work at SC, PHC/CHC areas and hospital. People are most important resource of an organization.

What is Motivation?

Motivation is goal-directed or goal-oriented behaviour. The motives are driving forces, which arouse and maintain activity and hence they determine the direction of behaviour of an individual. The concept of motivation must be understood by health team leaders and members because they are concerned with modification of people's behaviour. Recently the emphasis of whole science of communication has shifted to "behaviour change". Behaviour change communication is the crux. Changing reproductive behaviour and sexual behaviour are the key areas to limit the size or space children and to protect oneself against HIV and AIDS respectively. "Why do people behave the way they do?" The answer of this question lies in people's motivation. The driving force responsible for directing the behaviour of individuals is motivation. It is, therefore, important to understand and predict, and thereby control and modify their behaviour.

Definition

Motivation is a process that starts with a felt need, want, drive or impulse within an individual. Once the individual is able to satisfy the need/want, in the form of an incentive the drive is reduced and a new need is felt. This process continues throughout life as needs and wants keep on occurring and changing in life process (Fig. 2.1).

Motives are driving forces such as felt needs, wants, drives and impulses. That simply means something within an individual that prompts behaviour.[1–3]

Strategies for Motivation

People are the most important resources of an organization. Unlike non-human resources, such as equipment and finances, people want to participate, achieve, and want recognition and be motivated. Motivate people to get best out of them. Learn what motivates them. The seven main motivators are:

1 ***Achievement:*** Most people like to do things well. They like to succeed. Achievement or success is very important matter for an individual (success begets success). Satisfaction in success and in getting things done well comes largely from achieving, hence achievement is a big motivating factor.

A good team leader helps the team members to achieve by giving them clear instructions, suitable training, facilities, and supplies they need for their work. Success has lot many fathers failure has none. If the health team fails to achieve, leader must share failures. Leader helps people to achieve work objectives.

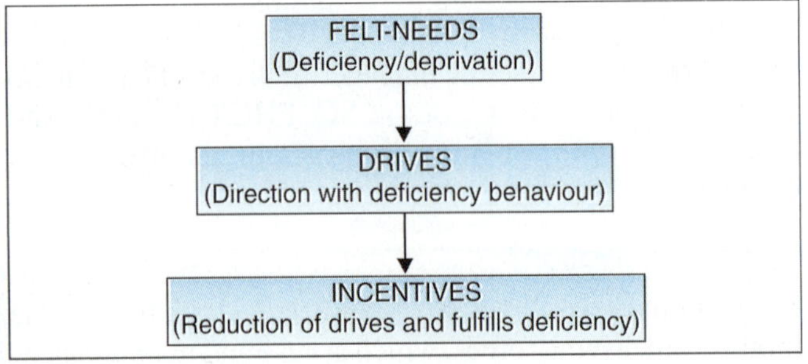

Fig. 2.1: Basic motivation process

2 ***Recognition:*** Giving recognition to people ensures them that their work is noticed and appreciated. Praise makes people feel good. It also makes them want to do a better job—so they can get more praise. "Give praise where praise is due." Acknowledging good performance by rewards to motivate people.

3 ***The work itself:*** The old saying that "work is worship" holds true for motivation. People like to do work that is constructive, that in their opinion is worthwhile and helpful to other people. Leader explains the value of work to his team repeatedly and supports them on the job.

4 ***Responsibility:*** Most people welcome responsibility, some people fear it. Most people like to make decisions about their lives and to accept the responsibility for doing so. Leader should delegate responsibility to subordinates (health workers for maternal and child health work at subcentre and in the village) and always help them to take responsibility to sustain their interest.

5 ***Advancement:*** Advancement or promotion in career is a form of recognition. Recognition without reward is not very convincing. People want recognition that comes in tangible form, such as an increase of salary or more responsibility, with freedom to use their own initiative, which leads to job satisfaction. Leader helps others to train for promotion and encourages increasing their knowledge and skills so that they are ready for promotion.

6 ***Self-improvement:*** People like to become mature, to develop as people. Many people make great sacrifices to improve themselves or to offer such opportunities to other members or their family. Team leader should 'give opportunities for self-development' by giving them learning resource material and help to improve and upgrade their skills by—on the job training and continuing education.

7 ***Job satisfaction and security:*** Job satisfaction is also a motivating factor. Job should be enriched from time to time, as the technology advances, to improve the quality of work and the job.

All these factors help in retention of manpower.

Maslow's Hierarchy of Needs

A motive, which has highest strength, is met first. People work on satisfying needs in an orderly fashion. The need that has the highest motive strength receives attention first. Maslow presents a theory that designates categories of needs and strengths when unsatisfied (Fig. 2.2).

According to "Maslow's theory", the physiological needs at the bottom of the pyramid in Fig. 2.2 are top priority motive strengths when unsatisfied. Physiological needs have highest priority until satisfied. Once physiological needs are satisfied, safety needs take priority. This format follows as the pyramid climbs to self-actualization, which is a

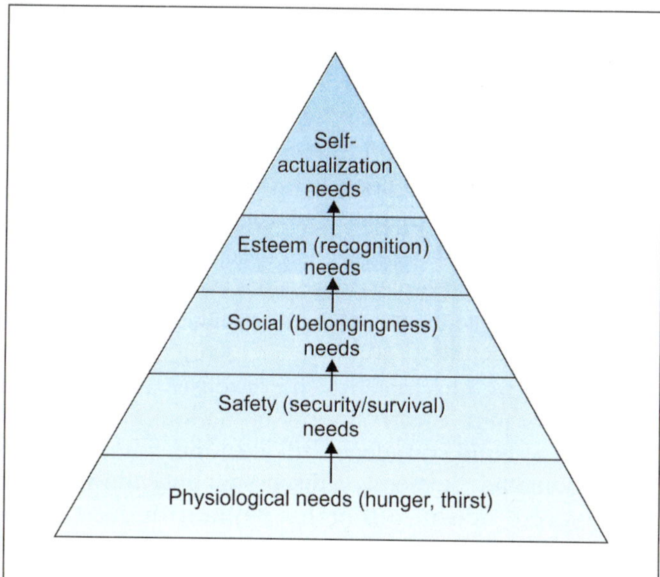

Fig. 2.2: Maslow's hierarchy of needs

priority only when other four needs are satisfied. It must be noted that all needs are present within an individual, the priority of needs, however, shifts.

The old saying "you can lead a horse to water, but you cannot make it drink" is very true in case of motivation. The health leader may not be able to make someone behave in certain way. If the individual has an internal need, the sight of external goal increases the probability that behaviour aimed at goal attainment will follow, no guarantee, however, exists. For example, if the health worker, is provided with facilities, and is also well trained to perform his/her responsibilities, it is probable that he/she will be motivated to carry out the task effectively and efficiently but one cannot be absolutely sure.

A motivated person accomplishes goal in shorter time and produces quality work at lower cost. If the individual has positive experience, it serves as stimulus for motivating her/him to accomplish the task.

Common causes of dissatisfactions:

1 Inefficient administration.
2 Incompetent supervision.
3 Poor personal relationship.
4 Poor leadership qualities.
5 Low pay.
6 Bad working conditions.
7 Non-participation in plans of work.

GROUP DYNAMICS AND TEAM BUILDING

A health team at subcentre consists of health workers (male and female) traditional birth attendant, Anganwadi workers and health guides and in most situation other link workers (ASHAs) or NGO workers (Social workers). The team building is the responsibility of health manager. The team needs to meet together at regular interval for organized in-service training and review of progress of their work. Under the present circumstances, the sector meeting day is fixed in the block. On sector meeting day, 25–30 Anganwadi workers, 6 health workers female and equal number of male workers, health supervisor and Mukhya Sevika or ICDS supervisor, Child development and project officer (CDPO) and medical officer meet at sector headquarter once a month on fixed date. This is a unique opportunity to develop team or building teamwork, holding a continuing education session on a chosen problem observed by the supervisor or medical officer. This occasion is used to achieve maximum coordination and joint planning. In the group, all team members have a chance to express their feelings, narrate the successful experiences as also failures. The health manager (medical officer) and child development project officer participate and solve the problems to the extent possible and plan jointly the activities for the next month. The shortcomings as observed through monthly monitoring reports are discussed with health team, the work is coordinated and information of report is shared between team members. The health team finds a great opportunity to learn from peers experience, share the problems, and come out with solution. It is a great occasion for building team and mutual learning.

Further health team exists for the community at village level (AWWs, health workers, TBAs and ASHAs). The community has health needs and it is the function of the health team to respond to their health needs.[1–3]

No one person can acquire all the necessary skills, or have enough time to do everything that must be done to satisfy the needs of even a small community. Therefore, people have to work **in team** to get the work done.

The function of health team at village level is:

- To promote community participation.
- To consult the community or contact them on regular basis say once a month meeting with Panchayat or *Mahila Swasthya Sangh* to assess their health needs.
- To give responsibility to community on the problems which families and community can undertake themselves, such as sanitation and personal hygiene and improving their dietary habits.
- To elicit cooperation from other sectors or other functionaries, such as village chowkidar (for birth and death registration), school teachers and *Mahila Mandals* and *Sakshar Mahila* Smooh (SMS).
- The health team learns from community by listening and observing, by talking with community leaders to have first hand information on health practices—child rearing and feeding practices, health attitudes, values, beliefs and customs, family life and decision-making process in the family.

Ultimately, health team prepares village action plan or subcentre action plan to help people to meet their felt needs and organize community efforts to solve a problem. Health teams are not well trained to organize village community for self-help and the health manager must build capacity of health team in this area.

Group Discussion in Health Communication

Group discussion is a process in which a group of individuals come together; deliberate on an issue or problems so as to arrive at a solution or consensus opinion. In this process the group goals are jointly set, all the members participate and contribute to group discussion, usually facilitated by a leader, find solution, evaluate their effectiveness and finally try to arrive at a consensus.

Anganwadi workers and health workers have been made responsible to organize mother's meetings once a week and Mahila Swasthya Sangh meeting/VHSC meeting once a month at the village level. This has been done to enhance interpersonal communication for behaviour change on pressing problems, such as breastfeeding, illegal abortion or sex-selective abortions and PNDT Act, sex-ratio of under six children, anaemia and maternal mortality, safe pregnancy and safe delivery. Workers have seldom organized group meetings and they have seldom been adequately trained to organize meaningful group meetings. The purpose is not clear and end results are obscure. Hence, the health manager should take up this challenge to build capacity of health workers for organizing women groups, group formation, group dynamics, group discussion and ensuring their regular meetings at least once a month. Every month, a chosen subject is discussed by a group of women. It can be organized more frequently with the help of Anganwadi worker, traditional birth attendants and accredited social health activist (ASHA).

Essential Component of Group Meeting

The group size consists of 10–15 men or women of a locality. Priority should be women of economically weaker sections. The group could be homogeneous say—pregnant women, lactating mothers, women having children below two years of age, and adolescent girls. There could be heterogeneous group as well.

- The day/date of meeting should be well publicized and place should be well prepared for their reception.
- The meeting should be organized at familiar place, like Anganwadi centre, *Mahila Mandal* premises, or subcentre. It should be easily accessible.
- Make arrangement for sitting. Everyone in the group is equal. Prefer a circle or semicircle arrangement.
- Select a most pressing problem you wish to address or women feel to know/understand.
- Arrange or obtain learning resource material-printed material, posters and demonstration material if possible. Demonstration is best method in a group.
- Health workers should act as facilitators and not as teachers and they should not talk at people.
- Let women discuss the chosen problem themselves and arrive at a solution. Let women express different/divergent views on the chosen subject. The health workers should facilitate and ensure that everyone participates. Health worker's responsibility is to prepare notes or record salient points of discussion and provide supportive information on the subject.
- Prime role of the worker is to listen attentively all the viewpoints and discuss the various facilities made available at village Anganwadi centre, Subcentre and PHC.
- Worker should never forget that women themselves and family itself are very important resource to deal with the identified problem.
- The group must reach to a consensus decision and workers must ensure follow-up actions on decision made to build confidence amongst the women group. It should not be merely a discussion but followed by a concrete action either by women or by family themselves or with the supportive services available at various levels.
- Group discussion, which are purely theoretical are least effective. These can be made most productive and interactive by use of demonstration, women-to-women communication of a life experience, such as use of copper-T as spacing method, preparation for safe delivery, early breastfeeding initiation and exclusive breastfeeding, and immunization.
- The workers in group discussion should never sit on chair and act as teachers, they should sit with women on mat.
- It is better to identify a group leader on voluntary basis to conduct meeting and regulate time.
- Refreshment during group meeting is optional, it should be offered by community and women group leader and not by government expenses.

During the group discussion, if health manager or supervisor is available, it provides additional support and it enriches group discussion and status of discussion rises, but health manager must sit with women group and have face-to-face discussion.

In this manner, direct feedback can be obtained from group. Women are already busy and have least time for group discussion. This is big challenge. Only meaningful, informative and interactive group discussion lasting for 30–60 minutes time is enough. If women cannot come out because of busy work schedule, the smaller group meetings can be held during home visits to discuss the pressing problem and behaviour change.

Role of Members

Some members in the group dominate and do not give chance to other women to speak, this should be discouraged and controlled by group leader.

Some members keep silent and do not participate at all. Encourage such women to speak on the issue and tell them nothing is wrong or right. Other members obstruct and disturb the proceedings and they play negative roles, discourage this practice. Some women are quite positive they give information and seek more information and promote harmony in the group, some members may even be hostile and some are engaged in mutual discussions.

Interaction between group members and interaction of group members with the facilitator/resource person during group discussion is known as *group dynamics*. This can be shown by arrows (who interacted with whom and how many times). If arrows are connected it becomes a *sociogram*. Regular group discussions provide lot of feedback to improve the health services. The students can be given this exercise for better comprehension of group dynamics.

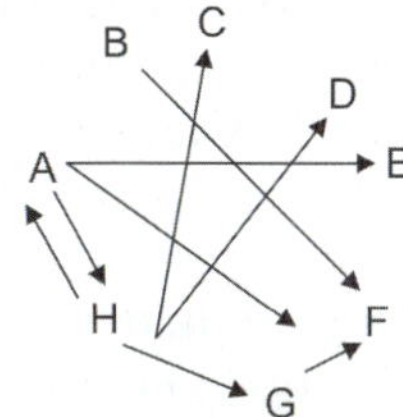

Group dynamics (Sociogram)

Focus-group discussion (*see* Chapter 19).

Fish Bowl

The group sits in two circles. Inner circle group members (FISH) deliberate a problem/issue to arrive at solution. The outer circle group members record, and observe the behaviour/interaction of each member of the inner circle group and later on present and discuss in the group. This is known as **fish bowl formation** in group discussion.

REFERENCES

1 Mathur SC. Organizational Behaviour and Community Health. 3rd ed. Jaipur: State Institute of Health and Family Welfare; 2001.

2 GOI. Manual for the training of trainers of health and family welfare training Institutes, New Delhi: Rural health division DGHS, GOI; 1996.

3 NIHFW. Management training module for medical officers (PHC). New Delhi: NIHFW; 1986.

BEHAVIOUR CHANGE COMMUNICATION (BCC)

Health Determinants

The most important determinants of health are *environment*, *behaviour*, *health services* and heredity to some extent.

"Behaviour" comes next to environment. "Behaviour" of an individual, family and community determines their "health", hence all efforts must be made to promote "healthy behaviours" to achieve the goal of "health in all".

Healthy actions on the part of individual, family and community should become part of life to prevent diseases and promote healthy life. That is why the "health education", "IEC" and "behaviour change communication" form an integral part and one of the essential component of all the national health programmes and primary health care in India. Communication of facts for life on reproductive and child health (RCH), communicable and non-communicable diseases has been adopted as one of the important strategy and means to prevent diseases by adopting healthy behaviours (Fig. 2.3).

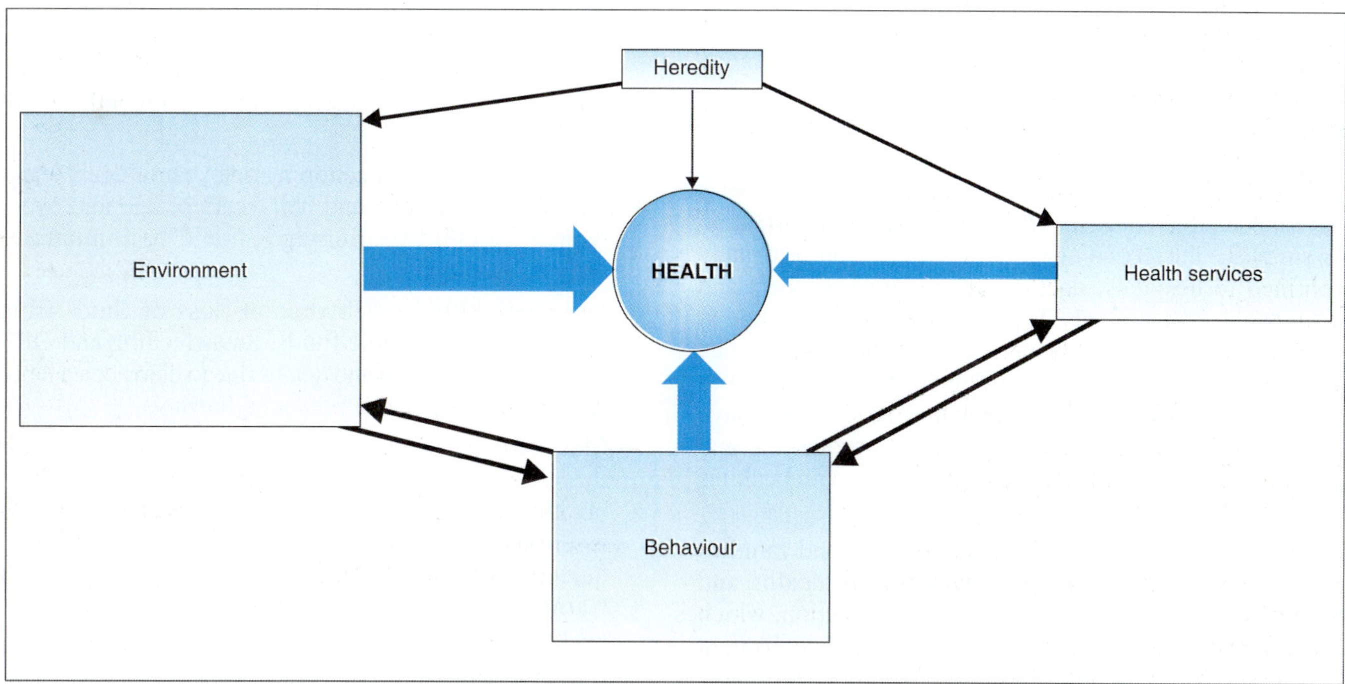

Fig. 2.3: Determinants of health (WHO)

2

"Health" remains a cherished goal to be attained by an individual, family and community. Goal is to achieve maximum level of positive health inclusive of all dimensions of health as defined by WHO.

"Education" is an important means and process to achieve the goal of "health".

Thus, health education concerns itself with process of change, its aim is to help individuals, families and communities to attain and maintain positive state of health by their own "efforts" and "action".[1]

Health Education—Definition

"Health education (HE) is a gradual process of learning that informs, motivates and helps people to adopt and maintain healthy practices and lifestyles. It also advocates environmental changes as needed from time to time to facilitate this goal and conducts professional training and research for achieving the same end."[1]

According to Lawrence W Green "Health education is any combination of learning opportunities designed to facilitate voluntary adoption of behaviour which will improve or maintain health".[2,3]

The main aims of health education are threefolds: First to *inform* and educate people the principles of hygiene and healthy living; second to *motivate* people to change their habits and ways of living and practices that are detrimental to health; and lastly to guide people into *action* about the medical and health services provided for their benefit and encourage them to *utilize* these services.

Health Information to People—Information for All

Information means knowledge, ideas, emotions, skills and data on health. The fundamental principle of Health Education is to provide or give scientific health information or knowledge to people, which would empower them for self-reliance and actions. Health knowledge is a power and great mean to improve their health. On health/disease knowledge explosion has occurred and health technologies have made rapid advance. The knowledge and information on simple health technologies and advances is unfortunately confined to hospitals, doctors, paramedical workers and other health professionals. The knowledge and information has not reached to those who need it most. The poor, illiterate and disadvantaged have been deprived of "vital health information and knowledge" which they need most to save their lives and of their children apart from promoting and maintaining their health. Adequate information on health is the right of everyone.

Information, which could enable parents and families to drastically reduce disease, malnutrition, deaths and disability among their children, is the information, which every parent should have. It is the information, which ought to be part of every family's basic stock of knowledge. It is information, which ought to be part of the normal way of bringing up children, and made available to every community through multiple channels. It is the information to which all families now have a right and almost all parents can put into practice, in some degree, at very low cost.

Information Revolution and Information for All

The coming decades should be observed as information revolution and communication (IRC) decades. All out, intensive efforts be made in these decades to create people movement for self-reliance in matters of health. Information which could enable individual, families and community, to reduce disease, malnutrition and deaths is the information which all must have. It is the information which ought to be made available to every community via the schools, the radio, the television, the newspaper, the religious leaders, the health workers and every other possible means of communication and support. In other words, it is an urgent task of mass communication to most needy, the poor. Task is too big for health sector alone, others have to join hands and intersectoral approach will pave the way.

The following are top ten messages adopted from facts for life (UNICEF) for action, which are most relevant to our country and we can add to these messages, the messages of lifestyles and chronic non-communicable diseases which are emerging fast in our country besides the epidemic of HIV/AIDS and accidents.[4,5]

1 The health of both women and children can be significantly improved by spacing births at least three years apart, by avoiding pregnancies before the age of 18 and after 35 and limiting the total number of pregnancies to two or less.

2 To have safe pregnancy by having adequate prenatal check ups and safe delivery by trained person.

3 Exclusive breastfeeding for first 6 months of life and adequate complementary feeding after 6 months of age by home available foods.

4 Complete all immunization by one year of age and get booster doses at one and half years of age and every woman in child bearing age should be immunized against tetanus.

5 Diarrhoea kills by dehydration (loss of fluids from body). Home available fluids, breastfeeding and ORS prevents dehydration and deaths due to diarrhoea. Handwashing before eating prevents diarrhoea.

6 Most coughs and colds get better on their own. But if the child with cough is having difficult and fast breathing and there is indrawing of chest, then the child is seriously ill and it is essential to go to a health facility quickly. A child with cough and cold should be kept warm, continue breastfeeding, give more fluids and continue feeding.

7 Children under three years have special feeding needs. They need to eat 5 to 6 times a day. Adequate feeding

of young children is essential for their growth. Fats and oil should be added along with vegetables. Whatever is cooked in home should be fed to child in enough quantities.

8 Many illnesses are caused by germs and germs enter the mouth. This can be prevented by clean eating, drinking safe water, and handwashing with soap and water and by using sanitary latrines.

9 After each episode of illness, one extra meal should be given to every child for a few days to make up the losses due to illness.

10 All girls and boys should be enrolled in schools at the age of 6.

Malaria, HIV/AIDS, injury prevention and disasters and emergencies are other areas.

We can add to these the messages on: Healthy lifestyles, such as no smoking, no alcohol, and regular exercise, maintaining appropriate weight, eating healthy diet, avoiding junk foods and regular brushing can prevent many illnesses (chronic diseases).

We have over 8.9 lakhs ASHAs, 13 lakh Anganwadi workers, 236034 health worker females, over 5,00,000 trained birth attendants, 153655 subcentres 25308 primary health centres and 5396 community health centres and infrastructure of Indian system of medicine and non-governmental organization to inform and educate people besides self-help groups and system of village Panchayats and Nagarpalikas. Thus, India has a massive infrastructure to reach rural and urban slums of the country. Apart from this, the system of elementary education is near universal to reach every village to cover the school children for inculcation of healthy lifestyles and healthy habits. If the knowledge and information is made available to target population and is acted upon, it will save millions of lives and disabilities. It is needed most in India.

The major task remains as how to communicate the available information and knowledge to individuals, parents, families and community in rural, tribal, and urban slum areas. Communication for behavioural change has become a major strategy in reproductive and child health as also for other national health programmes.

There is a distinct shift from earlier strategies. To begin with, the emphasis was laid on awareness generation, which was considered necessary but not sufficient. Awareness is no guarantee that it will lead onto behaviour change. In India, awareness on contraception is almost universal (100%) but only 56% of couples practice contraception. Therefore, in second phase—health education and extension education strategy was adopted in 3rd, 4th and 5th five-year plan period.

Subsequently, we adopted the strategy of information, education and communication (IEC). Of late we have adopted a strategy of communication for behaviour change, which is much more comprehensive.[6–8] The stages of evolution were as under:

Awareness Generation (by Mass Media)

↓

Health Education and Extension Education (Mass Media + Interpersonal Communication and Opinion Leaders Camps)

↓

Information Education and Communication (IEC)

↓

IEC provides information, does not specify what and how behaviours, attitudes and practices to be changed as also the outcomes

↓

Behaviour Change Communication is more specific and comprehensive

EVOLUTION OF HEALTH COMMUNICATION IN INDIA

The shift in policy can be summed-up as:

Past focus	*Present focus*
Awareness generation	Behaviour change
Instructive	Empowering
Generic approach	Specific information
Centralized plan of communication	Decentralized approach

Behaviour change communication is a dynamic process, which **specifies** the "behavior" to be changed within **specified time** as also **methods** and **outcomes** (*see* Table 2.2).

Learning Health Behaviour

Most of health behaviour is learned through:

Family

The foundation of learning is laid by the family and its environment.

The first school for child is the family. Family and parents have the responsibility to create healthy behaviour in their children. The behaviour of washing hands, wearing shoes, using toilets, brushing teeth and no smoking, dietary habits are developed and nurtured in the family and in home. Parents have to become ideal role models for their children. By the time the child is 5 years, over 80% of his brain gets developed.

Extra-familial Institutions

Anganwadi and Creche is an extra-familial institution where the young children learn a lot. Here learning is informal and through play way activities and it is joyful learning. Anganwadi workers provide varieties of stimuli and lay down further foundations of physical, mental and social development and motivate parents to provide learning stimuli at home. Habit of handwashing, brushing teeth, rinsing mouth, eating clean and eating enough, nail cutting, getting themselves weighed, use of toilet/sanitary latrine, drinking clean water and playing safe are promoted by AWWs apart from language and psychomotor development. It has positive influence on parents who continue what Anganwadi workers initiate and vice versa is also true. This is a first or initial step in education.[9]

School

It is a formal institution of learning. Elementary education infrastructure is universal. Learning in school is a cherished memory for lifelong period. The teachers are role models for the taughts. Universal elementary education, schooling of minimum of 8 years for everyone is a nation building activity apart from personality development and developing 'healthy lifestyles' and value system. It is *Sustainable development goal 4.* Personal hygiene (washing hands, brushing teeth, nail cutting, balanced diet, drinking clean water and no smoking, regular exercise, etc.) is best learnt in schools during an hour of socially useful and productive work (SUPW). Teachers leave an indelible impression on the minds of students.

Health and nutrition, reproductive health, adolescent health practices can be best improved and built in the schools through curriculum and extracurricular activities. Not only children learn themselves but also they act as ambassadors of health to their families and neighbourhood.

Learning through peers has great influence on the life of school children. The learning continues in colleges. Prevention of HIV/AIDS and reproductive health can be taught at appropriate age.

Population Education

It was an effort initiated under family welfare Programme by Government of India with an emphasis on life cycle approach—population education for the young. Its focus is young adolescents in schools, colleges and out of schools; systematic population education by formal and non-formal methods was one of the important planks of the revised family welfare strategy. In pursuance of the revised strategy, population education was introduced in the school education system, adult education programme and higher education system in the country with UNFPA assistance. Population education messages were included in the textbooks of schools through National Council of Education, Research and Training (NCERT). The emphasis was on population trends, raising the age of marriage, safe motherhood and spacing, child survival (ORT and immunization), antenatal and postnatal care with stress on women's status to counteract the son preference and to promote male responsibility.

Population education is a slow learning process. It shows how the size, composition and distribution of the population in an area is related to the welfare of the individual, the family and the community. It also shows the effects of changes in the size and composition of population brought about by births, deaths and migration (rural and urban) and how the population changes affect the physical and human resources.

Contents of population education: Guiding men and women in reproductive age group (15–49 years) besides decision makers in the family and opinion leaders in the community; improving their knowledge on contraception, developing favourable attitudes to enhance the acceptance of contraception of their choice. It focuses on family size and composition, problem of large sized family, sex of child, right age of marriage and child bearing, equal education opportunities for boys and girls, spacing of births, role and status of women, growth and development of children, feeding of children, economic value of small family and quality of life, existing services for maternal and child health including contraception and their utilization, population trends and problems, early childhood mortality, environments and population, relationship of availability of food, shelter, housing and education and employment with population, population policy and family planning programme in the country.

At Subcentre, PHC, CHC/Hospitals

These are the store houses of information and learning. The education and information is provided or targeted to specific groups like women in reproductive age group, eligible couples, pregnant and nursing mothers and young children. The focus of education is reproductive and child health besides the major killer diseases, their prevention by immunization and by other means. Adequate information depends upon the skills of person managing such institutions as also availability of information material in such situations. These institutions can enrich the process of education by demonstration and participation of mothers and families in the total process.

These institutions can provide organized information for action and are available to offer any clarification and remove doubts of the clients.

At Workplace

The owner or corporate house/industrial set-up or business organizations have the responsibility to provide health information to their staff. Peers have great influence on the behaviour of the person. Peer education holds the promise in these situations.

Adoption Process

Emerging out of interplay of ideas in a given environment, the communication leads individuals and communities to "action" passing through stages of awareness, interest, evaluation, trial and adoption. Thus the diffusion of new ideas and knowledge passes through distinct stages:

1 ***Awareness:*** In this stage, the person acquires new knowledge about the issue or his health need.

2 ***Interest:*** In the second stage, person develops interest and seeks more knowledge to solve the problem.

3 ***Evaluation:*** In this stage, the client evaluates the pros and cons of the decision involved, evaluates its usefulness to him or her and this may result in decision.

4 ***Trial:*** The method, idea, or skill is tried. The idea may be tried out on himself or a friend or other trusted source, such as relative. The person seeks the approval of friends and relatives at the trial stage. During the stage of trial, the health system should support the person in implementing the decision and see that he/she succeeds in the attempts. The support may include counselling, providing supplies and referral services.

5 ***Adoption:*** If the result of trial is good the method, idea, or practice is adopted for regular use.

COMMUNICATION IN HEALTH

Definition

Communication is a process of transfer of information (including ideas, emotions, knowledge-skills and data, etc.) from a person or persons to others. Daily in our life we perform activities of listening, speaking, reading or writing or take recourse of facial expression, gestures, movement of hands and arms, body movements and feelings. Spoken words are the most important means of communication. We call it oral or *verbal communication*. We also communicate through facial expressions, gestures and body movements, signals, which we call as *nonverbal communication*.[10]

Purpose and Goal

Communication has a purpose. Identify the behavior you would like from your audience. Single overriding communication objective (SOCO) guides the communication strategy. Purpose and goal of communication is to change behaviour of people. Promoting and adopting healthy behaviours, which improve and maintain health and discontinue behaviour, which is harmful to health.

Behaviour

It is an action or observable practice/practices in an individual, family and community. Most prevalent practices or behaviours can be classified into:[10]

Harmless: Such as wearing charms, amulets, worshipping and appeasing gods and goddesses. Leave these behaviours as such.

Good behaviours and best practices: *Best practices:* exclusive breastfeeding, immunization, washing hands, eating clean food, drinking safe water, spacing births and limiting the size of the family, using iodized salt, brushing teeth, and regular exercise, etc. These behaviours and practices are to be promoted through communication.

Harmful practices: Early marriages, bottle feeding, drinking unsafe water, tobacco use, chewing pan-masala, excessive use of alcohol, unprotected sex with stranger and physical inactivity are unhealthy behaviours hence need to be changed. We have to analyze all the behaviours and practices and put them into these categories for appropriate action.

Verbal or Oral Communication

Spoken words are often the most common means of communication. Oral method of communication is a weak method of communication. Some doctors and health workers are very good in speech and they articulate it so well that it leaves indelible impression on the minds of people. Most often, we "talk at people", it should be discouraged. This is authoritative communication "talking with people" by group discussion, demonstration of a good practice and having return demonstration are the examples of *participatory communication*. Discussing the results of growth monitoring with mothers is *participatory communication*. Verbal/oral communication, which is traditional or conventional method of communication, can be enriched by use of pictorial and action photographs and live situations like demonstration techniques, which leave good impression and motivate people to accept the things.

Nonverbal Communication

Body language and silence also communicates a lot and makes much more sense. You communicate through visual contacts, nodding your head, symbols, movement of your body parts, facial expressions, gestures, sadness and anger. Combining verbal and nonverbal skills is an art to enrich the process of communication. One should learn how to interpret body language.

Anganwadi worker in ICDS programme uses her skills of nonverbal communication for developing cognitive, affective and psychomotor domains in young children through play-way activities.

Elements of Communication Process

There are various elements of communication process; which are: *source* of information, *message* or content of information, *channel of information*, the *receiver* of information and *feedback*.

Source

The first element in the process of communication is the source. The source is the originator of the message. The source can be an individual, group of individuals or an institution or organization. The source of "*Hum do Hamare do*" message was the Government of India. The source should be credible, accessible, acceptable and legitimate. Source creates an idea (ideation) or chooses a piece of information for communication.

"Only 10–30% of ever married women in India had comprehensive knowledge of HIV/AIDS." The most important source of information on HIV/AIDS to these women was television (78.8%) followed by radio (41.5%).

About one-third of women who know AIDS also report receiving information on AIDS from friends and relatives. Health workers appeared to be marginal source of information on AIDS (3.6%).

Similarly, family planning messages disseminated through mass media were seen or heard by 60% of ever-married women in India. The most common source of message was again television. 44% of women reported having seen a family planning message on television and 38% heard on radio.[11] The major source of pulse polio immunization (PPI) happened to be Anganwadi workers.

Message

The message is an idea or information being communicated. The message is the intended action, which the source wishes the receiver to take. The message links the source and receiver. The message should be very simple, in local language and dialect, easily understandable and action oriented. The message should be pretested among the intended audience before being communicated. Too often, the messages are designed centrally and may not be relevant to specific situation. The messages and pictorials should be produced locally; should address both men and women and would be most effective if this is supported by adequate supportive services and information. For example, message "Get your child fully immunized before 12 months of age" will go well if vaccines are made available when the children need these with arrangement of safe injection. Further the message should address the most significant problem or needs of target groups with due respect to available services. Message creates demand and we must have arrangements to meet these demands.

Key Messages

1 Space the births at least three years apart—use spacing methods. Why? For healthy mother and healthy child, to improve chances of survival, to avoid low birth weight babies, to reduce anaemia in mothers, to reduce morbidity and mortality in mothers and children. The risk of death for young children is increased to 50% if interval between births is less than two years.
2 Becoming pregnant before 18 years and after 35 increases the health risk for both mother and child.
3 Know AIDS for no AIDS.
4 Prenatal sex determination is unlawful.
5 Sex test of fetus is illegal.
6 Diarrhoea can be killer.
7 Deaths due to diarrhoea can be prevented by giving plenty of fluids, home available fluids, ORS and feeding.
8 Breastfeeding is best for a child and a complete food for child up to 6 months of age.
9 Hypertension is a silent killer.
10 Use iodized salt only.
11 Tobacco kills, tobacco causes cancer.

Channel of Communication/Select Right Media

The channel is the means or vehicle by which the message or information travels from source to receiver/audience. The important channels of communication are media (television, radio, newspaper or print media), person-to-person, telephone, or satellite transmission. The choice of channel is important. To ensure maximum coverage of audience or receivers, more than one channel can be used to convey the message or information. Ownership of television in urban areas is 76.7% and in rural India is around 33.4% while radio ownership is maximum. Apart from mass media, interpersonal communication channel should be extensively used. Health workers should increase the frequency of home visits and contact with family and women in reproductive age group and adolescents. At the moment, 7–31 of women in rural and 10% of urban women have received a visit of health worker in the past one year which is quite distressing.

Receiver or Target Audience

Define your audience and their concern. *Seek first to understand then to be understood.* Who are the target audience or receiver of information and specific messages? Target audience needs to be segmented according to their knowledge, beliefs and practices, incidence and severity of illness or health problems, literacy level, economic level, geographic locations, media reach and social network. The audience or receiver is not the end point. Audience segmentation is seldom done. Examples of target audience are:

1 Currently pregnant women.
2 Married women with 1, 2 and 3 children.
3 Adolescent boys and girls.
4 Women with child below 6 months (lactating mothers).
5 Newly married couples.
6 Community leaders—men and women.
7 Health workers male and female and supervisors.
8 Women who have accepted IUD or satisfied customers.

Feedback

Feedback is an essential element of communication. Feedback is the reaction or response of the receiver to the source. Feedback from receiver helps the source to improve the message and information or its modification. An experienced and wise communicator is always keen to get a feedback and continuously modifies his message in the light of what he observes or hears from the intended audience. Without feedback, the communication is one-way traffic or one-way communication.

Case Study in Communication

In a group discussion, the feedback is obtained on the spot. We launched a programme of "Radio in support of mother and child development". Organized listening groups were formed with the help of AWWs, who acted as group *animators* (a local person chosen by community trained in communication who canvases from house to house and facilitates "mother's meeting"). After listening the broadcast programme, the reply paid letters received from AWWs (incorporating the views of mothers who listened the programme) helped us a lot to improve the programme. Continuous feedback from audience is seldom obtained hence it is weakest element in the system of communication. Continuous feedback guides the source and planner to improve the contents of message and better management of the programme.

ONE-WAY AND TWO-WAY COMMUNICATION MODELS

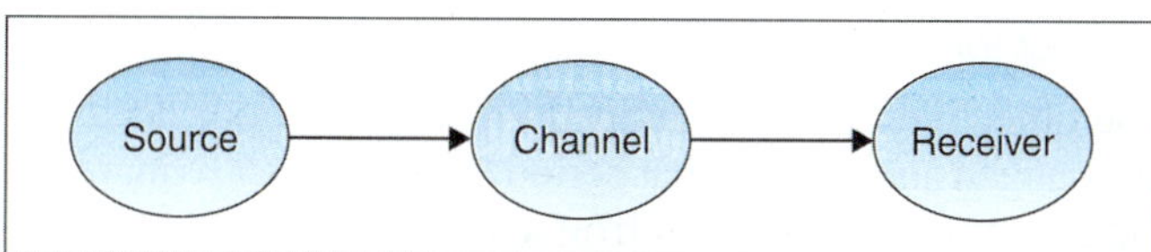

One-way Communication Model

i Systems that provide health information to the user (one-way communication)

ii Systems that tailor specific information to the user unique situation (customized communication)

iii Systems that allow the user to communicate and interact with health care providers or other users (two-way communication).

When the source is communicating the information to receiver or audience and there is no feedback it is one-way communication. It has many disadvantages.

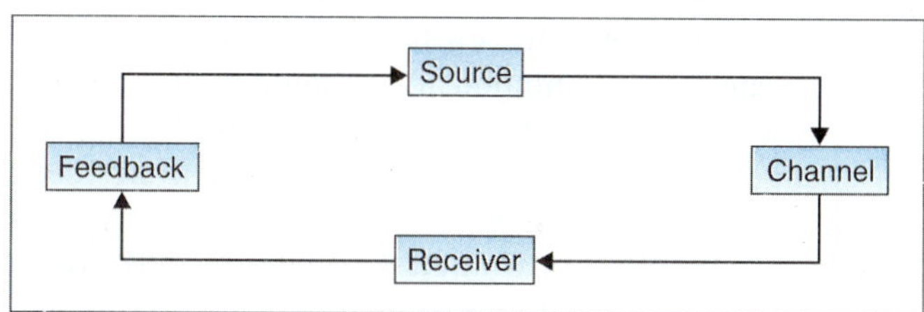

Two-way Communication Model

When there is feedback from receiver to the source it is two-way communication.

Example: When mothers are involved in growth monitoring and their reactions are obtained, it is two-way communication. When AWW weighs alone and mothers are not involved, it is one-way or no communication. Mass media is one-way communication most of the time. Interpersonal communication is two-way communication.

Strategies/Approaches in Communication

Three approaches are commonly used, individual, group and mass communication.

(A) Interpersonal (Individual Approach)[12]

It is one-to-one communication, which happens during home visits by health workers when they contact family and mother. It is most precise and specific communication dealing with the precise needs of an individual. It occurs in most friendly manner. It is also called interpersonal communication (IPC). It is most interactive and participatory.

Interpersonal communication skills of workers need to be sharpened through training and retraining in group dynamics, group discussions. Home visits programme of health workers, their beat programmes should focus attention on interpersonal communication based on individual's health needs and suggest home-based actions within the capacity of family. Every contact of worker with the people should have an element of need-based education. This should be the major strategy in the clinics and hospitals. Support health education material (printed and visuals) and case material or live situations can enrich the interpersonal communication process.

Enhancing Interpersonal Communication

Interpersonal communication can be enhanced by:

- Empowering *Mahila Swasthya Sanghs* (MSS) who could take responsibility of contacting married women in their neighbourhood on regular basis.
- ICDS functionaries like Anganwadi workers and health workers should be trained together and make joint home visits for interpersonal communication.
- Mahila Mandals and elected women Panchayat members and ASHAs can spearhead interpersonal communication in RCH programme to the best advantage of women in reproductive age group.

(B) Group Communication

When health worker female organizes a small group of *Mahila Swasthya Sangh* (10–20 women) she organizes a group discussion and group meets to discuss a common problem say problem of anaemia in pregnant women it is called group communication. All members of the group are encouraged to participate and express their views and come to an agreed upon solution for an identified problem. In a group discussion, group dynamics are important. Many methods are used in group communication, it could be a demonstration, discussion, an audio video show, organized listening and watching television, question answer, etc. It all depends upon the communication skills of health workers and their supervisors. Group communication with *Mahila Swasthya Sangh, Mahila Mandal*, Village Panchayats, self-help groups and adolescent girls and boys could be most rewarding experience. Health workers must be trained on how to organize a group communication.

Sitting in a circle and semicircle, on ground or on chairs, provides an opportunity of visual contacts and generates a sense of equality amongst all group members. In this arrangement, group members can see each other and can interact in a friendly manner. Regular Village Health Sanitation and Nutrition Committee meetings must be organized at Anganwadi Centre.

(C) Mass Communication

Radio, television, and print media (newspapers) reach and communicate masses and cover a wide geographical area and population in short time. The message can be disseminated to large population with a clear focus on target groups. This is known as mass communication. The mass communication is most cost-effective and is primarily used to generate awareness and impart knowledge to masses. It needs to be followed up and supplemented and supported with group and individual communication to facilitate the process of adoption and acceptance of a practice. Family planning programme used mass media to build up awareness and as a result, now the awareness about contraception is almost universal (100%). Similarly, pulse polio programme used mass media at national level to build a favourable climate and message through a popular actor (Amitabh Bachchan) ***Do Boond Zindgi Ki*** (two precious drops of polio vaccine for life) had a mass appeal for massive social mobilization. Similarly, message of honourable Prime Minister on polio had mass appeal. Mass communication must be supported by services and accessibility to quality services to achieve the desirable success.

Commercialization of media by producing audio-tapes and video-tapes for self-learning and learning at family level on the pattern of social marketing strategy can go a long way. Health education video libraries be established, to empower more people.

Communication Skills

Communication skills of health managers and workers and Anganwadi workers are crucial, critical and much depends on their training.

Listening to client is most important skill of communication. Listening means analyzing the mind of client and assessing their communication needs and understanding their profile.[13]

Speaking is another important skill. What to speak, how to speak when to speak and whom to speak is essential. It means the communicator should have latest knowledge and speak scientifically. Convey message which is sense making and has proven scientific evidence.

The other communication skills are *reading, writing* and *reasoning*.

Effects of Communication

The most important effect of communication is change in behaviour. It should result into change in behaviour or practice. There are three main effects of communication.

1. ***Thinking:*** The communication may lead to change in thinking and perception of an individual, group or community. It adds on the knowledge and builds "cognitive domain".
2. ***Feelings/attitude:*** This is second effect that the feelings (attitudes) may change. Negative attitudes may change to positive attitudes and often indicates an action that the individual may take.
3. ***Behaviour change:*** Change in action (practice). These are changes in overall behaviour, such as adopting a contraceptive, quit smoking, starts brushing teeth.

These three changes usually occur in sequence that is a change in knowledge precedes change in attitude which precedes change in behaviour, but not always; attitude change often follows an action.

Planning, Organizing, Implementation and Evaluation of Health Communication Programme

(a) Planning

The objectives must be defined—what behaviour needs to be changed and within what period? Example is "To increase the acceptance of condom from current level of 5.3 to 12% within a span of three years" could be objective. You must define objective for communication (single overriding communication objective (SOCO) to guide the strategy) as explained in Table 2.2: Matrix… .

(b) Communication Needs Assessment (CNA)

Assess the communication needs of, individuals, family and community in the area. This can be done by contacting the clients through routine visits and annual survey of eligible couples, or any opportunity of contact with mother or parents, such as immunization sessions. Communication needs are seldom assessed. Communication needs assessment (CNA) are to be listed client-wise, family-wise; so that these can be met **(a best practice)**.[12]

Example: Need of newborn is survival, breastfeeding, asepsis, clean cord. Communication should focus on these needs. Know the practices and list the harmful practices and change these harmful practices to **best practices,** focusing on most urgent ones, which save lives. In short know your people, know their knowledge, attitudes, practices, beliefs, myths, and misconceptions on the issues of MCH and family welfare and other areas.

(c) Define your Target Audience and their Concern

Identify the families, which need your help most. Weaker section of community or those families which have problems; families having pregnant women, infant and young children could be your target audience. Segment your audience based on their economic status, caste and literacy, practices/behaviour.

(d) Message

Message should be specific. It should not only generate awareness but also lead onto behaviour change. In family planning, messages on promoting the norms of small families are disseminated to build up an awareness rather than providing method specific information to clients. Provide information on all methods to promote informed choice. Adequate education material must be made available to communicate message to target groups.

(e) Tracking Clients

After messages have been given, these must be repeated and keep contacts with the clients to observe the effect of communication and measure your success and failure and learn lessons from those who have understood your message and who have changed their practices and who have adopted a method of contraception, etc. Sustained contacts with client build a mutual trust, increase understanding and generate confidence. Right now only 7.6 to 31% of families are being contacted by health workers in the rural settings, it means tracking of client is very low.

(f) Selecting Channel to Reach the Audience

Select appropriate channel of communication, such as televisions or radio, print media, women groups (MSS), person or persons whom you think to be most effective. It should reach to maximum number of clients; the intention is maximum coverage and channels chosen must be effective to carry the message to target audience. Always use multiple channels to enhance the coverage. Priority channel for each audience needs to be selected and planned.

Manage activities within the budget provided and train the staff for communication (particularly on communication skills and organization of groups and use of educational material).

(g) Evaluation

Finally, we need to evaluate the results of communication. The evaluation is done by the workers themselves during their home visits and contacts with the audience or clients, as also through annual survey and updating of couples or through district rapid surveys under RCH programme.

NFHS 1–4 have been undertaken nationwide surveys and provide useful information on evaluation of communication efforts. Similarly, behavioural surveillance surveys under National HIV/AIDS control programme provides useful information on evaluation for further action to improve the communication process. The process evaluation is most important.

The communication gaps and needs as identified by NFHS III were:

1. Among the women aged 20–24 years, almost one quarter married before 15 and 44.5% married before 18, the legal minimum age of marriage.
2. The total fertility rate was 2.98 in rural and 2.07 in urban area which indicates high fertility rates.
3. Teen age (15–19) contributes to 16% of total fertility.
4. Only 36.8% of children under 6 months of age were exclusively breastfed.
5. Early initiation of breastfeeding (< 1 hr) 33.5%.
6. Short birth interval was obvious as one birth out of every eight occurs within 18 months of previous birth.
7. Female sterilization is predominant method of contraception, men participation is low; only 1% of men accepted sterilization against 37.3% of women.
8. High maternal mortality rate of 212 per 100,000 live births.
9. Nearly 69% of mothers received three or more antenatal check ups.
10. Around 24% of deliveries are unsafe in India.
11. Postnatal care was provided only to 36.4% of mothers within 2 days of birth.
12. Nearly 40% of currently married women in India report at least one reproductive health problem (RTI).
13. Immunization coverage was far from universal, as 61% were fully immunized.
14. ORS use rate was only 43%.
15. 28% of births weigh under 2.5 kg.
16. 47.9% of men and 20.3% women used tabacco.

Table 2.2: Matrix of behaviour change communication to increase men participation

Area of concern	*Current behaviour or practice 2014*	*Expected behaviour in 2016*	*Target audience*	*Message*	*Media and channel*	*Indicator of change in 2016 (evaluation)*
Use of spacing methods by women	5% of women practice	10%	Currently married women with one child	Spacing births at least three years apart to improve the health of mother and survival of child	Interpersonal communication by health worker female • TV • MSS groups	• Percentage of women with one or two children who are using spacing methods (Annual survey data of workers)
Use of spacing methods by men (condom use)	5.3% of men use condom	12%	Currently married men with one child	Do	Interpersonal communication by health worker male • Opinion leaders • TV	• Percentage of men using condoms (Annual survey data of workers)

Thus, the communication needs are obvious. This tells us clearly, where we stand and what are the cardinal needs for behaviour change communication (BCC).

Responsibility of planning and evaluation lies with medical officer incharge of primary health centre and community health centre.

a The knowledge can be evaluated by asking standard questions about a specific problem.

b The attitudes can be evaluated by "Likert scale—a scale measuring the degree to which people agree or disagree with a statement; usually on a 3–, 5– or 7– point scale.

Example: Spacing births two years apart is good for the health of mother and survival of child (statement).

3 point scale: Agree..........neutral.........disagree

5 point scale: Strongly agree..... agree.... neutral... disagree.......strongly disagree.

c Practices can be evaluated by observations—like practice of washing hands, nail cutting, delivery room, cord cutting, cooking food and feeding practices.

National Communication Strategy in Reproductive and Child Health Programme (RCH)

The communication strategy aims to facilitate awareness, dissemination of information regarding availability of and access to quality health care within public health system. The key objective of the strategy is encourage a health seeking behaviour that is doable in the context in which people live. The strategy views recipients of health services as not merely passive *users* of services but key *participants* in generating demand for services.

The national strategy on communication under RCH programme lays stress on:[13, 14]

- Interpersonal communication for behaviour change at the field level.
- ***Decentralized planning for communication:*** Production of material and messages at state and district level. Districts will prepare their own plans for IEC.
- Use of mass media for advocacy and awareness.
- Increased involvement of non-governmental organizations (NGOs).
- Capacity building and training at all levels to undertake the newly developed tasks and thrust areas under RCH I and II.

  The responsibilities of central government, state and district have been defined. In the decentralization of IEC activities, the role of states and district is crucial.

Thrust areas for communication under RCH:

- Meeting the unmet needs of contraceptives, both for spacing and terminal methods.[14, 15]
- Improving maternal health.
- Raising chances of survival.
- Adolescent health.
- Implementation of PC—PNDT Act to achieve balanced child sex ratio.
- Coverage of urban slums and tribal areas.
- Newborn care.

In order to achieve the goals of RCH programme, the communication interventions have to focus on behaviour change. Accordingly, the matrix of behaviour change has been indicated under the RCH strategy on communication (Table 2.2).

The areas or issues to be focused are: unwanted fertility, unmet need of contraception, unsafe abortions, high maternal mortality, maternal morbidity, adolescent reproductive health, RTI/STI, infant mortality, drop in immunization coverage, newborn care, adverse child sex ratio, urban and tribal health.

COUNSELLING IN HEALTH AND DISEASE

COUNSELLING IN RCH AND OTHER PROGRAMMES

Concept of Counselling

Through counselling, you help clients make informed choices that suit them. For example, some clients are choosing family planning methods; other clients are deciding how to avoid sexually transmitted diseases. Young clients (adolescents) may be choosing whether to delay sexual activity. All these clients make better decisions with your help.

Definition

"Counselling is face to face communication by which you help the person to make decision or solve a problem. Counselling is a helping process aimed at problem-solving. It helps people to understand themselves better in terms of their own needs, strengths, limitations and the resources they can avail of. It brings about a change through supportive relationship aiming to make client independent through the interpersonal contact along with the opportunity to ask questions and to seek frequently needed help greatly."

Counselling Skills[16]

(A) Listen Actively

You have to listen actively. Attentive and active listening is essential. How to listen actively? Some guidelines are as under:

- Accept your clients as they are, treat him/her as an individual.
- Listen to what your client says and how they say it. Notice tone of the voice, choice of words, facial expressions and gestures **(best practice).**
- Keep silent sometimes. Give your clients time to think, ask questions and talk more at the client's speed.
- Listen to your client carefully instead of thinking what you are going to say next (Table 2.3).

Table 2.3: Sharing facts and feelings

	Share facts	*Share feelings*
Provider's job	• Give clear, accurate information that the client wants and needs • Help the client apply this information to his/her own life	• Care for client by showing understanding respect and honesty
Client's job	• Describe personal situation and health conditions • Ask questions and make sure of understanding	• Express attitudes, preferences, concerns, expectations and wishes

- Every now and then, repeat what you have heard. Then both you and your client know whether you have understood.
- Sit comfortably. Avoid distracting movements. Look directly at your clients when they speak, not at your papers or out of the window.
- Use words, such as "then"? "And" "Oh" these worlds encourage clients to keep talking.
- Show your interest and understanding at all times. Express empathy. Avoid judgment and opinion.

(B) Responding to Client's Feelings

Once you recognize client's feeling let them know in clear and simple words that you understand. This is called "reflecting feeling". Two examples are given hereunder. You cannot change client's feeling. Only they can do that, but when you reflect feeling, you are showing that you understand. You also are saying it is all right to feel that way (Fig. 2.4).

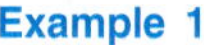

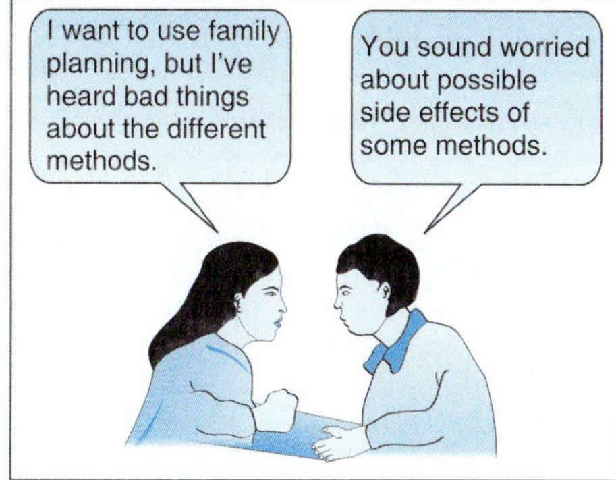

Example 2

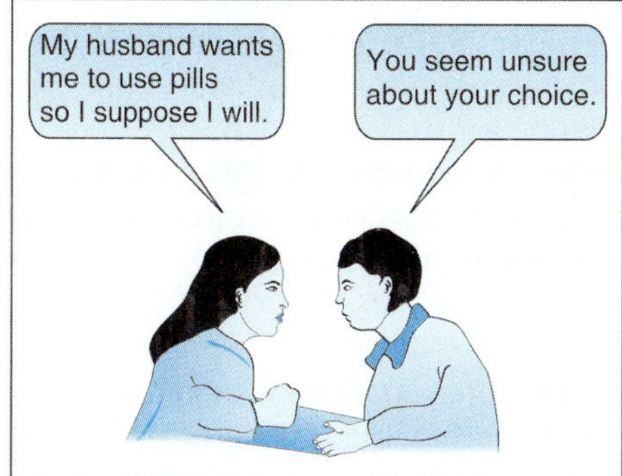

Fig. 2.4: Reflecting feelings

(C) Questioning

Asking question to understand clearly the clients problem or worries and help client go deeper into his/her own awareness or insight. The question is centered on the prime concern of the client and open-ended questions are better than close-ended.

(D) Paraphrasing and Interpretation

Repeating in one's own words 'what the client has said' to show one understands. Saying it in a few words, so that it gives a summary essence of client's words.

(E) Interpretation

Giving back to client the core or basic issue he/she is talking around or hinting at. Picking up what the client is feeling but not saying. This skill involves going to a slightly deeper level of the issue to point out the feeling of meaning or meanings, which are just below the surface of the client's awareness. Check with the client, if one's interpretation is correct.

GATHER Approach to Counselling about IUDs[17,18]

There are six steps to counselling. The provider can remember the steps using the English word "GATHER". The GATHER approach applies to all kinds of counselling.

G: *Greet clients:* The provider greets clients politely and gives them full attention.

A: *Ask clients about themselves:* The provider asks clients about their family planning needs and obtains information that will help the provider to advise and inform each client individually.

T: *Tell clients about family planning methods:* The provider lists the available family planning methods and clearly describes those that interest the client—how they work, advantages and disadvantages and possible side effects. Even clients who immediately express a preference for the IUD or some other method should know of other available methods for future reference and so they can inform friends and family members.

H: *Help clients choose a method:* Some women may have already decided that they want an IUD. Others may want advice and guidance from the provider. In either case, the provider helps the woman decide on a safe method that suits her needs and plans. If the method is not appropriate, the provider explains why and helps the client select another method. If there are reasons that another method would be preferable, the provider and client compare the risks and benefits of the IUD and of other contraceptive methods and consider the risks of an unintended pregnancy. The final decision to use an IUD—or any other method must be an informed choice made by the client. If possible, involving the husband in counselling is a good idea. In an African study, husbands' wishes accounted for many IUD removals after postpartum insertion.

E: *Explain how to use the IUD:* Once a woman decides to use an IUD, the provider explains:

- When, where, and how it will be inserted
- The common side effects
- The slight chance of more serious complications, expulsion, or unintended pregnancy
- Reasons to return to the clinic or see another provider
- When a copper or hormone releasing IUD should be replaced.

Women who understand that mild cramping and bleeding in the days following insertion and heavier menstrual periods while using an IUD are common and usually harmless will be less likely to have their IUDs removed unnecessarily.

It is helpful to give clients printed material to take home, particularly a card with the name and picture of the IUD, noting the date of insertion and time for removal (printed materials can help providers, too). During counselling and screening, flip charts, wall charts, cue cards, and checklists help providers maintain accuracy and remember what to cover and they help clients to understand.

The client should be told if and how she will be notified when it is time for the IUD to be replaced. The family planning program should keep records for each IUD user showing the type of IUD and when it was inserted. These records should be used to answer questions from women who have forgotten when to have their IUDs replaced and to follow-up users when the time for replacement approaches.

R: *Return for follow-up:* When a woman has an IUD inserted, she and the provider should plan for a follow-up visit 3 to 6 weeks later, after her next menses. While no further scheduled follow-up visits are required for the safe use of the IUD, the women should be strongly encouraged to return whenever she has questions or problems or if she wants the IUD removed. Also she should return as soon as possible if she notices any warning signs. The provider should be sure that the woman knows both when and where to seek medical care.

Counselling in HIV/AIDS

Counselling is concerned with preventing infection with HIV and its transmission to people from person living with HIV/AIDS.

The main steps of preventive counselling are to:

- Determine whether individual/group has high-risk behaviour pattern.
- Help people understand and acknowledge their high-risk behaviour patterns.
- Define with them how their lifestyle and self-image are linked to their behaviour.
- Help individuals define their potential for changing behaviour.
- Work with individuals to introduce and sustain the modified behaviour.

2

Health Promotion

This involves counselling those individuals having high-risk behaviour patterns but not aware of the magnitude and the nature of risk involved to their life. It aims at creating this change focusing on behaviour that presents a risk of HIV infection and reviewing ways of managing individual change.

Specific Protection

Those infected with HIV should be given instructions as to ways by which they can prevent the spread of infection to others. An attitude of understanding should be adopted as the fact that he has tested positive is traumatic enough to accept. Since behaviour change is going to be difficult, he should be asked to take certain precautions:

- Do not donate blood.
- Use condoms while having sexual intercourse.
- Do not share needles and syringes.

Psychosocial Support

People diagnosed with HIV infection related illness and those close to them are confronted by a multitude of problems and often need emotional support and/or practical support. People have anxieties regarding hospitalization and depression because of stigma attached to their conditions. Counselling should help those infected by HIV to live full and productive lives by enabling them to take charge of their lives and help in decision-making, thus enabling people to remain active in their work and in their education. Families and friends can help to reduce their dependence on health and social services and reduce their psychosocial problems.

Requirement of Counselling

Approaches to counselling will differ from individuals and groups depending upon the characteristics of the people being counselled and their social and family network. Certain points, which remain constant irrespective of the situation, are given below.

Rapport

The client must not be rushed with the news that he is HIV positive. Sufficient time should be taken to establish rapport with the client, so, as to understand his mental framework and basic level from where the counselling should be carried forward. This basic level will determine the number of sessions required by the person to take decision about his lifestyle.

Acceptance

The people infected by HIV should not be shunned on the basis of the behavioural patterns adopted by them. They should be treated with respect whatsoever their background or behaviour.

Accessibility

People found to be HIV positive are bound to develop anxieties and fears, which will be always raising some doubts in their minds. Therefore, counselling services should be available easily where the individual can approach at any time and get clarification.

Consistency and Accuracy

Any information provided through counselling should be consistent; therefore, the counsellor must equip himself with all the latest knowledge and management of HIV infection and disease so as to be able to clarify doubts/ uncertainties arising in the minds of the client. He should not pretend to know or acknowledge a thing when in doubt but try to clarify it.

Confidentiality

Being diagnosed HIV positive creates uncertainties in the mind of the clients. The counsellor should be able to gain the trust of the client and convince him that all information provided by him will be kept confidential.

What to Counsel?

As HIV infection is progressive, it is necessary that counselling should be undertaken regularly to understand what the client is going through due to the various changes occurring within him and those around him. The counsellor should also provide to the client necessary information regarding where he will be able to get medical support, community resources and what changes he can make in his lifestyles to cope with emerging needs.

Counselling before HIV Testing (Pretest Counselling)

Counselling before the test should provide the individuals being tested with information on technical aspects of screening and possible personal, medical, social, psychological and least implications of being tested positive or negative. The information should be simple and up to date. Testing should be organized in a way that minimizes the possibility of disclosure.

Issues in Pretest Counselling

Pretest counselling consists of two parts:

1. Personal history and assessment of risk.
   - Sexual behaviour multi-partners, prostitutes, unprotected sex, homosexuality, bisexuality.
   - Drug users.
   - Blood transfusion.
   - Organ transplant.
2. Assessment of factors and knowledge.
   - Why test is being requested?
   - What behaviour/symptoms are of concern to the client?
   - What the client knows about test and its uses?
   - What will the client do if test is positive or negative?
   - Beliefs regarding HIV transmission.
   - What roles will family play?

Counselling after HIV Testing (Post-testing Counselling)

If Result is Negative

The client may feel relief, however caution should be exercised as following exposure to HIV, there is a **window period** of 6–12 weeks between initial infection with HIV and the time when HIV antibodies can be detected in the blood. A blood test performed during the **window period** may yield a negative test result for antibodies. These cases may require further testing after 12 weeks. A negative test result becomes a certainty if 6 months have lapsed after last exposure. HIV infection can be prevented by avoiding high-risk behaviour, safe sex and avoiding sharing needles. In general, development of safe sex behaviour to be advocated to the client.

If Result is Positive

People diagnosed as having HIV infection should be told about their results privately and in confidence. Single test giving positive result does not necessary mean HIV infection. To establish HIV infection, *three tests* for antibodies based on different antigen methods are to test positive. Time should be allowed for the client to absorb the news. After a period of preliminary adjustment, the client should be given clear and factual explanation or what the news means. This does not mean speculating about prognosis of estimate about the time left to live but for providing support; and encouraging hope for achievable solutions to personal and practical problems that may result. The client must be informed where resources are available and possible treatment for some symptoms to HIV infection and efficacy of antiviral treatment.

Psychological Issues

The uncertainty involved when the individual comes to know he has tested positive are longevity of life, etc. Clarifications are to be given regarding the fears which arise related to illness, death, etc. Besides these, the individual feels at loss due to stigma attached by society and the speculation in the minds of people regarding the behaviour of those infected with the virus.

There is generalized anxiety regarding all aspects of life, anger and expression of the fact that he has tested positive; can even lead to suicidal thinking within the individual.

These numerous feelings can only be changed through counselling and giving correct information about the infection and disease and building the self-esteem and the positive thinking ability of the individual. Besides the individual who has tested positive, those dealing with them, i.e. the health workers and family face their share of fears and uncertainties regarding their getting the infection.

All those involved with those who have tested positive need to be given proper and full information so that they can provide the support, which the individual requires to be able to face their problem.

VOLUNTARY COUNSELLING AND TESTING CENTRES (VCTCs)

Now VCTCs have been renamed as Integrated Counselling and Testing Centres (ICTCs)

The HIV counselling and testing services, started in the year 1997, have been scaled up in the recent years. Today there are more than 15606 counselling and testing centres which are located at all levels of the public health care system (4818 Stand alone and 10788 Facility-based ICTCs). The earlier voluntary counselling and testing centres (VCTCs) and facilities providing prevention of parent-to-child transmission (PPTCT) of HIV/AIDS services are now remodelled as a hub to deliver integrated services to all clients under one roof renamed as "Integrated Counselling and Testing Centres" (ICTCs).

Though counselling and testing services have been implemented in India for the past sixteen years, not more than 25–30% of the people who are living with HIV/AIDS are aware of their HIV status. Under the National AIDS Control Programme Phase III (NACP-III), it was planned to have 22 million clients counselled and tested through ICTCs every year. An equal number of clients will be tested in the private sector.

What is an Integrated Counselling and Testing Centre?

An ICTC is a place where a person is counselled and tested for HIV, on his own free will or as advised by a medical provider. The main functions of ICTC include:

- Early detection of HIV.
- Provision of basic information on modes of transmission and prevention of HIV/AIDS for promoting behavioural change and reducing vulnerability/risk.
- Link people with other HIV prevention, care and treatment services.
- Outreach visits to the homes of HIV positive clients facing severe crisis.

ICTC can be located in the Obstetric and Gynae Department for pregnant women, or with tuberculosis microscopy centre for TB patients, at workplace, on national highways and in universities.

Voluntary counselling and testing (VCT) provides for all segments of the population, an opportunity to access complete and accurate information on HIV/AIDS.[19,20]

This is a critical entry point to prevention, care, support and treatment for all people, and particularly for those already infected and affected. VCT services enable the 'client' to confidentially explore and understand his or her risk of HIV infection, provides an opportunity to fully comprehend the implications of one's serostatus and to learn about precautions for one's protection and preventing the further spread of HIV infection. VCT facilitates personal, and more informed decisions about HIV testing. Counselling is client centered. This promotes trust between the counselor and the client. The client is helped to identify and understand the implications of a negative and positive result.

In the event of positive HIV test result, counselling strengthens strategies for coping with the immediate stress, possible stigma, psychological and social impacts. It provides referrals to appropriate facilities for care, support and treatment and promotes more informed choices for the future.

This common facility will remove fear, stigma and discrimination among the clients. The ICTCs have common television and video-based health education material that are screened continuously in the waiting area. Further two strategies are adopted in ICTCs for HIV testing—"opt out" and "opt in" strategy.

1. *Provider initiated counselling and testing*—"opt out". These clients are referred by health care providers. There are three varieties of patients who are offered provider-initiated counselling and testing:
   a. Patients who present at a health facility with symptoms suggestive of HIV infection (pneumonia, TB and persistent diarrhoea).
   b. Patients with STI/RTI.
   c. Pregnant women who register at antenatal clinic.

   In such cases the client is given basic information on HIV, and educated about testing for HIV. The counsellor will ask each client, "Do you wish to test for HIV or not?" The client can "opt out" or choose not to test for HIV. If a client does not "opt out" then he/she is tested for HIV.
2. *Client initiated counselling* and testing "opt in" or Direct walk in clients/self-referred clients.

   These clients who present themselves at the ICTC of their own free will based on their individual risk behaviour or information and advice received from a friend, sexual partner, or outreach worker or peer educator. Here the client is counselled for HIV and then "opts in" or actively agrees to be tested for HIV. Written consent has to be obtained from such clients before testing.

As per the National AIDS Prevention and Control Policy, all HIV tests are voluntary based on the clients consent, accompanied by counselling and confidentiality of the results.

VCT services have reached up to block level in high prevalence states. The moderate and low prevalence states are in the process of extending VCT services to district and subdistrict level.

Different Types of ICTCs

There are three types of ICTCs.

1. Fixed facility ICTCs
2. Mobile ICTCs
3. Public–private partnership ICTCs

A fixed facility ICTC can be of three types:

1. "Stand alone" ICTC having full time counsellor and a laboratory technician located in medical colleges and district and in some sub-district hospitals. It is envisaged under NACP-III to have such ICTCs established up to the level of CHC (block level).
2. "Facility-integrated" ICTC which does not have full time staff and provides HIV counselling and testing as a service along with other services. Such centre caters to small number of clients, below the block level in high prevalent states.
3. Public–private partnership ICTCs.

Core Staff

Depending upon resources available and size of VCTC/ICTCs the core staff could include:

1. VCTC incharge/VCTC manager (often a microbiologist).
2. Two trained counsellors (one male and one female) or ideally as per client load (Per counsellor 8–10 counselling sessions per day).
3. One trained laboratory technician.

Counselling in VCT consists of *pre-test* and *post-test* counselling. During pre-test counselling, the counsellor provides to the individual/couple an opportunity to explore and analyse their situation, and consider being tested for HIV. It facilitates more informed decisions about HIV testing. After the individual/couple has received accurate and complete information they reach an understanding about all that is involved. In the event that, after couselling, the individual decides to take the HIV test, VCT enables confidential HIV testing.

Post-test counselling: Consists of how to cope up with positive test and live positive life and share result with spouse and family members, notify partners and prevent transmission of HIV infection.

Peer Counselling

Peer counsellors are HIV positive men and women specially trained to hear the concerns of clients and offer support and referral services. A peer counsellor is an individual who is open about his/her HIV positive status and shares experiences with client and is willing to sustain his/her behaviour change and that of peers.

Peer counselling is a process that is carried out as a one to one interaction, followed by group interaction. During this process, experiential information is shared among the peer group to modify knowledge, attitude and beliefs to bring about change at the individual level. Counselling provided through this modality has a component of informality to it and addresses client issues through following processes:

- Sharing feelings about similar experiences and emotions.
- Sharing of information for availability of HIV/AIDS prevention, treatment and care services
- Narrating their success stories to the peers and conveying messages of positive living.
- Advocating on behalf of the clients rights.
- Supporting clients in becoming more involved in community activities.
- Enable clients to learn self-help skills.

Goals of Peer Counselling

- To modify the attitudes, beliefs and behaviour of persons with high-risk behaviour.
- To identify actions needed to achieve behaviour change.

REFERENCES

1 Somer AR. Preventive Medicine 1977; 6(3): 406.

2 IGNOU (2003). Communication for Behaviour Change Preventive MCH. Maidan Garhi; New Delhi: IGNOU; 2003.

3 IGNOU. Information Education and Communication PGDMCH-1 Preventive MCH. Maidan Garhi, New Delhi: IGNOU School of Health Sciences; 1998.

4 UNICEF, WHO, UNESCO, UNFPA, UNAIDS, WFP and the World Bank. "Facts for life", 3rd edition, 2002, UNICEF: House 73, Lodhi Estate, New Delhi.

5 UNICEF. The State of the World's Children 1987, 3UN Plaza (NY). UNICEF, Division of Public Affairs; 1987.

6 Ministry of Health and Family Welfare. Report of IEC strategy workshop for USAID assisted areas projects; 1984 Dec. 3–6; Taj Palace Hotel, New Delhi.

7 Govt. of India. Monitoring Communication Needs for Health and Family Welfare in USAID assisted area projects in Gujarat, Haryana, Himachal Pradesh, Maharashtra and Punjab. New Delhi: MOH and FW, GOI; 1986.

8 Govt. of India. RCH 2 and Family Planning Programme Implementation Plan (PIP). Nirman Bhavan, New Delhi: MOH and FW, Govt. of India; 2004.

9 Lal S. Newer Strategies in Health Education for 21st Century. The Journal of Applied Primary Health Care 1990; Oct.-Dec.

10 Hubley J. Communicating Health—an action guide to health education and health promotion. First edn, London: The Macmillan Press Ltd.

11 Indian Institute for Population Sciences and ORC Macro. National Family Health Survey (NFHS-2). Key Findings. Mumbai, IIPS; 1998–99.

12 Measham AR, Heaver AR. Directions in Development. Supplement to India's Family Welfare Programme, moving to reproductive and child health approach. Washington, DC: The World Bank, 1996.

13 GOI. National Communication Strategy for reproductive and child health programme. New Delhi: Department of Family Welfare IEC Division, MOH and FW, GOI; 2000.

14 Govt. of India. National Population Policy 2000. New Delhi: GOI; 2000.

15 Govt. of India. Training module on HIV infection and AIDS for medical officers. New Delhi: NACO, MOH and FW, Govt. of India; 2000.

16 Family Planning Programmes. New GATHER GUIDE to counselling. Population Reports 2000 Feb; J (48).

17 Intrauterine Devices—an update. The GATHER approach to counselling about IUD's. Population Reports, Jan 1997; 8(6).
18 Family Planning Programmes—informed choices in family planning helping people to decide. Population Reports. 2001 Aug; J (50).
19 GOI. Voluntary Counselling and Testing Operational Guidelines 2004, NACO, MOH and FW, GOI New Delhi 2004.
20 GOI—Operational Guidelines for Integrated Counselling and Testing Centres, July 2007, NACO, MOH and FW, Govt. of India New Delhi.

HEALTH ECONOMICS

The health has a price and the sickness has a cost. Resources are always scarce or limited and these have to be allocated to priority problems. Health economics studies the allocation of scarce resources to different areas of health sector to achieve the results. Hard choices have to be made. Economics is most famously defined as "the science which studies human behaviour as a relationship between ends and scarce means which have alternate uses". Health economics is concerned with the choices over how best to spend limited resources available for health care.

1 In absolute terms, the plan outlay spent on health care has been falling from plan to plan and from 2002 to 2007. During Tenth Plan period, it increased to 2.09% of the total outlay (Table 2.4).[1] for health and 1.83% for family planning and during XIth plan it further increased to 6.50%.
2 The public health investment in the country over the years has been comparatively low, and as a percentage of GDP has declined from 1.3% in 1990 to 0.9% in 1999.[1]
3 The aggregate expenditure in the health sector is 5.23% of the GDP (Year 2009). Out of this 21% of the aggregate expenditure is public health spending and rest 79% being out of pocket expenditure.
4 Government health expenditure on health (% of GDP): 1% from 2001 to 2005 and private health expenditure (% of GDP): 4%—WHO World Health Report, 2007.[2]
5 Per capita, public expenditure on health care financing is no more than ₹ 242 (2004–05).

India ranks low among developed countries in per capita health expenditure, despite the relatively developed and widespread infrastructure. A significant feature of health in India is its maldistribution in favour of urban, upper and middle classes and biased against the rural poor.

To meet the objectives of reducing various types of inequities and imbalances—inter-regional; across the rural-urban divide and between economic classes—the most cost-effective method would be to increase the sectoral outlay in the primary health sector. Such outlets afford access to a vast number of individuals, and also facilitate preventive and early stage curative initiative, which are cost-effective. In recognition of this public health principle, National Health Policy 2002 sets out an increased allocation of 55% of the total public health investment for the primary health sector, the secondary and tertiary health sectors being targeted for 35% and 10% respectively.[1]

The cost of secondary and tertiary care is going up day by day and it is enormous as in government teaching hospital. A hospital bed may cost ₹ 50000–75000 per annum. Most of this cost goes to salaries of staff (75%) and maintenance cost (water-electricity) which is around 20%.

Economic Impact of Tuberculosis in India

The burden of suffering caused by tuberculosis in India is enormous. TB is one of the India's biggest health and social problem—a problem that India can ill afford.

Man Days Lost due to Tuberculosis

Indian worker with tuberculosis lost an average of 83 work days because of disease. Considering that 2 million new cases are reported annually in India, the national loss per year works out to 166 million lost work days, at a cost of about $ 200 million (₹ 694 crore). In addition, the debts incurred by patients because of tuberculosis amounted to $ 120 million (₹ 416 crore).

If we add indirect cost, it is estimated that TB costs India ₹ 12,000 crores annually. Other non-disease cost due

Table 2.4: Pattern of investment in health and family welfare (central budgetary allocations percentage to total outlay)

Sector	*Investment as percentage of total plan investment*									
	IInd plan	*III*	*IV*	*V*	*VI*	*VII*	*VIII*	*IX*	*X*	*XI*
Health	3.01	2.63	2.13	1.93	1.87	1.88	1.75	2.31	2.09	6.50
Family welfare	0.11	0.29	1.76	1.25	1.04	1.81	1.50	1.76	1.83	

	Health expenditure as percentage of GDP												
	1961	*1971*	*1981*	*1986*	*1991*	*1995*	*1996*	*1997*	*1998*	*2000*	*2003*	*2005*	*2009*
Public	0.71	0.84	1.05	1.19	0.92	0.95	0.91	0.88	0.81	0.87	1.00	1.0	1.10
Private	2.25	2.60	4.06	3.61	2.88	3.04	3.07	3.00	3.30	4.76	5.60	4.0	4.13

to tuberculosis are 300,000 school dropouts due to parental TB. The costs to the patient for diagnosis and successful treatment averages US$ 100–150, more than half of the annual income of daily wage labourer.

Thus TB leads to poverty and poverty leads to tuberculosis and it exerts an enormous social and economic toll on India. More than 300,000 children leave school as a result of parental TB. More than 100,000 women are rejected by their families on account of TB. More than 80% of cases are in the economically productive age group (15–54 years), the economic and social costs to them and to their families are enormous.

Cost of Tobacco use

Tobacco is also an economic burden for the government. According to ICMR the cost of treating tobacco related disorders like Chronic, Obstructive Pulmonary Disease (CoPD); Coronary artery disease (CAD) and cancers in 2002–03 was ₹ 308.33 billion, which more than offsets all the benefits accruing in the form of revenue and employment generated (₹ 81.6 billion) by the tobacco industry.

Economic costs of tobacco use, which causes serious diseases was ₹ 104500 crores in 2011 for users aged 35–69 years, which translates into1.16% of the GDP, which is 12% more than the annual budget on health.

Macroeconomic impact of noncommunicable diseases in India accounts for an economic burden in the range of 5–10% of GDP, which affects development. Similarly, disease burden has marked effect at *household* and *family level* in terms of loss of wages and out of pocket expenses of illness (*microeconomics*):

Definition of cost: Economist defines cost as the value of resources used to produce something; including a specific health service or set of services (as in health programme).

Customer want "value for the money" spent on health intervention.

Knowing the cost-effectiveness of a health intervention—the net gain in health (compared with doing nothing) divided by the cost can be extremely useful for both public and private decision.

What is benefit: In economic language "benefits" strictly speaking refers only to "*outcomes*" that can be measured in terms of money. Outcomes are: Products and services (*output*), improved knowledge attitudes and practices (*effects*) and improvement in health status; reduction of morbidity and mortality and fertility, improvement of nutritional status (*impact*). *Effectiveness* or *effects* are outcomes in natural way that are not expressed in financial terms, such as number of lives saved by a health intervention or life years gained as a result of intervention or quality adjusted life years (QALY) gained or number of heart attacks prevented or number of cases due to a disease prevented or births averted.

Classification of Cost by Inputs

Costs are divided into direct and indirect. *Direct costs* are the resources used up in an intervention, such as drugs, hospitalization and transport, etc. *Indirect costs* are the reduction in productive potential because of an intervention, such as value of time used in seeking care (wage loss).

There are two important categories of resources, those that are used up in the course of a year and are usually purchased regularly (i.e. recurrent costs) and those that last longer than one year, such as buildings, vehicles and equipment (i.e. capital cost).

Capital Cost

- *Vehicles:* Bicycles, motorcycles, trucks.
- *Equipments:* Refrigerators, sterilizers, manufacturing machinery, scales and other equipment with a unit price of ₹ 5000 or more.
- *Buildings:* Space, health centres, hospitals, training schools administrative office and storage facilities.
- *Training:* Non-recurrent training activities for health personnel that occur only once or rarely.
- *Social mobilization:* Non-recurrent social mobilization activities, e.g. promotion publicity campaigns, that occur only once or rarely.

Recurrent Cost

- *Personnel (all types):* Supervisors, health workers, administrators, consultants, casual labour.
- *Supplies:* Drugs, vaccines, syringes, small equipment (unit cost less than ₹ 5000).
- *Vehicle operation and maintenance:* Petrol, diesel, lubricants, tyres, spare parts, registration and insurance.
- *Building operation and maintenance:* Electricity, water, heating, fuel, telephone, telex, insurance, cleaning, painting, repairs of electrical supply, appliances, plumbing, roofing, etc.
- Training recurrent (e.g. short in service courses).
- *Social mobilization:* Operation costs.
- Other operating costs not included above.

Costs

Opportunity Cost

Opportunity cost is a central notion in economic analysis. Simplest concept of opportunity cost is—Rupee spent on 'A' is Rupee denied to 'B'. It can be used to explain the consequences of choosing between two alternatives. If we have a choice of two effective treatments, A and B, but we have enough money for one of them. If the treatment A is funded rather than treatment B, the opportunity cost of funding A is the benefits we forgo in not choosing B, the next best alternative use of resources. Consider for example two possible interventions: a cancer screening programme (intervention A) and the next best alternative, a smoking cessation programme (intervention B). Only one of these intervention can be funded within the available budget. The opportunity cost of funding A can be thought of as the number of life years that would have been gained through smoking cessation programme. Opportunity cost reflect the fact that choices have to be made between interventions because of scarcity of resources.

Average Cost

It is the total cost for the intervention divided by the total number of units provided for the treatment, e.g. average cost of OPD treatment at PHC per patient per day.

Incremental Cost

Incremental cost is the difference in cost found between two interventions (i.e. the intervention and its comparator).

Marginal Cost

Marginal cost is an additional cost or extra cost of producing one unit of output or expanding a programme, e.g. additional cost of adding hepatitis B vaccine in universal immunization programme or increasing the length of stay in hospital by one day.

Methods of Economic Evaluation

Economic evaluations always consider benefits as well as costs. There are four main methods of economic evaluations:[2,3]

i Cost minimization analysis (CMA)

ii Cost-effectiveness analysis (CEA)

iii Cost utility analysis (CUA)

iv Cost benefit analysis (CBA)

I. Cost Minimization Analysis (CMA)

CMA compares the costs of different interventions that are assumed to provide equivalent benefits. A good example would be a comparison between a generic drug and a branded equivalent. If the assumption of equal effectiveness is established, the decision hinges on finding the least expensive way of obtaining that health benefit.

Here only the costs are compared and not the benefits. The cheaper intervention will provide the best value for the money, however, it is rare for two health care interventions to provide exactly the same benefits.

II. Cost-effectiveness Analysis (CEA)

Cost effectiveness in health care: The net gain in health or reduction in disease burden from a health intervention in relation to cost. It is measured in dollars per disability adjusted life year.

In cost-effectiveness analysis (CEA), benefits are measured in 'natural' units. For examples, these could be heart attacks avoided, or life years gained (i.e. the number of years by which life is extended as a result of intervention). Quality adjusted life years (QALY) gained is also used which is most comprehensive indicator of CEA.

The results of CEA are usually presented in the form of ratio (e.g. cost per life year gained or lives saved).

$$\text{Cost effective ratio (CER)} = \frac{\text{Cost}}{\text{Number of lives saved}}$$

Effectiveness is an expression of the desired effect of a programme, service or institution or support activity in reducing a health problem or improving the unsatisfactory health situation. Thus effectiveness measures the degree of attainment of predetermined objectives and targets of the programme, service or institution. The assessment of effectiveness is aimed at improving programme formulation or function and structure of health services and institutions through analysis of extent of attainment of their objectives.[3,4]

Population-based services like immunization, nutrition, fertility, tobacco and other drugs, the household and external environments (indoor air pollution safe water and sanitation, vector control) and HIV/AIDS are highly cost-effective. The public health package should include all these components.[5,6]

III. Cost Utility Analysis (CUA)

While cost-effective analysis is useful for health care technologies that impact on a 'single' outcome dimension (e.g. length of life), it is often the case that treatments impact both on quality and quantity of life (i.e. multi-dimensional). Cost utility analysis can be used to compare the costs and benefits of health technologies where this is the case. 'Utility' as used by economist refers to happiness or pleasure.

In CUA, benefits are measured in healthy years, to which a value has been attached. Unlike CEA, CUA is multidimensional and incorporates considerations of quality of life as well as quantity of life using a common unit. The most widely used measure of benefit in CUA is quality adjusted life years (QALY) but other measures include disability adjusted life years (DALYs) and healthy year equivalent.

$$\text{CUA} = \frac{\text{Cost}}{\text{QALY gained or DALYs averted}}$$

The results of cost-effectiveness and cost utility analyses can be expressed by many ways. If the benefits of drug A and drug B are equivalent, then the analysis is CMA and intervention with drug of lowest cost should be chosen. If an intervention is both cheaper and more effective than its comparator, the intervention is said to be dominant and should be chosen. Since it would provide larger benefits at a lower cost than its comparator. However, most commonly an intervention will be found to be more effective but it will also be more costly than the comparator. In order to make a decision on which treatment to select, the incremental cost-effectiveness ratio (ICER) should be calculated.

$$\text{ICER} = \frac{\text{Cost of A} - \text{Cost of B}}{\text{Effectiveness of A} - \text{Effectiveness of B}}$$

IV. Cost Benefit Analysis (CBA)

In CBA, the benefits are measured in monetary terms. The final result is expressed as net monetary gain (or loss) or cost benefit ratio.

$$\text{CBA} = \frac{\text{Cost in monetary terms}}{\text{Benefits in monetary terms}}$$

There are two main methods to measure health gains for CBA: the human capital approach and the willingness to pay approach.

Efficiency

It is output-input ratio or efficiency is an expression of relationships between the results obtained from health programme or activity and the efforts expended in terms of human, financial and other resources, health processes and technology, and time. The assessment of efficiency is aimed at improving implementation.

QALY

Quality adjusted life years (QALY): A quality adjusted life year (QALY) is a common measure of a benefit that combines quantity and quality of life. It is calculated by estimating the total number of life years gained from treatment and weighing each year with a quality of life score (or utility) to reflect the quality of life in that year. For example, a patient living for 10 years, but with quality of life of say, 0.7 on a scale of 0–1 (with 0 as death and 1 as perfect health), would live for seven (0.7 × 10) QALYs.

How the Utility Score is Obtained?

Utility score is a number generally between zero (representing death) and one (perfect health), utilities can be measured by using direct method, such as the "standard gamble" or "Time Trade off". Because these techniques are complex, simple method has been devised to obtain health state utilities. Generic health state questionnaire (e.g. Euroqol) asks respondent a number of simple health related questions and then convert the results into utilities using pre-scaled responses obtained by "standard gamble" or "time trade off" from a relevant reference group.

The standard gamble is a technique widely used in economics. It is based on the idea that something is only of value if we are prepared to give another thing up in order to get it. The respondent is asked to make a trade-off between the certainty of having a chronic disease for a period (t) and a gamble that has two possible alternatives: staying in good health for the same period or death. Finding the point where the respondent is indifferent between being in the chronic condition and the gamble provides us with a value that reflects the quality of life that the respondent attaches to chronic condition.

Time Trade off (TTO) techniques are based on concepts similar to the standard gamble. The respondent is asked how many years of life in a health state with a disease, he or she would be willing to give up to be in full health but for a shorter period. For example, the respondent may be asked if he or she would prefer to live five years in health state, with a specified chronic condition or three years in perfect health. The process goes on until the point, at which the respondent is indifferent between the two health states, is found.

Quality Adjusted Life Years

(Euroqol Group 1990) EQ-5D used multiattribute utility scales.[7] The EQ-5D uses five dimensions—mobility, self-care, usual activities, pain/discomfort and anxiety/depression. Each dimension has three levels of severity, thus enabling the EQ-5D to define 243 (3^5) different health states. Two extra health states, unconscious and dead have been added to have 245 possible health states descriptions to assess quality adjusted life years (QALYs) (Table 2.5).

This is administered in the form of Self Completed Questionnaire. Subjects are asked to define of their own.

Disability Adjusted Life Years (DALYs)

Given a common currency for measuring cost and a unit for measuring health effects, different interventions can be compared by what it costs to achieve additional year of healthy life. Outcomes are measured in the same unit of disability adjusted life years (DALYs) used to estimate disease burden. DALYs is another indicator

Table 2.5: Dimension of Euroqol EQ-5D[8]

Mobility
- I have no problem in walking about
- I have some problem in walking about
- I am confined to bed

Self-care
- I have no problem with self-care
- I have some problems washing or dressing myself
- I am unable to wash or dress myself

Usual activities
(*Examples:* Work, study, housework, family or leisure activities)
- I have no problems with performing my usual activities
- I have some problems with performing my usual activities
- I am unable to perform my usual activities

Pain/discomfort
- I have no pain or discomfort
- I have moderate pain or discomfort
- I have extreme pain or discomfort

Anxiety/depression
- I am not anxious or depressed
- I am moderately anxious or depressed
- I am extremely anxious or depressed

similar to QALYs, developed by World Bank and WHO to quantify the global burden of disease. Like a QALY, it incorporates both quantity and quality of life in a common measure. The main difference is that it measures losses of healthy life rather than life years gained. One DALY can be interpreted as equalling one year of healthy life lost.[4, 7]

DALY is thus a unit used for measuring both the global burden of disease and the effectiveness of health interventions, as indicated by reductions in the disease burden.

REFERENCES

1 Govt. of India (2002). Planning Commission Tenth Five-Year Plan. Govt. of India, New Delhi.

2 World Health Report (2007), WHO; Geneva.

3 http://www.nhs.co.uk. Retrieved on March 10, 2005.

4 WHO (1981) Health Programme Evaluation Guiding Principles for its application in the managerial process for national health development, WHO; Geneva.

5 World Development Report (1993). Investing in Health World Development Indicators. Oxford University Press, Oxford: New York: 1993.

6 Agha Khan Foundation (1993). Primary Health Care Management Advancement Programme. Assessing Information Needs Module 1, Facilitators Guide. Aga Khan Foundation. University Research Corporation Centre for Human Services.

7 WHO, UNICEF AKF (1994). Cost Analysis in Primary Health Care—a training manual for programme managers. WHO; Geneva.

8 Auld CM, Donaldson C, Mitton C, Shackley P. Health economics and public health. In: Detels R, McEwen J, Beaglehole R, Tanaka H (editors). Oxford Textbook of Public Health, 4th edn., New York: Oxford University Press; 2002; 877–902.

E-HEALTH (TELEMEDICINE)–E-GOVERNANCE

a **Establishment of National Medical College Network (NMCN):** Wherein 41 Govt Medical Colleges are being networked in first phase riding over NKN National Knowledge Network—high speed bandwidth connectivity with the purpose of e-Eduction and e-Healthcare delivery. National cum regional resource centre (SGPGI) Lucknow, five regional resource centres at AIMS, New Delhi, PGIMER, Chandigarh JIPMER, Puducherry, NEIGRIHMS, Shilong and KEM, Mumbai shall be networked for Tele-eduction, Tele-CME, Tele Specialist consultation, Tele follow-up and access to digital library.

b Utilization of space technology in Health Sector is being worked out.

c **M-Health for taboacco cessation:** As a part of the WHO 'be healthy be Mobile' initiative it is proposed to reach out to tobacco users who want to quit tobacco use through continuous messages on telephones (SMS).

d **National health portal (NHP)/voice portal:** Launched for providing information related to various issues of health, disease, lifestyle, first aid, directory services, health programmes, etc. through a toll free national number 1800–180—1104 in multiple languages.

e **Mobile apps for NHP:** Application have been developed to access the National Health Portal through mobile phones.

f **Kilkari:** It is an Interactive voice response (IVR) based mobile service that delivers time sensitive mobile messages (voice calls) about pregnancy and child birth directly to mobile phones of pregnant women and mothers of young children and their families.

g **Mobile academy:** It is anytime anywhere audio-training course on interpersonal communication skills that ASHA can access from her mobile phone.

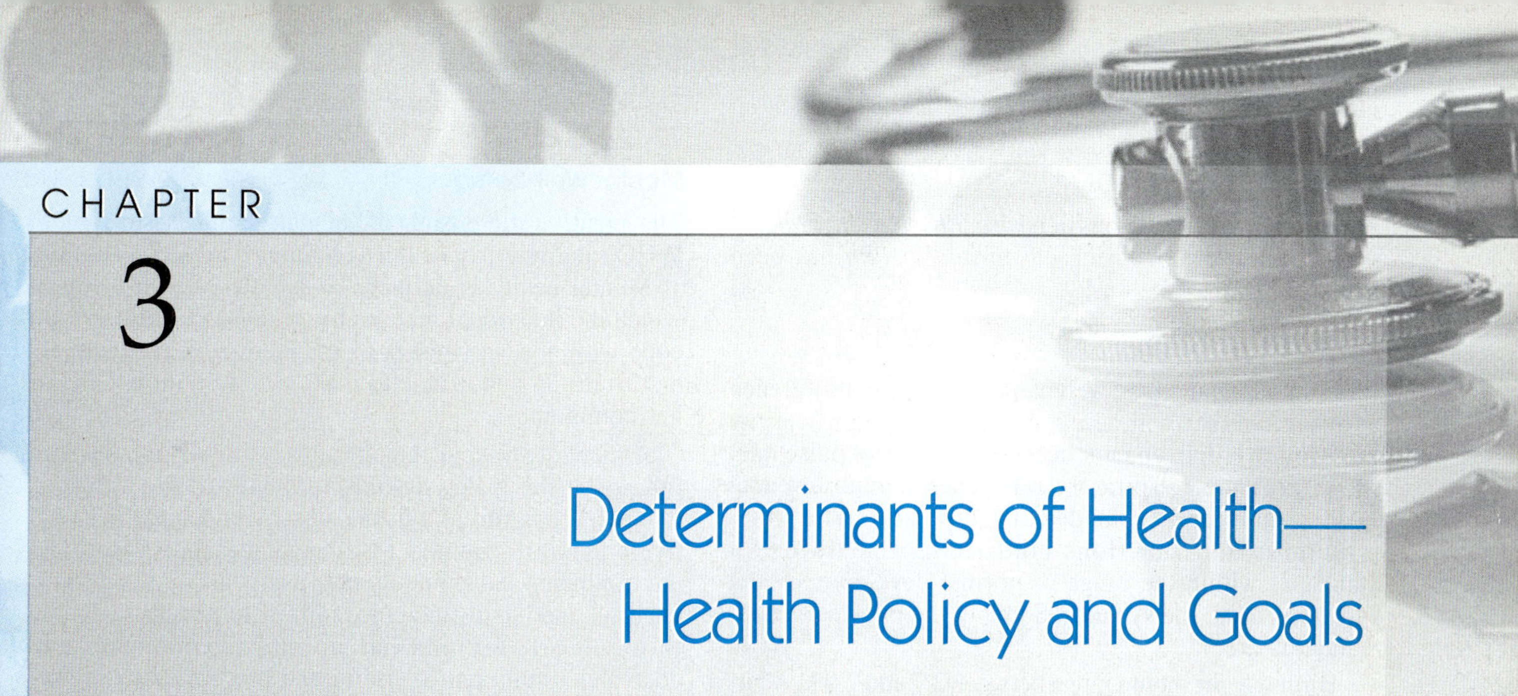

CHAPTER

3

Determinants of Health—Health Policy and Goals

DIMENSIONS AND DETERMINANTS OF HEALTH

"Health should be seen and believed as development function."

Health is difficult to define but easier to understand. To many of us, it may mean absence of disease or infirmity and to many it may mean sound body and sound mind and sound function of the body.

To an anatomist: Healthy body means it should confirm to normal anatomical structures.

To a physiologist: Health means normal body functions.

To a biochemist: It means normal biochemical levels/values.

To a pathologist: It means normal cellular make up.

To a geneticist: It means full realization of genetic potential.

Similarly, to a clinician it means no abnormality in structure and function and usually when a clinician fails to detect anything in a person by his clinical wisdom and laboratory tests he/she labels a person no abnormality detected (NAD).

To a psychiatrist: It means well adjusted and a balanced personality.

Definition

World Health Organization (WHO) has given a comprehensive definition of health which includes important dimensions, such as physical, mental and social health. WHO in its constitution has defined health in the largest sense of the term that states:

"**Health** is a state of complete physical, mental and social well-being and not merely the absence of disease or infirmity." WHO's 199 member states have endorsed this statement.[1] The Executive Board of the World Health Organization (WHO) proposed redefining 'health' as "a dynamic state of complete physical, mental, social and spiritual well-being, and not merely the absence of disease or infirmity" (WHO 1998).

WHO recognizes 'health' as a fundamental human right of an individual, family and community and it sets a most important social goal of attainment of highest possible standard of health by all nations or countries "without distinction of race, religion, political belief, economic or social condition". Realization of this goal requires the action of many other social and economic sectors in addition to health sector. Health is thus a multisectoral subject. Inter- and intra-sectoral coordination is essential to achieve the goal of health for all. In the international conference on primary health care jointly organized by the WHO and UNICEF in Alma Ata, USSR, in September 1978, fundamental principles of health were enunciated and a declaration was made; this declaration endorsed the earlier resolution of 30th World Health Assembly (1977).

"The attainment by all citizens of the world by the year 2000 of a level of health, that will permit them to lead a socially and economically productive life."[2]

This is popularly known as "Health for all" (HFA) and it is to be achieved through primary health care approach, in a spirit of social justice and as a part of overall development. Development of health is to be based on self-determination and self-reliance in health on the part of individual, the community and the nation. Ottawa Charter (1986) further lends support to health promotion by developing personal skills through education, strengthening community action by community participation, reorienting health services in favour of prevention and promotion, building healthy policy and creating supportive environments.

DIMENSIONS OF HEALTH

There are three dimensions of health: *Physical, mental* and *social*. A fourth dimension of *spiritual health* has been added.

Physical Well-being

It means adequate body weight, height and circumference as per age and sex with acceptable level of vision, hearing, locomotion or movements, acceptable levels of pulse rate, blood pressure, respiratory rate, chest circumference, head circumference, and waist hip ratio. The body structures and functions confirming to laid down standards within the range of normal development and functions of all the systems. Some of the physical health standards are:

- Birth weight should range between 2.7 and 2.9 kg "cut-off", level of low birth weight is 2.5 kg.
- Standard growth charts have been evolved to monitor growth of young children.

Body mass index: Normal range is 18.5–25 and waist hip ratio normal range is 0.6–0.9 and triceps skin fold thickness 12–15 mm and sub-scapular skin fold 18–20 mm.

Similarly, ideal weights as per age and height for male and female have been worked out. Reference Indian adult man and woman have been defined.

Reference Indian Adult Man and Woman (NNMB)

Reference man is in age group 18–29 years and weighs 60 kg with a height of 1.73 m with a BMI of 20.3 and is free from disease and physically fit for active work; on each working day, he is engaged in 8 hours of occupation which usually involves moderate activity, while when not at work he spends 8 hours in bed, 4–6 hours in sitting and moving about, 2 hours in walking and in active recreation or household duties.

Reference women is in age group 18–29 years, non-pregnant non-lactating (NPNL) and weighs 55 kg with a height of 1.6 m and a BMI of 21.2, is free from disease and physically fit for active work; on each working day she is engaged in 8 hours of occupation which usually involves moderate activity, while when not at work she spends 8 hours in bed, 4–6 hours in sitting and moving about, 2 hours in walking and in active recreation or household duties.

Reference Body Weight and Height

Reference weights and heights of Indians as under physical health are easier to understand and easier to measure. Periodical health examination and pre-placement health examination determine the level of health of an individual. We want best of physical health standards to be attained by all individuals and we are most particular for recruitment in army for physical standards apart from mental health.

Mental Well-being

The positive dimension of mental health is stressed in WHO's definition of health as contained in its constitution.

Mental health is defined "as a state of well-being in which the individual realizes his or her own abilities, can cope with normal stresses of life, can work productively and fruitfully and is able to make a contribution to his or her community".[3]

A mentally normal person has the ability to mix up with others, he/she makes friendship, behaves in a balanced manner, keeps himself tidy and observes adequate personal hygiene, well oriented to time, place and person and environments and is unduly not suspicious of others, he is cheerful and happy and enjoys life with a purpose and he thinks positively and has normal development and contributes fully and is useful and productive to society and nation. He or she is a balanced person and emotionally stable and realizes his shortcomings and strengths and abilities. People are judged by others. The friend circle or family members are the one's who can endorse the mental health status of an individual first of all.

Mental Ill-health

A person who behaves in a strange manner and people consider his behaviour as abnormal and strange or who stays aloof and is very quiet and does not talk or mix with people and is not interested in his personal hygiene and is a withdrawn person, and who claims to hear and see things which others do not see and hear and who is abnormally suspicious of others (abnormally suspicious and claiming that others are trying to harm him), who is unusually cheerful and boastful without reason and who is unusually sad, sits alone, feeling sad and crying without reason, person having suicidal tendency and the family members feel that a person is being possessed by spirits (Bhoots) and being influenced by evil spirits and a person who is slow in development and has delayed mental development are suspected to be suffering from mental ill-health.

Social Well-being

It is third dimension of health. It means ability of a person to adjust with others in his social life, at home, at work place and with people. Men interact with men and they interrelate and interdepend on each other and play their effective role in accordance with a situation. Essentially social well-being includes harmonius interrelation and interaction of human beings.

Social well-being is a composite function of income level, literacy, occupation and working conditions, marital harmony, institution of family, social groups and cultural and behavioural pattern of the society and stressful situation. Social well-being is conditioned by the influence of environments as well. Social well-being can be measured on a scale by taking into consideration indicators like income, literacy and occupation (as discussed under socioeconomic status of family).

Spiritual Well-being

The WHO at its 37th World Health Assembly has added the spiritual dimension to health. The recognition of this dimension speaks of the importance of multidimensional well-being of swasthya.

Spiritual health has been defined as "That part of the individual which reaches out and strives for meaning and purpose in life. It includes integrity, principles and ethics, the purpose in life, commitment to some higher beings and beliefs in concepts that are not subject to the state-of-the-art explanation."

Positive health: A person who enjoys all the four dimensions of health (physical, mental, social and spiritual) is said to be in a state of positive health. The concept of perfect positive health cannot become a reality because a person can never be in perfect state of all the four dimensions.

Medical Classification—Officers

Health of serving officers is continuously monitored through periodical medical check ups during the entire length of their service. Similarly periodical medical examination of Industrial workers in done regularly.

Medical Classification

Medical classification of serving officers is done by medical board after assessing his fitness under five factors, indicating by the code letter "SHAPE" which represent the following factors.

S Psychological
H Hearing
A Appendages
P Physical capacity
E Eyesight

Medical classification under the system is based on functional capacity of the individual as a whole for military duties. Thus classification done under this system enables the administrative authorities to assign appropriate assignment to officers depending upon their employment capacity. Functional capacity of an officer under each factor is denoted by numerals 1–5 against each code letter, indicating declining functional efficiency. The numerals are written next to the code letter, except that where an officer is in grade 1 in all factors, his categorization may be denoted by writing SHAPE-1 instead of writing S1 H1 A1 P1 E1. General evaluation of numerals is as under:

1 Fit for all duties anywhere.
2 Fit for all duties but may have limitations as to type of duties of employability. Employment restrictions are given separately by the medical board.
3 Excepting for 'S' factor fit for routine or sedentary duties but may have limitations of employability at high altitude (above 2700 mtr), extreme cold area/hilly terrain and for lone assignments for which specific recommendations are given.
4 Temporary unfit for military duties on account of hospitalization/sick leave.
5 Permanent unfit for military duties.

DETERMINANTS OF HEALTH

Health is a development function. Much more health comes through sectors other than health sector, such as water and sanitation (Environments) nutrition, literacy women and child development and lifestyles (behaviours). These are also known as determinants of health. Hence integration of health services with determinants of health (water and sanitation, nutrition, education and literacy, etc.) achieves better health. The National Health Mission adopts a synergistic approach by effective integration of *Health* concerns with determinants of good health, *viz.* of *nutrition*, *sanitation*, hygiene and safe drinking water through district action plan for health.[4]

Environment

This is considered to be the most important determinant and input to health. The environment is defined as "The aggregate of all external conditions and influences affecting the life and development of an organism, human behaviour and society". A composite of physical, economic pressures, culture and education contributes largely to the background to which one's genetic apparatus reacts. Harmonious environment relationship to man contributes to an improved state of health (Fig. 3.1).

Rightly so the national health planners have included in their agenda to control and improve the natural physical environments, e.g. **air**, **water** and **soil**.

Man-made Environment

In man-made environment or artificial environment are included items like **housing**, **transport**, **industries** and **communication**.

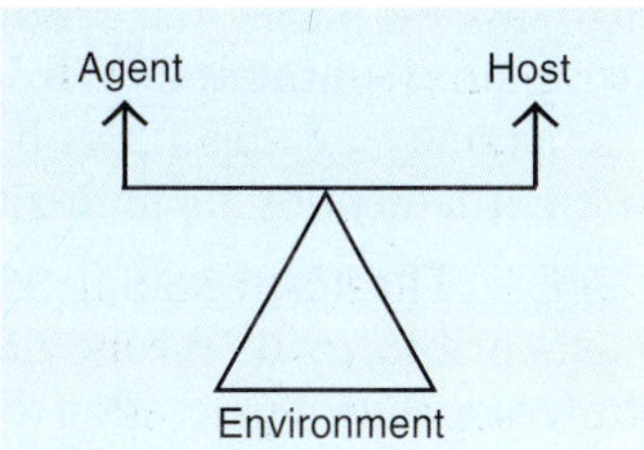

Environment forms the fulcrum in the chain of transmission (epidemiological triad) as shown in the diagram above. There is continuous interaction between agent, host and environment:

3

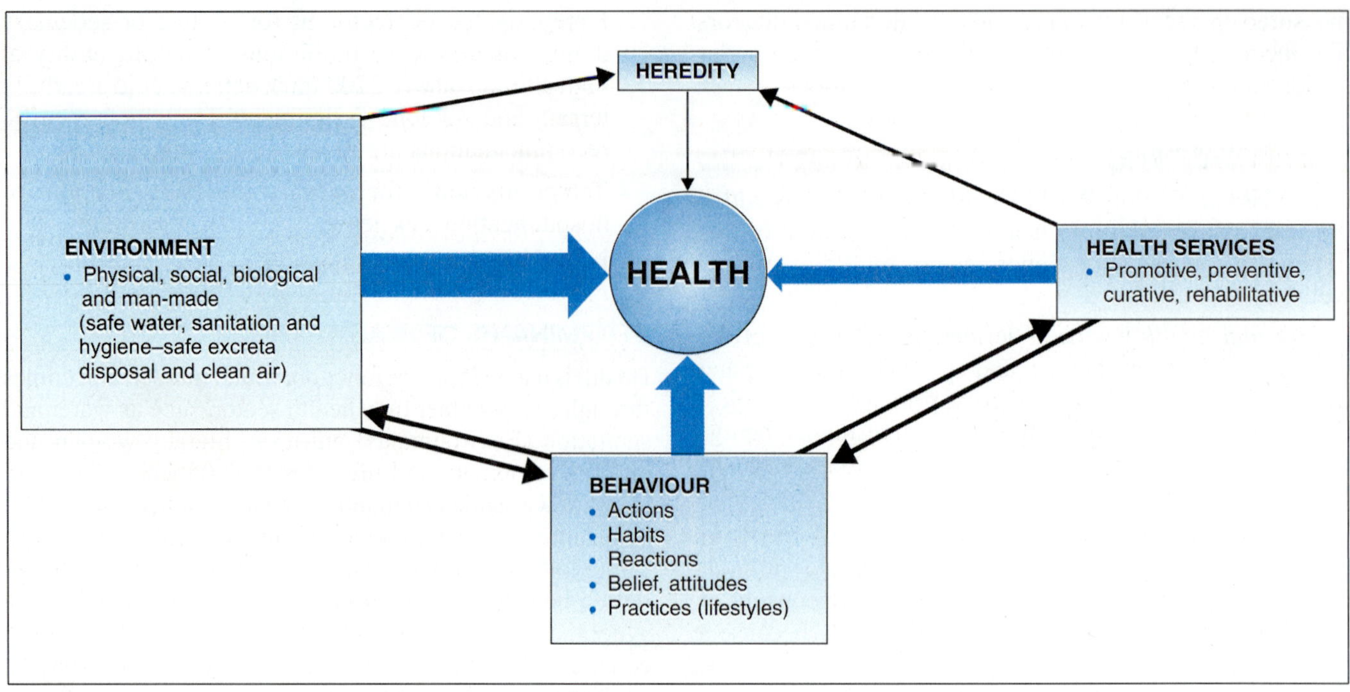

Fig. 3.1: Determinants of health (WHO*)

*The direction of the arrow indicates the direction of impact while the width of the arrow indicates the relative weight or importance of the input to health (WHO).

Agent ⇄ environment ⇄ host. If there is an equilibrium between agent, host and environment, the balance is maintained and the individual, family and community enjoys perfect health. If the environments become favourable for agent (disease producing stimulus/factors/conditions/microorganisms) the balance is tilted, health is disturbed and the result is disease or bad outcome. Treating and modification of environments favourable to human host promotes health and prevents diseases.

Over 80% of diseases are due to bad environments like unsafe water supply, wide spread insanitary conditions due to indiscriminate defecations, poor disposal of waste water, garbage and refuse apart from air pollution leads to wide spread filthy conditions and are perpetual threat to endemic diseases and outbreaks. Mosquitoes and fly breed enormously and pose threat to occurrence of several diseases. Environment is a global concern and all energies are now focused to save the planet (our earth) by improving the deteriorating environments. While talking of environments, community treatment has been successful by handling the environment by three methods:

1 *Socioeconomics:* The term social and economics although susceptible to different definitions are completely interdependent in relation to environment. Economic life is chief determinant of social existence, hence the term socioeconomics. The poor governments do not have enough money and so are the people of that government. *Poverty affects* the health in that productivity is lost due to partial disability. There is vicious circle because *people are poor as they are sick and sick because they are poor.* However, the high economics does not always assure good health. They may purchase things which impair health.

2 *Wealth distribution:* Remunerating jobs, freedom from unemployment provides for improving living standards which in turn can help provide personal and environmental health, these are considered purchasable commodities. Wealth ensures good housing facility, nourishment, clothing, recreation, good use of leisure, and all these contribute to health.

3 *Education:* Besides socioeconomics education is another variate for contribution to health. Educational progress conditions biological, domestic and technical progress. Its positive contribution to economic growth including health is recognized by all. Planning for education is thus considered planning for health and vice versa. "Education for all" and universal elementary education are the thrust areas which will contribute substantially to improved health for all including environments besides **health seeking behaviour.**

The Environment (Protection) Act of 1986 is an Umbrella Act for the *protection of the environment.* Relevant to the water environment, this Act has (among others) the following features:

- Nationwide programme for prevention, control and abatement of environmental pollution.
- Empower any person to enter, inspect, sample and test.
- Establish/recognize environmental laboratories.

- Regulate, close, prohibit industries, processes, and operations.
- Require Government organizations to furnish information, etc.

The Central Pollution Control Board (CPCB) is the national apex body for assessment, monitoring and control of water and air pollution. Well-managed and integrated water and sanitation programmes are crucial to health and development. A clean environment and adequate safe water are essential prerequisites for all children to grow and develop and attain good health. There is now distinct change in the strategy for promoting sanitation by the Government. The Central Rural Sanitation Programme now promotes sanitation as a seven component package: handling of drinking water, disposal of waste water, disposal of human excreta, disposal of garbage and animal excreta, home sanitation and food hygiene, personal hygiene and village sanitation. Investments for ensuring access to safe drinking water will bring the desired health benefits only when complemented by investment in all the seven components of sanitation.

A staggering 60% of Indians defecate in open risking the environments and leaving the excreta to seep through the soil and contaminate the water table and water bodies with pathogens which come back into food chain. This is a key causative factor behind the high prevalence of soil and water-borne diseases in rural India as also in urban slums. According to World Health Organization, 80% of all diseases, such as diarrhoea, cholera, typhoid fever infective hepatitis, vector borne diseases, etc. are caused due to lack of safe water and sanitation.

As per UNICEF 2015 data, only 40% of households have toilets. This percentage is lower in villages where only 28% use toilet (Table 3.1). Total sanitation campaign (TSC) is a sound beginning. Its objective are to bring about improvement in the general quality of life in rural areas, accelerate sanitation coverage and generate demand for toilets in all schools and Anganwadis in rural areas through awareness and education involving PRIs. *Nirmal Gram Puraskar* a National Award under total sanitation campaign has been launched on Feb. 24, 2005 by the Government. Panchayati Raj Institutions (PRIs) can look forward to get cash prizes ranging from 50,000 to 5,00,000 if:[5]

- All households in the village have access to toilets with full usage.
- There is no open defecation.
- All anganwadi centres have access to sanitation facilities.
- There is general cleanliness all around.

Table 3.1: Sanitation coverage year 2015

Country	Improved sanitation coverage (%)		
	Urban	Rural	Total
China	87	64	76
India	63	28	40
Iraq	86	84	86
Pakistan	83	51	64
Sri Lanka	88	97	95
World	**82**	**51**	**68**

Environment Being Compulsory Subject

50 hours compulsory core module course in *Environmental studies*, spread over to six months, at undergraduate level in all streams has been introduced by various universities in view of direction of the Hon'ble Supreme Court of India; with effect from 2004 to 2005. This course will enhance knowledge, skills and attitudes to environment. The syllabus is divided into eight units covering 50 lectures including field work activities of five lecture hours.

Behaviour (Fig. 3.1)

1 It is considered second largest area of determinant/input to one's health and at some places it is even higher than environment. Like most personally held values and beliefs, certain habits are first learnt from family, community and school, all of these play an important role in general behaviour pattern. In terms of satisfactory survival, one's behaviour may not be the most rational and will therefore require modification through effective behaviour change communication (BCC) in most of non communicable diseases.

2 Each society and indeed individual has cultural values, ideologies and interests relating to health and health services. The beliefs inimical to survival indicate need for health promoting changes in cultural pattern. But it may also be determined whether such changes are desirable or even tolerable. Behaviour change communication is to create healthy lifestyles, healthy habits, responsible reproductive behaviour, values of traditional and indigenous foods, safe sex and practice of personal hygiene to promote health and prevent diseases. Proper evaluation of beliefs, social values and motivation should determine the needed changes and in which way the services are to be provided to be acceptable.

3 Attitude change is a major change and may bring about permanent behavioural change (feeding young children, promotion of exclusive breastfeeding, feeding and eating habits—a core cultural variable, adequate diet for physical and mental alertness).

4 Primary values are respected and self-image is not destroyed.

5 Geographical social mobility and dissatisfaction foster change.

6 Attitudes are also related to utilization of services provided. Even for the existing services, the utilization rates are low at 50% or even less for antenatal care, use of iron and folic acid and vitamin A prophylaxis.

7 ***Habits:*** Habits die very hard. In the word 'HABIT' if you remove 'H' ABIT of it is there, if you further

remove 'A' BIT of it is there, if you remove 'B' IT is still there. It means to change habit you have to make lot of efforts.

Health Services

Availability, accessibility, affordability and acceptability of health services are considered an important determinant/ input to health. Health services utilization depends on quality of services offered as also faith and satisfaction derived from services apart from accessibility. Health services include promotive, preventive, curative and rehabilitative services available through various systems. Utilization of health services depends upon health behaviour and socioeconomic conditions (income, literacy and occupation).

Heredity

Genetic inheritance may provide the initial significant contribution to one's state of health, may be modified by environments and specifically by health services. Even before individual's birth, comprehensive health planning will need to include such aspects of health care as prenatal counselling and prenatal care; apart from marriage and genetic counselling.

Ecology of Health: Ecology is defined as mutual relationship between living organisms and their environment. Ecology of health is the study of relationship between variations in man's environments and his state of health.

Social Determinants of Health

These include early year's experiences, education, economic status, employment and decent work, housing and environment and effective systems of preventing and treating ill health. Actions on these determinants, such as—eradicating povery and hunger, ensuring food security, access to safe drinking water and sanitation, employment and decent work and social protection, protecting environments and delivering equitable economic growth will ensure economically productive and healthy society.

How to Achieve Goal of "Health"?

Public Health System Achieves Goal of Health by:

1. **Providing health services** (Promotive, preventive curative and rehabilitation services)
2. **Promoting healthy behaviours** and lifestyles (Eexclusive breastfeeding, handwashing, physical activity and avoid tobacco.
3. **Promoting healthy environments** (Household and external) water supply and sanitation, prevent indoor and outdoor air pollution, accidents and mosquito breeding .
4. **Implementing health legislation** against tobacco use and food adulteration.

Concept of Disease

The WHO has defined health, but not disease because of its variations, e.g. mild, moderate, severe, fatal, and disease without clinical manifestations. Definitions, given by Webster—"A condition in which the body health is impaired, a departure from a state of health, an alteration of human body interfering in performance of vital functions".

Morbidity: Any departure, subjective or objective, from a state of physiological or mental well-being, whether due to diseases, injury or impairment.

CONCEPT OF PUBLIC HEALTH

I. Public Health

- Winslow defined **public health** as "the art and science of preventing diseases, prolonging life, and promoting physical health and efficiency through organized community efforts."

  It means organizing health care systems, resources and infrastructure. Health management (Chapter 15) is an example of public health.
- WHO and Acheson report defined **public health** as, "the science and art of preventing diseases, prolonging life and promoting health through organized efforts of society."
- Focus of public health is total population.

II. Concept of Preventive Medicine

"It is the science and art of preventing diseases, prolonging life and promoting health."

Generally the preventive medicine focuses on individual health or groups, such as high-risk groups and advocates screening of high-risk groups/individuals. The concept can be extended to general population. This term and concept became popular in the United States of America.

In India we adopted the term of "Social and Preventive Medicine" or "Preventive and Social Medicine" and subsequently the term "Community Medicine" has been adopted.

III. Concept of Social Medicine

"Social Medicine is the study of socioeconomic, cultural, environmental and health services and genetic factors and conditions which influence the health of population". This term and concept became popular in United Kingdom during the industrial revolution.

IV. Community Medicine/Community Health

Last JM defined community medicine as "The field concerned with the study of health and disease in the population or a defined community or group. Its goal is to identify the health problems and needs of defined populations (community diagnosis) and to plan, implement and evaluate the extent to which health measures effectively meet these needs".

The Ottawa Charter (1986) is the pivot of principles and practices of health promotion. It recognizes the fundamental conditions and resources for health—peace, shelter, education, food income, a stable ecosystem, sustainable resources, social justice of equity. The Ottawa Charter on health promotion advocates five key strategies:

1 Building healthy public policy
2 Create supportive environments
3 Strengthen community action
4 Develop personal skills
5 Reorient health services.[6]

HEALTH INDICATORS

It is somewhat easier to define health for an individual or person or child or adolescent or youth but to define "community health" is somewhat more difficult. "Community health" parameters are different from health parameters of an individual. Community health can be measured through indicators of economics (gross national product, gross national income and per capita income), life expectancy, under five mortality, infant mortality, literacy level, composite index like human development index, and maternal mortality, etc.[7–9]

The other indicators of community health are environmental indicators, demographic, health services, health care utilization and health policy indicators.

A community is healthy when it enjoys sound health where disease and death rate is acceptably low, it is not threatened with bad environments and its economy is sound and the health practices are sound and based on scientific evidences. Its literacy levels are high and demographically it has balanced sex ratio and people live long, quality of life is good and human development index is high. A village is said to be healthy if it has safe source of improved water supply, safe method of waste water disposal, paved streets, disposal of garbage, refuse and animal excreta by manure pits, people use sanitary latrines, female literacy is high, girls enrolment is universal, deliveries are conducted by trained persons, birth rate and death rate are within acceptable limits, immunization coverage is high, children are well-nourished and housing condition is good.

INDICATORS OF QUALITY OF LIFE

Gross National Income (GNI) Per Capita Current US $ (Atlas Method)

Definition: The gross national income (GNI), formerly referred to as gross national product (GNP) measures the total domestic and foreign value added claimed by the resident producers, at a given period in time, usually a year expressed in current US dollars using World Bank Atlas method.

Limitations of GNI

Growth of GNP does not necessarily "trickle down" to the poor and Governments often struggle to intervene to ensure the distribution of economic progress to the poor but it percolates very slowly.

The GNI is concerned with production which is traded or monetarized, it does not reflect such factors as growing of food for family consumption or the unpaid labour of women or do it yourself building of homes, or local collection and consumption of water or firewood and varieties of activities in home settings in rural and urban areas.

Average income statistics fail to reflect real levels of "social income" provided by such Government financed services as health and education.

Large proportion of GNI does not enter world trade, official exchange rate cannot reflect domestic purchasing power.

Moreover, GNI is an average figure. GNI of India was 1570$ per annum per person in the year 2014.

Gross Domestic Product (GDP) Per Capita

Definition: The average per capita market value of the sum of gross values added of all resident institutional units engaged in production, for a given national economy, at a given period in time, usually a year, expressed in international dollars using purchasing power parity rates.

GDP measures the total output of goods and services for final use occurring within the domestic territory of a given country, it provides an aggregate measure of production. GDP for the year 2011 in India was 3620 $.

HUMAN DEVELOPMENT INDEX

The Human Development Index (HDI) remains an aggregate measure of progress in three dimensions—**health, education** and **income.** But in the HDR Report 2010, the indicators used to measure progress in education and income have been modified, and so is the way they are aggregated. In the knowledge dimension mean years of schooling—the years of schooling that a child can expect to receive given current enrolment rates. Mean years of schooling is estimated more frequently for most of the countries and can discriminate better among countries, while expected years of schooling is consistent with the reframing of this dimension in terms of years. To measure the standard of living, gross national income (GNI) per capita replaces gross domestic product (GDP) per capita. In a globalized world differences are often large between the income of a country's residents and its domestic production. Some of the income residents earn is sent abroad, some residents receive international remittances and some countries receive sizeable aid flows. India moved up from 134th to 130th position in the UNDP, HDI in 2015 because of improved life expectancy and GNI.

Table 3.2: Goalposts for the Human Development Index (HDI) 2010: Dimension-observed maximum, minimum and Indian value

Dimension	*Observed maximum*	*Minimum*	*India*
Life expectancy (years)	83.2 (Japan, 2010)	20	64.4
Mean years of schooling	13.2 (United States, 2000)	0	4.4
Expected years of schooling (years)	20.6 (Australia, 2002)	0	10.3
Combined education index	0.951 (New Zealand, 2010)	0	
Per capita income (PPP$)	108,211 (UAE, 1980)	163 (Zimbabwe, 1980)	3,337 (PPP $, 2008)

Given this framework (UNDP 2010), the sub-indices for the three different dimensions are worked out as follows:

Life expectancy index

$$= \frac{\text{Actual value} - \text{Minimum value}}{\text{Maximum value} - \text{Minimum value}}$$

Mean years of schooling index (a)

$$= \frac{\text{Actual value} - \text{Minimum value}}{\text{Maximum value} - \text{Minimum value}}$$

Expected years of schooling index (b)

$$= \frac{\text{Actual value} - \text{Minimum value}}{\text{Maximum value} - \text{Minimum value}}$$

$$\text{Education index} = \frac{(\sqrt{(a \times b)} - \text{Minimum value})}{\text{Maximum value} - \text{Minimum value}}$$

Income index

$$= \frac{\text{In (Actual value)} - \text{In (Minimum value)}}{\text{In (Maximum value)} - \text{In (Minimum value)}}$$

Human development index

$$= (I_{life}^{1/3} \times I_{education}^{1/3} \times I_{income}^{1/3})$$

The 2010 UNDP HDI entitled the Real Wealth of Nations: Pathways of Human Development focuses specifically on inequalities in human development attainments across countries. To quantify the potential loss because of such inequalities, the report introduces three new indices, viz. Inequality-adjusted Human Development Index (IHDI), Gender Inequality Index and Multi-dimensional Poverty Index.

Estimation of HDI for India

$$\text{Life expectancy index} = \frac{64.4 - 20}{83.2 - 20} = 0.702$$

Mean years of schooling index = (4.4 – 0)/(13.2 – 0) = 0.333

Expected years of schooling index = (10.3 – 0)/(20.6 – 0) = 0.5

Education index = (√(0.333 × 0.5) – 0)/(0.951 – 0) = 0.607

Income index = In (3337) – In (163)/(In (108211) – In (163) = 0.328

Human development index (India) in 2010

$$= (0.702^{1/3} \times 0.607^{1/3} \times 0.328^{1/3}) = 0.519$$

Another report published by the UNDP India office in 2011, after adjusting for inequality, found that the HDI falls by 32% at All-India level. This is more than the global average decline in HDI after adjustment is made for inequality, which is 22%. Among the states, decline is highest for Madhya Pradesh and lowest for Kerala, implying that the inequalities in human development are least in Kerala and highest in Madhya Pradesh followed by Chhattisgarh. Table 3.3 illustrates in the decline in HDI values after adjustment for inequality in different states of India.

In India, the Planning Commission has used a different methodology to estimate the human development and gender development indices at state level for different states, twice in 1996 and 2006 respectively.

This report uses 3 dimensions which measure the dimension of a long and healthy life (measured by infant mortality rate and life expectancy at age 1), education dimension (measured by 7 + Literacy Rate and Mean years of Education for 15 + age group) and a dimension for a decent living standard (measured by Estimated Earned Income per capita per annum).

PHYSICAL QUALITY OF LIFE INDEX

Physical quality of life index (PQLI) is one of the indicators used to measure the level of human development. This index takes into consideration of the following components:

- Infant mortality rate.
- Life expectancy at age one.
- Literacy rate.

For the lowest level of IMR of Kerala of 16 against the 90 of UP or MP, the score for Kerala would be 100 and for UP it would be only 5.6 where zero score is allotted to absolutely defined lowest performance and score of 100 denotes absolutely defined highest performance. After allocating the scores to each component, aggregate score of three components is averaged out. Each component has equal weightage. The PQLI is a composite index and measures social well-being of human development of a defined geographical territory. The PQLI does not include the component of GNP meaning thereby that economic development is not a prerequisite for human development. PQLI is not totally dependent upon economic development.[10,11]

MEASUREMENT OF HEALTH STATUS AND HEALTH INDICATORS

Since morbidity and mortality only relate to sick persons and persons who die. What about those who survive? The objective of nations all over the world is to improve the quality of life (physical, social and mental well-being). Therefore, the population or community health and development is judged through other indicators in addition to morbidity and mortality indicators. The quality of life of survival is judged through some of the following *indicators*, positive and negative both.

Policy Indicators

- Allocation of financial resources for health, e.g. allocation of percentage of budget on health and percentage of GDP spent on health.
- Percentage of public health investment on primary health care, secondary and tertiary health care.
- Policy on social insurance and coverage of most vulnerables and poor people.
- Equitable access to health services and equity in medical education and human resource development.
- Decentralized management of health institutions and delegation of authority to Panchayati Raj Institutions.
- Convergence and intersectoral coordination
- Public-private and NGOs partnership.
- Use of rational drugs and drug policy.
- Population norms for health facility and IPHA.

1. Basic Indicators[10,11]

Under-five mortality (negative indicator). India ranks at 47th place with under-five mortality of 52 (2012).

- Infant mortality rate (negative indicator)
- Neonatal mortality rate
- Gross national income (positive indicator)
- Life expectancy at birth (positive indicator)
- Total adult literacy (positive indicator)
- Net primary school enrolment ratio

2. Nutrition Indicators

- Percentage of infants with low birth weight
- Early initiation of breastfeeding (%)
- Exclusively breastfed up to 6 months (%)
- Introduction of solid, semisolid or soft foods at 6–8 months (%)
- Malnutrition prevalence in under-five (under weight, wasting and stunting).
- Vitamin A supplementation coverage
- Households consuming iodized salt.

Table 3.3: Human Development Index (HDI) and inequality adjusted HDI in Indian States

States	*HDI*	*IHDI*	*Ratio*	*Loss (%)*	*Rank*	*Rank*	*Difference*
Andhra Pradesh	0.485	0.332	0.685	31.55	11	12	–1
Assam	0.474	0.341	0.718	28.17	12	11	1
Bihar	0.447	0.303	0.679	32.06	18	16	2
Chhattisgarh	0.449	0.291	0.649	35.14	17	18	1
Gujarat	0.514	0.363	0.705	29.50	8	7	1
Haryana	0.545	0.375	0.688	31.18	5	6	–1
Himachal Pradesh	0.558	0.403	0.722	27.81	3	3	0
Jharkhand	0.464	0.308	0.663	33.67	15	14	1
Karnataka	0.508	0.353	0.696	30.44	10	9	1
Kerala	0.625	0.520	0.832	16.78	1	1	0
Madhya Pradesh	0.451	0.290	0.643	35.74	16	19	–3
Maharashtra	0.549	0.397	0.722	27.75	4	4	0
Odisha	0.442	0.296	0.669	33.11	19	17	2
Punjab	0.569	0.410	0.720	28.04	2	2	0
Rajasthan	0.468	0.308	0.660	34.02	14	13	1
Tamil Nadu	0.544	0.396	0.727	27.28	6	5	1
Uttar Pradesh	0.468	0.307	0.655	34.47	13	15	–2
Uttarakhand	0.515	0.345	0.670	33.03	7	10	–3
West Bengal	0.509	0.360	0.707	29.30	9	8	1
India	**0.504**	**0.343**	**0.680**	**32.00**			

3. Health Indicators

- Population using improved drinking water source.
- Percentage of population using adequate sanitation facilities.
- Percentage of routine vaccines financed by government.
- Immunization status of pregnant women and infant.
- ORS use rate and ARI management rate at health facility.
- Children sleeping under impregnated bed nets (%).
- Percentage of under-five with fever receiving antimalarial drugs.

4. HIV/AIDS

- Adults (15–49 years) prevalence rates.
- Estimated number of people living with HIV/AIDS.
- HIV prevalence among young people (15–24 years).
- Comprehensive knowledge of HIV (%).
- Women living with HIV (%).

5. Education

- Adult literacy rate
- Primary school gross enrolment ratio
- Net primary school enrolment ratio
- Primary school entrants reaching grade 5
- Secondary school gross enrolment ratio.

6. Demographic Indicators

Population, population annual growth rate, crude birth and death rate, life expectancy, total fertility rate, percentage of urban population, average annual growth rate of urban population (%).

7. Economic Indicators

GNI per capita, GDP per capita average annual growth rate, percentage of central government expenditure allocated to health, education and defence, and percentage of population below $ 1 a day.

8. Women

Life expectancy of female, women literacy, gross enrolment ratio for girls, contraceptive prevalence, antenatal care coverage, skilled attendant at delivery (%) and maternal mortality ratio and lifetime risk of maternal death.

9. Child Protection

Child labour (5–14 years), birth registration, female genital mutilation, and child marriage.

10. Adolescents

Adolescents indicators include—Adolescents as proportion of total population, marrital status, age at first birth, adolescent birth rate (15–19 years), attitudes towards domestic violence, secondary education and comprehensive HIV knowledge.

11. Equity

Equity indicators include Birth registration, skilled attendance at birth, underweight prevalence in children, immunization-measles coverage and use of improved sanitation facilities in poorest and richest 20%.

REFERENCES

1 WHO. Implementation of the global strategy for health for all by the year 2000. 2nd evaluation. Eighth report on World Health Situation 1993; 1: Geneva.

2 NIHFW. Health for All by 2000 AD. Problems, approaches and challenges. Technical Paper. New Delhi: NIHFW; 1983.

3 WHO. Strengthening mental health promotion. Fact Sheet 220. Geneva: WHO; 2001 Nov. 21.

4 National Rural Health Mission (2005–12).

5 UNICEF. The state of the World's children 2015 executive summary

6 WHO (1998 c). Resolution WHA 42.44 on health promotion to the fifty first World Health Assembly. WHO, Geneva.

7 UNICEF. Rights and opportunities. The situation of children and women in India, New Delhi: UNICEF; 1998.

8 UNDP. Human Development Report 2003; New York: UNDP; 2004.

9 UNICEF. 70 years for every child. The State of World Children 2016. A fair Chance for every child.

10 NFI. Bose A. Towards a Humane Development Report. NFI Bulletin 2002 Oct; 23 (4).

11 UNICEF. The State of the World's Children 2004 and 2008 and 2010, and 2016 Regional Office for SEA, New Delhi.

NATIONAL HEALTH POLICY (NHP)-2002

The policy means statement of intentions. National health policy (NHP) was formulated in 1983. The broad objectives of 1983 policy were to provide "Health for all" by the year 2000 AD, through "Universal primary health care". Attempt was made to restructure and reorganize the health care infrastructure to universalize primary health care. It was intended:

- To provide at least one trained birth attendant and one health guide (health volunteer) at village level or per 1000 population.
- One subcentre for 5000 population in plain areas and 3000 in tribal/hilly/difficult areas with one multipurpose health worker female and one MPHW male.
- To set-up one PHC for 30,000 population in plain area and 20,000 in tribal area with 4–6 beds manned by medical officer.

- One community health centre for 1,00,000–1,20,000 population in plain area and 80,000 population in tribal area with 30 beds to be manned by health specialists.
- Establishment of well-worked out referral system.
- Setting-up of speciality and superspeciality services.

There were significant achievements through the years but much remains to be done.

The morbidity and mortality levels in the country are still unacceptably high. The incidence of malaria stabilized at high level in 1990s. Over the years increasing levels of insecticide resistance have developed in the malaria vectors in many parts of the country, while the incidence of the more deadly *P. falciparum* malaria has risen to about 50% in the country as a whole. In respect of TB, the public health scenario has not shown any significant decline in the pool of infection in the community and there has been increasing trend of drug resistance in tuberculosis. A new and extremely virulent communicable disease—HIV/AIDS has emerged on the health scene since the declaration of NHP-1983. The common water-borne infections—gastroenteritis, cholera and hepatitis continue to contribute a high level of morbidity in the population.

"The lifestyle diseases"—diabetes, cancer and cardiovascular diseases burden has increased since 1983. The increase in life expectancy has increased the requirement for geriatric care. Similarly, the increasing burden of trauma cases is also a significant public health problem and micronutrient deficiency diseases are persisting at high level. In view of these developments after 1983 and many other developments, Health Policy has been revised and NHP-2002 has been formulated with the following objectives:

Objectives of NHP-2002

- The main objective of NHP-2002 is to achieve an acceptable standard of good health amongst the general population of the country.
- The central objective would be to ensure equitable access to health services.
- To increase public health investment through substantially increased contribution by Central Government.
- To enhance the participation of private and NGO sector in health services.
- Increased sectoral share of allocation for preventive and curative initiatives at the primary health care level.
- Emphasis will be laid on use of rational drugs within the allopathic system and appropriately supplemented with tried and tested system of traditional medicine.

Approach

The approach would be to increase access to the decentralized public health system by establishing new infrastructure in deficient area and by upgrading the infrastructure in the existing institutions. Goals to be achieved are indicated in Table 3.4.

Table 3.4: Goals to be achieved by 2015

Goal	Year
Eradicate polio and yaws	2005
Eliminate leprosy	2005
Eliminate kala-azar	2010
Eliminate lymphatic filariasis	2015
Achieve zero level growth of HIV/AIDS	2007
Reduce mortality by 50% on account of TB, malaria and other vector and water-borne diseases	2010
Reduce prevalence of blindness to 0.5%	2010
Reduce IMR to 30/1000 and MMR to 100/lakh	2010
Increase utilization of public health facilities from current level of < 20 to > 75%	2010
Establish an integrated system of surveillance, National health accounts and health statistics	2005
Increase health expenditure by Government as a % of GDP from the existing 0.9 to 2.0%	2010
Increase share of central grants to constitute at least 25% of total health spending	2010
Increase state sector health spending from 5.5 to 7% of the budget, and	2005
Further increase to 8% by	2010

FUNDAMENTAL DETERMINANTS WHICH IMPACT ON GOALS OF HEALTH POLICY

Financial Resources

Under the constitutional structure, health is the responsibility of the states. Principal contribution for the funding of public health services will be from the resources of the state. Financial conditions of the state is very poor.

The public health investment in the country over the years has been comparatively low and, as a percentage of GDP, has declined from 1.3% in 1990 to 0.9% in 1999. The aggregate expenditure in the health sector is 5.2% of GDP. Out of this, 17% of the aggregate is public health spending, the balance being out of pocket expenditure (patient have to spend themselves) (Table 3.5). India with higher expenditure on health and low public health expenditure has high under five mortality as compared to countries which have lower total health expenditure but higher proportion of public health expenditure.

Under the policy, it is planned to increase health sector expenditure to 6% of GDP, with 2% of GDP being

Table 3.5: Public health spending in select countries

Indicator	*% population with income of < $1 a day*	*Infant mortality rate/1000*	*% Health expenditure to GDP*	*% public expenditure on health to total health expenditure*
India	44.2	70	5.2	17.3
China	18.5	31	2.7	24.9
Sri Lanka	6.6	16	3	45.4
UK	–	6	5.8	96.9
USA	–	7	13.7	44.1

3

contributed as public health investment by the year 2010. The state government would also need to increase the commitment to the health sector. In the first phase, by 2005 the state would be expected to increase the commitment of their resources to 7% of their budget and in the second phase by 2010 to increase it to 8% of the budget. With the stepping up of the public health investment, the Central Government's contribution would rise to 25% from the existing 15% by 2010.

To meet the objective of reducing various types of inequities and imbalances—inter-regional; across the rural urban divide and between economic classes, the most cost effective method would be increase the sectoral outlay in the primary health sector. Such outlets afford access to vast number of individuals, and also facilitate preventive and early stage curative initiative, which are cost-effective. NHP-2002 sets out increased allocation of 55% of total public health investment for the primary health care sector, 35% of the public health budget will go for the secondary and 10% for tertiary health sectors respectively.

The health policy projects that the increased aggregate outlays for the primary health sector will be utilized for strengthening of existing health facilities and opening additional public health services outlets, consistent with the norms of such facilities.

Further it also recognizes the practical need for levying reasonable user charges for certain secondary and tertiary public health care services for those who can afford to pay.

Equity

While inadequate resource allocation led to suboptimal performance in public health in the country as a whole, there are wide variations or gaps in performance between states, rural and urban areas, rich and poor and men and women. These differentials impact directly on those sections of the society who bear the double burden of poverty and social discrimination (Tables 3.6 and 3.7).

To ensure equity in allocation and to minimize the differentials in health status, the following measures are proposed under the NPP-2002.

- ***Strengthen primary health care:*** Increased public health spending at the grass root level to strengthen primary health care system (SC-PHC-CHC).
- ***Provide for vulnerables:*** Special needs of socially vulnerable sections like scheduled tribes, nomadic communities, and urban slum dwellers. These groups need targeted programmes for improving their health status.
- ***Poor:*** There should be provision for social security for poor and vulnerable sections, who lose their life savings in attending to care and support of their families. NHP-2002 will promote social insurance schemes and encourage states to establish a sickness fund for covering the cost of treatment for families below poverty line on pilot basis and then enlarge it after gaining experience.

Table 3.7: Differentials in health status among socioeconomic groups

Indicator	*Infant mortality/ 1000*	*Under 5 mortality/ 1000*	*% children underweight*
India	**70**	**94.9**	**47**
Social inequity			
Scheduled castes	83	119.3	53.5
Scheduled tribes	84.2	126.6	55.9
Other disadvantaged	76	103.1	47.3
Others	61.8	82.6	41.1

Table 3.6: Differentials in health status among states

Sector	*Population BPL (%)*	*IMR/1000 Live births (1999-SRS)*	*< 5 mortality per 1000 (NHFS II)*	*Weight-for-age— % of children under 3 years (≤ 2SD)*	*MMR/Lakh (annual report 2000)*	*Leprosy cases per 10000 population*	*Malaria +ve cases in year 2000 (in thousands)*
India	26.1	70	94.9	47	408	3.7	2200
Rural	27.09	75	103.7	49.6	–	–	–
Urban	23.62	44	63.1	38.4	–	–	–
Better performing states							
Kerala	12.72	14	18.8	27	87	0.9	5.1
Maharashtra	25.02	48	58.1	50	135	3.1	138
TN	21.12	52	63.3	37	79	4.1	56
Low performing states							
Odisha	47.15	97	104.4	54	498	7.05	483
Bihar	42.60	63	105.1	54	707	11.83	132
Rajasthan	15.28	81	114.9	51	607	0.8	53
UP	31.15	84	122.5	52	707	4.3	99
MP	37.43	90	137.6	55	498	3.83	528

- ***Strengthening of public health delivery system:*** The serious gaps in infrastructure (manpower, supplies equipment, medicines, building, etc.) act as big impediment in delivering health care to people living in rural areas in the country. Increased commitment of resources for primary health care is of prime necessity in strengthening the delivery system. Shortage of doctors in primary health care institutions can be met by organizing a cadre of Licentiates of Medical Practitioners (LMPs) or using doctors of Indian system of medicine. The states can hire doctors on contractual basis to remove deficiency.
- ***Drugs at PHC:*** A big disincentive for people in rural areas to access primary health care is the absence of drugs and other consumables in many of these centres. To set this right, NHP-2002 would commit financial resources from the Central Government for funding of the drug and equipment costs of primary health centres through a simplified procedure.
- ***Flow of funds:*** There are impediments in flow of resources from the Central Governments to programmes operated at the field level like the national disease control programmes. Formation of state and district societies would facilitate direct transfer of funds from Central Government to the operating units at the field level without the usual budgetary constraints. Societies mode helps flow of funds directly to peripheral units and avoids delays.

Role of States

Decentralization

Under constitutional provisions, "States" have the primary responsibility to provide health care to its people. However, the health care delivery system in many states remain largely centralized at the departmental level in spite of the strong and effective presence of institutions of local self-government at village, block and district levels. *Decentralized management* of health institutions especially those at the primary level through Panchayati Raj Institutions (PRIs) and Nagarpalikas is strongly advocated in NHP-2002. Flow of central funds to states for public health programmes should be effectively linked to performance of the states in the area of decentralization of programme management to the PRIs.

Decentralization of programme management should also be reinforced by convergence of all vertical public health programmes at the district level and below. This would avoid duplication of efforts in areas like IEC, training and supervision, etc.

Convergence

The health care functionaries at the field level now operate under various departmental authorities with control at the state level. There is need to bring in convergence in their work, though it may not be possible to bring them under one administrative umbrella. Personnel like Anganwadi workers, ANMs, male health workers, link volunteers, etc. can be brought on a common platform for effective delivery of health care at the primary care level.

School Health

States should also accord priority to school health programmes aiming at preventive health education, regular health check ups and promotion of health seeking behaviour among school children. Investment of resources in school health programmes would have a long-term impact on the general health status of the people and may reduce the requirement of public health spending substantially.

Intersectoral Coordination

The states should also try to bring in effective linkages with other social sectors like education, water supply, sanitation, and nutrition which are also contributory factors to improving the general health status of the community. Convergence of socially relevant programmes in these sectors with the health sector would bring in greater effectiveness in implementation.

Private Sector

The states should actively involve private sector in public health programmes. Medical practitioners in the private sectors can be effective implementers of national programmes for reduction/control of communicable diseases, spreading awareness of non-communicable diseases and promote healthy lifestyles among the people. NGOs and community-based organizations should find an increasingly important role in the public health programmes for social mobilization through health education campaigns.

Private sector is the dominant provider of health care services with a substantial share of 80% in outpatient treatment and 55% in inpatient care. But due to absence of regulatory mechanism, the quality of services is variable and there is lack of accountability among the private sector health care providers. NHP-2002 envisages strong and effective regulatory mechanism for private sector health care institutions and diagnostic facilities by enactment of a statute. The law will spell out the minimum statutory requirement for setting up a health care institution and establish qualitative standards to bring in accountability. With this effective control, the tertiary care can largely be left to private sector. With proper financial incentives, the private sector can be helped in channelising the resources to priority areas of clinical care and management at the tertiary level.

Human Resource Development

As in other areas, there is serious imbalance in availability of qualified medical practitioners, nursing and paramedical personnel across the country. NHP-2002 envisages financial support to *under-served* states in the country for providing medical education through establishment of medical/dental colleges, nursing colleges and other health care institutions. The Central Government should be able to provide adequate resources to these states for promoting centres of medical education.

Need for specialists in public health and family medicine: The present education system is heavily accented towards clinical care at the expense of public health.

NHP-2002 will try to give primacy to public health in medical education. Adequate incentives will be provided for young medical aspirants to choose public health as carrier. The policy envisages the progressive implementation of mandatory norms to raise the proportion of postgraduate seats in these disciplines in medical training institutions, to reach a stage wherein 1/4th of the seats are ear marked for these disciplines. Public health needs qualified *managers* and not merely *clinicians.*

Urban Health

The NHP-2002 envisages setting up of an organized urban primary health care structure. The structure conceived under NHP-2002 is a two-tiered one: the primary centre is seen as the first tier, covering a population of one lakh, with a dispensary providing an OPD facility and essential drugs, to enable access to all national health programmes; and a second tier of urban health organization at the level of the government general hospital, where referral is made from the primary centre. The funding for the urban primary health system will be jointly borne by the local self-government institutions and the state and central government. The policy also envisages the establishment of fully equipped "hub-spoke" trauma care networks in large urban areas to reduce accident mortality.

Use of Generic Drugs and Vaccines

The policy emphasizes the need for basing treatment regimens, in both public and private domain, on a limited number of essential drugs of "generic nature". In public health system, this would be enforced by prohibiting the use of proprietary drugs except in special circumstances. The list of essential drugs would no doubt have to be reviewed periodically. To encourage the use of only essential drugs in the private sector, the imposition of fiscal disincentives would be resorted to. The sale of irrational combinations of drugs would be prohibited through drug standard statute.

Uninterrupted supply of vaccines will be ensured at an affordable price for universal immunization.

Women's Health

NHP-2002 envisages the identification of specific programmes targeted at women's health. The policy commits the highest priority of the central government to the funding of the identified programmes related to women's health. Also the policy recognizes the need to review the staffing norms of the public health administration to meet the specific requirements of women in more comprehensive manner.

Mental Health

NHP-2002 envisages a network of decentralized mental health services for ameliorating the more common categories of disorders. The programme outline for such diseases would involve the diagnosis of common disorders, and the prescription of common therapeutic drugs by general duty medical staff, and upgrading physical infrastructure of mental health institutions at central government expense so as to secure the human rights.

Research

There would be adequate investment in areas like biotechnology, genomic-based drug development, molecular biology, etc. Research in vaccines and therapeutic drugs for important diseases like HIV/AIDS, cancer, multi-drug resistant TB would be actively promoted by the government. The Indian Council of Medical Research would play increasing vital role in promoting biomedical research and transfer of technology to the manufacturing sector. The country should also develop technical competence in the area of patent regimens and in filing product patents for interventions.

Disease Surveillance and Response

Even though vast sums of money have been spent on control of communicable diseases, they continue to take their toll through outbreaks in various parts of the country. In most of the cases, lives could be saved if the response was to be quick and effective. In the absence of proper surveillance and reporting system, valuable lives are lost in outbreaks of even curable diseases like malaria, JE, and cholera. The surveillance systems of polio and HIV/AIDS have demonstrated that the centre and the states can build an effective response to control diseases by getting critical and timely information. NHP-2002 would strive to build an integrated disease surveillance system for the entire country initially for communicable diseases which will later be expanded to include non-communicable diseases also. An effective networking of public health laboratories with health care institutions to provide results of samples is an important component of an effective surveillance system.

In addition, development of a proper management information system would lead to establishment of reliable national health accounts which will be one of the priority of NHP-2002.

Information Education and Communication

Public health programmes need strong visibility. In a country with around 35% illiterate population, effective communication on public health-related issues is a big challenge. The NHP-2002 would strive to develop a national IEC strategy for health communication, health education programmes, specially tailor-made to rural and illiterate populace. All the national health programmes should have a very strong component of IEC which should be implemented not only through Government media but also through NGO and community-based organization. Promotion of healthy lifestyles is incumbent upon provision of health messages targeted at different groups like women, students, youth, and migrant workers.

Population Stabilization

The population policy 2000 sets certain sociodemographic goals for 2010, which are also relevant to the National Health Policy in 2002. Prevention and control of communicable diseases, containing the spread of HIV/AIDS, universal immunization, addressing the unmet needs for basic reproductive and other health services, supplies and infrastructure are goals which run like a common thread in both the policies. The objective of NHP-2002 is to achieve acceptable standard of good health among the general population of the country can be attained through these sociodemographic goals set in the population policy. Improving the general health status of the populace in our country will itself be a contributory factor for population stabilization.

The health needs of the country are enormous and financial resources and managerial capacity fall short. In this situation, NHP-2002 has had to make hard choices between various priorities and options. NHP-2002 does not claim to be a road map for meeting all the health needs of the population of the country. Broadly speaking the NHP-2002 focuses on enhanced funding and organizational restructuring of the national public health initiatives to increase equitable access to health facilities. Policy focuses on those diseases which contribute to high disease burden; TB, malaria, and blindness and HIV/AIDS.

Government and private sector programme planners will have to design separate schemes for the needs of women, children, geriatrics, tribals and other socio-economically under-served sections. An adequate disaster management plan has to be in place to effectively cope up with situation arising from natural and man made calamities.

NHP gives primacy to "equity" as also to primary health care and provisioning of *essential drugs* at the level of PHC through central government funding.

The policy broadly envisages a greater contribution from the central budget for the delivery of public health services at the state level.

National Health Policy 2015 (Draft)

Goal: To attain the highest possible level of good health—"Health in all" as complement to "Health for All".

Objectives

i. To improve population health status
ii. To achieve significant reduction in out of pocket expenditure (OOP).
iii. To assure universal availability of free comprehensive primary health care as an entitlement.
iv. Universal access to free essential drugs, diagnostics and emergency services
v. Affordable secondary and tertiary health care services
vi. Influence growth of private health care industry.

Policy Directions

Increase public health expenditure to the level of 2.5% of GDP. Major source of financing would remain general taxation.

The seven key policy shifts

1. From **selective Primary Health Care** to comprehensive Primary Health care that has continuity with higher levels, i.e. secondary and tertiary care.
2. **In Secondary and Tertiary Care:** From an input oriented budget line financing to output/outcomes based strategic purchasing care from public/private hospitals.
3. **In Public Hospitals:** From users fees and cost recovery to assured free drugs, diagnostics and emergency services to all.
4. **Infrastructure and Human Resource Development:** From normative approach to targeted approaches to reach under-served areas.
5. **Urban Health:** From token under-financed services to assured interventions that reach the urban poor and establish linkages with national health programmes.
6. **In National Health Programmes:** Integration with Health Systems for effectiveness.
7. **In AYUSH:** From stand alone AYUSH to three dimensional mainstreaming. (Co-location of AYUSH, availability of standard medicines and protocols and Yoga.

Seven Key Priority Areas

- Swachh Bharat Abhiyan—Reduction of water and vector borne diseases
- Balanced and healthy diet—To reduce malnutrition
- Addressing tobacco, alcohol and substance abuse
- Rail and road traffic accidents and injuries
- Action against gender violence and sex discrimination
- Safety at work pace
- Reducing indoor and outdoor air pollution.

REFERENCES

1. Ministry of health and family welfare December 2014, National Health Policy 2015 (Draft).

3

CHAPTER

4

Population Stabilization and Declining Child Sex Ratio

"Greatest asset of nation is its people."

DEMOGRAPHY OF INDIA AND POPULATION PROBLEM—CENSUS 2011

India is a country of striking demographic diversity. Substantial differences are visible between states in achievement of basic demographic indices. The five states Bihar, MP, Odisha, Rajasthan, and UP that currently constitute nearly 44 percent of total population of India, are projected to comprise 48 percent of total population by 2016. In other words, these states alone will contribute an estimated 55 percent increase in population during the period 1996–2016 and beyond. Demographic outcome in these states will determine the timing and size of population at which India achieves population stabilization at "low birth rate–low death rate" from current intermediate transition stage of "high birth rate–low death rate" by repositioning family planning programme.

Population stabilization is to be achieved by implementation of reproductive and child health strategies universally with focus on increasing female literacy and status of women, decreasing infant and maternal mortality, improved health, nutrition, livelihood and ecological security for shared decision-making by couples.

Demography is defined as composition and distribution of human population and changes in its size and composition over different time-periods. Population increases/decreases because of births, deaths and migration.

Population Census

"Population **Census** is the total process of collecting, compiling, analyzing or otherwise disseminating demographic, economic and social data pertaining, at a specific time, of all persons in a country or a **well-defined** part of a country". Census is conducted once in ten years in India.

Current world population crossed the mark of 7.3 billion (2015) and is expected to rise to 8.9 billion by 2050, according to UN estimates. China, India and the United States are projected to remain three most populous countries for the next three centuries. China followed controversial policy of one child norm to reduce the population growth rate to 0.6%.

SIZE OF POPULATION AS PER CENSUS—2011

With 2.4% of geographic land area, India has to support 17.5% of world population. It took several thousands years (5000 given here for the sake of convenience) before our population reached 500 million in 1966. India took 64 years to achieve first doubling from 238 (1901) million to 474 million in the year 1964.[1] The second doubling took only 34 years. Within a span of 34 years, the population got doubled and reached to the mark of 1000 million in May, 2000. As per census 2011 India is now home to 1210 million people[2] (Fig. 4.1). This phenomenon in the history of demography in India has been described as "population explosion". During the first phase 1901 to 1921, the increase was very little as birth rate and death rate were

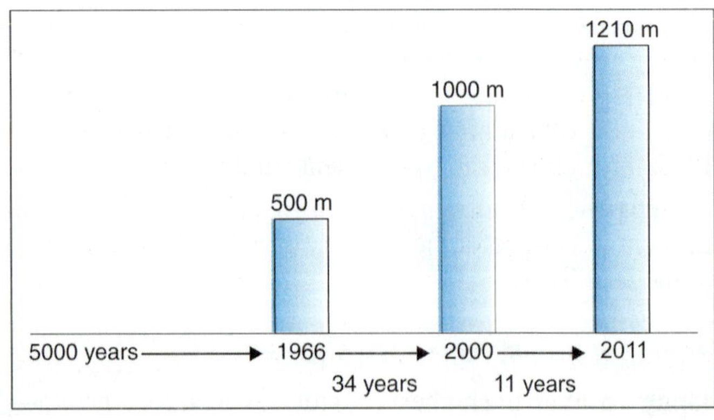

Fig. 4.1: Population explosion

very high and almost equal at 48 and 47 and increase was only one per 1000 per year. During the second phase of demographic transition from 1921 to 1951, the increase was slow and steady and India reached to the mark of 361 million as a result of decline in death rates. During the third phase of demographic transition 1951–2001, there was rapid growth of population in India and within a span of 50 years we increased almost three times. During this phase, there was steep decline in death rates and fertility rates also declined but at a slow pace (Figs 4.2 and 4.3).

Problem—Population Size

India is a country of diversity with 29 States and 7 Union Territories and 671 districts varying in language, social customs and traditions. There are regions in the country with health profile comparable to developed countries and there are others that are way behind.

In India, population size is the key issue and major significant problem. It is the single most important problem in the country. India way back, in 1951 recognized the interrelationship between population and socioeconomic

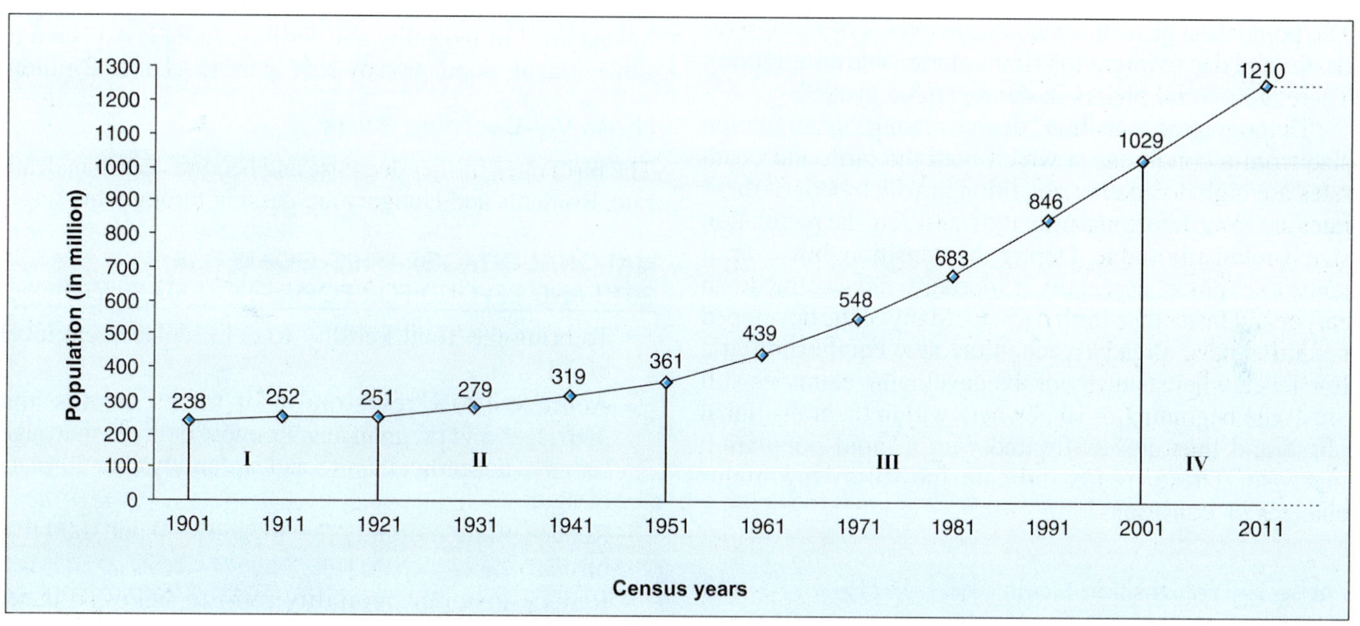

Fig. 4.2: Population growth and phases of demographic transition in India

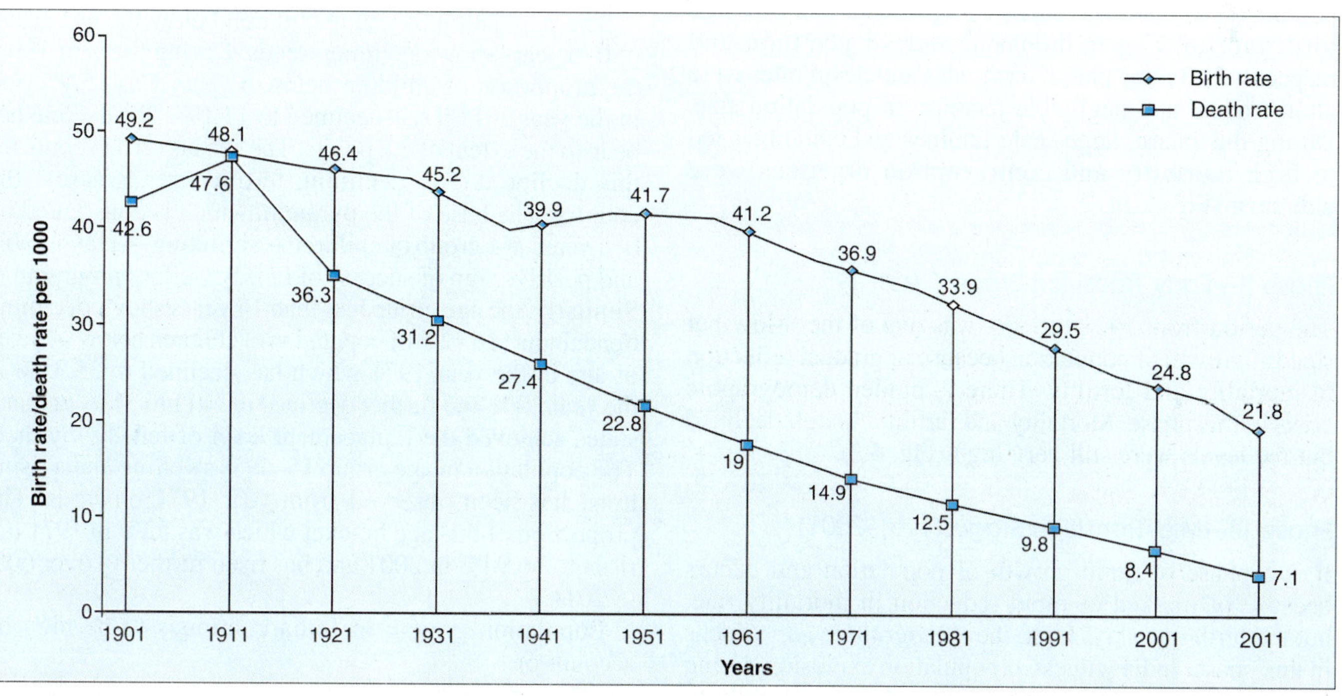

Fig. 4.3: Demographic transition in India

development. Thus, the integration of population policies into the development process is now being increasingly recognized for "human resource development". Population neutralizes all the developments and because of these reasons, India was the first country in the world to launch official programme of National Family Planning Programme (NFPP) in the year 1951 to reduce birth rate and to stabilize the population at a level consistent with the requirement of national economy.

DEMOGRAPHIC TRANSITION

The population growth occurs due to excess of births over deaths and due to migration (immigration and emigration). There are several phases in demographic cycle.

"Demographic transition" denotes change in population size from a condition, in which both the birth and death rates are high, to another condition in which both of these rates are low. Before and after the transition, the population size is relatively stable. During the transition, however, it tends to explode, especially if mortality rates come down earlier and faster than birth rates do. Many of the developed countries have already reached the new equilibrium at a low level, whereas many of the developing countries still are at the beginning or somewhere within the transitional phase and thus are confronted with a rapid population increase. These trends indicate the following major changes or transitions.

Phase I—Pretransition Stage (1901-1921)

The year 1921 is considered as "great divide" in the demographic history of India.[1] During 1911–1921, the population of India was *stable* at high death rate and high birth rate of 47 per thousand and 48 per thousand respectively. In this phase, birth rates and death rates were almost equal and negligible increase in population size. During this phase, large scale famines and epidemics led to high mortality and contraception practices were unknown (Fig. 4.2).

Phase II—Early Transition Stage (1921-1951)

The period from 1921 to 1951 was one of the "slow but steady" growth of population because of gradual reduction in mortality and fertility. There is hidden demographic crisis in this phase. Mortality and fertility though declined but the levels were still very high (Fig. 4.2).

Phase III—Mid-Transition Stage (1951-2001)

It is a phase of rapid growth of population and occurs because of marked or rapid reduction in mortality rate, but the birth rate stays high, the *demographic gap* widens in this phase. India witnessed population explosion during this phase and continues to be in this phase—"High birth rate and low death rate" (Figs 4.2 and 4.3).

Phase IV—Late Transition Stage (2001-2021)

Mortality or death rate further falls and comes to minimal level because of development, birth rates also declines and *demographic gap* is somewhat narrowed and population grows at slow speed. India is likely to reach this stage by 2021 when replacement level of fertility is achieved.[3] Twenty-three states/UTs in India have already achieved the replacement level of fertility.

Phase V—Post-transition Stage

The "birth rates and death rates are low"– at optimal level and are nearly equal and the population becomes *stable* at lowest level of mortality and fertility. India is expected to achieve stable population by 2056 at the level of 1.62 billion.

Phase VI—Declining Phase

The birth rates further decrease and become less than death rate. Romania and Hungary are passing through this stage.

NATIONAL DEMOGRAPHIC GOALS FOR 2010 AND BEYOND FOR POPULATION STABILIZATION

- To bring the Total Fertility Rate to replacement level of 2.1.
- Achieve 100% registration of births, deaths and marriages and pregnancies. Promote delayed marriage for girls, not earlier than 18 and preferably after 20 years of age.
- Reduce infant mortality rate to below 30 per 1000 live births.
- Reduce maternal mortality ratio to below 100 per 100,000 live births.
- Achieve population stabilization by 2045.

The population of young children below the age group of 0–6 years show declining trends. During the year 1991, the proportion of children below 6 years was 15.9% and in the year 2011 it has declined to 13.1%. The decline has been to the extent of 2.8 points. The census (2011) confirms this decline due to declining fertility trends across the country. The base of the pyramid, which is constituted by 0–4 years age group of children is shrinking—a favourable and positive sign of success of family welfare programme. Similarly, the age group less than 14 years shows declining trend; India had 42% of population of children below 14 years of age in the year 1971 which has declined to 35.35% in the year 2001 and further declined in 2011 to 31%, as many states achieved the replacement level of fertility by then. The population in age group 15–59 is swelling and a rising trend has been observed from year 1971 onwards. The proportion of this age bracket which was 52% in 1971 has risen to 56.94% in 2001 and has risen further to over 60% in 2011.

Population growth in India continues to be high on account of:

- The large size of the population in the reproductive age group is mainly responsible for population growth (estimated contribution 58%). An addition of 417.2 million in years 1991–2016 is anticipated despite substantial reduction in family size in several states including those, which have already achieved replacement level of TFR. This momentum of increase in population will continue for some more years because high TFR in the past have resulted in a large proportion of population being currently in their reproductive years. It is imperative that the reproductive age group adopts without further delay or exception the "small family" norm for the reason that about 45% of population increase is contributed by births above two children per family.

- Higher fertility due to unmet needs for contraception (estimated contribution 20%).
- High wanted fertility due to high infant mortality rate (estimated contribution 20%).

Our population has increased from 230 million in 1901 to 1210 million in 2011 and has crossed 1274 million in July 2015. It is now growing by 18 million each year and likely to reach 1339 million by 2021. We have to ensure food supply, water and other amenities for this massive population.

Stabilization of Population

Stable population: A population that has been growing at a constant rate over a number of years.

Stationary population: A population with no migration and for which crude birth rate is equal to crude death rate.

Zero population growth: Absence of growth in the population.

India launched the world's first national Family Planning Programme in 1952 for reducing birth rates "to stabilize the population at a level consistent with the requirement of national economy". The programme has been respositioned to not only achieve population stabilization but also to promote reproductive health and reduce maternal, infant and child mortality and morbidity.

Stabilizing population is essential requirement for promoting sustainable development with more equitable distribution. The vast number of people in India can be greatest asset if they are provided with means to lead healthy and economically productive lives. Population stabilization is a multisectoral endeavour requiring constant and effective dialogue among a diversity of stakeholders and coordination at all levels of the government and society. Spread of education and literacy, availability of affordable reproductive and child health services, convergence of service delivery at village level, participation of women in paid work force, together with steady, equitable improvement in family income will facilitate early achievement of sociodemographic goals and population stabilization.

National population policy (NPP) provides framework for achieving goals to meet the reproductive and child health needs of the people of India.

The total fertility in the country stands at 2.3 as against the expected level of 2.1. The current projection shows that we are likely to reach a replacement level of fertility by the year 2021 and stabilization of population by 2056 at the level of 1620 million with the present growth rate.

Distribution of Population

Uttar Pradesh is most populous state in the country, followed by Maharashtra, Bihar, West Bengal and Andhra Pradesh (Table 4.1).

Table 4.1: Distribution of population of major states in India, 2011

States	*Population in million*	*State*	*Population in million*
Andhra Pradesh	84.6	Karnataka	61.1
Assam	31.1	Kerala	33.3
		Madhya Pradesh	72.5
Bihar	103.8	Maharashtra	112.3
Chandigarh	10.5	Delhi	16.7
Chhattisgarh	25.5	Odisha	41.9
Gujarat	60.3	Punjab	27.7
Haryana	25.3	Rajasthan	68.6
		Tamil Nadu	72.1
Himachal Pradesh	6.8	UP	199.5
J & K	12.5	Uttarakhand	10.1
Jharkhand	32.9	West Bengal	91.3
India			**1210**

URBAN RURAL DISTRIBUTION (Table 4.2)

Nearly 31% of population of the country is urban and the remaining 69% is rural population. According to this distribution, it is evident that majority of India's population lives in rural areas spread over to 550,000 villages and many of these villages are difficult to access. Priority of allocation of resources including health must focus on rural areas to have adequate demographic impact. As per

Table 4.2: Trends in urban population in India, 1901–2011

Year	*Percentage of urban population to total population*
1901	10.84
1911	10.29
1921	11.18
1931	11.99
1941	13.86
1951	17.29
1961	17.97
1971	19.91
1981	23.33
1991	25.71
2001	27.8
2011	31.16

demographic norms, 69% of resources must flow to rural areas. Present scenario indicates that much more resources are concentrated in urban areas and quality of life is better in urban areas as most facilities are located in urban areas. The development indicators, fertility indicators, morbidity and mortality indicators are much better in urban areas than rural areas. The pace of urbanization in India is one of the lowest in the world. The urban population is growing in India at a slow pace and it is leading to unplanned urban growth resulting into urban slum areas with deplorable conditions. The plight of urban slum dweller may be worse than rural area. Statistic of urban slum may be statistic of shame in most slums. Urban poor people living in slum areas need to have organized services including health services. Though multiple health agencies work and are available in urban areas, yet the poorer are deprived of these facilities because of poverty and ignorance. Demographically, urban slums are deprived areas.

AGE AND SEX COMPOSITION (Table 4.3)

The large size of the population in the reproductive age group—15–49 years (married females), which counts to over 205 million eligible couples responsible for population growth and 56% of them are currently effectively protected by contraceptives. Urgent steps are required to make contraception more widely available, accessible and affordable in rural and urban areas. The age pyramid reveals a story of high fertility and high mortality in younger age groups. The population above the age of 60 will rise to higher proportion to demand the geriatric services (services for the aged). India has to gear up itself to provide resources for the services of aged people. The demographic trend will determine epidemiological trend of chronic diseases and burden of disease due to non-communicable diseases (Table 4.3).

Table 4.3: Population by age and sex (census 2011) (% to total population)

Age	India	Male	Female
0–4	9.58	4.84	4.74
5–9	10.48	5.47	5.01
10–14	10.96	5.73	5.23
15–19	9.95	5.28	4.67
20–24	9.20	4.75	4.45
25–29	8.37	4.24	4.13
30–34	7.31	3.68	3.63
35–39	7.03	3.54	3.49
40–44	5.98	3.10	2.88
45–49	5.14	2.65	2.49
50–54	3.95	2.09	1.86
55–59	3.23	1.60	1.63
60–64	3.11	1.54	1.57
65–69	2.18	1.06	1.12
70–74	1.58	0.79	0.79
75–79	0.76	0.37	0.39
80+	0.93	0.43	0.50
Age not recorded	0.36	0.19	0.17
Total percent	**100.0**	**51.35**	**48.75**

Population Pyramid of India

It has broad-based pyramidal population: with broad base at the bottom and tapering towards the top, indicating the effect of mortality in successive age groups. Nearly 31% of population is composed of children, below 14 years of age (Census 2011). The young structure of the population highlights the phenomenon of continued population growth in the country.

Thus, the dominant character of India's age and sex pyramid is high fertility rate, high mortality in younger age and females in reproductive age group and high dependency ratio in addition to growing proportion of people above 60 years of age (Fig. 4.4).

The age distribution of the population of India is projected to change by 2016 and these changes should determine allocation of resources in policy interventions. The population below 14 years of age (currently 31%) is projected to decline to 28% by 2016. The population in the age group 15–59 (currently 60%) is projected to increase to nearly 64% by 2016. The age group 60+ years is projected to increase from current level of 8.5% to nearly 9% by 2016. Thus, India will face the burden of chronic diseases and epidemic of non-communicable diseases due to increase in population of aged as a result of increased life expectancy. The pyramid would change its shape and a bulge will appear in its middle to signify enormous number of people in age group 15–59 to participate in reproduction pool.

Still the young age structure of the population holds the potential for the rapid population growth in the future unless special measures for more accelerated reduction in fertility are undertaken. These young children would add to the population of eligible couples in reproductive age group.

The demographic transition in India will lead onto "epidemiologic transition" that is a long-term shift in mortality and disease patterns whereby large scale epidemics of infectious and parasitic diseases disappear and come under control and India will face the epidemic of degenerative and man-made diseases, due to lifestyle changes, air pollution and accidents. The disease pattern and mortality pattern in India by 2050 will change drastically and non-communicable diseases will take over, people will live longer and problem of management of elderly people will come to the fore.

Demographic dividend: Over 65% of India's Population is below 35 years of age. To harness the potentials of this segment for development is a challenging task. This in real sense is a demographic dividend for India's all round development.

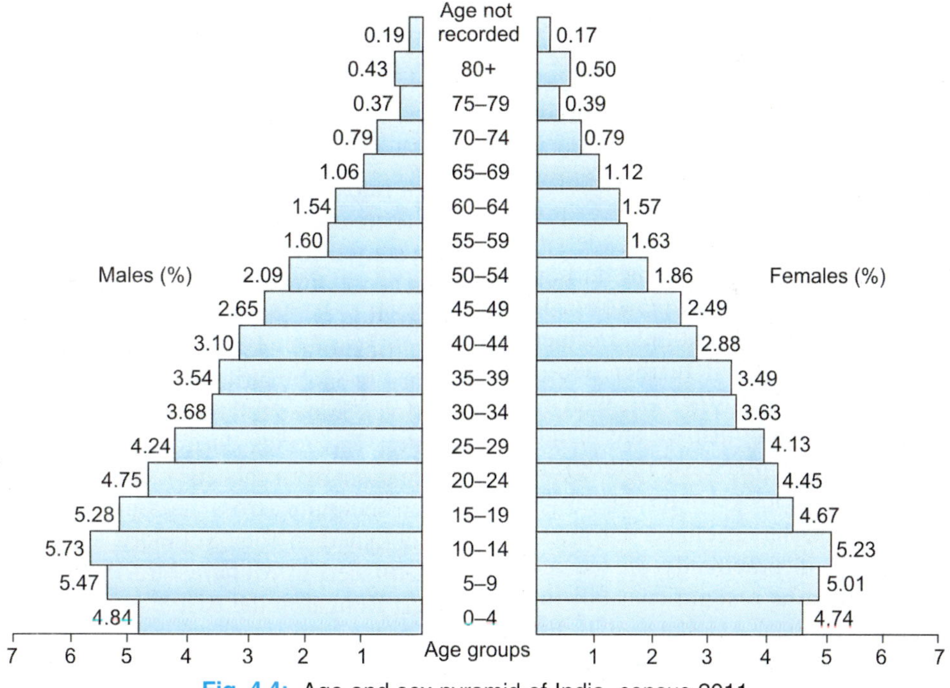

Fig. 4.4: Age and sex pyramid of India, census 2011

DENSITY OF POPULATION IN INDIA

Density of population is related to human activity. Density tends to be more in urban areas as compared to rural areas. Density of population is maximum in urban slums. Chances of spread of respiratory infections are maximum in dense population. Survival of young children in dense population is threatened with acute respiratory infections. Tuberculosis prevalence is much more in dense population. The average density of population per square km in India is 382. Delhi has the highest density of 11,297. Some of the areas have sparse population, and the terrains are difficult and access to population becomes difficult in such areas. Villages and hamlets are small and distances are too much to reach the services.

GROWTH RATE OF POPULATION (Fig. 4.5)

Natural growth rate: It is the difference between the birth rate and death rate, was estimated as 1.47% per annum in 2011 against a high of 1.64% in 2001. Between 2001 and 2011 we added whooping 181 million people.

Positive Sign

India can smile at slowing of its population growth rates, which were indicated by census 1991. The growth rate of population has further declined in the year 2001 and 2011.

India's population as on the midnight of February 28–March 1, 2011 stood at 1,21,01,93,422, i.e. 1210 million higher than the 1192 million projection made by the experts. This makes India the second most populous

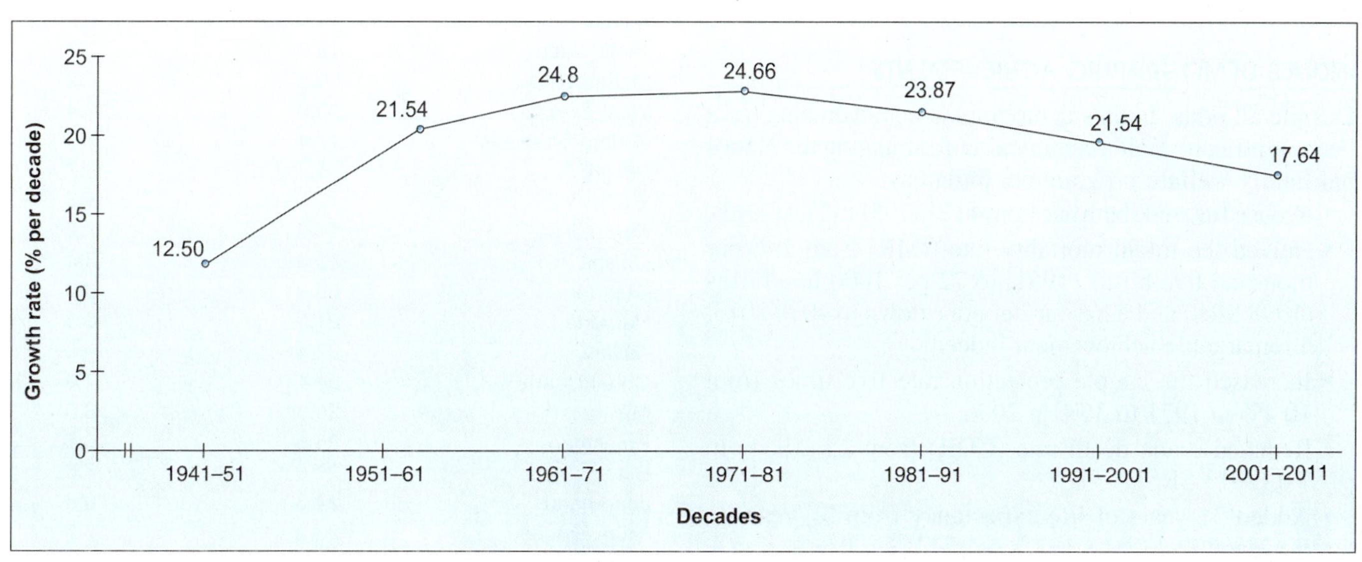

Fig. 4.5: Trends in decadal population growth rate, India, 1941–51 to 2001–2011

country in the world, behind China (1341 million on Nov. 2010), and way ahead of the next most populous country the United States of America (308.7 million in April 2010). However, the growth rate of population has come down in India during the decades since census 1991. The decadal growth rate in the decade 2001–2011 was 17.64% lowest ever growth rate after independence. This is 3.90% points lower than the growth rate of 21.54% in the decade 1991–2001, it is in-fact lowest intercensus growth rate during the period 1951–2011. Maximum decadal growth rate of 24.8% was recorded in the decade 1961–71 and this declined to 23.87 in the decade 1981–91 and it further declined favourably to the mark of 21.54 in 1991–2001, which is a favourable declining trend indicating that we are marching ahead and entering in another phase of demographic transition of achieving replacement level of fertility by 2021.

The population growth rate has declined during 2011 as compared to 1991–2001 in practically all the major states. For the first time, there is a significant fall in the growth rate of population in the EAG states (UP, Bihar, Rajasthan, Uttarakhand, Jharkhand, MP, Chhattisgarh and Odisha), after decades of stagnation.

Dependency Ratio

Definition: Economically dependent population is defined as sum of the population under 15 years of age plus population of 65 years of age and over, and economically productive population is defined as the population in age group 15–64 years. The dependency ratio is average number of economically dependant population per 100 economically productive population.

The broad base of pyramid of India indicates the high dependency ratio (i.e. the number of persons in the age group 0–14 and 65+ per 100 persons in the age group 15–64). Nearly 35 percent of population is dependent on 65% of 15–64 persons in India. Real dependency ratio may be much higher because of unemployed youth and disabled people in age bracket 15–64 years.

INDIA'S DEMOGRAPHIC ACHIEVEMENTS

Despite all odds, India's demographic achievements have been significant. Half a century after formulating the National family welfare programme, India has:

- Reduced its crude birth rate from 40.8 in 1951 to 21.4 (2013).
- Halved the infant mortality rate (IMR) from 146 per thousand live births (1951) to 72 per 1000 live births (1998 SRS) and it has further gone down to 40 in 2013, a remarkable achievement indeed
- Increased the couple protection rate five times from 10.4% in 1971 to 56% in 2006.
- Reduced crude death rate (CDR) from 25 (1951) to 7.0 (2013 SRS).
- Added 31 years of life expectancy from 37 years to 68 years.
- Reduced total fertility rate from 6.0 (1951) to 2.4 (2012).

DEMOGRAPHIC PROFILE

India is following the demographic transition pattern of all developing countries from initial levels of "high birth rate – high death rate" to the current intermediate transition stage of "high birth rates – low death rates" which leads to high rates of population growth.

There are positive signs that the broad base of pyramid has started shrinking. Census 2011 notes "in a population that is not affected by huge changes in age structure, adult migration or child mortality between two points of time, a significant fall in population of children in age group 0–6 years broadly indicative of fall in fertility during the period". Such a fall has occurred in a number of states and Union Territories during 2001–2011. There is thus confirmation from the 2011 census that fertility rates have been declining across the country. The decline appears well established in four Southern states and reasonably well established in Maharashtra in the west and Odisha and West Bengal in the east.[4,5]

INTER-STATE DIFFERENCES IN FERTILITY (BIRTH RATES)

India is country of striking demographic diversity. Substantial differences are visible between states in the achievement of basic demographic indices (Table 4.4).

Highest birth rates have been observed in the state of Uttar Pradesh, Bihar, Rajasthan and Madhya Pradesh. This had led to significant disparity on current population size and potential to influence population increases in future. These differences stem largely from poverty, illiteracy and inadequate access to health and family welfare services, which coexist and reinforce each others.

Table 4.4: Crude birth and death rates in major states of India, 2013 (SRS Sept. 2014)

States	Birth rate	Death rate
Kerala	14.7	6.9
Tamil Nadu	15.6	7.3
Maharashtra	16.5	6.2
West Bengal	16.0	6.4
Andhra Pradesh	17.4	7.3
Punjab	15.7	6.7
J & K	17.5	5.3
Karnataka	18.3	7.0
Odisha	19.6	8.4
Gujarat	20.8	6.5
Haryana	21.3	6.3
Assam	22.4	7.8
Chhattisgarh	24.4	7.9
MP	26.3	8.0
Rajasthan	25.6	6.5
Bihar	27.6	6.6
Jharkhand	24.6	6.8
Uttar Pradesh	27.2	7.7
India	**21.4**	**7.0**

TOTAL FERTILITY RATE

Twenty-three States/Union Territories (UTs) have already reached below replacement levels of fertility and 10 states are approaching fast to replacement levels of fertility (Table 4.5).[4–6]

Table 4.5: Total Fertility Rates (TFR) in various states, 2012

TFR Levels/categorizations	*States*
TFR of 2.1 or less **Non High Focus States** for FP (23 States and UTs)	Odisha 2.1, Karnataka 1.9, J & K 1.9, Kerala 1.8, TN 1.7, AP 1.8, WB 1.7, Punjab 1.7 Himachal Pradesh 1.7, Delhi 1.8, Maharashtra 1.8, Other States and UTs
TFR Rate of 2.2 to 2.9 **High Focus States** for FP (11 States)	Jharkhand 2.8, Arunachal 2.3, Chhattisgarh 2.7, Uttarakhand 2.6, Assam 2.4, Haryana 2.3, Gujarat 2.3, Rajasthan 2.9, MP 2.9, Meghalya 2.9, Dadra and Nagar Haveli 2.9
TFR of 3 and above **Very High Focus States** for FP (2 States)	Bihar 3.5, UP 3.3

Since the pace of achievement of TFR varies from state to state. We have to ensure differential strategies in different areas to achieve the desired TFR. High Focus Approach has been adopted by Govt of India.

Impact of High Focus Approach of Govt of India: Government of India has categorized states as per the TFR level as **very high focus** (more than or equal to 3.0), **high focus** (more than 2.1 and less than 3.0), **and non high focus** (less than or equal to 2.1).

SEX RATIO

India shares a distinctive feature of South Asian and Chinese population as regards the sex ratio, with a country's old deficit of females.

(a) THE OVERALL POPULATION SEX RATIO

The number of female per thousand males has been showing a secular decline, from 972 in 1901 to 933 in the year 2001. The sex ratio represents the survival scene of women. It has registered a very marginal improvement from 927 in the 1991 to 933 in the 2001 census. This is a welcome feature of 2001 census results (Table 4.6). It remains to be seen whether the observed increase in sex ratio between 1991 and 2001, constitutes a reversal of secular trend of decline or is just a chance phenomenon like the four point increase between 1971 and 1981, which was followed by 7 points decline between 1981 and 1991. Overall sex ratio at national level has increased by 7 points since census 2001 to reach 940 in census 2011. Kerala has highest female sex ratio of 1084. The sex ratio has improved in a number of major states between 2001 and 2011. These include all the Southern States, Odisha, West Bengal, Madhya Pradesh, Chhattisgarh, Bihar, Jharkhand, Uttar Pradesh, Uttarakhand, Rajasthan and Assam. But it is worrisome to note that the sex ratio has declined in three major states Gujarat, J & K and Bihar an already low level in Punjab. One also notes decline in Himachal Pradesh and Haryana. Haryana has the lowest female sex ratio of 830 in the country.

Table 4.6: Secular trends of sex ratio in India, 1901 to 2011

Years	*Sex ratio*	*Years*	*Sex ratio*
1901	972	1961	941
1911	964	1971	930
1921	955	1981	934
1931	950	1991	927
1941	945	2001	933
1951	946	2011	940

There has been slight increase in proportion of female population of the country from 48.26% in 2001 to 48.46% in 2011. Yet, the demographic divide between women and men continues to exist till date. Out of total population of 1210 million, we have 586.4 million population of female and 623.7 million males, it means some 37.3 million female are missing in India.[7,8]

Reasons for consistently low levels of sex ratio are:[8,9]

- Son preference
- Neglect of gril child resulting in higher mortality at younger age.
- Female infanticide, female foeticide
- Higher maternal mortality
- Male bias in enumeration to some extent
- Easy availability of sex determination tests and abortion services may also be proving to be catalyst in the process, which may be further stimulated by pre-conception sex selection facilities
- Biased Family Planning Programme—Undergoing sterilization after two male/one male child.
- Rapid fertility decline.
- Social problems—Dowry problem, insecurity for girls, sexual-abuse, etc. all of these make girl child as unwanted child.

Sex determination techniques have been in use in India since 1975 primarily for determination of genetic abnormalities. However, these techniques were widely misused to determine sex of the foetus and subsequent elimination if the foetus was found to be female.

DISTURBING SIGNS OF DEMOGRAPHY

(b) Child Sex Ratio—CSR (0-6 Years)

One of the most disturbing feature of demography is adverse sex ratio of female children as revealed through census 2011. Though the overall proportion of 0–6 children has been declining in India, a favourable trend indeed to attribute to the success of family welfare programme intervention, however declining female child sex ratio or juvenile sex ratio (JSR) over the years is a disturbing trend. The most alarming and disturbing aspect of census 2011 report is sharp fall in sex ratio of female children (0–6 years) from 927 in 2001 to 914 in 2011, a significant decline of 13 points. The decline is even sharper in several states. Haryana, Punjab, Delhi and Chandigarh lead the dubious club, with adverse child sex ratio of 830, 846, 886 and 867 repectively. The bottom-most districts on child sex ratio lie in Haryana—Jhajjar being worst in India with meager 774 girls per 1000 boys followed by Mahendragarh at 778.

However increasing trend in child sex ratio was seen in states/UTs, viz. Punjab, Haryana, Himachal Pradesh, Gujarat, Mizoram, Chandigarh, Tamil Nadu and Andaman and Nicobar islands, but in all the remaining 21 states/UTs child sex ratio showed decline over the census 2001 (Table 4.7)[10].

The general decline in the juvenile sex ratio (JSR) practically across the entire country must be viewed with concern. There is enough evidence from the field to indicate alarming spread of practice of female foeticide not only in the contiguous belt of Punjab, Chandigarh, Haryana, Uttarakhand, Himachal Pradesh, but also in Maharashtra and Gujarat, even more worrisome, in the much vaunted South, where the female fetus and infant were earlier not thought to be at great risk. In Tamil Nadu, for instance there is considerable evidence of the practice of female foeticide.

Child sex ratio (CSR) reflects both pre-birth and post-birth discrimination against girls. Therefore sex ratio at birth (SRB) is considered to be more accurate and a refined indicator of the extent of sex selection.

(c) Sex Ratio at Birth (SRB)

Natural sex ratio at birth in India is 105 male per 100 female births. SRB is not influenced by post birth factors, such as

Table 4.7: Adverse ratio of 0–6 female children

State	*1991*	*2001*	*2011*
J & K	–	941	859
Punjab	875	798	846
Haryana	879	819	830
Chandigarh	899	845	867
HP	951	896	906
Maharashtra	946	913	883
Delhi	915	868	866
Rajasthan	916	909	883
UP	927	916	899
Uttarakhand	948	908	886
AP	975	961	943
Karnataka	960	946	943
Tamil Nadu	948	942	946
Kerala	958	960	959
Bihar	953	942	933
Odisha	967	953	934
MP	941	932	912
Gujarat	928	883	886
All India	**945**	**927**	**914**

mortality or neglect. The SRB for India for 2009–11 was estimated at 906 girls for every 1000 boys.

Goal of 12th Plan: Raise the sex ratio for age group 0–6 from 914 to 950 by the end of plan.[11]

EXPECTATION OF LIFE AT BIRTH (Table 4.8)

Expectation of life is used as an indicator of human development and countries are judged and graded on life expectancy. India has made considerable demographic gains over the years.

Table 4.8: Expectation of life at birth (India)

Census years	*Male*	*Female*
1901	23.63	23.96
1951	32.45	31.66
1971	46.40	44.70
1980	54.10	54.70
1991	58.10	58.60
1992	58.60	59.00
1995	59.40	60.40
1996–2001	62.30	65.27
2001–2006	63.87	66.91
2006–2011	65.65	67.67
2011–2016	67.04	69.18

Source: RGI

The life expectancy over the years in India has improved significantly. Life expectancy which was just 37 years in 1951 has risen to 68 years in 2013. Since the life expectancy will rise further, India will face the problems of chronic and non-communicable diseases. Currently we in India are facing double disease burden, communicable diseases and emerging lifestyle diseases or non-communicable diseases.

LITERACY AND FERTILITY RATE

The results of census 2011 indicate significant increase in literacy rates and number of literate persons. The literacy has been defined as the ability to read and write with understanding in any language and it is determined for persons aged 7 years and above. Overall, literacy level of India was reported to be 74%, which is 9 points gain over literacy level of 2001 (65.38%). The female literacy level has increased to 65.46% from 54.16% in the year 2001, thus a gain of nearly 11 points. Kerala leads the way ahead of all the states with literacy of 93.9%. The male-female gap in literacy has declined to 16.68 percentage points, the lowest since the 1951 census. There is reduction in the gender gap in literacy levels in all the states and union territories. The biggest improvement in literacy has occurred in the state of Chhattisgarh, Rajasthan and MP.

Contraception acceptance or limiting the family size, spacing births at least three years apart is a function of literacy of parents and more so of women. If women are literate, their marriages will be at right age and their

Table 4.9: Literacy, fertility and sex ratio in major States and UTs-2012, India

States	*Literacy (2011 census) (%)*	*TFR-2012*	*Birth rate (SRS-2012)*	*Sex ratio (0–6 years)*
Andhra Pradesh	67.66	1.8	17.5	943
Assam	73.18	2.2	22.5	957
Bihar	63.82	2.5	27.7	933
Chandigarh	86.43	1.8	14.8	867
Chhattisgarh	71.04	2.7	24.5	964
Delhi	86.34	1.6	17.3	866
Gujarat	79.31	2.2	21.1	886
Haryana	76.64	2.1	21.6	830
Himachal Pradesh	83.78	1.7	16.2	906
J & K	68.74	1.6	17.6	859
Jharkhand	67.63	2.3	24.7	943
Karnataka	75.60	1.9	18.5	943
Kerala	93.91	1.8	14.9	959
MP	70.63	2.8	26.6	912
Maharashtra	82.91	1.8	16.6	883
Odisha	73.75	2.0	19.9	934
Punjab	76.68	1.7	15.9	846
Rajasthan	67.06	2.5	25.9	883
Tamil Nadu	80.33	1.7	15.7	946
Tripura	87.75	–	13.9	953
UP	69.72	2.9	27.4	899
Uttarakhand	79.63	2.6	18.5	886
West Bengal	77.08	1.7	16.1	950
India	**74.04**	**2.4**	**21.6**	**914**

reproductive behaviour will change and they will have optimal total fertility rate and thereby the demography of a place would change as has happened in Kerala. Literacy is the best contraceptive to make positive impact on fertility (Table 4.9).

MORTALITY IN INDIA

The crude death rates over the years have declined from 25 in the year 1951 to 7.0 in the year 2013. Similarly, infant mortality has declined to 40 and under five mortality has been reduced to 49, but these levels are unacceptably high. By 2020 India would have 9.3 million premature deaths before the age of 70—more than any other country—if its 2010 death rate continues. Maternal mortality, neonatal mortality and perinatal mortality continues to be unacceptably high. These have been picked up as thrust areas for aggressive actions at the community level. It is expected that with increase in standards of living and quality of life, the mortality will come down to acceptable level.

The mortality is maximum or highest in the early childhood period, during infancy and children between 1–4 years of age. Mortality is least in age bracket 5–19 years, which is considered to be the healthiest period of life. Mortality tends to higher in female in reproductive age group (15–49 years) and thereafter the mortality rates go on increasing as the age advances (Table 4.10). Young children and old people are most vulnerable to death. Thus,

Table 4.10: Age and sex specific death rates in India, 2013

Age group	*Male*	*Female*	*Combined*
Below 1	42.0	43.5	42.7
0–4	10.9	12.1	11.5
5–9	1.0	1.0	1.0
10–14	0.8	0.6	0.7
15–19	1.1	1.1	1.1
20–24	1.9	1.6	1.8
25–29	2.1	1.5	1.8
30–34	2.7	1.5	2.1
35–39	3.8	1.9	2.8
40–44	5.2	2.5	3.9
45–49	7.5	3.8	5.7
50–54	10.3	5.4	8.0
55–59	17.2	9.7	13.1
60–64	24.7	17.8	21.3
65–69	37.3	29.2	33.1
70–74	56.6	43.7	49.9
75–79	75.5	61.9	68.3
80–84	103.9	96.8	100.2
85+	173.4	151.8	161.3
All ages (crude death rate)	7.7	6.4	7.0

Source: Sample Registration System Registrar General, India (2014).

4

the prime need of young infant is survival and development. The determinants of high mortality during infancy are high reproduction and prematurity due to repeated pregnancies. The other determinant is environment, which exposes the children to diarrhoea, respiratory infections and injuries. Lifestyle diseases and non-communicable diseases take heavy toll beyond the age of 50 but more young people die of coronary heart disease in India than in developed countries. New emerging epidemics of HIV and accidents take a heavy toll of life.

Premature Deaths

By 2030, India will witness 9.3 million premature deaths before age 70–more than any other country, if its 2010 death rate continues.

Of these, 1.5 million will occur before age of five, 2.7 million at age five to 49 and 5.1 million at age 50 to 69.

The research stresses India needs rapid progress, not only to reduce child mortality, but also tuberculosis malaria and deaths from chronic diseases and non-communicable diseases which are are made more common by tobacco use. With current rate of progress, deaths in India before age of 70 would fall only by 31% by 2030 short of suggested 40% target. Between 2000 and 2010 Indian death rate fell 30% before the age of five, 15% during ages 5–49, and 12% during ages 50–69. Overall death rates in India below age 70 fell by 17%.

The rising population disturbs all the norms. In health and ICDS sector, the rising population has increased the demand of subcentres, primary health centres and community health centres and district hospitals. The population norms are difficult to meet because of rising costs. Further, the population is spread over to small villages, which are remote and not easily accessible. The coverage of services is affected badly due to rapid increase in population. Similarly, increasing slum population poses serious problems to establish primary health care services. Quality is the casualty in view of rapid increase in population. It is difficult to provide sustained quality services because of sheer number of clients who always outnumber against the meagre resources.

FERTILITY INDICATORS

High fertility is a serious problem in India. The fertility can be measured by following indicators:
(1) Age at effective marriage (AEM), (2) Crude birth rate, (3) General fertility rate, (4) Age specific fertility rate, (5) Total fertility rate, (6) Gross reproductive rate, (7) Net reproduction rate, (8) Parity, (9) Birth interval, (10) Child women ratio, and (11) Eligible couples.

Age at Effective Marriage (AEM)

4

The mean age at effective marriage is the age at consummation of marriage. At the national level, the mean age at effective marriage for female in the year 2012 was 21.2 years. The state level data show variation in AEM. It was highest in J & K (24.6) followed by Kerala (22.9), Delhi and Tamil Nadu (22.9 and 22.4), Himachal Pardesh (22.4) in 2012. Rajasthan has the lowest AEM (20.6). AEM determines the number of children born by women. The AEM in respect of more than 16.5% of female was below 18 years while 35% were married below 20 years of age.

Crude Birth Rate (CBR)[12]

Crude birth rate is the most commonly used and simplest measure of fertility. It is computed regularly by sample registration system (SRS) every year for rural and urban areas; for different states of India.

Crude birthrate has come down from 23.8 in 2005 to 21.4 in the year 2012

Years	2005	2009	2011	2012	2013
CBR	23.8	22.5	21.8	21.6	21.4

Computation

CBR is the number of live births per 1000 population per year.

$$\text{CBR} = \frac{\text{Live births in one year}}{\text{Mid-year population in that year}} \times 1000$$

CBR are higher in rural and urban slum areas. States like UP, Bihar, Rajasthan, and MP have higher crude birth rates: above 27 per 1000 population.

Limitations

It is called crude because the whole population is used as denominator, but the fact remains that only females in reproductive age group (15–49 years) are able to produce children. Generally, girls below 15 and women above 49 years of age are unable to produce children.

General Fertility Rate (GFR)

It is refined measure of fertility. Only women in reproductive age group of 15–49 years of age are able to produce children, is used as denominator in this rate. Accordingly, GFR is calculated by:

$$\text{GFR} = \frac{\text{Live births in the year}}{\text{Women in reproductive age group (15–49 years)}} \times 1000 = 100$$

Since women in reproductive age group are approximately 25.75% of the total population, therefore, the level of GFR in India is around 80, i.e. four times that of CBR.[13]

Example:

$$\text{GFR} = \frac{\text{Live births in the year 2012 in India were 26 million}}{\text{Women in reproductive age group in that year 334 million}} \times 1000 = 80$$

At the level of subcentre or PHC, GFR can be calculated by dividing the total number of live births in a year by total number of eligible couples (15–49 years married women). However, fertility rate varies with the age of women and age at marriage.

Age Specific Fertility Rate (ASFR) and Age Specific Marital Fertility Rate (ASMFR)

It is used to measure the reproductive performance of women of a given age. The ASFR is defined as the number of children born to women in the specific age group per 1000 women in that age group and ASMFR is the number of children born to married women in the specific age group per 1000 women in the same age group.

$$\text{ASFR} = \frac{\text{Number of live births to women of specified age or age group in a year}}{\text{Mid-year population of the specified age or age group}} \times 1000$$

During the year 2012, the ASFR of women in age bracket 20–24 years was highest at 191.9, while in the age bracket 40–44 it was around 8.2. There is thus marked difference in fertility levels in different age brackets (Table 4.11).[14] ASFR is, however, not a summary index of overall fertility level of the whole population.

Table 4.11: ASFR (India) 2012—SRS

Age group	Urban	Rural	India
15–19	16.7	36.3	31.5
20–24	140.4	210.6	191.9
25–29	131.4	164.8	154.6
30–34	55.6	68.3	64.5
35–39	15.4	27.5	23.9
40–44	3.7	10.1	8.2
45–49	0.8	2.8	2.2

Implications: Age group 20–24 years should be prime focus for spacing and limiting child births. Spacing methods need to be promoted and priority for contraception should be younger couples (20–24 years of age) with 2 or less children.

Total Fertility Rate (TFR)

It is used as standardized index for the overall fertility level. It overcomes the limitations of the crude birth rate and general fertility rate.

The TFR means the average number of children that would be born per woman if she was to live to the end of her child bearing years (15–49 years) and bear children at each age in accordance with prevailing age specific fertility rates, or else TFR is average number of children born to woman during her lifetime.

Computation

Total fertility rate is arrived at by sum of all age specific fertility rates for each year of age from 15 to 49 years. It is average number of children that a synthetic cohort of women would have at the end of reproductive period, if there was no mortality among the women. Synthetic birth cohort is artificial birth cohort, composed of cross-sectional sample of the women in reproductive age group.

During the year 1951, the TFR in India was 6.0. The current level of TFR is 2.3 (Table 4.12). We wish to bring it down to the level of 2.1 by repositioning Family Planning Programme. This in other words means two child norm. Twenty-three States and UTs in India have already achieved replacement levels of fertility with TFR of less than or equal to 2.1. These states are Kerala, AP, TN, Punjab, Delhi, HP, West Bengal, Karnataka and Maharashtra (Table 4.5). On the other hand in states like UP, Bihar, Rajasthan and MP, the high TFR of more than three has been reported; which means differential strategies for contraception and regulating fertility are needed for these states to achieve the desired level of TFR.[15–18]

Table 4.12: Trends in TFR in India (UNICEF)

Year	TFR
1951	6.0
1970	5.6
1990	4.0
2005	2.9
2006	2.8
2007	2.7
2008	2.6
2009	2.6
2010	2.5
2012	2.4
2014	2.3

Gross Reproductive Rate (GRR) in the Year 2012

The GRR means total number of female children born to a woman throughout the span of reproduction (15–49 years of age). Assumption here is that no female dies, and lives up to full span of reproduction and produces children at prevailing fertility rates. This rate is about half of TFR and in India it is nearly 1.3, it means that on an average 1.3 daughters are born per woman. Pool of daughters born to women will determine the future pool of women in reproductive age group. Sex selective abortions and sex selective sterilizations have disturbed this rate.

Net Reproduction Rate (NRR)

While GRR assumes that no woman will die during her reproductive span, the NRR takes into consideration the mortality effects in women of reproductive age group. In essence, NRR is similar to GRR but it is adjusted for mortality in women. NRR is really replacement index. NRR 1 or unity means that a woman is replaced by another woman in her lifetime. Currently NRR in India is 1.2. NRR 1 is equivalent to TFR of 2.1. The National Health Mission has set the goal of achieving NRR 1 by 2017 or TFR of 2.1 by 2017 by different strategies, protecting effectively over 60% of eligible couples.

Parity

Parity means number of live births/living children. High parity is a problem in India which reflects high level of fertility. In a subcentre population, 46% of eligible couples in the year 2003 were of parity three and above, 26% had parity two, 17% were of parity one and the remaining 11% were of parity zero. Thus in that area high level of improvident maternity (parity three or more) prevailed; which speaks of high fertility rates. Similarly, urban slum areas have high improvident maternity rate (birth orders 3 and 4).

Implication: High *improvident maternity* of over 25.7 was evident in India, which means high fertility. In UP and Bihar, improvident maternity was nearly 33.4% to 40% (Table 4.13). Different methods of contraception are required based on parity of couples. Subcentre ANMs routinely generate these data and they can determine priority couples for contraception.

Table 4.13: Percentage distribution of current live births by birth order in India and major states (SRS, 2012)

India and states	Birth orders			
	1st	2nd	3rd	4th and above
India	43.2	31.4	13.8	11.6
UP	37.1	29.5	16.9	16.5
Bihar	34.4	25.6	17.9	22.0
Jharkhand	35.8	29.4	17.8	17.0
Rajasthan	37.9	30.0	16.1	16.0
Chhattisgarh	43.1	32.2	16.2	8.6
MP	41.6	32.7	14.1	11.6

Source: SRS statistical report 2012. Report No. 2 of 2013.

Birth Interval

This is the time interval between two consecutive births.

Birth interval is expressed as *closed* and *open* birth interval.

Closed birth interval: Interval between two successive births.

Open birth interval: Interval between the last birth and the date of study.

Spacing births at least three years apart by using spacing methods is good for health and survival of mothers and children. The risk of death for young children is increased to 50% if interval between births is less than 2 years. Short birth interval was obvious in India, as one birth out of every eight occurred within 18 months of previous birth (NFHS-2).[16]

Child—Woman Ratio (CWR)

This is the ratio of 0–4 years children to women in reproductive age group (15–49). If this ratio is high it means fertility rate of the area is high. In the year 2001, the child women ratio in India was 10.7:50.6. Infant mortality and maternal mortality affect this ratio. This indicator is generally used if no other indicator is available.

4

0–4 years age group constitutes the base of population pyramid, if it is broad it signifies high fertility which is true for population pyramid of India. Of late (census 2011), the base has begun to shrink which is positive sign and it speaks of success of family welfare programme in India.[19]

Eligible Couples (ECs)

All currently married women between 15 and 49 years age group are listed as eligible couples by all the health workers and updated every year. Thus, the proportion of eligible couples stands worked out at the level of subcentre. There will be at least 150–180 such couples per 1000 population. Over the years, the proportion of ECs should decline. If the proportion of ECs is high the fertility level is also high due to unmet needs of contraception. Large pool of ECs in India is responsible for high fertility rate and population growth to the extent of 60%.

Contraceptive Prevalence Rate (CPR)[18]

Contraceptive prevalence rate is percentage of women between 15 and 49 years who are practicing or whose sexual partners are practicing, any form of contraception. During the year 2012–13 CPR was 54.8%.

Out of 205 million of ECs in the year 2011 only 44% were effectively protected (using contraception). ECs have to be disaggregated parity wise and age wise to focus on young couples for spacing and limiting the size of the family by contraception. *Effective couple protection rate* of more than 60% is required to achieve NRR of 1 or TFR of 2.1. Protecting couples of high parity with sterilization or other means of contraception will have little demographic impact. In some states, paradox of high couple protection rate and high birth rate was observed due to over-reporting or inflation of reports to complete the targets. Sterilization of women who already have 3–4 children will have little demographic impact.

Couple Protection Rate (CPR)

It is defined as the percent of eligible couples effectively protected against child birth by one or the other approved method of family planning.

- *Number of couples protected effectively* can be arrived at by taking 100% for sterilization, and oral pills, 95% for IUD users and 50% for CC users.[20]
- *Equivalent sterilization* can be calculated by adding the number of sterilizations, 1/3 the number of IUD insertions, 1/18 the number of equivalent CC users and 1/9 of equivalent oral pill users.[21] Under the national programme, one beneficiary for oral pills is a woman who completes 13 cycles and for CC user one beneficiary is a person who uses 72 pieces of condoms.

According to NFHS III, 48.5% of ECs were using modern contraceptives (Female sterilization 37.3%, male sterilization 1%, condoms 5.3%, IUD 1.8%, pills 3.1%) and traditional methods were used by 7.8%.[22] Therefore, to bring down birth rate significantly, it would be necessary to provide effective contraceptive coverage to about 75% of eligible couples. Spacing methods need to be promoted vigorously.

REFERENCES

1 GOI. India's Population Demographic Scenario. New Delhi: Department of Family Welfare MOH and FW; 1990.
2 www.censusindia.gov.in/2011 census/Age-level—Data/India/Age-data. XIs. Single year age Data—C13 Table (India/States/UTs.
3 Imhof AE. Can India learn lessons from Europe's Demographic and Epidemiologic Transitions. Ind J Comm Med 1986; Vol. 2(2).
4 GOI. Centre Calling Census 2001. Provisional results Jan-Apr. 2001, New Delhi: Department of Family Welfare.
5 Bose A. First Result of census of India, 2001—Population Scan. Health for the Millions, 2001.
6 GOI. National Population Policy, 2000.
7 GOI. Reproductive and Child Health News Letter Vol. 4(2). New Delhi: RCH Prog. Department of Family Welfare; 2001.
8 Lal S, Vashisht BM, Punia MS. Down with low child sex ratio. Ind J Comm Med 2002; 27(1).
9 UNICEF. Rights and opportunities. The situation of children and women in India. New Delhi: UNICEF, India Country Office; 1998.
10 NFI. Bose A. Towards a Humane Development Report. NFI Bulletin 2002 Oct; 23(4).
11 Planning Commission—Report of steering committee on Health for the 12th five year plan February 2012.
12 GOI-RGI (2006–2007) SRS Bulletin, volume 41 No. 1 to volume 47 No. 1 October 2006 to 2014. Registrar General of India, New Delhi.
13 WHO. Teaching Health Statistics. Lessons and seminars outline. Second Edition by Lwanga SK, Cho Yook Tye, O. Ayeni World Health Organization, Geneva, 1999.
14 GOI. RGI. Report No 3 of 2014 SRS statistical Report 2014. Office of the RGI 2/A Mansingh Road, New Delhi.
15 GOI. National population Policy, 2000. Dept of FW, MOH and FW, GOI; New Delhi.
16 IIPS. National Family Health Survey-2, Mumbai, India, 2002.
17 GOI. Working paper series, paper no. 2/2000 Planning Commission, GOI; New Delhi.
18 UNICEF: The State of the World's Children 2007 and 2008 and 2015 UNICEF, Lodi Estate, New Delhi.
19 GOI. Age group wise distribution of male and female population in India, Census 2001.
20 GOI. Family Welfare Programme in India. Year Book 2001, pp 201, Dept of FW, MOH and FW. GOI, New Delhi.
21 GOI. Family Welfare Programme in India. Year Book 1990–91, pp 163, Dept of FW. MOH and FW. GOI, New Delhi.
22 IIPS National Family Health Survey-3, 2005–06 Mumbai, India.

MATERNAL MORTALITY

Maternal mortality is an indicator of state of maternal health services, status of women, women's health and above all the development of nation. Women are half of the nation and half of the power; their concerns must be addressed on priority basis. Maternal mortality ratio (MMR) has been included in the Millennium Development Goals (MDG). Target of MDG is to reduce MMR by three quarters between 1990 and 2015. March 8th is observed as international women's day every year to affirm our commitment to women's health and development.

Definition

A maternal death is defined as the death of woman while pregnant or within 42 days of termination of the pregnancy, irrespective of the duration and site of pregnancy, from any cause related to or aggravated by the pregnancy or its management but not from accidental or incidental causes (ICD-10).[1]

Late Maternal Death

A late maternal death is the death of a woman from direct or indirect obstetric causes more than 42 days but less than one year after termination of pregnancy.

Pregnancy-related Death

A pregnancy-related death is death of a woman while pregnant or within 42 days of termination of pregnancy, irrespective of the cause of death.

Maternal deaths are divided into two groups:

(a) Direct Obstetric Deaths

Direct obstetric deaths are those, resulting from obstetric complications of the pregnant state (during pregnancy, labour and puerperium) from interventions, omissions, incorrect treatment or from chain of events resulting from any of the above. Most maternal deaths are related to obstetric complications—including haemorrhage (usually postpartum haemorrhage), sepsis, eclampsia and prolonged or obstructed labour and complications of abortion.

(b) Indirect Obstetric Deaths

Indirect obstetric deaths are those, resulting from previous existing disease or diseases that developed during pregnancy and which were not due to direct obstetric causes, but which was aggravated by physiological effect of pregnancy (ICD-10)—anaemia, malaria, HIV, AIDS and cardiovascular diseases.

Problem of MMR

Global Problem: A Statistic of Shame

Though the safe motherhood initiative was launched way back in 1987 at Nairobi (Kenya), more than 5,36,000 women continue to die globally each year due to pregnancy related causes (estimates for 2005).

In the South-East Asia Region, Nepal and Bangladesh have the dubious distinction of having highest MMR, while Thailand and Sri Lanka have the lowest MMR (UNICEF 2015). Over 40% of all maternal deaths occur in SEAR. Pregnancy, related deaths constitute the leading cause of loss of healthy lives among women of reproductive age group in South-East Asia region. In India, women are 100 times more likely to die due to pregnancy than their counterparts in developed world (Tables 4.14 and 4.15).[2,3]

Table 4.14: World scenario of MMR

Country/region	*Population 2013 (million)*	*MMR*
India	1252	180
China	1385	25
USA	320	13
Sweden	9.5	4
Least developed countries	1835	420
World	7122	210

MMR per 100,000 live births

Table 4.15: Adjusted maternal mortality ratio (MMR) in countries of the South-East Asia Region-2015, UNICEF

Country	*Reported 2009–2013*	*Adjusted 2013*
Bangladesh	210	170
Pakistan	250	170
Bhutan	150	120
DPR Korea	77	87
India	180	190
Indonesia	360	190
Maldives	140	31
Myanmar	320	200
Nepal	280	190
Sri Lanka	31	29
Thailand	12	26

Problem of MMR in India

India alone contributed 15 percent of global maternal deaths. Lifetime risk of maternal death in India was one in 220 as against one in 5800 in UK.

Data on MMR is available at national level, which has been generated through special studies/surveys (Table 4.16).

The national level maternal mortality ratio—MMR is unacceptably high when compared with some of the neighbouring countries in the region. India had the dubious distinction of having very high MMR rate of 400–500 per 1,00,000 live births. According to international estimates India's maternal mortality ratio, stood at 450 per 1,00,000 live births in 2005. Special bulletin on MMR in India from 2004–06 by SRS brought out in 2009 estimates level of MMR at 254. This has been derived by pooling the three year data to yield reliable estimates of maternal mortality. During the period 2004–06 to 2011–13 the MMR declined from 254 to 167 which is well short of 12th plan goal of 100. Besides Kerala (66), Tamil Nadu (90) and Maharashtra (87) have realized the MDG targets of 109 in 2007–09. The major burden of MMR is in EAG states, where the average MMR was 308 and continues to be high. As per recent SRS data of 2011–13 high MMR was observed in Assam (300), Bihar (208), Jharkhand (278), MP (221), Chhattisgarh (275), Odisha (222), Rajasthan (244), UP (285) and Uttarakhand (188) respectively.

Table 4.16: Estimates of maternal deaths per 100,000 live births in India[4–8]

Years	*Rural*	*Urban*	*Total*
1990*	–	405	405
1992–93 NFHS-1	434	385	424**
1998–99 NFHS-2	619	267	540**
1992 Rohtak, Haryana	475	–	475
1998 RGI SRS	–	–	407
2000 WHO/UNFPA/UNICEF	–	–	540
2002 UNICEF	–	–	540
2005 WHO, UNICEF, UNFPA	–	–	450
1997–03 SRS			301
2004–06 SRS			254
2007–2009 SRS			212
2010–12 SRS			178
2011–13 SRS			167

*ICMR Task Force (1990)
**The 95% confidence interval for MMR ranges from 428 to 653 for NFHS-2 and from 324 to 524 for NFHS-1 hence difference between NFHS-1 and NFHS-2 estimates is statistically not significant

Besides SRS "Sisterhood method" has been used to capture levels of maternal mortality. This method makes use of data obtained from female respondents in a sample survey on the number of ever married sisters they had, the number who were currently alive and the number who died while pregnant, during child birth or during six weeks after delivery. This reduces cost and sample size. The method generates information on long past maternal mortality. In the absence of MMR data at state/district level other indicators of maternal health status like antenatal check-up, institutional deliveries and delivery by trained personnel, etc. are used.

National estimates do not tell the story of variation of MMR in different states. India being large country and there are several inequalities between regions and states and within the state there are variations in the districts as development and facilities vary. Statewise data on MMR is available through SRS as states have limited capacity to collect such data and similarly no data on MMR is available at district level.

The disaggregated data in India indicates that some of the states like Assam, UP, MP. Rajasthan and Odisha are having very high MMR needing differential strategies and focused attention (Table 4.17). RCH programme is flexible to meet these needs and augment the resources of these states through empowered action groups (EAG).

4

Table 4.17: Estimates of MMR from 1989–99 to 2011–13 for India—major states

States	*1998–99*	*2001–03*	*2004–06*	*2007–09*	*2011–13*
AP	341	195	154	134	92
MP	601	379	335	269	221
Assam	762	490	480	390	300
Odisha	552	358	303	258	222
Bihar	714	371	312	261	208
Rajasthan	526	445	388	318	244
Gujarat	393	172	160	148	112
Tamil Nadu	284	134	111	97	79
Haryana	468	162	186	153	127
Uttar Pradesh	737	517	440	359	285
Karnataka	364	228	213	178	133
West Bengal	451	194	141	145	113
Kerala	262	110	95	81	61
Maharashtra	365	149	130	104	68
Punjab	199	178	192	172	141
India	**466**	**301**	**254**	**212**	**167**

AP: Andhra Pradesh, MP: Madhya Pradesh

In India according to SRS estimates, 0.55% of all deaths n the country are due to maternal causes. Though the roportion is small but it is very critical. Similarly, maternal leaths are 4% of total deaths in women in reproductive ge group (15–49).

Causes of Maternal Mortality (Fig. 4.6)

Three delays analysis of causes of maternal deaths adopted y WHO Include:

Delay 1: Delay in recognizing the problem and delay in leciding to seek care

Delay 2: Delay in reaching the health facility

Delay 3: Delay in receiving the adequate treatment once a voman has arrived at health facility.

Causes of maternal mortality are well known and these ave not changed much over the time. Looking at these auses, it can be stated that most of the maternal deaths are preventable by suitable intervention. Over 80% of maternal deaths are due to *direct obstetrical causes*, i.e. related with pregnancy and indirect causes, such as anaemia, malaria, jaundice, hypertension, tuberculosis, gestational diabetes during pregnancy are responsible for 20% of maternal deaths (Fig. 4.6 and Table 4.18).

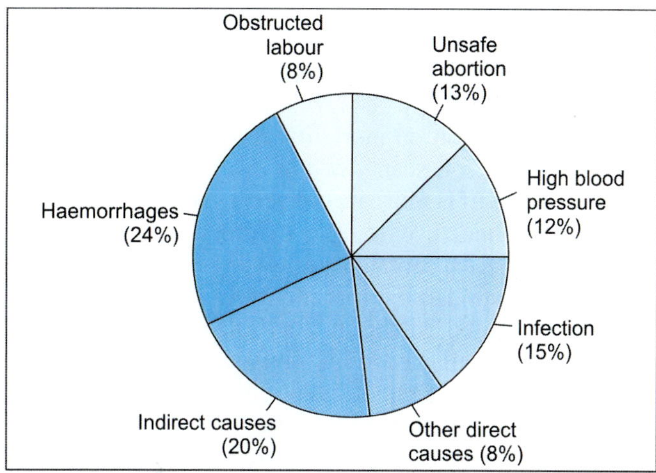

Fig. 4.6: Causes of maternal mortality (2000–2003)—World Health Report-2005

WORLD HEALTH REPORT-2005

In the World Health Report-2005—"Make every mother and child count" WHO estimated that about 536,000 die in pregnancy or childbirth per year, more than 3 million babies are stillborn and more than 4 million newborn die within the first a few days or weeks of life and altogether 10.6 million children a year die before their fifth birthday. WHO estimates that out of total of 136 million births a year worldwide, less than two-thirds of women in less developed countries and only one-third in the least developed countries have their babies delivered by a skilled attendant. "Make every mother and child count" New Delhi, India was used as major launching pad to achieve millennium development goals (MDGs) of improving maternal and child health by the year 2015.

Table 4.18: Obstetrical causes of maternal mortality[3]

Causes	*SRS (RGI) 1998 (%)*	*WHO 2005 (%)*
Haemorrhages or severe bleeding	29	24
Infection/sepsis	16	15
Unsafe abortion	9	13
Eclampsia/hypertension	8	12
Obstructed labour	10	8
Other direct causes (ectopic pregnancy, embolism, anaesthesia related)	9	8
Indirect causes (anaemia, malaria, heart disease, diabetes and jaundice)	19	20
Total	**100**	**100**

Source: WHO SEARO-2001 and World Health Report-2005.

Goal

Goal is to reduce maternal mortality ratio below 100 per 100,000 live births by 2017.[4,9,10] and below 70 by 2030.

The information on mortality during reproductive age group is either too scanty or not available at all through routine reports of health care delivery system. In the system of primary health care, the primary health centres, community health centres and district health organization do not generate data on this indicator. Bhore Committee (1946) estimated MMR of 20/1000 live births. These estimates were reflected in first five-year plan. The national health policy document of 1983 relied on hospital figures to estimate MMR around 4–5 per thousand live births. The child survival and safe motherhood programme too relied on hospital data on maternal mortality and quoted a rate of 5.0 per thousand. Hospital MMRs are not indicators for general risk of maternal death in India. Women in serious conditions reach hospitals and often the hospital MMRs are much higher than the rate in the population at large. But hospital MMR provides accurate causes of death. Now annual Health Surveys generate MMR state wise and region wise (2011 to 2013).

A hospital MMR is the number of maternal deaths taking place in the hospital divided by the number of live births taking place in the same institution during the same period.

Measuring Maternal Mortality

$$\text{Maternal mortality ratio} = \frac{\text{Maternal deaths}}{\text{Live births}} \times 100{,}000$$

$$\text{Maternal mortality rate} = \frac{\text{Maternal deaths}}{\text{Women in reproductive age group}} \times 100{,}000$$

There are various ways to measure maternal mortality:

1. Maternal deaths per 100,000 live births (*maternal mortality ratio*). This is most commonly used measure. It expresses risk of death among women once they are pregnant. Although it is often called the maternal mortality rate, it is not really a rate because the numerator (maternal deaths) is not part of the denominator.
2. *Maternal mortality rate* is maternal deaths per 100,000 women of reproductive age per year.
3. Lifetime risk of maternal death in India is one in 220.

The maternal mortality rate indicates the impact of maternal deaths on the population of women of reproductive age (usually defined as ages 15–49).

Maternal mortality is not merely a health disadvantage, it is a matter of social injustice. Low social and economic status of girls and women limit their access to education, good nutrition, as well as money to pay for health care and family planning services. The extent of maternal mortality is an indicator of disparity and inequity in access to appropriate health care and nutrition services, throughout a lifetime, and particularly during pregnancy and childbirth.

4

RISK FACTORS OR UNDERLYING CONDITIONS FOR MATERNAL MORTALITY IN INDIA[11-13]

Knowledge on underlying conditions of maternal deaths is essential for effective application of interventions to reduce the maternal deaths or prevent the maternal deaths. In India, following epidemiological risk factors or underlying conditions have been identified.

Early Marriages

In India, nearly 17% of girls marry below the age of 18, the minimum legal age of marriage, resulting in a typical reproductive pattern of "too early, too frequent, too many". They start bearing children at early age and bear frequently and bear too many children. Around 26.6% of births occur at interval of less than 24 months, which result in high maternal and high infant mortality, more so in rural areas.

High Fertility

Repeated pregnancies and too closely spaced pregnancies result in unacceptable high fertility in India and more pregnancies means more danger and more risk. Too many pregnancies are risky for mothers who themselves are poorly nourished and each pregnancy costs them heavily in terms of nutrition. Though the total fertility rate has declined from 6.0 (1951) to 2.3 (2014) but many regions and states continue to have high fertility which endangers the lives of women in reproductive age group. In high fertility states, number of children born per women may be 5 or even more. Having more than 3 children increases the health risks of pregnancy and childbirth and these become much greater after the fourth pregnancy.

Anaemia and Malnutrition

Anaemia is rampant during adolescent period and over 58% of pregnant women may be anaemic and many of them are severely anaemic having haemoglobin less than 7 g%. Anaemic mothers are exposed to the risk of toxaemias, pre-eclampsia and haemorrhage after delivery and even to infections after delivery. Tracking of severely anaemic mothers is in place now. Story of anaemia begins during early childhood, continues during adolescence and becomes much more serious when women become pregnant. In the process, the "women die" to give birth. Severely anaemic mothers should not become pregnant and they must improve their anaemia first. Around 20% of maternal deaths are due to anaemia alone. We can certainly reduce this part of mortality by *adequate diet* and supplements of iron and folic-acid tablets by tracking every pregnancy.

Teenage Pregnancies and Pregnancies beyond 35 Years

Becoming pregnant before the age of 18 and after the age of 35 increases the health risks for both mother and child. Teenage pregnancies are risky pregnancies and similar he pregnancies over 35 years are risky. Hence a woman hould bear children in the age group 24–30 which is most afe.

Jnwanted Pregnancies

Jnwanted pregnancies and pregnancies out of wedlock re risky pregnancies both for mother and child, as these re often terminated by illegally induced abortions, vhich are unsafe and life-threatening most of the times.

llegal Abortions (Unsafe Abortions)

'ractice of illegal induced abortions in India is quite revalent. Around 9% of maternal mortality is due to nsafe abortions itself. Data on abortions is too scanty and nany of the abortions are done by quacks and through llegal means. Though the Government has provided afeguards for abortions through Medical Termination of 'regnancy Act but services for safe abortions are not vailable at PHCs or in urban slums.

Jnsafe Pregnancies

Each year 30 million women get pregnant and 26 million abies are born. Pregnancies which are ill-timed, too losely spaced, pregnancies to severely anaemic mothers nd teenaged pregnancies and pregnancies over the age of 5 are unsafe pregnancies.

Every year in India over 47000 women die from roblems linked to pregnancy and childbirth leaving ehind many motherless children. Making pregnancy safe an reduce maternal deaths. Content, coverage and quality f antenatal services are poor although 69% of antenatal nothers have been covered for *antenatal care services*—vho received three check ups (UNICEF-2009 CES) but nly 26% could receive full antenatal care services. Severe bstetric complications can be reduced/minimized by good ntenatal care and making pregnancies safe. Hence ssential obstetric care for all pregnant women (which at he moment is weak) is essential, as all pregnant women re at risk from obstetric complications.

Jnsafe Deliveries

Nearly 81% of deliveries in India are safe (UNICEF 2009). Around 52.3% deliveries in India occur at home in rural nd even in urban slum areas (NHP–2012–13). These eliveries are attended by trained/untrained birth ttendants. Share of institutional deliveries has increased o 78%. Deliveries attended by untrained persons and *nclean deliveries* stand to the increased risk of maternal nortality. Delivery practices of untrained birth attendants nd some of the trained birth attendants may be dangerous nd life-threatening. Recognition of danger signs during abour or delivery is essential for timely action. Target to chieve 80% of institutional deliveries and 100% deliveries y trained persons by 2015 or even earlier is a step in the ight direction to reduce maternal deaths. Skilled birth attendants (SBA) training has been intensified to promote safe deliveries at home and in institution.

Home Delivery Practices—Case Study

Over 52.3% of deliveries are home deliveries in India. In some areas, the proportion of home deliveries may be 95% or even more. Home deliveries are preferred and are advantageous to the family and government resources are limited. If all mothers decide to deliver in hospitals or institutions we will run short of resources and run into problems. However, the policy is to encourage institutional deliveries. Hospital stay after institutional delivery is very short as most mothers return home before 48 hours. In India for quite sometime, the home deliveries will continue to be popular in rural and urban slum areas. Some of the common home delivery practices in rural areas are:

- Home deliveries are conducted by traditional birth attendants (trained and untrained). Training of dais is variable and inadequate.
- Practices of these birth-attendants, such as non-washing of hands, use of unclean blade, unclean tie, unclean surface and covering umbilical cord with dirty linen, are harmful practices.
- All dais pointed out that the delivery is considered to be an impure or dirty process and hence the family or mother-in-law selects a discarded room secluded from all possible avenues of light and air. Most often the room selected happened to be a store house, a fodder house or a rear most room in the house, full of darkness and dust. The selection of the room is purposive as delivery is considered to be impure process and air and light are believed to be harmful for mother and newborn.
- Women is confined to the delivery cell after delivery at least for a period varying from 10 to 40 days and all physiological functions happen in this cell.
- Most often floor of the room chosen happens to be kutcha, and deliveries are done on unclean floor. Discarded gunny bag or old clothes are laid on floor, as cushion. This arrangement is to the satisfaction of birth attendants as it facilitates the disposal of products of labour.
- Disposable delivery kits (DDKs) are seldom provided to birth attendants and so is the status of delivery kits. Delivery kits provided to health worker female remain as an ornament to be handed over and taken over once the workers get transferred. It is therefore kept intact and seldom used by health worker female. As a policy matter, these delivery kits should be handed over to trained skilled birth attendants.
- In such a situation, the cord cutting material and cord tie material is whatever available in that situation.
- Antenatal care utilization by pregnant women tends to be low and over 80% of pregnant women tend to be anaemic. Post-delivery practices also leave much to be desired and same holds true to newborn care practices.

Care after Delivery (Postnatal Care)

Since 53% of deliveries occur in home in rural settings and many of the deliveries in urban areas too occur in home and the care immediately after delivery is available to only 36–45% of mothers (NFHS-3 and CES 2009). The postnatal care in rural areas and urban slums is negligible by health personnels, it is left to traditional birth attendants. We do know that over 60% of maternal deaths occur after birth and more than half of these take place within one day of delivery and it is sufficient hint to make sure that *puerperium* is *safe* and postnatal care is sound. Early contact with mothers and babies is critical, ideally within 24 or at the most 48 hours of birth for the first visit instead of more common visit six weeks after birth.

Women Workload

The women in Indian scenario are beast of burden and their prime function is work and work and produce children. Women workload in the farm/field, and home is energy sapping. They fetch water, fuel, fodder and work in the farm, to ground food, cook food, clean the house and care children. Energy consumption is low against heavy expenditure. Even during pregnancy, they keep on working and excessive workload makes pregnancy unsafe and risky.

Women Status (Gender Disparity)

Women status in India is low, their literacy is low, mortality level is high and social disparities and gender biases are too many which put them at risk. Information to women is low as access to modern media—newspaper, television and schooling is low which puts them to disadvantageous position to strive for self-help and self-care and utilization of services for themselves and their children. Most maternal deaths occur in economically weaker sections, illiterate and poor families. Poverty is inter-linked, universally to health.

Accessibility to Services

Services like first referral unit (FRU) and even services at PHC and CHC have not developed to the extent desired to take care of emergency obstetric care. Obstetric emergencies like obstructed labour, haemorrhages, eclampsia are life-threatening. Sometimes the access to these services may be difficult because of poor roads and lack of availability of transport. 12–15% of all deliveries may need obstetric emergency services and hence FRU should be accessible within 2 hours of travel time.

Urban/Rural Differential

MMR is higher for rural areas and it may be worst for remote rural areas because of poor access to services and least developed facilities of primary health care. Urban areas have better access to hospitals, nursing homes and private practitioners and non-governmental organizations. Institutional deliveries are more for urban areas and hence more safe deliveries and reduced risks of maternal morbidity and mortality except in urban slums.

Poor Referral Services and Transport Services

The referral services and support (functional FRUs) is sub optimal in rural areas and urban slums. Therefore the management of obstetrical emergencies is poor. Analysis has shown that 60% of maternal deaths occur during the postnatal period, 25% during antenatal period and 15% during labour and abortion. These data indicate early recognition of obstetrical complications and transportation of mothers to appropriate facility within two hours, can be life-saving by providing **referral transport services.**

Prevention of Maternal Deaths[14–19]

About 50% of maternal deaths could be prevented if women have access to essential maternity and basic health care services under RMNCH + A approach.

Promotion of Maternal and Child Health has been one of the most important objectives of the Family Welfare Programme in India. Maternal mortality can be reduced by following major strategies of:

- i Essential obstetric and newborn care services for all pregnant women (make pregnancy safe).
- ii Provision of emergency obstetric and newborn care at FRUs and referral hospitals.
- iii Skilled attendance at every birth—make delivery safe
- iv Postnatal care—make postnatal period safe.
- v Safe Abortion services/medical termination of pregnancy
- vi Prevention, management and control of RTIs and STIs
- vii Adolescent health.
- viii Community action and referral transport
- ix Fertility regulation

Continuum of maternal, newborn and child health care across life cycle—during adolescence, pre-pregnancy, pregnancy, at birth, neonatal, postnatal, infancy and childhood, connecting care giving between household, community and health facilities can reduce maternal, newborn and child deaths significantly.

Essential Obstetric Care for All Pregnant Women (Make Pregnancy Safe) Track all Pregnancies

Essential obstetric services to all pregnant women makes pregnancy safer and avoid risks, identify the danger signs and avoid *delay* by seeking health services at the earliest from nearest health facility. This includes quality antenatal care including prevention and treatment of anemia, institutional/safe delivery services and postnatal care. To provide essential Obstetric care services Government of India is Operationalizing the PHCs for 24 × 7 services and also training the SNs/LHVs/ANMs in skilled attendance at birth.

Tracking Every Pregnant Women by Name (By Mother and Child Tracking System) for Quality Services

Quality ANC includes minimum of 4 antenatal check ups. Components of good quality antenatal care include—early recognition and registration of pregnancy in first trimester, weight and height record, abdominal examination, blood test, urine test, blood grouping, Rh factor and VDRL test (where facilities exist) blood pressure measurement, consumption of iron and folic acid tablets for 100 days, calcium supplementation besides screening for gestational diabetes and hypothyroidism and tetanus immunization. The system of *tracking all pregnant women* and children to *ensure* timely antenatal and postnatal care, safe delivery and universal immunization of children with priority to weaker sections.

Prophylaxis and Treatment of Nutritional Anemia

Around 20% of maternal mortality is due to anaemia (indirect cause). Around 57.8% of pregnant women and 63.2% of lactating mothers are anaemic (NFHS-3). Adequate diet including iron rich foods (green leafy vegetables) is the sustainable solution. Under the programme all pregnant and lactating women are provided with one tablet (containing 100 mg of elemental iron and 0.5 mg of folic acid) daily for 100 days. Those who have severe anaemia (Hb less than 7 g) are provided with double dose of these tablets besides tracking these women. **Deworming** of pregnant women after first trimester is done to reduce worm load.

Convergence of services between ICDS and health sector on monthly village health and sanitation day can enhance registration of all pregnant women. The key strategy is care for the mother and newborn has to be provided from conception to the first 42 days after delivery at the home/community levels, institutions where delivery takes place and again at home after discharge from the facility.

Safe Deliveries—Make Delivery Safe

Shift the focus from institutional deliveries to safe deliveries and ensure that all deliveries are attended by skilled birth attendants/health workers. Involve private practitioners for safe deliveries through "Vande Mataram" scheme.

Strategy is to promote institutional deliveries and provision of 24 hours delivery services at PHC: under RCH-II, all the CHCs and 50% of PHCs are being operationalized for providing round the clock delivery services by placing at least 3–5 staff nurses and one medical officer in these facilities. This level provides Basic Emergency Obstetric and Newborn Care (BEmONC).

Skilled Attendance at Every Birth—New Initiative

Providing skilled attendance at every birth both, at community and institutional level can reduce maternal deaths. Currently skilled birth attendance rate reported as 78.7% in 2013–14.

Skilled Birth Attendant (SBA): It is defined as "an accredited health professional, such as midwife, doctor or nurses—who has been educated and trained to achieve proficiency in the skills needed to manage normal pregnancies, child birth and immediate postnatal period and in the identification, management and referral of complications in women and newborns." Government of India considers the "Skilled Birth Attendant" as a person who can handle common obstetric and neonatal emergencies, recognizes when a situation reaches a point beyond his/her capability and refers the woman or the newborn to an FRU/appropriate facility without delay.[20] The govt has initiated SBA resident training at district level for LHVs, ANMs and Staff Nurses. The duration of training varies from 3 to 6 weeks. The Govt of India has taken policy decision to make them competent for undertaking certain life-saving measures, such as:

- Permission to use uterotonic drugs for prevention of PPH.
- A new initiative of prevention of postpartum haemorrhages through community based advance distribution of **Misoprostol** by ASHAs/ANMs has been launched in the districts with high home deliveries rate.
- Permission to use drugs in emergency situations prior to referral for stabilizing the patient.
- Permission to perform basic procedures at community level in emergency situations at subcentre and PHC.

SBAs have been Trained to use Partograph

Partograph: It is a graphic record of progress of labour and condition of pregnant women and foetus. Dilatation of cervix, Pulse and BP, foetal heart rate are recorded on standard graph. There are two lines on graph one is *alert line* and second is *action line* with a gap of four hours between two. If cervical dilatation is progressing well the plotting line will remain on the left of alert line. In prolonged labour the plotting line moves to the right of *alert line* and such women should be referred to hospital at this point so that women can reach hospital before *action line* is reached, i.e. within four hours.

Making Home Delivery Safe

While we continue to promote institutional deliveries, we have a "responsibility to help families choosing to give birth at home to have a safe and clean labour, delivery and postpartum experience". The single most important component making a home delivery safe is ensuring that SBA attends the delivery. The second most important component is to have a plan for referral if complication arise.

Janani Suraksha Yojna (JSY)

National maternity benefit scheme from nutrition improving initiative has been modified to JSY.

JSY was launched in April 2005. The scheme has the dual objectives of reducing maternal and infant mortality by promoting safe and institutional deliveries and 48 hours stay at hospital among the poor women. Cash incentive (conditional cash transfer) are provided to the beneficiary belonging to below poverty line (BPL) families and also to village link worker/ASHA for coming to the institution for delivery and also the cost of transportation, etc. Benefits are graded in nature and vary from high performing to low performing states (HPS and LPS); and also from rural to urban areas. The funds for JSY have been given to MPHWF for disbursement. The JSY is 100% centrally sponsored through the RCH flexi-pool mechanism.

The scheme focuses on poor women of states having low institutional delivery rate namely the states of UP, Uttarakhand, Bihar, Jharkhand, MP, Chhattisgarh, Assam, Odisha, Rajasthan, J & K, while these states have been classified as low performing states (LPS), the remaining states have been named as high performing states (HPS).

Scales of cash assistance for institutional delivery under JSY

Area	LPS	HPS
Rural area		
(a) Mother's package	₹ 1400	₹ 700
(b) ASHA's package	₹ 600	600*
Urban area		
(a) Mother's package	1000	Rs 600
(b) ASHA's package	400	400*

*ASHA package of ₹ 600 in rural area include ₹ 300 for ANC component and ₹ 300 for facilitating institutional delivery. ASHA component of ₹ 400 in urban area is ₹ 200 for ANC and ₹ 200 for delivery.

Provision of hiring services of experts in Government medical facility for C section and payment of ₹ 1500 per case to hired specialist has been provided for.

Eligibility for Low Performing States (LPS)

All pregnant including those from women belonging to BPL, SC and ST families delivering in the Government health centres like Sub-centre, PHC/CHC/FRU or the general ward of district and state hospitals or accredited private health institutions.[21]

Eligibility for High Performing States (HPS)

All BPL pregnant women aged 19 years and above and all women from SC and ST families. The cash incentive for institutional delivery would be limited to 2 live births.[20]

JSY has increased access to antenatal and postnatal care.

In HPS and LPS states all such BPL pregnant women, prefering to deliver at home are entitled to cash assistance of ₹ 500/- per delivery. The conditionalities of age of pregnant women, i.e. 19 years or above and only up to two children have been removed w.e.f 8.5.2013. Implementation of scheme varies from state to state. Most mothers (50%) stay at hospital less than 24 hours against policy of 48 hours stay after delivery.

Programme monitoring: Programme monitoring need to track experiences and outcomes of women rather than only disbursement of cash.

Strengthening Delivery Points

More than 17000 'delivery points'—at SC, PHC, CHC, DH have been identified to allocate resources for comprehensive RMNCH + A services.

Delivery—Huts

For safe deliveries at village level, delivery huts have been constructed, attached with subcentre. There is arrangement for running water, electricity, equipment and facilities for safe delivery. Additional MPHW (F) and a helper has been posted to conduct safe deliveries in order to reduce deaths due to complications.

Janani Shishu Suraksha Karyakram (JSSK)

It was launched in Jan 2011. The initiative envisages free and cashless services to all pregnant women, delivering in government health institutions, as well as to sick neonates. Free entitlement include drugs and consumables, blood, free diagnostics, diet and free transport services including caesarean section. Assured package benefit extended to sick children up to age of one year.

Provision of Comprehensive Emergency Obstetric and Newborn Care (CEmONC) at FRUs (Level 3)

Management of life-threatening conditions like haemorrhages, sepsis and obstructed labour in time can save the life of many women. Provision of Emergency Obstetric and Neonatal Care at FRUs has been provided by operationalizing all FRUs in the country. Provision of adequate and timely Comprehensive Emergency Obstetric and Newborn Care (CEmONC) has been recognized globally as the most important intervention for saving life of pregnant women who may develop complications during pregnancy or child birth or after birth. The operationalization of First Referral Units (FRUs) at sub-district level or at CHCs for providing CEmONC to pregnant women is a critical strategy of RCH-II, which needs focused attention. Critical components of FRUs are manpower, anaesthesia, blood storage facilities, facilities for C section and newborn care apart from referral linkages.

Referral Services at Both Community and Institutional Levels

Establishing referral linkages between the community and FRUs is an essential component for utization of services particularly during emergencies. Since emergencies during the process of birth cannot be predicted, it is essential to place effective referral linkages which can be accessed by pregnant women in cases of obstetric emergency within **two hours of travel time.**

Referral Linkage and Transport (21000 Ambulances) has been provided through JSY in case of complications requiring surgery and blood transfusion.

Multiskilling: To fill the gap of trained manpower at FRUs the GOI has taken a policy decision and is implementing 18 weeks programme for training of MBBS doctors in life-saving skills—anaesthesia skills and 16 weeks training programme in emergency obstetric management skills including caesarean section.

Postnatal Care for Mothers and Newborn

Ensuring postnatal care within first 24 hours of delivery and subsequent home visits on day 3, 7th and 42th are the important components for identification and management of emergencies arising during postnatal period (engorged breasts, bleeding and sepsis). This strategy will reduce maternal mortality. The ANMs, LHVs and staff nurses are being made aware of and also oriented for tackling emergencies identified during these visits. The Policy document recommend duration of stay after delivery at least 48 hours at the institute and 6 hours at sub-centre.

Safe Abortion Service/Medical Termination of Pregnancies

Comprehensive Abortion Care (CAC)

Unsafe abortions account for 8–10% of maternal deaths in India. The MTP Act 1971 provides for legal and safe abortions services however availability and accessibility to safe abortion services is a challenge. Facilities for safe abortions services have been made available at 24 × 7 PHCs, FRUs and District Hospitals. Medical officers have been trained to provide CAC at PHCs. ANMs, ASHAs and field functionaries and RMNCH + A counsellors provide confidential counselling for MTP and post abortion family planning methods.

Training of Obstetrician and Gynaecologist faculty of medical colleges in the latest technology as well as non clinical aspects of comprehensive abortion care has been imparted.

At community level: Spread awareness regarding safe MTP services besides confidential counselling for safe abortions by ANMs, ASHAs and RMNCH + A Counsellors.

Most MTPs (75%) are being done in private health sector, hence encourage **Private** and **NGO** sector to establish quality MTP services.

Prevention, Management and Control of RTIs and STIs

STIs poses a major public health problem and adversely affects the reproductive health of poor and untreated women. Some of the RTIs are associated with poor pregnancy outcome and high morbidity in neonates and infants. The prevalence of RTI/STI is estimated to be 6% in adults in India and around 40% of women have symptoms of STDs at any given point of time. STIs as co-factor for HIV is well known. Under RCH II prevention, early detection and effective management of common lower reproductive tract infections have been included as a component of essential care through existing primary health care at sub-district level, i.e. in at least 50% of PHCs and all FRUs. Prevention and management of RTI/STI in pregnant women as per national guidelines on syndromic management can go a long way to prevent maternal morbidity and better outcome of pregnancy.

Adolescent Reproductive and Sexual Health (ARSH)

It is a new initiative under RCH-II. Prevent anaemia during adolescence period itself through adequate diet at home and IFA supplementation. Prevent tetanus by ensuring TT 10 and TT 16 in schools and out of school girls and provide information to adolescent girls on the reproductive health (on the issues of menstrual hygiene, age of marriage and child bearing, contraception and risk of anaemia, risks of marriage before 18 years and bearing children after 35 years). Prepare adolescents for safe motherhood. ARSH has been expanded to *Rashtriya Kishor Swasthya Karyakram* (RKSK).

Community Action—Households and Community

Since half of the women dying of pregnancy related causes die at *home*. Community and home level response is essential to prevent these deaths, to recognize the danger signs or early complications themselves and take rapid action for treatment. Education of people, mothers, community volunteer and traditional birth attendants on danger signs is essential to ensure appropriate action at community level. ASHA under National Rural Health Mission may help enhance community support. Danger signs include any bleeding in pregnancy, swelling of the body, seizures, high fever, jaundice, severe anaemia, and medical disorders (diabetes, heart disease TB, and hypertension).

Fertility Regulation

To reduce number of pregnancies, controlling fertility by contraception and having fewer pregnancies can save lives. Contraception and spacing birth at least three years apart and limiting the number of pregnancies and childbirth to two on voluntary basis and meeting the unmet needs could cut maternal mortality by one-third. Contraception and fertility regulation saves lives of mothers and improves quality of their life.

Right age of marriage and childbirth not only saves mothers lives but also it improves the lives of young children. Minimum level of literacy and universal elementary education of girls (*Sarva Shiksha Abhiyan*) and promoting their literacy and functional literacy of girls out of schools and adolescent health can lead to safe-motherhood and delaying of marriage. Promote delayed marriage for girls, not earlier than age 18 and preferably after 20 years of age.

Policy Issues

The initiative of "Safe-motherhood" envisaged at Nairobi in 1987 focused attention on women's health in reproductive period and on maternal mortality. Global programmes for safe motherhood got initiated. International Conference on Population and Development (ICPD, Cairo-1994), the Fourth World Conference on Women (Beijing 1995), and the joint WHO/UNFPA/UNICEF/World Bank statement on reduction of maternal mortality, all drew attention on the crucial issue. In India, the National Task Force on maternal morbidity and mortality was set-up in 1987 and child survival and safe motherhood programme was started in 1992. Goals of reduction of maternal mortality were set way back in 1983 under National Health Policy but these could not be achieved. Population Policy-2000 set a goal of reducing MMR below 100 by 2010. Thus, the maternal mortality has been an important issue and policy has been defined to reduce it through Reproductive and Child Health Programme. World Health Report-2005, SRS, 2006, 2009, 2011–13, countdown to 2015 initiative and Sustainable Development Goals have further drawn the attention on high MMR and its reduction to below 70 by 2030.[22–26]

New Initiative: Maternal Death Review (MDR)

It has been decided to review every maternal death at the facility level and in the community through formation of MDR committees at district level and task force at state level. The purpose of review is to find gaps in the service delivery and to take corrective actions to improve the quality of services to reduce material mortality and morbidity.

Mother and Child Tracking System (MCTS)

Web enabled mother and child tracking system (MCTS) is being used to register and track every pregnant women, neonate, infant and child by name for quality ANC, INC, PNC, FP, immunization (full maternal and child health services). The objective of MCTS is to ensure maximum coverage and thereby to reduce maternal, infant and child mortality. MCTS also helps in generation of work plan for field staff for providing full range of services on time. MCTS has been integrated with material death review. Mother and child tracking **facilitation centre** has been set up at NIHFW to validate data entered in MCTS. This centre guides and helps both the beneficiaries and service providers.

REFERENCES

1 WHO. International Classification of Diseases. ICD-10. Geneva: WHO; 1993.

2 Bala Subramanian K. Indian Institute of Health and Family Welfare. Demographic situation and reproductive child health in India. Indian Institute of Health and Family Welfare, Hyderabad. In Press Sep. 2004.

3 WHO. Making Pregnancy Safer. Towards better maternal and Perinatal health. South-East Asia Region, New Delhi: WHO; 2001.

4 Government of India. National Population Policy 2000. New Delhi: GOI; 2000.

5 Indian Institute of Population Sciences and ORC Macro. National Family Health Survey 2-1998–99. Mumbai: IIPS and ORC Macro; 2002.

6 ICMR. Collaborative study on Highrisk Pregnancies and Maternal mortality. New Delhi: ICMR; 1990.

7 Lal S, Satpathy S, Khanna P, Vashisht BMS, Kumar S. Problem of Mortality in women of reproductive age in rural area of Haryana. Ind J Maternal and Child Health 1995; 6(1): 17–21.

8 WHO/UNICEF/UNFPA. Maternal mortality in 2000–Estimates. Geneva: WHO/UNICEF/UNFPA; 2000.

9 Government of India. 10th Five Year Plan 2002–2007. New Delhi: GOI; 2002.

10 United Nations. Platform for action summary – obstacles, strategies and action. Proceedings of 4th World Conference on Women; 1995 Sept. 4–15; Beijing, China.

11 MOH and FW. National Child survival and safe motherhood programme. Programme Interventions. New Delhi: MOH and FW/GOI; 1992.

12 MOH and FW. Task force on maternal mortality and morbidity. New Delhi: MOH and FW/GOI; 1987.

13 WHO. Safe Motherhood—India backs maternal record. Geneva: WHO; 1990.

14 Deborah M. Centre of Population and family health. Safe motherhood programme and options and issues—prevention of maternal mortality. Geneva: WHO; 1986.

15 WHO. Maternal mortality: Helping women off the road to death. Based on the report of the international meeting on the prevention of maternal mortality. WHO Chronicle 1986; 40(5): 175–83.

16 MOH and FW. Safe motherhood—major causes of maternal mortality are preventable. New Delhi: MOH and FW/.GOI; 1995.

17 WHO. Mother baby package—implementing safe motherhood in countries, maternal health and safe motherhood programmes. Geneva: Division of family health organization, WHO; 1994.

18 GOI. Basic guide to reproductive and child health programme for use by NGOs, training institutions and health functionaries.

19 UNICEF. Facts for life—a communication challenge. New Delhi: India country office. UNICEF; 1990.

20 GOI. NRHM guidelines for ANC and skilled Attendance at birth by ANMs and LHVs, MOH and FW, New Delhi, 2005.

21 GOI. NRHM *Janani Suraksha Yojna*—Safe Motherhood–New Delhi, 2006.

22 WHO. World Health Report. Geneva: WHO; 2005.

23 Government of India. SRS Maternal Mortality in India, 1997–2003 and 2004–06, 2010–12, and 2011–13. Trends, causes and risk factors. Office of Registrar General of India.

24 UNICEF. The State of World's Children 2008, 2009, and 2015 Child Survival, UNICEF.
25 GOI. Special Bulletin on MMR in India, 2004–06, SRS office of RGI, India. R.K. Puram, New Delhi, April 2009.
26 GOI. NRHM, April 2010. Operational Guidelines on Maternal and Newborn Health. MOH and FW, GOI.

INFANT AND CHILD MORTALITY

Infant mortality is a most sensitive and reliable indicator of health status of a country or geographical area. Infant mortality rate (IMR) has been used in combination with other parameters to assess the physical quality of life index and Human Dvelopment Index. It is used to assess the impact of maternal and child health services. Therefore, reduction of IMR is a global goal and all health policies in India including National Health Policy of 1983, NPP of 2000, NHP-2002, and MDGs have focussed on this indicator.

$$\text{Definition of infant mortality rate (IMR)} = \frac{\text{No. of deaths under one year of age per annum}}{\text{No. of live births in the same period}} \times 1000$$

Infant mortality rate – probability of dying between birth and exactly one year of age expressed per 1000 live births.

PROBLEM OF IMR IN ASIA (Table 4.19)

Chances of survival during first year of life depend upon where one is born. Most births occurring in Japan have much better survival as compared to babies born in India or Pakistan or Bangladesh. Infant mortality rates are highest in Pakistan in the region of Asia. There are possibilities that high infant mortality rate can be reduced even without achieving marvels in economic development, the best example in India is the state of Kerala; where low infant mortality of 12 has been achieved by measures like female literacy, low fertility rate, access to quality health services, increasing woman status and over 90% deliveries in institutions. Fertility or birth rates are also very low in Kerala (14.6 per 1000). This model in India has shown the way to achieve maximum gains and ensure better quality of life even within limited economic development.

Table 4.19: Estimate of IMR for selected countries in Asia (2013).[1,2]

Country	IMR	Country	IMR
Pakistan	69	Thailand	11
India	40	Sri Lanka	8
Bangladesh	33	Malaysia	7
Indonesia	25	Japan	2
Philippines	24	Kerala (India)	12
China	11		

Source: UNICEF (2015)

INFANT MORTALITY IN INDIA

India halved its infant mortality rate (IMR) from a high of 146 (1951) to 74 in the year 1995 and it has been further reduced to 40 in 2013 a significant achievement indeed. It means better survival of children in the first year of life (Table 4.20). Decline after 2004 is very slow.

The trends of infant mortality is declining favourably in India; but still the IMR is unacceptably high as compared to many other countries and hopefully we meet the target in near future (Table 4.20).

Table 4.20: Trends of IMR in India

Year	*IMR*	*Year*	*IMR*
1951	146	2006	57
1971	129	2007	55
1980	114	2008	53
1985	97	2009	50
1990	80	2010	47
1995	74	2011	44
2002	63	2012	42
2005	58	2013	40

Source: SRS (RGI)

Goal

Goal was to reduce IMR to less than 25/1000 by the year 2017. We are moving in the right direction.

Problem

India's IMR of 40 at national level hides the shades and grades of IMR in many geographical areas of states (Table 4.21).[3] Rural IMR is higher than urban and similarly female IMR is higher than male IMR, both in rural and urban area.

Geographical Variations (Table 4.21)

There are wide interstate variations in IMR in the country. Madhya Pradesh, Assam, Odisha and UP have the highest IMR in the country, while it is lowest in the State of Kerala. Extra energies and focused interventions and differential strategies are needed in these states to reduce IMR to favourable and acceptable level. 27 states and union territories have achieved IMR of less than 40 by 2013. Similarly, IMR needs to be worked out for each district to have focused attention to reduce it favourably. The state level estimates of IMR are given by sample registration scheme (SRS); regrettably district level IMR estimates are not available for local and focal planning of reduction of incidence of IMR; district households rapid surveys generate some data but it is inadequate. Registrar General of India has now launched Annual Health Surveys (AHS) to generate IMR data at district level from 2010 onwards.

Table 4.21: Infant mortality rates for selected states in India 2013 (SRS-2014)

States	Total	Rural	Urban
Delhi	24	35	22
Assam	54	56	32
Kerala	12	13	9
Tamil Nadu	21	24	17
Maharashtra	24	29	16
Gujarat	36	43	22
West Bengal	31	32	26
Uttar Pradesh	50	53	38
Punjab	26	28	23
Haryana	41	44	32
Karnataka	31	34	24
Rajasthan	47	51	30
Andhra Pradesh	39	44	29
Madhya Pradesh	54	57	37
Chhattisgarh	46	47	38
Bihar	42	42	33
Jharkhand	37	39	28
Odisha	51	53	38
J & K	41	44	32
India	**40**	**44**	**27**

Source: SRS RGI-2013

Factors and conditions of high infant mortality can be classified into following categories:

1. Maternal Factors

Maternal age, age of marriage, age at childbirth, order of birth, birth interval, premature birth and low birth weight babies, maternal nutrition (anaemia), maternal diseases (diabetes, hypertension, heart disease, etc.) influence infant mortality.

2. Environmental Factors

Unhygienic conditions, selection of unhygienic room for delivery; unclean hands, unclean food, and unsafe water, air pollution, indoor air pollution, and unsafe excreta disposal influence infant mortality to a great extent.

3. Cultural Factors and Practices

- Lack of immunization.
- Delivery room—discarded and unclean darkest room is chosen for delivery which may lead to infections.
- Delayed initiation of breastfeeding; delayed weaning, inadequate feeding, restriction of food during illnesses like diarrhoea and acute respiratory infections and fevers.
- Discrimination between girls and boys in feeding and treatment seeking behaviour.
- Nonacceptance of contraception, early marriages (teenage marriages).

4. Social and Economic Factors

Poverty, illiteracy, economically weaker sections in general and illiterate women seek services less often and lack information on services and prevention of diseases by simple actions.

Some of the leading factors of IMR are discussed.

Rural-urban Distribution

Rural IMR is higher in India as compared with urban area. Rural IMR is 1.70 times higher than urban areas. This speaks of disparity that exists between rural and urban areas. Though there has been decline in the ratio of rural to urban IMR, yet the rural rates of IMR are significantly higher than urban rates in all the states of India. The differential tends to narrow down as the level of infant mortality declines (Table 4.21).

But all is not well in urban areas. If urban IMR is further split into IMR in urban slums versus non-slums, the IMR rate tends to be worse in urban slum areas and even may be much higher than rural IMR rates or national averages. The IMR in urban slums of Delhi and Bombay and even in other slum areas of bigger cities is much higher than non-slum areas. This evidence indicates that much more focus attentions are needed to develop measures and interventions in urban slum areas. Priority must be given to urban slums.

Sex Distribution (Gender)

IMR is higher for girls than boys in many states of India, particularly Rajasthan, Assam, Chhattisgarh and Gujarat. This speaks of neglect of female births, less care, less nutrition and neglect during illness could be the most probable reasons. Cultural practices come in the way. If a female child is borne, the couple goes for next pregnancy at the earliest, denying the female child adequate care and breastfeeding and female children are less often taken to hospitals or health facility and male children are considered precious and care for male children is sought more often and promptly as compared to female child.

Socioeconomic Background

The IMR in India varies considerably between various groups with different socioeconomic background. The IMR is higher in scheduled castes and scheduled tribes. Health services must reach to these sections on priority basis to reduce the incidence of low birth weight and IMR.

Other Epidemiological Factors

High Fertility Rates

India still has high fertility rate. 26 million birth are occurring every year. Fertility is much higher in many states and many districts of the country show much higher birth rate than India's crude birth rate of 21.4. The states of Madhya Pardesh, Rajasthan, Bihar and Uttar Pradesh have birth rates more than 26 and these are the states which have high infant mortality as well.

High-wanted fertility is due to high infant mortality rate (IMR) and this factor alone is responsible for population growth (estimated contribution about 20%).

Repeated childbirths are seen as an insurance against multiple infant and child deaths and accordingly, high infant mortality results in high fertility. More infant deaths mean more births.

Acceptance of contraception is still low in many areas, though the overall contraceptive prevalence rate in the country has increased to 56%.

Place of Birth and Type of Birth Attendant

Birth occurring in homes and by untrained birth attendants have higher risk of infant mortality, higher rates of complications, more morbidity in mothers and young children as compared to institutional deliveries. Therefore the goal is to achieve safe deliveries by skilled birth attendants and by increasing the institutional deliveries to 80% to reduce perinatal, neonatal and postneonatal deaths.

Age of Mother

Births occurring to very young mothers (teenage pregnancies) and very old mothers above the age of 35 years stand to the high-risk of mortality while births occurring between 25 and 29 years have low mortality.

Skilled Birth Attendant at the Time of Birth

Chances of survival are better if the birth is attended by skilled birth attendant, deliveries in the hands of untrained birth attendants are unsafe and it leads to more infant mortality. One of the strategy to reduce infant deaths is to train skilled birth attendants at least one for each village, more the better. Continuing education and retraining birth attendants on safe delivery saves many lives and ensures survival.

Legitimate/Illegitimate Birth

Illegitimate births have low chances of survival and face more mortality because of neglect and non-acceptability of such unwanted births out of wedlock.

Spacing of Births

Births which are spaced closely are likely to be low birth weights and have more chances of mortality as compared to births which are spaced at least three years apart. Spacing ensures healthy children and better survival after birth.

Birth Order

The first birth order and birth order 4 and above have higher risk of infant mortality.

Multiple Births

Twin pregnancy or multiple births are exposed to the risk of high mortality as these births tend to be of low birth weights, thriving and feeding of multiple births is a problem.

MAJOR CAUSES OF INFANT MORTALITY

These are shown in Table 4.22 and most of these are preventable. The principal causes of infant mortality are: Perinatal conditions (prematurity and low birth weight, sepsis, asphyxia and trauma) pneumonia, diarrhoeal diseases, parasitic diseases and congenital anamolies.

Component of Infant Mortality

Infant mortality consists of two components:[6,7]

i Neonatal mortality

ii Postneonatal mortality.

Neonatal Mortality

Over two-thirds of all deaths during infancy occur during neonatal period, i.e. within first 28 days of life and most of neonatal deaths (75%) occur in the first week of life itself.

$$\text{Neonatal death rate} = \frac{\text{Deaths among live births during the first 28 completed days of life}}{\text{No. of live births in the same period}} \times 1000$$

Table 4.22: Causes of infant mortality in India: 2010–13

Rank	Cause of death	Deaths (%)		
		Male	Female	Person
1.	Prematurity and low birth weight	35.6	36.4	35.9
2.	Pneumonia	17.0	16.8	16.9
3.	Birth asphyxia and birth trauma	10.7	9.1	9.9
4.	Other noncommunicable diseases	8.2	7.5	7.9
5.	Diarrhoeal diseases	6.2	7.3	6.7
6.	Ill defined or cause unknown	4.4	4.9	4.6
7.	Congenital anomalies	4.8	4.3	4.6
8.	Acute bacterial sepsis	4.2	4.3	4.2
9.	Injuries	2.0	2.1	2.1
10.	Fever of unknown origin	1.7	1.8	1.7
	All other remaining causes	5.2	5.7	5.4
	Total	100.0	100.0	100.0

Neonatal mortality rate – probability of dying during the first 28 completed days of life, expressed per 1000 live births.

Neonatal mortality has two parts:

$$\text{Early neonatal death rate} = \frac{\text{Deaths occurring from birth to seven days after birth}}{\text{No. of live births in the same period}} \times 1000$$

$$\text{Late neonatal death rate} = \frac{\text{Deaths from the eighth days after birth to 28 completed days after birth}}{\text{No. of live births in the same period}} \times 1000$$

Postneonatal Mortality

These are deaths after 28 completed days up to 364 days of life (Table 4.23).

$$\text{Postneonatal death} = \frac{\text{No. of deaths of infants between 28 days and under one year per annum}}{\text{No. of live births in the same period}} \times 1000$$

Trends of different components of IMR

Components	2005	2006	2007	2008	2009	2012
Early neonatal mortality	28	28	29	27	27	23
Neonatal mortality	37	37	36	35	34	29
Postneonatal mortality	22	20	19	18	16	13
Infant mortality	58	57	55	53	50	42

Neonatal mortality which is almost two-thirds of IMR is around 29 which is unacceptably higher than neighbouring countries like Nepal, Bangladesh, Bhutan and Sri Lanka.

Two-thirds of all neonatal deaths occur in the first seven days after birth. The major causes of neonatal deaths are premature birth, asphyxia and sepsis. Therefore, essential newborn care for all is a must in all settings, priority should be for those areas showing high IMR and NNMR, urban slums and rural areas and identified states and regions (Table 4.23).

Both neonatal and postneonatal mortality have declined but the postneonatal mortality has declined faster, whereas neonatal mortality has declined slowly and is still very high. It is nearly two-thirds of the infant mortality. Proportion of NNM has not changed over the years. However, NNM has declined 50% from 60 in 1986 to 29 in the year 2012[8, 9] and 28 in the year 2013.

Causes of Neonatal Deaths (2012) (Fig. 4.7)

4 Neonatal deaths constitute 53% of under five deaths. Major causes of neonatal mortality are preterm deaths or prematurity (35%), severe infection (33%), birth asphyxia

Table 4.23: Neonatal and postneonatal mortality rates (NMR and PNMR) in India, 1972–2013

Year	Neonatal mortality rate	Postneonatal mortality rate	% NNM*
1972	72	68	51
1973	68	66	51
1974	70	56	56
1975	78	62	56
1976	77	52	60
1977	80	50	62
1978	77	50	61
1979	77	52	60
1980	76	48	61
1981	70	41	63
1982	67	38	64
1984	66	38	63
1985	60	37	62
1986	60	37	62
1989	57	38	60
1990	56	27	66
1991	53	29	64
1992	51	29	63
1993	50	26	65
1995	48	26	65
1996	47	25	66
1997	46	25	65
1998	45	27	62
1999	45	24	65
2001	40	26	60
2003	37	23	61
2005	37	22	62
2006	37	20	65
2007	36	19	66
2008	35	18	66
2009	34	16	68
2010	33	14	69.3
2012	29	13	69.0
2013	28	12	70.0

Source: SRS, (RGI) Government of India[3,8]
*Percentage of neonatal deaths to total infant deaths.

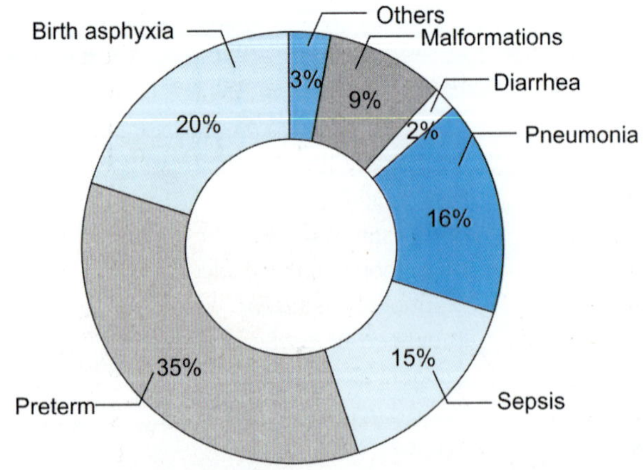

Source: Liu et al, Lancet 2012 Statistical Report

Fig. 4.7: Causes of neonatal deaths in India

and trauma (20%), congenital anomalies (9%), and others (3%). Causes are well known and these are amenable to prevention.

STILLBIRTH RATES (SBR) (Table 4.24)

Stillbirth or Fetal Death (Dead Born Fetus)

Death of foetus after 28 completed weeks of pregnancy, or the birth of a dead foetus which weighs over 1000 g or is more than 35 cm body length.

Table 4.24: Trends of stillbirth rate in India

Year	Total	Urban	Rural
1986	10.2	9.0	10.5
1987	12.9	9.8	13.6
1988	13.5	11.7	13.9
1989	12.7	11.2	13.1
1990	11.8	11.0	11.9
1991	10.7	9.6	10.9
1992	12.0	10.0	12.0
1993	10.5	9.3	10.8
1994	8.9	15.2	7.3
1996	9.0	9.0	9.0
1998	8.7	7.9	8.9
1999	10.0	8.0	11.0
2005	9.0	8.0	9.0
2006	9.0	8.0	9.0
2007	9.0	8.0	9.0
2008	8.0	–	–
2009	8.0	–	–
2010	7	7	7
2012	5	5	5

Source: SRS (RGI)

Significance

Stillbirth is an indicator of pregnancy wastage as also coverage and quality of maternal health services in an area.

Fetal death is death prior to the complete expulsion or extraction from its mother of a product of conception, irrespective of the duration of pregnancy, the death is indicated by the fact that after such separation the fetus does not breathe or show any evidence of life, such as beating of the heart, pulsation of the umbilical cord, or definite movements of voluntary muscles.

Stillbirth rate in India is around 5%. It means 5% of pregnancies get wasted due to various factors. Most of the factors are maternal and predominant of these are—maternal malnutrition, RTI and STI in women, malpresentation, obstructed labour and haemorrhage.

Stillbirth Rates: The estimated stillbirth rate (SBR) in the country is 22 per 1000 live births (Lancet 2011). The SBR from Sample Registration System (SRS) however requires careful interpretation because of under-estimation due to unreliable pregnancy history for women and misclassification of deaths. Denominator used in SRS is total births (live births + stillbirths).

Calculation

$$\text{Stillbirth rate} = \frac{\text{Fetal deaths of 28 completed weeks of gestation and more in a year}}{\text{Total births (live and stillbirths) during the same period}} \times 1000$$

PERINATAL MORTALITY

Perinatal period commences at 22 completed weeks (154 days) of gestation (the time when birth weight is normally 500 g) and ends seven completed days after birth.

For the purpose of international comparison, "Standard perinatal statistics" in which both the numerator and denominator of all rates are restricted to fetuses and infants weighing 1000 g or more (or where birth weight is not available), the corresponding gestational age (28 weeks) or body length (35 cm crown heel) should be ascertained. This rate is most difficult to arrive at:

$$\text{Perinatal mortality rate} = \frac{\text{Late fetal and early neonatal deaths weighing over 1000 g at birth}}{\text{Total live births weighing over 1000 g at birth}} \times 1000$$

OR

$$\text{PMR} = \frac{\text{Deaths occurring after 28 completed weeks of gestation (stillbirths) and up to seven completed days (early neonatal deaths) after birth}}{\text{Total live births in the same year}} \times 1000$$

The perinatal mortality rates are significant to capture late fetal deaths and early neonatal deaths and to ensure favourable outcome of pregnancy and survival of child after birth by adequate maternal care and neonatal care.

Up to year 2000, the perinatal mortality in India has not declined much and was stable at high level of more than 40. There is 9 point decline in PMR from 37in the year 2005 to 28 in the year 2012 which is a good sign hopefully the declining trend is maintained (Table 4.25). It indicates that neonatal services during first 7 days of life have improved. It also signifies that low birth weight incidence and particularly very low birth weight incidence has not much changed over the years. To make any further dent in perinatal mortality, the health and nutritional status of women must improve, anaemia must be controlled and prevented and adolescent health component needs to be strengthened and similarly postnatal care and delivery practices need to be improved. Newborn care component has been added under RCH programme but the component of neonatal care during first 7 days of life is very weak in the system of primary health care set-up.

Table 4.25: Perinatal mortality rate (PMR) in India, 1986–2012

Year	Total	Urban	Rural
1986	48.1	32.7	51.8
1987	50.1	32.4	54.4
1988	49.6	34.5	53.1
1989	47.2	31.0	50.9
1990	48.4	34.0	51.7
1991	46.0	32.7	49.1
1992	48.0	34.0	50.0
1993	44.2	31.0	47.9
1994	42.5	38.7	43.3
1996	44.0	32.0	46.0
1997	43.2	29.1	46.3
1998	42.0	29.3	45.2
1999	44.0	30.0	47.0
2000	40	26.0	44.0
2005	37	24	37
2006	37	24	41
2007	37	24	41
2009	35	23	39
2010	28	21	29
2012	28	17	31

Source: SRS (RGI)

AGE SPECIFIC MORTALITY RATE—CHILD MORTALITY RATE

Child (0–4) mortality rate (CMR) is defined as the number of deaths of children in the age 0–4 years per thousand population in the same age group.

$$\text{Age specific (0–4 years) mortality rate} = \frac{\text{Death of 0–4 years children in a year}}{\text{Population of 0–4 years children}} \times 1000$$

At the national level, CMR was 11.5 in the year 2012 while the goal is to bring down CMR to 10 per thousand children in the age group 0–4. The child mortality trends have shown a declining trend from 41.2/1000 in 1981 to 11.5 in the year 2012.

The highest child mortality rate was recorded in Madhya Pradesh (21.4) closely followed by UP (20.1), Assam (19.0), Kerala with 2.6 CMR is best performing state.

National Health Policy-1983 set the goal of reduction of child mortality rate from prevalent rate of 40 at that time, to less than 10 by 2000 but this target could not be achieved. Child mortality continues to be high. The SRS estimates of child mortality are presented in Table 4.26.

Rural child mortality is almost double than the urban areas. It means that survival chances of children in urban areas are high as compared to rural areas, because of better health facilities available in urban areas. This urban rural divide needs to be plugged and it holds true for all mortalities.

Mortality between 1 and 4 years reflects the effects of both malnutrition and common infectious diseases on child health. Girls die at the rate of 50% higher than boys do. This is evident from the adverse ratio of under six children in India as million of girls are missing. The census 2011 indicated

Table 4.26: Trends of child mortality rate in India (0–4 years age group)

Year	CMR	Urban	Rural
1981	41.2	20.4	45.5
1986	36.6	20.9	40.8
1987	35.2	18.0	39.4
1988	33.3	18.7	35.7
1989	29.9	16.9	33.2
1990	26.3	15.1	29.1
1992	26.5	15.6	29.1
1993	23.7	13.4	26.6
1994	23.9	15.7	26.1
1995	24.2	15.0	26.5
1996	23.9	14.2	26.2
1997	23.9	13.1	25.6
1998	22.5	12.8	24.8
1999	20.4	11.7	22.9
2001	19.3	10.3	19.7
2004	17.0	10.1	17.1
2005	17.3	10.3	17.3
2006	17.0	10.7	16.3
2007	16.0	9.6	18.0
2009	14.1	8.7	15.7
2010	13.3	7.8	14.9
2011	12.2	7.4	13.6
2012	11.5	7.0	12.8

SRS (RGI) of India and NFHS-3

914 girls against 1000 boys (in age 0–6 years) and this ratio is much worse in Northern states and disaggregation of data by districts unfold much worse stories and tales of foeticides and increased girl child mortality. Girls die in numbers for exceeding boys in rural and urban areas.

This is due to disparity between boys and girls and it begins at family and in the community.

UNDER-FIVE MORTALITY IN INDIA

Under-five mortality is the probability of dying between birth and exactly five years of age expressed per 1000 live births (Table 4.27). Millennium Development Goal 4 seeks to reduce under-5 mortality (infant and child mortality) rate by two-thirds between 1990 and 2015.

$$\text{U5MR} = \frac{\text{Deaths up to five years of age in a year}}{\text{Live births during the same period}} \times 1000$$

U5MR in India is declining favourably. The under-five mortality has been used as an overall indicator of development of a nation. The level of U5MR declined to 48 in 2013 and India was ranked at 49th from bottom in the world. India contributes 21% of Global U5MR.

Causes of Deaths in Under-5 Children

According to World Health Statistics 2010, almost 90% all deaths among children under-five years of age are

Table 4.27: Under-5 mortality rate in India

Year	U5 MR
1960	242
1970	202
1990	123
1999	98
2002	93
2005	74
2006	76
2007	72
2008	69
2009	64
2011	55
2012	52
2013	48

Source: UNICEF

attributable to just six conditions. These are acute neonatal conditions (mainly preterm births, birth asphyxia and infections) which account for 53% of the total; lower respiratory infection, mostly pneumonia 15%, diarrhoea 12%, malaria 8%, measles 3%, injuries 3%, and HIV/AIDS 2%. Most of these deaths are avoidable by simple affordable, and effective methods. They include oral rehydration therapy, antibiotics, antimalarial drugs and use of insecticide treated bednets, Vitamin A and other micronutrients, promotion of breastfeeding, immunization and skilled care during pregnancy and childbirth. The report stresses "Continuum of care" approach for MNCH (maternal, newborn and child health) that begins before pregnancy and extends through childbirth and into baby's childhood. For optimum safety, every mother without exception, needs professional care (Fig. 4.8).

UNICEF has advocated the use of under-5 mortality rate (U5MR) as an overall indicator of development, not only for child but also of the entire society. It has since emerged as both the composite indicator of well-being in children as well as quality of life in a society.

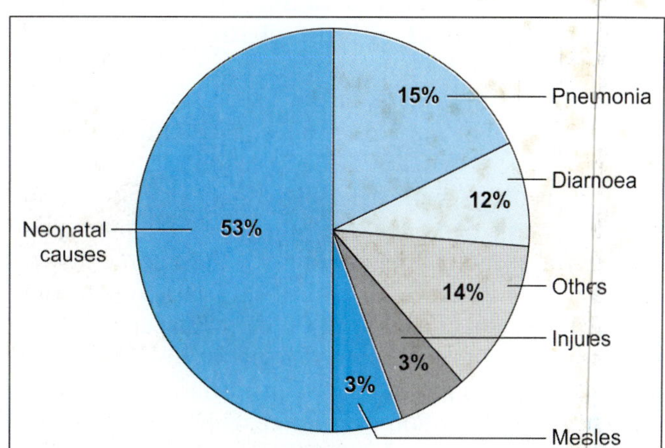

Fig. 4.8: Causes of deaths in children under-5 years 2012)

U5MR captures both child survival and health conditions of children through first five years of life.

UNICEF has chosen U5MR way back in 1987 as a composite indicator for development and considered it a much better indicator of human development than GDP. Since then the countries are being graded on the level of U5MR in descending order of their U5MR. During the year 2002, the U5MR in India was at 93 and India was ranked at 140 out of 193 countries, meaning thereby that the U5MR was unacceptably very high. It declined to 48 in the year 2013 against the target of 42 by 2015, a favourable sign of development.[10–11]

The U5MR reflects the nutritional and health knowledge of mothers, the level of immunization and ORT use, the availability of maternal and child health services (including prenatal care), income and food availability in the family, the availability of clean water and safe sanitation and overall safety of the child's environment. The U5MR is therefore chosen by UNICEF as its single most important indicator of the state of a nation's children. U5MR is the best available single indicator of social development overall, as most of the factors which it distils are indicative of the meeting of the essential needs of the human beings as they are of the particular well-being of children. The average annual reduction rate (AARR) in the levels of U5MR and illiteracy serves as a useful "speedometer" for progress against these key social indicators expressed above.

Goal is to reduce U5MR to 42 by 2015. India has achieved U5MR of 59 in 2010 and 48 in 2013.

Under-5 mortality rates were very high in the State of Madhya Pradesh, Uttar Pradesh, Odisha, Bihar, Ragasthan and these states lag behind overall development in India. Differential strategies are to be evolved for these states. Since the U5MR is an indicator of overall development, it measures the level of development in various states of India. Kerala is best state according to this rating (Table 4.28).

Table 4.28: State-wise under-five mortality rates in India 2013

State	Rate	State	Rate
India	48	West Bengal	38
Delhi	28	Andhra Pradesh	43
Haryana	48	Assam	75
Himachal Pradesh	43	Chhattisgarh	55
Jammu & Kashmir	43	Meghalaya	70.5
Punjab	34	Jharkhand	50
Rajasthan	59	Gujarat	48
Madhya Pradesh	73	Maharashtra	28
Uttar Pradesh	68	Karnataka	37
Bihar	57	Kerala	13
Odisha	68	Tamil Nadu	24

Source: SRS 2013

The Child Development Index (CDI) was developed in 2009 by Indicus Analyticus for UNICEF India. The CDI is based on three categories of indicators—Health and Nutrition, Cognitive Development and Education, and Safety and overall Child Development. The CDI is calculated using an additive approach where all the variable are normalized (to give them comparable ranges) and a simple arithmetic mean is used to calculate the index for each of three categories. The three indices are then averaged and thus each category is given an equal weightage to arrive at composite index (CDI) for each district and for each state in India.

i Health and nutrition category include—Infant mortality rate, immunization rate, oral rehydration therapy use rate, percentage of women 15–19 who have begun child bearing, percentage of children under-five who are underweight and percentage of households using iodized salt.

ii Cognitive development and education category include child literacy rate, primary and middle transition index.

iii Safety and overall child development category include—gender ratio (0–6 years), percentage of households with improved source of drinking water, percentage of households with toilet facility and percentage of crimes targeting women and percentage of crimes that are violent.

Child Survival Index [12]

The basic measure of infant and child survival is the under-five mortality rate or U5MR (number of deaths under the age of five, per 1000 live births). A child survival rate per 1000 can be simply calculated by subtracting the U5MR from 1000 and dividing this figure by 10 shows the percentage of those who survive to the age of five. In India the child survival index during year 2007 to the age of five was 92.8.

$$\text{Child Survival Index (India)} = \frac{1000-72}{10} = 92.8$$

It means over 92.8 of children survive to the age of 5 and 7.2 die before the age of five. In Sweden, Switzerland and Norway, over 99% survive to the age of five. India has to go a long way to achieve this mark.

Child Death Review: All neonatal postneonatal and child deaths will be notified, investigated for causes at community and facility level for better planning and interventions.

PREVENTION OF PREMATURITY AND LOW BIRTH WEIGHT BABIES (LBW)

Around 30% of the country's total annual births are LBW (birth weight less than 2500 g). Public health interventions to reduce low birth weight babies include: avoiding teenage pregnancies by marrying after attaining 20 years of age, improve nutritional status of women (young girls, adolescents, pre-pregnancy period and during pregnancy) particularly correcting anaemia by adequate diet and IFA supplements, full antenatal care, essential obstetrical care for all pregnant women, malaria prophylaxis, spacing births at least three years apart and limiting the size of family.

Other preventive strategies for reduction of IMR and child mortality include: aseptic delivery, delivery by skilled birth attendant at home and at institution and essential postpartum care of newborn and mother, exclusive breastfeeding, immunization against killer diseases, growth monitoring and infant and young child feeding as per national guidelines to prevent malnutrition in children and to improve environments to prevent diarrhoeal diseases and acute respiratory infections.

NATIONAL STRATEGIES TO REDUCE IMR AND CHILD MORTALITY

Goal: To reduce Infant Mortality below 25 by 2017

- To reduce Child Mortality below 10 by 2015.
- To reduce Neonatal mortality and still birthrate to less than 10 by 2030.

Strategies (interventions)

1. **Essential newborn and neonatal care at home and at all health facilities as explained below.**
2. **Infant and young child feeding:** Early initiation of breastfeeding—within one hour of birth and exclusive breastfeeding till 6 months of age with complementary feeding after 6 months along with continued breast-feeding till the age of 2 years is the single most preventive intervention for child survival and reducing IMR.
3. **Integrated management of neonatal and childhood illness (IMNCI) and facility based integrated management of childhood illness (F-IMNCI):** IMNCI includes pre-service and in-service training of providers, improving health systems, community and family level care to reduce IMR and childhood mortality. F-IMCI is the integration of facility based care package with the IMNCI package, to empower the health personnel with the skills to manage the newborn and childhood illness at the community level as well as at the facility. F-IMNCI focuses on in-patient management of major causes of neonatal and childhood mortality, such as asphyxia, sepsis, low birth weight and pneumonia, diarrhoea, malaria, meningitis and severe malnutrition in children. F-IMNCI is available at CHCs, FRUs and 24 × 7 PHCs where deliveries are taking place.

4. **Reduction in mortality and morbidity due to pneumonia and diarrhoeal diseases (ending preventable deaths by 2025):**
Integrated Action Plan for Pneumonia and Diarrhoea (IAPPD).
(a) *Childhood diarrhoea:* Accounts for 14% of mortality in newborn and children under 5 years. In order to control diarrhoeal diseases Govt. of India has adopted WHO guidelines. Goal is to reduce mortality to less than 1 per 1000 live births.
   - Low osmolarity oral rehydration therapy along with home available fluids and continued feeding during diarrhoea are the key strategies to prevent dehydration and deaths due to diarrhoeal diseases.
   - Zinc has been used as an adjunct to ORS management of diarrhoea. Addition of zinc results in reduction of the number and severity of episodes and duration of diarrhoea.

(b) *Acute respiratory infections (ARIs):* Pneumonia is responsible for 15% of deaths in newborn and children under five years. Early diagnosis and appropriate case management by rational use of antibiotics remain one of the most effective strategy to prevent deaths due to pneumonia. Goal is to reduce pneumonia mortality to less than 3 per 1000 live births by 2025.

5. **Universal immunization programme (UIP):** Under UIP of India providing vaccination to prevent killer diseases—diphtheria, pertussis, tetanus neonatorum, polio, measles, severe form of childhood tuberculosis, hepatitis B and Hib disease. Measles vaccine 2nd dose as part of routine immunization has been introduced in the country. Pentavalent vaccine has been introduced recently in UIP in limited areas.
6. **Growth monitoring and supplementary nutrition under ICDS:** To prevent malnutrition and promote growth.
7. **Supplementation with micronutrients for prevention and control of anaemia in children as also vitamin A prophylaxis.**
8. **Nutrition rehabilitation centres (NRCs):** For treating severe acute malnutrition (SAM). Severe acute malnutrition is an important contributory factor for most deaths in children. For treatment of SAM, NRCs are being set up to manage SAM and counsel mother and caregivers on feeding at home.
9. **Contraception:** Promoting at least three years of spacing between births and limiting the number of children promotes child survival and survival of mother and this also prevents low birth weight babies apart from maternal deaths.
10. **Female literacy drive (*Sarva Siksha Abhiyaan*).**
11. **Adolescent reproductive and sexual health.**
12. **Environmental sanitation (safe drinking water and safe disposal of human and animal excreta)**
System of tracking has been evolved to track all mothers and children for above mentioned interventions.

ESSENTIAL NEWBORN CARE

1. Facility Based Newborn and Child Care[14]

Neonatal mortality contributes about two-thirds of all infant deaths and about half of all under-five deaths. Infant mortality has declined from 58 per thousand live births in 2004 to 40 per thousands live births in 2013. However, there is slow progress in reducing neonatal mortality which declined from 37 in 2004 to 29 in 2012. Deaths in the first weak of life has shown least progress. It has been estimated that health facility based interventions can reduce neonatal mortality by as much as 25–30% (Lancet 365:977–88).

Newborn Care at Different Levels

Health facility levels	All newborns at birth	Sick newborns
• Primary health centres/subcentres Identified as MCH level I	Newborn care corner in labour room	Prompt referral
• Community health centres/first referral units—MCH level II	Newborn care corner in labour room and in operation theatre	Newborn stabilization unit (NBSU)
• District hospital—MCH level III	Do	Special newborn care unit (SNCU)

(a) Newborn Care Corner (NBCC)—Level I

This is a space within the delivery room in any health facility where immediate care is provided to all newborns at birth. This area is *mandatory* for all health facilities where deliveries are conducted. This level provides care of normal newborn above 2500 g at birth—for prevention of infection, provision of warmth, resuscitation, Early initiation of breastfeeding, weighing the newborn besides immunization. This level also identifies *sick newborn for prompt referral*.

(b) Newborn Stabilization Unit (NBSU)—Level II

Neonatal Stabilization unit is a facility within or in close proximity of maternity ward where sick and low birth weight newborns can be cared for short period. It is 4 beded units. All First Referral Units (FRUs/CHCs) need to have a Neonatal Stabilization Unit, in addition to the newborn care corner. This level provides all the services as of level I plus it provides care of sick newborn like, management of low birth weight infant ≥1800 g with no other complications; phototherapy for newborns with hyper-bilirubinemia, management of newborn sepsis, besides stabilization of referrals of sick newborns and those with very low birth weight (rooming in), also referral services and immunization.

(c) Special Newborn Care Unit (SNCU)—Level III

Special newborn care unit (SNCU) is a unit in the Vicinity of labour room which provides special care for **sick newborns.** Any facility with more than 3000 deliveries per year should have a SNCU (most district hospitals, and hospitals attached with medical colleges would fulfill this criteria). Besides essential newborn care this facility provides care of sick newborn, manages low birth weight infants < 1800 g, manages all sick newborn (except those requiring mechanical ventilation and major surgical intervention), besides follow-up of babies discharged from the unit and care to high-risk newborn, referral services and immunization. The minimum number of beds for SNCU at district is 12.

(d) Janani Shishu Suraksha Karyakram (JSSK)

Free Service-Guarantee and Elimination of out of pocket expenses: Implemented across the country entitles all pregnant women delivering in public health institutions to absolutely free and no expense delivery including caesarian section.

- Absolutely free treatment for all sick children (first 30 days of life) in public health institutions, now the benefits have been extended till one year of age.
- Benefits also extended for complications during antenatal, intranatal and postnatal periods.
- Free assured transport (ambulance service from home to health facility, inter-facility transfer in case of referral and drop back.)

District Early Intervention Centres (DEIC)

Follow-up of sick newborn after discharge from newborn facilities can be taken up at DEIC that are under Rashtriya *Bal Swasthya Karyakram* (RBSK), a newly announced scheme launched in 2013.

(e) Navjat Shishu Suraksha Karyakram (NSSK)[15]

NSSK aims at training health personnel in basic newborn care and resuscitation has been launched to address care at birth issues, i.e. prevention of hypothermia, prevention of infection, early initiation of breastfeeding and basic newborn resuscitation. Essential newborn care and resuscitation is an important starting point for any neonatal programme and is required to ensure the best possible start in life. The objective of this new initiative is to have a trained health person in basic newborn care and resuscitation at *every delivery* point. Delivery points are being strengthened in terms of human resources, equipment for providing comprehensive range of MCH and FP services.

2. Home Based Newborn Care (HBNC) and Home Based Postnatal Care (HBPNC)—Rationale

Around 25–40% pregnant women deliver in homes, and those women delivering in institutions/hospitals return home after 48 hours of delivery and nearly 50% return to home before 48 hours. Even while we continue to promote institutional deliveries we have a "responsibility to help family choosing to give birth at home to have safe and clean labour, delivery, postpartum experience and care to all newborn babies". It is now well established that community newborn care significantly impacts the newborn mortality. To improve care in the community, the IMNCI was launched in India in 2003. At the same time the effectiveness of home based newborn care was established by Dr Abhay Bang through trained community health workers in the tribal area of Gadchiroli district in Maharashtra.[16]

Objective: The major objective of HBNC and HBPNC is to reduce neonatal mortality and morbidity apart from reducing maternal morbidity and mortality.

Key activities: Essential Care of every newborn and postnatal mother (mother baby cohort) through a series of home visits by a trained health worker in the first six weeks of life and in most states this health worker is ASHA. Six home visits in case of institutional deliveries (Day 3, 7, 14, 21, 28 and 42), seven home visits in the case of home delivery (Day 1, 3, 7, 14, 21, 28 and 42). An examination of every newborn for prematurity and low birth weight, ensuring that birth weight is recorded on the mother and child protection card (MCP) and ensure early initiation of breastfeeding[17]:

- Delay bathing up to 7 days in all newborns
- Ensuring that newborn is immunized with BCG, first dose of OPV, DPT and entered into MCP card.
- Ensuring birth registration.
- Ensuring mother and newborn are safe until the 42nd day of delivery.
- Extra home visits for low birth weight babies by ASHA and ANM and referral for appropriate care.
- Early identification of illness in the newborn for referral and appropriate home care and follow-up of sick newborns after discharge from hospital/facilities.
- Counseling the mother on breastfeeding, warmth, care of the baby, immunization, postpartum complications and enabling referrals apart from adopting an appropriate family planning method.

ASHA is required to mobilize all pregnant mothers to ensure that they receive full package of antenatal care. The 8th to 9th month visit is used for preparing the family for birth, motivating mother and family members for institutional delivery.

Payment/incentive: ASHA is paid ₹ 250 for conducting home visits for the care of newborn and postnatal mothers. The payment are made on 45th day after validation by facilitator (ANM). The ASHA is supported and guided by the health system which is directly responsible for newborn and child survival. Support of ANM and medical officers is essential for responsive referals which will add to the credibility and improve the performance of ASHA.

4

INDIA NEWBORN ACTION PLAN (INAP) SEPT 2014

INAP aligns with the Global Every Newborn Action Plan (GENAP) launched in June 2014 at 67th world Health Assembly to advance the Global strategy for Women's and Children's Health. The INAP is to be implemented within the existing RMNCH + A framework.

Goals: Two specific goals of INAP are:

i Ending preventable newborn deaths to achieve single digit "Neonatal Mortality Rate" (NMR less than 10) by 2030 from current level of 29.

ii Ending preventable stillbirths to achieve "Single Digit Stillbirth Rate" (SBR less than 10) by 2030 from current level of 22 per thousand live births. The development of INAP has provided an opportunity to review and strengthen the specific newborn health interventions listed under RMNCH + A.

Strategic Intervention Packages: The recently launched Lancet Every Newborn series estimated that million of newborn deaths could be prevented each year by evidence based high impact interventions. These interventions have been grouped into six packages corresponding to the various life stages of newborn. High coverage (90%) of available interventions package by 2025 could prevent almost 75% of newborn deaths, one-third of stillbirths and half of maternal deaths.

The package with greatest impact on neonatal mortality (in decreasing order) include:

i Care during labour and child birth.
ii Care of small and sick newborn.
iii Care of healthy newborn
iv Immediate newborn care
v Preconception and antenatal care
vi Care beyond newborn survival.

Package 1: Preconception and Antenatal Care

Adolescent pregnancies have a higher risk of adverse birth outcomes, with a 50% increased risk of stillbirths and neonatal deaths. Adolescent and maternal undernutrition, anaemia, interpregnancy interval less than 12 month have been linked to low birth weight babies and small for gestational age (SGA) babies. Importance of antenatal care for improved neonatal and perinatal outcome is well established. Health intervention before conception, such as adolescent friendly health services (nutrition and reproductive health counselling), immunization, prophylaxis for anaemia delaying age of marriage and age at first pregnancy, birth spacing and counselling for birth preparedness, multiple micronutrient supplementation (IFA and iodine), antenatal screening for management of mild to moderate and severe anaemia, pregnancy induced hypertention, diabetes, hypothyroidism eclampsia, pre-eclampsia, can reduce maternal and neonatal mortality. Prevention against malaria by intermmitent prophylaxis and use of long lasting insecticidal bednets in endemic areas.

Package 2: Care During Labour and Child-birth—Most Critical

i Care during labour and childbirth have the potential to reduce stillbirths by a third.

ii Basic emergency obstetric care can reduce intrapartum related neonatal deaths by 40%.

iii Comprehensive emergency obstetric care can also reduce neonatal mortality by 40%.

iv Whereas skilled attendance at birth alone without access to emergency care has a smaller effect at 25%.

v Antenatal corticosteroids use to manage preterm labour not only reduces neonatal deaths by 31% but this intervention is also associated with reduced need to specialized care for newborn, such as ventilators, etc.

Use of Antenatal Corticosteroids in Preterm Labour (Under Specific Conditions by ANM)

Out of 26 million live births 3.5 million are born Preterm. Around 35% of neonates die because they are preterm babies, i.e. borne alive before 37 weeks of pregnancy. Most common cause of death among preterm babies less than 34 weeks is Respiratory Distress Syndrome (RDS). This is an acute lung disease due to surfactant deficiency in the lungs which lead to atelactasis and subsequent failure of gas exchange. RDS can be prevented by administering injection corticosteroids to pregnant woman.

Objective: To reduce morbidity and mortality in preterm births.

- A single course comprising of four doses of injection Dexamethasone 6 mg each at 12 hours interval by intramuscular route to be given to all pregnant women going to preterm labour (24–34 weeks of gestation).
- ANM's will administer pre-referral dose and refer the case to higher facility.
- Quality antenatal care, skilled attendance at birth, kangaroo mother care for preterm and low birth weight babies will continue to contribute towards reducing the morbidity and mortality in preterm babies.

vi Antibiotic administration for premature rupture of membrane (PROM) reduces early onset of postnatal sepsis.

vii Clean birth practices especially handwashing with soap and water by birth attendant has been found to reduce mortality due to sepsis in births at home (15%), facilities (27%) and during postnatal period (40%).

Package 3: Immediate Newborn Care

Essential care for all newborn, this includes: delayed cord clamping (1–3 minutes after birth), interventions to prevent hypothermia (immediate drying, head covering, skin to skin care, avoidance of bathing during the first 24 hours), early initiation and exclusive breastfeeding,

4

hygiene to prevent infections, vitamin K at birth, neonatal resuscitation to babies who do not breathe at birth and advanced neonatal resuscitation. About 10% of newborns require assistance to breathe at birth, while only 1% need advanced newborn resuscitation. Birth asphyxia contributes to 20% of all neonatal deaths.

Package 4: Care of Healthy Newborn

Community based interventions can significantly improve child survival. These include (I) Home based newborn care (HBNC) by home visits till six weeks by trained ASHA focusing on: counselling, prevention of hypothermia, cord care, early identification of danger signs, prompt and appropriate referral, (II) exclusive breastfeeding (III) clean postnatal practices (IV) immunization–BCG, OPV and Hepatitis B.

Injection Vitamin K Prophylaxis at Birth (in Facilities)

Vitamin K administration to infants soon after births is an effective, safe and sustainable approach to prevent vitamin K deficiency bleeding (VKDB)

All newborns delivered in the facilities at all levels (both public and private) should be given vitamin K injection within 24 hours of birth by intramuscular injection.

Dose: Birth weight 1000 gm or more: 1 mg

Birth weight less than 1000 gm 0.5 mg

Package 5: Care of Small and Sick Newborn

Small babies due to preterm birth or small for gestational age (SGA) or a combination of both run high-risk of death. Significant intervention include (I) Thermal care and feeding support for home deliveries, (II) Integrated management of newborn and child illness (IMNCI) and use of oral antibiotics, (III) Full supportive care at block and district level in: Newborn stabilization Unit (NBSU) at block level (CHC and first referral unit). Sick newborn care unit at district level by special newborn care unit (SNCU), (IV) Intensive care services, Neonatal intensive care unit (NICU) at regional level for assisted ventilation, surfactant use, and surgery. (V) Injectable Gentamicin by ANMs for sepsis as pre-referral dose and completion of antibiotic course in case referral is refused/not possible "OR" as advised by treating physician.

Use of Gentamicin by ANM's for Management of Sepsis in Young Infants under Specific Conditions

Objective: Objective of treatment is to reduce neonatal deaths due to Sepsis and Pneumonia.

As per SRS 2013 neonatal mortality accounts for 70% of total infant deaths and 56% of total under five deaths.

According to Lancet 2012 estimates neonatal infections or sepsis constitute 33% of neonatal deaths. Improved survival of young infants (0–2 months) depends greatly on the prevention, detection and treatment of systemic infections (sepsis and pneumonia).

Under IMNCI all ANM's have been well trained to recognize signs of suspected sepsis or possible serious becterial infection in young infants and provide pre-referral treatment:

- ANM's should administer pre-referral dose of injection Gentamicin along with oral Amoxycillin to young infants (0–2 monts).
- If the infant has not completed the course of either of the antibiotic following discharge from a health facility the ANM will complete the course of treatment.
- If referral is not possible or refused—under this special situation where referral is not possible or is refused the ANM will continue to give treatment for 7 days. Dose of Gentamicin is 5 mg/kg/once a day for seven days by intramuscular injection. Dose of Amoxycillin is 25 mg/kg/day twice a day orally for 7 days.

Kangaroo Mother Care (KMC) and Optimal Feeding of Low Birth Weight Babies (LBW)

KMC is simple method of care for low birth weight babies that includes early and prolonged skin to skin contact with the mother or substitute caregiver and exclusive and frequent breastfeeding.

Components: KMC has two components

1. Prolonged skin to skin contact
2. Exclusive breastfeeding.

WHO recommends skin to skin care immediately after delivery for **every newborn,** irrespective of birth weight to ensure warmth and early initiation of breastfeeding. In delivery room KMC is meant for stable LBW infants and denotes a sustained long duration skin to skin contact.

Duration-short: 4 hours daily. Extended: 5–8 hours daily. Long: 9–12 hours daily.

Priority: Though all LBW infants should be provided KMC but considering the huge burden at facilities, priority must be given to infants with weight less than 2000 g.

The two Prerequisites of KMC:

- Support to mother in hospital and at home
- Post discharge follow-up.

Benefits of KMC

- Reduces risk of hypothermia
- Promotes lactation and weight gain
- Reduces infections and hospital stay
- Better bonding between mother and newborn.

Steps in Providing KMC

- Counsel the mother/caregiver, provide privacy to mother. Request the mother to sit or recline comfortably.
- Undress the baby gently except for cap, nappy and socks.
- Place the baby prone to mother's chest in an upright position with the head slightly extended, between the

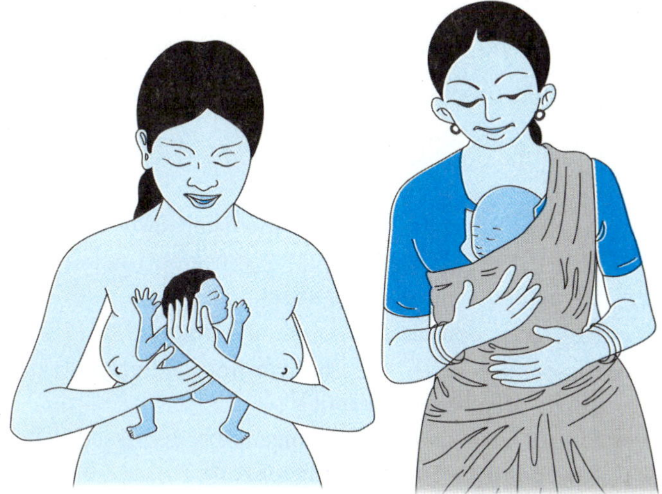

Fig. 4.9: KMC position

breasts in skin to skin contact in frog like position, turn baby's head to one side to keep airway clear. Support the baby's bottom with sling/binder.

- Cover the baby with mother's pallu or gown, wrap the baby-mother duo with an added blanket or shawl depending upon the room temperature.
- Advise mother to breastfeed LBW babies frequently (every 2 hours)–exclusive breastfeeding be promoted up to 6 months. Alternate method of feeding when direct breastfeeding is not possible are feeding tube, spoon, paladai or cup.
- Ensure warm room temperature maintained between 25–28°C.
- Advise mother to provide KMC for at least one hour per session. The length of skin to skin contact should be as long as possible.
- **Where?** KMC can be provided at Home, at Special Newborn Care Unit (SNCU), postnatal ward or neonatal ward.

Discontinuation: Often an infant is taken off KMC when the weight is around 2500 grams.

Package 6: Care Beyond Newborn Survival

Interventions to care for newborns beyond their survival include:

i. Screening for birth defects, failure to thrive and developmental delays
ii. Follow-up visits of SNCU discharged babies till one year of age, small and low birth weight babies till 2 years of age.
iii. Management of birth defects–diagnosis, and treatment including surgery at higher level of facility.

REFERENCES

1 UNICEF. The State of the World's Children. New York: UNICEF; 2004.

2 Indian Institute of Health and Family Welfare. Balasubramanian K. Demographic situation and reproductive and child health in India. Hyderabad: IIHFW; 2004.

3 RGI. SRS Bulletin 2004 to 2005. Apr. New Delhi. RGI GOI; 2004 to 2006, 2008 to 2014.

4 UNICEF. The State of the World's Children. New York: UNICEF; 1998.

5 Lal S, Kumar V, Vashisht BMS, Malik JS, Punia MS. Surveillance of vital events in rural areas. IJCM 1998; 23(4).

6 WHO. International Classification of Diseases 1975. Revision Vol. I. Geneva: WHO, 1977.

7 WHO. International Classification of diseases 1993. 10th Revision Vol. 1. Geneva: WHO; 1993.

8 CBHI. Health Information of India 2000 and 2001. New Delhi: DGHS. MOH and FW, GOI; 2001.

9 MOH and FW. National Population Policy 2000. New Delhi: Dept. of Family Welfare. MOH and FW, GOI; 2000.

10 MOH and FW. National Child Survival and Safe Motherhood Programme. Programme Interventions Safe Motherhood, Newborn Care, New Delhi: MCH Division, MOH and FW, GOI; 1994.

11 UNICEF. The State of the World's Children. Women and Children. The double dividend of equality UNICEF. 2007 to 2015.

12 UNICEF. The State of the World's Children. New York: Division of Information and Public Affairs, UNICEF; 1987.

13 GOI, WHO and UNICEF (September 2014) Integrated Action Plan for pneumonia and diarrhoea (IAPPD).

14 Government of India, MOH and FW. Facility Based Newborn Care Operational Guidelines 2011.

15 Bang AG, Bang RA, Baitule BS, Reddy MH, Deshmukh MD. Effect of home based neonatal care and management of sepsis on neonatal mortality: field trial in rural India. The Lancet 1999 Dec;354:1955–61.

16 Government of India, MOH and FW. Home based Newborn Care Operational Guidelines 2011.

17 Government of India, MOH and FW. Annual Report 2011–2014.

CONTRACEPTIVES IN NATIONAL FAMILY WELFARE PROGRAMME

The National Family Welfare Programme was initiated in 1952 and expanded with increasing efforts and inputs in successive plans, the crude birth rate is still 21.4 per 1000 population (SRS-2013) with annual growth rate of 1.47% which is still very high. Total fertility rate (TFR) has declined steadily to level of 2.3 in 2013. It is estimated that only 54.8% of currently married women use contraceptive methods of which only about 11% are using spacing methods. By far, the most popular method of contraception is sterilization which is adopted by 35.8% of women. Among sterilizations, about 99% are on women with men contributing very little. Although the contraceptive prevalence rate (CPR) has increased from

22.8% in 1981 to 54.8% in 2012–13, the impact in reduction of birth rate has not been as significant. This is because most of the couples who accepted sterilization, already had 3 or more children. Therefore, to bring down the birth rate significantly, it would be necessary to provide effective contraceptive coverage to about 75% of couples; special attention being given to younger couples with 2 or less children through the promotion of spacing methods (Table 4.29).[1]

Table 4.29: Trends of contraceptive use rate in India by currently married women, age 15–49

Methods	*NFHS-1 92–93*	*NFHS-2 98–99*	*NFHS-3 2005–06*	*DLHS 2012–13*
Any method	40.7	48.2	56.3	54.8
Any modern method	36.5	42.8	48.5	48.2
Female sterilization	27.4	34.1	37.3	35.8
Male sterilization	3.5	1.9	1.0	1.1
IUD	1.9	1.6	1.8	1.8
Pill	1.2	2.1	3.1	3.6
Condom	2.4	3.1	5.3	5.5

Figures are in percentages source: NFHS and NHP 2015

PEARL INDEX

The use effectiveness of a contraceptive depends upon the client and the method. The Pearl index, universally accepted measure of contraceptive efficacy, is the pregnancy rate per 100 women years of use of a given contraceptive method. It is calculated as below:[2]

$$\text{Pearl index} = \frac{\text{No. of pregnancies}}{\text{Cycles of use}} \times 1200$$

Failure-rate of Contraceptive

The corrected Pearl index is calculated in the same manner, but reflects only those pregnancies which are attributable to failure of the contraceptive method used.

Services for Eligible Couples

Promoting use of contraceptive methods among eligible couples is important to prevent unwanted pregnancies. Couple should be able to choose from various contraceptive methods including condoms, oral pills, IUDs, male and female sterilization.

Safe services for medical termination of pregnancies should be encouraged for women desiring abortions.

Emphasis should be on informed choices of contraception.

Adopt the principle of GATHER approach in promoting contraceptive practices.

Assess the contraceptive needs of eligible couples by contacting all eligible couples and ensuring services at Subcentre, PHC, CHC or District level facility.

Greet the clients, ask their needs, tell about different methods—their advantages and disadvantages. Help the client to choose suitable method. Explain how to use the method and return visit of follow-up.[3]

The whole process is helping the client to choose a method:

G = Greet the clients, make them comfortable—respect them

A = Assess their needs–listen to them and show concern

T = Tell different methods of contraception—their advantages and disadvantages

H = Help the client to choose suitable method

E = Explain how to use the method—demonstrate effectively on model or TV

R = Return visit or follow-up needs be discussed. The whole process is to help the clients.

Currently, the following methods are available under the National Family Welfare Programme to the acceptors of family planning:

BIRTH CONTROL METHODS

a. Spacing Methods—Reversible Methods

There has been a shift in the family planning approach to promote spacing rather than just terminal methods of family planning. RMNCH dedicated counselors are being placed in district hospitals and at the facilities with high case load to promote spacing methods.

- Condom for spacing births and prevention from STI/RTI/HIV/AIDS
- Oral pills—oral contraceptive pills
- IUD (intrauterine devices)
- Diaphragms and spermicides

b. Terminal Methods (Sterilization)

- Vasectomy (including no scalpel vasectomy)
- Tubectomy (by minilap of laparoscopic method)

Condom

Most male condoms are made of latex while some are made of polyurethane. Male condoms are of two types—non-lubricated and lubricated.

Condom is the most widely known and used barrier device by the males around the world. In India, it is marketed by the name Nirodh. Condom protects both men and women from sexually transmitted diseases including HIV/AIDS. Government of India has made available three brands of condoms: New lubricated Nirodh, deluxe Nirodh and super deluxe Nirodh. These are available in the market under Social Marketing Scheme at a subsidized rate. Nirodh is also available free in all government hospitals, community health centres, primary health centers and subcentres. Use effectiveness of condom is 88%. Failure rate is quite high having Pearl index of 12. It diminishes sensation leading to impairment of pleasure, and may occasionally cause reactions. Only 6% of men in India are using condom inspite of its easy availability and accessibility.

To increase the availability of condom to the users and to promote the use of condom, distributors of condoms may charge sales promotion incentive at 10 paise per piece of deluxe/super deluxe variety of Nirodh and at 3 paise per piece sold in case of new lubricated variety.

To increase the access and use of condom, condom vending machines (CVMs) have been installed at prominent points. Under condom social marketing programme condom promotion programme has been scaled up in 370 high HIV prevalence and high fertility districts in states.

Female Condom (FC)

Female condoms are made of polyurethane. One advantage of it over male condom is that its size and shape enables it to cover the wider surface area, including some of the external genitalia, thus it may offer additional protection against infections that can be transmitted by contact with skin, normally not covered by male condom. However, female condom is expensive. It is freely available in open market but not yet included in the National Family Welfare Programme. It ensures protection from HIV/STD/RTI, besides spacing births. National AIDS Control Programme under social marketing programme is implementing FC programme in Andhra Pradesh, Tamil Nadu, West Bengal and Maharashtra.

RMNCH + A counselors are being placed at various facilities to promote contraception.

Oral Pills

At present, about 70 million women worldwide use oral pills. In India, only 4% of women in reproductive age group use oral pills. The pills are available under the National Family Welfare Programme under two brand names:

i **Mala-N:** For free distribution through Government hospitals, community health centres, primary health centres and subcentres. Composition of Mala-N is Levonorgestrel IP 0.15 mg and Ethinyloestradiol IP 0.03 mg.

ii **Mala-D:** Under the social marketing scheme through chemist shops, grocery shops, pan shops, etc. at a highly subsidized price of ₹ 2/- per packet. A sales promotion incentive of 25.0 paise is provided to the marketing companies/NGOs. In order to further promote the use of the pill, these companies have also been allowed to sell oral pills of their own brand name. Such brands are available in the market as 'Ecroz'; 'Pearl', 'Moti' 'Choice', etc. at a price ranging from ₹ 3 to 7 per cycle. Composition of Mala-D is D-norgestrol 0.5 mg and Ethynyloestradiol 0.04 mg. Each packet of Mala-N and Mala-D contains 28 pills (21 white hormonal contraceptive pills and 7 black coloured iron pills). Use effectiveness of oral pills is very high—99.2%. Mala-D and Mala-N are to be started on 5th day of menstrual cycle and thereafter to be taken regularly till desired.

Weekly Oral Pill: Centchroman

A weekly oral pill developed by Central Drug Research Institute, Lucknow, is a non-steroidal and non-hormonal contraceptive pill which is virtually free from side effects like nausea, vomiting, dizziness or other systemic effects like weight gain, thrombotic episodes, etc. It can be given to all women of reproductive age group who want to space their children.

The first tablet is to be taken orally on the first day of the menstrual cycle and thereafter twice a week, three days apart and on the same day every week, for three months followed by once a week same day every week, for as long as contraceptive protection is desired.

Centchroman is being manufactured in India by M/s Hindustan Latex Limited. It is marketed under the name of 'Saheli' or Novex and is freely available in the market. Each tablet contains 30 mg Centchroman.

Since1995, it is being subsidized under social marketing programme. The pill is now available in the market at ₹ 2 per tablet.

Intrauterine Device (IUD)—Key Spacing Method

Promotion of spacing methods (Interval IUCD and Postpartum IUCD). IUCD is a key spacing method and in 2006 Government of India launched "Repositioning IUCD in National Family welfare Programme" IUCD 375 provides protection for 5 years.

IUD 380A is one of the most effective reversible contraceptive method and once inserted it remains effective for 10 years. It is a one time convenient spacing method for preventing pregnancy and does not interfere with sexual desire or intercourse. Yet only 2% of currently married women use IUD as a method of preventing pregnancy. Three common reasons for low IUD use in India are; first the women are not being clearly advised about minor inconveniences expected for first few weeks which are not the reasons for IUD removal. Secondly, the skill of the ANM is inadequate which leads to early removal of IUD. Thirdly, the women are not being screened for STI/RTI. IUD insertion in such woman leads to substantial complications leading to early removal. The most common side effects are alteration in normal menstrual pattern like prolonged bleeding, cramps in abdomen, etc. The normal menstrual pattern, however, returns within 3–6 months of use in most women. To address the unmet need in IUD fixed day static services (FDS) for IUD insertion has been provided at the level of subcentre and PHC (at least two days in a week).

Different Types of IUDs[4, 5]

- *First generation IUDs:* Lippes loop introduced in 1965.
- *Second generation IUCDs:*
  - –Earlier device: CU-7 and CUT-200
  - –Newer device: TCu-200B, TCu-380A
  - –Nova T: (Multiload devices) (MLCu-250, MLCu-375)

- *Third generation IUCDs:*
  These are hormonal devices, such as:
  – Progestasert
  – LNG 20 (Mirena Levonova)

Copper T-375

Cu IUCD 375 with effectiveness of 5 years as a short-term spacing method has been introduced.

Copper-T-380A

An advanced version of IUD, i.e. Cu-T-380A has been introduced in the national family welfare programme in 2003–04. This has longer life of placement in the body and thus provides protection from pregnancy for a period of about 10 years. It has replaced the earlier Cu-T-200B.

Effectiveness

Use effectiveness of copper T is 97–99%. With most devices, pregnancy rates range from less than 1 to 3 per 100 women per year. Among widely used Copper IUDs, three are most effective–The TCu-380A, TCu-220C and MLCu-375 with TCu-380A being the most effective of these having effective life of 10 years from the date of insertion. Pregnancy rates for all major IUDs are less than 1% per 100 women per year.

Timing of Insertion and Follow-up

IUD insertion is safe and effective at any time during the menstrual cycle. Conventional practice is insertion during the first five days of menstrual cycle. Thus when it is reasonably sure that woman is not pregnant, the best time to insert IUD is when she comes to the health centre to request it. Postpartum insertion and post-abortion insertion can be safely undertaken. "Fixed day services" are being made available at all levels of health facilities. The acceptors need to return for follow-up visits after 1, 3 and 6 months of insertion.

Use Rate

Current use rate of IUD is only 1.8% in India. One of the main reason of underutilization of IUD in India is that many health service providers and potential clients lack accurate, up to date information about the IUD.

Postpartum Family Planning (PPFP) Services

Immediate postpartum intrauterine contraceptive device (PPIUCD) insertion of IUCD (CuT-380A) is a new intervention introduced in the country to address high unmet needs of spacing during postpartum period. Postpartum sterilization of female has also increased by this intervention.

New Initiatives—Contraceptives at Doorstep

To improve access to contraceptives by eligible couples a scheme to deliver contraceptives at doorstep is being implemented in the entire country. Services of ASHA are being used. The packs of contraceptives are marketed as "GOI supply for home delivery by ASHA". ₹ 1 for pack of 3 condom and ₹ 1 for a cycle of OCPs and ₹ 2 for pack of one tablet of Emergency Contraceptive Packet (ECP).

ENSURING SPACING AT BIRTH

Services of ASHAs are being used for counselling newly married couples to space births three years apart and delay the first birth by 2 years in newly married couples.

Alternate Method of Training in IUCD[6]

Lady medical officers, Medical officers, Health workers female, Supervisors and staff nurses have been trained for IUDs insertion. A versatile training tool—ZOE Gynecologic Simulator pelvic model has been used for demonstration and practice of IUD insertion and removal by health professionals. It is full size model of adult female lower torso (abdomen and pelvis),[4,5] incorporating adult learning principles and humanistic training techniques started in 2007.

Diaphragms and Spermicides

A rubber diaphragm is inserted into the vagina prior to intercourse where it covers the cervix completely. To increase the effectiveness, a spermicidal jelly is used along with it.

Merits

More reliable than the rhythm or withdrawal method.

Drawback

Failure rate is quite high. Pearl index is 15. Needs elaborate preparation before the sex act and may occasionally cause local reaction.

Sterilization (Male) No Scalpel Vasectomy

The Department of Family Welfare is implementing UNFPA's supported, **'no scalpel vasectomy'** project to promote male participation in the National Family Welfare Programme. "No scalpel vasectomy" is a new technique of performing male sterilization, which is very simple and easy to perform without any stitch or cut and with least complications. The project has been under implementation since January, 1998. Till date, the project has covered 20 states in the country holding NSV training courses in 186 districts, performing 44,038 NSV operations, training 506 doctors in NSV technique and 39 certified trainers who would further train doctors in NSV. The main objective of the project is to make available the NSV technique at the periphery for men to avail. The progress of the project has been very good with the national average for male sterilization increasing from 1.9% in 1997 to 2.5% in 1996 and it has further improved to 5.6% in 2009–10[7–8].

In case of male sterilization eligible couple is considered to be 'inactive' after 4 months.

Sterilization (Female)

In early 70s, the share of female sterilization to total sterilization done was 50–60%. Gradually, however, over the years, because of various misconceptions like vasectomy leads to impotence and decrease in virility and also possibly because of introduction of new technique of conducting female sterilizations, the percentage of female sterilizations increased, so much so that now more than 99% of sterilizations done, are female sterilizations. It may not be out of place to mention that male sterilization is not only a safe and effective method with much less complications but it does not affect male potency or sexual ability. On an average, maximum number of sterilizations are done when the age of females is within 28–37 years, an age when they already have, on an average 3–4 children, i.e. when they have completed their desired family size. It is because of this disparity that though the couple protection rate has been increasing, there has not been sufficiently large effect on the demographic impact. In order to achieve a net reproduction rate of unity, it is necessary to ensure that people being sterilized have only two children, sterilization will affect the birth rate much more if most cases are performed after the couple has two children. National Family Health Survey–4 notes the trend of feminization in sterilization is persisting and flourishing.

Types of Female Sterilization

Minilap: Mini-laprotomy involves making a small incision in the abdomen. The fallopian tubes are brought to incision to be cut or blocked. It can be performed by trained MBBS doctors.

Laproscopic: Laproscopy involves inserting a long thin tube with a lens in it into the abdomen through a small incision. This laproscope enables the doctor to see and block or cut the fallopian tubes in the abdomen. It can be done by trained and certified gynaecologist or surgeon.

One of the prominent reasons for people not opting sterilization is that they cannot go to hospital for sterilization and hope to have it done on the same day since mostly sterilization facilities are not available at health centres daily. To avoid this difficulty, *camp approach* was started and still is the main mechanism in many states. However, since camps too do not have a predictable schedule, the arrangement in terms of sanitation and aseptic conditions are below acceptable level and the after care also is almost absent. The quality also suffers in sterilization camps because of the need to complete all the cases on the same day. Therefore, decision has been made to offer sterilization services in all district hospitals, sub district hospitals once a week on fixed day, at CHC/Block PHC once a fortnight and at 24 × 7 PHC once a month on fixed day. The objective of fixed day static service is to make conscious shift from camp approach to regular services apart from making health facilities self sufficient and increase coverage. In case of Female Sterilization eligible couple is considered "inactive" after 2 months.

Injectable Contraceptives

Injectable contraceptives are used in a large number of countries throughout the world.

Under national family planning programme following new choices have been introduced now:

1 POP: Progesterone only pill for lactating mothers.

2 DMPA (Depomedroxyprogesterone acetate)—also known as depoprovera—given as a three monthly injection. Both DMPA and NET-EN act essentially by:
   - Inhibiting ovulation
   - Increasing viscosity of the cervical secretions thus forming a barrier to spermatozoa
   - Changing the rate of ovum transport
   - Making the endometrium less suitable for implantation.

The effectiveness is very high. Average pregnancy rate or failure rate is 0.7 or less per 100 women per year.[7]

Emergency Contraceptive (EC) Pill

The term emergency contraception refers to methods that can prevent pregnancy when used shortly after unprotected intercourse. They are also sometimes known as morning after pills. Dr. Ellertson focussed on three regimens currently available in clinical practice.[9]

1 The Yuzpe regimen consists of tablets of combined oral contraceptives and reduces the chances of pregnancy by about 75%. The failure rate is about 2%. The regimen must be started within 72 hours of unprotected sex and involves the equivalent of four tablets of Mala-D followed by four more tablets 12 hours later. Brands that have been studied include Ovral, Lo-ovral, Levlen and Eugyron.

2 The Levonorgestrel only regimen, consists of 0.75 mg levonorgestrel taken within 48 hours of unprotected intercourse and repeated after 12 hours. This regimen shows comparable efficacy with fewer side effects.

3 Copper releasing IUDs Cu-T-380A can also prevent pregnancy when inserted up to 5 or even 7 days after unprotected intercourse. They are highly effective, preventing more than 99% of the pregnancies that would have been expected without treatment.

EC may merit a place as backup in case of rape, burst condoms, failed withdrawal attempts or non-use of another method. The EC has been introduced in the National Family Welfare Programme in the year 2002–03. Emergency contraceptive pills (E pills) are used within 72 hours of unplanned/unprotected sex.

Natural Methods—Coitus Interruptus

This is the oldest of the useful methods. The male withdraws the penis before ejaculation so that the semen is not deposited in the female genital passage. No external aid required. No religious objection.

Drawback

High failure rate: Pearl index is 25.

Calls for a great deal of will power and hence psychologically unsuitable.

Rhythm Method

The basic principle of this method is avoidance of coitus during the time of ovulation. Sexual intercourse during relatively *safe period* in the menstrual cycle prevents pregnancy. Each woman determines her own safe period.

Service Delivery Points

All the spacing methods, viz. IUCDs, OCPs, and condoms are available at the Public Health Facilities beginning from subcentre level. Additionally OCPs, condoms and emergency contraceptive pills are available at the village level through trained ASHAs. Permanent methods are generally available at Primary Health Centre level and above. Laprascopic sterilization is offered at CHCs and above.

Salient Features of the Family Planning Programme

- More emphasis on spacing methods
- Availability of services on fixed day static services
- Emphasis on Minilap tubectomy services
- Increasing male participation and promoting NSV
- Ensuring Quality Care in Family Planning services by establishing quality Assurance Committees
- Accreditation of more private/NGO facilities to increase provider base for FP Service (PPP)
- Compensation scheme for sterilizatin acceptors for loss of wages to the beneficiary and to service provider
- 'National Family Planning Indemnity Scheme' under which clients are indemnified in the eventualities of deaths, complications and failures following sterilization. The providers/accredited institutions are indemnified against litigations in those eventualities.

SOCIAL MARKETING PROGRAMME (SMP) IN HEALTH AND FAMILY WELFARE

The NPP 2000 stressed the need to formulate and implement Social Marketing schemes for advocating "Products and Services" through partnerships between the voluntary sector, non-governmental organization and the private corporate sector, Government, Panchayati Raj Institutions and the community. This will reduce the unmet needs of contraceptives and family welfare services.

What is Social Marketing?

Social marketing applies commercial marketing skills and technologies to the analysis, planning, execution and evaluation of programmes designed to influence the voluntary behaviour of target groups in order to improve their personal well-being and that of their society.[10]

Objectives

i Objective of SMP is to increase the number of outlets of services or products, such as condoms, oral pills, ORS, MTP and CUT.

ii To improve the quality of services and products.

iii To involve or enhance partnership between government and private sector.

iv To improve the access to services of family welfare.

Scope

SMP techniques are used to promote the products and services of family welfare.

Apart from this, the SMPs are also used to change the attitudes and behaviour in areas like smoking, use of seat belts, drug abuse, heart disease and other chronic diseases associated with lifestyles.

Approach

The SMP recognizes the "Consumer" as "king" of services and ensures consumer consultation about the product and services suiting to his/her need. It analyses the needs of consumers, their felt needs, likes and dislikes and satisfaction level. This early "consumer consultation" is called feed-forward by Manoff. It attempts to define in what the consumer is interested, what do they think and what are their reactions about presentations of products or idea or service.

The view point and concern of clients is ascertained through various techniques, such as focus group, discussions, interviews and surveys.

In conclusion, it is the *precise delivery* of *precise product* or *service*, *precise idea*, to *precise client* at the *precise time* of their *precise need*. This is social marketing's primary tactic, a focus on priority need, when, where and for whom it is essential. In SMP, primary *focus* is on the *consumer*—on learning what people want and need in terms of social behaviour and services.

In government service set-up, this approach is seldom stressed and this sector most of the time considers only providing services, ideas, products, *pushing these as directives*, seldom consults the consumer and works on a strategy to "Take or leave it basis".

INFORMATION—EDUCATION AND COMMUNICATION (IEC)

While IEC creates health seeking behaviour, social marketing facilitates the practice of such behaviour by promoting, distributing and selling socially beneficial tangible products, services, ideas at affordable cost to low income group people. Consumer can access these through wide range of private outlets.

Planning of Social Marketing Programme in India

Planning of SMP requires a consumer focus by addressing the different elements of the "marketing mix", i.e. *the concept of product, its price, distribution place, its promotion, partnership involved and policy environment (six Ps).*

Product

People must perceive the problem and need of contraception. The SMP analyses such needs and perception of clients and thereafter SMP for RCH provides a diverse range of products, such as condoms, oral pills, sanitary napkins for girls and services, such as medical termination of pregnancy and to practices, such as breastfeeding, oral rehydration therapy (ORT). The product under SMP is distinguished and bears a special label or logo.

Price

Price of product should be affordable by the poor also—both in rural and urban settings.

Place

Place of selling or outlets of products must be identified and known to people. It could be through *Mahila Swasthya Sangh* in RCH or through women's organization or through grocery shops or a pharmacy or chemist.

Promotion

Promotion of sale of product is through mass media–advertisement, publicity and interpersonal communication. The focus is to create sustained demand.

Partnership Involved

The partnership in SMP under RCH is essential as no single agency in a diverse country like India can provide or make impact. Key partnership between private sector, NGOs and government is essential.

Policy Environments

The government policy must encourage and support the SMP to sustain the practice or behaviour initiated by SMP.

Achievements of SMP in India[10, 11]

1 The social marketing of condoms increased from 16 million pieces in 1968–69 to 648.91 million pieces in 2012–13. Condoms marketed under SMP represent one-third of the total condoms distributed in India.

2 The social marketing of oral contraceptive pills (OCP) increased from 7.24 lakh cycles in 1987–88 to 376.82 lakh cycles in 2012–13, i.e. one-third of the total oral contraceptives distributed annually in India through social marketing.

3 Since the introduction of the SMP in 1968, for condom promotion and that for oral pills in 1987, awareness regarding condoms and oral contraceptive pill has substantially increased, and is reflected in declining total fertility rates and increased contraceptive prevalence rates from 10.4% in 1951 to 56% in the year 2005–06.[10]

4 SMP has helped to change the choices and options within each product (condom and the OCP) for the consumer.

5 Social marketing pilot project in rural India: In Madhya Pradesh, a trust of Hindustan Latex Limited, and in Uttar Pradesh, by the State Innovation in Family Planning Services Agency (SIFPSA) have been successful in demonstrating the feasibility of social marketing in rural area. Lot of field is open in rural area for SMP.

6 The brand name "NIRODH" (GOI-owned brand) also distributed through social marketing, has become a generic name for condom in India.

7 National Aids Control Programme is Promoting use of Condoms through SMP.

National Strategies on SMP in India[10, 11]

- Maximal use of public health infrastructure in rural and urban areas. As till now SMP largely confined to urban areas—make use of Subcentres, PHCs, CHCs and Indian system of medicine as outlets for SMP.
- Expand the basket of products—add diverse brands of condoms, low dose oral pills because usage of contraceptive in India has been quite low; this step may increase usage of spacing methods.
- Enhance partnership between private, NGO and government for SMP products.
- ***Introduce services:*** Social franchises: In India private sector provides higher profit curative services only. Motivate this sector to support national health goals and provide preventive services to weaker sections at affordable cost.
- Promote Information Education and Communication for SMP. The overall thrust of SMP is to accelerate achievement of sociodemographic goals of National Population Policy (NPP)-2000.

Under the social marketing programme both condoms and oral pills are made available to people at highly subsidized rates, through diverse outlets. The social marketing organization are given Deluxe NIRODH condom at ₹ 2 per packet of 5 pieces and this is sold at ₹ 3 per packet of 5 pieces to consumers. One cycle of oral pills is given to social marketing organization at ₹ 1.6 and is sold to consumer at ₹ 3 per cycle under the brand name of "MALA-D"

REFERENCES

1 IIPS National Family Health Survey 1–2 and 3 IIPS, Mumbai, India, 2005–2006.

2 MOH and FW. Report of WHO assisted workshops of "A" type Postpartum centres for development of training module and guidelines for practice of contraceptive technology and MTP for Medical Officers of Primary Health Centres. MOH and FW, New Delhi, 1987.

3 Population Reports. New GATHER Guide to Counselling. Series J, Number 48 Family Planning Programme Feb. 2000. Vol. XXVI No. 4.

4 Population Reports IUD's—An Update. Intrauterine Devices Vol. XXII, No. 5, Series B, Number 6, January 1997.

5 GOI. Reference manual on the IUD 380A for the Nursing personnel. MOH and FW, Government of India December 2007; Nirman Bhavan, New Delhi.

6 GOI. Alternative methodology of Training in IUD. Facilitator's Guide MOH and FW. Government of India October 2007.

7 Contraceptions – Background Document of National Population Policy-2000. Government of India, New Delhi.

8 Basic Guide to Reproductive and Child Health Programme for use by NGO's training institutions and health functionaries Department of Family Welfare Government of India.

9 The Population Council Regional Workshop on Emergency Contraception December 1996 at Lucknow organized by the Population Council. The Population Council Regional Office South and East Asia. India Habitat, Lodhi Road, New Delhi, India.

10 Government of India. National Strategy for Social Marketing. Department of Family Welfare. MOH and FW Government of India. Draft 05 March 2001.

11. GOI MOH and FP Annual report 2013–14.

CHAPTER

5

Reproductive and Child Health, Policy and Programmes in India

MATERNAL AND CHILD HEALTH (MCH) SERVICES

In India, women in reproductive age group (15–49 years) and children (below 15 years) constitute nearly 54% of the total population. They comprise the vulnerable section of the population due to risks connected with childbearing in case of women; and growth, development and survival in case of infants and children. Reduction of infant and childhood mortality, maternal mortality and improvement in maternal health care are the major goals stated in the National Health Policy-1983, National Population Policy-2000, National Health Policy-2002, National Rural Health Mission-2005 Millennium Development Goals, Family Planning Summit 2020 and others. The MCH is an overriding priority area for the policy makers and planners in India.

SITUATION OF MATERNAL HEALTH IN INDIA

About 17% of the girls get married by the age of 18 resulting in teen age risky pregnancies. Every year in India, roughly 30 million women experience pregnancy and 26 million have live births. Every year over 46500 pregnancy related maternal deaths occur in the country. Million more suffer pregnancy related ill health. Coverage of full antenatal care in India remains around 26.5% with variable quality of antenatal care. Nearly 81% of deliveries are attended by skilled birth attendants and nearly 25–40% of deliveries happen in homes. Postnatal care tends to be low at 36% (NFHS-3).

India has the dubious distinction of having unacceptable very high maternal mortality and in some states like Assam, Uttar Pradesh and Rajasthan it is much higher. Rural areas experience high maternal mortality in comparison to urban areas. Causes of maternal deaths (anaemia, haemorrhages abortions, toxaemia, puerperal sepsis and malposition, etc.) are well known and are largely preventable. For every woman who dies, approximately 20 more women suffer injuries, infections and disability in pregnancy or childbirth.

Out of 11 million abortions in India, the estimated illegal induced abortions (unsafe abortions) are in the range of 6–7 million, and sex selective abortions account for approximately 11%.

Thirty-five percent of ever married women report reproductive tract infection (RTI). Literacy levels amongst women are low and less women are exposed to media and thereby women lack health information. Women workload is energy sapping and malnutrition (anaemia) is rampant in women (over 58% of pregnant women, lactating mothers and adolescent girls have anaemia).

Major Health Problems of Women

- High maternal mortality
- Malnutrition in women and adolescent (anaemia)
- Early marriage
- Teenage pregnancies
- High fertility and high level of unmet needs of contraceptives besides infertility
- Reproductive tract infections (RTIs)
- Unsafe abortions
- Unsafe deliveries
- Low level of coverage of antenatal care and variable quality of antenatal care
- Low level of coverage of postnatal care
- Excessive workload
- Illiteracy, poverty and lack of information
- Low status of women
- Adverse female sex ratio
- Poor referral services (inadequate first referral units).
- Breast and cervical cancers

SITUATION OF CHILD HEALTH IN INDIA

Each year around 26 million babies are born in India, around 5% of them do not even survive to 5 years of age. Neonatal mortality, infant mortality and childhood mortality continues to be unacceptably high. Causes of childhood mortality are well known (prematurity, sepsis, asphyxia, diarrhoea, acute respiratory infections and fever are largely preventable and curable).

One-third of babies born in India tend to be of low birth weight (less than 2500 g). Over 29% of children below the age of 5 are underweight and 39% stunted reflecting widespread or rampant malnutrition during early years of life. Because of poor environments, overcrowding and indoor air pollution, the young children are exposed to the risk of killer diseases like acute respiratory infections, diarrhoeal diseases, measles and fevers.

Feeding practices in many young children are not appropriate and consequently malnutrition threatens the lives of these children. Neonatal care is negligible or poor in rural and urban slum areas.

Major Health Problems of Children

- Low birth weight babies (22–28%)
- Inadequate newborn care
- High level of neonatal, infant and under-five mortality
- Lack of essential neonatal care
- Wrong beliefs and faulty feeding practices
- Malnutrition (underweight, stunting and wasting)
- Acute respiratory infections
- Diarrhoeal diseases
- Low level of coverage of measles immunization
- Discrimination against girl child (gender disparity)
- Adverse child sex ratio
- Low level of enrolment and retention in schools for girls
- Unorganized school health and adolescent health services
- Childhood impairment, disability and handicap are quite high
- Street children face several hardships apart from behavioural problems.

EVOLUTION OF MATERNAL AND CHILD HEALTH SERVICES IN INDIA

Maternal and child health services have been one of the pivotal functions of the primary health centres and subcentres ever since the primary health centres and subcentres were conceived way back in 1952. To begin with, three *maternal and child health subcentres* were placed under one PHC and subsequently three more *family planning subcentres* were added under the PHC making a total of six subcentres. Gradually, the number of subcentres increased, under the minimum needs programme, ICDS programme and as a result of universalization of primary health care under National Health Policy, 1983. As of now one subcentre is available for 5000 population in rural areas and for 3000 population in tribal areas.

After eradication of smallpox in the year 1978, the expanded programme of immunization was launched which focused on children up to 5 years and pregnant women.

National Health Policy 1983 focussed the attention on high morbidity and mortality in infants, young children and mothers and accordingly it formulated 17 goals to be achieved by 2000 AD. Out of 17 goals, 13 goals related to maternal and child health. In 1985, Universal Immunization Programme (UIP) was started and focus shifted to infants and pregnant women. Eradications of poliomyelitis and elimination of tetanus neonatorum were the focused strategies in 1990s.

System of ICDS (1975 onward) laid foundations for convergence of maternal and child health services at the Anganwadi centres at village level. For quite some time maternal health services occupied a back seat and so much so "M" was the missed opportunity. Out of "MCH" programme, i.e. mothers (M) were not covered by any meaningful programme.

Coverage under Universal Immunization Programme (UIP) for pregnant women and infants increased significantly well over 79% and this provided encouragement to use the base of UIP for integrating other services for mother and child development.

Accordingly, the programme of child survival and safe motherhood (CSSM) was started in 1992 to integrate UIP + Family planning + MCH. The process of integration and convergence was further enhanced by launching of reproductive and child health (RCH) services in the year 1997. The National Health Policy (2002), Millennium Development Goals and National Rural Health Mission further committed to enhance the maternal and child health services and programmes.

In view of these developments, the infrastructure for the delivery of maternal and child health services was reorganized at various levels. The health teams were reoriented by providing in service short-term training to improve their skills. Essential supports in the form of essential drugs, essential equipment and supplies were made available at various levels. Referral services were also upgraded.

Maternal and Child Health Services/Programmes

- Maternal and child health in 1952 was one of the function of Primary Health Centre.
- National Family Planning Programme
- Medical Termination of Pregnancy Act
- Integrated National Family Planning and MCH Programme
- Integrated Child Development Services Scheme (ICDS)

- Expanded programme of immunisation
- Universal Immunisation Programme
- Child Survival and Safe Motherhood Programme (CSSM)
- Reproductive and Child Health Programme (RCH).
- National Rural Health Mission
- National Health Mission
- *Vande Mataram* Scheme
- *Janani Suraksha Yojna* (JSY)
- School Health and Adolescent Health Programme.
- Janani Shishu Suraksha Karyakram
- RM NCH + A approach
- Early detection of cervical and breast cancers and treatment
- Management of infertility and menopause problems
- Referral services including referral transport
- Implementation of Preconception and Prenatal Diagnostic Techniques (PC and PNDT)
- Behaviour change communication.

Child Health Services/Programmes

Tracking every child for package of services is the goal.

- Facility Based Newborn and Child Care:
  - a Special Newborn Care Units (SNCU) at district level and Newborn Intensive Care Unit (NICU) at regional level.
  - b Newborn stabilization units at CHC/FRU
  - c Newborn care corners attached to labour room/OT
  - d Facility based Integrated Management of Neonatal and Childhood Illness (F-IMNCI)
- *Home based care of newborn (HBCN)*
- Navjat Shishu Suraksha Karyakram (NSSK)
- Integrated Management of Neonatal and Childhood Illness (IMNCI) and pre-service and in-service training under IMNCI
- Universal immunisation programme
- Early detection and management of acute respiratory infection, diarrhoea and other infections
- Infant and young child feeding including promotion of breastfeeding and exclusive breastfeeding
- Management of children with severe acute malnutrition
- Vitamin A supplementation and iron and folic acid supplementation
- Integrated child development services (ICDS)
- School Health Services (Programme)
- Rashtriya Bal Swasthya Karyakram (RBSK)
- India's Newborn Action Plan – 2014
- Rashtriya Kishor Swasthya Karyakram
- Management of special problems like disability and behavioural problems
- Referral services
- Behaviour change communication.

Delivery of Maternal and Child Health (MCH) Services

The three tier rural health system in India is well-structured. The MCH services are being delivered through organized infrastructure.

Rural Areas

Level 1: Through network of Subcentres, PHCs not functioning as 24 × 7 and home deliveries by skilled birth attendant (SBA)—Elementary obstetric and neonatal care.

Level 2: By 24 × 7 PHCs and CHCs other than FRUs—Basic obstetric and neonatal care.

Level 3: FRUs and district and subdistrict hospitals or referral hospital and selected CHCs—provide comprehensive obstetric and neonatal care.

- By private practitioners
- By non-governmental organizations.

Urban Areas

Unlike the rural areas, the cities and towns do not have a well-structured health system.

Maternal and child health services are being provided through district hospitals, urban health posts/centres, nursing homes, private practitioners and system of hospitals. Most urban slums have ICDS infrastructure besides urban health centres, postpartum centres, maternity centres and maternity homes run by Municipal Corporations or Red Cross Society apart from philanthropists and charitable organizations as also India population projects and Non-Governmental Organizations.

Thus in urban area, multiple health agencies are available with little coordination to deliver MCH services. Urban slum population have poor access to MCH services. Urban RCH centres were set-up.

Tribal Areas

Tribal people constitute 8.2% of the country's total population, i.e. 84 million. They have poor access to the health services. Population norms for SC, PHC and CHC have been relaxed for tribal areas. Besides government health infrastructure, several NGOs are working in tribal areas to provide MCH services. RCH-2 gives priority to tribal areas.

CHILD SURVIVAL AND SAFE MOTHERHOOD PROGRAMME (CSSM), 1992–1997

The child survival and safe motherhood (CSSM) programme was launched on *Sadbhavna Diwas* on 20 August 1992 by the President of India. The CSSM programme underlines the high priority to the various programmes for improving the health status of women and children and the reduction of maternal, infant and child morbidity and mortality rates. The CSSM programme is directed at achieving 9 of the 17 goals of the National Health Policy 1983 (Table 5.1) which are related to maternal and child health as stated above.[1] CSSM was built on the edifice of UIP. CSSM integrates UIP + Family planning + MCH. Thus, UIP became UIP + programme in 1992.

Table 5.1: National Health Policy 1983 MCH Goals

CSSM goals	*Current level (1992)*	*2000*
A. Reduction of mortality rate		
1 Infant mortality rate (1992)	79	≤ 60
2 Perinatal mortality rate (1990)	48.4	35
3 Child (0–4 yrs) mortality rate (1990)	26.3	10
4 Maternal mortality ratio (Est. 1992)	4	2
B. Reduction in the proportion of LBW (%)		
1 Under weight babies (Est. 1992)	30	10
C. Services (%) Coverage		
1 Immunization—Infant	85.8	85
2 Pregnant women	79.4	100
3 Deliveries by trained personnel (1990)	44.1	100
4 Antenatal care (Est. 1992)	79	100
D. Prevention of blindness due to Vit. A deficiency		
• Incidence of blindness (%)	NA	0.3

The major causes of infant and child mortality are—prematurity, severe infection, birth asphyxia, acute respiratory infections, diarrhoeal diseases, fever, vaccine preventable diseases (in places where the immunization coverage has not reached optimal levels) and inadequate maternal and newborn care. The major causes of maternal deaths are anaemia, haemorrhage, toxaemia, septicaemia, obstructed labour and illegal abortions.

The interventions for reducing morbidity and mortality in children include: *Essential newborn care*, immunization, oral *rehydration therapy*, *treatment of pneumonia* and *vitamin A prophylaxis.*

Interventions to reduce maternal mortality are: TT immunization, prevention and treatment of anaemia, training of traditional birth attendants and provision of disposable delivery kits (DDK) for promoting clean deliveries, promotion of institutional deliveries and strengthening of health care institutions for maternal care, treatment of maternal complications, management of obstetric emergencies and promotion of birth spacing.

The programme addresses the major causes of morbidity and mortality in women and children which are preventable by readily available cost-effective interventions. Many of these interventions were ongoing under the maternal and child health (MCH) programme but now being integrated under CSSM. Coverage levels have increased and quality of services improved through supply of additional equipment, regular supply of essential drugs and retraining of medical and paramedical personnel. *The treatment of ARI, newborn care, and strengthening of emergency obstetric services were the new thrust areas.* The access established under the immunization programme is being utilized to extend and intensify other services related to mother and child health. The efficacy of interventions combined with a systematic expansion of services for universal access by 1996–97, makes the set goals under the National Health Policy, feasible and realistic.

In the districts under the CSSM, retraining of the medical and paramedical personnel was undertaken to ensure high quality of services and an integrated implementation of field activities. Drugs and equipment kits were provided to all districts under CSSM to ensure availability of essential supplies in adequate quantities.

SUBCENTRE DRUG KITS under CSSM
(Twice a year to each subcentre)

Drug Kit A (for all districts under CSSM)	
• IFA (large)	15,000 tablets (100 mg)
• IFA (small)	13,000 tablets (20 mg)
• Vitamin A solution	12 bottles (100 ml each) (1 ml = 1 lakh IU)
• Cotrimoxazole	1000 tablets (paediatric)
• ORS packets	150 packets
Drug Kit B (for safe motherhood districts)	
• Methyl ergometrine	500 tablets (0.125 mg)
• Chlorpheniramine	400 tablets (4 mg)
• Paracetamol	500 tablets (500 mg)
• Anti-spasmodic tablets	250 tablets
• Inj. methyl ergometrine	5 ampoules (0.2 mg/ml)
• Mebendazole	300 tablets (100 mg)
• Chloramphenicol (1%)	500 eye applicaps
• Cetrimide powder	5 packets (125 gm each)
• Povidone ointment (5%)	5 tubes (tubes of 25 gm)
• Cotton bandage	120 rolls (4 cm × 4 metres)
• Cotton absorbent	One roll (500 gm)

THE PACKAGE OF SERVICES under CSSM

1. For the children
- Essential newborn care
- Immunization
- Appropriate management of diarrhoea
- Appropriate management of ARI
- Vitamin A prophylaxis

2. For the mothers
- Immunization
- Prevention and treatment of anaemia
- Antenatal care and early identification of maternal complications
- Deliveries by trained personnel
- Promotion of institutional deliveries
- Management of obstetric emergencies
- Birth spacing
- Training of traditional birth attendants and provision of disposable delivery kits for promoting clean deliveries by observing five cleans (**clean surface, clean hands, clean blade, clean tie and clean cord stump** without any applicant)

Reporting forms for surveillance of all the childhood diseases and monitoring of performance of the interventions under the CSSM programme have been integrated. Vaccination coverage evaluation surveys for assessment of the immunization programme have been expanded to include other interventions like ORT, pneumonia treatment, breastfeeding and birth spacing.

The child survival and safe motherhood programme has been phased over a 5-year period. The implementation of the CSSM programme was started in August 1992–93 in 51 districts and the expansion to all the districts completed by 1996–97.

In the states of Assam, Bihar, Madhya Pradesh, Odisha, Rajasthan and Uttar Pradesh which have very high maternal mortality rates, additional inputs were provided to upgrade existing health facilities in the rural areas for the management of obstetric emergencies. These first referral units (FRUs) for providing emergency obstetric care were established in 219 districts over a 5-year period. In each district, 4–6 rural health institutions were covered. The state health authorities in other states have been encouraged to mobilize resources and upgrade health facilities for strengthening the management of obstetric emergencies. Essential obstetric care being an important intervention to be promoted in all the districts.[2,3]

CSSM programme laid down foundation of Newborn Care and FRUs at the National Level.

REFERENCES

1 GOI (1994) National Child Survival and Safe Motherhood Programme. MCH division Department of Family Welfare Government of India.

2 GOI (1993). CSSM Review A newsletter on the Child Survival and Safe Motherhood Programme Issue No. 9, September 1993. MOH and FW, New Delhi.

3 IGNOU. Maternal and Child Health Services PGDMCH-1. Preventive MCH. Indira Gandhi National Open University School of Health Sciences. Maidan Garhi, New Delhi –1997.

INTEGRATED CHILD DEVELOPMENT SERVICES (ICDS)

Integrated child development services (ICDS) scheme was launched on 2nd October, 1975 as a follow-up measure of National Policy for Children, formulated in 1974.[1,2]

Development of children is the first priority on country's development agenda, not because they are most vulnerable, but because they are our supreme assets and also the future human resources of the country. Therefore, the foundations of lifelong learning and human development are necessarily to be laid down in the very critical years of the childhood. ICDS programme is essentially *human resource development programme* and it adopts life cycle approach. Prime focus in on mother.

The ICDS has covered many milestones since its inception in 1975, today ICDS is globally recognized as one of the world's largest and most unique community based out-reach system of promoting early childhood care for survival, growth and development.[3,4] The Nodal Ministry of ICDS is Human Resource Development or Social Welfare Department. The major objectives of ICDS are:

1 To lay the foundation for overall development of child (physical, social and psychological development).
2 To improve the nutritional and health status of children below the age of six, pregnant and lactating mother and adolescent girls.
3 Reduce the incidence of mortality, morbidity, malnutrition and school dropouts.
4 Achieve effective coordination of policy and implementation among various departments to promote child development.
5 Enhance the capability of mother to look after the normal health, nutritional and development needs of the child, through proper community education.
6 Improving the health and nutritional status of adolescent girls.

These objectives are being achieved through package of following services. The services relate to *health*; *education* and *nutritional* (HEN) *components*.

Health Services

These include: Immunization, health check-ups, treatment of ailments and referral services, besides health and nutrition education.

Nutritional Services

Supplementary nutrition/feeding, growth monitoring and promotion, nutrition and health education.

Education Services

Early Childhood Care Education and Development: It includes:

a Early care and stimulation for younger children under 3 years.
b Early joyful learning opportunities to children in the 3–6 age group (Preschool Non-Formal Education).

Supportive Services and Convergence of other supportive services, such as safe drinking water, environmental sanitation, women's empowerment programmes, non-formal education and adult literacy.

Package of core services has been redesigned and following new components have been added in 12th plan (Table 5.2).

- Child care and nutrition counselling service for pregnant and breastfeeding mothers of 0–3 years children has been introduced as one of the core services.
- Early stimulation and detection of developmental delays.

Table 5.2: Core package of services under ICDS mission

	Services	Service standards
1	Early Childhood Care Education and Development (ECCED)	4 hours session per day Monthly fixed ECCE day
2.	Supplementary Nutrition	300 days in a year
3.	Care and Nutrition Counselling	
	(a) Growth monitoring and promotion including development (mile stones)	0–3 years once a month 3–5 years every 3 month
	(b) Infant and young child feeding and counseling	Home visits at cirtical contact points
	(c) Lactation support	Regular quarterly parents meet
	(d) Maternal care counseling	
	(e) Nutrition and health and hygiene education	One session per month
	(f) Community based management of severely and moderately underweight children	Improvement in nutritional status
4.	Health services	Monthly Fixed VHND • Full immunization • Regular health check ups
5.	Community participation and mobilization	Quarterly AWC management committee meeting Quarterly meeting VHSNCs

- Community based care for under-nourished children.
- Tracking of pregnant women and children on mother and child protection card.
- Redefining—Preschool education, as Early Childhood Care and Education (ECCE).

Target Groups/Beneficiaries

The following are targeted for package of services:

- Children under 6 years of age. *Priority is for children under 3 years of age*. Second priority is for children between 3 and 6 years age group.
- Pregnant and lactating mothers.
- Women in reproductive age group (15–49 years).
- Adolescent girls (10–19 years).

Heart of ICDS System—Anganwadi

The Anganwadi (AW), literally means courtyard play centre, is a child care centre, located within the village or urban slum area. It is the focal point for delivery of services at the community level to children below 6 years of age, pregnant women, nursing mothers and adolescent girls. Anganwadi centre functions for 6 hours (including 4 hours of ECCED and SNP, 2 hours for home visits) per day.

Besides this, the Anganwadi centre is a meeting ground where women and mother groups can come together with other community-based workers to promote awareness and joint action for child development and women's empowerment; hence AW is the heart of ICDS. Over 1342126 Anganwadi centres were operational as on 22nd September 2014.

Anganwadi Worker (AWW)

5

AWW is the key functionary or key volunteer at Anganwadi centre to provide the package of services. The Anganwadi worker is middle or matriculate married women, resident of the same village or community—chosen by the community and has received three months training for child and mother development. Duration of basic training of AWW has been reduced from 3 months to 52 days (45 working days and further reduced to 30 days).[5–9] The revised curriculum consists of 75% core subjects and 25% state specific areas. She has been given one female helper to support or assist her functions. Thus, the base of the ICDS is honorary worker drawn from the community and chosen by people who works for their own people as she is one of them, who understands their culture, practices, needs and resources.

Job Functions of AWW

Each Anganwadi worker has been assigned a geographical area of about 400–800 (80–160 houses) population in rural/urban slum and in tribal area the population is 300–800. Even small hamlets of 150–400 population have mini Anganwadi center. Her job functions are:

A. Planning and Implementation of ICDS

1. Village or urban slum mapping—to know her area.
2. Rapport building with community right from beginning.
3. Conducting community survey and enlisting beneficiaries keeping household records of each family, children 0–6 years, children at risk, below poverty line households expectant and nursing mothers and adolescent girls.
4. Registration of marriages, pregnant women, births and deaths.

B. Service Delivery

1. Preparation and distribution of supplementary nutrition for children 6 months to 6 years, nursing mothers pregnant women, and adolescent girls.
2. Growth monitoring.
3. Assisting health staff in immunization and health check-ups. She motivates mothers for immunization.
4. Referral services.
5. Detection of disability among children.
6. Providing treatment for common ailments.
7. Integrated management of neonatal and childhood illnesses.
8. Health and nutrition education of adolescent girls, women and community.
9. Organizing non-formal preschool education activities.
10. Anganwadi worker as facilitator of ASHA: Depot holder of medicine kit and contraceptives for ASHA and will guide ASHA in organizing health day.
11. Assists CDPO and supervisors in implementation of KSY and national programme for adolescent girls.[10]

C. Information Education and Communication

Communicate with and counsel parents, families and communities besides organizing awareness campaigns.

D. Community Contacts

1. Mobilize community and elicit community participation.
2. Maintain liaison with Panchayat, primary schools, Mahila Mandals and health functionaries.

E. Management and Administration

Management of Anganwadi centre, maintenance of records and registers and preparation of reports.

THE ICDS TEAM AND ORGANIZATION

- The ICDS team consists of Anganwadi workers, ASHA, helpers at village level, supervisors (Mukhya Sevikas) one for 25 AWWs at circle level and child development project officers (CDPOs) one for one lakh population at block level. In large sized rural and urban projects, additional CDPOs are also part of the team.
- The female health workers, male health workers at subcentres, health supervisors and medical officers of PHCs form a team with social welfare/women and child development functionaries to implement ICDS programme and provide integrated services. Of necessity, the ICDS functions have to be integrated with health services.

Package of Services and Participants (Table 5.2)

ICDS is unique because all basic sectoral services related to early childhood care, preschool *education*, *nutrition* and *health* converge and are delivered under one roof at Anganwadi centre.

The convergence of services by ANM, AWW and ASHA are essential to address the interrelated needs of children and women in a comprehensive and cost-effective manner.[11,12] The spectrum of services has been expanded during 12th plan period.

1. EARLY CHILDHOOD CARE AND EDUCATION (ECCE)

It is one of the core service in ICDS.

ECCE: This Component of ICDS includes two types of services of 4 hours session:

i. Early psychosocial stimulation (EPSS) for children below 3 years (free play and lot of adult child interaction) a home based programme.
ii. Non-formal preschool education (NFPSE) for children 3–6 years, redefining NFPSE to ECCE.

EPSS: It aims to provide learning opportunities and know his/her environments for holistic development. It is meant for under three children. It is a programme of close interaction between the child and the mother or caregivers with the help of AWWs. It is mainly home based activity.

NFPSE/ECCE: It is a programme for 3–6 years children at Anganwadi. It is child centred programme which follows play way activity approach. It is mainly Anganwadi based and reinforced at home by home visits.

The early childhood care and education (ECCE) is an activity to promote physical, social and psychological development of young children. It lays foundations for all-round development. This is the first step in the ladder of education. ECCE is considered as most important and pivotal activity. In ICDS, ECCE is done through play-way daily activities visibly sustained for 4 hours a day preceded by snacks and followed by supplementary nutrition, growth monitoring and other related interventions. Children learn by playing and undertaking creative activities with the help of Anganwadi worker who provides learning stimuli and arranges material for play-way and creative activities. Children have lot of curiosity and they eagerly explore and satisfy their curiosity. Varieties of games and ECCE activities are organized at the Anganwadi and a special kit material has been provided to all Anganwadis. It brings and keeps young children at the Anganwadi centre—an activity that motivates parents and communities.

Focus of ECCE is total development of child, in the age range up to 6 years from the under privileged groups. It combines physical, mental and social development by organized activities (Age appropriate activities for ECCE as per norms and quality standards). The early learning component of the ICDS is a significant input for providing a sound foundation for cumulative lifelong learning and development. It also contributes to universalization of primary education by providing to the child the necessary preparation for primary schooling and offering substitute care to younger siblings thus freeing the older ones especially girls to attend school. Currently, preschool component of ICDS is very weak.

Some of the positive outcomes of ECCE have been learning of language, recognition of common objects, colour, size and shape discrimination, concept of heavy and light, waiting for their turn, sitting in rows and circle, mixing with each other, competition and cooperation, sharing and healthy lifestyles, such as washing hands, brushing, and eating clean food, etc.

Regular monthly fixed ECCE day should be observed at Anganwadi as 'Balbodh Divas'.

Elementary education for all, i.e. *Sarva Shiksha Abhiyan* (SSA) aims at universalization of elementary education up to 8 years of schooling. Under SSA, importance has been given to preschool learning and early childhood care and its role in improving participation of children in schools. Also there is an emphasis on convergence between SSA and ICDS with an effort to strengthen the preschool education component of ICDS.[13]

Under the National Education Policy, the district primary education programme has established pre-primary education wing covering children 4–6 years of age and providing mid-day meal.[11] This step reduces the workload of Anganwadi workers as shifting preschool education programme to teachers provides more time to AWW to *focus attention* to mothers and young *children below the age of three*.

2. SUPPLEMENTARY NUTRITION

Supplementary feeding is given to pregnant women, nursing mothers and children between 6 months and 6 years of age and selected adolescent girls (Table 5.3). Priority is given to low income families and moderately underweight children and all children who attend Anganwadi for non-formal preschool education. These beneficiaries avail supplementary feeding support for 300 days in a year. Over 84.94 million children and 19.56 million mothers are receiving supplementary feeding. By providing supplementary feeding, the Anganwadi worker attempts to bridge the caloric gap between the recommended daily allowance (RDA) and average daily intake (ADI) of children and women, in low income and disadvantaged communities. The objective is only supplementing and not substituting for family food. It also provides an important contact opportunity with pregnant women and mothers of infants and young children, to promote improved behavioural actions for care of pregnant women and young children. This provides a crucial opportunity to counsel pregnant women, enabling utilization of key services, i.e. antenatal care, immunization, iron and folic acid supplementation and improved care, adequate extra food and rest during pregnancy; exclusive breastfeeding and introduction of complementary food at right age. Special care is taken to reach children below the age of 3 years. The type of food varies from state to state, but usually consists of a hot meal cooked at the Anganwadi, containing a varied combination of pulses, cereals, oil, vegetables and sugar/iodized salt. Some states provide ready to eat meal; containing the same ingredients. There is flexibility in the selection of food items; to respond to local needs. The expenditure towards supplementary feeding is met by the state under the plan budget. The nursing mothers are provided food up to 6 months after delivery to help meet increased requirement during this period.

Table 5.3: Norms for supplementary nutrition in ICDS

Recipients	*Calories*	*Grams of protein*
• Children (6–72 months)	500	12–15
• Severely underweight children	800	20–25
• Adolescent girls	600	18–20
• Pregnant and nursing mothers	600	18–20

The supplementary nutrition acts as a spring board to develop other activities, such as improving attendance at Anganwadi, eating clean, washing hands, development of non-formal education besides developing healthy lifestyles. It should not be perceived as "feeding Programme". It seldom improves malnutrition because of many problems, such as sharing and not eating enough food at home or missing a meal at home as also problem of acceptance of food. Supplementary feed is no guarantee to improve nutritional status. Move than half of ICDS budget is spent on SNP.

Decentralization of supplementary feeding: The supplementary feeding activity has been decentralized now. The money of supplementary feeding has been given to village level coordination committee, chaired by Mahila Panch. Now local recipes are prepared at the village. Village people (self-help groups) have greater say now and they themselves decide local recipes. Usually a hot meal is cooked at Anganwadi based on a mix of pulses, cereals, oil, vegetable, sugar and iodised salt. ₹ 6, 9 and 7 per day is spent on supplementary feeding for child, severely underweight child and pregnant women respectively.

Incorporation of green leafy vegetables, seasonal fruits, milk, egg in the supplementary feeding under ICDS, needs to be promoted and community educated on the importance of these foods.

Micronutrient Supplementation

National prophylaxis programme for prevention of blindness caused by vitamin. A deficiency and control of nutritional anaemia among mothers and children, are two direct interventions integrated in ICDS. Dietary promotion of foods rich in vitamin A, iron, and folic acid and vitamin C is an important part of nutrition and health education and targeted supplementation is also provided. At 9 months of age 1,00,000 IU of vitamin A solution is administered along with measles immunization.

Children in the age group of 1–5 are provided 2,00,000 IU of vitamin A solution every 6 months with priority given to children under 3 years of age. Similarly, iron and folic acid tablets supplements are given to pregnant women and children for prophylaxis and treatment of anaemia.

THERAPEUTIC NUTRITION

It is given to treat severe malnutrition, i.e. severely underweight children (weight-for-age below –3SD of median). Therapeutic food is given as per revised scale or adequate eating/feeding at home is to be encouraged or special supplementary feeding is advised. Domiciliary management helps and these children are also referred to Nutrition Rehabilitation Centre (NRC).

3. CARE AND NUTRITION COUNSELLING SERVICES

A new initiative under ICDS as one of the core services, targeting mothers of children under 3 years, pregnant and Lactating mothers. Objective of this activity is to enhance the child care abilities/capacities of mother and or care givers to look after the health and nutritional needs of children within the family environments. Following interventions are in place to achieve this:

a. **Infant and Young Child Feeding (IYCF):** Promotion and counselling: One to one counselling for optimal breastfeeding practices linked to growth monitoring. One to one counselling on complementary feeding to ensure adequate food intake by home visits and follow-up.

b. **Monitoring and promotion of child growth and development:** Growth and deveopment monitoring and nutrition surveillance is one of the vital services under ICDS. Family retained Mother and Child Protection Cards are being used by AWW to monitor growth and early detection of delayed developmental milestones.

c. **Lactation support:** Support for early initiation and exclusive breastfeeding.

d. **Maternal care and counselling:** Early registration of pregnancy, 4 or more ANCs, institutional delivery and postnatal care, counselling on diet, rest, IFA compliance during home visit, monitoring weight gain, examination of pallor and oedema and any other danger signs, home based counselling for essential newborn care and counselling on spacing.

e. **Nutrition, Health and Hygiene Education (NHHE):** Targeting pregnant and lactating and other caregivers, community and family by organising monthly health and nutrition education sessions, education on improved caring practices—feeding, health and hygiene and behaviour change communication to promote healthy eating during pregnancy, lactation and adolescence and early childhood period, promoting local foods by food demonstration, celebration of nutrition week and breastfeeding week and ICDS day.

f. **Community based care and management of underweight children:** This activity targets moderately and severely underweight children and their mothers/caregivers for:

- 100% weighing of all eligible children and identification of underweight children and referral to Nutrition Rehabilitation Centre (NRC).
- Community based management of severely and moderately under-weight children: **Sneha Shivirs** for mothers for 12 days at AWCs, followed by 18 days of home practice and monitoring weight gain after 12 days and 18 days. Those severely underweight children with medical complications are referred to Nutrition Rehabilitation Centre (NRC).

4. HEALTH SERVICES

Health centre and subcentre staff have their obligatory responsibility to provide maternal and child health services in geographical area of PHC covering 30,000 population. Providing maternal and child services in an area with the help of ICDS infrastructure becomes much more easier as system of Anganwadi workers prepare mothers and children, motivate them to utilize services. Since mothers and children come to Anganwadi that becomes the focal point for delivery of services. The health component of ICDS comprises health check-ups, immunization, referral services, and nutrition and health education.

i. Health Check-ups

This includes health check-up and growth monitoring of children under 6 years of age, pregnant and lactating, mothers as per norms laid down. At the Anganwadi, children, adolescent girls, pregnant women and nursing mothers are examined at regular intervals by health worker (female), and health supervisors with the supportive supervision of medical officers. Infants and young children below 3 years of age is a priority group for weighing, health check-ups and management of sicknesses like diarrhoea, fevers and respiratory infections and worm infestation, etc. Anganwadi centre based screening and early intervention services under Rashtriya Bal Swasthya Karyakram has been initiated in Feb 2013.

ii. Referral Services

During the health check-ups and growth monitoring, sick and malnourished children, in need of prompt medical attention, are provided referral services through subcentre, female health workers or through nearby PHCs by medical officers. The Anganwadi worker has also been trained to detect disabilities in young children. She enlists all such cases in a special register and refers them to medical officer. The effectiveness of this service depends upon timely action. The referral support services are weakest or just minimal that is why people turn to private sector for treatment of illnesses in mother and children and for other disease as well. Early response at home, at Anganwadi and at health subcentre and helth facility is most critical and it saves many deaths due to diarrhoea, respiratory infections and fevers.

iii. Immunizations

AWW mobilizes mothers and children and identifies all pregnant women at the earliest and registers all the births occurring in her area, motivates them and informs them the place and date of immunization. It is better to plan immunization activities with ICDS system and AWWs. Immunizations are done by health workers and their supervisors as AWWs have not been trained for the task of injection and immunization procedures. Coverage of immunization for pregnant women and infants can be increased with the help of Anganwadi workers. Anganwadi workers help in organization of outreach session and she maintains perfect records of immunizations and she knows the left over children and pregnant women in her area.

iv. Management of Childhood Illnesses

Anganwadi workers have been provided with drug kit for managing diarrhoea, anaemia, fever, worm infestation, minor cuts and injuries. She also holds contraceptives, vitamin A solution, iron and folic acid tablets besides other drugs. She is depot holder of medicine kit of ASHA. She has been trained in IMNCI strategy.

GROWTH AND DEVELOPMENT MONITORING AND PROMOTION

New WHO growth standards for girls and boys have been introduced in ICDS. Growth monitoring and nutrition surveillance are two important activities that are in operation in ICDS. Children below the age of three are weighed once a month and children between 3 and 6 years are weighed once in three months. Mother and child protection session or immunization session held on fixed days, when mothers and children come to avail services, is the best opportunity for growth monitoring and promotion of growth. Result of growth and development monitoring must be shared and communicated to mother, best is let mothers themselves weigh their children and know the status of nutrition of their child for appropriate actions. Weight-for-age growth charts are maintained for all children below 6 years of age. This helps to detect growth faltering and also would help identify children in various categories like normal, moderately underweight and severely underweight children. The concept of community-based nutrition surveillance has also been introduced in ICDS. A community chart for nutrition status monitoring is maintained at each Anganwadi. This chart reflects the nutrition status of all children registered with Anganwadi at any given point of time.

Community-based monitoring has been further strengthened by use of ICDS NRHM Mother and Child Protection Card (MCPC) which is retained by the family which incorporates new WHO child growth and development standards.

Growth monitoring is a time consuming activity, it is productive only when mothers are involved and action is taken by them promptly. Children below 3 or 2 years are left over as they are to be weighed in their homes. Most often the growth monitoring is done to report the nutritional status to higher levels which defeats the very purpose of growth monitoring. Growth monitoring without involving mothers is futile and serves no purpose. Growth monitoring is very important epidemiological tool to learn growth and to ensure adequate growth and initiate appropriate timely actions and measure their impact continuously. Health department should have more concern and commitment for growth monitoring which is preventive strategy for malnutrition. Monitoring of developmental milestones will also be undertaken from now onward, integrated with growth monitoring.

5. COMMUNITY MOBILIZATION/PARTICIPATION

This component aims at enhancing community participation and ownership in ICDS programme. Powers have been given to Panchayati Raj Institutions (PRIs) and Local Bodies in the implementation of the ICDS. These institutions have been involved in selection of Anganwadi workers, supervision and monitoring, location, construction and maintenance of the ICDS centres. Village health, Sanitation and Nutrition Committee has been involved in management and supervision of ICDS programme at the village level. Prime position have been given for involvement and Participation of PRIs and Local Bodies at village, block, district, state and national levels. Similarly NGOs and voluntary associations have been involved in ICDS programme. However, this component is weak and needs further strengthening.

VILLAGE HEALTH NUTRITION AND SANITATION DAY

ASHA along with Anganwadi workers and Auxiliary Nurse Midwife (ANM), self-help group and community-based organizations, PRIs, and preraks of continuing education centres organizes village health, nutrition and sanitation day (VHND) once a month on fixed day at the Anganwadi centres. This day is used for provision of immunization, ante/postnatal check-ups and services related to mother, child, and adolescents health care, including nutrition. This generates awareness and leads to increased utilization of services besides promoting convergence. Drawing up and implementation of local village plan and meeting of village health committee also happens on that day. Fixed monthly Early Childhood Care and Education (ECCE) day *Balbodh Divas* can be combined with VHND.

6. ADOLESCENT GIRL'S SCHEME IN ICDS[14]

Adolescent girl's scheme has been redesigned as *Kishori Shakti Yojna* (KSY). The KSY aims at improving the nutrition and health status of adolescent girls and promoting self-development, awareness of health, hygiene, nutrition, and family life and child care.[14]

Initially the KSY covered 2000 ICDS projects and it has been expanded further to cover all ICDS projects. A new comprehensive scheme for adolescent girls called SABLA has been implemented in 200 districts replacing KSY.

TRAINING OF ANGANWADI WORKERS

The national training component for ICDS is an innovative strategy. The ICDS programme has increased its coverage over the last 40 years. The content and quality of services under ICDS depends largely on the skill and competence of over 13.4 lacs AWWs and their helpers besides 50,000 supervisors and more than 10,000 CDPOs and ACDPOs. Responding to this need led to birth of UDISHA—the new dawn in training. It is a national initiative of quality improvement through training and communication through a large scale movement of social mobilization and empowerment. UDISHA has given a new thrust to training of child care functionaries and caregivers education. Its holistic approach is reflected in a new child centered curriculum structured along the life cycle and development continuum of child.[6,7]

UDISHA gives primacy to parents/families and community for child development, protection and survival, new curriculum is based on life cycle approach and emphasizes on skill and competency building, laying stress on decentralized training at states and field—learning by doing and teams training is to be strived. The duration of basic training has been reduced to 32 days in 2004. The training follows a design of modular training but much depends upon the implementation of the proposed modular training and the trainers. In our opinion, the best learning occurs in the community and best design of training is community to AWW and AWW to AWW and over and above teams training where AWW and ANMs (health workers female) undergo training together.

CONTINUING EDUCATION

The ICDS deserves credit for innovations. One time training of 3 months and now reduced to 32 days is not enough. On the job training on continuous basis and regular orientation training once a month is considered essential. On the job, training is provided by supervisors and health worker female while one day orientation training once a month is the responsibility of medical officer and child development project officer.[15] Sector meeting is the best opportunity for continuing education and training, planning of activities for the next month, reviewing the performance, preparation of reports and solving the problems of the workers. Sector meeting is regularly held once a month in the last week of the month at a designated place (sector headquarter village) where 20–25 Anganwadi workers and all the female and male health workers (5–6 female health workers), health supervisors, ICDS supervisors, medical officer of PHC and CDPO meet together to review the activities of the programme. Monthly monitoring reports are prepared in this meeting and activities for the next month are planned together by consultation process. AWWs are provided continuing education essentially problem-based and issue-based and learning by doing is attempted. The subject of learning is identified by the workers and training needs assessment (TNA) is based on the field supervision and deficiency in the performance/ skill as also newer areas like adolescent health, women empowerment, gender issues, girls enrolment, adverse sex ratio and implementation of PNDT Act, etc.

ACHIEVEMENT OF ICDS[16-23]

- ICDS is now a universal programme covering rural, tribal and urban slum areas reaching unreached and underprivileged. It is strongly rooted in the community and has a strong community base.
- It is a massive outreach programme for women and child development with our own resources—an indigenous pride and programme acknowledged the world over.
- The spectrum of services and coverage of services for mother and children have increased many folds due to ICDS.
- AWWs have been recognized as the biggest strength of ICDS who are a force to be recognized for massive social mobilization and community contacts.
- ICDS has provided AWW as companion to ANM (female health workers) who can now work fearlessly in the village and in the community. A new health team at village level has emerged and it draws strength from each other.
- In spite of several weaknesses (inadequate coverage of under three years children, inadequate community participation) the programme has inner strengths.
- ICDS is the finest example of intersectoral coordination in operation and achieving results.
- ICDS has shown the way of innovative designs of domiciliary and community-based care for neonates, infants, children and women. It has many untapped potentials.
- ICDS is a strong advocacy base for women and children. The constituency of ICDS is urban poor, tribal areas and rural disadvantaged women and children.[24]

Conclusion

In the light of experience gained over the last 38 years the task of ICDS will not only be confined to feeding and teaching young children. Its contents will be enriched to cover adolescent girls and to ensure women empowerment and building capacity of family, caregivers and community.[24] ICDS belongs to community and community ownership will be strived by all means by information.

UNIVERSALIZATION OF ICDS WITH QUALITY AND EQUITY

ICDS has been universalized and it has become a familiar name and has been recognized the world over. In view of Supreme Court ruling of April 2004 and Government commitment in the National Common Minimum Programme, it has led to the decision to **universalize the integrated child development services** (ICDS) scheme; with a target of providing a functional Anganwadi in every settlement. Population norms for setting up of AWCs and Mini AWCs have been revised under third phase of universalization of ICDS scheme:

- One Anganwadi centre for 400–800 population in rural/urban project, 2 AWCs for 800–1600, 3 AWCs for 1600–2400 and thereafter in multiples of 800 one AW Centre.
- One Anganwadi centre for 300–800 in tribal project.
- One mini, AWC for 150–400 population in rural/urban project.
- One mini, AWC for 150–300 population in tribal riverine, desert and hilly areas.[25–27]

It covers almost all blocks and most urban slums. 7075 ICDS projects have been sanctioned and 7067 were fully operational as on 22nd September 2014.

ICDS Strengthening and restructuring in 12th Plan

Monitorable outcomes of ICDS restructuring: ICDS restructuring aims to achieve three monitorable outcomes by the end of 12th Five-Year Plan (2017)

- Prevent and reduce young child undernutrition (% underweight 0–3 years) by 10 percentage points.
- Enhance early development and learning outcome in all children 0–6 years of age.
- Improve care and nutrition of girls and women and reduce anaemia prevalence in young children, girls and women by one fifth. In order to achieve the above monitorable goals following reforms will be undertaken mainly as new initiatives to transform and energise the ICDS system.

Salient Features

i Continued implementation of ICDS in 12th Five-year plan in Mission mode along the lines of NRHM and SSA (*Sarva Shiksha Abhiyan*).

ii Redesigning and reinforcing of revised package of ICDS services to focus on under 3 children; Maternal Care, Early Childhood Care and Education (ECCE).

iii Rolling out strengthened and restructured ICDS in three years beginning with 200 high burden districts in 2012–13, additional 200 districts in second year and remaining 243 districts in third year of plan period.

Reforms in ICDS

i. Programmatic Reforms

Repositioning the Anganwadi centre as a "vibrant, child friendly Early Childhood Development (ECD) centre" (*Baal Vikas Kendra*) which will be owned by women in the community. This will have life cycle approach. This will have expanded/redesigned services, extended duration (6 hours), with an additional Anganwadi Worker (AWW) initially in 200 high burden districts with piloting of creche services in 5% of AWCs. Second AWW cum child care and Nurtrition Counsellor will focus on *0–3 years children* and counsel parents and caregivers of 0–3 years. Core intervention include home based guidance for parents, early childhood care and education (ECCE), early stimulation, early screening of developmental delays, optimal infant and young child feeding practices, monthly monitoring and promotion of child growth and developmental milestones and fixed village ECCE day besides supplementary nutrition, early registration of all pregnant women, 4 or more ANCs, institutional delivery and postnatal care, as also counselling on breastfeeding, complementary feeding, home based counselling for essential newborn care and spacing methods by home visits at cirtical contact points – newborn, postnatal and neonatal care (Days 1, 3, 7, 14, 21, 28 and 42).

- *Redesigning and Reinforcing of the Package* of ICDS services, including a new component of child care and Nutrition counselling for mothers of children under three years.
- *Enhancing Nutritional Impact* with revised nutrition and feeding norms, cost indexation of SNP. SNEHA SHIVIRS for community based prevention and care of severely undernourished children. This includes 12 days Nutrition care and counselling sessions at AWCs for mothers of undernourished children followed by 18 days of home practice.
- *Strengthening Early Childhood Care and Education (ECCE)* by redefining Preschool Education to ECCE; with additional and trained human resources and introduction of a developmentally appropriate curriculum framework with joyful learning methodologies.
- *Convergence with Flagship Programmes:* Convergence with NRHM, SSA and TSC, MGNREG Act and other schemes will be harnessed.
- *Community Mobilization and Monitoring:* Community based monitoring through ICDS NRHM Joint Mother and Child Protection Card.

II. Management Reforms

- Decentralized Programme Planning and monitoring in implementation systems with a result framework and flexible architecture.
- Improved human resource management for women and child development.

- Training and capacity building
- Strengthening civil society partnerships for operating up to 10% of the ICDS Projects.
- Increased public accountability by strengthening the role of PRIs, urban local bodies and village level functionaries in overseeing AWC functioning by **VHSNCs** and Anganwadi Management Committees.
- Ensuring Convergence with related sectors.
- Colocation of Anganwadi centres in schools.
- *Strengthening ICDS Management Information System* (MIS)
- Improved Financial Management system with linkages to outcome and social audits, provision of untied funds with empowerment for local action.

III. Institutional Reforms

Institutional Reforms aim at transforming ICDS into "Mission Mode", decentralized programme with flexible implementation framework with monitorable outcomes. Preparation of state district, sub-district programme implementation plans (PIP) on local needs.

- Capacity building through National/State ICDS Mission resource centres.
- Devolution of powers to PRIs and urban local bodies with untied funds, as also community ownership of ICDS.

IV. Enhancing Financial Resources

REFERENCES

1 GOI. Integrated Child Development Services Scheme. New Delhi: Department of Social Welfare Ministry of Education and Social Welfare GOI; 1976.

2 GOI. National Policy for Children. New Delhi: Ministry of Social Welfare; 1984.

3 GOI. Integrated Child Development Services. New Delhi: Department of Women and Child Development Ministry of HRD; 2000.

4 GOI. ICDS a compendium of guidelines. New Delhi: Department of Women and Child Development Ministry of HRD; 2000.

5 NIPCCD. Syllabus for job training of Anganwadi workers of ICDS programme. New Delhi: NIPCCD; 1989.

6 NIPCCD. UDISHA Syllabus for job training of Anganwadi workers. New Delhi: NIPCCD; 2003.

7 GOI. UDISHA The National Training Component for ICDS Building human resources for meeting women and child development goals. New Delhi: Department of Women and Child Development; 2000.

8 NIPCCD. Guidebook for Anganwadi workers training centres. New Delhi; NIPCCD; 1985.

9 NIPCCD. Organized job training of Anganwadi workers – Guidelines for instructors. New Delhi; NIPCCD; 1999.

10 NIPCCD. Handbook for Anganwadi workers, April 2006 NIPCCD. 5, Siri Institutional Area Hauz Khas, New Delhi.

11 GOI. National Policy of Education 1986, (revised 1992). New Delhi: Ministry of HRD GOI; 1992.

12 National Population Policy 2000. New Delhi: MOH and FW GOI; 2000.

13 Planning Commission. Twelfth Five-Year Plan 2012–17 Vol. II – Sectoral Policies and Programmes. New Delhi: MOH and FW GOI; 2012.

14 GOI. Reaching adolescent girls – Kishori Shakti Yojna and other initiatives. New Delhi: Department of women and child Ministry of HRD; 2002.

15 Lal S, Vani SN, Srivastava BC. ICDS Orientation Course for Medical Officers (a guide for consultants). Report of Central Technical Committee on Health and Nutrition. New Delhi: AIIMS; 1983.

16 Tandon BN. ICDS Evaluation and Research 1975–88. New Delhi: Central Technical Committee. Department of Women and Child Development Ministry of HRD GOI; 1990.

17 Central Technical Committee. ICDS – Survey Evaluation and Research. New Delhi: CTC; 1995.

18 NIPCCD. National Evaluation of ICDS. New Delhi: NIPCCD; 1992.

19 GOI. A Data Sheet – Fifteen Years of ICDS. New Delhi: Department of Women and Child Development; 1990.

20 Tandon BN. Participation of Medical Colleges in National Health Programmes – Experiments in India. NFI Bulletin 1986; 7(3).

21 Lal S, Sachar RK. Past, present and future of ICDS. Ind. J. Maternal and Child Health 2003; 4(1): 19–24.

22 Nutrition Foundation of India. Integrated Child Development Services – A study of some aspects of the system. Scientific Report No. 7.

23 NIPCCD. Three Decades of ICDS—An Appraisal 2006 NIPCCD 5, Siri Institutional Area Hauz Khas New Delhi.

24 GOI. National Policy for the Empowerment of Women. New Delhi: Department of Women and Child Development Ministry of HRD; 2001.

25 Government of India and UNICEF. National consultation of State, WCD Ministers and Secretaries on "ICDS Universalization with quality" held on 6–7 July 2005 at New Delhi organized by DWCD Ministry of Human Resource Development Government of India.

26 DWCD. Universalization of ICDS scheme. DWCD News letter "Sampark" vol. 1, issue 1, page, 17 New Delhi, 2005.

27 GOI, Ministry of Women and Child Development. ICDS Mission (2012). The Broad Framework for Implementation.

REPRODUCTIVE AND CHILD HEALTH (RCH) PROGRAMMES

The overriding objective of economic and social development is to improve the quality of lives that people lead, to enhance their well-being and to provide them with opportunities and choices to become productive assets in society.

NATIONAL FAMILY PLANNING PROGRAMME (NFPP)

EVOLUTION OF NEPP

The contraception services were clinic based to begin with and "extension approach" was adopted in the third five-year plan. From 1952–62 network of family planning clinics was established in the hospitals and hence it was known as "hospital-based and clinic-based approach" wherein contraception, counselling services besides information on methods to limit size of family and spacing between births were provided. During the "extension approach" information, education and services were expanded to cover the whole country.

"Lippes loop" (Intrauterine device) was introduced into the programme in the year 1965, it was an important armamentarium in the programme. During the year 1975–76, a new type of IUD known as "Cu-T 200" was introduced into national family planning programme. Statement on national population policy on the floor of Parliament was made way back in 1976 by Dr. Karan Singh the then Union Health and Family Welfare Minister. Important features of the statement were to raise the age of marriage to 18 years for girls and 21 years for boys and freezing the seats of Parliament Constituencies on the basis of Census 1971.[1]

National Family Planning Programme was renamed as National Family Welfare Programme in 1977. Female sterilization was the major thrust area of the programme and men participation was marginal in sterilization.

National Health Policy was adopted in 1983 and demographic goals of achieving net reproduction rate of unity (one) and birth rate of 21 by the end of century was intended, which could not be achieved.[2]

National Family Welfare Programme was integrated with maternal and child health programme during the fourth plan period.[1]

After successful eradication of smallpox in the year 1978, the expanded programme of immunization (EPI) was launched which became ultimately universal immunization programme (UIP) in 1985 and the process of integration of family planning, maternal and child health and UIP was further continued by launching child survival and safe motherhood programme (CSSM) in the year 1992.[3] The CSSM was MCH + Family planning + UIP. The interventions were focussed sharply with the objective of reducing infant mortality, maternal mortality and reducing the maternal and childhood morbidity to enhance the child survival and safe motherhood.

What went wrong with Family Welfare Programme? India's Family Planning/Welfare Programme had a *single objective* to *reduce fertility* as quickly as possible. The programme strategy was contraceptive targets and cash incentive to acceptors and providers. It was highly centralized. Targets to each state were allotted by the centre, and states allocated targets to districts. It promoted method specific contraception—sterilization. It resulted into inflation of performance statistics, but quality of services were compromised.[4]

Subsequently in the year 1994 landmark International Conference on Population and Development (ICPD) was held at Cairo where 180 countries of the world participated and recommended that the spectrum of services be enlarged, to cover total reproduction period and this conference recommended the strategy of "Reproductive and child health". India launched reproductive and child health (RCH) programme in the year 1996 to carry forward the process of integration of services. RCH means integration of CSSM + Family planning + prevention and treatment of reproductive tract infections including sexually transmitted infections including HIV/AIDS + Adolescent health.[5–9] Phase I of RCH was launched in 1997 and then came the National Population Policy in 2000.

Revised National Health Policy was adopted in year 2002. In the year 2005, phase II of reproductive and child health was launched to achieve the stated goals of 10th plan, Millennium Development Goals (MDGs), goats of National Health Policy of 2002, and the goals of National Rural Health Mission. Revised MDGs-2008 includes "universal access to Reproductive health by 2015".[10]

Based on the assessment of status of implementations of the programme of Action of ICPD the framework of actions for the follow-up programme of ICPD beyond 2014, it highlights to further strengthen health systems to provide universal access to sexual and reproductive health and rights and understanding of the implications of population dynamics as critical foundations for sustainable development goals.

With its Historic initation in 1952, NFPP primarily aimed at population stabilization and the strategy was to regulate births by providing fertility control methods both for limiting and spacing. The programme has been repositioned not only to achieve population stabilization but also to reduce maternal mortality, infant and child mortality. The promotion of maternal and child health has been one of the most important objectives of Family Welfare Programme in India, besides population stabilization. National Population Policy was adopted in 2000.

- **The Immediate Objective of National Population Policy** was to address the unmet needs of contraception, health care infrastructure, health personnel, and to provide an integrated service delivery for basic reproductive and child health care, with special focus on states facing the biggest sociodemographic challenges.

- **The medium-term objective was to bring** the Total Fertility Rate (TFR) to replacement level (2.1), through convergence and intersectoral linkages.
- **The long-term objective was** to achieve a stable population by 2045, at a level consistent with the requirement of sustainable economic growth, social development and environmental protection.

INTERVENTIONS

Many interventions are in position now:

- Family Planning services in public health sector include: **Limiting methods** (minilap, laparoscopic sterilization, no scalpel vasectomy) and **spacing methods** includes—IUD 380A, and IUD 375, oral contraceptives, condoms besides emergency contraception.
- Quality assurance in Family Planning by providing new standard guidelines, regular monitoring of sterilization services, conducting medical audit and improving skills by regular training programmes.
- Introduction of IUD 380A in the programme (10 years protection) and IUD 375 (5 years protection).
- Male participation in Planned Parenthood including no scalpel vasectomy and package of incentives to acceptors of sterilization.
- Introduction to newer contraceptives like injectable contraceptives—Cyclofem.
- Ensuring family planning services at all levels of health care delivery service—at village—subcentres, PHC and CHC which have been strengthened now by NRHM.
- Revised compensation scheme for acceptors of sterilization service for loss of wages.
- National Family Planning insurance scheme: National Family Planning Indemnity Scheme:

Government of India has launched National Family Planning insurance scheme in November 2005 as a promotional and motivational measure for compensation to the acceptors of sterilization or his/her nominee in the unlikely event of his/her death, failure or complications following a sterilization operation. The scheme also provides for indemnity insurance cover to Medical Officers of the facilities and accredited institutions against litigations.

- Another reproductive need to be addressed is the fertility promotion for infertile couples who constitute nearly 10–15% of the total couples in India.

Assisted Reproductive Techniques (ART) for Infertility

As per WHO data the prevalence of infertility in various countries including India is around 10–15%. There has been increased demand for assisted reproduction from these infertile couples. This has led to mushrooming of infertility clinics and in many of these centres the quality of services is questionable. The national guidelines on ART have been developed by ICMR and National Academy of Medical Sciences.

- Contraceptives in the National Family Welfare Programme (*see* Chapter 4).

Achievements

- The birth rate has been brought down to 21.4 by 2013 and total fertility rate to 2.3 by the year 2014. However, there still remains a huge unmet need of 21.5% (DLHS-3) for family planning methods. The unmet need varies from state to state. The main reasons for high unmet needs and unwanted fertility are:
- Non-availability of quality services
- Lack of skilled providers
- Gender biased programme with poor male participation.

International Conference on Population and Development in 1994 recognized the relevance of population stabilization by integrating the various health determinants to ensure population development and enhance quality of life.

India launched national family planning programme in 1952 and was the first country in the world to do so. The objective was to reduce the birth rate to the extent necessary "to stabilize the population at a level consistent with the requirement of national economy".

REPRODUCTIVE AND CHILD HEALTH (RCH) PHASE I (1997–2005)

The RCH approach has been defined as "*People have the ability to reproduce and regulate their fertility, women are able to go through pregnancy and childbirth safely, the outcome of pregnancies is successful in terms of maternal and infant survival and well-being and couples are able to have sexual relations free of fear of pregnancy and of contracting diseases*" (Fathalla, 1988). This concept is in keeping with the evolution of an integrated approach to the programmes, aimed at improving the health status of young women and children, which has been going on in the country. It is obviously sensible that integrated RCH programme would help in reducing the cost of inputs to some extent because overlapping of expenditure would no longer be necessary and integrated implementation would optimise outcomes at the field level. During the 9th plan, the RCH programme, accordingly, integrated all the related programmes of the 8th plan. The concept of RCH is to provide to the beneficiaries *need-based, client-centred, demand driven, high quality* and *integrated* RCH *services* by adopting 'life cycle approach'. The RCH programme is a composite programme incorporating the inputs of the government of India as well as funding support from external donor agencies including World Bank and the European Commission.[11]

It is a legitimate right of the citizens to be able to experience sound reproductive and child health and therefore, the RCH programme will seek to provide relevant services for assuring reproductive and child health to all citizens. However, RCH is even more relevant for attaining the objective of stable population for the country. The overall objective since the beginning has been that the population of the country should be stabilised at a level consistent with the requirement of national development. It is now well established that parents keep the family size small if they are assured about the health and longevity (survival) of the children and there is no better assurance of good health and longevity of the children than health care for the mothers and for young children. Therefore, RCH programme by ensuring small families also ensures stable population in the medium and long-term, though in the short-term, population is controlled by use of spacing methods and terminal methods for avoiding unwanted pregnancies. Therefore, the overall strategy of the government of India (department of family welfare) is to simultaneously strive for obtaining reproductive and child health arrangements for the whole of the country's population and to promote and make available contraceptive/terminal methods for desirous couples. It also needs to be observed that the measures through the health system alone do not and cannot assure success in either ensuring reproductive and child health or in controlling population.

The **RCH programme** incorporates the components covered under the child survival and safe motherhood programme (CSSM) and includes two additional components, one relating to reproductive tract infection (RTI) including sexually transmitted infections (STIs) and other relating to adolescent reproductive and sexual health. The main highlights of the RCH programme are:

i The programme integrates all interventions of fertility regulation, maternal and child health with reproductive health of both men and women.

ii The services to be provided will be *client centred, demand driven high quality* and based on the *needs* of the *community arrived* at through decentralised participatory planning and the *target free approach.*

iii The programme envisages upgradation of the level of facilities for providing various interventions and quality of care. The first referral units (FRUs) being set-up at sub-district level will provide comprehensive emergency obstetric and newborn care (CoEmONC). Similarly, RCH facilities in PHCs will be substantially upgraded.

iv The programme will improve access of the community to various services which are commonly required.

v Life cycle approach—continuum of services.

PARADIGM SHIFT—MOVING TO A REPRODUCTIVE AND CHILD HEALTH APPROACH

The Government of India made historical reform in family planning programme and thereby continued the process of reforms in health sector. It was a *Turning Point* in FP programme. The major policy shift was announced in 1996 (Table 5.5). The salient features of historical landmark shift were:

1 ***Target free approach:*** Doing away targets allocation for family planning by the Central Government/State Government.

2 ***Decentralization of planning, training and funding:*** Delegation of responsibilities to local bodies (Panchayats and Nagarpalikas) and delegation of authority and funds to local bodies. It is reversal of "top down" to "bottom up" approach (Fig. 5.1).

3 ***Community needs based planning:*** Community needs assessment approach (CNAA): Community consultation or consultation of people or clients by health workers to ascertain their needs and work out targets themselves at local level.

4 **Improved quality** of clinical services and **coverage**.

5 **Sustainability** of infrastructure and work-force to provide benefits for the present as well as future.

6 **More efficient financial management** especially ways of linking funding to performance, i.e. perform an activity or achieve work completion and get money or funds.

7 **Client satisfaction**, i.e. focus on consumer or client.

8 **Full range of maternal and child** health services including RTIs/STIs and HIV/AIDS and adolescent health by "life cycle approach".

9 **Listening** to client and accountability to clients. Helping them to achieve small family norms themselves.

10 Family planning performance in district was not to be used to rank or assess the administration.

Essentially, the *paradigm shift* means need-based, client centered, demand-driven quality services, planning with consultation of people, local planning and funds available with the people or at the lowest level (District, Block, PHC and Subcentres) for immediate action. It is planning with the people by the people and for the people. *Coverage, quality* of services and *client satisfaction* are the hallmark of such a shift. *Spectrum* of services has been enlarged and access to services increased.

Programme Interventions

The RCH programme has been implemented based on differential approach as it has been realized that a 'one size fits all' may not suffice. Inputs in all the districts have not been kept uniform because efficient delivery will depend on the capacity of the health system in the district. Therefore, basic facilities are strengthened and streamlined specially in the *weaker districts* as the better-off districts already have such facilities and the more sophisticated facilities are proposed for the relatively advanced districts which have acquired the capability to make use of them effectively. All the districts have been categorised into categories A (58), B (184) and C (265), on the basis of crude birth rate and female literacy rate which reasonably reflect the RCH status of the district. The districts have been covered in a phased manner over three years. The nationally uniform and differentiated RCH interventions would be as stated in Tables 5.4 and 5.5.

COMPONENTS OF REPRODUCTIVE AND CHILD HEALTH PROGRAMME[11]

Components of RCH programme:

1 Community needs assessment approach (CNAA) and decentralized participatory planning (DPP)
2 Integrated package of services for mother and child

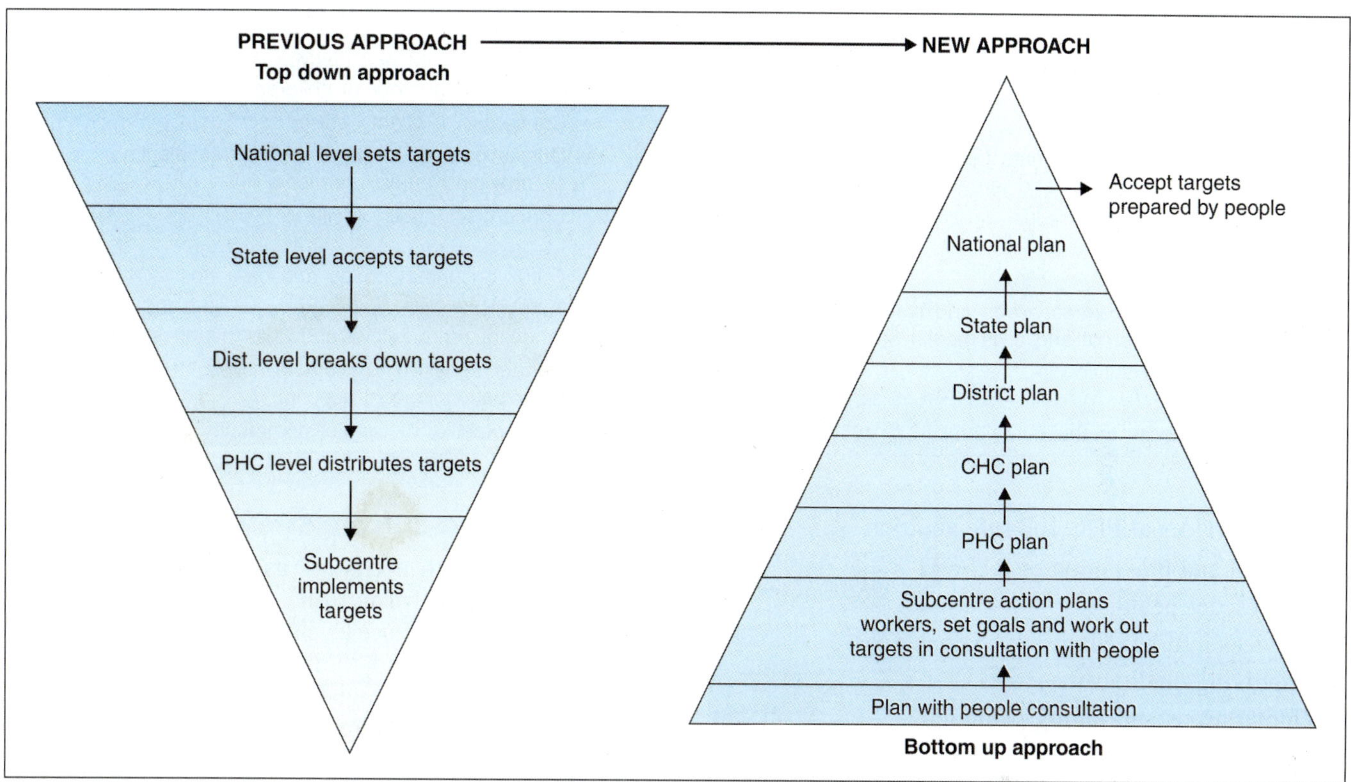

Fig. 5.1: Paradigm shift

Table 5.4: RCH interventions

Interventions in all districts	Interventions in selected states/districts
• Child survival interventions (as available under CSSM programme) • Safe motherhood interventions (as available under CSSM programme) • Facilitation for operationalisation of target free approach • Institutional development • Integrated training package • Modified management information system • IEC activities and counselling on health, sexuality and gender • Urban and tribal areas RCH package and ANM kits at subcentres • District sub-projects under local capacity enhancement • RTI/STI clinics at district hospitals (where not available) • Facility for safe abortions at PHCs by providing equipment, contractual doctors, etc. • Enhanced community participation through Panchayat, women's groups and NGOs • Minor civil works • Provision for Lab technicians for laboratory diagnosis of RTI/STI and essential obstetric care • Adolescent health and reproductive hygiene	• Screening and treatment of RTI/STI • Emergency obstetric care at selected FRUs by providing drugs • Essential obstetric care by providing drugs and PHN/staff nurse at PHCs • Additional ANM at subcentres in the selected districts for ensuring MCH care • Improved delivery services and emergency care by providing equipment kits, IUD insertions and ANM kits at subcentres • Rental to contracted PHNs/ANMs, not provided Government accommodation • Facility of referral transport for pregnant women during emergency to the nearest referral centre

5

Table 5.5: Paradigm shift

Family welfare approach	*RCH approach*
• Top down approach	• Bottom up approach (community needs assessment approach)
• Target and technology driven	• Human and social development centred
• Centralized planning	• Need-based decentralized and participatory planning—act locally and support nationally
• Promoted contraceptive specific method (mainly sterilization)	• Helps clients to help themselves to space or limit the number of children
• Method centred	• Consumer or client centred
• Quantity centred to inflate targets and to achieve numbers and targets	• Quality centred to improve client satisfaction by providing quality services
• Single objective to reduce fertility as quickly as possible	• Concern for quality of life
• Focus on targets	• Focus on unmet needs and demands
• Focussed on contraceptives and limited range of maternal and child health services	• Focused on "life cycle approach" and full range of reproductive and child health services
• Gender insensitive	• Gender sensitive to promote men's participation in contraception
• Accountability to the bureaucracy	• Accountability to clients, community and workers

3 MTP services at PHC and safe abortion
4 Control and prevention of RTI/STI
5 Adolescent health
6 Services in urban slums and Tribal areas
7 Improving quality of services
8 Unmet needs and family planning
9 Communication strategy in RCH
10 Gender sensitiveness
11 Greater involvement of Panchayati Raj institutions, non-governmental organizations and community
12 Civil works, Dai training and RCH Camps.

1. COMMUNITY NEEDS ASSESSMENT APPROACH (CNAA) OR TARGET FREE APPROACH

Target free approach has been repositioned as "Community needs assessment approach". In this approach under RCH programme, the health workers work out the targets for themselves by a process of consultation with clients and community in their respective areas.[12] Health workers plan the services at village level every year and submit subcentre action plans to respective primary health centre. The aggregation of village plans lead onto subcentres action plan, aggregation of subcentres action plans constitute "Primary health centre plan" and aggregation of PHCs plans lead onto CHCs plan and district action plan is an aggregate of all CHCs plans. These plans will help to work out the requirements of all materials and supplies for the population to be served at each level.

Subcentre action plans are vital as the process of CNAA begins at the level of village and subcentre. This is decentralized participatory planning (DPP).

How the Needs of RCH are Assessed by Workers?

Generally the health needs are assessed on the basis of epidemiological information, such as contraceptive prevalence rates/acceptance levels, number of births, number of eligible couples and their status of acceptance of contraceptive services, registration of pregnant women, lactating mothers and children below five years of age apart from disease burden. These events need to be continuously updated by *surveillance mechanism*. Health workers must ensure registration of all marriages, pregnancies, births and eligible couples on continuous basis in the assigned area. It is most desirable that the registration of pregnancy, births and deaths should be 100% and the total area population must be covered. Needs are also determined by utilization of services by the clients, as also from the past year performance.

Health workers assess the needs of pregnant women, infant and young children, nursing mothers and eligible couples by way of regular contacting and identification of these beneficiaries, registration of beneficiaries and their continuous updating by home visits, periodic surveys, as and when they get an opportunity to contact these beneficiaries during outreach session and subcentre clinic or at Anganwadi centre. Needs of each and every family and individual member are assessed by the health workers by **household survey.**

Needs of pregnant mothers: Safe pregnancy—antenatal check-ups and early recognition of danger signals, prevention and treatment of anaemia and immunization against tetanus and safe delivery are their prime needs, besides adequate diet.

Needs of nursing mothers: Postnatal care, prevention of infection, care of breast, adequate diet, prophylaxis and treatment for anaemia, spacing births, and limiting size of family are their prime needs.

Need of newborn and infant: Survival, breastfeeding, exclusive breastfeeding, immunization, adequate feeding, growth, and integrated management of childhood illnesses, vitamin A prophylaxis.

Needs of 1–5 years: Immunization, growth and development by adequate feeding, vitamin A and iron and folic acid. Prophylaxis and treatment of anaemia, prevention and control of acute respiratory infection, diarrhoeal diseases, malaria and worm infestations, prevention of accidents and injuries, preschool education or early childhood care and education.

Needs of 5–14 years: Education and schooling, immunization, personal hygiene, development of healthy lifestyles, prevention of accidents and injuries, family life education.

Needs of adolescents: Health information is the prime need of adolescents. Adequate diet, menstural hygiene, prevention of anaemia, tetanus toxoid, prevention of RTI/STI. HIV/AIDS besides family life education.

Needs of eligible couples (15–49) years: Contraception to space births and limit the size of family. Prevention and control of RTI/STI including HIV, and management of infertility (reproductive health).

Community needs: Safe water, safe excreta disposal, waste water disposal, garbage disposal, all weather roads and health facility. Right age of marriage of girls, schools, and organized men and women groups.

Health needs are felt by people and expressed in the form of demands. The people demand hospitals, health centres, doctors, drugs, and other facilities. The felt needs must be met, through adequate and quality services. The best compromise is to start where the felt needs and real needs overlap.

Generally, the priority demands with the people are roads, electricity, water, schools, veterinary services for cattle and hospitals/health services come last of all.

Preparation of Subcentre Action Plan—Decentralized Participatory Planning (DPP)

People first. Planning of services actually begins at grassroot levels in consultation with households, families and village Panchayat, *Mahila Swasthya Sangh* (MSS), school teachers, village birth attendant, Anganwadi workers and registered practitioners.

The first step in the process is to work out the service **needs** or requirements on the basis of information as elaborated above.

The needs or requirements of maternal and child health and Family Planning services can be ascertained by:

i Preparing household records of all families in the area by annual surveys on household register. The household surveys are conducted once in a year in the month of February or March.

ii From the household surveys the health workers work out the total population, eligible couples, pregnant women, infants and young children. One time survey is not enough as marriages, pregnancy and births, disease events go on occurring in the population or area and these events needs to be continuously recognized and registered (*surveillance*) by the health teams working at the level of village and subcentre.

The subcentre action plan is most important document and has sound epidemiological basis of planning work, determining the workload, work schedule, coverage of services, reporting of services, monitoring of services, self-evaluation of performance and improvement of work.

Subcentre may have 4–10 villages under its jurisdiction, all events are to be registered and recorded village-wise to determine the number of clients who need our services. Knowing only the number of clients is not enough. It must be known where they are? In which household they are? Who are the young couples? How many eligibles couples belong to weaker section? Hence contacting clients in their *homes/household on regular basis* to meet their needs is an essential step. Home visits on regular basis to locate clients and contacting them for varied MCH services forms the basis of action plan at subcentre. Action plan should ensure contact with all clients with *fixed schedule* on *regular basis*. One such practical method evolved over the time is "home visits" to cover the entire area in 3–4 months time.

The second method to contact the clients is through "outreach session" on immunization. Yet, another method of contact is receiving clients at *"subcentre clinic"* or meeting clients at Anganwadi centre or meeting them during intensive campaigns or on Village Health Sanitation, and Nutrition Day (VHSND). Sustained contacts on regular basis are essential to know the clients and their needs to meet their needs and to develop confidence and their satisfaction.

iii Through these methods—(*survey, surveillance* and *regular contacts*), workers are able to develop annual subcentre action plan and project the number of clients to be provided services during the year.

iv The workers themselves give or allot targets to themselves for immunizations, *family planning* and *maternal and child health*. Every month they report the coverage and performance.

v Since the task of preparing of subcentre action plan by workers themselves is a new beginning it is a challenging work for health workers and medical officers, who are not used to such things. All along and throughout their life they have worked on the basis of what is told to them or whatever targets come and plan comes from above or higher levels. They have developed a culture to obey and do whatever comes from higher level. This is a new beginning to plan for themselves and use the *science of epidemiology* at local level to evolve a sensible action plan.

vi Developing functional linkages with ICDS system (Anganwadi workers) helps to assess the community needs as also validate the subcentre action plans. Developing linkages with traditional birth attendants, ASHAs and village Panchayats (village chowkidar) help to register events timely for appropriate actions. Health workers would prepare better action plans if they work with and work through Anganwadi workers and ICDS system, which is now universal in India. Having joint home visits, joint surveys and joint reports, integrated work schedule means better action plan and better work and better quality of services for mother and child.

vii Since, this is a new culture, the medical officers, health supervisors and health workers have temptations to work out the magic figures of clients by application of formulae to assumed population, which should be avoided and discouraged, workers should use their own data.

Adequate training and retraining of medical officers and health team on "Community needs assessment approach" is essential.

District training teams need to be oriented well. Subcentre action plans have not taken off well in the RCH phase I, hopefully these are put to operation in the phase II of RCH. Decentralized action plans at the subcentre level are vital and all efforts must be made to revitalize these. The concept of subcentre action plan should be included in the basic curriculum of multipurpose health workers (female and male) as also in the curriculum of undergraduates. Village health sanitation and nutrition committee under NRHM will initiate village health plan for each village and aggregation of village plans will lead to subcentre PHC and block plan. The block plans would eventually converge into district action plans (DAP) which would thereafter converge into State plans.

The *Operational Guidelines* on *Maternal* and *Newborn Health* (April 2010) under NRHM is a major effort to address the problem of maternal and neonatal mortality. The service delivery framework identifies three levels.

Level 1: Consists of deliveries conducted by skilled birth attendants (SBA) in all subcentres, PHCs not functioning as 24 × 7. Newborn corner in all facilities and home deliveries assisted by SBA would also be included under safe deliveries at this level. This level provides essential obstetric and neonatal care at community level.

Level 2: Consists of 24 × 7 PHCs, CHCs other than FRUs or stabilization unit or private nursing homes with equivalent facilities, which provides basic obstetric and neonatal care and basic emergency obstetric and newborn care (BEmONC) at institutional level. This manages low birth weight babies above 1800 g.

Level 3: Consists of FRUs, Districts and Subdistricts or referral hospitals (public and private) and selected CHCs, special newborn care unit which provides comprehensive emergency obstetric and newborn care (CEmONC). This level manages low birth weight babies below 1800 g. It can manage obstetric complications including C—section and blood transfusion.

Strengthening of *Delivery Points*: Depending upon the number of deliveries at level 1, 2, and 3, these *deliver points* need to be strengthened for Providing Comprehensive Reproductive maternal and Child Health Services.

2. INTEGRATED PACKAGE OF SERVICES FOR MOTHERS AND CHILDREN

Essential Obstetric Care (EOC) for all Pregnant Women EOC Includes—Antenatal Care, Safe Delivery and Post-natal Care Including Newborn Care

Quality Antental Care Includes—Minimum 4 Check-ups

Tracking Every Pregnant Women and Child by name. Early recognition and registration of all pregnancies ideally within first trimester (before 12th week of pregnancy) and ensuring minimum four antenatal check ups. First visit to antenatal clinic within 12 weeks, 2nd visit between 14th and 26th week, 3rd at 28th to 34th week and 4th between 34 week and full term.[13,14]

Antental care-package: The antenatal care package includes counseling for birth, emergency preparedness, preparation for newborn care, breastfeeding, nutrition, family planning counseling and information about post-partum family planning methods. Early registration of pregnancy, physical and abdominal examination, weighing, measuring height taking blood pressure, breast examination, urine and blood examination for pregnancy test, albumin, sugar, haemoglobin and RH factor, VDRL and blood grouping (where facilities exist). This is done for early detection of danger signs and complications which can develop at any time in any pregnant women. (Danger Signs include swelling over feet, severe anaemia, bleeding, excessive weight gain, Jaindice, etc.). Besides check ups ensure that all pregnant women receive two doses of tetanus toxoid or a booster dose of tetanus toxoid, folic acid supplementation in the first trimester, iron and folic acid tablets from 12 weeks onwards for 100 days for prevention and treatment of anaemia and deworming after first trimester, Tablet calcium, Vit. C and B_{12}. Linkages with nearest ICTC or PPTCT centre for voluntary counseling and HIV testing are essential for 90% coverage.

- The testing kits for early detection of pregnancy are available under the package. Pregnancy test kits (Nishchay) should be made accessible to all women in reproductive age group including adolescent girls (unmarried and married). Early diagnosis of pregnancy has many advantages: It facilitates early registration for antenatal care as well as safe termination of unwanted pregnancies.

Preventive use of Folic Acid in Periconception Period

Promoting use of folic acid in planned pregnancies during the periconception period (3 months before and 3 months after conception) for prevention of neural tube defects and other congenital anomalies may be adopted by states as preventive measure.

- **Under Prevention of Parent to Child Transmission (PPTCT)** programme all pregnant women who are diagnosed with HIV are linked with HIV services for prevention of HIV transmission to newborn babies.
- **Management of severely anaemic women:** ANM and PHC medical officer incharge are the nodal officers for line listing of severely anaemic women, tracking and management of these pregnant women during and after pregnancy and child birth has been started now. In malaria endemic areas there is provision for providing Long Lasting Insecticide Treated Nets (LLIN) under the NVBDCP.
- **Implementation of Preconception and Prenatal Diagnostic Techniques (PC & PNDT):** Female sex ratio at birth and in age group of 0–6 years continue to be unfavourable. Implementation of this Act is essential to have an optimal sex ratio at birth.

Intranatal Care (Safe Delivery)

- Promotion of institutional deliveries
- Provision of 24 hours delivery services at PHC
- Skilled attendance (SBA) at home and institutional deliveries
- Appropriate and prompt referral and transport system
- Promotion of safe home deliveries
- Essential newborn care
- Strengthening of "*delivery points*".

Safe Deliveries

a. **Skilled obstetric care:** It is considered to be the single most critical intervention for ensuring safe motherhood and improved perinatal mortality. Training for Skilled Birth Attendance include:
   - 10 days for medical officess in Basic Emergency Obstetric Care (BEMOC); and
   - 3 weeks for ANM/LHV/Staff Nurses in Skilled Birth Attendance
b. **Demand Generation for Skilled Obstetric Care—*Janani Suraksha Yojna* (JSY)** has provision of conditional cash transfer to pregnant women for institutional delivery and care during delivery and immediate postpartum period. Other features related to JSY are:
   - Promotion of 48 hours stay at health facility for the well-being and survival of mother and newborn.
   - Focus on motivating mother/family for adoption of postpartum family planning methods and counseling on exclusive breastfeeding, immunization and child care practices.
c. **Essential newborn care and resuscitation:** Essential newborn care and resuscitation is significant in preventing neonatal deaths and illnesses. It improves access to quality emergency care for the sick child. Newborn care corners are being established at all delivery points which have skilled birth attendants who are also trained on Navjaat Shishu Suraksha Karyakram (NSSK).
d. **Operationalizing delivery points:** Health facility located across the health system are now assessed against a minimum bench mark of performance (number of deliveries conducted per month as one of the parameters of service utilisation, more than 3 deliveries per month in SC; > 10 per month in PHC, > 20 per month in CHC, > 50 per month in SDH/DH) are designated as "Delivery Points", norms have been relaxed for North Eastern States, Himachal and J & K. The delivery points are to be prioritized for the allocation of resources (infrastructure, human resources, drugs and supplies, referral transport, etc.) in order to make available comprehensive RMNCH + A services at these facilities.
e. **Maternal and child health wings (MCH Wings):** 100/50/30 beded Maternal and Child Health Wings are being established at high case load facilities in order to expand the public health care infrastructure and quality of care for mothers and newborns.
f. **Multiskilling of doctors in public health system:** It is being undertaken to address the shortage of specialists.

Postpartum Care for Mother and Newborn

Three quarters of all maternal deaths occur from complications either during or immediate postpartum period. Similarly around three quarters of neonatal deaths take place in the first week with up to half of these occuring within 24 hours of birth.

Provision of 48 hours stay at the health facility in case of institutional delivery, with dietary services is essential so that both the mother and newborn are under medical observation to deal with any life-threatening complications, such as haemorrhage, sepsis and engorged breasts. Post-natal period is critical period when most neonatal and maternal deaths (75%) take place.

Postnatal **home visits** to both mother and baby are made by ASHA, AWW's and ANM's:

- In all cases–at least **3 postnatal visits** to mother and 6 postnatal visits to the newborn within 6 weeks of delivery/birth.
- In case of home deliveries–an additional first visit within 24 hours of birth (a total of 7 neonatal visits and 4 postnatal visits to mother).

These visits are useful for identification and management of emergencies occurring during postnatal period. ANMs, LHVs and staff Nurses are being trained for managing emergencies identified during these visits, as also for referrals to higher level. These visits ensure:

- Initiation of early breastfeeding within an hour of birth.
- Counselling on diet and rest, hygiene, contraception, essential newborn case (resuscitation of newborn with asphyxia, prevention of hypothermia prevention of infections exclusive breast feeding and referral of sick newborn, infant and young child feeding and immunization—OPV, BCG and hepatitis B). Spacing births at least 3 years apart and limiting family size.

Postpartum IUCD Insertion

There has been shift in family planning approach to promote spacing rather than just terminal method (sterilization). Inter pregnancy interval of at least 3 years is known to improve pregnancy outcomes in terms of birth weight and overall survival of the newborn as also build up necessary reserves of mother. Immediate Postpartum Intrauterine Contraceptive Device (PPIUCD)—insertion of IUCD (CuT 380 A) is a new initiative introduced in the country to address high unmet needs of spacing during postpartum period by placement of trained providers for Postpartum IUCD (PPIUCD) insertion at district and sub-district hospital besides expansion of PPIUCD services to health facilities up to subcentre level. Dedicated RMNCH + A counsellors have been placed in public health facilities for counselling at high case load facilities.

Hygiene during pregnancy, delivery and postpartum: Observing strict hygiene and infection prevention protocols should be followed while providing services to mothers; newborns and children. Handwashing before examination, initiation of breastfeeding and cord care. Observe 5 cleans during home delivery—clean surface, clean hands, clean place, clean cord and clean cord tie.

Emergency Obstetric Care at CHC/FRU/District

It is an important intervention for preventing *maternal* and *infant mortality* and *morbidity*. The complications of pregnancy, such as anaemia, haemorrhages, obstructed labour, sepsis are major causes of maternal mortality and morbidity, if these complications are detected early and managed appropriately, maternal mortality and morbidity will be reduced substantially. If minimum four check-ups by ANM at antenatal and 3 at postnatal stage are ensured by competent supervision, most of such cases can be detected and attended before they become life-threatening. The ANM is expected to refer cases of complication during pregnancy or at the time of delivery or after delivery to primary health centres (PHCs) or first referral units (FRUs) or District hospital. Expected referral rate is around 15 percent.

What is First Referral Unit (FRU)?

The purpose of FRU is to prevent maternal and infant deaths. The FRUs were set-up under CSSM and have been expanded and strengthened under RCH. First referral units have been set-up at community health centres or sub-district hospital. At FRU, we have the facilities of operation theatre, C-section, newborn care, and blood transfusion facility and specialist in obstetric and gynae, anaesthesia and paediatrics. In identified FRUs, necessary equipment and emergency obstetric drug kits have been provided to deal with emergencies. If regular specialists are not available, these can be hired on contractual basis. The sub-district hospitals, CHCs and FRUs are entitled to hire services of private anaesthetists for conducting emergency operations for which they are to be paid ₹ 1500 per case.

The progress of setting up of FRUs has been very slow. The FRUs are non-functional more so in category B and category C districts, which are weak in their performance, it is a matter of deep concern as maternal mortality continues to be very high in these districts. Steps should be taken to operationalize the identified FRUs at the earliest by district RCH societies and through public private-partnership or by non-governmental organizations.

To build-up capacity of FRUs for looking after the needs of emergency obstetric care and RTIs/STIs, the districts have been assisted to engage two laboratory technicians on contractual basis for doing routine blood, urine and RTIs/STIs tests.

In FRUs the thrust should be on **critical components** of FRUs, such as surgical intervention (C-section), newborn care and blood storage facilities, man power and referral linkages.

- Referral services at both Community and Institutional level: Establishing referral linkages between the community and FRUs is essential component for utilization of services particularly during emergencies. Since emergencies during the birth process cannot be predicted it is essential to ensure access of referral services to all pregnant women.
- Accessibility: FRU should be accessible within 2 hours of travel time.
- Training of MBBS Doctor in lifesaving anaesthesia skills and obstetric management skills to provide emergency obstetric care to save lives of women.

National Ambulance Services

NRHM has supported free ambulance with basic life support services to provide patients transport in every nook and corner of the country connected with toll free number 102, 104 and 108. Over 16000 basic and emergency patient transport vehicles have been provided under NRHM.

Besides these, over 5778 vehicles have been empanelled to transport patients particularly pregnant women and sick infants from home to public health facilities and back. Call centres have been set up by states for effective patient transport system. This step reduces delay in reaching health facility and prevents maternal and infant deaths.

5

3. MEDICAL TERMINATION OF PREGNANCY (MTP)

Medical termination of pregnancy is permissible under certain conditions laid down in the Medical Termination of Pregnancy Act, 1971. However, MTP should not be a mechanism for restricting family size, or for avoiding unwanted births in routine.

Although officially the figures for MTP in the country are only one million in a year but various experts and studies have estimated the actual number may be in the range of eleven million or even more per year. Such MTPs (unsafe illegal abortions) in the hands of untrained, unqualified, quacks and unexperienced persons result in maternal deaths and morbidity on large scale. Around 8–10% of maternal mortality in the country is due to unsafe abortions alone.

Under the RCH programme, the medical officers have been trained for MTPs and MTP equipment has been provided to trained medical officers to conduct the MTPs at the level of PHCs/CHCs and district hospitals where operation theatres and trained doctors are available.

To supplement these arrangements, the government of India has given a liberty to district health society to engage trained medical officers to conduct MTPs at PHC once a week or once a fortnight and payment of ₹ 500 per day is permissible to such doctors engaged for MTPs.

Equipment of MTP has been provided to non-governmental organizations also to promote safe abortions. Training facilities for MTP have been set-up by the government. Most MTPs are done in private sector.

Problem of Unsafe Abortions

Unsafe abortion is a public health problem in India as it is one of the important cause of maternal mortality in India besides maternal morbidity. Around eleven million women seek abortions every year. Out of eleven million abortions, 6–7 million are illegal abortions. 15,000–20,000 deaths due to illegal abortions have been reported per year.[15] Abortion is legal in India under MTP Act, 1971.

What is Abortion?

Abortion has been defined by WHO: Termination of pregnancy before the fetus becomes viable or capable of living independently. Abortion can be spontaneous or induced.

In India, six states have the highest number of abortions. These states are—Assam, Bihar, Madhya Pradesh, Odisha, Uttar Pradesh and West Bengal.

Indian women seek abortion throughout the reproductive period. Adolescents; both married and unmarried seek abortion services in significant number. A substantial number of unwanted pregnancies among adolescents result from forced sexual intercourse. As adolescents have less access to reproductive health information and services compared to older married counterparts and they are more likely to delay recognizing pregnancy and seeking care. They are more likely to seek care from unsafe providers.

India's second trimester abortion rate is high at 10%. The risk of complications following second trimester abortion is much higher for physiological reasons.

Illegal abortions are done by unscientific and dangerous techniques by vaginal and oral methods. Sticks, roots and foreign bodies are introduced into vagina, which result into life-threatening complications like infections and excessive bleeding, perforation of uterus or injury to bowel.

Why do women seek abortions: Women seek abortions for a variety of reasons, such as unwanted pregnancy, health problem during pregnancy, pregnancy at older age, extramarital pregnancy, pregnancy on account of rape, etc. Sex selective abortions are commonly sought. Strong son preference and easy availability of prenatal diagnostic techniques have resulted in increase use of prenatal sex determination tests even among rural poor. Many private clinics offer both sex determination and abortion services. Despite the Prenatal Diagnostic Techniques (Regulation and Prevention of Misuse) Act, 1994, the practice of sex determination is rampant.

Contraceptive failure can also lead to unwanted pregnancies and these can be terminated legally.

What is MTP?

Medical termination of pregnancy (MTP) is a reproductive health measure that enables women to "opt out" of an unwanted/unintended pregnancy without endangering her life and well-being. Ensuring women's access to safe abortion services is an essential component of ensuring women's right to safeguard their health. Safe abortion is one of the components of RCH programme.

India legalized medical termination of pregnancy on broad sociomedical grounds through the MTP Act, 1971. The aim of the Act was to reduce maternal mortality and morbidity due to illegal abortions.

Conditions under which pregnancy can be terminated under MTP Act: **Medical grounds:** Where the continuation of pregnancy might endanger the life of pregnant women or cause grave injury to the physical and mental health (such as severe heart disease, renal disease, psychiatric disorders, severe hypertension).

Eugenic: Where there is substantial risk of the child being born with serious handicaps due to physical or mental abnormalities.

Humanitarian: Where pregnancy is the result of rape.

Socioeconomic: If a women who already have too many children and with an unplanned pregnancy who cannot support another child.

Failure of contraceptives: When pregnancy occurs due to failure of contraceptive.

The written consent of the guardian is necessary before performing abortions in women under 18 years of age and in lunatics even if they are older than 18 years.

Person who can Perform Abortion

Act provides for termination of pregnancy up to 20 weeks. Registered medical practitioner trained in MTP can perform MTP. Single doctor can terminate pregnancy below 12 weeks, however where pregnancy exceeds 12 weeks and not more than 20 weeks the opinion of two medical practitioners is necessary to terminate pregnancy. The Act stipulates that no termination of pregnancy shall be performed at any place other than a hospital established and maintained by the government or the place approved for the purpose of this Act. PNDT authority at district level is civil surgeon or chief medical officer of the district.

MTP under RCH Programme

MTP is an important component of the RCH programme, which was launched in 1996. Under RCH, it is envisaged to improve MTP facilities and their utilization. MTP can be performed at all District hospitals, Sub-district hospitals, CHCs and in all PHCs where there are operation theatres and doctors trained in MTP procedures. The CuT can be safely inserted concurrently with first trimester medical termination of pregnancy and after first menstrual period following spontaneous/medical/ second trimester abortion.

4. REPRODUCTIVE TRACT INFECTIONS/STIs

Annual incidence of RTI is 5% in India. This is a problem of public health importance as 30–40% of women suffer silently with RTI. Different studies indicate variable prevalence because of different methodologies adopted.

HIV is killer STD. RTIs can lead to infertility, ectopic pregnancy, foetal wastage, preterm deliveries, low birth weight babies or by infecting newborns during delivery.

Under the RCH programme, all district hospitals and selected FRUs have been assisted for setting up of RTI/ STI clinics. Drugs for RTI and STI have been provided at the PHC level. Family health awareness campaign organized under National HIV/AIDS programme is partial solution to the problem of RTI and STI. However, most clients turn to private practitioners for their treatment, therefore the need to involve private practitioners is essential to control the RTI/STIs in the community. (For more details *see* sexually transmitted diseases.)

Priority Family Plannig Services—*see* Chapter 4.

SERVICES FOR CHILDREN UNDER RCH

Essential Newborn Care

Proportion of neonatal mortality has not much changed over the years and it contributes over two-thirds of infant mortality. The high incidence of low birth weight babies is a common contributory factor in neonatal deaths. The major causes of neonatal mortality have been identified as hypothermia, asphyxia and infections. Therefore essential newborn care was included as an important component of child services under CSSM and it has been retained as an important intervention under RCH programme.

Institutional Care of Newborn

Under RCH programme, the medical officers of District hospital, CHC and PHC have been trained by national neonatology forum for newborn care. Newborn care corners at all delivery points, newborn stabilizing units at CHCs , sick newborn care units at district level and intensive newborn care units at regional level have been established for newborn care.

Community-based Care of Newborn

However, *community-based care* of *newborn* has been considered vital as 25–40% deliveries occur in home, hence the need of essential newborn care at community level is must to save the life of newborn. Training of traditional birth attendant and health workers at the village level has been undertaken under RCH programme. Essential newborn care like keeping the baby warm, initiating breastfeeding at the earliest, clean cord, care of cord, keeping the environments clean, and weighing of babies soon after birth to identify high-risk neonates for referral can prevent many deaths in newborn. The Government of India has recently approved the implementation of home-based newborn care (HBNC) based on the Gadchiroli model to prevent neonatal sepsis and manage neonatal sepsis and childhood pneumonia.

Home visits are to be provided to every newborn starting with first visit on the day of birth followed by visits on day 3 and 7. 14, 21, 28 and on 42nd day to reduce IMR and MMR. (See India Newborn Action Plan)

Postnatal care and newborn care component at the moment is most weakest component of RCH.

The other important services for children include:

Infant and Young Child Feeding (IYCF)

- Exclusive breastfeeding must be encouraged for the first 6 months as it is the best food for child for adequate growth and prevention against diarrhoea. Start complementary feeding at 6 months while continue to breastfeed at least two years could prevent more than 10% deaths.
- Special care for very low birth weight (less than 1800 gm) babies at FRUs or subdistrict and district hospital.
- **Immunization for children** as under universal immunization programme (OPV, BCG, Hepatitis B at birth).
- Vitamin A prophylaxis up to 3 years of age and now extended up to 5 years of age.
- Iron and folic acid prophylaxis and control of anaemia.
- Integrated management of newborn and childhood illness (IMNCI) is a new initiative and it is being implemented to cover newborn and young children. The killer diseases like acute respiratory infection,

diarrhoeal diseases, malaria, measles malnutrition and fever if managed well by adequate response at household level and under primary health care set-up can save lives of neonates and young children.

- India's Newborn Action Plan.
- Navjat Shishu Suraksha Karyakram.
- Janani Shishu Suraksha Karyakram.
- School health and adolescents health services.
- Rashtriya Bal Swasthya Karyakram (National Child Health Programme).
- Rashtriya Kishor Swasthya Karyakram (RKSK).
- ICDS services.
- Behaviour change communication for child health.

5. SPECIAL PROGRAMME FOR ADOLESCENT HEALTH

Adolescents (10–19 years age group) constitute over one-fifth of India's population hence a large segment of population. They enter in reproductive cycle at early age, hence needs to be attended. The special needs of this segment have not been addressed adequately in the past.

6. ADDITIONAL PROGRAMMES FOR URBAN SLUMS AND TRIBAL AREAS

The percentage of total population living in urban areas has increased from 20% in 1970 to 28% in year 2001. and 31% in 2011. Nearly 30–40% of urban population lives in urban slum areas with deplorable living conditions. Nearly 90–100 million people are living in urban slums in India.

Reproductive health needs of this segment are enormous as the fertility rates are high and access to services is poor and acceptability of contraceptive is low.

For providing Family Welfare and MCH services in urban areas, Urban Family Welfare Centres (UFWCs) have been sanctioned in the country. In order to improve out-reach service delivery system in urban slums, Urban Revamping Scheme has been introduced. The scheme of revamping of urban family welfare services envisages reorganization of existing UFWCs. Now 1083 UFWCs have been reorganized to 871 Health Posts.

Though the health indices of urban population are better than those of rural population, however, conditions of urban slums may be worse than rural areas. Urban migration will result in rapid growth of urban slums. The risk factors for slum population are overcrowding, poor sanitation, lack of access to safe drinking water supply and safe disposal of human excreta and widespread environmental pollution.

It is evident that majority of hospitals and beds, doctors, are available in urban areas, yet the urban slum population is deprived of organized health services. This is a paradoxical situation. Unlike rural health services there have been little effort to provide planned and organized primary, secondary and tertiary care services in urban areas.

New Focus

To address the health needs of urban poor National Urban Health Mission (NUHM) has been set up in January 2008.

Goals: To improve the health of urban poor.

7. IMPROVING QUALITY OF SERVICES IN RCH

Provision of good quality care is the crux of RCH programme. Quality has not been given adequate attention in family welfare programme. This is one of the reason that why people have not availed family welfare services to the desired extent. Good quality of care ensures satisfied clients, who in turn come back for services if they are satisfied.

What is quality of care: Quality care means care as per specific standard or norm or quality of care is what we want for ourselves and our family. The manner in which the client is treated determines quality of care. The dimentions of good quality care are:

i ***Access to services:*** Physical access near to home, economic access means affordability and social access means acceptability of service.

ii ***Service delivery:*** Promoting informed choice. Let the client choose the service after adequate information and knowledge. Need-based service delivery and providing follow-up care improves quality.

iii ***Interpersonal communication:*** Listening to client is essential and spending time with client, friendly and cooperative attitude of health workers and consultants, caring for clients privacy and dignity enhances quality of care.

iv ***Technical factors:*** Technical competence of service providers, usage of good quality equipment and drugs, maintain highest standards of hygiene.

v ***Social factors:*** Gender sensitive service provision, more Lady doctors encouraging male participation in contraception, increased role of men in the programme.

vi ***Client's perspective:*** Waiting time of client should be minimum, the reception facility and waiting time should be well utilized. There should be good seating and physical arrangements, such as water and toilet.

vii ***Safety:*** Safety means minimizing the risk of injury, infection and harmful side effects by ensuring safety of procedures.

Example: Registration of pregnant women will be measured not in numbers registered but the numbers registered before 12 weeks of pregnancy.

Quality will be judged if accurate abdominal examination and palpation done, accurate BP recorded and pregnant mother weighed, fundal height recorded accurately and appropriate advice given.

Indicators of quality have been used in RCH programme in terms of number of pregnant women given four antenatal check ups, number of children fully immunized, percentage of institutional deliveries, number of high-risk mothers referred, ORS use rate, exclusive breastfeeding rates, etc.

Promotion of Quality Services under RCH—Strategies

RCH programme has imparted skill-based training, provided standard medicine kits and equipment, besides standard treatment protocols at various levels, promoted institutional deliveries and has done away the targets, emphasized on client consultation and people participation in planning. All these measures tend to enhance the quality of MCH and family welfare services. Accountability is to the people now. Indian Public Health Standards have been prescribed now to improve quality of services at all levels.

8. UNMET NEED OF FAMILY PLANNING

India launched National Family Planning Programme in 1952. The major strategy was to regulate births by providing fertility control methods—both for limiting and for spacing throughout the country.

Women who want to postpone or avoid childbearing and also report that they are not using contraception (including use by their partners) are defined as having an unmet need.

Health survey like NFHS 1, 2 and 3 have measured the extent of unmet needs in India.

1 For unmet needs group includes all fecund women who are married, sexually active able to produce children (fecund) and are not using any method of contraception and who do not either want to have any more children or want to postpone their next birth for at least two more years.

Those who want to have no more children are considered to have unmet need for limiting births, while those who want more children but not at least two more years are considered to have an unmet need for spacing births.

2 The unmet need group also includes all pregnant married women whose pregnancies are unwanted or mistimed and who became pregnant because they were not using contraception.

3 Similarly, women who recently have given birth but are not yet at risk of becoming pregnant because they are amenorrhoeic postpartum, are considered to have an unmet need if their pregnancies were unintended.

Extent of Unmet Needs

Of estimated 334 million women of reproductive age group (15–49 years), about one in five have an unmet need of family planning; that is they are sexually active and want to avoid pregnancy but are not using contraception (Table 5.6).

The unmet needs of contraception in India are as high as 25% and it is one of the major reason of population growth and high fertility. NFHS-3 indicates total unmet needs of 13.2%, including 6% for spacing.

Table 5.6: Unmet needs in India (percentage eligible couples)

Method of contraception	*Rapid household survey 1999–2000*	*NFHS-1*	*NFHS-2*	*NFHS-3*
Spacing	10.7	11.0	8.3	6.4
Terminal	14.6	8.5	7.5	6.8
Total	**25.3**	**19.5**	**15.8**	**13.2**

Under RCH programme, priority is to meet the unmet needs and reduce the level of unmet needs.

Reasons for unmet needs could be due to inadequate or deficient health infrastructure and difficult access and non-availability of contraceptives or lack of information or side effects, or combination of these factors. Improvement of quality of family welfare services will promote acceptance and bring about reduction in unmet need for contraception. Similarly easy access to health facility, adequate infrastructure, trained personnel, regular service and proper counselling will reduce unmet need.

9. COMMUNICATION STRATEGY IN RCH

In India, awareness of contraception is nearly 100% or universal but acceptance is around 56%. To bridge the gap between awareness and practice of contraception, national communication strategy for RCH programme has been evolved by Government of India. The goal of the communication strategy is to encourage individuals, families and communities to make informed decisions concerning reproductive and child health through a programme of health communication, which facilitates behaviour change. The focus of the strategy is *behaviour change communication.*

The key elements of the strategy are:

i Emphasis is being laid on interpersonal communication for behaviour change, to encourage community participation through *Mahila Swasthya Sangh* (MSS) in villages. ANM is the member secretary of MSS. Workers will organize women group meetings and make home visits to identify the communication needs of the eligible couples and on the basis of these needs they will motivate individual couples and their family to adopt the specific contraceptive method as per their choice.

ii Multiple channels of communication will be used.

iii IEC activities will be planned locally at PHC level, it means these will be area specific (according to needs of the area and clients). The focus of communication would be on unwanted fertility (unmet needs of contraception, unsafe abortions), maternal health (high maternal mortality, high maternal morbidity), adolescent reproductive health, RTI/STI care, child health, immunization coverage and newborn care.

iv The process of communication has been decentralized for planning and developing education material and messages, at local level (District/State).

10. GENDER SENSITIVITY

Gender sensitivity is an important consideration in provision of good quality care. Making the RCH programme gender sensitive or responsive to the needs of women must be an important concern for everyone involved in planning and implementation. The following strategies will make programme gender sensitive:

- Focussing on women health problems, such as RTI.
- Encouraging male participation in family planning.
- Popularization of no scalpel vasectomy and male sterilization.
- Keeping clinic open at time suitable to women.
- Training in gender sensitivity for service providers.
- Getting women feedback in monitoring.
- Encouraging involvement of Panchayats that now have one-third women members.
- Preparing the mindset of community and masses through massive education drive about the place of women in society. Educating people about male and female childbirth, females are not to be blamed for bearing girls as it is determined by X and Y chromosomes of men.
- Recruiting more lady medical officers for RCH services.

11. GREATER INVOLVEMENT OF PANCHAYATI RAJ INSTITUTIONS, NON-GOVERNMENTAL ORGANIZATIONS AND COMMUNITY

Greater involvement of Panchayati Raj Institutions (PRIs) non-governmental organizations and community under RCH programme is envisaged for decentralized planning, to enhance client satisfaction and to improve the quality and coverage of services as also to increase acceptability and utilization of services.

State Committee on Voluntary Action (SCOVA)

Decentralization of Fund Flow

These have been set-up under RCH programme. RCH funds are released to SCOVA for quick action and smooth functioning. SCOVA is registered society with state Chief Secretary as its Chairman and state Health Secretary as its Vice-Chairman. These SCOVAs have been strengthened with the provision of contractual staff. District RCH societies were set up for district health planning.

12. CIVIL WORKS UNDER RCH

The RCH programme initiative to establish and strengthen the FRUs as also district hospitals, in order to promote institutional deliveries and provide essential obstetrical care and MTP services. Following works were undertaken.

1. ₹ 10 lakh per CHC (District hospital was also provided ₹ 10 lakh) have been provided for operation theatre component or labour room have been constructed and provided water supply and electricity where these were deficient and facilities for existing labour rooms and operation theatres were improved under RCH. Up to 33% of NRHM Funds in high focus states can be used for infrastructure development.
2. Districts were provided flexibility to select CHC and adjust the spending of amount within the limits.
3. ₹ 10 lakh to each district was provided for minor civil works, providing water supply or electric facility in the PHCs or their upgradation if it was already provided in part. This money was also available for upgradation of facilities in labour rooms or repairs in the PHCs if needed.

Decentralized in-service Training

District training centres (DTCs) have been established under RCH programme for in-service training or orientation of health functionaries on RCH strategies. 1–2 weeks skill-based training has been imparted to all health functionaries. Specialized skill-based training in MTP and no scalpel vasectomy have also been undertaken. Similarly, specialized management and training in information education and communication skills has also been conducted.

Dai Training Programme under RCH

RCH has taken up birth attendant training programme in 142 districts of states, which had less than 30% of institutional deliveries, for safe deliveries. Dais selected at local level have been trained in their own environments at the level of CHC.

RCH Camps/Mobile-Medial Units

RCH camps have been organized under the programme with the objective of ensuring higher level RCH services (sterilization and MTP, etc.) in underutilized PHCs or in remote communities. The results have not been encouraging. National Mobile Medical Units (NMMUs) have been provided in 418 districts for outreach services.

Drugs for RCH services: Drug kit A, drug kit B, midwifery kit and equipment kit that have been provided under CSSM programme are being continued under RCH programme.

EUROPEAN COMMISSION (EC) FAMILY WELFARE SECTOR INVESTMENT PROGRAMME (SIP)

In India the health sector is covered by three departments within the Ministry of Health and Family Welfare: Department of health, Department of Family Welfare (DOFW) and the Department of Indian Systems of Medicine and Homeopathy. The EC programme will support the Government of India 9th five-year plan policies of "Paradigm shift" stated below:

- Community needs assessment approach for planning.
- Integrated reproductive and child health (RCH) package.

- Client oriented approach to family planning, with greater choice of methods and more male participation.
- Improve quality of clinical services.
- Introduction of access, quality and impact indicators
- Managerial and financial decentralization.
- Community participation.

In order to further the process of reform in India's Health and Family Welfare as set out in the Government of India publication, The "Paradigm Shift" European Commission (EC) is providing grant assistance of 200 million European Currency Units (ECU).[15] The primary objective is to enhance central, state and district capacities in implementing the family welfare system, policy reform and the community needs assessment approach (CNAA). The EC and health and family welfare programme essentially aimed to operationalize the "Paradigm Shift" by assisting Government of India and states to implement stated policy approaches and achieve desired goals.

The SIP will support at bringing about structural, systemic, and operational reforms. The major thrust is reform in health and family welfare, such as:

- Decentralized planning of RCH at district level
- Setting up of district RCH societies for fund release
- User charges
- Contracting staff
- Reforms in management information system
- Community participation.

European Commission has provided untied grant but stresses on performance-based expenditure. It lays set of benchmarks; by assessing need, complete it and get the fund. The most visible part of EC assistance has been:

- Collection of user charges and retention of these charges at local level for improvement of services.
- Contractual staff appointment by district societies and easy fund flow mechanism. Local plans of giving funds to local level for repairs, purchase of essential items for improving quality of RCH services at the level of Subcentre, PHC, CHC and District hospital.

Thus RCH programme is a turning point as it makes a start from grass root level, initiates work plan in consultation with the people, makes workers accountable to people, changes service priority from "sterilization" to range of integrated maternal and child health services, moves away from numerical method specific targets to client satisfaction and their needs and places emphasis on quality of services and client satisfaction.[16,17] National Rural Health Mission further reinforces the concept of village plan by Village Health and Sanitation Committee[18].

REFERENCES

1 Gupta JP, Sinha NK, Bardhan A. Evolution of family welfare programme in India. Vol. I-II. New Delhi: NIHFW; 1992.

2 GOI. National Health Policy 1983. New Delhi: MOH and FW GOI; 1983.

3 GOI. National child survival and safe motherhood programme. New Delhi: MOH and FW GOI; 1992.

4 GOI. Manual on target free approach (TFA) in family welfare programme. New Delhi: MOH and FW GOI; 1996.

5 GOI. National Population Policy 2000. New Delhi: MOH and FW GOI; 2000.

6 Measham AR, Heaver RA. Directions in development–India's family welfare programme moving to reproductive and child health approach. New York: The World Bank; 1996.

7 Measham AR, Heaver RA. Directions in development–Supplements to India's family welfare programme moving to reproductive and child health approach. New York: The World Bank; 1996.

8 GOI. Annual report 2002–03. New Delhi: MOH and FW, GOI; 2003.

9 GOI. Annual report 2003–04. New Delhi: MOH and FW, GOI; 2004.

10 UNICEF. The State of the World's Children 2009.

11 GOI. Basic guide to reproductive and child health program for use by NGOs, training institutions and health functionaries. New Delhi: MOH and FW, GOI; 1997.

12 GOI. Manual on Community Needs Assessment Approach (CNAA) in family welfare programme. New Delhi: MOH and FW, GOI; 1998.

13 GOI. National Rural Health Mission, Meeting People's Health needs in rural areas. Framework for implementation 2005–2012.

14 GOI. Guidelines for ANC and Skilled Attendance at Birth, by ANMs and LHVs. MOH and FW, New Delhi, 2005.

15 GOI. Health and Family Welfare Sector Investment Programme–Supported by European Commission. New Delhi: MOH and FW, GOI.

16 GOI. Reproductive and Child Health Newsletter Vol 4: (2) August 2001: MOH and FW, GOI; New Delhi.

17 Lal S. A turning point in national family welfare programme. Moving to target free reproductive and child health approach. Ind J Comm Med 1997 Apr-June; 22(2): 1–4.

18. United Nations Economic and Social Council, Commission on Population and Development Forty seventh section, 7–11 April 2014.

REPRODUCTIVE AND CHILD HEALTH II (RCH II, 2005–2012)

All components included in RCH I will continue with rectification of weaknesses as observed during the implementation phase.

RCH Phase I continued from 1997 to 2005. RCH Phase II started in 2005 and continued till 2012.

The RCH II is the flagship programme of the Government of India on reproductive child and maternal health under

National Rural Health Mission (NRHM). The Programme has been reoriented and revitalized to give it a pro-outcome and pro-poor focus[1].

RCH is principal vehicle and major component of NRHM aimed at reducing Maternal Mortality Ratio to 100/100,000, infant mortality to 30/1000 live births and total fertility to 2.1. Against these goals, IMR of 42/1000 live births (SRS 2012), MMR of 178/100,000 live births and TFR of 2.4 (SRS 2012) has been achieved. The approach to population stabilization is to provide quality health services in remote rural areas along with wide range of contraceptive choice to meet the unmet needs of these services (including delivery, safe abortions, treatment of reproductive tract infections and Family Planning Services to ensure full reproductive choices to women). The strategy also focuses to promote male participation in family planning.

Under RCH II it is envisaged that 50% of PHCs and all the CHCs would be made operational as 24-hour delivery centres; in phased manner; by the year 2012. These centres would be responsible for providing basic emergency obstetric care and essential newborn care and basic newborn resuscitation services round the clock. Besides these all, the FRUs will also be made operational for providing emergency obstetric care by the end of RCH II.

RCH II operates under the umbrella of NRHM and its key characters are:

Adoption of Sector Wide Approach in Family Welfare Sector: The programme is envisaged as an umbrella programme by integrating all the related and interlinked as also stand alone schemes (sanitation and hygiene, nutrition, safe drinking water, women and child development, elementary education, Panchayati Raj and rural development) into a single composite programme. Family welfare programme is being viewed as development programme and hence *convergence* and linkages of all *related sectors* and their goals are essential.

Rationalization of existing budget heads and creation of a flexible funding pool: Flexible financing is the key strategy by providing untied funds to every level—to the village health and sanitation committee, to Subcentre, to PHC, to CHC and district in addition to resource envelope to each district and state Programme Implementation Plan.

Donor convergence: Funds will be pooled from all the donors to simplify the process of accessing.

State ownership and decentralized planning and programme implementation: RCH II programme design and implementation strategy is accordingly wedded to adopting a decentralized process under which extensive consultations were held with each state/union territory on the programme design. The programme invited each state/union territory to prepare its own programme implementation plan (PIP) based upon situational analysis of ground realities and requirements. The states have been encouraged to evolve *district plans* with the clear objective of each district having its own plan as per schedule to be laid down by the states/UTs themselves.

Institutional strengthening at district, state and central level for effective programme implementation: Institutional capacity has been the major constraint for translation of policy intentions into actions at national, state and district levels. The decentralized and macro-management approach places the onus of planning, implementation, monitoring and evaluation more squarely on the states than ever before. The new approach requires a change of mindset as well as different skill set at the central level, to this end state and district level programme management units (PMUs) comprising of skilled personnel (professionals) on hiring/contract basis have been established under RCH II.

Results framework and monitoring: "Results orientation" is an important paradigm shift envisaged in RCH-II programme. The RCH II vision articulates "improving access, use and quality of RCH services, especially for the poor and underserved populations", as an important outcome of the programme. The logical framework is being used as a tool to define *outcomes at* the planning stage and subsequently for monitoring, which ensures that for each programme intervention there is an outcome as well as objectively verifiable indicator.

Public private partnership: It is recognized that besides the Government of India, the state Governments and development partners, the private sector is also an important stakeholder in the programme. The programme accordingly solicits the involvement of private sector participants.

Programme funding: The programme would receive funding from three sources: The Government of India, pooled funding from DFID/World Bank/UNFPA and funding from other development partners (including EC, USAID, UNICEF and UNFPA).

- **Performance based funding:** To ensure adherence to programme objectives, reward good performance and support weak performers through enhanced technical assistance.
- **Convergence:** Both intersectoral and intrasectoral to optimize utilization of resources as well as institutional facilities.

The RCH II programme implementation was governed by the following:[2–5]

- Immediate and medium term goals of NPP, 2000.
- The National Health Policy-2002.
- The millennium development goals (MDG).
- The tenth and eleventh plan goals.

NEW AREAS/COMPONENTS AND STRATEGIES IN RCH II

Differential approach is adopted for implementation of RCH II programme in EAG states based on the level of infant mortality rate, and institutional deliveries. Strengthening of the health systems will be the focus to close the gaps. Newer interventions/strategies are as under:

Strategies New Interventions

i Integrated management of neonatal and childhood illness (IMNCI) introduction in phased manner.

ii Adolescent reproductive and sexual health initiative for adolescent friendly health services and counselling during routine subcentre clinics and once a week clinic at PHC/CHC on fixed day.

iii Strengthening of social marketing of contraceptives in rural areas, through rural health practitioners and community mobilization through satisfied acceptor couples.

iv Urban health: Provision of quality integrated primary health care services to urban poor by establishing 'urban health centre—1:100,000 population with two medical officers, 3–4 ANMs, one laboratory assistant, one public health nurse/lady health visitor, one clerk and one chowkidar and a peon.

Second tier referral centre: It could be district hospital/maternity home/private and NGO nursing home (by public–private partnership).

v Tribal health will be given primacy.

vi Establishing newborn care corner in phased manner in the existing FRUs/CHCs/PHCs/subcentres and priority will be given to Empowered Action Group States.

vii Hospital generated waste management/infection management and environment protection.

viii Incorporation of new areas (adolescent health, urban primary health care infrastructure, tribal health, adverse sex ratio in different states, PNDT Act) in the matrix of priorities for *behaviour change communication* strategy (BCC).

ix Revamping of training in RCH at various levels especially training under newer areas incorporated under RCH II.

REFERENCES

1 WHO. World Health Report 2003. Shaping the future. Geneva: WHO; 2003.

2 Planning Commission. Tenth five-year plan 2002–07. Vol II. New Delhi: Planning Commission GOI; 2002.

3 GOI. National Population Policy 2000. New Delhi: MOH and FW GOI; 2000.

4 NFHS-3 IIPS, Mumbai, India, 2005–06.

5 GOI. RCH II and family planning – programme implementation plan (PIP). New Delhi: MOH and FW GOI; 2004.

NATIONAL RURAL HEALTH MISSION (NRHM) 2005–2012

The National Rural Health Mission (2005–12) seeks to provide effective health care to rural population throughout the country with special focus on 18 states, which have weak public health indicators and/or weak infrastructure.

NRHM is a flagship programme of Government of India. Under its umbrella it integrates all related and stand alone programmes in the health sector including: RCH phase II, National Vector-borne Diseases, National Leprosy Eradication, National Iodine Deficiency Disorders, Revised National Tuberculosis Control Programme, National Blindness Control, National Mental Health Programme, national Programme for Prevention and Control of CDC and Strokes, National Programme for Care of Elderly, Integrated Diseases Surveillance, AYUSH schemes in hospitals and dispensaries and thrust areas under NRHM (ASHA, Village Health Sanitation and Nutrition Committees, strengthening of Subcentres, PHCs, CHCs, Sub-district and District Hospitals, Untied grant at village, SC, PHC, CHC, besides annual maintenance grant, state and district Health Societies, community monitoring, essential drugs at SC, PHC, CHC, Intersectoral convergence, Mobile Medical Units and facility and household surveys, District Health Action Plan, etc.).

Aim: The NRHM *aims* to provide accessible, affordable, accountable quality health care through a functional public health system. It also seeks to reduce maternal mortality ratio, infant mortality rate and total fertility rate. The key features of NRHM include: making the public health delivery system *fully functional* and accountable to the community, *human* resources management, community involvement, decentralization, rigorous monitoring and evaluation against Indian Public Health Standards, convergence of health and related programmes form village level upwards, innovations and flexible financing as also interventions for improving the health indicators.[1]

The NRHM represents a major departure from the past, in that Central Government health financing is now directed to the development of *state health systems* rather than being confined to a select number of national health programmes. NRHM provides a unique opportunity to states to build a partnership and carry out necessary reforms in health sector with more resources.

District and State Programme implementation Plans (PIPs) form the basis to suit the diverse needs of states and regions. NRHM has set a new standard of partnership with states where it is the state that determines what is needed to reform the public sector health system. The architectural corrections envisaged under NRHM are organized around five pillars each of which is made-up of a number of overlapping core strategies.

NRHM—5 MAIN APPROACHES

a **Increasing participation and ownership by the community (decentralization):** This means transfer of funds, functions and functionaries to Panchayati Raj Institutions (PRIs). Further this is sought to be achieved through an (i) increased role for PRIs in the ASHA programme, (ii) village health sanitation and nutrition committee, (iii) constitution of *Rogi Kalyan Samitis/* hospital development committee or users groups and (iv) *district health society* for decentralized district and village health planning with PRIs and People, (v) community monitoring system and through a greater space for NGO participation.

b **Indian public health standards (IPHS):** Setting of standards and norms helps in monitoring and evaluation. The prescription of the IPHS marks one of the most important core strategies of the NRHM. Once the norms and standards are in place, the challenge lies in identifying facility wise gaps in infrastructure human resources, equipment drugs supplies and above all in service outcomes. The *facility survey* identifies the *gaps* and funding is directed to *closing* the *gaps* so identified. IPHS have been adopted for Subcentres, Primary Health Centres and Community Health Centres and District Hospitals. The objectives of IPHS are:

i To provide minimum package of assured services.

ii To achieve and maintain acceptable standards of quality of services.

iii To make the services more responsive and sensitive to the needs of the community to enhance client satisfaction.

IPHS now specify what services would be delivered, what physical infrastructure (building and space for service) is needed, what manpower is required, what equipment and essential drugs and materials are needed. These standards would thus help monitor progress and improve the functioning of the facility. The IPHS have been worked out on the basis of population norms, patient/client load per day and levels of utilization of services, e.g. bed occupancy rate and coverage level of services. The setting up of standards is a dynamic process, if the level of utilization goes up and bed occupancy increases the norms can be revised. *Standard treatment protocols* for national health programmes and locally endemic diseases are the "heart" of quality and cost of the care.

c **Improved programme management through capacity building:** The core of this is professionalizing management by building up management and Public health skills in the existing workforce, supplemented by inclusion of management personnel into the system (States/District Programme Manager, IT Professionals and Accounts Professionals). Programme management units at state, district and block level have been set up by engaging programme managers with MBA, qualification, chartered accountant and data entry operators for improved programme management—Right from the national level, NRHM visualizes a sustained process of capacity development of management of programme through, National Health System Resource Centre, and State Health System Resource Centre, who help as technical resource for capacity building in district planning process and improving service delivery in health sector.

d **Flexible financing:** "The supply side financing" means government spends on health as being provider of health services, creates infrastructure and manpower and pays salaries to deliver services to people "free" of cost. In NRHM flexible financing is the hall mark so that service guarantee as spelled out in IPHS can be made available. The central strategy of this pillar is the provision of untied funds to every level—to the village health and sanitation committee, to the subcentre, to the PHC, to the CHC and district hospital. Even the strategy of providing resource envelope to each district and state which the district/state is to use against an approved plan that it develops is an unprecidented level of financial flexibility. *Financial packages for demand side financing* and various forms of risk pooling where money follows the patient are also major strategies declared by the NRHM. The *Janani Suraksha Yojna* is one major, almost overwhelming example of "demand side financing option" where the funding is to the user of services. The beneficiary is free to choose between private sector provider or public sector provider. It is envisaged that the hospital care system moves towards a fully funded universal social health insurance scheme. The programmes under erstwhile Department of Health and Family Welfare and Department of Ayush were not being run in an integrated manner. As a result the *transfer of funds* to the states *under different budget* heads at different points of time vertically hampered flexibility. It also led to duplication of efforts, and thereby wastage of scarce resources. From XIth plan onwards, instead of different budget heads the state would get budget under *single NRHM budget head*. This would provide the states much needed flexibility to direct the funds to those areas where they are needed most.

e **Innovations in human resources management for health sector:** *Contractual appointment* route to immediately fill human resource gaps as well as ensuring availability of locally resident health staff/ workers, incentives to staff posted in difficult and underserved areas, multi-skilling of doctors and staff, mainstreaming and integration with AYUSH are examples of innovations that seeks to find new solutions to old problems for optimal use of human resources. Accreditation and developing Public Private Partnership in health care is yet another approach under NRHM. Expansion of technical and professional education and increasing access to weaker sections to such education is also a core strategy.

Vision

- To provide effective health care to rural population throughout country with special focus on 18 states having weak infrastructure. These 18 states are Arunachal Pradesh, Assam, Bihar, Chhattisgarh, Himachal Pradesh, Nagaland, Jharkhand, Jammu and Kashmir, Manipur, Mizoram, Meghalaya, MP, Odisha, Rajasthan, Sikkim, Tripura, Uttarakhand and Uttar Pradesh.[2]
- To raise public spending on health from 0.9% of GDP to 2–3 % of GDP.
- It aims to undertake architectural correction of the health system to enable it to handle the increased allocation as promised under the National Common Minimum Programme (CMP) and promote policies that strengthen public health management and service delivery in the country.
- Provision of accredited social (female) health activist (ASHA) in each village health team.
- To revitalize local health traditions and mainstreaming of AYUSH (Indian System of Medicine—Ayurveda, Unani, Sidha and Homeopathy).
- Effective integration of health concerns with determinants of health like sanitation and hygiene, nutrition, and safe drinking water through district plan of health.
- Decentralization of programmes for district management of health.
- To improve access to rural people, especially poor women and children to equitable, affordable, accountable effective primary health care.

Goals

- NRHM would help achieve goals set under National Health Policy, population policy and the sustainable development goals and vision 2020.
- Reduction of infant mortality and maternal mortality.
- Reduction of total fertility.
- Universal access to public health services, such as women health, child health, water, sanitation and hygiene, immunization and nutrition.
- Prevention and control of communicable and non-communicable diseases including locally endemic diseases.
- Access to integrated comprehensive primary health care.
- Population stabilization, gender and demographic balance.
- Revitalize local health traditions and mainstreaming of AYUSH.
- Promotion of healthy lifestyles.

These are similar to essential elements of primary health care.

Most of these goals are stated in NPP—2000 and NHP—2002, also in RCH II, 10th Five-Year Plan, 11th Five-Year Plan and vision 2020.

Core Strategies of NRHM

- Training and enhancing capacity of Panchayati Raj Institutions (PRIs) to own control and manage public health services.
- Promote access to improved health care at household level through accredited social health activist (ASHA).
- Health plan for each village through *village health* and *sanitation committee* (VHSC).
- Strengthening of subcentres through an untied fund to enable local planning and action and more multipurpose workers (MPWs)/subcentres as per population norms.
- Strengthening of existing PHCs and CHCs and provision of 30–50 bedded CHC per lakh of population for improved curative care to a normative standard (Indian Public Health Standards—defining personnel, equipment and management standards).
- Preparation and implementation of intersectoral district health action plan prepared by the district health mission including drinking water, sanitation, hygiene and nutrition.[2]
- Integration of vertical health and family welfare programmes at national, state, district and block level.
- Technical support to national, state and district health mission for public health management.
- Strengthening capacities for data collection, assessment and review for evidence-based planning, monitoring and supervision.
- Formulation of transparent policies for deployment and career development of human resources for health.
- Developing capacities for preventive health care at all levels for promoting healthy lifestyles, reduction in consumption of tobacco and alcohol, etc.
- Promoting non-profit sector in underserved areas.
- Mobile Medical Units in every district to improve outreach services in un-served and underserved areas.

Supplementary Strategies

- Regulation of private sector including the informal rural practitioners to ensure availability of quality services to citizens at reasonable **cost.**
- Promotion of public private partnership for achieving public health goals.
- Mainstreaming of AYUSH—revitalising local health traditions.
- Reorienting medical education to support rural health issues including regulation of medical care and ethics.
- Effective and viable risk pooling and *social health insurance* to provide health security to the poor by ensuring accessible, affordable, accountable and good quality hospital care.

Plan of Action for NRHM

The plan of action includes increasing public expenditure on health, reducing regional inbalance in health infrastructure, pooling resources, integration of organizational structures, optimization of health manpower, decentralization and district management of health programmes, community participation and ownership of assets, induction of management and financial personnel into district health system and operationalization of CHCs into FRUs meeting public health standards in each block of the country. Ten components of NRHM are as follow:

Component (A): Accredited Social Health Activist (ASHA)—Community Health Volunteers

- Every village to have a female accredited social health activist (ASHA)—chosen by and accountable to village Panchayat to act as the interface between the community and the public health system.[3]
- ASHA would be trained women community health volunteer at village level.
- ASHA would act as a bridge between the ANM and the village and be accountable to Panchayat.
- She will be honorary volunteer, receiving performance-based compensation for promoting universal immunization, referral and escort services for RCH, construction of household toilets, and the other national health care delivery programmes.
- She will facilitate preparation and implementation of the village health action plan along with Anganwadi Worker, ANM, and functionaries of other departments and self-help group members under the leadership of village Panchayat.
- ASHA will take steps to create awareness and provide information to the community on determinants of health, such as nutrition, basic sanitation and hygienic practices, healthy living and working conditions, information on existing health services and the need for timely utilization of health and family welfare services.
- She will counsel women on birth preparedness, importance of safe delivery, breastfeeding and complementary feeding, immunization, contraception and prevention of common infections including reproductive tract infection/sexually transmitted infection (RTI/STI, HIV/AIDS) and care of the young children.
- ASHA will mobilize the community and facilitate them in accessing health and health-related services available at the village/subcentre/primary health centres, such as immunization, antenatal check-up (ANC), postnatal check-up (PNC), family planning services, ICDS, sanitation and other services being provided by the Government on VHSN day once a month.
- She will work with local health committees of Panchayats to develop a comprehensive village health plan.
- She will escort/accompany pregnant women and children requiring treatment/admission to the nearest pre-identified health facility, i.e. primary health centre/community health center/first referral unit. She provides home based newborn care (HBNC).
- ASHA will provide primary medical care for most common ailments, such as diarrhoea, fevers, and first aid for minor injuries. She will be a provider of directly observed treatment short-course (DOTS) under revised national tuberculosis control programme. She will also act as a depot holder for essential provisions being made available to every habitation like oral rehydration therapy (ORT), iron folic acid tablets (IFA), chloroquine, disposable delivery kits (DDK), oral pills and condoms, etc. A drug kit has been provided to each ASHA.
- She will inform about the births and deaths in her village and any unusual health problems/disease outbreaks in the community to the subcentres/primary health centre.
- Participation in National Filaria Day.
- Identify the cases of skin patch with loss of sensation and bring them to the notice of health worker male/ females ensure that all the patients of leprosy are taking regular treatment.
- Fulfillment of all these roles by ASHA is envisaged through continuous training and upgradation of her skills.

Component (B): Strengthening of Subcentres

- Each subcentre has been provided an untied fund for local action (₹ 10000 per annum). This fund will be deposited in a joint bank account of the ANM and Sarpanch and operated by the ANM, in consultation with the village health committee.
- Supply of essential drugs, both allopathic and AYUSH to the subcentres besides necessary equipment.
- Sanction of new subcentres as per 2001 population norms and additional health workers male and female and upgrading existing subcentres, including building for subcentres functioning in rented premises.
- To upgrade quality of services as per IPHS.

Component (C): Strengthening of Primary Health Centres (PHCs)

Mission aims at strengthening PHCs for quality preventive, promotive, curative, supervisory and outreach services through:

i Adequate and regular supply of essential quality drugs and equipment including auto-disable syringes for immunization.

ii Provision of 24-hour services at least in 50% of PHCs by mainstreaming AYUSH manpower.

iii Observance of Indian Public Health Standards, and standard treatment guidelines and protocols.

iv Provision of second doctor at PHC (one male and one female doctor) in case of additional outlays and intensification of ongoing communicable disease control programme, new programmes for control of non-communicable diseases and upgradation of 100% of PHCs for 24 hours services.

v *Rogi Kalyan Samiti* for each PHC.

vi Provision of untied and maintenance funds.

vii Citizen's charter at each PHC.

Component (D): Strengthening Community Health Centres (CHCs)

For referral care: The key strategy of mission is:

- Operationalising of existing CHCs (30–50 beds) as 24-hour first referral units including posting of anaesthetist.
- To set-up or creation of new CHCs to meet population norms of 2001 census and bearing their recurring costs.
- To upgrade quality of services as per Indian Public Health Standard.
- Develop, display and ensure compliance of citizen's charter at CHC.
- Promotion of stakeholder committees (*Rogi Kalyan Samitis*) for hospital management.
- Untied funds for local action.

Component (E): District Health Action Plan (DHAP)

One of the core strategy of NRHM is preparation and implementation of an intersector District Health Plan by District Health Mission, including drinking water, sanitation, hygiene and nutrition, early childhood development, female literacy and women empowerment, etc.

The District Health Action Plan would be the main instrument for planning, intersectoral convergence, implementation and monitoring of activities under NRHM. Rather than funds being allocated to the states for implementing programmes **designed** and **approved** by the **Government of India Level** the states have been encouraged to prepare their perspective and annual plans which in turn would be based on the district plans. What is District Health Action Plan (DHAP)? It is local planning and village is the primary unit for planning. Village plans leads to subcentre plan and aggregation thereof leads to Primary Health Centre Plans, and community Health Centres Plans and district health action plans. Each institution should have its annual action plan. DHAP covers the main features of the district, situation analysis, village, block and district level consultations, objectives, matrix of key strategies (interventions) and activities, costing, time frame, responsibility level, monitoring and evaluation and budget/unit cost for each activity.

The District Health Mission under the Zila Parishad would get the district plan prepared covering health as well as other determinants of health. Components of district health plan include: new interventions under NRHM, RCH II, strengthening of immunization, disease control/ surveillance programmes and intersectoral convergence including nutrition, safe drinking water and sanitation. 636 DHAP have been finalized.

Household and facility survey should provide basis for mapping diversity and defining baseline, periodic surveys would thereafter be taken up on annual basis to track the improvements in the facility as well as improvements in the health indicators. Village Health Register is a tool for planning regarding all incidents and people's health needs round the year. Village Health Plans, reflecting local health needs have to be aggregated at Gram Panchayat, cluster and block levels to ultimately feed into District Health Plan.

Component (F): Convergence or Synergies with other Departments

Convergence means working together or coming together or coordinating two or more sectors to produce a combined effect greater than the sum of their separate effects.

The indicators of health depend as much on drinking water, sanitation, nutrition, female literacy, early childhood development and women empowerment, etc. as they do on hospitals and functional health systems. Realizing the importance of wider determinants of health, NRHM seeks to adopt a **convergent approach** for intervention under the umbrella of district plan. The **Anganwadi** Centre under ICDS and **School System** at the village level will be the principal hubs for health action. Likewise, wherever village committees have been effectively constituted for drinking water, sanitation, ICDS, etc. NRHM will attempt to move towards one common **village health** and sanitation committee covering all these activities. Panchayati Raj Institutions will be fully involved in this convergent approach to coordinate various functions and functionaries at the village level (ICDS, education, agriculture rural development, and self-help groups). Village action plan and district action plan will be major instruments for intersectoral convergence actions. While substantial spending in each of these sector will be by concerned department, the Village Health Plan/District Plan will provide an opportunity to some catalytic resources for convergent action. NRHM household surveys through ANMs, ASHAs and AWWs will target availability of drinking water, smokeless chullah, livelihood, toilets and other issues in order to allow a framework for effective convergent action in the Village Health Plans by promotion of sanitary latrines in households, schools and Anganwadis as also drinking water through *Total Sanitation Campaign*. The success of convergent action would depend upon quality fo district planning process. Village is the first level of convergence of programmes of all the Ministries.

Component (G): Strengthening Disease Control Programmes

National disease control programmes for malaria, Japanese encephalitis, dengue and chikungunya, kala-azar, filaria, TB, leprosy, blindness and iodine deficiency and integrated disease surveillance programme shall be integrated under the mission, for *improved* programme delivery.

- New initiative will be launched for control of non-communicable diseases (NCD).
- Disease surveillance system at village level will be strengthened.
- Supply of generic drugs (both AYUSH and Allopathic) for common ailments at village, SC, PHC/CHC.
- Provision of mobile medical unit at district level for improved outreach services and control of outbreaks.

Component (H): People Public-Private Partnership (PPPP) for Public Health Goals

The non-governmental health sectors accounts for nearly 80% of health expenditure in India. In the absence of effective public health system majority of the households seek health care from non-governmental sector.

A variety of partnerships are being pursued under the existing programmes of the ministry, especially the RCH II and independently by the states with their own resources. *Contracting* is the predominant model of PPPP in India. Under this system states are trying *contract in*, *contract out*, outsourcing, management of hospital facilities by leading NGOs, hiring staff, service delivery, including family planning services, MTP, treatment of STI/RTI, etc. Franchising and social marketing of contraceptives are already built into the Family Welfare Programmes. The immunization and polio eradication programme effectively make use of partnership with WHO, UNICEF, the Rotary International, NGOs, etc. *Under Janani Suraksha Yojna* (JSY) Private facilities have been accredited for institutional deliveries. The disease control programme (tuberculosis leprosy, blindness, cancer, malaria, HIV and AIDS, etc.) make use of NGO partnership in a big way.

The professional bodies like FOGSI, IMA, IAPSM, IAPH, and IAP have been involved in building awareness, advocacy, training programmes and mass campaigns. The growth of private hospitals—not for profit centres and diagnostic centre was also encouraged by central and state governments by offering tax exemptions and lands on concessional rates, in return for provision of free treatment for the poor as a certain proportion (30%) of outpatients and (40%) inpatients. Apart from subsidies, private corporate hospitals receive huge amounts of public funds in the form of reimbursements from public sector undertakings, the central and the state governments for treating their employees. Involvement of people and civil society is the key in PPPP.

The NRHM attempts to provide people friendly regulation framework that promotes ethical practice in the non-governmental sector. Such efforts involve system of accreditation, standard treatment protocols, training and upgradation of skills of non-governmental providers which are likely to improve quality of services.

Component (I): New Health Finance Mechanism

- Progressively, the district health missions to move towards paying hospitals for services by way of reimbursement, on the principle of "money follows the patient".
- Standardization of services—out-patient, in-patient, surgical interventions and costs will be done periodically by committee of experts in each state.
- All existing CHCs to have wage component paid on monthly basis. Other recurrent costs may be reimbursed for services rendered from district health fund. Over the mission period, the CHC may move towards all costs, including wages reimbursed for services rendered.
- Community-based health insurance schemes (CBHI) will be encouraged.

Component (J): Reorienting Health/Medical Education to Support Rural Health Issues

- Promoting new medical colleges in deficient states.
- Correct undue emphasis on specialization and tertiary care with more emphasis on preventive aspect of health and primary health care.
- Offering short-term courses in anaesthesia and emergency obstetric care to medical officers.
- Universal continuing medical education programme in the medical community.
- Strengthening of nursing colleges and ANMs training centres.

Suggestion for setting up of commission for excellence in health care (Medical Grant Commission) and national institute for public health management, etc.

Institutional Mechanism

- Merger of multiple vertical societies and constitution of district and state mission.
- Merger of Departments in the Health and Family Welfare Sector and appoinment of State Mission Director.
- Constitution of village health and sanitation committee at village level (consisting of panchayat representatives, ANM, Anganwadi worker, teacher, ASHA, and community health volunteer), and hospital management committee (*Rogi Kalyan Samiti*) for community management of public hospitals.
- District health mission under the leadership of Zila Parishad with district health head as convener, State health mission, national mission and empowered programme committee chaired by secretary health and family welfare to be executive body of the mission.

The mission would require two distinct support mechanisms:

- Programme management support centre for strengthening management systems.
- Health trust of India proposed as a knowledge institution, to be repository of innovation—research and documentation, health information system, planning, monitoring, evaluation, etc.

Table 5.7: Paradigm shift due to NRHM[5]

Moves from	To
1. Current Public expenditure on Health 0.9% of GDP	1. Increased Public expenditure 2–3% of GDP by 2012. States will also make a matching increase.
2. Inflexible Financing	2. Flexible Financing—untied grant at village, subcentre PHC, CHC and District level for local actions and full packages for plans developed at district level.
3. Financial outlays	3. Outcomes—Result-oriented
4. Dysfunctional health infrastructure	4. Fully Functional Health Facilities at village, subcentre, PHC, CHC and district hospital.
5. No standards prescribed for quality	5. Indian Public Health Standards for Physical infrastructure, human resources, equipment, drugs and supplies and service outcomes.
6. Central Govt. Financing Confined to select **Programmes or Programme** Disease Centric—fragmented approach	6. Financing now is directed to Development of state **health systems**. System Centric approach
7. Time consuming recruitment system and inadequate provision of human resources	7. Contractual appointments, local residency and incentives to staff working in difficult areas, additional human resources.
8. Low level of Community Participation	8. Increasing Community Participation by way of Village health and sanitation committee, ASHA Programme, Hospital Management Committee or *Rogi Kalyan Samiti* and Funds, Functions and Functionaries given to people with citizen's charter at each facility.
9. Poor management capacity	9. Improved Management capacity by building up management and public health skills in existing workforce along with induction of management personnel into the system.
10. Lack of convergence	10. Integrating vertical health and Family Welfare programmes at National, State, Block and District level.
11. Centralized planning and evaluation	11. Decentralized District Health Action Plans are the major instruments to achieve intersectoral coordination, implementation, monitoring and evaluation of programme.

The Mission is expected to achieve the goals set under the National Health Policy, National Population Policy, Goals of Xth and XIth Five-Year Plans and Millennium Development Goals besides vision 2020.

NRHM tries to achieve these goals by making the health system fully functional and credible at all the levels by decentralized district plans with full participation of community, user groups and NGO; with substantial financial support at all levels.

States would sign memorandum of understanding indicating their commitment to increase contribution to public health budget (by 10% each year), increased devolution to Panchayati Raj institutions as per 73rd constitution Amendment Act and performance benchmarks for release of funds.

Achievements of NRHM[4]

- More than 8.96 lakh ASHAs are connecting households to health facilities. The presence of community volunteers on this unprecedented scale has resulted in people's growing pressure on utilization of services from public sector health system.[5]
- The untied grants to subcentres has given a new confidence to ANMs in the field who are far better equipped now with blood pressure apparatus, stethoscope and weighting machines, etc. Now they can actually undertake a proper antenatal care and other health care services.
- NRHM has provided an opportunity to provide cashless hospitalized services to the poor through *Rogi Kalyan Samiti* resources.
- Over 5.12 lakh *village-health nutrition and sanitation committees* have been constituted and untied money of ₹ 10,000 per annum provided for local health action.
- Subcentres have been strengthened by way of providing untied money of ₹ 10000 per annum and second ANM at Subcentre.
- NRHM has benefited below poverty line women for safe delivery. *Janani Suraksha Yojna* (JSY) is in operation to promote institutional and safe deliveries.
- Delivery huts have been constructed to promote safe delivery at village level. Second ANM at delivery hut has been posted apart from one helper.
- PHCs and CHCs have been strengthened by provision of untied fund of ₹ 25,000 per annum per PHC and ₹ 50,000 per annum per CHC.
- An amount of ₹ 20 lakh per CHC has been provided for its upgradation as per Indian public healh standards and ₹ 20 lakh to district hospital for upgradation as per. Indian Public Health Standards (IPHS).
- District level plans have been formulated by 636 districts.

- District programme management units have been set up besides Citizen's charters at facility level.
- Upgrading of CHCs, PHCs and SCs as per Indian public health standards (IPHS) in terms of manpower, equipment, space and services has begun to improve quality of services.
- District, state and national health mission constituted.
- Public–private partnership with NGOs and private practitioners has begun.
- Considerable reduction of out of pocket expenditure from 72% to 60%.
- Indigenous system of medicine: AYUSH has been promoted and services set-up at district level.
- What functions and responsibilities are taken up by village health nutrition and sanitation committee and mothers meetings constituted under the umbrella of NRHM are to be keenly watched.
- First referral units (FRUs) for 24-hour referral services and PHCs for 24-hour referral services are progressing at very slow speed.

Thus money-wise, the primary health care has been supported considerably, hopefully it makes impact in due course of time.

Impact of NRHM

The information system to measure the process and impact of the NRHM including Family Welfare Programme includes:

- Service statistics through HMIS and Routine monitoring.
- Sample Registration system and Population census.
- Large scale surveys (NFHS, DLHS, Facility surveys and Annual Health Surveys.
- Area specific survey by Population Research centres.
- Other surveys by National and International agencies.
- Field evaluation through Regional evaluation teams.

India's Annual Health Surveys (AHS)—2010–13

The country's first ever district level health surveys of 2010–13 conducted by MOH and FW in collaboration with the Registrar General of India across Assam and Eight Empowered Action Group (EAG) States—Rajasthan, UP, Uttarakhand, Bihar, Jharkhand, Odisha, MP and Chhattisgarh covering 20.1 million persons in 284 districts of the country. It provides data on 161 indicators for focused policy planning which was hitherto based on the Sample Registration System. The report listed 100 bottom most districts, 45 in UP, 27 in MP, 7 in Assam, 6 in Bihar, 7 in Rajasthan, 6 in Odisha, one each in Chhattisgarh and Uttarakhand (baseline data).

Data indicate rampant child marriages: every 6th marriage in girls in rural Rajasthan, and in Bihar and every 8th in Jharkhand is before the legal age of 18 years. The surveys show that the unmet needs for contraceptive is high ranging from 12.6% in Rajasthan to 38.5% in Bihar; 98 districts report India's poor progress in population stabilization. In six of the eight high population states women continue to bear more than three children each. Only 35 of the 284 districts in high population states have so far met population stabilization goal of Total Fertility Rate (TER) of 2.1. High TFR in Bihar 3.5, UP 3.3, Rajasthan 2.9, Madhya Pradesh 3.0, Jharkhand 2.7, and Assam 2.4 is disturbing observation. This is the largest survey in the world. Now the district level data on maternal and child health indicators are available for planning and evaluation of various programmes at district level.

Health and NRHM in 12th Five-Year Plan, 2012–17

Universal Health Coverage

Rolling Out Universal Health Coverage (UnHC)—A New Strategy. 12th Plan strives to establish system of UnHC over the next two plans periods which will "Ensure equitable access for all Indian Citizens in any part of the country, regardless of income level, social status, gender, caste or religion to affordable, accountable and appropriate, assured quality health services (promotive, preventive, curative and rehabilitative) as well as services addressing wider determinants (water, sanitation, nutrition and education) of health delivered to individuals and population with the government being guarantor and enabler, although not necessarily the only provider of health and related services".

Various UnHC models will be pilot tested by the states (at least one district of each state). Cashless delivery of an Essential Health Package (EHP) to all, ought to be the basic component of all the models. Outpatient Care and medicines (essential medicines) will be a priority and every UHC Model will include for full and free access to essential drugs. EHP of National Health Programmes will be entirely funded and provided by the government and no fee of any kind will be levied on primary health care services.

- EHP will be delivered by mix of Government and Private Providers. Private sector will be contracted only for critical gaps filling.
- Define clinical services at different levels in an Essential Health package (EHP) which the government would finance and ensure provision through public health system supplemented by contracted in Private Providers.
- The Universal Provision of high impact, Preventive and Public health interventions which the Government would universally provide (including all national health programme services).
- Frame a national core of Essential Health Package for outpatient and inpatient care for uniform adoption in pilot projects.
- It is possible to use the platform of *Rashtriya Swasthya Bima Yojna* (RSBY) and expand the package of services under RSBY into EHP with the vision of replacing an insurance based system with a tax funded UnHC

system over a period of time. RBSY has now been shifted under MOH and FW as an integral part of National Health Mission (NHM).

NATIONAL HEALTH MISSION (NHM)

- The NHM is the primary vehicle to move towards Universal. Health coverage. It has two sub-missions– National Rural Health Mission and National Urban Health Mission. To address health needs of the urban poor, mission document on National Urban Health Mission has been approved in January 2008. Theme of World Health Day 2010 "Urban Health Matters" is a strong advocacy for urban health. After the success of the NRHM, the nation now wants to expand the scope of Health services in towns also (for urban poor in urban areas). The NRHM has been converted into National Health Mission, which would cover all villages and towns in the country. The NHM now extends all over the country both in urban and rural areas and promotes universal access to continuum of cashless health services from primary to tertiary care. Services will be delivered with seamless integration between primary, secondary and tertiary levels of care. The gains of the flagship programme of NRHM will be strengthened under the umbrella of NHM which will have universal coverage. The focus or thrust on covering rural areas and rural population will continue.
- 12th Plan envisages increase in public spending on **core health** from 1.04% of GDP in 2011–12 to 1.87% of GDP by the end of 12th Plan with 70% of the budget to be spent for primary health care (HLEG). Principle source of financing would be general tax revenues, supplemented by partnership with private sector and contribution by corporates as a part of their Corporate Social Responsibility (CSR).[6]

The NHM will incorporate the following core principles: Universal Health Coverage, Achieving quality standards by adopting revised Indian Public Health Standards, Continuum of Care by networking of institutions like Medical Colleges, District Hospitals, CHC, PHC and SCs linked with each other, Decentralized planning at District, Block, CHC, PHC and Village level and Prioritization of services (Maternal and Child health, Universal Immunization coverage, Family welfare, Communicable and Non-communicable disease control and Prevention, Focus on Dedicated Public Health Cadre in States, and Behaviour change communication).

12th Plan lays stress on Effective Governance System by use of structure of NHM, accountability for outcomes at all levels, adequate human resources for health care delivery, conversion of district hospitals and CHCs as knowledge centres/teaching centres, enhancing community participation and strengthening of health systems and mainstreaming of AYUSH systems.

Goals and Outcome Indicators by 2017 (12th FYP)

1 Reduce infant mortality rate to 25
2 Reduce maternal mortality rate to 100
3 Reduction of Total Fertility Rate to 2.1
4 Reduce prevalence of undernutrition in children under 3 years to 27%
5 Reduction of anaemia among women (15–49 years) to 28%
6 Raise child sex ratio from 914 to 950
7 Prevention and reduction of burden of communicable and non-communicable disease and injuries.
8 Reduction of poor household's out of pocket expenditure from 71% to 50%. State wise targets for IMR, MMR and anaemia have been set.

IMPROVING MATERNAL AND CHILD HEALTH THROUGH RMNCH + A APPROACH

Life cycle approach adopted under National Rural Health Mission is referred to as RMNCH + A approach. RMNCH + A stands for Reproductive, Maternal, Newborn, Child and Adolescent health.

Principles of RMNCH + A

- **Health System Strengthening:** Infrastructure, human resources, drugs commodities and transport.
- Evidence based interventions: High impact simple interventions for various stages in life cycle.
- **Convergence with other sectors:** Women and Child Development, Education, Water and sanitation and nutrition.
- Priority of interventions in high burden districts.
- Integrated monitoring through, Mother and Child Tracking System and Score cards.

The RMNCH + A approach in fact renews its commitment to the strategies adopted under Natioal Health Mission and Reproductive and Child Health (RCH–Phase I and Phase II) to achieve speedily the millenium development goal 4 and 5, vision 2020 and goals of 12th plan period as elaborated above.

The Critical Life Points

The critical life points for service delivery are adolescence, pre-pregnancy, pregnancy, birth, postpartum, neonatal, infancy and childhood.

The Essential Package and Services/Interventions

The high impact simple interventions to save lives of newborn and mothers within the continuum of RMNCH + A approach include:

i Adequate nutrition: Girls and women must receive adequate nutrition **from birth** through **childhood** and into **adolescence,** womenhood and their potential childbearing years.

ii Adolescent health

iii Antenatal care package (4 ANCs).

iv Skilled assistance at **delivery.**

v Basic and comprehensive emergency obstetric and newborn care

vi Postnatal and newborn care: Home based and facility based (at newborn stabilization unit and special newborn care units). Integrated management of neonatal and childhood-illness.

vii Improved household practices and behaviours (Healthy practices for mother and newborn care): Clean delivery-clean surface, clean blade, clean tie clean cord, clean hands, promotion of early initiation and exclusive breastfeeding and appropriate infant and young child feeding practices.

viii Child health screening and early intervention services (Rashtriya Bal Swasthya Karyakram)

ix Family planning interventions—contraception (spacing and terminal methods and comprehensive Abortion care services) as also management of RTI/STI

x Convergence with determinants of health: Water, sanitation, hygiene, nutrition education and empowerment of women.

Focus: RMNCH + A approach essentially focuses on major causes of mortality among women and children as well as delay in accessing and utilization of health care services.

Priority: 184 Low performing districts have been identified as high priority districts–where the burden of maternal and child mortality is high. The other priority is most vulnerable populations/areas–hilly and remote places, tribal and desert areas, weaker sections and urban poor.

- **The key delivery modes for services are:** Family/household and community, Outreach and Outpatient and Health facilities (PHC, CHC, District level and Medical Colleges, etc.)
- **The supportive environment:** This requires respect and rights of women and children; quality education; exploitation, discrimination and violence; equal participation in home, community, social and political life; emporverment of women; and greater involvement of men in maternal and child care.
- **Continuum of care under RMNCH + A—across time and location:** Continuum of care aims to integrate maternal, newborn, and child health care. Its central premise is: essential services for mothers, newborns and children are most effective when these are delivered in an integrated packages at critical points across life cycle of mother and children in a dynamic health system.

An effective continuum of care connects essential maternal newborn and child health packages through pregnancy, childbirth, postnatal and newborn periods, and into childhood and adolescence. The advantage is that each stage builds on the success of the previous stage. For example, providing integrated services to adolescent girls means fewer unintended or poorly timed pregnancies. Skilled care before, during and immediate after birth reduces the risk of death and disability for both mother and the baby. Continued care for children supports their right to health. An effective continuum of care also addresses gaps in care, whether at home, community, health centre or hospital. To be effective continuum of health care must forge strong links between the household/family, the community and quality outreach and clinical services at primary health facilities which in turn have strong connection to a district hospital.

The Household and Community are places where child care and maternal care **practices** and care **seeking behaviours** are learned and supported by community. Delivering comprehensive health care for mother and children requires preventive measures as well as management/treatment of illness.

Prevention essentially requires behaviour changes that begins in the household and family and can gain support of community. At a later stage the behaviour is influenced by peers in school and in company of preschool children, neighbour and friends. For example, improvement in nutrition, are often the result of breastfeeding practices and infant and young child feeding in the family. Use of sanitary latrines, hygienic practices, such as washing hands, gender discrimination begins at family, learned by individual and reinforced by community. Mobilizing the community to support improved health practices, demand generation for quality health services and ownership of programme; can go a long way to reduce morbidity and mortality in children and mothers.

The first response to illness like diarrhoea, cough and difficult breathing comes through mother and family or caregivers and similarly seeking early care during pregnancy, deciding place of birth and hygienic practices during and after delivery rest with family, *hence integrating household/family and community with the dynamic system of health care is an imperative in continuum* of RMNCH + A approach.

Daksh: To improve the skills of health care providers and to enhance their capacity to provide quality RMNCH + A, five National **skills** lab "Daksh" with the support from Liverpool School of tropical medicine have been set up.

REFERENCES

1 GOI. National Rural Health Mission (NRHM) Mission document. New Delhi: MOH and FW GOI; 2005.

2 GOI. Broad framework for preparation of District action plans August 2006. MOH and FW GOI. New Delhi.

3 GOI. Accredited Social Health Activist (ASHA). Guidelines, New Delhi: MOH and FW GOI; 2005.

5

4 GOI: MOH and FW Annual Report 2007–08, NRHM, GOI.
5 GOI. NRHM five years of NRHM, 2005–10 Bringing people back to public system. MOH and FW GOI, New Delhi, April 2010.
6 Planning Commission 12th Five-year plan 2012–17.

INTEGRATED MANAGEMENT OF NEONATAL AND CHILDHOOD ILLNESS (IMNCI)

Every year about 8.75 million children die before reaching their fifth birthday and over 70% of these deaths occur in developing world. The major killers diseases happen to be newborn deaths—under one month (41%), pneumonia (14%), diarrhoea (14%), measles (1%), malaria (8%), HIV/AIDS (2%), and others (13%). Malnutrition affects 35% of children. These diseases occur in combination most often (World Health Statistics 2010, Fig. 5.2).[1]

Over three-fourths of all 2.3 million deaths in India in 2005 were caused by five conditions: Pneumonia, prematurity and low birth weight, diarrhoeal diseases, neonatal infections, and birth asphyxia and birth trauma. (Million Death Study-Lancet Nov 12, 2010).

What is IMNCI?

Integrated management of neonate and childhood illness is a *strategy* for reducing mortality and morbidity associated with major causes of childhood illness. This strategy was developed by WHO and UNICEF in 1992. It has curative, preventive and promotive components.[2, 3]

- The curative component addresses syndromic approach to management of life-threatening conditions focusing on diarrhoea, pneumonia, measles and malaria as well as management of severe acute malnutrition and nutrition counselling.
- Health promotive and preventive measures include breastfeeding, nutrition counselling, vitamin A and iron supplementation, immunization and periodical deworming including hygiene and sanitation.

Target

All children under five years of age (in two age brackets children below 2 months and children between 2 months up to 5 years of age). Not only sick but all children below five years of age are targeted for interventions.

Implementation Principles

It is not a vertical programme. It is an *integrated strategy* that incorporates many of the elements of diarrhoeal disease and ARI control programmes and some of the child-oriented aspects of malaria control, nutrition and

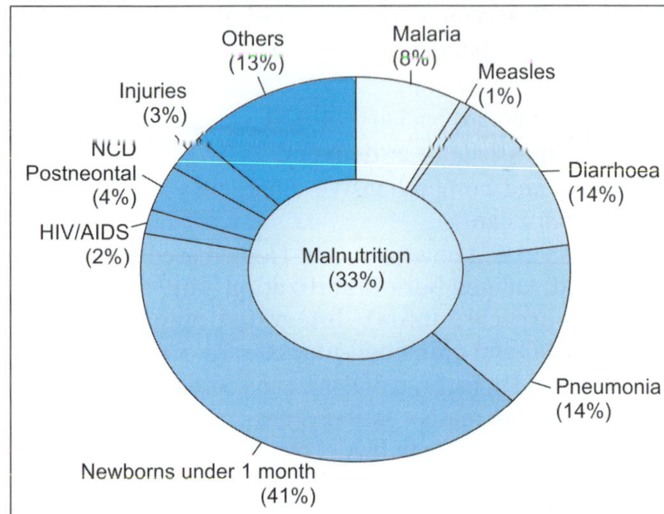

Fig. 5.2: Distribution of 8.795 million deaths among children less than 5 years old in 193 countries in 2008[1]

other related programmes, such as universal immunization, and essential drugs under primary health care programme. In essence it is an evidence-based *syndromic approach* to case management.

Main Components of IMNCI Strategy

The strategy has four main components:

i Improving case management skills of health care staff.
ii Improving overall health systems.
iii Improving family and community health practices.
iv Collaboration/coordination with other departments like PRIs, Self-help groups, *Mahila Swasthya Sangh* and ICDS.

The first two components of the strategy are facility-based IMNCI and the third and fourth are community-based IMNCI.

i. Improving Case Management Skills of Health Care Staff and AWWs

This is achieved by in-service skill based training. Medical officers and front line workers have been trained in the strategies of IMNCI by participatory methods of training.

ii. Improving Overall Health Systems

a Ensuring the availability of essential drugs and other supplies covered under IMNCI.
b Improvement of referral system. Make identified referral facility fully functional. In the Indian Context under NRHM, Subcentres, PHCs and CHCs are being made fully functional and *upgraded* to the levels of Indian Public Health Standards. However, upgradation of CHCs to the level of FRUs to provide comprehensive Emergency Obstetric and Neonatal care is very slow and there are 81% of vacancies of specialists in CHCs hence referral services support is very weak.

c Ensuring public-private partnership.
d Ensuring supervision and monitoring through follow up visits.

iii. Improving Family and Community Health Care Practices

Promoting healthy behaviours, such as breastfeeding, exculsive breastfeeding, illness recognition, early care seeking and compliance of care at home, counseling of caregivers during home visits and on overall health promotion and Community Participation. *Home based Newborn Care* and *Postnatal Care* Programme-2011: Series of *home visits* by ASHA or AWW or other health worker on days 1, 3, 7, 14, 21, 28, and 42nd day for home deliveries and on days 3, 7, 14, 21, 28, and 42nd for institutional deliveries for care of Newborn babies and postnatal mothers have begun.

iv. Collaborating/Coordination with other Departments

Effective implementation of IMNCI is possible only with the total involvement of ANM and Anganwadi workers of ICDS and grass-root functionaries of other sectors (Self- help group and PRIs). Community ownership and participation is of paramount importance.

Depending upon child's age, various clinical signs and symptoms differ in their degree of reliability and diagnostic value and importance. Therefore, IMNCI guidelines recommend case management procedures based on two age categories:

- Young infants up to 2 months
- Children age 2 months up to 5 years.

Principles of Integrated Care

The IMNCI guidelines are based on the following principles:

1 All sick young infants up to 2 months must be *assessed* for "*Possible serious bacterial infection* and *jaundice*". Then they must be routinely assessed for major symptom—"*diarrhoea*".

2 All sick children aged 2 months up to 5 years must be examined for "general danger signs" which indicate the need for immediate referral or admission to hospital. They must then be routinely *assessed for major symptoms*: cough or difficult breathing, diarrhoea, fever and ear problem.

3 All sick infants and children up to 5 years must also be routinely *assessed for nutritional* and *immunization status, feeding problems*, and *other potential problems*.

Only a *limited number of carefully selected clinical signs* are used, based on their sensitivity and specificity to detect disease. These signs were selected considering the conditions and realities of first level health facility.

A combination of individual signs leads to an infant's or a child's *classification*(s) or *syndrome rather than a diagnosis*. Classification(s) indicate the severity of condition(s). They call for specific actions based on whether the young infant or the child (a) should be urgently referred to another level of care, (b) requires specific treatments (such as, antibiotics or antimalarial treatment), or (c) may be safely managed at home. The classifications are colour coded. A child with "Pink" classification needs urgent attention, complete the assessment and *pre-referral treatment* immediately so that referral is not delayed. "Pink" suggests hospital referral or admission, "yellow" indicates initiation of specific treatment, at outpatient health facility, and "green" calls for home management.[4–5]

The IMNCI guidelines address *most, but not all, of the major reasons a sick infant or child is brought to a clinic*. An infant or child returning with chronic problems or less common illnesses may require special care. The guidelines do not describe the care at birth and the management of trauma or other acute emergencies due to accidents or injuries.

- IMNCI management procedures use a *limited number of essential drugs* and *encourage active participation of caretakers in the treatment* of infants and children.[6]
- An essential component of the IMNCI guidelines is *counselling of caretakers* about home care, including feeding, fluids and when to return to a health facility.

Case Management Process

The case management process is presented in Flowcharts 5.1 to 5.6. These charts describe the following steps:

a Assess the young infant or child
b Classify the illness
c Identify the treatment
d Treat the young infant or child
e Counsel the mother/caregiver
f Give follow-up care

a "Assess the young infant or child" means, asking, looking, listening and feeling (symptoms and signs).

b "Classify the illness means" making a decision on the severity of the illness. You can select a category or "classification" for each of the child's major symptoms which corresponds to severity of the disease. It is again stressed that the *classifications are not specific disease* diagnosis, instead these are categories used to determine severity of condition for management at appropriate level.

c The charts recommend appropriate treatment for each classification. When using this process, selecting a classification on the chart is sufficient to allow you to "identify treatment" for a young infant or child. For example, a young infant with the classification *possible serious bacterial infection* could have pneumonia, septicaemia or meningitis.

Flowchart 5.1: ASSESS AND CLASSIFY THE SICK YOUNG INFANT AGE UP TO 2 MONTHS

ASSESS: Ask the mother what young infant's problems are? Use all boxes that match infant's symptoms

CLASSIFY: A child with a **Pink** classification needs **URGENT** attention, complete the assessment and pre-referral treatment immediately so that referral is not delayed. Check for possible bacterial infection/jaundice

ASK: • Has the infant had convulsions?

LOOK, LISTEN, FEEL:

- Count the breaths in one minute.
- Repeat the count if elevated.
- Look for severe chest indrawing.
- Look for nasal flaring.
- Look and listen for grunting.
- Look and feel for bulging fontanelle.

} Young infant must be calm

- Look for pus draining from the ear. • Look at the umbilicus. Is it red or draining pus?
- Look for skin pustules. Are there 10 or more skin pustules or a big boil?
- Measure axillary temperature (if not possible, feel for fever or low body temperature).
- See if the young infant is lethargic or unconscious.
- Look at the young infant's movements. Are they less than normal? • Look for jaundice? Are the palms and soles yellow?

Classify All Young Infants

SIGNS	CLASSIFY AS	IDENTIFY TREATMENT (Urgent pre-referral treatment in bold print)
• Convulsions or • Fast breathing (60 breaths per minute or more) or • Severe chest indrawing or • Nasal flaring or • Grunting or • Bugling fontanelle or • 10 or more skin pustules or a big boil or • If axillary temperature 37.5°C or above (or feels hot to touch) or temperature less than 36.5°C (or feels cold to touch) or • Lethargic or unconscious or • Less than normal movements or not able to feed	**POSSIBLE SERIOUS BACTERIAL INFECTION**	• **Give first dose of intramuscular gentamicin and amoxycillin**[6] • **Treat to prevent low blood sugar.** • **Warm the young infant by skin to skin contact if temperature less than 36.5°C (or feels cold to touch) while arranging referral.** • **Advise mother how to keep the young infant warm on the way to the hospital.** • **Refer URGENTLY to hospital*.**
• Umbilicus red or draining pus or • Pus discharge from ear or • <10 skin pustules.	**LOCAL BACTERIAL INFECTION**	• **Give oral cotrimoxazole or amoxycillin for 5 days.** • Teach mother to treat local infections at home. • Follow-up in 2 days.

And if the infant has jaundice

SIGNS	CLASSIFY AS	IDENTIFY TREATMENT
• Palms and soles yellow or • Age <24 hours or • Age 14 days or more	**SEVERE JAUNDICE**	• **Treat to prevent low blood sugar.** • **Warm the young infant by skin to skin contact if temperature less than 36.5°C (or feels cold to touch) while arranging referral.** • **Advise mother how to keep the young infant warm on the way to the hospital.** • **Refer URGENTLY to hospital*.**
• Palms and soles not yellow	**JAUNDICE**	• Advise mother to give home care for the young infant. • Advise mother when to return immediately. • Follow-up in 2 days.

And if the temp. is between 35.5 and 36.4°C

SIGNS	CLASSIFY AS	IDENTIFY TREATMENT
• Temperature between 35.5 and 36.4°C	**LOW BODY TEMPERATURE**	• Warm the young infant using skin to skin contact for one hour and REASSESS. If no improvement, refer. • Treat to prevent low blood sugar.

* If referral is not possible, treat the young infant and counsel the parents

Flowchart 5.2: YOUNG INFANT AGE UP TO 2 MONTHS

THEN ASK: Does the young infant has diarrhoea?

1. **IF YES, ASK**
   - For how long? Is there blood in stool?

   LOOK AND FEEL
   - Look at the young infant's general condition. Is the infant lethargic or unconscious? Restless or irritable.
   - Look for sunken eyes. • Pinch the skin of abdomen. Does it go back: Very slowly (longer than 2 seconds)? Slowly?

   What is diarrhoea in a young infant?

   If the stools have changed from usual pattern and are many and watery (more water than fecal matter). The normal frequent or loose stools of a breastfed baby are not diarrhoea.

Classify Diarrhoea for Dehydration

SIGNS	CLASSIFY AS	IDENTIFY TREATMENT
Two of the following signs: • Lethargic or unconscious. • Sunken eyes. • Skin pinch goes back very slowly.	**SEVERE DEHYDRATION**	• **Give first dose of intramuscular ampicillin and gentamicin.** **–If infant also has low weight or another severe classification:** ▪ **Refer URGENTLY to hospital with mother giving frequent sips of ORS on the way*.** ▪ **Advise mother to continue breastfeeding.** ▪ **Advise mother how to keep the young infant warm on the way to the hospital.** *OR* • If infant does not have low weight or any other severe classification: – Give fluid for severe dehydration (Plan C) and then refer to hospital after rehydration.
Two of the following signs: • Restless, irritable • Sunken eyes. • Skin pinch goes back slowly.	**SOME DEHYDRATION**	• **If infant also has low weight or another severe classification:** – **Give first dose of intramuscular ampicillin and gentamicin.** – **Refer URGENTLY to hospital with mother giving frequent sips of ORS on the way*.** – **Advise mother to continue breastfeeding.** – **Advise mother how to keep the young infant warm on the way to the hospital.** • If infant does not have low weight or another severe classification: – Give fluids for some dehydration (Plan B) – Advise mother when to return immediately. – Follow-up in 2 days.
Not enough signs to classify as some or severe dehydration.	**NO DEHYDRATION**	• Give fluids to treat diarrhoea at home (Plan A) • Advise mother when to return immediately. • Follow-up in 5 days if not improving.

And if Diarrhoea of 14 days or more

Diarrhoea lasting 14 days or more.	**SEVERE PERSISTENT DIARRHOEA**	• Give first dose of intramuscular ampicillin and gentamicin if the young infant has low weight, dehydration or another severe classification. • Treat to prevent low blood sugar. • Advise how to keep infant warm on the way to the hospital. • Refer to hospital*.

And if there is blood in stool

Blood in stool	**SEVERE DYSENTERY**	• Give first dose of intramuscular ampicillin and gentamicin if the young infant has low weight, dehydration or another severe classification. • Treat to prevent low blood sugar. • Advise how to keep infant warm on the way to hospital. • Refer to hospital*.

* If referral is not possible, treat the young infant and counsel the mother.

5

Flowchart 5.3: CHECK FOR FEEDING PROBLEM AND MALNUTRITION (Age up to 2 months)

ASK, LOOK, AND FEEL

- Is there any difficulty in feeding? Is the infant breastfed? Yes, how many times in 24 hours?
- Does the infant usually receive any other food or drink? If yes, how often?
- What do you use to feed the infant?
- **If AN INFANT:** Has any difficulty in feeding or is breastfeeding less than 8 times in 24 hours or is taking any other foods or drinks, or is low weight-for-age and has no indication to refer urgently to hospital.

LOOK, FEEL: Determine weight-for-age

ASSESS BREASTFEEDING: • Has the infant breastfed in the previous hour? Is the infant able to attach?

If the infant has not fed in the previous hour, ask the mother to put her infant to breast. Observe the breastfeed for 4 minutes. (If the infant was fed during the last hour, ask the mother if she can wait and tell you when the infant is willing to feed again.)

_ No attachment at all. _ Not well attached. _ Good attachment.

TO CHECK THE ATTACHMENT, LOOK FOR: • Chin touching breast. • Mouth wide open. • Lower lip turned outward.

- More areola visible above than below the mouth. (All of these signs should be present if the attachment is good.)
- Is the infant suckling effectively (that is, slow deep sucks, sometimes pausing)? Not suckling at all, not suckling effectively, suckling effectively.
- Clear a blocked nose if it interferes with breastfeeding. • Look for ulcers or white patches in the mouth (Thrush).
- Does the mother have pain while breastfeeding? If yes look and feel for: Flat or inverted nipples, or sore nipples, engorged breasts or breast abscess.

Classify Feeding

SIGNS	CLASSIFY AS	IDENTIFY TREATMENT
• Not able to feed or • No attachment at all or • Not suckling at all or • Very low weight-for-age.	**NOT ABLE TO FEED POSSIBLE SERIOUS BACTERIAL INFECTION OR SEVERE MALNUTRITION**	• Give first dose of intramuscular ampicillin and gentamicin. • Treat to prevent low blood sugar. • Warm the young infant by skin to skin contact if temperature less than 36.5°C (or feels cold to touch) while arranging referral. • Advise mother how to keep the young infant warm on the way to the hospital. • Refer URGENTLY to hospital*.
• Not well attached to breast or • Not suckling effectively or • Less than 8 breastfeeds in 24 hours or • Receives other foods or drinks or • Thrush (ulcers or white patches in mouth) or • Low weight-for-age *OR* • Breasts or nipple problems	**FEEDING PROBLEM OR LOW WEIGHT-FOR-AGE**	• If not well attached or not suckling effectively, teach correct positioning and attachment. • If breastfeeding less than 8 times in 24 hours, advise to increase frequency of feeding. • If receiving other foods or drinks, counsel mother about breastfeeding more, reducing other foods or drinks, and using a cup and spoon. – If not breastfeeding at all advise mother about giving locally appropriate animal milk and teach the mother to feed with a cup and spoon. • If thrush, teach the mother to treat thrush at home. • If low weight-for-age, teach the mother how to keep the young infant with low weight warm at home. • If breast or nipple problem, teach the mother to treat breast or nipple problems. • Advise mother to give home care for the young infant. • Advise mother when to return immediately. • Follow-up any feeding problem or thrush in 2 days. • Follow-up low weight-for-age in 14 days.
• Not low weight-for-age and no other signs of inadequate feeding.	**NO FEEDING PROBLEM**	• Advise mother to give home care for the young infant. • Advise mother when to return immediately. • Praise mother for feeding the infant well.

* If referral is not possible, treat the young infant and counsel the parents.

Flowchart 5.4: ASSESS AND CLASSIFY THE SICK CHILD AGE 2 MONTHS UP TO 5 YEARS

ASK THE MOTHER WHAT THE CHILD'S PROBLEMS ARE?

- Determine if this is an initial or follow-up visit for this problem.
  - If follow-up visit, use the follow-up instructions on treat the child chart.
  - If initial visit, assess the child as follows:

CHECK FOR GENERAL DANGER SIGNS

ASK:

- Is the child able to drink or breastfeed?
- Does the child vomit everything?
- Has the child has convulsions?

LOOK:

- See if the child is lethargic or unconscious.

A child with any general danger sign needs urgent attention; complete the assessment and any pre-referral treatment immediately so that referral is not delayed.

THEN ASK ABOUT MAIN SYMPTOMS: Does the child have cough or difficult breathing?

IF YES, ASK: • For how long?

LOOK, LISTEN:

- Count the breaths in one minute.
- Look for chest indrawing.
- Look and listen for stridor.

} (Child must be calm)

Classify Cough or Difficult Breathing

SIGNS	CLASSIFY AS	IDENTIFY TREATMENT (Urgent pre-referral treatments are in bold print)
• Any general danger sign or • Chest indrawing or • Stridor in calm child.	**SEVERE PNEUMONIA OR VERY SEVERE DISEASE**	**• Give first dose of injectable chloramphenicol (If not possible give oral amoxycillin).** **• Refer URGENTLY to hospital*.**
• Fast breathing is If the child is 2 months up to 12 months: 50 breaths per minute or more 12 months up to 5 years: 40 breaths per minute or more	**PNEUMONIA**	• Give cotrimoxazole for 5 days. • Soothe the throat and relieve the cough with a safe remedy if child is 6 months or older. • Advise mother when to return immediately. • Follow-up in 2 days.
No signs of pneumonia or very severe disease.	**NO PNEUMONIA COUGH OR COLD**	• If coughing more than 30 days, refer for assessment. • Soothe the throat and relieve the cough with a safe home remedy if child is 6 months or older. • Advise mother when to return immediately. • Follow-up in 5 days if not improving.

* If referral is not possible, treat the child and counsel the mother/parents.

Flowchart 5.5: SICK CHILD AGE 2 MONTHS UP TO 5 YEARS

DOES THE CHILD HAVE DIARRHOEA?

IF YES, ASK:

- For how long?
- Is there blood in the stool?

LOOK AND FEEL:

- Look at the child's general condition. Is the child lethargic or unconscious? Restless and irritable?
- Look for sunken eyes.
- Offer the child fluid. Is the child:
  - Not able to drink or drinking poorly?
  - Drinking eagerly, thirsty?
- Pinch the skin of the abdomen. Does it go back:
  - Very slowly (longer than 2 seconds)?
  - Slowly?

Classify Diarrhoea for— Dehydration— Persistent Dirrhoea and Dysentery

SIGNS	CLASSIFY AS	IDENTIFY TREATMENT
Two of the following signs: • Lethargic or unconscious. • Sunken eyes. • Not able to drink or drinking poorly. • Skin pinch goes back very slowly.	**SEVERE DEHYDRATION**	• If child has no other severe classification. – Give fluid for severe dehydration (Plan C). • **If child also has another severe classification: Refer URGENTLY to hospital with mother giving frequent sips of ORS on the way*. Advise the mother to continue breastfeeding.** • **If child is 2 years or older and there is cholera in your area, give doxycycline for cholera.**
Two of the following signs: • Restless, irritable • Sunken eyes • Drinks eagerly, thirsty • Skin pinch goes back slowly.	**SOME DEHYDRATION**	• Give fluid and food for some dehydration (Plan B) and zinc supplements. • **If child also has another severe classification: Refer URGENTLY to hospital with mother giving frequent sips of ORS on the way. Advise the mother to continue breastfeeding*.** • Advise mother when to return immediately. • Follow-up in 5 days if not improving.
Not enough signs to classify as some or severe dehydration.	**NO DEHYDRATION**	• Give fluid and food to treat diarrhoea at home (Plan A) and zinc supplements. • Advise mother when to return immediately. • Follow-up in 5 days if not improving.

And if Diarrhoea 14 days or more

SIGNS	CLASSIFY AS	IDENTIFY TREATMENT
• Dehydration present.	**SEVERE PERSISTENT DIARRHOEA**	• **Treat dehydration before referral unless the child has another severe classification.** • **Refer to hospital.**
• No dehydration.	**PERSISTENT DIARRHOEA**	• Advise the mother on feeding a child who has PERSISTENT DIARRHOEA. • Give single dose of vitamin A. • Give zinc sulphate 20 mg daily for 14 days. • Follow-up in 5 days.

And if blood in stool

SIGNS	CLASSIFY AS	IDENTIFY TREATMENT
• Blood in the stool.	**DYSENTERY**	• **Treat for 5 days with ciprofloxacin, treat dehydration give zinc.** • Follow-up in 2 days.

* If referral is not possible, treat the child and counsel the mother/parents.

Flowchart 5.6: SICK CHILD AGE 2 MONTHS UP TO 5 YEARS

DOES THE CHILD HAVE FEVER? (by history or feels hot or temperature 37.5°C or above)

IF YES: Decide Malaria Risk: High/Low

THEN ASK: • Fever for how long? • If more than 7 days, has fever been present everyday? • Has the child had measles within the last 3 months?

LOOK AND FEEL: • Look or feel for stiff neck. • Look and feel for bulging fontanelle. • Look for runny nose.

Look for signs of MEASLES: • Generalized rash and • One of these: cough, runny nose, or red eyes.

If the child has measles now or within the last 3 months: Look for mouth ulcers. Are they deep and extensive? Look for pus draining from the eye. Look for clouding of the cornea.

Classify Fever—High Malaria Risk Area

SIGNS	CLASSIFY AS	IDENTIFY TREATMENT
• Any general danger sign or • Stiff neck or • Bulging fontanelle.	**VERY SEVERE FEBRILE DISEASE**	• **Give first dose of IM quinine after making a blood smear.** • **Give first dose of IV or IM chloramphenicol (if not possible, give oral amoxycillin).** • **Treat the child to prevent low blood sugar.** • **Give one dose of Paracetamol in clinic for high fever (temp. 38.5°C or above)** • **Refer URGENTLY to hospital*.**
• Fever (by history or feels hot or temperature 37.5°C or above).	**MALARIA**	• **Give oral antimalarials for HIGH malaria risk area after making a blood smear.** • **Give one dose of paracetamol in clinic for high fever (temp. 38.5°C or above)** • Advise mother when to return immediately. • Follow-up in 2 days if fever persists. • If fever is present everyday for more than 7 days, refer for assessment.

Low Malaria Risk Area

SIGNS	CLASSIFY AS	IDENTIFY TREATMENT
• Any general danger sign or • Stiff neck or • Bulging fontanelle.	**VERY SEVERE FEBRILE DISEASE**	• **Give first dose of IM quinine after making a blood smear.** • **Give first dose of IV or IM chloramphenicol (if not possible, give oral amoxycillin).** • **Treat the child to prevent low blood sugar.** • **Give one dose of paracetamol in clinic for high fever (temp. 38.5°C or above)** • **Refer URGENTLY to hospital*.**
• NO runny nose and NO measles and NO other cause of fever.	**MALARIA**	• **Give oral antimalarials for LOW malaria risk area after making a blood smear.** • **Give one dose of paracetamol in clinic for high fever (temp. 38.5°C or above)** • Advise mother when to return immediately. • Follow-up in 2 days if fever persists. • If fever is present everyday for more than 7 days, refer for assessment.
• Runny nose PRESENT or • Measles PRESENT or • Other cause of fever PRESENT	**FEVER MALARIA UNLIKELY**	• **Give one dose of paracetamol in clinic for high fever (temp. 38.5°C or above).** • Advise mother when to return immediately. • Follow-up in 2 days if fever persists. • If fever is present everyday for more than 7 days, refer for assessment.

If Measles now Within Last 3 Months, Classify

SIGNS	CLASSIFY AS	IDENTIFY TREATMENT
• Any general danger sign or • Clouding of cornea or • Deep or extensive mouth ulcers.	**SEVERE COMPLICATED MEASLES**	• **Give first dose of vitamin A.** • **Give first dose of injectable chloramphenicol (if not possible, give oral amoxycillin).** • **If clouding of the cornea or pus draining from the eye, apply tetracycline eye ointment.** • **Refer URGENTLY to hospital*.**
• Pus draining from the eye or • Mouth ulcers.	**MEASLES WITH EYE OR MOUTH COMPLICATIONS**	• Give first dose of vitamin A. • If pus draining from the eye, treat eye infection with tetracycline eye ointment. • If mouth ulcers, treat with gentian violet. • Follow-up in 2 days.
• Measles now or within the last 3 months.	**MEASLES**	• Give first dose of vitamin A.

* If referral is not possible, treat the child and counsel the parents.

d "The treatment listed for *possible serious bacterial infection* will be appropriate because they have been chosen to cover the most important diseases included in this classification".

e **Counselling the mother or caregivers.** A child who is seen at clinic needs to continue treatment, feeding and fluids at home. Good communication skills are required for counselling. Give information, demonstrate the practice and let them practice. Counselling is required on:

- Feeding and fluids of young children during illness
- Recognition of danger signs and return immediately for care
- When to return for immunization
- Counsel the mother about her own health.
- Praise the mother/caregiver for what they have done well.

f **Give follow-up care:** Some sick children will need to return for follow-up care. At a follow-up visit see if the child is improving on the drug or other treatment that was prescribed. Give follow up care when the child returns to the facility and if necessary reassess the child for new problem. If the child does not have a new problem use the IMNCI follow-up instructions for each specific problem (pneumonia, diarrhoea, fever, malaria, measles, dysentery and feeding, etc.).

Implementation of IMNCI in India

In India the IMCI has been implemented as an Integrated Management of Neonatal and Childhood Illness (IMNCI). National Population Policy, 2000 incorporated the strategy of IMCI.

IMNCI strategy encompasses a range of interventions to prevent and manage five major childhood illnesses, i.e. Acute respiratory infections, diarrhoea, measles, malaria and malnutrition and the major causes of neonatal mortality—prematurity and sepsis. It focuses on preventive, promotive and curative aspects, i.e. it gives a holistic outlook to the programme.

Management algorithms of the young infant up to 2 months and children from 2 months to 5 years have been reproduced. In—service training itself will take long time (2–3 years time). It is better to build these modules/charts in the initial or recruit training of multipurpose health workers, medical undergraduates, postgraduates and nursing graduates for better results.

Up to 2014 over five hundred districts all over the country have initiated the implementation of IMNCI. Under RCH II IMNCI is the key component or strategy. The Government of India has recently approved the implementation of home based newborn care (HBNC) based on Gadchiroli model; where appreciable decline in infant mortality rates has been documented on the basis of work done by SEARCH; an NGO.

Special newborn care unit (SNCU). Sick children screened and referred to health facilities equipped better to handle sick children by setting up of SNCU at district hospitals, stabilization units at CHCs and newborn care corners at all facilities offering delivery facilities is thus a key activity.

F-IMNCI: It is the integration of the facility-based care package with the IMNCI package, to enable the health personnel with the skills to manage newborn and childhood illness at the community level as well as at the facility.

REFERENCES

1 Black, et al. Causes of death, World Health Statistics 2010, WHO. Lancet 2010, 375:1969–87.
2 World Health Organization, World Health Report 1999 Making a difference. Geneva, WHO, 1999.
3 World Health Organization and UNICEF. Integrated Management of Neonatal and Childhood Illness. Physician Chart Booklet. Ministry of Health and Family Welfare. Government of India, 2003.
4 UNICEF. Community IMCI: A strategy for accelerating child survival and development interventions. Discussion paper. UNICEF-New York, September 2001. WHO, improving family and community practices. A component of IMCI strategy.
5 WHO, UNICEF and GOI MOH and FW. Integrated management of neonatal and childhood illness MOH and GOI. New Delhi, 2005.
6 MOH and FW, GOI. Operational Guidelines: use of Gentamicin by ANMs for management of sepsis in young infants under situation, Feb 2014.

SCHOOL HEALTH PROGRAMME (SHP)

School Health Programme (SHP) in India has a long history. In British, India, a modest start was made in Baroda (Gujarat) in 1909 to start health check-ups for school going children. Thereafter, in 1946 Bhore Committee identified the school children as vulnerable group and indicated target group for health services. School health services constituted as one of the essential function of the PHC which were set-up in the country as part of community development block from 1952 onwards. Recognizing the significance and importance of SHP the Government of India constituted a school health committee in 1960 and it submitted its report and made valuable recommendations for SHP in India.[1] However, the services were confined to health check-ups, school meals and some selective immunizations (notably smallpox vaccination). Applied nutrition programme (ANP) promoted the concept of kitchen garden and school garden for growing and consumption of protective foods, probably the idea was to promote learning values of protective foods and significance of adequate diet for growing children. School health services were evaluated by National Institute of Health and Family Welfare in 1980s and a set of recommendations emerged, and to pursue these recommendations intensive school health education programme was launched in primary schools as a Pilot Project in 10 states by Central Health Education Bureau (CHEB) in 1989, wherein "child to child" and "youth to child" model demonstrated varying degree of success in three years period.[2] The Govermment of India launched school heath scheme in 1996–97.

The National Health Policy, 2002 intends targeting school and college students to improve the general level of awareness with regard to health promoting behaviour.[3]

An operational framework of school health programme has been formulated and circulated to states by NRHM and states have introduced SHP from the year 2008. NRHM provides for school health check-ups and school health education programme.

SIGNIFICANCE

National Education Policy of 1986 and National Health Policy of 1983 identified twin objectives of "Education for all and Health for all".[4,5] Universal elementary education (UEE) is an important vehicle for human resource development in India. Nation is striving to achieve the target of UEE through intensive programme of *Sarva Shiksha Abhiyan* (SSA).[6] "Right to Eduction Act" (RTE) April 2010 makes free elementary eduction as fundamental right of all 6–14 year old children in India. About 34.5 million Children are out of school (31st March 2015).

1. School children 5–14 years constitute around 21.4% of total population. There were 312 million children between 5–14 years of age.
2. They are most captive group and you can mould their behaviour, during the formative years of life; the way you like.
3. They can be used as resource for communication of ideas and values to their families and neighbourhood. Nation has used school children for IPPI and for several other drives.
4. The mortality is least in this age group. But growth and development continues during these years at rapid pace which needs to be supervised and supported. The diseases, defects deficiency and development delays which are common in school children consist of:
5. Malnutrition—underweight in rural and urban slum areas including anaemia and overweight in urban area is an emerging problem. Malnutrition and ill health are major causes of low school enrolment and high absenteeism. Other problems are:
   - Caries teeth—60–80% have caries teeth.
   - Refractive errors and visual problems.
   - Ear, nose and throat problems.
   - Skin diseases (ringworm—pyoderma and scabies).
   - Worm infestation.
   - Learning disorders and behavioural problems, smoking, substance use and disorders of psychological development: autism, behavioural and emotional problems, e.g. attention deficit hyperactivity disorders or conduct disorders.
   - Iodine deficiency disorders.
   - Injuries.
   - Postural defects.
   - Local endemic diseases including Rheumatic and Congenital heart diseases.
   - Impairments—visual hearing and locomotor.

Most of diseases are related to poor personal hygiene, behavioural problems and unhealthy lifestyles.

OBJECTIVES OF SCHOOL HEALTH PROGRAMME (SHP)

In view of the problems, the objective of SHP should be:

1. To inculcate healthy habits and lifestyles to promote healthy behaviour and to learn values of hygiene and oral health.
2. To protect them against some specific diseases like tetanus, diphtheria and pertussis by immunization.
3. To promote health seeking behaviour, to detect the defects, diseases, deficiency and disability at the earliest and ensure prompt treatment by periodical check-up.
4. Training of teachers for school health activities.
5. To establish parent-teachers associations and regular contacts for counselling.
6. To promote healthy environment in school with the active participation of school children which include safe water, safe disposal of human excreta, waste water and garbage disposal and protection of environments.

FOCUS

The prime focus in school health services is school going children of 5–14 years age group, however some components of SHP extend beyond that age group for example, immunization, adolescent health and population education or family life education to cover adolescent age group; up to the age of 19 years.

COMPONENTS OF SHP

These are health promotion by education, mid-day meal, environmental sanitation, periodic health check-ups including oral health, school immunizations, mass deworming, capacity building for screening and adolescent health.

Health Promotion by Education and Learning Values

Health education like general education, is concerned with change in knowledge, attitude and behaviour. Moulding behaviour and practices during formative years of life is much easier. School children are important groups for changing behaviour, establishing healthy behaviours and practice of healthy behaviours as also adopting healthy lifestyles. Hygiene can be learnt by actual practice and cannot be just taught by sermons or lectures. School teachers lead by good examples. "Child to Child" programme in schools and "Youth to Child" model in school means senior class students mind the healthy habits of younger children and take responsibility for forming and practice of healthy habits like washing hands, brushing teeth, eating clean food, drinking clean water, use of toilets and eating healthy foods and disposal of waste water and refuse. Teachers should become good role models for their students to leave permanent impression on the minds of students. One hour time or one period devoted to socially useful and productive work (SUPW) can be used for physical, creative and development activities for demonstration and practice of healthy habits and healthy lifestyles. Many lifestyle diseases have their origin in childhood. **Unhealthy eating habits** (Junk foods and carbonated drinks) and lack **of physical** activity among children leads to lifestyle diseases like obesity, diabetes and heart diseases later in life. This calls for need to educate children about the ill effects of unhealthy snacking. The school teachers themselves can provide a lead. Learning values and hygiene this way costs nothing and promotes healthy behaviour. These models when implemented sincerely produce desired effects much faster.[7–9]

"Cleanliness is next to Godliness" is a common saying mere teaching of cleanliness of body and surroundings is not enough unless it is effectively demonstrated and maintained by teachers and students themselves in schools, by homes and family and in the community. Essential and obligatory "five cleans" to be observed and practiced daily include clean hands before eating, clean mouth and teeth, clean food, clean water and clean environments. Basic training, orientation and reorientation training as also continuing education of teachers and regular contacts with parents and Panchayati Raj Institutions (PRIs) on sustainable basis are essential to improve hygiene and sanitation. Health workers can reinforce these messages on their home visits and regular contacts with people and leaders once they are making annual subcentre action plan or village health plans. Health, hygiene, and sanitation goes far beyond the area of teaching as a lesson or subject, but the same can be better learnt through activities and demonstrations on oral health and hygiene by the students themselves in an organized manner. Linking school health activities with the village and community life and ways of life can usher in better learning of values towards healthy living.

Although school curriculum (CBSE) consists of chapters on hygiene and health education but emphasis is not laid on their practical aspects. These chapters must be translated to practice and action to inculcate scientific temper and creative activities apart from learning values of health and hygiene. The teachers should attempt to give health projects to students based on curriculum and children should have a pride in completing such projects.[10,11]

Health Education Material

The material on health education should be displayed and used for providing health education informing them about available services. Whatever material on education comes to PHC/CHC must be made available to school teachers for dissemination of health education messages.

Health education material to be developed jointly by the health and education department on relevant and important topics and printed by education department. Additional material would be created by students/peer educators through competitive and creative activities.

National Population Education Programme (NPEP) in Eduction Sector by NCERT[12]

Since its launch in 1980, the NPEP is working to attain the institutionalization of population education in the education system of the country. The population education programme in school has been implemented as "population and development education in schools". The overriding objective of the project has been the institutionalization of population education in the content and process of school education. The project has been implemented by NCERT at the national level and SCERTs at the state and UTs level.

Role of Teachers in Health Education and Counseling

"Health education for all" is an essential component and it can only succeed if teachers take this onerous responsibility. The role of primary school teachers in health and other aspects of education is pivotal. The teacher's task should go beyond imparting of basic knowledge to include equipping children with skills and shaping attitudes towards learning.

In India there are school teachers in most villages and their number is five times more than health workers. Teachers when committed and trained can be an invaluable resource for health education both in school and in the community. The twin goals of "Education for all and Health for all" are inseparably linked. Good health is essential for effective learning and education is a means of empowering children and adults to attain and maintain health and ensure well-being. In essence, teachers must practice what they teach in school. Most of the time the messages conveyed by the teachers are in conflict with the actual practice or situation. Teaching cleanliness in dirty school or classroom is demotivating. Quit smoking makes a little impact if teachers themselves continue smoking. Therefore, teachers must practice the values before the taughts, who will emulate their respective teachers in later life. Behavioural problems can be identified by the teachers for *counselling activity*.

Role of Parents[9]

Parents have to be equal and rather more than equal partners in building health behaviours of the young one's as parents are the supreme teachers in the family set-up. Parents and teachers must meet periodically for counselling. Children learn the values of hygiene and practice of hygienic habits in the family. What home or a household does, influence the behaviour of young children far more than any government set-up or school system.

Implementation of School Health Programme

The School Health Committee (consisting of 4 teachers from school and a student from each class/grade/standard, selected parents and community members are members of parent–teacher association) constituted by principal/head master holds the prime responsibility for implementation of School Health Programme. The committee meets every month to plan, audit and monitor progress. School health coordinator (trained teacher) assists the health committee. School health clubs can be constituted to involve students and teachers.

Mid-day Meal (MDM) in Schools

The focus of mid-day meal programme are children between 6 and 11 years or primary school children.[6] Now it covers middle schools also (6–14 years).

Objective

1 To increase enrolment and retention as a step toward universal elementary education (UEE).
2 The primary aim of school meal programme is to improve health and encourage sound dietary habits among children.[6]
3 The other objective is to improve nutritional status and tackle micronutrient deficiency.
4 It is used as spring board to develop other activities like washing hands, brushing teeth and eating clean and nourishing foods, besides increasing enrolment and retention.

The ideal school meal should provide approximately one-third of the dietary and nutritional requirement of children.

What We Have?

The national programme of nutritional support to primary education commonly known as the mid-day meal. Programme was launched in 1995. It aims to give a boost to universalization of primary education by increasing enrolment, retention and attendance and simultaneously improving the nutritional status of students in primary classes. Under the scheme, cooked meals are to be served with calorie value equivalent to 100 g of wheat or rice per student per school day for 200 days in a year. Tamil Nadu provided a successful lead in mid-day meal scheme. The scheme has been successful in increasing enrolment as well as retention of students but has not achieved the target of nation wide coverage.[6] Food grains are supplied by central government free of cost. Two rupees per child per day are allocated for cooking of which one rupee should come from the state government.

Mid-day meal programme was being implemented in different style. At the end of the month, all the enrolled children of primary school classes were distributed 3 kg of raw cereals (rice or wheat) and children carry this ration to home. What happens to this, *no body* knows. It is inadequate to supplement one-third of calories per day. To some extent, it has improved the attendance in schools, but it is more or less a ritual and attendance improved only on the day of its distribution.[6] A Supreme Court order in 2001 makes it obligatory for states to provide cooked meals instead of dry rations within the stipulated time frame. As of now the cooked meals are being provided, with obligatory use of iodized salt.

Selling of eatables outside the premises of schools should be effectively controlled by teachers. The apex food regulator had recently framed guidelines to curb the sale of *Junk foods* and *carbonated drinks on* the school premises. School health programme must be revised and converged with MDM and MDM itself merged with SSA (*Sarva Shiksha Abhiyan*). Applied nutrition programme was rooted in schools to promote consumption of protective foods. Kitchen gardens in school and indeed maintenance of gardens/fruit trees in school premises has been used in many schools to improve concept of improved nutrition, a love for nature, and interest in gardening.

Environmental Sanitation in Schools

National school sanitation initiative and school sanitation rating were launched in July 2011 to promote sanitation.

Safe drinking water in schools and safe disposal of human excreta apart from clean and healthy physical environments is essential component of SHP. National water supply and sanitation programme accords high priority for safe drinking water in schools. The government of India has launched school water supply and sanitation and hygiene education programme (SSHE) through the Ministry of Rural Development under ARWS (Accelerated Rural Water Supply and Sanitation) and SSA (*Sarva Shiksha Abhiyan*) only 44% of rural schools have water supply facilities. The teachers are responsible to chlorinate the source of water in the school; clean storage of water, use of ladle and washing hands before eating. The role of health department is to train teachers and students on the technique of chlorination, supply bleaching powder or halogen tablets on regular basis. Inculcating habit of drinking chlorinated water in schools has made its impact in the community as well. School children successfully chlorinated drinking water at their home and motivated their parents to regularly drink chlorinated water. Testing of residual chlorine by *orthotoluidine* solution can be a fun with students and establishing scientific temper amongst school children and school teachers. Looking a drop of dirty water under the microscope could be a stimulus for thinking. Demonstrating a dirty water and clean water and how the water becomes dirty is an important exercise for school children. Similarly, taking students to local water works and demonstrating the process of water purification can build favourable attitudes.

Promotion of rural latrines programme focused more often at schools and preschool children at Anganwadi centre. Sanitary latrines in rural areas is the most slow activity as no more than 33% of village homes have some kind of sanitary latrines. School latrine programme has not met with much success. Right to Education forum shows that 40% of schools in India lack separate toilets for girls. Sanitary latrines have been installed by some well to do in the villages, but in general these are not valued by the families and community. Thus, whatever is taught in school gets diminished at home and in the village as the practice of indiscriminate human excreta disposal is widespread through open defecation and environments become unfriendly or filthy leading to wide spread worm infestation and infection.

Tree plantation drive has been quite vigorous in schools and this activity has added values in the lives of children for environmental protection by planting more trees. Trees are used for shade and to ward off sun and heat apart from other advantages. Cleanliness drives are part and parcel of the socially useful and productive work. School building should be simple and safe, attractive and sanitary. In selecting the location of a school, consideration should be given to sufficiency of space for buildings and playgrounds, availability of safe water supply, possibility of drainage and sanitation.

In rural areas, the school buildings are mostly constructed by village Panchayats (PRI), these are simple, constructed with local material, but are ill-planned. Furniture is mostly not available. Most private school buildings have come-up now on the outskirts of villages and it has been attracting lot of children and parents prefer to get their children enrolled in these schools.

The situation of urban area is much better in terms of buildings, water supply and sanitation. There is now tendency to set-up schools outside crowded urban localities to the country side. Design of school buildings and furniture in schools prevents postural defects and improves visual acuity.

Periodic Health Check-ups or Screening Including Oral Health and Remedial Measures

5

The system of community health centres and primary health centres and subcentres hold the responsibility of school health check-ups. The health check-ups are undertaken for primary school children (6–11 years). Millions of health check-ups were done in July, 1996 on the directive and desire of Hon'ble Prime Minister of India by involving paramedical workers.[13] Health check-ups are mostly perfunctory as there is no follow-up for correction of defects or treatment of illnesses detected. The common diseases/defects, deficiencies, delayed millstones detected during these check-ups are managed by ensuring appropriate referral support of District Early Intervention Centre (DEIC) community health centre or primary health centre. Ideally there should be one-day clinic for school health services at CHC or PHC or at the district. The referral support should be established for correction of refractive errors, treatment and prevention of caries, atraumatic restorative techniques for dental problems, deworming and treatment of other defects. At the school level, teachers have some funds in primary schools earmarked for purchase of medicine kit to manage minor injuries and minor illnesses.

The ophthalmic assistants posted at PHCs ensure some kind of regular refraction to detect refractive errors and correction of vision by glasses, but this is not adequate. School teachers can use 6/9 optotype to categorize the children with refractive errors to—normal or abnormal. Parents are seldom involved in these check-ups.

Teachers themselves have the ability to identify the children with physical defects. Rapid screening by teacher helps in identification of children with defects/disease or children who lag behind, which can be confirmed by doctors to save time. Focused attention can be given to these children for early treatment to limit the disability. Parents must be involved in the health check-up exercise.

The leading causes of morbidity in rural school children were malnutrition (underweight and anaemia), Obesity, oro-dental problems, refractive errors, skin diseases (Pyoderma ringworm, scabies and dermatitis), worm infestation, ear, nose and throat problem and postural defects and injuries besides learning disorders.

A total of 13,89,873 school children were examined in Haryana in Dec. 2003 of which 2,71,737 (19.5%) were found defective for one problem or another. The spectrum of health problems among these defective children included:

i Micronutrient deficiency disorders (anaemia, night blindness and stomatitis) 91,728 (33.8%).

ii Problems of orodental hygiene (caries, pyorrhoea): 77,732 (28.7%).

iii Eye problems (defective vision, squint and others) 29,487 (10.87%).

iv Skin problems (scabies, ringworm and others) 24493 (9.03%).

v Worm infestation (roundworm, threadworm and others): 14,640 (5.4%).

vi ENT problems (tonsils, nasal voice, defective hearing, and others): 13,852 (5.1%).

vii Postural defects: 414 (0.15%) (Fig. 5.3).

viii Behavioural problems and others 19,391 (7.0%).

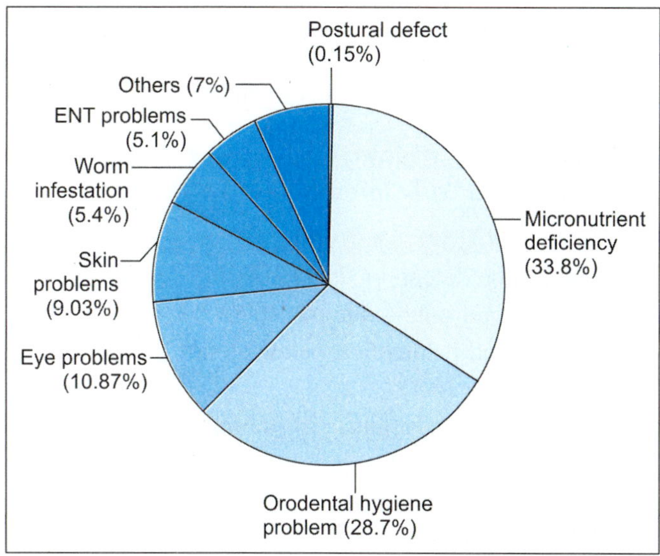

Fig. 5.3: Diseases, deficiency and defects in school children

A massive school health campaign (*Indira Bal Swasthya Yojna*) was lauched in Haryana in 2010–11 covering nearly 11 lakh children between 6 and 12 years, over 9 lakh of 0–6 years children and over 10 lakh of 12–18 years children. Major problems identified in 6–12 years children consisted of anaemia (57%), oro-dental problems (10.3%), respiratory and abdominal problems (9.5%), clinical signs of malnutrition (5.1%), skin problems (1.8%), impairments in 1.5% (visual impairment 1.2%, hearing orthopedic and mental retardation 0.3%) and other problems 14.8%. The spectrum and magnitude of problems has not much changed between 1996 and 2010.

Health check-ups including oral health check-ups without action are useless and meaningless. Health check-ups without parents are also meaningless. Some urban private schools offer regular check-up and ensure follow-up activities and there is regular visit of school medical officer. In government set-up, the health check-ups are done just in isolation. Several states have now adopted policy for free treatment of all children.

Periodicity

Complete health check-ups at school entry and after completing primary school education are essential. Annual health examination of all primary schools may not be feasible.

Records of Health Check-ups

The records of health check-ups for each student must be maintained by the school teachers. This helps them to contact parents and to ensure follow-up actions. Actions necessary on the part of school teachers must be ensured and documented as part of school health activities and records. These records help the medical officer to verify the improvement after treatment and monitoring the progress of the condition. Standard Health cards have been developed by many states.

School Immunization Programme

The schedule of school immunization consists of:

- DPT at school entry to children aged 5 years.
- TT at 10 years of age.
- TT at 16 years of age.
- JE vaccine in selected areas: Japanese encephalitis is endemic in some areas. Children in age group 1–15 years of age are being targeted for JE vaccine. Single dose of 0.5 ml is given by subcutaneous route.

The primary health centres and urban health set-up ensure regular coverage of DPT and TT immunization covering children who are 5 years, 10 and 16 years. Children who are out of school remains a problem in the programme. These children can be covered by involving ICDS system to cover adolescent girls also by involving nonformal education instructors or involving NGOs. Educating school children and teachers on vaccine preventable disease is essential. Teachers and parents must be informed well before taking up immunization activities in schools. Proper records must be maintained at school to avoid unnecessary repetition and to ensure adequate coverage. In due course of time, other vaccines, such as typhoid vaccine and some other vaccines (Measles and Rubella) may be introduced in the programme after assessing their needs on epidemiological basis. Measles catch up campaign has been launched to cover 9 months to 10 years children in seventeen states.

Mass-Deworming and IFA Supplements for Children and Adolescents (One Year to 19 Years)

Directly observed therapy with one chewable tablet of Albendazole 400 mg is being administered to children and adolescents on one particular day once every 6 months. National Deworming Day was observed on 10th Feb 2015–2016 in the country and mass deworming was done in schools. 270 million children were covered. Iron and folic acid tablets are given to each child once a weak under supervision under the National Programme.[14] Indira Bal Swasthya Yojna was merged with *Rashtriya Bal Swasthya Karyakram* in the year 2013 February[15] which is much more comprehensive.

Capacity Building for Health Screening

Since the role of school teachers is pivotal, their training and continuing education must be pursued with vigour and concern. The basic training programme of teachers covers most of the area of child learning, the teachers are provided in-service training for school health activities. The in-service training of primary school teachers is done by medical officers and senior medical officers of primary health centres and CHCs respectively. At times, joint training of teachers, *Mahila Swasthya Sangh* members, Panchayat members, health workers, Anganwadi workers and traditional birth attendants has been done at ground level. The purpose of their training is to motivate school teachers to play their effective and assigned role and responsibility of ensuring good health and clean environments conducive for education/learning for human resource development. Besides short-term training, the medical officer and health workers maintain regular contact with teachers for school health activities.[15–16] At least one teacher from each school has been trained as nodal teacher for programme of health screening, education and remedial actions and follow-up. Gradually all teachers would be trained and they will maintain class-wise records. Periodical training of medical officers, nurses and paramedical workers for 1–3 days is being undertaken.

Adolescent Health

Adolescent health programme is a component of reproductive and child health (RCH). The department of family welfare has supported setting up of adolescent friendly health clinics (AFHC) in selected PHCs, CHCs and hospitals/medical colleges of state on pilot basis. Self-learning modules for adolescents have been produced by Ministry of Youth Affairs and Sports. NSS units and *Nehru Yuva Kendras Sangathan* have been involved in imparting training on life skills. Good school health programme can reach many of the adolescents in the country.[17–19]

Other National Health Programmes in School Health

District Mental Health Programme (DMHP) has now incorporated school mental health services like life skills education in schools and counseling services. Similarly, under National Tobacco Control Programme and National Programme for deafness and National Programme on Control of Blindness and Anaemia, besides total sanitation campaign school children are being targeted.

RASHTRIYA BAL SWASTHYA KARYAKRAM (RBSK): Child Health Screening and Early Intervention Services under NRHM[15]. (Early Detection and Free Treatment)

Aim: RBSK is a new initiative aimed at screening over 270 million children from 0–18 years for 4 Ds–defects at birth, diseases, deficiencies and developmental delays including disabilities. Children diagnosed with illnesses shall receive follow-up including surgeries at tertiary level, free of cost under NRHM.

Objective: The objective of RBSK is to improve overall quality of life of children through early detection of defect, disease, deficiency, disability and developmental delays for prompt treatment and follow-up to reduce the severety and progression of these conditions to impairment.

Screening Programme: Screening will cover 30 identified health conditions for early detection, free treatment and management. These conditions include:

Identified Health Conditions for Child Health Screening and Early Intervention Services

Defects at Birth—6–7% births

1 Neural tube defect—4.7 per 1000
2 Down's syndrome—one per 1000
3 Cleft lip and palate/cleft palate alone
4 Talipes (club foot)
5 Developmental dysplasia of the hip
6 Congenital cataract
7 Congenital deafness
8 Congenital heart diseases
9 Retinopathy of prematurity

Deficiencies—39% Stunted

10 Anaemia especially severe anaemia
11 Vitamin A deficiency (bitot spot)
12 Vitamin D deficiency (rickets)
13 Severe acute malnutrition—3–6%
14 Goiter

Childhood Diseases

15 Skin conditions (scabies, fungal infection and eczema)
16 Otitis media
17 Rheumatic heart disease—1.5 per 1000
18 Reactive airway disease—4.75%
19 Convulsive disorders
20 Dental caries—50–60%

Developmental Delays and Disabilities

21 Vision impairment
22 Hearing impairment
23 Neuro-motor impairment
24 Motor delay
25 Cognitive delay
26 Language delay
27 Behaviour disorder (autism)
28 Learning disorder
29 Attention deficit hyperactivity disorder
30 Congenital hypothyroidism, sickle cell anaemia, beta thalassemia (optional)—1–17 per 1000.

Secreening Programme for Newborn

- Facility based newborn screening at public health facilities in institutional deliveries
- Community based newborn screening (0–6 weeks) at home by ASHAs for babies born at home

1 **For children 6 weeks to 6 years:** Anganwadi based screening by dedicated mobile health teams
2 **For children 6 years to 18 years:** Government and Government aided schools based screening by dedicated mobile health teams.

Frequency

The screening of children in the Anganwadi Centres would be conducted at least twice a year and at least once a year for school children to begin with.

Mobile Health Team Compositon

The mobile Health Team consists of four members–two doctors (AYUSH) one male and one female, one ANM/ staff nurse and one pharmacist/lab technician/ophthalmic assistant.

District Early Intervention Center (DEIC): An early intervention center has been established at District Hospital. The purpose of DEIC is to provide referral support, care and treatment free of cost to children detected with health conditions during health screening. The team at DEIC would consist of a paediatrician, a medical officer, a dental doctor, a physiotherapist, audiologist and speech therapist, psychologist, optometrist, social worker, lab technician, dental technician and a manager apart from a data entry operator. The manager carries out mapping of tertiary care facilities in Government institutions for ensuring adequate referral support.

At the **block level** health teams reach out to adolescents in classes VI–XII (adolescents) in government and government aided schools through RBSK.

It provides an important entry point for this team to engage with adolescents on a range of relevant health issues. These can include responding to common sexual and reproductive health queries and concerns, identifying and addressing mental health conditions, such as depression, healthy lifestyles practices, such as good foods and nutrition, physical activity, avoiding substance misuse (alcohol, tobacco, gutka among the most common ones). The visit of the block team is an opportunity to discuss the IFA supplementation—its benefits and necessity to maintain compliance with recommended dosages and weekly schedule; and informing children about the dietary sources of iron and calcium + dietary diversification.

REFERENCES

1 GOI. Final Report of school health committee. New Delhi: GOI; 1961.

2 Central Health Education Bureau. Intensive health education for primary school children (partners in primary health care)—guidelines for implementation. New Delhi: DGHS, MOH and FW; 1989.

3 GOI. National Health policy, 2002. New Delhi: MOH and FW, GOI; 2002.

4 GOI. National policy on education. New Delhi: Ministry of HRD, GOI; 1986.

5 GOI. National health policy 1983. New Delhi: MOH and FW GOI; 1983.

6 Planning Commission. Tenth Five-Year Plan. New Delhi: GOI; 2002.

7 Lal S. Health and development of school children. Ind J Comm Med 1998; 23(1): 3–6.

8 Lal S. Learning values and promotion of health in rural primary schools. Ind J Comm Med 2001; 26(1): 3–7.

9 Barbara A. Education for all. Mother and Children. American Public Health Association Bulletin on infant feeding and maternal nutrition 1990; 9(2).

10 NCERT. The curriculum guide on nutrition; health education and environmental sanitation in primary schools. New Delhi: NCERT; 1976.

11 UNICEF. Rights and opportunities—The situation of children and women in India. New Delhi: UNICEF India Country Office; 1998.

12 GOI. Annual report 1991–92. New Delhi: MOH and FW, GOI; 1992.

13 GOI. Special health check-ups for primary school children. Manual for health workers and school teachers. New Delhi: MCH division department of health and family welfare; 1996.

14 Government of Haryana. Director general of Health services of Haryana. Mass deworming of Primary School Children No 41/37-III E-07/310-49 Dated 30.1.2007. Panchkula.

15 *Rashtriya Bal Swasthya Karyakram*. Child Health Screening and Early Interventions Services under NRHM: MOH and FW GOI; 2013

16 GOI. A commitment to the child. New Delhi: Department of women and child development. GOI; 1992.

17 GOI. Health manpower planning, production and management report of expert committee. New Delhi: MOH and FW, GOI; 1987.

18 GOI. Draft RCH II and Family Planning Program Implementation Plan (PIP). New Delhi: MOH and FW, GOI; 2004.

19 GOI. School Health Proramme. MOH and FW, Govt of India.

ADOLESCENT HEALTH

WHO has defined adolescents as persons in the 10–19 years age group, while "Youth" has been defined as the 15–24 years age group. "Young people" is a combination of these two overlapping groups covering the range of 10–24 years.[1] Healthy adolescence is the cherished goal.

This phase of life cycle is marked by special characters which include:

- Rapid physical growth and development
- Physical social and psychological maturity.
- Sexual maturity and onset of sexual activity.
- Beginning of menstrual cycle in girls and onset of reproduction cycle.

- Experimentation.
- Development of adult mental processes and adult identity (want to establish their own identity).
- Transition from total socioeconomic dependence to relative independence.
- Underserved population group.

Demography

Adolescents between 10 and 19 years of age account for nearly one-fifth of the world's population. Adolescents constitute 20% of the total population in India. There are approximately 253 million adolescents in India in the age group 10–19 (2011). The sex ratio of adolescent girls in 10–19 age group has declined from 897 in 1981 to 880 in 2011. Female comprise almost 47% and males 53% of the total adolescent population.

Main Stages

1. Early adolescence (10–14 years) characterized by rapid growth (growth spurt) and development of secondary sexual characters.
2. Middle adolescence (15–17 years) striving for independence and identity and relationship with peers and opposite sex and experimentation.
3. Late adolescence (18–19 years) almost an adult.[1]

Puberty

Girls begin to show pubertal changes earlier than boys. Reproductive organs start maturing during puberty, human beings are able to reproduce after puberty. At puberty, the girls begin to ovulate and menstruate and boys begin to produce sperms and ejaculate.

In boys, testosterone hormone is responsible for hair growth on pubis and face, deep voice, growth of penis and testes and production of semen. In girls oestrogen hormone is responsible for development of breasts, pubic hair, rounding of hips and menstruation.[2] There are many stigmas, myths, beliefs and unhygienic practices during menstruation.

Adolescent Health

This period is the most healthiest period of life in one's life cycle. The morbidity and mortality is least, however during this period the adolescents gain up to 50% of their adult weight and 50% of their adult skeletal mass.

Health needs of the adolescents are tremendous and these have seldom been met as there is no comprehensive organized programme for adolescent health in India.

Needs of Adolescents

1. Their prime need is correct and complete information, on health, menstruation and its hygiene, right age of marriage, reproduction, nutrition, growth and development, puberty, sexuality and HIV/AIDS, STDs/STI, safe sex, contraception and substance misuse.
2. Adequate diet for growth and development.
3. Healthy lifestyles: Physical activity and no drugs.
4. Education and health.
5. Supportive environments.
6. Counselling.

Major Interventions/Strategies for Adolescents

Knowledge and information of adolescents tend to be poor on several issues mentioned above or they have erroneous impressions, myths and misconceptions related to sexual and reproductive health. Moreover, they tend to collect half baked knowledge from their peers, which is seldom factual or scientific.

Improve Nutrition

1. *Anaemia malnutrition and obesity:* Over 89% of girls are anaemic and one-third of boys and girls have chronic energy malnutrition. Poor nutrition is cited as an important cause of delay in onset of puberty in Indian adolescents. Due to poor dietary intakes, and discrimination of girls, these girls tend to develop as short-statured females with low body weights and produce low birth weight babies. These adolescents stand to the risk of diabetes, cardio-vascular diseases and cancer in later life.

***Oral health problems like*:** Caries teeth due to cariogenic foods, junk foods and unhealthy lifestyles.

2. *Adolescent Reproductive and Sexual Health (ARSH):*

a. *Early marriages:* Over 30% of girls get married below the legal age of marriage (18 years) when their pelvises are small, uterus and cervix is immature, body weight is less. The UNICEF State of World Children Report 2013 reveals 30% of adolescent girls get married in the 15–18 age group. The girls enter into early reproduction and it becomes a story of too early, too quick and too many children apart from poor outcome of teenage pregnancy in terms of low birth weight babies or these teen agers may seek illegal abortions.

b. *Reduce teenage pregnancies:* Teenage pregnancies in adolescents are risky pregnancies and over 16–19% of total pregnancies are teenage pregnancies. This threatens the life of pregnant teenage and leads to increased maternal mortality (NFHS-3). Nearly 27 percent of adolescents have unmet need for contraception. Adolescent fertility rates (AFR), i.e. number of birth per 1000 women aged 15–19 is 39 which is highest for India in South Asia.

c. *Unwanted pregnancies and illegal abortions:* Teenage pregnancies may be unwanted or may occur in unmarried girls and consequently illegal abortions are sought which may be life-threatening. Hence provide comprehensive abortion care services.

d. *STIs and STDs:* Because of early initiation of sexual activity (premarital sex) without use of condoms the adolescents are exposed to the risk of acquiring and transmission of STIs including HIV. Contraceptive acceptance (condom use) is poor in adolescents or they are reluctant to use it.

e. *HIV/AIDS:* 40% of new HIV infections occur in young people in age group 15–24, because of unsafe/unprotected sex and early sexual initiation and premarital sexual relationships. Sexual abuse of boys and girls like rape, trafficking for prostitution, and homosexuality are quite frequent.

3. *Conditions (risk factors) for noncommunicable diseases (NCD):* Problem of obesity is emerging in urban adolescents because of unhealthy eating, eating junk foods and fast-foods as also physical inactivity. One-fifth (20%) of Indian children above the age of eight are obese and overweight as per new national survey on physical fitness. One in ten adolescents and young adult in Delhi is clinically obese and 5% have high blood pressure because over 80% of them were physically inactive.

4. *Prevent substance misuse:* Adolescents start experimenting with their lives and indulge in unhealthy lifestyles like tobacco use, alcohol use and abuse of drugs apart from premarital sex, under the influence of peer pressure. Self-awareness, critical thinking, decision-making, effective communication, coping with stress are some of the life skills required to remain away from drugs and learning to say "No" to drugs/smoking and alcohol. National tobacco control programme focuses on adolescents in schools and colleges.

5. *Prevention of Injuries and Violence:* Unintentional injuries (accidents, sports injuries) and intentional injuries (suicide and homicide) are very common causes of adolescent morbidity and mortality. Adolescents are involved in fatal road traffic accidents and the incidence of trauma is much higher because of high speed driving and driving without licence and risky driving, non-use of helmets and violation of safety rules and mixing driving with alcohol.

6. *Enhance Mental Health:* Significant proportion of adolescents have behavioural problems–suicidal tendencies, anxiety, indulging in crime and violence, sexual abuse, pre-marital sex and drug abuse. District mental health programme addresses these needs through school and college counselling services apart from life skills training. Life skills are a vehicle for health and mental health promotion and lay the foundation for good health and mental well-being-adolescent wellness.

7. *School dropouts:* Many of the girls and boys are "dropouts" from schools and only one-third continue up to matric and beyond due to economic compulsions.

SOCIAL FACTORS IN ADOLESCENT HEALTH AND DEVELOPMENT—CASE STUDY

Parents perceptions, awareness attitudes and ambition about adolescents in respect of menstruation, ideal age of marriage, health risks associated with early marriage and childbirth and food distribution within family are critical. Many parents want their sons to study as long as they desire but for daughter 9th or 10th grade is considered enough and only 2–6% of rural mothers desired their daughters to have graduation and postgraduation. Many boys and girls of economically weaker sections are school dropouts or school enrolment is low and they start working for family or outside family and literacy levels tend to be low and information on health and development very poor. Most common reason for not favouring higher education for girls included; economic considerations/compulsions, using girls for household and economic activities and prefer to marry them at young age and no facility for higher education in the same village. While most daughters (96%) were found to communicate with their mothers but only 15% of mothers talked to their daughters on the subject of menstrual cycle, as they felt shy to talk on this subject or felt that their daughters were too young to be talked about on this issue. "Talking about menstruation is still a taboo" Opinion of nutritious food distribution within family did not find favour for girls, which corroborated with real practice as well. Though 50–60% of mothers favoured marriage of their daughters above the age of 18 but in practice over 97% of marriages occurred below the age of 18, it was a paradox.[3] Health seeking behaviour for adolescents was in favour of boys and girls were neglected.

NATIONAL PROGRAMMES AND POLICY FOR ADOLESCENT HEALTH AND DEVELOPMENT

There are many programmes, which focus on the needs of adolescents but these programmes are not comprehensive.

Ministry of Youth Affairs and Sports (MOYAS)

MOYAS has been designated as nodal ministry for adolescent related interventions. Under the National Youth Policy-2003, adolescents feature as a special group. The ministry is implementing the adolesscent health and development project in collaboration with UNFPA, which focuses on:

- Advocacy on adolescent issues, with focus on reproductive and sexual health and life skills education.
- Strengthening of *Nehru Yuva Kendra Sangathan* (NYKS).
- National Service Scheme (NSS) and Rajiv Gandhi National Institute of Youth Development and NGOs for implementing adolescent related programmes.[4]

The MOYAS has developed Facilitator's Manual on Adolescent Health and Development in the year 2006 and have undertaken training of teachers and distributed learning resource material in the form of 12 modules to various NSS units, NYKS, parents, community and students. This would focus on core life skills for adolescent health and development. "Life skills are the abilities for adaptive and positive behaviour that enables individuals to deal effectively with the demands and challenges of everyday life" (WHO). Core life skills—self-awareness, critical thinking, decision-making, effective communication, coping with stress, empathy, creative thinking, problem-solving, interpersonal relationship and coping with emotions. These modules will impart need-based information to adolescent for developing balanced personality, healthy lifestyles and appropriate behaviours in the long run. The modular information is imparted to adolescents through NSS units, NYKS, peer groups and parents.

RASHTRIYA KISHOR SWASTHYA KARYAKRAM (RKSK)[5, 6]

Adolescent reproductive and sexual health (ARSH) programme has been expanded from limited reproductive and sexual health to wider areas under Rashtriya Kishor Swasthya Karyakram (RKSK). There is paradigm shift now from clinic based services to promotion and prevention and reaching adolescents in their own environments such as **schools** and **communities**.

RKSK was launched in the year 2014. The new adolescent health (AH) strategy focuses on universal coverage of all adolescents, i.e. males and females, urban and rural, in schools and out of schools, married and unmarried and vulnerables and underserved. 7Cs: These seven critical components are: Coverage, content, communities, clinics, counselling, communication and convergence. Major seven strategic priorities include:

1. Nutrition
2. Adolescent Reproductive and Sexual Health (ARSH)
3. Noncommunicable diseases (healthy lifestyles)
4. Prevention of substance misuse
5. Prevention of injuries and violence
6. Exhance mental health
7. School dropouts

Key Interventions/Strategies

A. Community based interventions:
   - Peer Education (PE)
   - Quarterly Adolescent Health Day (AHD)
   - Weekly Iron and Folic acid Supplementation (WIFS)
   - Menstrual Hygiene Scheme (MHS)

B. Facility based interventions:
   - Strengthening Adolescent Friendly Health Clinics (AFHCs)

C. Convergence—Inter and intrasectoral convergence

D. Social and behaviour change communication with focus on interpersonal communication:

A. Community Based Interventions

Peer Education (PE)

Information and Education for Health Promotion: The prime need of adolescents is information and skill to use the information. Standard information package for adolescents have been prepared and provided in peer education kits (PEK). Peer education model is most successful.

The PE programme aims to ensure that adolescents benefit from regular and sustained peer education covering nutrition, reproductive and sexual health, risk factors for non communicable diseases, substance misuse, injuries and violence, and mental health. This is expected to improve life skills, knowledge and aptitude of adolescents.

Key Features of PE

PE is adolescent to adolescent programme. 2 male and 2 female peer educators selected in every village or per 1000 population or urban ward (slum areas). Each male and female PE form a group of 15–20 boys and girls respectively from their community and conduct weekly one to two hour participatory sessions using peer education kits which include standard books having a curriculum for PE sessions and games.

- PE ensures that adolescents attend the regular sessions and participate in Adolescent Health Day (AHD)
- Peer educators refer adolescents to Adolescent Friendly Health Clinics (AFHCs)
- PE constitute adolescent health club at sub-centre level under the overall guidance of health workers male and female; these clubs meet once a month to discuss issues of adolescents and get support from subcentres
- Peer educators are expected to maintain a diary to record activities of various sessions for review and reports.

Adolescent Health Day (AHD)

AHD is to be organized in every village/ward once every quarter on a convenient day (preferably on sunday) following the Village Health and Nutrition Day (VHND); in SABLA districts, this day should coincide with existing Kishori Diwas. On this day apart from adolescents, school teachers, parents and members of PRI, ASHAs, AWWs, Medical officer incharge and counsellors also participate. On this day health check ups of all adolescents is done and required services provided (imformation, and commodities–IFA, sanitary napkins, albendazole, anti-spasmodic tablets, contraceptives and referral services).

National Iron + Initiative

a. **The weekly iron and folic acid supplementation (WIFS):** Programme covers adolescents enrolled in class VI to XII of government, government aided and municipal schools as well as out of school girl's. The programme envisages:
   - Supervised administration of weekly IFA supplements of 100 mg elemental iron and 500 mcg folic acid.
   - Screening of target groups for moderate and severe anaemia and referral to an appropriate health facility.

- Biannual deworming (Albendazole 400 mg).
- Information and counselling for improving dietary intake and preventive actions for intestinal worm infestation.

Goal: To reduce anaemia in adolescent boys and girls from current level of 56% to 30% by 2017.

b. Scheme for Promotion of Menstrual Hygiene: Among adolescent girls (10–19 years) in rural India. The scheme aims to increase awareness among adolescent girls on Menstrual Hygiene, increase access to and use of high quality sanitary napkins to adolescent girls in rural areas and ensure safe dispossal of sanitary napkins in an environment friendly manner. Under the scheme sanitary napkins (NRHM brand "Free days") are being sold to adolescent girls at ₹ 6 for a pack of 6 napkins in the village by the ASHA worker.

B. Facility Based Interventions

Adolescent Friendly Health Clinics (AFHCs)

The aim of AFHCs is to provide information, clinical and counselling services to adolescents through existing health system. Both the Peer Education Programme and AHD should lead to referrals to AFHCs which would provide comprehensive services. AFHCs have been set up at the following levels of three-tier existing health care delivery system:

Level 1 Subcentre: Walk in services at sub-health centre by multipurpose health workers who provide basic package of promotive, preventive and curative services-screening for anaemia, obesity, blood pressure, IFA tablets, contraceptives and counselling and sanitary napkins besides albendazole tablets.

Level 2: Weekly dedicated AFHC at primary health centre by Medical officer and ANMs.

Level 3: Daily AFHC at Community Health Centre/District Hospital/Sub-district Hospital/Medical College by Medical Officers/Specialists and Counsellors (male and female and other support staff). Additional manpower in terms of Dedicated Medical officers, Dedicated counsellors, Staff nurses have been provided for services at level 3.

Services at AFHCs

Information (IEC and Interpersonal Communication): Communication is key component of adolescent health. Counselling on nutrition, puberty related concerns, menstrual disorders, personal hygiene, menstrual hygiene, use of sanitary napkins, use of contraceptives, abortion, sexual concerns, depression, sexual abuse, gender violence, substance misuse and promoting healthy behaviours to prevent noncommunicable diseases.

Clinical/Curative Services: Screening for obesity, anaemia, blood pressure, diabetes, antenatal care for pregnant adolescents, management of menstrual disorders, iron deficiency anaemia, management of common adolescent health problems: sexual and reproductive health issues (RTI, STIs, HIV/AIDS, unwanted pregnancy), depression/anxiety/low self-esteem and substance abuse. Make link with other services, such as ICTC, deaddiction centres, ICDS, School education and social workers.

Commodities: Provision of sanitary napkins, contraceptives, weekly iron and folic acid supplementation, albendazole and other medicines as also pregrancy testing kits.

C. Intersectoral Coordination/Convergence

- Intersectoral—Within health and family welfare Reproductive and Child Health (RCH), *Rashtrya Bal Swasthya Karyakram*, National tobacco control, National Mental Health, Noncommunicable diseases, National HIV and Aids control programme.
- Intrasectoral convergence with other departments/ schemes—women and child development (ICDS, *Kishori Shakti Yojna*, Human Resource Development, Adolescent Education Programme, Mid-day-meal and Youth Affairs and Sports).

D. Communication Strategy

Adolescent health and development is primarily a communication strategy to ensure that all adolescents have access to information and counselling services on 6 priority areas. *National communication strategy* for *adolescents'* has been developed in collaboration with UNICEF reproductive health. The strategic framework for health communication among adolescents, which will facilitate responsible behaviour, includes increasing knowledge and awareness on reproductive health issues and delayed age of marriage. The key tenets of the strategy for behaviour change are interpersonal communication, advocacy interventions by use of mass media, decentralization of IEC to states and districts, increased involvement of NGOs and private sector and capacity building at all the levels.

Adolescents require information and skills. Access to age and sex appropriate information and health and counseling services is necessary, but information alone is not sufficient. In addition to information they need life skills to use the information. GATHER approach for counseling helps adolescents to practice decision they make.[10–13]

School Health Programme

It is a major programme. More than half of the adolescents are in schools and can be reached for health, nutrition and population education programmes. The major component is health check-up, tetanus toxoid at age 10 and tetanus toxoid at age 16 to prevent tetanus. Immunization for hepatitis B and Rubella if MMR not given in childhood. Apart from this, adolescents (11–18 years) now are being targeted for iron and folic acid tablets under national anaemia control programme through reproductive and child health programme. Reaching health information and information on reproduction, sexual behaviour and population education, remain a poor programme as the school health activities are not the priority as a programme. Most of the information on health, nutrition and reproduction is built into the curriculum but it is not disseminated by teachers in practical or action terms. Teachers training is critical to reach adolescents in the school. A good school health programme could be rich source of information to adolescents for actions and developing *healthy lifestyles.*

For prevention and control of noncommunicable diseases.

National HIV/AIDS Control Programme (NACP)

Adolescent Education Programme is key intervention to build the skills of young people and help them to cope with negative peer pressure, develop positive behaviour, improve sexual health and prevent HIV infections under the programme "sixteen hours" sessions are scheduled during the academic sessions in classes IX and XI. NACP has launched massive Adolescent Health Education Programme on life skills education covering 112000 high schools. National AIDS control programme in India has produced a training package titled "AIDS education in schools". Some elementary aspects of HIV/AIDS have been included in the NCERT textbooks. The programme reached mainly to urban schools, rural schools were not covered. The teachers shy away from talking sexuality and reproduction in view of traditions and cultural sensitivity of society. It brought out that teachers training and advocacy among parents are of crucial importance.

University Talk AIDS Programme was launched way back in 1991 for creating awareness on HIV/AIDS among students and youth in schools, colleges and universities. 3.5 million students have been made aware about AIDS and 4044 institutions have been covered. This massive programme built favourable attitudes for voluntary blood donation as also prevention against AIDS. The credit goes to the department of Youth Affairs and Sports, Ministry of Human Resource Development and National Service Scheme (NSS). The NSS has brought out manual in 7 languages for students on AIDS and sexuality to serve as learning resource material. The critical comments on AIDS education in schools and colleges are that the programme focuses on urban youths and spread effect of AIDS knowledge through youths was limited to colleges and schools only.

Evaluation surveys in many parts of the country revealed different story altogether, as the major sources of information to youth and adult population on the issues of HIV/AIDS were television and radio as also print media. Health workers were mentioned as sources of knowledge only by 25% of young people. Teachers were not at all mentioned as source of knowledge and students' peers were seldom mentioned as source of information.

Reaching Out of School Adolescent Girls

Integrated child development services (ICDS) in 1991–92 launched programme for adolescent girls (AG) and this programme has now expanded to cover 2000 projects, and it has been given a new name *Kishori Shakti Yojna* (KSY), a new initiative started in the year 2000 AD. KSY has been now extended to cover all ICDS projects. The objectives of the scheme are as follows:[7–9]

1 To improve the nutritional and health status of girls in the age group 11–18 years.
2 To provide the required literacy and numeracy skills through the nonformal stream of education, to stimulate a desire for more social exposure and knowledge and help them improve their decision-making capabilities.
3 To train and equip the adolescent girls to improve/upgrade home-based and vocational skills.
4 To promote awareness of health, hygiene, nutrition and family welfare, home management and child care, and to motivate them to marry after attaining 18 years and if possible, even later.
5 To gain a better understanding of their environment-related social issues and the impact on their lives.
6 To encourage adolescent girls to initiate various activities to be productive and useful members of the society.

Adolescent Girls (AG) Schemes

There are two schemes:

Scheme-I: Girl to girl approach

Scheme-II: *Balika Mandal.*

Beneficiaries

Scheme I: Girl to Girl Approach

This has been designed for AG in the age group 11–15 years belonging to families with income level below ₹ 6400/- per annum and school dropouts in urban and in the rural areas.

Three girls are selected per Anganwadi and attached to the local Anaganwadi centre for 6 months duration for learning and training. These girls act as resource person for other girls in their neighbourhood.

Interventions

The focal point of services is an Anganwadi. These girls are provided supplementary nutrition equivalent to the entitlement of pregnant/lactating women six days a week.

Simple and practical messages are provided on preventive health, hygiene, nutrition, working of Anganwadi centres and family life education. This is provided through initial three days training programme, followed by six continuing education sessions of one day each, every month. This exercise is aimed at building confidence and encouraging adolescent girls to become active participants in the development process. Anganwadi workers act as role models for these girls.

Scheme II: Balika Mandal

All eligible girls in the age bracket 11–18 years irrespective of income levels of the family are eligible to receive assistance in this scheme, preference is given to 11–15 years age group. In each community development block and urban ICDS areas 10% of total Anganwadi centres are selected to serve as *Balika Mandals*. 20 girls in the age bracket 11–18 are identified. These, girls are enrolled for a period of 6 months in *Balika Mandal*. Thus in a year each *Balika Mandal* will reach out to 40 adolescent girls.

Interventions

- These girls are provided supplementary nutrition for 6 days in a week to provide 600 calories and 18–20 g of protein.
- Activities cover the areas of personal hygiene, environmental sanitation, nutrition, home nursing, first aid, communicable diseases, vaccine preventable diseases, family life, child care and development and the impact of constitutional rights on the quality of life.
- Participate in creative activities and recreation. Learning through sharing of experiences and discussions on issues that affect their lives.
- Training in vocational skills/agro-based skills/ household related appropriate technology.

The Anganwadi worker is regular honorary instructor for the *Balika Mandal* and provides general education and literacy to adolescent girls. She is also responsible for overseeing the work related to skills improvement/ upgradation.

Kishori Shakti Yojna (KSY) has much wider scope than the earlier AG scheme and involves the entire network of Government of state/union territory and district as well as supportive skills of local self-Government.

Training

Under the AG scheme, a 9-days training programme has been designed for selected girls, 3 days training period is spent at circle headquarter and remaining 6 days are devoted for continuing education, spread over to 6 months. The training is conducted by supervisors. There are 10 themes for training—environmental sanitation, nutrition, home nursing, first aid, family life education, child development, legal rights of women, home economics, positive attitudes and motivation.

THE RAJIV GANDHI SCHEME FOR EMPOWERMENT OF ADOLESCENT GIRLS (RGSEAG)—SABLA

The ministry of Women and Child Development Government of India, in the year 2000 launched *Kishori Shakti Yojna* (KSY) Scheme. Thereafter, the Nutrition Programme for Adolescent Girls (NPAG) was initiated as a pilot project in the year 2002–03 in 51 identified districts across the country to address the problem of undernutrition among AGs. Under this programme, 6 kg of free food grain per beneficiary per month was given to undernourished girls. Though both these schemes have influenced the lives of AGs to an extent, but have not shown the desired impact. Therefore a new comprehensive scheme, called Rajiv Gandhi Scheme for Empowerment of Adolescent Girls or SABLA, merging the erstwhile KSY and NPAG schemes has been formulated to address the multidimensional problem of AGs. SABLA has been implemented in 200 selected districts replacing KSY and NPAG, in rest of districts KSY continues as before. Districts have been chosen on the basis of high dropout rate of AGs from school-over 50%, low female literacy rate, marriage of girls before the age of 18 years (over 20%) and female work participation. The coverage of SABLA Scheme is likely to be expanded in near feature.

Objectives of SABLA

i To enable self development and empowerment of AGs.
ii To improve their nutrition and health status.
iii To generate awareness among AGs about health, hygiene, nutrition, Adolescent Reproductive and Sexual Health (ARSH) and family and child care.
iv To upgrade their home-based skills and vocational skills.
v Mainstreaming out of school AGs into formal/non-formal education.
vi To inform and guide them about existing public services, such as PHC, CHC, Bank, Police station, etc.

The scheme covers all out of school AGs in the age group of 11–18 years in selected 200 districts on pilot basis. The target group has been further sub-divided into two categories 11–14 and 14–18 years for age appropriate attention to components of ARSH and family matters.

Modalities of the Scheme

1 Formation of *Kishori Smooh* (KS): A Group, 15–25 out of school AGs from the village/area of AWW will be formed at the Anganwadi centre. The AGs will select three leaders of their choice for a year from within the KS. These selected girls will be called 'Sakhi' (one girl) and Sahelis (two girls). Each of three selected girls will have a term of four months as "Sakhi" on rotation basis. Thus, each KS will be headed by 'Sakhi' and Sahelis who will be imparted training and provided a training kit to guide and help KS in the area of: Health, Nutrition, Adolescent Reproductive and Sexual Health (ARSH) and Life Skills. Modular design of training has been adopted.

Time-Table: Planned activities for two hours per day for three days in a week at the Anganwadi centre or at any other convenient place. These sessions will be conducted by resource persons.

Services: For 11–14 years out of school girls and 14–18 years out of school and in school girls:

Nutrition component: Take home ration (THR) or hot cooked meal.

Other components for out of school adolescent girls (2–3 times a week) and in school girls (11–18 years).

a 11–18 years—IFA supplementation and nutrition and health education.
   - Health check-up and referral services
   - Counseling/guidance on family welfare, ARSH, child care practices.
   - Life skill education and accessing public services

b 16–18 years

Vocational training under national skill development Programme.

Kishori Divas: Once in three months on a fixed day. On this day the AWWs, with the help of health functionaries, including medical officer, ANMs, ASHAs, will mobilize AGs and their families especially mothers to assemble at Anganwadi to interact freely with ICDS. Village Health Nutrition and Sanitation Committee members will also be involved in the programme. General health check-up, nutrition and health education, counselling/behaviour change communication for promoting best practices among adolescents and family will be the prime focus.

Mixed group interaction for school going and out of school AGs would be held twice a month when schools are working and more frequently during school vacations (once a week).

The National Population Policy-2000, National Health Policy, 2002 identifies the adolescent girls as underserved group for priority intervention.

Issues of adolescent girls and boys need to be addressed separately, self-help groups in rural areas, NGOs and voluntary organizations apart from public sector can be most effective. These should strive for:

Registration of marriages and age of girls at marriage should become a routine record with subcentre to enforce the Child Marriage Restraint Act (1976) with a view to reduce the incidence of teenage pregnancies and preventing marriages of girls below the legally permissible age of 18.

The government of India agreed to the principle of compulsory registration of marriages, however, failure to get marriage registered will not invalidate marriage [Convention on elimination of all forms of discrimination against women (CEDAW)].[13]

Women development functionaries in rural areas like *Gram Sevikas, Mukhya Sevikas* should take the responsibility to organize adolescent groups along with *Mahila Mandals* to generate awareness among rural adolescents. Similar tasks can be entrusted to female volunteers of national service scheme in urban slums as also some adopted villages. *Mahila Swasthya Sanghs* (organized women groups) in rural areas could take up this onerous task and health workers female and Anganwadi workers could act as group animators.[14–17]

Different sectors like health and family welfare, women and child development, education, social welfare, human resource development, youth affair and sports and information and broadcasting do address one or the other component of adolescent needs but these tend to work in isolation. These programmes and efforts need to be integrated in terms of finances and other resources. Best way to integrate is through institutional mechanism of schools and nonformal system of education.

REFERENCES

1 UNFPA for UN system in India; Adolescents in India – A Profile. Sept. 2000 – Lodi Estate; New Delhi, India.
2 UNICEF. Adolecence – A time that matters. New York: UNICEF Division of Communication, United Nations; 2002.
3 Lal S. Mother's perception and ambitions about their daughters in rural areas. Ind J Comm Med 1992; 12(1): 22–8.
4 GOI. Facilitator's Mannual on Adolescent Health and Development Ministry of Youth Affairs and Sports (2006); GOI and UNFPA, New Delhi.
5 GOI. Implementation Guide on RCH II ARSH Strategy, for State and District Programme Managers, MOH and FW New, Delhi 2006–07.
6 GOI. Rashtriya Kishor Swasthya Karyakram (RKSK) operational framework, translating strategy into programme Adolescent Health Division, MOH and FW January 2014.
7 GOI. Reaching adolescent girls – *Kishori Shakti Yojna* and other initiatives. New Delhi: Department of Women and Child Development Ministry of HRD; 2002.
8 NIPCCD. Schemes for adolescent girls launched. NIPCCD Newsletter; 12: 4–6.
9 NIPCCD. Adolescent girls scheme – an evaluation. New Delhi: National Institute of Public Cooperation and Child Development; 2000.
10 GOI. Ministry of Women and Child Development. 'Rajiv Gandhi Scheme for empowerment of Adolescent Girls—SABLA. Implementation Guidelines' December 2010, New Delhi.
11 NIHFW. Reproductive and child health manual for health worker female – integrated skill training. New Delhi: MOH and FW, GOI; 2001.
12 Planning Commission. Ninth five-year plan 1997–2002 volume II–Thematic issues and sectoral programme. New Delhi: GOI; 1997.
13 Convention on the Elimination of all forms of Discrimination Against Women (CEDAW). Ratified by India on 25.6.93.
14 GOI. National Communication strategy for reproductive and child health project. New Delhi: MOH and FW GOI-2000.
15 NIPCCD. Programmes and functionaries reaching women Indian Women in development. NIPCCD Bulletin 1989; 2 (7).

16 International Institute of Population sciences/ORC Macro. National Family Health Survey II 1998–99. Mumbai: IIPS/ ORC Macro; 2002.

17 GOI. National Policy for empowerment of women 2001. New Delhi; Department of women and child development MOH and FW; 2001.

GENDER ISSUES AND WOMEN EMPOWERMENT

SUSTAINABLE DEVELOPMENT GOAL 5

- Achieve gender equality and empower all women and girls
- End all forms of discrimination, violence and harmful practices against women and girls.

What is gender? Gender is socially constructed by roles and responsibilities, attributes, behaviour and values, assigned to woman and man, boy and girl in a given culture and location by society. Gender is variable and can change from time to time and culture to culture. The way boys and girls socialize to be 'feminine' or 'masculine' is called gendering. Gender equality focuses on changes for both men and women. However, it is not sex, but gender that has far greater impact on women's health. Patriarchal (male dominance and authority) and wide spread discriminatory practices in the community like "Son Syndrome"—Son preferences, birth of a girl child is unwelcome, girl child unwanted, girl child as lesser child and liability, sex selective abortions, female infanticide, differential feeding practices, health seeking behaviour, depriving education to girls, getting them married at an early age, food distribution within family, "tripple burden"—work within home, outside home and child rearing, no control over resources and money, decision makers are men, violence against women (domestic violence, dowry deaths, honour killing, rape, trafficking of girls and women, sexual harassment, etc.), poor access to media, **stereotype** image of women in society have significant impact on women's health and health care system and are key determinant of ill health of women.

Gender and sex are taken as synonymous which is not true. Sex is determined biologically and sex identifies the biological differences between women and men and is genetically determined. Females have two X chromosomes and males have one X and one Y chromosome. Hence, spermatozoon (not the ovum) is the sex determinant. Females are always blamed for infertility and birth of girl child. Only a very small proportion of differences in roles assigned to men and women can be attributed to biological and physical differences based on sex. For example, pregnancy, childbirth and differences in physiology can be attributed to sex-related characteristics.

Gender equity is the process of being fair to both men and women. Equity leads to equality. Equality means that women and men enjoy the same status within the society. It does not mean that the men and women are the same, but rather that their similarities and differences are recognized and equally valued. Gender equality means that women and men experience equal conditions for realizing their full human rights and have the opportunity to contribute to and benefit from national, political and economic, social and cultural development.

In India, constitution not only grants equality to women, but also empowers State to adopt measures of positive discrimination in favour of women. From 5th plan onwards there has been marked shift in the approach to women's issues from welfare to development. Women development is the key issue for population stabilization and child health apart from their own health.

Gender roles are determined in the family and conditioned by the environments. It is important to understand how we learn to be boys or girls to become women and men, how we define masculine and faminine behaviour, how we are taught activities regarded as appropriate for our sex and the ways in which we relate to one another. These begin at the family level and in peers in schools. Most discrimination begins at family level and get widely adopted as practice at the community level.[1] There is strong son preference or "son syndrome" as male children are considered assets while female children are considered as liability. Sons are considered essential for old age economic and social security for parents, continuity of lineage and to perform last religious rites and for these reason all families pray; Oh God! *"Grant the birth of son here and daughter elsewhere*" Certain activities are exclusively done and performed by women and some are exclusively assigned to men. These activities needs to be looked critically as gender issues to be addressed on the basis of science and culture. However, it is not sex, but gender that has far greater impact on women's health. Patriarchal system—where male dominate in decision-making and authority, defines the life patterns and culture.

INEQUALITIES

Gender Development Index (GDI) in India

India ranks among the world's worst as far as gender gap index is concerned. The world economic forum has placed India at 114 position among 142 countries in its 2014 global gender gap index. Gender based disparity in the country have shown a decline over a period of ten years; The GDI scores estimated for India were 0.514 in 1996 and 0.590 in 2006 showing an increase of 0.076 points. Gender empowerment index increased from 0.416 in 1996 to 0.497 in 2006. UNDP Report of 2011 puts the value of gender equality HDI at 0.617. Health, Literacy and Standard of living that constitute GDI which is HDI also reflect increase over the decade.[1] Women are 48.46% of the total population against 51.54% of men in India (2011 census).

This shows demographic imbalance between women and men. This is further confirmed by declining sex ratio ever since 1901. Unfavourable sex ratio of 940 for female further confirms the low proportion of females. The sex ratio represents the low proportion of females.

The sex ratio represents the survival scene of women; it means lesser women survive as compared to men in India except in Kerala where women ratio is much more favourable. This is an indicator of low status of women in India.

Gender Biased Sex Selection

Adverse Child Sex Ratio: 0–6 Years Age Group

Gender biased sex selection is a discriminatory practice against girls that is a result of a complex web of socio-economic and cultural factors. The most dominant contributory factors seem to be preference for son, rapid fertility decline and access to technology and its misuse.

Adverse sex ratio is indicative of wide ranging gender discrimination in the country and is powerful indicator of social health of society.

The most disturbing finding of census 2011 is declining child sex ratio in almost all states and the only exception is honourable state of Kerala. Child sex ratio has come down from 927 in 2001 to 914 in 2011 and worst child sex ratio has been recorded in economically well to do states like Haryana, Punjab, Maharashtra and Gujarat. Haryana recorded child sex ratio of 820, while Punjab recorded 793. This is attributable to sex selective abortions (foeticides) through sex determination, as also to female infanticide in some states. It also unfolds the story of high mortality in girls during early childhood and sex selective sterilization and some faults in female count (it is negligible factor).[2]

Expectation of Life

India has made significant progress and added over 29 years to life expectancy. During the year 1951, life expectancy was just 37 years and during 2011 it has risen to 66 years for men and for female it is still higher at 67.7 years. The expectation of life for female has been rising steadily.

High Maternal Mortality

The maternal mortality ratio in India stays very high at 167 per hundred thousand live births. It is a reflection of high fertility and less care during and after delivery. High maternal mortality is an indicator of poor maternal health services.

Nutrition and Women

Women eat less and last of all in the family. Food distribution within the family is an important issue. The feeding practices for female children, adolescent girls are discriminatory and consequences are poor nutritional status of young girls. Over 58% of adolescent girls and pregnant women silently suffer from anaemia and half of children under-five are anaemic. Poor nutrition has intergenerational effects. Women who themselves are anaemic bear low birth weight babies and they themselves are at risk of dying once they become pregnant. Dietary practices for girls and women are unfavourable as compared to men.

Literacy

Women's education is critical for meeting the country's demographic and health goals. High level of women's education are consistently associated with lower fertility and infant mortality and with better nutrition and health of women and children. One of the significant result of census 2011 is increase in overall literacy to the extent of 74%. Literacy rate in men is better at 82.5% as compared to 65.46% in female. In some situations the female literacy may be much lower than average figure of 65.46%. Enrolment ratio, retention and continuation rate of schooling in female tends to be low and low literacy of girls and women is a discriminatory practice and significant inequality in the society. Girls are thought to be "Praya dhan" (someone else's property) hence investment in terms of education is low. Parents arrange early marriages of girls and girls are used as caregivers to their young brothers or sisters or share the workload in home with the mother and thus are deprived of schooling. Proportion of girls who attained secondary education was 23.6% as against 50.4% for boys. In labour force participation women make-up 32.8% work force as against 81.1% men. Girls usually suffer the triple burden of household, schoolwork and work outside the home, paid or unpaid. Low literacy; early marriage and early pregnancy puts them to added risk in their life. Low literacy of female means less of information or lack of information on health, development and advancement and prevention of diseases; a permanent disadvantage in life.

Decision-Making and Control over Resources

Women's control over economic resources is far less than that of men. They are paid less for wage work. While 85% of ever married women participate in decisions about what to cook, only about half participate in decisions about their own health care. Most women need permission (or are not allowed at all) to go to market (68%) or to visit friends or relatives (76%). Only 60% have access to some money that they can use as they wish. Autonomy of women is somewhat high in Himachal Pradesh, Punjab and North-Eastern States and it is relatively low in the State of Rajasthan, UP, MP, and Bihar. Women do not have control over money and only few hold bank or postal account in their names. In Kerala and Manipur, women enjoy far greater freedom than women in other states. The extent of women political representation is, however, limited.[3] The number of women in parliament has increased to 10.7%

and move for 40% reservation is gaining strength. India is among top 20 best performing countries on political empowerment sub-index.

Domestic Violence

Incidence of crimes and violence against women (physical, mental, domestic, rape and sexual violence, honour killing, forced prostitution and trafficking and sexual harassment, etc. is rising. Domestic violence is widespread phenomenon. Wife beating is quite frequent. Extreme degree of violence like dowry deaths appear in the media at regular intervals, but domestic violence seldom get reported or notified. Almost 3 out of 5 women (56%) believe that wife beating is justified for at least one of the six specific reasons: on account of neglect of house or children, showing disrespect for in-laws, going out without permission, if suspected to be unfaithful, when food is not cooked properly or if the wife does not bring money or other expected items from her parents. Rural and illiterate women are more likely to accept wife beating for any reason than their urban, educated counterparts. About one-fourth of illiterate women report being beaten and at least one-third of poorer women report beatings.[3]

Sex Differential in Childhood Mortality and Rearing

Although male mortality exceeds female mortality at every age in most countries. In countries where the overall mortality rate is high, the female mortality often exceeds male mortality during childhood and throughout child-bearing years. In India, excess female mortality among children is evident at ages beyond the first month of life. During the postnatal period (age 1–11 months) female mortality exceeds than male mortality by 10%. After the age one year, sex differentials in mortality are even greater. The female child mortality rate is one and a half times than male child mortality rate (NFHS-2). The female disadvantage in survival from age one to exact age five years is evident in both urban and rural areas, but it is much more severe in rural than in urban areas. These data on child mortality show disturbing trend and pattern where girls die in numbers for exceeding boys.

Girls are unwelcome. Birth of girl child in family is unwelcome and bringing up of girls is considered or thought to be "watering in neighbourer garden". Discrimination in rearing, feeding and care during illness leads to more severe malnutrition in girls and more death in girls during early childhood period.[4] Discrimination starts even before birth as girls are not allowed to be born by adopting sex selective termination by well to do families.

WOMEN WORKLOAD

Women grow most of the developing world food, market most of the crops, fetch most of its water, collect most of its fuel, feed most of its animals, weed most of its fields. And when their work outside the home is done, they light the third world's fires, cook its meals, clean its compounds, wash its clothes, shop for its needs and they bear children, rear children and do a variety of household chores. The message is clear that men must share the workload of women to enhance the health status of women and children.

Women workload in home, farm and field is quite heavy and it is seldom recognized. Women do much more work than their men counterpart. Women are never found resting, they keep on working and workload is quite energy sapping. They spend more energy on fetching water, fuels, fodder, washing clothes, cooking and farm work which is tremendous apart from taking care of children. On the top of it, they eat last and eat least and consequently suffer in silence from anaemia and malnutrition.

Employment of women for paid work has raised their status and position in the community apart from generating additional income, which is in the hands of mothers for better food, clothing and care of the child. Work outside home makes women more confident and increases their awareness and opens up whole set of options.

Participation of Women in Contraception

Men participation in contraception is quite low. Women bear the brunt of sterilization. Female sterilization is the predominant method of contraception in India.

Out of 54.8% of acceptors of contraception 35.8% was the share of female sterilization, pills and IUD acceptors were 3.6 and 1.8% respectively, condom use rate was just 5.3% and share of male sterilization was low at 1% (DLHS 2012–13). 7.8% used traditional methods. Women have least control on their fertility or for that matter even in choosing a contraceptive for themselves. Cultural and family influences lead on to use of a specific contraceptive. How many children are to be born, is decided by family or husband in most situations. Reduction of fertility and improvement in health and nutrition of adults and children at the household level are all often perceived to be responsibility of women.

Women have no say on the issue of protecting themselves from sexually transmitted diseases, including HIV, which could be transmitted to them through their own husbands, especially those men with multiple sexual partners.

Exposure to Mass Media

Women have less exposure to mass media as compared to men and hence are not well informed on many issues. Television and radio are home based popular media but women have poor access to these media and hence are deprived of vital information on life processes and development.

Policies and Programmes for Women Development

The 9th plan clearly stated the 'Women's Component Plan'–30% of funds were sought to be earmarked for women related sectors. All departments were instructed to open Gender Budget cells in 2005. As a part of this all RCH II and NRHM programmes are required to do a gender budgeting.

The GOI has taken several policy measures to reduce gender bias. The practice of gender budgeting in health will be made mandatory in all programmes of the centre and states. The performance of different health programmes will be judged on the basis of gender disaggregated data. All reports of PHC and ICDS must be genderwise (morbidity, mortality, nutrition and use of services).

There have been significant transformations in India:

National policy for the empowerment of women was adopted in 2001 but before this policy there have been significant transformations.[5]

The 73rd and 74th Constitutional Amendment Acts were passed in December 1992 and became law in April 1993. These two Acts entail major changes. They provide for direct election of all seats of Panchayats and Nagar Palikas at village, block and Zila Parishad as well as, at the ward, town and city levels. The most far reaching measure is reservation under the Act for women. Not less than one-third of the total seats and the offices of chairpersons at each level will be reserved for women. Also seats will be reserved for members of scheduled castes and scheduled tribes in accordance with, their representation in the population. Of the 475 Zila Parishads in the country, 158 are being chaired by women. At block level out of 51,000 members of Block Samitis, 17,000 are women. In addition nearly one-third of the Mayors of the municipalities are women. The women has been mainstreamed politically for decision-making.

Economic Empowerment—Women in Poverty

Women in poverty comprise nearly 70% of population living below poverty line and are very often in situation of extreme poverty. Women's control over economic resources is far less than that of men. Forty percent of benefits under *Sawaranjayanti Gram Swarojgar Yojna* (SGSY) have been earmarked for women but in practice, the benefits are not reaching women in the same proportion. Development of women and children in rural areas (DWCRA) has been merged under SGSY. Self-help groups have been formed to help women. Women to women programmes are best run by women organization. Generating income through group activities, and land reforms legislations will address 89.5% of women work-force who are landless and poor who have no inheritance rights either for land or other product assets. Distribution of surplus land will be done amongst women of these groups. Women's training in agriculture sector like fisheries, poultry, animal husbandry and horticulture has been undertaken on priority basis in proportion to their numbers. The first National Agriculture Policy announced in July, 2000 seeks to mainstream gender concerns in agriculture. Innumerable income generation activities have been launched by the Government to improve the economic status of women in organized sector, hopefully the women get hold on their income and are emancipated from poverty and exploitation. Unorganized sector is very large and it can make the things different.

Social Empowerment of Women

Health sector has implemented National Health Policy of 1983, National Population Policy 2000 and National Health Policy-2002 (Revised) and National Nutrition Policy to reduce the infant and maternal mortality as also to address, gender issues in health. PNDT (Prenatal Diagnostic Techniques (Regulation and Prevention of Misuse) Act, 1994 has been enforced to prevent sex selective abortions and improve sex ratio at birth.

Focuses of Eleventh and 12th Five-Year Plan

Developing clear targets of natural sex ratio at birth (SRB) which is 105 males per 100 females and link financial benefits to states that have improved SRB. From 2007 onwards Annual Health Survey will include estimates of SRB at the district level. Planning commission will obtain independent estimates of the SRB at the district level each year and include indicators on improvement in sex ratio at birth for arriving at decisions on plan assistance of states. The 11th and 12th five-year plan goal is to achieve 0–6 years sex ratio of 950 by the end of 2017.

Increased access to contraception and increased men participation in family planning programme should be the focus in near future to remove gender disparity.

Education and Literacy

The bold decision to declare "education as the fundamental right" (in April 2010) reflects the Government's concern and commitment to ensure the right of children (6–14 years) to free and compulsory elementary education to fulfil the constitutional commitment of "education for all". India has 34 million children out of school as on 31st March 2015. Through the specially targeted programme of *Sarva Shiksha Abhiyan* (SSA); launched in 2001, effort is being made to reach the unreached women and girl child.[6] The tenth plan focused to consolidate the gains to achieve the set goal of "education for women equality" as advocated by National Policy on Education 1986 (revised in 1992) by reducing the gender gaps at the secondary and higher education levels. Already low female literacy pockets have been identified and women and girl children belonging to the socially disadvantaged groups will have preference over others; as they lag behind the rest of population with female literacy rates as low as 5 to 10% while the national average of female literacy stands at 65.46% in 2011. Easy and equal access to all women and girls for education through enabling environment to meet the goal of "education for all" is a progressive step.

Similarly, vocational education at secondary educational level for women is another important priority area under the National Education Policy by establishing more women Industrial Training Institutions (ITIs).

Special incentives have been provided to increase the enrolment and retention of girls children in schools through free textbooks, scholarships, free supply of uniforms, mid-day meals flexible school timings attached hostels and crèches and lifelong learning through correspondence courses, distance learning and self-study programmes for girls who dropout from formal system of schooling.

Media

Media must be used to portray positive images consistent with human dignity of girls and women. Massive awareness and education on gender issues can be addressed through mass media with the help of subject experts. The steps have been initiated to remove gender bias and gender stereotypes in the curricula, textbooks and learning material: Promote gender sensitization of teachers, also appointing more women teachers at primary level.

Environment Conservation

Women have been involved in conservation and restoration of environment and control of environmental degradation. Efficient use of nonconventional energy sources, like solar energy, biogas, fuel efficient stoves, smokeless chullah (stoves) and other rural applications to preserve the environment. These are environmental friendly activities which needs to be promoted to save women energies and protect environment. Women can play useful role for planning and conservations of forest and to promote social forestry. Women friendly *technologies* are in progress to reduce their *drudgery* apart from involving men and increasing their participation.

Legislation Support for Women

There are several legislative support measures for women. Like the Immoral Traffic (prevention) Act. The Dowry Prohibition Act, 1961, The Indecent Representation of Women (Prohibition) Act, 1986. The Commission of Sati (Prevention) Act, 1987 to safeguard the interest of women. There are several women related legislations but their implementation is quite tardy. Twelfth plan, hopefully implements all these in favour of women.

Gender discrimination and disparity between boys and girls, men and women ultimately begins and ends at the "family level". Family is the most important institution which transmit the values and attitudes to their offsprings to bring change in the mindset of their sons and daughters, men and women to root out the gender disparity and develop respect for each other and tolerance to each others. Family and community should play dominant role to do away these disparities, the legislations come later and people come first. Changing societal attitudes and community practices by active participation and involvement of men and women, is the core strategy of women empowerment. It is the choice of family or community to have gender equality for prosperous lives of women and men.[7–9]

Yet, despite substantial gains in women's empowerment since the convention on the elimination of all forms of discrimination against women (CEDAW) adopted by the UN General Assembly in 1979, as ratified by India on 25.6.93, gender discrimination continues.[10] Achieving Gender equality and empowering all women and girls will move all the sustainable development goals forward.[11]

Under national policy for empowerment of women 2001 each state Government has prepared action plan to implement multisectoral endeavours for gender justice and women empowerment (It is sustainable Development Goal-5).

Disparity between boys and girls is ultimately a family, or at the most a community choice.

BETI BACHAO BETI PADHAO (BBBP) SCHEME

Census 2011, reveals the extensive and significant decline in child sex ratio (CSR) of 0–6 years recording an all time, low of 914 girls for every 1000 boys. 13 out of 35 states and UTs have CSR lower than the national average of 914 girls.

In order to address the issues of declining child sex ratio and promoting girls education in India, the Ministry of Women and Child Development has taken an initiative of "Beti Bachao, Beti Padhao" to improve child sex ratio, promote the importance of girl child and highlight the benefit of educating girl child by formulating various policies, programmes and legislations concerning women and children. Government has selected 100 gender critical districts in the country to:

- Raise awareness and provide insight into the current situation.
- Provide strategies and tools for grass root level functionaries to improve the declining CSR.

Ministry of Women and Child Development is designated as the nodal ministry for this initiative, supported by MOH and FW, Ministry of Human Resource Development, and Ministry of Information and Broadcasting. Overall objective of BBBP is to improve declining CSR and promoting education for girls. The specific objectives are:

- Prevent gender biased sex selective elimination.
- Ensure survival and protection of girl child
- Ensure education of girl child.

Multipronged approach to improve CSR should involve youth, adolescents, men, PRIs, community leaders, judiciary and media for achieving behavior change. Since it is an issue of traditional attitudes and awareness generation, advocacy will continue to be a major plank of the BBBP strategy in addition to stricter implementation of PC PNDT Act.

REFERENCES

1 Hindustan Times, Saturday, January 23, 2010. India's gender gap narrowing. Disparity in literacy, health declined in 10 years: GOI, Study.

2 Gender Training on women's empowerment. Dec. 1,2003. Reading material. Organized by women's Development Division NIPCCD, 5, Siri, Institutional Area, Hauz Khas, New Delhi.

3 IIPS India. NFHS-2 Key Findings. IIPS Mumbai, 1998–99.

4 Green MI. Watering the neighbour's garden. Investing in adolescent girls in India. Population Council South East Asia working Paper No. 7, New Delhi.

5 National Policy for the empowerment of women 2001. Department of Women and Child Development, Ministry of Human Resource Development, Government of India.

6 Government of India. Planning Commission. 10th Five-Year Plan 2002–2007. Policies and Programmes for women and development.

7 UNICEF. Rights and opportunities. The situation of children and women in India. UNICEF. India Country office, New Delhi 1998.

8 UNICEF. Facts for life. A communication challenge. Indian ed. New Delhi: UNICEF India Country Office.

9 GOI Strategic Initiatives for Inclusive Development. An Approach to the 11th Five-Year Plan GOI. Planning commission Yojna Bhavan, New Delhi 2006.

10 Women–Equal Partners. Convention on the Elimination of all forms of Discrimination Against Women (CEDAW). As ratified by India on 25.6.93.

11 United Nations General Assembly, September 2015 Transforming our World: the 2030 Agenda for sustainable development.

NATIONAL POPULATION POLICY (NPP)-2000

Milestones in evolution of the population policy in India:

1 Bhore Committee Report was submitted in 1946.
2 Family Planning Programme was launched in 1952.
3 Statement on National Population Policy was made in 1976.
4 Policy statement on Family Welfare Programme was made in 1977.

   Both (3 and 4) statements were laid on the table of the house in Parliament but never discussed or adopted.

5 National Health Policy of 1983 emphasized the need for "securing the small family norm, through voluntary efforts and moving towards goal of population stabilization while adopting the health policy, parliament emphasized the need for a separate National Population Policy.
6 The National Development Council (NDC) appointed a committee on population with Shri Karunakaran as chairman in 1991. The report of this committee was endorsed by NDC in 1993.
7 An expert group headed by Dr M.S. Swaminathan was asked to prepare a draft of a National Population Policy.
8 Another draft of National Population Policy was finalized and placed before the cabinet in 1999. National Population Policy (NPP) was finally adopted in the year 2000.

Policy

Policy means statement of intentions and time frame to achieve the set goals.

Major goal: To improve quality of life and stabilize population.

Objectives of NPP

- The immediate objective of NPP-2000 is to address the "unmet needs" of contraception, health care infrastructure, and health care personnel and to provide integrated service delivery for basic reproductive and child health care.
- The medium term objective is to bring total fertility rate (TFR) to 2.1 (replacement level).
- Long-term objective is to achieve a stable population by 2045 at a level consistent with the requirements of sustainable economic growth social development and environmental protection.[1]

NATIONAL SOCIODEMOGRAPHIC GOALS

1 Address the unmet needs for basic reproductive and child health services, supplies and infrastructure.
2 Make school education up to age 14 free and compulsory, and reduce dropouts at primary and secondary school levels to below 20% for both boys and girls.
3 Reduce infant mortality rate to below 30 per 1000 live births.
4 Reduce maternal mortality ratio to below 100 per 100,000 live births.
5 Achieve universal immunization of children against all vaccine preventable diseases.
6 Promote delayed marriage for girls, not earlier than age 18 and preferably after 20 years of age.
7 Achieve 80% institutional deliveries and 100% deliveries by trained persons.
8 Achieve universal access to information/counselling, and services for fertility regulation and contraception with a wide basket of choices.
9 Achieve 100% registration of births, deaths, marriages and pregnancies.
10 Contain the spread of acquired immunodeficiency syndrome (AIDS), and promote greater integration between the management of reproductive tract infection (RTI) and sexually transmitted infections (STI) and the national AIDS control organization.
11 Prevent and control communicable diseases.

12 Integrate Indian Systems of Medicine (ISM) in the provision of reproductive and child health services, and in reaching out to households.
13 Promote vigorously the small family norm to achieve replacement level of TFR.
14 Bring about convergence in implementation of related social sector programs so that family welfare becomes a people centred programme.

STRATEGIC THEMES

- Decentralized planning and programme implementation: 73rd and 74th Constitutional Amendment Act, 1992 made *health*, *family welfare* and *education* a responsibility of village Panchayats and Nagarpalikas respectively. The Panchayati Raj Institutions (PRIs) are important means of decentralized planning and programme implementation in the context of NPP 2000. Delegate administrative and financial powers to PRIs.
- Convergence of service delivery at village level.
- Empowering women for improved health and nutrition.
- Child health and survival.
- Meeting the unmet needs for family welfare services.
- Underserved population groups—(a) urban slums, (b) tribal communities, hill area population and migrant population, (c) adolescents, (d) increased participation of men in planned parenthood.
- Diverse health care providers.
- Collaboration with and commitments from Non-Governmental Organizations (NGOs) and the private sector.
- Mainstreaming Indian System of Medicine and Homeopathy.
- Contraceptive technology and research on reproductive and child health.
- Providing for the older population.
- Information, education and communication.

LEGISLATION

As a motivational measure, in order to enable state governments to fearlessly and effectively pursue the agenda for population stabilization contained in the NPP-2000, one legislation is considered necessary. It is recommended that 42nd Constitutional Amendment that freezes till 2001, the number of seats to the Lok Sabha and Rajya Sabha based on 1971 census be extended up to 2026.

Public Support

Enlisting support for small family norm by political, community, business, professional and religious leaders, media and film stars, sports personalities and opinion makers will enhance its acceptance.

NEW STRUCTURES

Population problem is multisectoral endeavour. This requires multisectoral coordination of planning and implementation between health and family welfare on the one hand, along with schemes for education, nutrition, women and child development, safe drinking water, sanitation, rural roads, communications, transportation, housing, forestry development, environmental protection and urban development. The following structures are recommended:

- National Population Commission.
- State/UT Commissions on Population
- Coordination Cell in Planning Commission.
- Technology Mission in the Department of Family Welfare.

FUNDING

In order to implement immediately the action plan, it would be necessary to double the annual plan budget of the Department of Family Welfare to enable government to address the shortfall in unmet needs of health care infrastructure, services and supplies. The annual budget of Family Welfare for the year 1999–2000 was 2920 crores, half of this gets spent on non-plan activities (recurring expenditures for maintenance of health care infrastructure in the states and UTs, and towards salaries). Only 50% is available for genuine plan activities including procurement of supplies and equipment.

PROMOTIONAL AND MOTIVATIONAL MEASURES FOR ADOPTION OF SMALL FAMILY NORMS

The following promotional and motivational measures will be undertaken:

1 Rewarding Panchayat and Zila Parishad for exemplary performance.
2 The ***"Balika Samridhi Yojna"*** run by department of Women and Child Development to promote survival and care of girl child, will continue. A cash incentive of ₹ 500 is awarded at birth of the girl child of birth order 1 or 2.
3 ***Maternity benefit scheme:*** Cash incentive of ₹ 500 to mothers who have their first child after 19 years of age for birth of first and second child only.
4 Family welfare health linked insurance plan for couples below poverty line.
5 Setting-up of revolving fund for income generating activities by village self-help groups.
6 Opening-up of crèches and child-care centres.
7 Enlarging the basket of contraceptives.
8 Facilities for safe abortion will be strengthened and expanded.
9 Strict Enforcement of Child Marriage Restraint Act, 1976.
10 Strict Enforcement of Prenatal Diagnostic Technique Act, 1994.
11 Soft loan to ensure mobility of ANMs.
12 Social marketing schemes for contraceptives.
13 Ambulance services to transport referral high-risk women to encourage village level organization by providing soft loans.

The vast number of people in India can be its greatest asset if they are provided with means to lead healthy and economically productive lives. In the new millennium, nations are judged by the well-being of their people, by level of health, nutrition and education, by civil and political liberties. Success will be achieved if the action plan contained in the NPP-2000 is pursued as a national movement.

NATIONAL POPULATION POLICY 2000 ACTION PLAN

Decentralization Planning and Programme Implementation and Convergence of Services at Village Level

Since 33% of Elected Panchayat seats are reserved for woman, representative committees of Panchayats (headed by elected woman member) should be formed to promote gender sensitive, multisectoral agenda for population stabilization, that will "think plan and act locally, and support nationally".

1 By utilizing self-help groups to organize and provide basic services for reproductive and child health (RCH) with ongoing integrated child development scheme (ICDS).

   Once a fortnight these *self-help acceptor groups* meet and provide at one place 6 different services for (i) registration of births, deaths, marriages and pregnancy; (ii) weighing of children under five years and recording the weight on standard growth chart; (iii) counselling and advocacy for contraception, plus free supply of contraceptives; (iv) preventive care with availability of basic medicines for common ailments: antipyretics for fevers, ORT/ORS for childhood diarrhoea together with standardised indigenous medicines; (v) nutrition supplements and (vi) advocacy and encouragement for the continued enrolment of children in school up to age 14. One health staff appointed by Panchayat will be suitably trained to provide guidance.

2 Meaningful decentralization will result only if the convergence of the national family welfare programme with the ICDS programme is strengthened. At village level, the Anganwadi centre may become the focal point for basic care activities, contraceptive counselling and supply, nutrition education and supplementation as well as preschool activities. The Anganwadi centre can also function as depot for ORS/basic medicines and contraceptive.

3 Establishment of maternity hut in each village for safe delivery. Panchayat may appoint competent and mature midwife.

4 Trained birth attendants as well as vast pool of traditional dais should be made familiar with emergency and referral procedures. This will greatly assist the ANMs.

5 Provide a wider basket of choices of contraception.

Empowering Women for Improved Health and Nutrition

- Cluster services for women and children at the same place.
- Open more child-care centres in rural areas and urban slums, i.e. establish Anganwadis or crèches where woman can leave her children in safe hands for care and development. This will encourage women to participate in development process.
- To empower women to pursue programme of social afforestation to facilitate easy access to firewood, fodder. Increased access to potable water. This will reduce long absence from home and need for large number of children to perform such tasks.
- Promote energy saving devices, such as solar cookers, provision of sanitary latrines, or extension of telephone lines; this will empower woman and households.
- Strengthen the referral network between SC, PHC, CHC and District hospital in management of obstetric and neonatal complications to reduce maternal and infant mortality.
- Establish mechanism of maternal and perinatal death audit from village level upwards.
- Ensure adequate transportation from village level upwards of mothers having obstetrical complications.
- Improve the accessibility and quality of maternal and child health services—through deployment of community midwives and additional health providers at village level, training, improved supervision and provision of standard equipment and medicines and physical facilities.
- Monitoring of maternal and child health services at each level. ANM should be responsible for registering every pregnancy and childbirth in her area.
- Providing universal antenatal and postnatal services.
- Improve technical skills of maternal and child healthcare providers by on the job training to all category of workers and birth attendants.
- Improve information education and communication at community level.
- Universalization of ICDS and convergence of maternal and child health services.
- Include STD/RTI and HIV/AIDS prevention, screening, and management in maternal and child health services.
- Develop health package for adolescents.
- Expand the availability of safe-abortion services at PHC level and CHC level. District civil surgeon should be the authority to register abortion clinics. Provide MTP training to medical officers and include MTP in the curriculum of all categories of workers and doctors.
- Establishing first referral unit at subdistrict level and community health centre and make them functional.
- Ensure the efficient functioning of first referral units, i.e. 30 bedded hospital at block levels (CHC) to bring down maternal mortality and IMR. Augment

availability of specialists in these units by increasing seats in medical institutions and acquiring postgraduate qualifications through National Board of examination and open universities like IGNOU. As an incentive, seats will be reserved for those in-service medical graduates who are willing to abide by a bond to serve for 5 yeas at FRU after completion of PG course. State would sanction the posts of specialists at FRUs.

- Create national network of public-private and NGO centres identified by a common logo for delivering RCH services free to any client. The provider will be compensated for the service provided. The end user can choose the provider of service.

CHILD HEALTH AND SURVIVAL

- Essential neonatal care at community level and at PHC, CHC and hospitals.
- Set-up national technical committee on neonatal care to align programme and project interventions with newly emerging technologies in neonatal and perinatal care.
- Train health personnel for integrated management of childhood illnesses (IMCI).
- Pursue rigorously the pulse polio-campaign to eradicate polio.
- Ensure 100% coverage of routine immunizations in particular tetanus and measles.
- Promote delayed marriage of girls not earlier than 18 years and preferably after 20 years of age by compulsory education of girls and vocational training for girls.
- Reduction of maternal malnutrition, morbidity and mortality by ensuring availability of supplies equipment at village level and subcentre.
- Expand the ICDS to include children between 6 and 9 years of age to promote 100% of school enrolment particularly for girls.

MEETING THE UNMET NEEDS FOR FAMILY WELFARE SERVICES

- Unmet need for contraceptive is estimated at 28%.
- Establishing adequate number of Sub-centres, PHCs, CHCs as per norms to complete their deficiency, provide manpower, equipment, medicines and supplies (contraceptives, laparoscopes, tubal ring, vaccines and RCH drugs).
- Formulate and implement social marketing schemes.
- Improve facilities for referral transportation at Panchayat, Zila Parishad and PHCs. Increase mobility of ANMs to increase coverage.
- Encourage local level organization and NGO to start ambulance services for transportation of women needing emergency care.
- Opening up of chemist shops at village level through loan facility.

UNDERSERVED POPULATION GROUPS

Urban Slums

Finalize comprehensive *urban health* strategy. Facilitate service delivery centres in *urban slums* to provide comprehensive basic health, reproductive and child health services by NGOs and private sector including corporate sector.

- Promote network of retired government doctors, paramedicals and nonmedical personnel who may function as health care providers on remunerative terms.
- Initiate specially targeted information education and communication activities in urban slums.
- Promote intersectoral coordination in urban slums to enhance services.
- Streamline the referral systems and linkages between primary-secondary and tertiary levels of health care in urban areas.

Tribal Communities, Hill Area Population and Displaced and Migrant Populations

NGO sector may be encouraged to organize system of preventive and curative health care in these areas. Promote indigenous system of medicine. Sensitization of providers to the needs of tribal areas.

Adolescents

Ensure for adolescent's access to information, counselling and services including reproductive health services. Strengthen PHCs and subcentres to provide counselling to adolescents on spacing and right age of marriage.

- Provide for adolescents the package of nutrition services available under ICDS programme.
- Enforce the Child Marriage Restraint Act, 1976 to reduce incidence of teenage marriages.
- Provide integrated intervention in pockets with unmet needs in the urban slums, remote rural areas, tribal area and border districts.

Increase Participation of Men in Planned Parenthood

- Currently 99% sterilizations are tubectomies. Repopularize vasectomies in particular-no-scalpel vasectomy.
- Focus attention on men in the information and education campaign to promote small family norms.
- Continuing education and training at all levels to promote use of no-scalpel vasectomy. Include this in the syllabi.

DIVERSE HEALTH CARE PROVIDERS

Public-Private Partnership

Involve private practitioners and assign satellite population of 5000 to provide RCH services and compensate them adequately for providing these services. One year contract at a time be given.

- Revival of licentiate of medical practitioners.
- Include RCH strategies into the curriculum of under/postgraduates, nursing and paramedical professional courses, syllabi and curriculum.

Collaboration with and Commitment from Non-Government Sector

Collaboration with voluntary sector and NGO in clinical services, for motivation of village level self-help groups and social marketing will be encouraged.

Collaboration with and Commitment from Industry

Collaboration with industrial sector for strengthening of the management information system in seven most deficient states at PHCs and Subcentre level by electronic data entry machines, to reduce the load on ANMs, in social marketing of RCH services, transportation, providing RCH services to their own employees, managing primary schools for children and outreach of basic reproductive and child care services.

Mainstreaming of Indian Systems of Medicine and Homeopathy

Providing orientation and training in respect of RCH programme for qualified doctors in Indian system of medicine and utilize their services, institutions and their time tested practices and medicines.

Contraceptive Technology and Research on RCH

Promote RCH research in consultation with Indian Council of Medical Research and the network of academic and research institutions. The International Institute of Population Sciences and the Population Research Centres will continue to review the programme and monitor the indicators of RCH services to provide feedback to the programme. Research areas would include contraceptive technology, CNAA approach, new models of neonatal care, convergence of services, public–private partnership, and newer technologies in vaccines.

Providing for Older Population

Sensitize, train and equip rural and urban health centres and hospitals towards providing geriatric health care. Encourage NGOs and voluntary organizations to make the elderly economically self-reliant. Tax benefits could be explored as an encouragement for children to look after their aged parents.

Information Education and Communication

Converge IEC efforts across the social sectors. Achieve coordination between family welfare and education sector to promote cause of literacy.

Involve all other departments like rural development, social welfare, transport, cooperative and education with special reference to schools to improve clarity and focus on the IEC efforts. Coverage and outreach of IEC activities can be extended by using elected leaders, opinion makers and religious leaders. Utilize radio and television as also indigenous media on the issues of small family norms. National communication strategies in RCH have been evolved and presented elsewhere. National Health Mission, 2012 provides a framework to implement NPP and National Health Policy-2002 and 2015 (Drafted).

Jansankhya Sthirata Kosh (JSK)

The objective of JSK is to facilitate the attainment of the goals of National Population Policy-2000 and support projects, schemes, initiatives and innovative ideas designed to help population stabilization both in the government and voluntary sector. It can generate resources through government and voluntary sectors contributions (from individuals, industry, trade organizations and other legal entities) in furtherance of the national cause of population stabilization.

JSK has Undertaken a Number of Initiatives for Population Stabilization

- **PRERNA strategy:** Aim is to delay the age of marriage of girls and space the births 3 years apart. Girls married after 19 years of age and giving birth to first child after at least 2 years of marriage are given incentive of ₹ 10000 to ₹ 12000. The scheme is meant for BPL families.
- **SANTUSHTI strategy:** Accredited Private Nursing Home/Hospital can sign a tripartite (state health society as first party, accredited private health facility as second party and JSK as third party) memorandum of understanding. Such hospitals and nursing homes are entitled for incentives for performing tubectomy and vasectomy operations.
- **JSK** has also set up National Helpline in India to provide reliable information on reproductive, and sexual health, contraception, pregnancy and child health issues.

REFERENCE

1 Government of India. National Population Policy 2000 GOI MOH and FW, New Delhi.

CHAPTER

6

Applied Nutrition Programmes and Intervention

NUTRIENTS AND THEIR REQUIREMENT

Goal 1: United Nations "Sustainable Development Goals" seek to eradicate extreme poverty for all people everywhere, currently measured as people living on less than $ 1.25 a day. By 2030 reduce at least by half the proportion of men, women and children of all ages living in poverty in all its dimensions according to national definitions.

Goal 2: End hunger, achieve food security and improved nutrition and sustainable agriculture. By 2030 end all forms of malnutrition, including achieving, by 2025, the internationally agreed targets on stunting and wasting in children under 5 years of age.

Nation has passed Food Security bill-"food for all" in 2013 to provide food grains at subsidised rate to BPL families. This law entitles 820 million people in India to food at an affordable cost.

Famines and starvation in India were common features before independence. India was food deficit country for about two decades after independence. India has not only become self-sufficient in food production but now has surplus food grains and enough of buffer stocks of over 60 million tonnes. The food grains production has increased to the level of 212.9 million tonnes in 2001–02 from 89.36 million tonnes in 1964–65 (Table 6.1). There was dilemma and paradox, that we had vast stocks of food grains but shortages were faced in some parts. Malnutrition persists as over 42% of young children being underweight, while the food rots in the open. Adequate access to food was not there because of poverty and inadequate and weak public distribution system (PDS).[1]

Due to green revolution, the food grain production has not only kept pace with fast growing population, but the widespread severe forms of malnutrition (marasmus, kwashiorkor and keratomalacia) have declined substantially in India and prosperity has been achieved. In 2002, India had massive reserve grain stocks of 63 million tonnes, much of which was exported at a loss. But today wheat stocks are almost zero and the government has decided to import three million tonnes. India has gone from food surplus to food deficits. Because its population has risen, while food production has stagnated or fallen for 6 years (Table 6.1). Grain output in 2005–06 is estimated to be no higher than the 209 million tonnes reached 6 years ago. Wheat production peaked at 76.4 million tonnes in 1999 and then declined. The output of pulses has stagnated at 13–14 million tonnes. Only coarse grain production has risen a bit, thanks to new hybrid variety.[2] Stagnant grain production is attributable to environmental degradation due to excessive pumping of ground water with free power

Table 6.1: Food grain output (million tonnes) trends from 2001 to 2012

Commodity	*2001–02*	*2002–03*	*2003–04*	*2004–05*	*2006–07*	*2011–12*
Rice	93.3	71.8	88.3	85.3	93	104
Wheat	72.8	65.8	72.1	72.0	76	94
Coarse grain	33.4	26.1	38.1	33.9	34	42
Pulses	13.4	11.1	14.9	13.4	14	17
Total	**212.9**	**174.8**	**213.5**	**204.6**	**217**	**257**

Source: Twelfth plan working group on Agriculture Statistics.

supply. During the year 2010–11 record food production of 235.8 million metric tonnes was achieved and at the end of 2009 India had a buffer stock of 206 lakh tonnes of wheat and 257 lakh tonnes of rice. In the year 2013–14 food production has crossed 264 million metric tonnes. India will need to produce 450 million tones of food grains in 2050 to be able to feed its population.

Besides undernutrition, we now have emerging problem of obesity and "lifestyle diseases", India is thus facing double burden of malnutrition, i.e. we have the problem of **overnutrition** as also **undernutrition**.

Major Nutrition Related Public Health Problems

1 Chronic energy *deficiency* and undernutrition (protein calorie malnutrition).
2 Micronutrient deficiency (hidden hunger) which includes:
   a Anaemia due to iron and folate deficiency.
   b Iodine deficiency disorders (IDDs)
   c Vitamin A deficiency.
   d Zinc deficiency.
3 Chronic energy *excess* and obesity.

Reference Indian Adult Man and Woman (NNMB)

Reference man is in age group 18–29 years and weighs 60 kg with a height of 1.73 m with a BMI of 20.3 and is free from disease and physically fit for active work; on each working day, he is engaged in 8 hours of occupation which usually involves moderate activity, while when not at work he spends 8 hours in bed, 4–6 hours in sitting and moving about, 2 hours in walking and in active recreation or household duties.

Reference woman is in age group 18–29 years, non-pregnant non-lactating (NPNL) and weighs 55 kg with a height of 1.6 m and a BMI of 21.2, is free from disease and physically fit for active work; on each working day she is engaged in 8 hours of occupation which usually involves moderate activity, while when not at work she spends 8 hours in bed, 4–6 hours in sitting and moving about, 2 hours in walking and in active recreation or household duties.

Reference body weight of Indians of different age groups are given in Tables 6.2 and 6.3.

Table 6.2: Reference body weights (kg) of Indians for computing RDA, 2010

	Age (yrs)	*Reference body weights (kg)*
Infants	0–6 m	5.4
	6–12 m	8.4
Children	1–3	12.9
	4–6	18.0
	7–9	25.1
Boys	10–12	34.3
	13–15	47.6
	16–17	55.4
Girls	10–12	35.0
	13–15	46.6
	16–17	52.1
Adult man	18–29	60
Adult woman	18–29	55

Table 6.3: 95th centile values of weight and height by age and gender: Rural India (16 states) (NNMB and INP)

Age (yrs)	*Males*		*Females*	
	Height (cm)	*Weight (kg)*	*Height (cm)*	*Weight (kg)*
1+	82.4	11.2	81.6	10.7
2+	90.7	13.0	89.8	12.6
3+	99.1	14.8	98.2	14.4
4+	105.7	16.5	105.1	16.0
5+	111.5	18.2	111.0	17.7
6+	118.5	20.4	117.5	20.0
7+	124.3	22.7	123.6	22.3
8+	130.1	25.2	129.2	25.0
9+	134.6	28.0	135.0	27.6
10+	140.0	30.8	140.0	31.2
11+	144.8	34.1	145.3	34.8
12+	151.1	38.0	150.2	39.0
13+	157.0	43.3	153.8	43.4
14+	163.0	48.0	157.0	47.1
15+	166.3	51.5	158.8	49.4
16+	168.3	54.3	159.7	51.3
17+	170.0	56.5	160.2	52.8
18–19	171.3	58.4	161.1	53.8
20–24	172.5	60.5	160.7	54.8
25–29	172.3	62.0	161.0	56.1

Dietary Principles

The available food stuffs are broadly classified as cereals, pulses, nuts and oil seeds, vegetables, fruits, milk and milk products and flesh foods. These foods contain substances known as nutrients which perform various functions.

The nutrients include proteins, fats, carbohydrates, vitamins, minerals and salt. Foods are classified sometimes as protein rich foods, carbohydrates rich foods, etc. Oil and ghee provide mostly fat while sugar is purely a source of carbohydrate.

Proteins, fats and carbohydrates are also sometimes called "proximate principles". They are oxidized in the body to provide the energy required for various activities of life. Together with water, proximate principles form the main bulk of foods.[3]

Proteins

Proteins are building blocks and are chief substances in the cells of the body. Protein is required by the body for growth, replacement of body tissues as also for synthesis of enzymes, haemoglobin, hormones, antibodies and breast milk. Proteins are made of amino acids. Some of the amino acids are "essential amino acids" which cannot be synthesized by the body and hence have to be supplied from dietary sources. These essential amino acids are isoleucine, leucine, lysine, methionine, phenylalanine, tryptophan, threonine and valine. The presence of essential amino acid determines the quality of proteins.

Biological value of protein depends upon amino acid content and its digestibility. Animal proteins have high biological value as compared to vegetable proteins. Cereal proteins are rich in methionine but poor in amino acid-lysine, while pulse proteins are rich in lysine but poor in methionine. Combination of cereals and pulses (Dal-Roti) can enhance their value and it has mutual supplementary effect, and deficiency of one amino acid in one food stuff can be made good by another. Therefore, eating mixed cereals and cereals plus pulses is nutritionally advantageous as it achieves balancing of amino acid content of food.

Egg and milk proteins are used as reference proteins. Biological value of egg protein is 94, milk 84, meat 74, fish 76 and that of rice, wheat and Bengal gram is 68, 65 and 68 respectively.

RDA for protein are roughly 1 g per kg body weight. Young children, pregnant women, and lactating women require more proteins (Tables 6.4 and 6.5).[4] Proteins normally should supply 10–12% energy.

Table 6.4: Protein requirement during pregnancy and lactation (ICMR-2010)

Group	*Daily additional requirement (g)*	*Total daily requirement (g)*
Pregnant women	23	78
Lactating mother		
0–6 months	19	74
6–12 months	13	68

Table 6.5: Protein requirement g/kg of infants

Age in months	*Daily requirement (g/kg/day)*
0–6	1.16
6–12	1.69

Carbohydrates and Energy

Carbohydrates are main source of energy (about 60%) to the body. Carbohydrates are glucose, cane-sugar, and starch. Food-grains are largely composed of starch. Food stuffs like cane-sugar and glucose are pure carbohydrates. Being cheap source of energy carbohydrates form the bulk of an Indian diet. Energy deficiency is primarily food deficiency. Major cause of undernutrition is energy deficiency or less food Intake. Energy requirements for different age groups as per ICMR 2010 are given in Tables 6.6 to 6.8, and 6.10.

Besides starch and other digestible carbohydrates, many foods contain cellulose and hemicellulose, gums, pectins and lignins which are also carbohydrates. These types of carbohydrates are called 'fibre' or roughage or unavailable carbohydrates to the body, as these are not digested in the human digestive system and are voided as such. These are designated as "dietary fibre" and have important role to play in diet, such as removal of waste, prevent constipation and increasing contraction of muscular wall of the gut.[5] Leafy vegetables, fruits and spices are rich in dietary fibre besides whole cereals. Dietary fibres make food bulky. Dietary fibres prevent obesity, cardiovascular diseases and cancer. Lack of adequate dietary fibre in diets containing refined foods, leads to constipation and colon cancer. Some of dietary fibre like gums, mucilages in our diets have shown to lower blood cholesterol and blood glucose. The daily diet of an adult should contain minimum 20–35 g of dietary fibre.

Table 6.6: Energy requirement of reference Indian man and woman (kcal/day) (ICMR-2010)

Sex	*Body wt (kg)*	*Activity*		
		Sedentary	*Moderate*	*Heavy*
Man	60	2320	2730	3490
Woman	55	1900	2230	2850

Table 6.7: Energy requirement of infants

Age	*Requirement kcal/kg/day*
0–6 months	92
6–12 months	80

Table 6.8: Energy requirement of children (kcal/day)

Age in years	*Energy requirement*	
1–3	1060	
4–6	1350	
7–9	1690	
	Boys	Girls
10–12	2190	2010
13–15	2750	2330
16–17	3020	2440

Energy

Practical nutrition work often involves the assessment of calories needs of group or persons. In such cases, it is usual to assess the needs of women and children in terms of those of the average man by applying various coefficients to the different age and sex groups. In the following scale which is suggested for practical nutrition work in India, the calorie consumption of an average adult male doing sedentary work is taken as one unit and other coefficients are worked out on the basis of calories requirements as shown in Table 6.9. One unit of Coefficient corresponds to energy requirement of 2318 kcal/day. It must be emphasized that the scale of coefficient is somewhat arbitrary one and concern only for calories. It is not meant to be applied in assessing the needs of other nutrients.

With the help of food consumption tables, the calorie contents of diets can be worked out and compared with suggested requirements. In dealing with a group of mixed age and sex composition, the number of "consumption

Table 6.9: Age-wise and sex-wise calorie coefficient consumption unit

Person/age	Calorie coefficient consumption unit[3]
Adult male (sedentary worker)	1.0
Adult male (moderate worker)	1.2
Adult male (heavy worker)	1.6
Adult female (sedentary worker)	0.8
Adult female (moderate worker)	0.9
Adult female (heavy worker)	1.2
Adolescents 12–21 years	1.0
Children 9–12 years	0.8
Children 7–9 years	0.7
Children 5–7 years	0.6
Children 3–5 years	0.5
Children 1–3 years	0.4

units" (or adult man value) in the group is first calculated. For example, a family consisting of father doing sedentary work, mother of three children aged 10, 8 and 6 years has an "adult man value" or consumption units (calculated on the above scale), comes out to be 3.9 (i.e. 1.0 + 0.8 + 0.8 + 0.7 + 0.6) and the minimum daily calorie requirement would be 2318 × 3.9 = 9040. It is necessary to draw up a diet schedule for this family supplying approximately 9040 calories. It is safer to err on the side of excess by 100–200 calories to allow the waste of all kinds.

Fats

Fats and oils are concentrated source of energy and increases the energy density of the diet. It supplies per unit weight more than double the energy provided by either protein or carbohydrate. 1 g of fat yields 9 kcal, 1 g of protein and 1 g of carbohydrate yields 4 kcal each. 1 g of dietary fibre yields 2 kcal.

Dairy fats, such as butter and ghee contain significant amount of vitamins A (retinol) and D as do some marine oils. These vitamins are not present in vegetable oils. Almost all vegetable oils contain vitamin E and are richest source of this vitamin in many diets. A few oils, e.g. redpalm oil contains substantial amount of carotenoids (provitamin A) which can also be found in many vegetables and fruits. Hydrogenated oil (Vanaspati) now popular in India as a cooking medium, does not normally contain vitamins. Vitamins A used to be added to vanaspati at a level of 50 IU/g and it was mandatory. However, this compulsory requirement is now withdrawn.

Functions of Dietary Fats

Fats are source of concentrated energy, essential for cell structure and membrane functions, as a source of essential fatty acids (EFA) (linolenic and linoleic acids), for cell structure and prostaglandin synthesis, as a vehicle for oil soluble vitamins and essential for control of blood lipids. In addition, fat contributes to the palatability of food and is important in cooking and food processing. Fat in the diet also helps in the absorption of beta-carotene and other fat soluble vitamins. While a minimum amount of fat has to be present in the diet to meet the requirement of two unsaturated EFAs (linoleic and linolenic acid), excess of fat in the diet is considered harmful. Hence, the minimum level, the

Table 6.10: Recommended Dietary Allowances (RDA) for energy, protein, fat, minerals, and vitamins for Indians (2010)

Group	Particulars	Body wt. kg	Net energy kcal/day	Protein g/d	Fat g/d visible fat	Calcium mg/d	Iron mg/d	Vit.A µg/d Retinol	Vit.A µg/d β-carotene	Thiamin mg/d	Riboflavin mg/d	Nicotinic acid mg/d	Vit. B_6 mg/d	Ascorbic acid mg/d	Folic acid µg/d	Vit. B_{12} µg/d
Man	Sedentary work		2320		25					1.2	1.4	16				
	Moderate work	60	2730	60	30	600	17	600	4800	1.4	1.6	18	2.0	40	200	1.0
	Heavy work		3490		40					1.7	2.1	21				
Woman	Sedentary work		1900		20					1.0	1.1	12				
	Moderate work		2230	55.0	25	600	21	600	4800	1.1	1.3	14	2.0	40	200	1.0
	Heavy work		2850		30					1.4	1.7	16				
	Pregnant woman	55	+350	78	30	1200	35	800	6400	+0.2	+0.3	+2	2.5	60	500	1.2
	Lactation															
	0–6 months		+600	74	30	1200	21	950	7600	+0.3	+0.4	+4	2.5	80	300	1.5
	6–12 months		+520	68	30					+0.2	+0.3	+3	2.5			
Infants	0–6 months	5.4	92/kg	1.16/kg		500	46 µg/kg/day			0.2	0.3	710 µg/kg	0.1	25	25	0.2
	6–12 months	8.4	80/kg	1.69/kg	19		05	350	2800	0.3	0.4	650 µg/kg	0.4			
Children	1–3 years	12.9	1060	16.7	27		09	400	3200	0.5	0.6	8	0.9		80	
	4–6 years	18.0	1350	20.1	25	600	13			0.7	0.8	11	0.9	40	100	0.2–1.0
	7–9 years	25.1	1690	29.5	30		16	600	4800	0.8	1.0	13	1.6		120	
Boys	10–12 years	34.3	2190	39.9	35	800	21			1.1	1.3	15	1.6	40	140	0.2–1.0
Girls	10–12 years	35.0	2010	40.4	35	800	27			1.0	1.2	13	1.6			
Boys	13–15 years	47.6	2750	54.3	45	800	32	600	4800	1.4	1.6	16	2.0	40	150	0.2–1.0
Girls	13–15 years	46.6	2330	51.9	40	800	27			1.2	1.4	14	2.0			
Boys	16–17 years	55.4	3020	61.5	50	800	28			1.5	1.8	17	2.0	40	200	0.2–1.0
Girls	16–17 years	52.1	2440	55.5	35	800	26			1.0	1.2	14	2.0			

desirable level, and the safe upper limit of fat intake has to be considered.

Visible and Invisible Fats

Visible fats are those which have been separated from animal tissues, milk, oil seeds, nuts or other vegetable sources, e.g. butter, ghee, groundnut, mustard, coconut and sunflower oils. They are used to produce shortening, margarine, salad oil, butter, etc. *Visible fats* are largely triglycerides, the common fatty acids present in visible fats are palmitic acid, stearic acid, oleic acid and linolenic acid.

Invisible fats are fats present as integral components of food or those which have not been separated from their original source and are therefore consumed as part of the tissues in the diet principally as meat, fish, poultry, dairy products, cereals, pulses nuts and vegetables. *Invisible fats* in diets are around 60% or more.[5] *Invisible fats* of plant foods are good sources of oleic acid, linoleic acid (LA) and α-linolenic acid (ALA). While in most foods LA predominates, legumes, green leafy vegetables and spices contain high proportion of ALA. The invisible fats from pulses and cereals alone contribute as much as 6 energy% or 16 g of invisible fat.

Quality of Fats and Safety Levels of Consumption[5]

Daily intake of fat should be such that it contributes not more than 20–30% of energy/calories in the diet. Considering the EFA requirements of different groups and knowing that the invisible fat in a cereal-based diet can meet more than half the linoleic acid requirements of an adult, a minimal intake of 20–40 g *visible fat* is recommended for adult male and female per day with higher levels of 25–30 and 35–50 g for young children and adolescents and 30 g visible fat per day for pregnant and lactating women respectively. It should be in the form of an oil containing at least 20% of linoleic acid. Apart from providing the essential fatty acid, *visible fat* in the diet has other desirable functions, such as improving the palatability and increasing the caloric density of the diet. A higher caloric density in the diet is essential for feeding young children so as to provide the needed calories.

Mustard oil (Brassica oil) contains erucic acid which should be reduced by blending with other oils. Reuse of refined oil over and again in deep frying operation makes it harmful due to release of certain toxic substances.

Saturated fatty acids (SFA): Stearic acid and short-chain fatty acid.

Unsaturated fatty acids: Lauric and myristic acid. These raise the level of cholesterol, however, stearic acid and some short-chain fatty acids do not raise the level of cholesterol.

Monounsaturated fatty acids (MUFA): Oleic acid. Oleic acid is monounsaturated fatty acid. It lowers blood cholesterol as effectively as essential fatty acid—linoleic acid. It also lowers serum triglycerides (VLDL).

Polyunsaturated fatty acids (PUFA) are linolenic and linoleic acid. These lower blood cholestrol level.

Quality of Fat—Essential Fatty Acids

Besides being a concentrated source of energy, fats are also a source of essential fatty acids (EFA). Fats are made up of fatty acids which include saturated fatty acids like palmitic and stearic, monosaturated fatty acids like oleic and polyunsaturated fatty acids (PUFA) like linoleic (Lin) and linolenic (Len). The latter two cannot be synthesized in the body and have to be supplied through dietary fats. These are known as essential fatty acids (EFA). Dietary fats with an appropriate proportion of saturated, monosaturated, and polyunsaturated fatty acids (PUFA) components have been considered as most desirable—1.0:1.5 : 1.0 [NFI-21(4), Oct., 2000]. EFA lowers the levels of cholesterol and triglycerides and hence protective against cardiovascular diseases. It raises the levels of protective lipids (HDL) and lowers the levels of dangerous lipid (LDL). Soya bean oil is high quality vegetable oil which contains EFA with cholesterol lowering function. A moderate consumption within the recommended dietary fat intake levels provides optimum health benefits. EFA also decreases thrombotic tendency of blood platelets. Fats like ghee, hydrogenated fats (vanaspati) and coconut oil are saturated and are poor sources of EFA. Other edible oils (rice bran and soya bean) are better sources of EFA (Table 6.11).

The *invisible fats* present in many Indian food materials have a high linoleic acid content. The average Indian diet predominantly based on cereals and some pulses including the diets of poor income groups carry sufficient linoleic acid levels and a proportion of linolenic acid as well. Although their diet may contain very low amount of *visible fat*, the quantity of EFA and the levels of invisible fats compensate for the lack (Table 6.11).

Fat Intake in India

Daily intake of visible fat varies from 6 to 22 g/day per consumption unit in rural India. In many states, as much as quarter of population may not have any visible fat at all in their diets. In urban area, in middle and upper income group, fat intake ranges from 22 to 45 g which is much higher than rural area where per capita availability of fat is worked out to be 15–17 g/day.

Upper Limit of Fat

Although a *minimal* intake of 12 g of *visible fat* can meet the requirement of EFA, a higher level of intake of 25 g/day is *desirable* to provide energy density and palatibility to the diet. Fat intake above a certain level is also undesirable, being associated with hazard like cardiovascular diseases and obesity.

Even in a predominantly cereal based diet would Contribute 15 g *invisible fat*, 50% of which would be EFA.

Table 6.11: Linoleic (Lin) and linolenic (Len) acid content of edible oils (g/100 g)

Oil	Lin	Len	Total EFA
Ghee	1.6	0.5	2.1
Coconut	2.0	–	2.0
Vanaspati	3.4	–	3.4
Palmolein	10.3	0.3	10.6
Rape/Mustard	18.1	14.5	32.6
Groundnut	29.9	–	29.9
Rice Bran Oil	34.3	1.4	35.7
Sesame (Til)	44.5	–	44.5
Cotton seed	50.9	–	50.9
Corn oil	57.4	–	57.4
Sunflower	66.2	Trace	66.2
Soya bean	50.7	6.5	57.2
Safflower	73.5	–	73.5

This with 20–40 g of *visible fat*, should meet EFA requirement of all age groups. However, the *upper limit* of *fat* in the diet should not exceed 30% calories—about 60 g/day. Total calories from visible fat should not exceed 10%.

Transfats (Hidden Fat)

Transfat in commercially fried and processed food is more hazardous than dietary cholesterol. Transfat is formed from chemical process known as "partial hydrogenation of vegetable oils" used to convert liquid oils into semi-solid form. The body is unable to breakdown transfat causing it to accumulate in the body. Transfat has been part of the urban diet for decades, enhancing the taste and shelf-life of popular packaged food products. The cheap and harmful oil is used in most processed foods, such as biscuits, instant noodles to deep fried *samosas* and *french fries*; *fried chickens*, frozen food cookies and candy, cake and pancake mixes, hard margarine is loaded with trans and saturated fats. While saturated fat—found in butter, cheese, red meat, and coconut and palm oil—raises cholesterol levels, transfat harms you further. It increases low density lipoprotein (LDL or bad cholesterol) and lowers heart protecting high density lipoprotein (HDL or good cholesterol). WHO recommends that transfats should not be consumed at all. From September 1, 2007 the use of transfats will have to be clearly listed on the food labels of all products manufactured in India.[6]

Vitamins and Minerals

Vitamins and minerals are protective nutrients and have specific metabolic functions in the body. They do not provide energy. Daily requirement of vitamin A (retinol), vitamin D, thiamine riboflavin, nicotinic acid (niacin), pyridoxine, vitamin B_{12}, vitamin C are given in Table 6.10. Important mineral/metals include—calcium, phosphorus, iron and magnesium and trace elements are—iodine, zinc, copper, chromium, cobalt, manganese, arsenic, fluoride and molybdenum.

FOOD GROUPS

Cereals

Rice, wheat and millets (Jowar, Bajra, Ragi, etc.) are the main cereal grains consumed in India. Cereals are the most widely eaten staples. These are cheapest sources of calories and they constitute as much as 70–80% of the calories in the diets of majority of the population in our country. In view of the large amounts in which cereals are included in the diet, they form important sources of nutrients in an average Indian diet. Most cereal grains contain 6–12% proteins and in general cereal proteins are deficient in the essential amino acid—lysine, which limits the protein quality of cereals. Rice protein, however, is richer in lysine compared to other cereal proteins and for this reason rice protein is of better quality.

Cereals are an excellent basis for the diet of young children in India, however because of their bulky nature the child is unable to eat enough hence cannot meet the energy requirement of young children. Energy density of cereals can be increased by adding fats and oils in cereal preparations.

Whole cereal grains are important sources of B-complex vitamins especially thiamine and nicotinic acid. Since these vitamins are present in the cereal grain in the outer bran layers, the vitamin content of the finished product depends upon the removal of the outer layers. Excessive milling of rice and excessive polishing of rice removes outer covering and hence decreases the thiamine content of rice. Parboiled rice on the other hand contains significant amount of thiamine because during the course of parboiling in which paddy is subjected to steaming or boiling in water, the vitamin seeps into the inner portions of the grain so that even if the grain is milled and polished, significant amount of vitamins are still retained in the grain. Cereal grains do not contain vitamin A except yellow maize which contains some amount of β-carotene. The total fat content in cereals vary from 2 to 5%. Considering the amount of cereals consumed, it is estimated that fat present in cereals in our diet can meet more than 50% of essential fatty acid requirement. Cereals together with pulses can nearly meet the EFA of adult. On an average 470 g of cereals were available per person per day in India (2011–12).

Whole wheat flour contains more B vitamins, iron and calcium than white flour. Whole wheat also contains more phytates and "dietary fibre" which interferes with the absorption of iron and calcium. Cereals are deliberately withheld in the diet of young children because of wrong beliefs.

Pulses (Legumes)

Pulses are rich in proteins. Pulse proteins, however, are of relatively low biological value because of deficiency of the essential amino acid—methionine. Red gram is deficient in tryptophan also, however, pulse proteins are rich in lysine and they are therefore of good supplementary value to cereal diets. Eight parts of cereals and one part of pulses make good combination and supplement. The lysine deficient in cereals is made good by the lysine present in pulses and thus, the overall biological value of cereal pulse diet is better. Pulses are rich in B vitamin, especially thiamine and folic acid. Sprouted pulses especially sprouted green gram and Bengal gram become rich source of vitamin C and folic acid. Most pulses contains 18–20% of proteins and soya bean contains 40% of proteins. Pulses with their higher content of total fat (visible and invisible) contribute along with cereals to meet the essential fatty acids needs of an adult. On an average 29 g of pulses per capita per day is the availability in India.

Legumes

Legumes contain some natural toxins but usually this is removed by soaking or in normal cooking procedures. *Khesari dal* (*Lathyrus sativus*) contains toxin BOAA (β-oxalyl amino alanine) which can be removed by soaking the pulse in water for sometime before cooking. Legumes are good for young children provided these are cooked and finely mashed and can be mixed with other food items. Trypsin inhibitor is present in soya bean which can be removed by soaking soya bean in water overnight and cooking thereafter.

Soya bean oil is excellent source of EFA and tocopherol (vitamin E) and this makes it high quality vegetable oil.

Nuts and Oil Seeds

Like pulses, nuts and oil seeds are also rich in proteins and in addition they contain fat (almond, cashewnut, groundnuts contain 20–25% protein) so they are rich in calories also (570–650 calories per 100 g). Most of oil seeds produced in the country are used for extraction of edible oil and the cakes left after extraction are richer in proteins. Off flavour can be removed and cakes can be made suitable for human consumption. Oil seeds proteins are of low biological values because of relative deficiency of amino acid—methionine. Sesame protein, however, is relatively richer in this amino acid as also the sunflower seed protein.

When nuts are stored for long time a fungus *Aspergillus flavus* grows on nuts and produces aflatoxin and this toxin may cause liver damage thus only clean and wholesome groundnuts should be used as food.

Green Leafy Vegetables (GLV)

Many types of green leaves, such as palak, amaranth, fenugreek leaves, drumstick leaves, mint, coriander, mustard leaves, colocasia leaves, raddish and turnip leaves as also Chenopodium (bathua) are rich sources of iron, β-carotene, vitamin C, riboflavin and folic acid and calcium. Besides these vitamins and minerals, green leafy vegetables provide "dietary fibre"and antioxidants. Green leafy vegetables are therefore inexpensive sources of many nutrients which are essential for growth and maintenance of health. Green leafy vegetables can be grown in kitchen garden or in farm and field, some grow wild, their consumption should be promoted. Distressingly intake of GLV in Indian diet is no more than 15 g per day/CU against the recommended daily intake of 50–100 g per day. In place of fruits, green leafy vegetables should be recommended for poor families to improve their diet.

Root vegetables: Root vegetables are tapioca, potato, sweet potato, carrots, yam and colocasia. They all are rich in carbohydrate and provide energy. Carrots and some varieties of yam are also rich in β-carotene and food like potato contains significant amount of vitamin C. At times of cereal shortages, root vegetables can serve as an emergency food in famines and drought.

Other vegetables: These include brinjals, lady fingers, French beans, gourds, pumpkins. Some of these are rich sources of vitamins and minerals besides dietary fibre.

Fruits: Fresh fruits are generally good sources of vitamin C and amla is especially rich source of this vitamin. Yellow fruits like mango and papaya contain β-carotene in addition and dried fruits like dates and raisins are rich sources of iron. The commonly used banana is a fruit rich in carbohydrate and therefore yields energy also. If the green leafy vegetables are included in the diet in sufficient quantities, the need for fruit as an essential item in the diet is much reduced. Fruits also contain pectins (dietary fibre) which provide bulk to the diet and helps bowel movement, reduce blood sugar of cholestrol levels.

Bioactive Phytochemicals

Bioactive phytochemicals include dietary fibre, antioxidants and detoxifying agents. These are present in fruits and vegetables. These are non-nutrient chemicals but have significant role in prevention of diseases, such as colon cancer, diabetes, cardiovascular diseases, cataract and gallstones, constipation and diverticulosis.

Dietary Fibre (DF)

Dietary fibre is the remanent of the edible part of plants and analogues carbohydrates that are resistant to digestion and absorption in the human small intestine with complete or partial fermentation in the human large intestine. It includes: polysaccharides, oligosaccharides, lignin and associated plant substances. Dietary fibre exhibits one or more of either laxation (fecal bulking and softening, increased frequency and or regularity), blood cholesterol attenuation and or blood glucose attenuation. There has been overwhelming evidence that dietary fibre is essential to maintain body weight and composition, blood level of sugar (low glycaemic index), triglycerides and cholesterol. Glycaemic index of blood is defined as the area under two hours blood glucose response curve (AUC) following the ingestion of a fixed portion of test carbohydrate (usually 50 g either glucose or white bread) as a proportion (%) of AUC of the standard.

DF is further divided into Insoluble Dietary Fibre (IDF) and Soluble Dietary Fibre (SDF). The sum of these two fractions is also known as Total Dietary Fibre (TDF). The IDF fractions are—cellulose, lignin and some portion of hemicelluloses. The cereals, seeds, beans, many fruits and vegetables, bran and whole grains are food sources of insoluble dietary fibre. IDF is composed of structural components of plant cell. The SDF fraction are—pectins gums, β-glucans, mucilages of major portion of hemicelluloses. Soluble dietary fibre is derived from "maltodextrins", inulin (from wheat, onion, banana and chicory) or oligofructose. While the IDF is known to reduce constipation and diverticulosis, the SDF is effective in delaying the *absorption of glucose* and delay the *secretion of insulin* as also *lower lipid level* and *cholestrol* levels by binding bile salts, removing bile acids and neutral sterols by excretion through faeces and inhibit cholesterol biosynthesis.

Fenugreek seeds (methi seeds) which have high levels of IDF (48.6%) and SDF (20.0 g%) is very effective in reducing blood glucose and cholesterol levels. Since TDF contributes bulk to diets, it may help in reducing energy intake and thus useful for reducing obesity. Adverse effect of DF include prevention of absorption of trace minerals like iron. The dietary fibre consists of wide range of complex polysaccharides, such as cellulose, hemicellulose, pectins, gums, mucins and lignins with different chemical physicochemical and physiological properties. These have biological functions, such as water holding capacity, delay in nutrient absorption and binding toxins and bile acids besides lowering of blood cholestrol and lipids and reducing incidence of coronary heart disease, type II diabetes and obesity. The suggested intake of TDF is 20–35 g/day or 40 g/2000 kcal in diet is considered reasonably safe.

Antioxidants

Dietary antioxidants include nutrients, such as β-carotene, provitamin A, ascorbic acid—vitamin C, tocopherols, tocotrienols, riboflavin, sulphur amino acids, cysteine and methionine and selenium. Similarly, non-nutrient antioxidants are various carotenoids, flavinoids, Anthracyanins and indoles. These agents remove free radicals, such as oxygen (O_2^-), superoxide, hydroxyl, peroxide and lipid peroxide. These agents inhibit lipid peroxidation. These agents lower cholesterol level and promote HDL levels, prevent cancer, cardiovascular diseases and cataract. Phytochemicals also help in detoxification, i.e. detoxification of drugs, toxicants, carcinogens and mutagens. Antioxidants are present in green leafy vegetables, plant foods and fruits like papaya, turmeric, palm oil, amla and guava.

Milk and Milk Products

Milk is ideal food for infants and children and is a good supplementary food for adults. It contains proteins (3.2–4.3%) of good quality and also other nutrients in proper proportion and it is thus a complete food. Milk is rich in calcium. It is however, deficient in vitamin C and iron. Human milk contains more lactose and buffalo milk contains more fat as compared to cow's milk. Curd has the same nutritive value as that of milk. The nutrient contents of dried milk is more or less the same as that of milk on a moisture free basis. Milk consumption should be promoted. White revolution and operation "flood" has led to increased production and consumption of milk and milk products. Milk is available in various forms because of advance in technologies. Cow's and buffalo's milk contain 3.2 and 4.3% proteins respectively while human milk contains 1.1% protein.

Sugar and Jaggery

Sugar and jaggery are mainly sources of energy, though jaggery contains iron in addition. Frequent consumption of sugar in between meals increases the incidence of caries and excessive consumption may lead to obesity.

Flesh Foods

Flesh foods, such as fish and meat are rich in proteins of high biological value and in B vitamins, especially vitamin B_{12} is contained only in foods of animal origin and not in plant foods. Protein content of flesh foods is around 20%. Flesh foods are generally not good sources of vitamin A; but liver which is very rich in vitamin A is an exception. Fish is a good source of calcium, especially small varieties which are consumed whole. Fish also contain polyunsaturated fatty acids which protect against cardiovascular diseases. Haem iron of flesh foods is better absorbed than non-haem iron.

Eggs

Egg is a rich source of nutrients except vitamin C. The protein present in egg is considered to be perfect protein and because of its high biological value and digestibility, the egg protein is used in nutrition work as a *reference protein*. Protein content of egg is 13.3%. Raw egg-white contains a protein known as avidin, which renderes the vitamin biotin unavailable to the body. Duck egg contains trypsin inhibitor, heating and boiling destroys both avidin and the trypsin inhibitor.

Condiments and Spices

These are used as seasoning or flavouring agents in food to increase their acceptability. Some of the condiments like chillies and coriander are good sources of carotene. Green chillies supply vitamin C and turmeric and tamarind are fair sources of antioxidants and iron. Many of the condiments and spices are used in small quantities hence do not add substantially to the nutritive value of the diet.

Salt

Salt is universally consumed. Salt intake in India is 10–15 g per person per day. Salt is being universally iodated to eliminate IDDs. Now NIN recommends 6 g of salt consumption per person pre day.

CHARACTERISTIC OF AN AVERAGE INDIAN DIET

The Indian diets are highly cereal-based, particularly of the weaker economic sections. In the case of majority of population, cereals form almost the bulk of diet and constitute the major source, if not the only source of nutrients and provide 80% of energy. These diets are deficient in pulses, green leafy vegetables, oils and fats as also fruits. Most staple used are—rice in Southern parts and wheat in North India but the trend of mixed cereals consumption is emerging. The diets of even poor people which consist of predominant cereals and have little or no visible fats consist significant quantities of invisible fats. The invisible fat from cereals and pulses alone contributes as much as 6 energy% or 16 g of invisible fat in adult diet-that provides 2400 kcal. In average Indian diet in many parts of the country, the total visible plus invisible fat contributes about 15% of the dietary energy. Cereals are deliberately withheld from the diets of infants and young children or given in small quantities (inadequate amounts). Varied kinds of dietary beliefs and practices are prevalent in the community which lead to malnutrition in young children besides wide spread infections due to bad environments and poor personal hygiene.

These diets can be improved by eating mixed cereals or by adding coarse cereals (millets) as also locally grown leafy vegetables, butter milk and increased use of pulses and local fruits. Cheap flesh foods if available locally (such as fish) can be encouraged. Cost of balanced diet is prohibitive. Use of health facilities to supplement iron and folic acid as also vitamin A nutrient and supplementary feeding through Anganwadi can help to some extent but the people have to develop self-reliance to improve their diets.

Another improvement which can be effected is improvement of cooking practices, not to discard cooking water. It is advisable to use minimum quantity of water or to utilize cooking liquor in either soups or gravies. It is not advisable to peel and cut the vegetables long before they are ready for boiling. Excessive washing of rice should be avoided to save vitamin B (thiamine). The rice conjee, which is strained away after cooking also carries with thiamine and nicotinic acid. Tamarind when added to cooking water preserves vitamins.

Balanced diet: A balanced diet is defined as one which provides all the nutrients in proper proportion (carbohydrates, proteins, fats, vitamins and minerals and salt) to meet human requirements for different physiological functions—growth, pregnancy, lactation and maintainence of body weight and body functions. The amount of each nutrient needed for an individual depends on age, body weight and physiological status.

Balanced Diet (Moderately Active Man) ICMR-NIN

Food composition	Amount g/day
Cereals and millets	400
Animal food[1]	60
Pulses (legumes)[1]	80
Green leafy vegetables	50
Other vegetables	150
Roots and tubers	100
Fruits	100
Milk	300 ml
Oil and fat	30
Sugar and jaggery	40
Nuts and oil seeds	25

[1] Protein content depends on the type of protein containing foods. Pulses can be replaced with animal foods (egg, meat, fish and chicken) for non-vegetarians to meet the requirements.

This diet provides 2730 kcal, 80 g of protein, 30 g of visible fats, 850 mg calcium, 20 mg iron, 12 mg zinc, 600 μg vitamin A, 2.0 mg Vit B_1, 1.5 mg riboflavin, 20 mg niacin, 2.0 mg Vit B_6, 80 mg Vit C, 250 μg folate and 0.40 μg Vit B_{12}.

Common Dietary Beliefs and Practices in India

Many dietary beliefs and practices are strongly held by individual, family and community, in almost all the regions or different parts of the country. Some of these beliefs and practices are detrimental or harmful and produce malnutrition in young children, pregnant women and lactating mothers. Some of the dietary beliefs and indigenous practices are good, hence need to be promoted. Some of the common prevalent dietary beliefs and practices are being elaborated:

The concept of hot and 'cold' foods is widely prevalent, similarly some foods are considered 'heavy' and others as 'light'. These concepts and beliefs affect food choices and many dietary restrictions are imposed on the diets of young infants, children, pregnant women and lactating mothers and consequently the undernutrition or malnutrition develops in vulnerable groups.

Jaggery, sugar, halwa, groundnuts, almonds, coconut, raisins, palm dates, fried foods, mangoes, millets, maize, eggs, and meat are believed to be 'hot' and heat producing foods and related with occurrence of abortion, hence avoided by pregnant women. Papaya is strongly suspected to cause abortion, hence not touched by any pregnant women. Buttermilk, curd, milk, green grams, green leafy vegetable, barley flour, and apple are labelled as 'cold' foods hence encouraged during pregnancy.

Black grams, beans, halwa (sweetened wheat porridge), whole buffalo milk and ghee (animal fat) are generally believed to be 'heavy' foods, being associated with indigestion and colic hence avoided by mothers and discouraged during illness like fever, diarrhoea and respiratory infections. Rice + green gram dal, curd, wheat porridge (dalia), sago porridge, bread slices, diluted milk, butter milk are believed to be 'light' foods hence encouraged during pregnancy and ailment like diarrhoea, fevers and respiratory infections.

Rice, potatoes, cauliflower are commonly believed to be 'wind' producing foods and for that reason are seasoned with variety of condiments to the likes of individual and family. Cucumber, and watermelon are considered to be cold and windy foods and suspected to cause joint pains, body aches, etc. Such strong beliefs are entertained by most families over generations and have become way of life.

Ghee is valued most nutritious and is encouraged in the diet of adults and working men, while cereals and ghee and green leafy vegetables are considered bad for young children and associated with, cough, protuberance of abdomen, and bad for liver, hence avoided or given in very small quantities. Parents believe that young child cannot digest cereals and green leafy vegetables. Whole milk is diluted several times as it is thought to be heavy for young children. It is a common practice to add four parts of water to one part of milk. Several dietary restrictions are imposed during diarrhoea, fever and respiratory infection. Similarly, nursing mothers are forbidden to eat pulses, green leafy vegetables, Bengal grams, cereals and milk for variable period. Ghee, sugar and jaggery and coconut are encouraged with the belief that these foods help in evacuation of secretions of uterus and helps involution of uterus.

It must be realized that many of these beliefs and practices are deep rooted, and it may not be possible to fully modify the attitudes and change the behaviours in a short period of time. Under the circumstances, we can achieve the desired objectives to a large extent if we build on these beliefs and practices and incorporate positive messages without any cultural conflict.

By suggesting suitable combination of the so-called 'hot food' with cold food and of heavy food with light foods in desired proportions, we could overcome the usual objections.

Seasoning of so-called cold foods with condiments like cumin, ginger, onion, dalchini, pepper, cloves and cardamom, was exploited fully to reduce the effect of 'cold' and 'windy' foods. Mothers did not hesitate to try such food combinations. Use of curd, rice and green gram dal (Khichri) is acceptable during acute watery diarrhoeal episodes and we promoted its use to prevent and treat dehydration. Mothers agreed to give plenty of water and use ORS solution as also weak tea during diarrhoea.

Knowing these dietary beliefs and practices helps to effect changes in behaviour by nutrition education programme. Encourage foods which are liked most. Since most families and mothers believe that diarrhoea occurs due to teething problem and associated with hot and cold weather, one should act and advice accordingly. Curd, butter milk and light foods (rice + green grams) which are culturally acceptable must be encouraged. One must respect culture, beliefs, traditions and effect minimum changes to improve the nutrition of young children, pregnant women and lactating mothers. Good dietary practices, such as breastfeeding, eating mixed cereals, consumption of green leafy vegetables by pregnant women should be promoted. Indigenous recipes must be encouraged as these are time tested and most nutritious. Knowledge of dietary beliefs, practices, taboos helps to formulate a better nutrition education programme.

Junk Foods

Globalization has brought a lot of changes in food habits of children and adolescents, "Junk food" refers to "empty calories" lacking in ideal nutrients and mainly consists of excess of sugar, salt and fats. Most urban population, youth in particular thrive on junk foods, which are refined carbohydrates rich in calories, low in vitamins and dietary fibre. These foods contain lot of calories and lot of saturated fat. Salted snack food, candy, gum, most sweet desserts, fried fast foods and carbonated beverages are considered by most as junk foods.[7]

Junk foods and fast foods are not only calorigenic but leads to obesity and rise of low density lipids and fall of high density lipids (or good cholesterol). The centre has recently asked state governments to ban the sale of junk foods and carbonated drinks on the school premises. Good quality foods like dal, roti, sprouts and green leafy vegetables should be promoted as mid-day meal.

UNDERNUTRITION DURING INFANCY

Birth weight: The first weight of the fetus or newborn obtained after birth.

Low birth weight (LBW): Less than 2500 g (up to and including 2499 g).

Very low birth weight: Less than 1500 g (up to and including 1499 g).

Extremely low birth weight: Less than 1000 g (up to and including 999 g).[8]

One-third (30–33%) of the babies born in India were low birth weight babies (undernourished in the womb) who weighed less than 2.5 kg. According to NFHS-3 data 22% of babies born in India were of low birth weight, while according to UNICEF (2012) report 28% of births were low birth weight (Table 6.12). Those babies have a poor start of life cycle and are exposed to the risk of morbidity

Table 6.12: Percentage of infants with low birth weight*		
South Asia	1994	2009–13
Bangladesh	50	22
India	33	28
Nepal	26	18
Pakistan	25	32
Sri Lanka	25	17

*Human development report: UNDP Oxford University Press, 1994 and the state of World Children 2009 and 2012.

and mortality. Average birth weight in India has not much improved (Table 6.12).[9] In India, an average birth weight ranges from 2.7 to 2.9 kg.

The problem of LBW in India is widespread and multifactorial. A newborn baby can be LBW because of two reasons:

- Preterm
- Intrauterine growth retardation (IUGR)

Intrauterine growth retardation (IUGR) is a problem of great magnitude. Over two-thirds of babies are *small* for *gestational age* (SGA), i.e. they are full term babies, from 37 completed weeks to less than 42 completed weeks (259–293 days) of gestation and remaining one-third are born *pre-term*, i.e. less than 37 completed weeks of gestation (less than 259 days).

The first important cause of malnutrition is—low birth weight itself—a form of malnutrition, which began in mother's womb. Low birth weight is associated with poor growth during infancy and thereafter throughout childhood period.

Retrospectively, low birth weight reflects poor nutritional and health status of women during pregnancy, adolescence and during childhood period.

Low birth weight is reflection of maternal and foetal malnutrition.[10] The problem of LBW is multidimensional.

Prevention of LBW: Public health interventions to reduce the incidence of LBW are avoid teenage pregnancies, improve the nutritional status of women, correct anaemia in pregnancy, full antenatal care, rest during pregnancy, malaria prophylaxis and treatment in endemic areas besides improving literacy, spacing births at least two years apart and limiting the size of family.

Needs of infant are (0–6 months of life): Survival, adequate growth and development and prevention of infections.

Strategies for prevention of malnutrition during infancy are: Exclusive breastfeeding up to 6 months of age, complementary feeding, immunization, growth monitoring and integrated management of illness.

Exclusive breastfeeding: Promotion of universal exclusive breastfeeding is the national policy and it has been incorporated in reproductive and child health (RCH) programme as also in integrated child development services (ICDS). WHO in its guidelines recommends exclusive breastfeeding for the 6 months rather than the first 4–6 months.

Promotion of exclusive breastfeeding until the age of 6 months in developing countries through existing primary health care services is feasible, reduces the risk of diarrhoea and does not lead to growth faltering.[11]

What is Exclusive Breastfeeding?

Exclusive breastfeeding implies giving newborn infants no food or drink other than breast milk (including milk expressed or from wet nurse). It allows the infant to receive drops, syrups (vitamins and minerals, medicines). It does not allow the infant to receive anything else.[12] WHO global data bank gives various definitions which are reproduced below in Table 6.13.

Breastfeeding Promotion

International code of marketing of breast milk substitutes was adopted by WHO in 1981 and subsequently Indian National Code for Protection and promotion of breastfeeding was evolved by Government of India.[13,14] These

Table 6.13: Definition of infant feeding

Category of infant feeding	Requires that the infant receives	Allows the infant to receive	Does not allow the infant to receive
Exclusive breastfeeding	Breast milk (including milk expressed or from wet nurse)	Drops, syrups (vitamins, minerals, medicines)	Anything else
Predominant breastfeeding	Breast milk (including milk expressed or from wet nurse) as the predominant Source of nourishment	Liquids (water, and water-based drinks, fruit juice, ORS), ritual fluids and drops, syrups (vitamins, minerals, medicines)	Anything else (in particular, non-human milk, food based fluids)
Complementary feeding	Breast milk and solid or semisolid foods	Any food or liquid including non-human milk	–
Breastfeeding	Breast milk	Any food or liquid including non-human milk	–
Bottle feeding	Any liquid or semi-solid food from a Bottle with nipple/teat	Any food or liquid including non-human milk. Also allows breast milk by bottle	–

6

codes aimed at provision of safe and adequate nutrition to infants by protection and promotion of breastfeeding and by ensuring proper use of breast milk substitutes when these are necessary.

The code applies to the marketing and practices related thereto of following products:

Breast milk substitutes including infant formula, other milk products, foods and beverages, including bottle fed complementary foods; feeding bottle and teats.

In India, the breastfeeding is 'universal practice'. Let it be promoted and preserved. It is best practice and offers the young infant best feed. Most mothers in India continue breastfeeding up to 2 years or even beyond it; is also best practice for child survival and adequate growth.

From Universal Breastfeeding to Exclusive Breastfeeding

Exclusive breastfeeding in Indian culture is nothing new. It was advocated by UNICEF and WHO in 1989 and thereafter in 1992 by Baby Friendly Hospital Initiative (BFHI) and subsequently World Health Assembly (WHA 54: 2; 18) May, 2001 adopted the resolution to approve exclusive breastfeeding for first 6 months.[12–15]

Benefits of Exclusive Breastfeeding

- It ensures intake of colostrum.
- Provides optimal and adequate nutrition.
- No water supplementation is required.
- Reduces risk of various infectious and noninfectious diseases.
- Contributes to better intelligence.
- Promotes emotional development between mother and baby.
- Prevents breast problems in mothers.
- Reduces risk of breast and ovarian cancer; iron deficiency anaemia.
- Helps in birth spacing.

Goals of 10th Plan

- Enhance early initiation of breastfeeding (colostrum feeding) from the current level of 15.8 to 50%.
- Enhance the exclusive breastfeeding rate for children up to age of 6 months from the current rate of 55.2 to 80%.
- Enhance the complementary feeding rate at 6 months from the current level of 33.5 to 75%.[1]

Infant Feeding Practices in India: NFHS-2 and 3

Recently the NFHS-3 (2005–06) data provided cardinal information on breastfeeding practices in India.

Breastfeeding initiation: Breastfeeding is "life line" for newborn babies, should be started immediately after birth. In our culture, several ceremonies are performed, these should be performed quickly and breastfeeding should be commenced immediately after birth.

Although breastfeeding after birth is nearly universal practice in India, very few children are put on breastfeeding immediately after birth. Only 23.4% of newborn babies were put on breastfeeding within one hour of birth and only 37% of mothers initiated breastfeeding within one day. Nearly two-thirds of women (63%) squeezed the first milk from the breast (discarded colostrum) before they began breastfeeding (NFHS-2). Thus initiation of breastfeeding is delayed and newborn is deprived of most nutritious feed and energy.

Exclusive Breastfeeding—Recent Report

Only 44.6% of mothers initiated breastfeeding within one hour after birth. In India, 64% of children till 6 months of age were exclusively breastfed and the remaining children (36%) received breastfeeding plus fluids and supplementary feeds. As 64% of children were exclusively fed on breast at 6 months of age and thus over 36% of children were exposed to the risk of infections—predominant being diarrhoeal diseases. The introduction of supplementary foods before 6 months of age may put infants at risk of malnutrition because other liquids and solids are nutritiously inferior to breast milk. Consumption of liquids and solid mashed foods at an early age also increases children's exposure to pathogens and consequently puts them at a greater risk of diarrhoea (NFHS-3).

Bottle Feeding

Practice of bottle feeding is prevalent in 16% of mothers this is also a risk factor for diarrhoea and malnutrition in young children.

Feeding Low Birth Weight (LBW) Babies

Mother's milk is the best food for low birth weight babies. The borderline, term, and growth retarded LBW babies can suckle fairly well at the breast and should be fed on demand. Breast milk saves the lives of LBW babies and ensures growth and development. Mothers need to be adequately supported and even weak babies can suck and can be optimally fed on breast. Breast milk is enough for their requirement, no supplementary foods are needed. However, LBW and other high-risk infants who cannot suckle should be given expressed breast milk in preference to formula feeds by appropriate techniques. Mothers can be helped to express their milk every 3 hours and feeding the expressed milk to the baby with a cup and spoon or if necessary by nasogastric tube, helping the baby to suckle at mother's breast, which helps the babies to develop the ability to suck besides stimulating maternal milk production. Keeping LBW baby with mother 24 hours a day and breastfeeding regularly have been quite helpful (Kangaroo mother care). Breast milk offers nutritional advantage to LBW babies because of its higher proteins, essential fatty acids and electrolyte concentration helps increase in weight. Formula foods are no better for LBW babies.

Ten Steps to Successful Breastfeeding (WHO-UNICEF and BFHI)[15]

Every facility providing maternity services and care for newborn infants should:

1 Have a written breastfeeding policy that is routinely communicated to all health care staff.
2 Train all health care staff in skills necessary to implement this policy.
3 Inform all pregnant women about the benefits and management of breastfeeding.
4 Help mothers initiate breastfeeding within half an hour of birth.
5 Show mothers how to breastfed, and how to maintain lactation even if they are separated from their infants.
6 Give newborn infants no food or drink other than breast milk unless medically indicated.
7 Practise rooming in-allow mothers and infants to remain together—24 hours a day.
8 Encourage breastfeeding on demand.
9 Give no artificial teats or pacifiers (also called dummies or soothers) to breastfeeding infants.
10 Foster the establishment of breastfeeding support groups and refer mothers to them on discharge from the hospital or clinic.
   - Eliminate any support by the manufacturers of infant formula/infant food or feeding bottles.
   - Prohibit distribution of free and low cost supplies of breast milk substitutes.
   - Provide additional lactation assistance to mother of special cases: LBW, and caesarean section.
   - Assure a safe, healthy and positive birthing experience for the mother and infant.

What we have Done in India?

Baby Friendly Hospital Initiative (BFHI), launched by UNICEF and WHO now recommends that infant should be given only breast milk for first 6 months of their life. Most babies do not require any other foods or liquids during this period. Water supplementation or prelacteal meals are unnecessary and dangerous. Use of non-nutritive liquids is associated with decline in breast milk intake.

India has a written policy on infant feeding (national guidelines on infant and young child feeding). However, policy on infant and young child feeding has been revised in 2004 which advocates exclusive breastfeeding for first 6 months, and continuation of breastfeeding up to 2 years of age or beyond and promoting feeding of colostrum.[16,17]

The Government of India has taken positive and effective legal measures to protect breastfeeding from the commercial influence and support women at work. The infant milk substitutes, feeding bottles and infant foods (regulation of production, supply and distribution) Act, 1992 (Infant Milk Substitutes Act) and cable TV Network Amendment Act, 2000 and Maternity Benefit Act of 26 weeks of maternity leave are the examples of supporting women and promoting exclusive breastfeeding. Infant, milk substitute (IMS) Act has been further strengthened through "IMS Amendment Act, 2003" enhancing the protective level.

Breastfeeding during Illness in Young Children

Breast milk is most easily digestible food for an ill baby. Breastfeeding is beneficial in common infantile ailments including diarrhoea and acute respiratory infections. Breastfeeding should be continued during such illnesses. The child may suckle less vigorously or for a shorter time and should receive the feed at more frequent intervals. Exclusive breastfed babies have least chances of developing diarrhoea.

Maternal Illness and Breastfeeding

Most common maternal illnesses do not require discontinuation of breastfeeding. Breastfeeding is recommended even with mastitis, breast abscess and other infections, illnesses including urinary tract infections, tuberculosis, HIV positive mothers, hepatitis and other viral illnesses. If initiation of breastfeeding is delayed for one or two days, it can result into breast abscess because of milk stasis. Initiation of breastfeeding immediately after birth is important and helpful and benefits both mother and infant. As soon as the infant starts suckling at the breast, the hormone oxytocin is released, resulting in uterine contraction that facilitates expulsion of the placenta and reduces the risk of postpartum haemorrhage. It also helps in faster involution of uterus.

Colostrum: First milk is rich in nutrients. It is recommended that first breast milk (colostrum) should be given to the child rather than squeezed from the breast and discarded because it provides natural immunity to the child.

Breastmilk Substitutes

If a mother cannot for some reason exclusively breastfed her young child below 6 months, e.g. a working mother, her expressed milk should be given to the child in preference to formula milk. If it is unavoidable to give non-human milk during first 6 months of life, undiluted milk normally consumed by the family should be utilized. Of course such situations rarely arise. For infants, part of excessive fat in buffalo's milk should be removed by separating the cream from milk after boiling and cooling to room temperature.

Breastfeeding and Fertility

Breastfeeding helps spacing children and it is known to the mankind since ancient times. Full and exclusive breastfeeding for first 6 months serves as contraceptive; this method may not have absolute efficacy but it does play an important role in spacing births and preventing pregnancies. Cu-T is highly advisable contraceptive in the postpartum period.

Continue Frequent Breastfeeding up to 2 Years of Age or Beyond

In India in addition to exclusive breastfeeding till six months, continued breastfeeding beyond 6 months up to 2 years or beyond along with other good practices like addition of safe, hygienic adequate and timely complementary food is important to prevent malnutrition in young children. Breast milk provides 413, 379 and 346 kcal/day at 6–8, 9–11 and 12–23 months of age. Since, NFHS-2 indicates that 15.6% of infants are underweight at 0–6 months, 43.3% at 6–11 months and 63.4% at 12–23 months hence breastfeeding is a saviour and prevents malnutrition by providing additional energy.

The global strategy on infant and young child feeding has been adopted by World Health Assembly Resolution (55.25/May 2002) which endorses exclusive breastfeeding and urges the nations to evolve policy on infant and young child feeding and action plans.[18–20]

Exclusive breastfeeding for first six months is a strategy to lower neonatal and postneonatal infant mortality and this strategy assumes significance for LBW as most LBW babies survive with exclusive breastfeeding and more would die if exclusive breastfeeding was not there—Breastfeeding and Promotion Network of India (BPNI).[20]

WHO Indicators of Breastfeeding Practices

These include: Ever breastfed rate, exclusive breastfeeding rate and the timely complementary feeding rate. The exclusive breastfeeding rate is defined as proportion of infants under age 6 months who receive only breast milk.

Timely complementary feeding rate is the proportion of infants aged 6–9 months who receive both breast milk and solid or semisolid food.

The continued breastfeeding rate through one year of age is the proportion of children aged 12–15 months who are still breastfed. Continued breastfeeding rate until two years of age is proportion of children aged 20–23 months who are still breastfed.

The bottle feeding rate is proportion of infants who are using a bottle with a nipple.

HIV and Breastfeeding

The increasing threat of perinatal transmission resulting in an alarming incidence of pediatric AIDS cases is posing a challenge globally. HIV in industrialized countries is a clear contraindication to breastfeeding. An update review of incidence of mother to baby transmission of HIV through breastfeeding in 1997 estimates that the risk is only 12–14%. In a developing country like ours where the hazards of bottle feeding with formula milk have been well documented including repeated diarrhoeal episodes and consequent malnutrition and deaths during infancy. All mothers should be explained this risk and decision after informed choices should rest with the mother. When children born to women with HIV/AIDS can be ensured uninterrupted access to nutritionally adequate breast milk substitutes that are safely/hygienically prepared and fed to young children are at less risk of disease and death (UNICEF and WHO) if they are not breastfed. More research is needed on this subject.[21]

Protecting, Promoting and Supporting Breastfeeding

Protection means having legal framework and protecting breastfeeding women from commercial influence. Promotion means giving full information to women and families about benefits and advantages of breastfeeding and support means women receive skilled support of health workers, community workers and community.[22]

Health workers should focus on exclusive breastfeeding for first 6 months and continued breastfeeding for up to 2 years along with appropriate and timely complementary foods that are started at the age of 6 months. Mothers need information support during antenatal, delivery and postnatal period. All contacts during these stages should impart information on breastfeeding and prepare mothers for the act of breastfeeding. Home visits, clinic visits and hospital situations should promote information on breastfeeding. These steps would translate UNICEF and WHO initiative of 1989 to protect, promote and support breastfeeding globally into meaningful action.

National Guidelines on Promotion of Infant and Young Child Feeding (2004)

These guidelines have been prepared by food and nutrition board of the department of women and child development based on the global strategy on infant and young child feeding adopted during the 55th World Health Assembly. The appropriate infant and young child feeding practices include:[23]

- i Early initiation of breastfeeding within half an hour of birth.
- ii Feeding of colostrum.
- iii Exclusive breastfeeding for the first 6 months.
- iv Introduction of complementary feeding at 6 months of age.
- v Staple cereal of the family should be used to make the first food for infant.
- vi Encourage time tested traditional foods (Khichdi, Dalia, Kheer, Upma, Dokhla, etc.).
- vii Encourage foods which are routinely cooked in the family.
- viii Energy density of infant foods should be increased by adding teaspoonful of oil or ghee in every feed or by adding sugar and Jaggery.
- ix Infant and young child should be fed 5–6 times a day.
- x Continue breastfeeding up to the age of two years or beyond.

xi Appropriate feeding during and after illness.

xii ***HIV and breastfeeding:*** The absolute risk of HIV transmission through breastfeeding for more than one year is 10–20%. HIV positive mothers should receive counselling on risk and benefits of various feeding options.

xiii Growth monitoring and promotion.

xiv Feeding in difficult circumstances.

REFERENCES

1 GOI. Tenth Five-Year Plan 2002–07. Vol II: New Delhi: GOI; 2002.

2 Sunday Times of India, Bangalore April 30, 2006 'Swaminomics'. S Anklesaria Aiyar "India the new commodity gluton."

3 ICMR. Nutritive values of Indian Foods. 2007, National Institute of Nutrition, Hyderabad.

4 ICMR. Nutrient requirements and recommended dietary allowances for Indians. ICMR; 1992, New Delhi.

5 FAO. Joint FAO/WHO report 1977 Sept. Rome: Food and Agriculture Organisation of United Nations; 1977; p. 44.

6 Sanchita Sharma. Fat lot of Harm. Sunday Hindustan Times, Chandigarh, March 18, 2007.

7 Pai JS. Impact of Junk Foods on obesty and nutritional intake. "In touch". Heinz Nutrition Foundation India. Vol 7, Number 3, October-December, 2005.

8 WHO. International Classification of Diseases (ICD-10). Geneva: WHO; 1993.

9 NIHFW. Newsletter 2002 July-Sept.; 3(3).

10 Swaminathan MS. Ensuring access to balanced diets and safe drinking water. NFI Bulletin 2003; 3(2).

11 Bhandari N, Bahl R, Mazumdar S, Martines J, Black RE, Bhan MK and other members of Infant Feeding Study Group. Effect of community based promotion of exclusive breastfeeding on diarrhoeal illness. Lancet 2003; 361: 1418–23.

12 Gupta A, Mathur GP, Jindal T, Dadhich JP. Breastfeeding. BPNI Technical Info Series-2, 2003.

13 WHO. International code on marketing of breast milk substitutes. Geneva: WHO; 1981.

14 GOI. Indian National code for protection and promotion of breastfeeding. New Delhi: Ministry of Social Welfare GOI; 1983.

15 WHO/UNICEF. Protecting, promoting and supporting breastfeeding—The special role of maternity services. Geneva: WHO; 1989.

16 GOI. National guidelines on infant feeding. New Delhi: Food and Nutrition Board. Deptt. of Women and Child Development Ministry of HRD; 1992.

17 GOI. Strategic guidelines for breastfeeding and complementary feeding, policy options for government. New Delhi: National Technical Committee on Child Health (NTCCH). MOH and FW (GOI); 2000.

18 Gupta A. National trends in breastfeeding and effective strategies to improve breastfeeding rates. J of Neonatology 2002 July-Sept.;16(3):4–14.

19 Infant and young child feeding – from policy to practice. Proceedings of Asia Pacific Conference on breastfeeding and National Convention of BPNI; 2003 Nov. 30-Dec. 3; India Habitat Centre, New Delhi.

20 BPNI. Infants and young child feeding. Nutrition of the young child during first two years; 2001; New Delhi.

21 International Baby Food Action Network (IBFAN). Geneva Infant Feeding Association (GIFA). Rea MF, Cattaneo A, Peck R, Lhotska L. editors. Breastfeeding beliefs. HIV, Infant feeding and maternal and child health. June 2002; 34.

22 Lal S, Goomer R. Incidence of low birth weights in rural ICDS block. Ind J Maternal and Child Health 1994;5(3): 76–9.

23 Govt. of India. National guidelines on infant and young child feeding. Ministry of Human Resource Development, Department of Women and Child Development—Food and Nutrition Board, Govt. of India, 2004.

MALNUTRITION IN YOUNG CHILDREN

Preschool children are most vulnerable to the effect of undernutrition because of rapid growth and thus their nutritional status is considered to be sensitive indicator of community health.

In South Asia region, the problem of undernutrition is widespread and in many countries like Bangladesh, Bhutan, India, Maldives, Nepal and Pakistan prevalence of stunting is high ranging from 30 to 63%.

FAO estimates that world wide 800 million children, women and men are undernourished and malnourished. Over 2 billion suffer from "hidden hunger". Table 6.14 shows malnutrition in young children in India and world.

India and Malnutrition (Protein Energy Malnutrition)

India has been a world leader in the science of nutrition and has to its credit several innovations. It has achieved marvels in food production—achieving self-sufficiency, yet India is home to over one-third of the stunted/ wasted children of the world who have protein energy malnutrition manifested by: (i) underweight—less

Table 6.14: Malnutrition in young children—India and World

Country	*Prevalence* (%)
India	44
Nepal	29
Bangladesh	37
Ethiopia	29
Pakistan	32
Somalia	33
Thailand	9
Malaysia	13
China	3
USA	1
Australia	0

Source: UNICEF–2015.

weight-for-age, (ii) stunted—short for their height, and (iii) thin or wasted—low weight-for-height or acute undernutrition.

The Global Hunger Index (GHI) released annually since 2006 combines three equally weighted indicators into one index: (a) under-nourishment (inadequate feeding), (b) child underweight and (c) child mortality. With the largest hungry population in the world, India ranks 66 among 105 countries in the 2012 Global Hunger Index.

The Hunger and Nutrition Commitment Index (HANCI) lunched in 2013 compares the performance of 45 developing countries using 22 indicators of political commitment to reduce hunger and malnutrition. Overall on HANCI India is ranked 20th below Brazil (4th) China (22nd) and South Africa (23rd). According to HANCI, there is low commitment of GOI towards addressing the problem of stunting in children below 5 years of age.

EPIDEMIOLOGY OF PROTEIN ENERGY MALNUTRITION (PEM)

Prevalence

National family health survey (NFHS-2 and 3), NNMB and India nutrition profile data indicate that nearly 50% of children below 5 years of age in India have protein energy malnutrition of varied severity.

Recent national survey reveal the 26.4% of under-5 children are **underweight**, 38.7% are **stunted** and 15.1 are acutely malnourished (**wasted**). More importantly 4.6% of children suffered severe acute malnutrition (SAM).

The HUNGaMA (Hunger and Malnutrition) Survey[1]

This survey captured 109093 children under five year of age in 2011 in 100 districts across nine states conducted by Nandi foundation Hyderabad. Voices of over 74000 mothers were also heard first ever. Study indicates that child malnutrition was wide spread across states and 100 focus districts of Bihar, Jharkhand, Madhya Pradesh, Odisha, Rajasthan and UP. The focus districts were selected from the bottom of child development district index developed for UNICEF India 2009.

Over 42% of children under-five were underweight 16.4% were severely underweight and nearly 59% were stunted and 34% were severely stunted. Over 11% had wasting. Even the best districts manifest the problem of underweight and stunting (Table 6.15). Now proportion of underweight below 3 years has declined from 52% in 1990 to 33% in 2015.

Trend of Clinical Signs

From 1975–79 to 1996–97, the clinical signs of PEM have declined significantly. Marasmus has declined from 1.3 to 0.6%, kwashiorkor from 0.4 to 0.1%, Bitots spots have come down from 1.8 to 0.8% and angular stomatitis from 5.8 to 2% whereas oedema has, almost, been eliminated.

Geographical Distribution (NFHS-4-2015-16)

PEM is a widespread problem in all the states of India, however, the worst affected states due to severe PEM are; Bihar, Madhya Pradesh, Karnataka Maharashtra, AP, and Meghalya, Uttarakhand, Haryana and West Bengal respectively as shown in Table 6.16. These are the most populous states of the country and all other health indicators are also low in these states; hence special efforts are required in these states to mitigate the problem of undernutrition. Due priority should be given to these states.

Table 6.16: Prevalence (%) of malnutrition in under five children in different states (NFHS-4) 2015–16

States	*Underweight*	*Stunting*	*Wasted*
Bihar	43.9	48.3	20.8
MP	42.8	42.0	25.8
Maharashtra	36.0	34.4	25.6
Karnataka	35.2	36.2	26.1
Andhra Pradesh	33.1	32.5	17.8
West Bengal	31.5	32.5	20.3
Haryana	29.4	34.0	21.2
Uttarakhand	26.6	33.5	19.5
Meghalya	29.0	43.8	15.3
Tripura	24.1	24.3	16.8

Table 6.15: Trends in prevalence (%) of underweight, stunting and wasting in children below five years of age in India[2–7]

Indicator	*NNMB 1975–79*	*NNMB 1988–90*	*Ind. Nut Profile 1998*	*NFHS-1 1992–93*	*NFHS-2 1998–99*	*NFHS-3 2005–06*	*HUNGaMA 2011*	*NFHS-4*
Weight-for-age								
Underweight < –2SD	77.5	68.6	49.2	51.5	42.7	43	42.0	29.4
Severely underweight < –3SD	38.0	26.6	20.3	20.6	17.6	15.8	16.4	–
Height-for-age								
Stunted < –2SD	78.6	65.1	56.5	52.0	51.0	48	59.0	38.7
Severely stunted < –3SD	53.3	36.8	36.4	28.9	27.7	22.0	34.0	–
Weight-for-height								
Wasted < –2SD	18.1	19.9	20.0	17.5	19.7	20	11.4	15.1
Severely wasted < –3SD	2.9	2.4	7.1	3.2	6.7	6.4	3.3	4.6
n =	**6428**	**13422**	**46457**	**25578**	**24215**	**26541**	**109093**	

Ind. nut profile and NFHS data pertain to children under 3 years of age.

Rural/Urban Distribution

Higher proportions of rural children are suffering from PEM as compared to urban areas. Urban slum areas have as much prevalence of PEM as in rural areas and more often the situation of PEM in urban slum areas may be worse than rural areas because of poor living conditions and presence of all the risk factors for malnutrition.

Gender and PEM

Usually prevalence of severe malnutrition is much more in young girls as compared to young boys below 5 years of age. This is due to differential child rearing practices observed including feeding and health care seeking behaviour.

Age Group Affected and Feeding Practices

It has been observed that the prevalence of PEM is lowest in children below the age of 6 months. The prevalence levels are at peak in age group 12–23 months and thereafter it is maintained around that level. Critical age at which undernutrition starts is around 6 months and growth faltering is at peak in second year of life, hence growth monitoring programme which aims at prevention of undernutrition must cover these children at home and discuss with mother the growth of respective child. Growth monitoring should be integrated with routine outreach sessions of immunization.

PEM is much more common in age group 6–24 months. Reasons for this are quite obvious. Up to 6 months, the babies thrive well on breast milk which is adequate for normal growth and development, thereafter the baby needs supplementary feeds in addition to breastfeeding. Most mothers delay the weaning (giving complementary or supplementary foods) in young children and secondly the quantities of foods given are quite inadequate for normal growth and development. Cereals are deliberately not encouraged or are given in very small quantities.

Seasonal Variations

Malnutrition is maximum when children are less cared for or left under the care of mother substitutes during peak harvesting period. April and May, or September–October when mothers are away for long hours of work in the field.

Table 6.17: Prevalence of severe acute malnutrition (SAM) NFHS–4 (2015–16)

Prevalence levels	*States*
Less than 5%	Manipur 2.2, AP 4.4
5–7%	Sikkim 5.9, Tripura 6.3, Pudducherry 6.4, WB 6.5, Meghalaya 6.5
7–9%	Bihar 7, AN 7.5, AP 7.9, Uttarakhand 9, Haryana 9
More than 9%	Karnataka 10.5, Goa 9.5, Maharashtra 9.4, MP 9.2

In north India, malnutrition is maximum during summer and that is the peak season for diarrhoeal diseases as well. Diarrhoea is one of the most important nutritional leak; it drains away fluids and nutrients from the body. Withholding of foods and liquids worsens the nutritional status and exposes the children to high mortality.

Literacy and Castes

Undernutrition in children below 4 years is higher in economically weaker sections (scheduled castes and scheduled tribes). There is strong correlation between the educational level of the mother and the child's nutritional status.

Secular Trends of PEM

Severe forms of PEM have diminished. The NNMB data shows declining trends of prevalence of PEM (underweight and stunting) including severe underweight—below 3SD. There is almost 1% decline per annum. NFHS and ICDS data also have shown declining trends of undernutrition. However, prevalence of wasting and severe wasting has stagnated overtime (Tables 6.15 and 6.17).

Small remains small: Stunted children, severely malnourished and low birth weight babies may grow as stunted adults thus poorly contributing to the economy and low levels of scholastic attainment and poor work capacity.

Mortality due to PEM

Malnutrition contributes directly or indirectly to 35% of all deaths in young children. Those who are severely malnourished have 15–20% more chances of dying as compared to well-nourished children.

Poverty

Undernutrition has no correlation with per capita income. 28% of people in India live below poverty line but level of undernutrition in India is much higher at 50% or over. Latest poverty estimate by planning commission is 38% (2009). Poverty alone cannot explain this level of malnutrition. Even poorest of poor have enough of grains for young children, e.g. breastfeeding and 50 to 120 g of cereals per young child per day is affordable. Economic intervention or giving employment to below poverty line to raise their income is necessary but not sufficient to improve nutritional status of young children and mothers.[7]

Household Food Security

Similarly increasing food production and availability of food at household level is essential but not sufficient to improve nutrition. Food grain production has risen from 89 million tonnes in 1965 to 264 million tonnes in 2013–14 and in the past we had enough of buffer stocks of 60 million tonnes. Every home has enough of grains but brains (best practices) are essential for food distribution within the family and improving dietary practices. Best of food is available in home and farms. Govt. of India spends 24000 crores for subsidized food grains for below poverty line people through Targeted Public Distribution System. Food production and distribution is no guarantee of good nutrition.

Food availability at the household level is seldom a problem. A young child requires 120 g of complementary food (rice or cereal) to obtain enough of calories and nutrients. Problem is that cereal-based complementary foods are bulky and it needs to be made energy dense by addition of oil and ghee and frequency of feeding should be 5–6 times per day.

Causes of PEM—Inadequate Feeding and Infections

(a) Inadequate Feeding and Delayed Weaning or Starting of Complementary Food

Exclusive breastfeeding should be adequate for a child up to 6 months of age. Data on growth monitoring indicates that the growth of many children falters earlier, reflecting either inadequate or partial breastfeeding practice (inadequate feeding and less frequency, inadequate diet of lactating mother and introduction of non-nutritive food through bottle or other means which decreases the flow of breast milk). Most mothers do not give adequate quantities of food to their young children beyond 6 months of age. NFHS-3 data indicates that only 55.8% of breastfed children aged 6–9 months receive solid or semisolid food.

(b) Infections and Environments

Unclean food, utensils and dirty hands unsafe water and unsafe excreta disposal leads to infections and most common being diarrhoea and worm infestation. Repeated attacks of diarrhoea and acute respiratory infections lowers the nutritional status. Continuing feeding during illness and more diet during convalescence period is essential for catch up growth. Adequate eating during illness reduces the severity of illness and gives energy to the body, leading to fast recovery.

High Fertility—Low Birth Interval

India has high fertility rates. Large sized families and closely spaced births and higher birth orders are exposed to the risk of low birth weight babies and more malnutrition of women in child bearing age because of repeated pregnancies on account of early marriages and non-acceptance of contraception.

Spectrum of PEM

6

The spectrum of protein energy malnutrition is quite wide. It begins with inadequate birth weights (22–28% of newborns have birth weight below 2.5 kg), passes through the period of growth faltering or inadequate weight gains during infancy and in second and third year of life. Inadequate growth and growth faltering is the earlier sign and mothers can best judge this and if this is supported by growth monitoring programme, the growth faltering can be detected at the earliest. The advanced stages of malnutrition like marasmus or typical kwashiorkor (which is now rare) is the end spectrum of PEM; 30–40% of young children are moderately underweight while 16% are severely underweight. Detect the malnutrition at the earliest by growth monitoring and correct it at the earliest.

By the time, the overt clinical signs of malnutrition appear it is too late a stage of undernutrition. Marasmus is just the tip of the 'iceberg' of overall prevalence and problem of undernutrition.

MEASURING CHILD NUTRITION

Anthropometric measurements are the mainstay of assessment of PEM or undernutrition or overnutrition. WHO, ICDS, NNMB, NFHS and India nutrition profile all have used anthropometric measurements. Commonly used measurements are:

1 Weight-for-age to assess degree of "underweight"—an indicator of acute malnutrition.
2 Height-for-age to assess degree of "stunting"—an indicator of chronic malnutrition.
3 Weight-for-height to assess degree of "wasting"—an indicator of current malnutrition.

Each of the three nutrition indicators is expressed in standard deviation units (Z Scores) from the median of reference population.

In April 2006, the WHO has released the WHO Child Growth Standards replacing NCHS standards. These standards establish breastfed infants as the normative growth model. The weight-for-age measurement can be viewed as summary indicator of a child's nutritional status and a composite of both wasting and stunting.

Clinical Signs of Malnutrition

Deficiency signs appear late and can be recognized by health workers. Most important signs are anaemia, goitre, vitamin A deficiency (Bitot spots), angular stomatitis, signs of rickets, oedema of the feet, and marasmus or wasting and obesity.

Subclinical Malnutrition

Biochemical changes can be detected by laboratory tests. Haemoglobin estimation, serum level of retinol, iron, vitamins, urinary iodine can be estimated. These tests are done for specific purposes. Laboratory facilities require trained manpower and usually these facilities are not available.

DIETARY SURVEYS

Dietary surveys are done to assess the dietary intakes; qualitatively and quantitatively with a view to improve the dietary practices and improve the diets.

Assessment of Nutritional Status by Anthropometric Measurements

The most commonly used measurements are body weight, height or length and mid upper arm circumference and fat fold at triceps.

Weight-for-Age

Weight-for-age is the robust parameter, most widely used and practical method to monitor growth and assess the nutritional status of young children. It is most sensitive and simple measurement which indicates improvement or deterioration of nutritional status. Weight-for-age measures current as well as past nutritional status. Single measurement is not sufficient to decide the nutritional status, it is much better to have serial weights at an interval of one month during first 3 years of life and thereafter once in 3 months. It is the direction of growth which matters most. Weighing children and putting it on growth charts makes the invisible malnutrition visible much before the clinical signs of malnutrition become visible. The system of ICDS which is world's largest outreach programme for mothers and children is using growth charts for growth monitoring and promotion.

Height-for-Age (HFA)

Height of an individual is determined by genetic and environmental factors (adequate diet and infections). Height once gained is not lost. Height-for-age measures chronic malnutrition (stunting) or long standing malnutrition. If the height-for-age is low the child is called *stunted.*

Weight-for-Height

This measurement is useful to assess current nutritional status or *wasting*. This is age independent measurement.

Mid Upper Arm Circumference (MUAC)

MUAC is age independent measurement to assess the nutritional status. The mid arm circumference does not vary much between ages one and five. It is simple, does not require any sophisticated equipment and is acceptable. MUAC can be measured by simple tape (fibre glass tape) or by tricolour tape. The cut-off level is 13.5 cm. Children in age group 1–5 years who have MUAC of 13.5 cm or above are considered as normals. Children having MUAC between 12.5 and 13.5 are classified as moderately malnourished while those below 12.5 cm are classified as severely malnourished. Recently, it has been suggested that MUAC of 11.5 cm should be used to pick up severely malnourished children. MUAC is used to screen malnutrition or nutritional status rapidly by paramedical workers, AWWs and even by mothers. QUAC stick (arm circumference and height) can also be used to assess nutritional status.

Classification of Degree of PEM (Fig. 6.1a)

Underweight: Means children aged 0–59 months who are below minus two standard deviations and severely underweight means below minus 3SD from median weight-for-age of WHO child growth standards, 2006.

Stunting: Children aged 0–59 months who are below minus two standard deviations from median height-for-age of the WHO reference population are called *stunted* and those who are below minus three standard deviations from median height-for-age are called *severely stunted.*

Wasting: Children aged 0–59 months who are below minus two standard deviations from median weight-for-height of the WHO reference population are called *wasted* and those who are below three standard deviations from median weight-for-height are called *severely wasted* children (Severe Acute Malnutrition—SAM).

PREVENTION AND CONTROL OF PROTEIN ENERGY MALNUTRITION

The problem of protein energy malnutrition is a complex problem and involves many sectors, i.e. the people, households, the governmental and non-governmental organizations. Essentially, it involves:

i Adequate eating or enough food for young children at home, improving dietary and hygienic practices.
ii Prevention and control of common infections in children.
ii Use of iodated salt only by all and specific nutrients.

Essentially, integrated approach is required to mitigate malnutrition. Mother holds the key position for prevention and improvement of nutrition of young children.

Management of PEM

To begin with we laid heavy emphasis on "proteins" to tackle the problem of PEM, but soon we realized that the major issue was "food gap" or energy gap for PEM and hence emphasis shifted to adequate or sufficient eating of food to mitigate the problem of PEM.

1 ***Breastfeeding:*** Initiation of breastfeeding soon after delivery, exclusive breastfeeding for first 6 months of life and continuation of breastfeeding up to 2 years or longer prevents malnutrition and ensure adequate growth and development. In India, steps have been taken for protection and promotion of breastfeeding by implementation of Infant Milk Substitutes Act, 1992.
2 ***Complementary feeding:*** At 6 months, in addition to breastfeeding, adequate complementary food should be introduced to meet the nutritional requirements for adequate growth. Food cooked at home should be given

to young children. Best nutritious foods are available in home and farm. Sufficient household food security exists in family. Infant and young child feeding guidelines should be followed in letters and spirit.

3 ***Immunization:*** Children should be given all immunization at right age. Measles immunization prevents malnutrition and first mega dose (1 lakh IU) of vitamin A should be given along with measles immunization.

4 ***Control of infections:*** Hygienic practices, like washing hands, clean food; use of safe drinking water and safe disposal of human excreta prevents diarrhoeal diseases and worm infestation and thereby it prevents nutritional leaks in young children. If the child develops diarrhoea, the first response should be enough of home available fluids and ORS and continuation of breastfeeding. Feeding in young children will prevent deaths and this also prevents malnutrition and ensures early recovery. Feeding during diarrhoea should continue. Increased frequency of feeding after diarrhoea helps catch up growth in young children. Periodical deworming in young children is being done on National Deworming day to cover 1–19 years old.

5 ***Supplementary feeding programmes:*** Home foods are best foods. Supplementary nutrition programme for children, pregnant and lactating mothers and adolescent girls are there under integrated child development services (ICDS). These foods are supplementary only, unless the child eats enough of food at home the supplementary feeding at Anganwadi will not help. Severely malnourished children get double the amount of supplementary food from Anganwadi (therapeutic feeding). Supplementary feeding programme of ICDS has extensive coverage of children under 6 years of age, but it is difficult to say if it leads to improvement of malnutrition in young children. Targeted supplementary nutrition and therapeutic nutrition to most vulnerable children and poor section of people or below poverty line families can be helpful. Supplementary nutrition programmes (SNP) have been used as "Spring board" to attract children and mothers to increase the attendance, to develop other activities like nonformal education and creative activities, growth monitoring (to be more precise weighing children, involving mothers, to demonstrate clean eating, developing good habits like washing hands and brushing teeth, to educate mother on preparation of recipes apart from cooking and testing of acceptability of food items).

6 ***Specific nutrient supplementation*** (iron and folic acid and vitamin A prophylaxis) helps to mitigate micronutrient deficiency in children, pregnant and lactating women and adolescent girls.

7 ***Management of children with severe acute malnutrition (SAM):*** SAM can be categorized into: SAM with medical complications and SAM without medical complications.

Nutrition rehabilitation centres (NRCs): Inpatient management of SAM with complications can reduce the mortality in young children. NRCs have been set up at District and FRU/CHC level. However, NRCs cannot handle 8 million load of SAM of which 85–90% do no have medical complications. Hence community based programme for management of SAM should be in place where home and family takes responsibility.[8]

8 ***Nutrition of adolescents, pregnant women and lactating mothers:*** Malnutrition have intergenerational effects. Improving nutrition of adolescent girls and boys should become prime concern and it should be considered as good investment. Adequate nutrition to young girls is of paramount concern to prepare them for safe motherhood. Nutrition education and supplementation of iron and folic acid to adolescents is essential to prevent and treat anaemia and to ensure good reproductive health. Right age of marriage and adequate nutrition of pregnant women will prevent low birth weight babies and also lower the maternal morbidity and mortality. Adequate nutrition of lactating women ensures adequate breast milk, so essential for child survival, growth and development. Women nutrition and women development ultimately helps healthy child growth.

9 ***Food production and distribution:*** India has achieved marvels in food production, to achieve not only self-sufficiency but have adequate buffer food stocks, through green revolution, white revolution and blue revolution. Food grain production of over 257 million tonnes during the year 2011, ensures reasonable food security at national level and the programmes of poverty alleviation and targeted public distribution system further ensure food security at "household level" through increased purchasing power and access to highly subsidized food grains. Thus, graduating from "food security" to "household food security" to "nutrition and health security" of all and more so of vulnerable becomes a prime task and agenda.

10 ***Public distribution system and targeted public distribution system (Food Security Act, 2013):*** Public distribution system (PDS) has become targeted public distribution system (TPDS) and covers below poverty line families. With a network of 4.62 lakh fair price shops (FPS) distributing commodities and spending more than 30,000 crores annually to reach about 160 million families. The PDS in India is perhaps the largest distribution network in the world. TPDS provides 25 kg of rice or wheat per month at 50% of economic cost (₹ 3/kg for rice and ₹ 2/kg for wheat). Besides this 35 kg of food grain is provided to the poorest of poor families under the *Antyodaya Anna Yojna* at a highly subsidized rates. Coarse grains will be provided at ₹ 1 per kg.[8]

Annapurna Yojna: Under this scheme, old destitude individuals who are not receiving old age pension are entitled to 10 kg of grain per month free of cost.

Though the government has taken all possible steps to make available food grains to the poorest of poor, it has however, been observed that off-take of food grain under BPL category has not gone beyond 55% during the preceding two years. On the one hand, we have one of the largest public distribution system in the world with government spending over ₹ 30,000 crores on food subsidy, yet many people are going without adequate food and half of young child population (0–5 years) suffer from malnutrition. This is a paradoxical situation, which speaks of "poverty" in "plenty". Many of the states are unable to lift the food stocks collected by the central Government due to their poor financial health and political will. Thus, the record production of food grains and adequate buffer stocks are no guarantee against malnutrition.

11 ***Mahatama Gandhi National Rural Employment Guarantee Act and Scheme:*** To increase food security and purchasing power as per Act any adult in rural area who applies for work is entitled to being employed on public works within 15 days. The work guarantee is limited to 100 days per household per year.

12 ***Fight against hidden hunger (micronutrient deficiency)*** should focus on food-based approach. Fighting micronutrient deficiency through food fortification technology is yet another gimmick to divert the attention of common man to obtain micronutrients through fortified foods rather than promoting local initiatives. It is killing of local initiatives and capacity to fight the scourge of anaemias, vitamin A deficiency, through consumption of green leafy vegetables and locally grown fruits and vegetables. Delivering micronutrients through lozenges, sugar, oil, wheat flour, and other ready to eat foods appears to be a trap to eliminate local capacities and initiatives in a systematic manner, apart from changing dietary habits of people and promoting a particular product, which may have deleterious effect in the long run. Micronutrients supplementation programme of vitamin A and IFA should be focused and targeted to children in age group of 1–3 years and universal iodized salt consumption should be strived at.

13 Though we have world reputed National Institute of Nutrition in India, universities, food and nutrition board, home-science colleges and medical colleges, district training centres apart from regional training centres and NIPCCD to train manpower on nutrition and health. We have enough of ready made nutritionists, besides information technologies like mass media and print media and evidence/database on nutrition, but still we are not able to communicate effectively with the mother or household who ultimate need our help to translate nutrition knowledge into action. **The whole science of nutrition is effective communication strategy for behaviour change.** Invariably, too much of technical knowledge and all book recipes are handed over to mothers for improving dietary practices which are in conflict with the, cultural and economic conditions of family hence seldom acted upon. Local workers can communicate best of nutrition messages provided they are imparted good training in their locale. Learning resource and communication material on nutrition is so much variable that there are conflicting messages and contents thereof. Standard communication material on nutrition needs to be evolved and acted upon in curriculum of all categories of professionals and workers. Local data and worker's own data and information must be put to use to increase the ownership and measure the success of **best practices adopted at local level/household level and success must be attributed to mothers/parents**.

14 ***Population control and stabilization:*** India was the first country in the world to formulate a National Family Welfare Programme in 1952. The objective of the policy was "Reducing birth rate" to the extent necessary to stabilize the population at a level consistent with the requirement of national economy. National population policy 2000 agenda is being pursued speedily to bring down birth rate to 21 by 2015. Unless we control the numbers, the problem of malnutrition will continue.

Having fewer number of children, spacing births at least 2 years apart will prevent low birth weight babies and improve the nutritional status of women and their quality of life as also quality of life of children. Every household has voluntarily to decide the number of children they wish to have.

15 The National Nutrition Policy adopted in 1993 advocated comprehensive intersectoral strategy for alleviating the multifaceted problem of malnutrition. National plan of action on nutrition launched in 1995 has not resulted into actions on the ground level and most of the sectoral commitments are on paper. The National Nutrition Policy was adopted in 1993 and national nutrition goals for the year 2000 were formulated.

***GOAL of 12th plan*:** Reduce malnutrition among children of age group 0–3 to half of its present level.[9–10]

Our response to malnutrition and undernutrition: Right from the beginning we heavily relied on feeding programmes and over emphasized on "protein component" but the wisdom soon prevailed and we realized that the real culprit was "food gap" rather than protein gap. Our energies and resources got diverted towards growing and producing more of animal's and vegetable proteins; through applied nutrition programme. Standard teaching and training programmes also adhered to protein protocol. Subject of nutrition drew the attention of planners in successive five-year plan and it was considered as an important area of "minimum need programme" under Fifth Five-Year Plan. Food and nutrition was embodied as one of the essential element of primary health care.[11]

Malnutrition is to be fought through integrated health, nutrition and educational activities focused on vulnerables and BPL families. Convergence of services at village level through integrated child development services and self-help groups of women and village Panchayats holds much more promise. Building capacities of mothers and women at household level through integrated efforts can enhance the nutritional status of women and children. *Promotion of breastfeeding, exclusive breastfeeding up to 6 months of age, adequate home available supplementary feeding along with breastfeeding, eating clean along with washing hands and immunization at right age and household response to diarrhoea and acute respiratory infections can ensure adequate growth and health of young children.*

ICDS programme laid more stress on detection and reporting of malnutrition by weighing children, rather than preventing malnutrition through supporting mothers and building their capacities at household level. Wherever the Anganwadi workers adopted this strategy the results were obvious and success was sure. Mothers and Anganwadi workers together were winner to ensure healthy growth of young children. Mothers attributed the success to adequate feeding and adequate household response to illness, along with utilization of health services.

REFERENCES

1. HUNGaMA Survey 2011. India by Nandi Foundation, Hyderabed, India.
2. IIPS. National Family Health Survey-2 and 3. Mumbai: International Institute of Population Sciences; 2002 and 2006.
3. Nutrition foundation of India. NFI Bulletin 2003;24(2): New Delhi.
4. Sachdev HPS. Nutritional Status of Children and Women in India: Recent trends. NFI Bulletin 1997;18(3): New Delhi.
5. Lal S. Combating malnutrition in India through community efforts. Ind J Comm Med 2003;28(3):99–106.
6. Central Technical Committee on IMCD. Integrated Child Development Services – Survey Evaluation and Research 1975–1995. New Delhi, R.K. Puram: CTC; 1996.
7. GOI. India Nutrition Profile. New Delhi: Department of Women and Child Development; 1998.
8. Government of India MOH and FW (2011) operational Guidelines on Facility Based Management of Children with Severe Acute Malnutrition.
9. Planning Commission (GOI). 10th Five-Year Plan. New Delhi; Govt. of India; 2002–2007.
10. GOI Planning Commission 12th Five-Year Plan (2012 to 2017).
11. WHO. The Health Aspects of food and Nutrition. Manual for Developing Countries in Western Pacific Region of WHO. Manila: WHO; 1979.

GROWTH MONITORING AND NUTRITION SURVEILLANCE

GROWTH MONITORING

Definition

Growth monitoring means regular weighing of young children at agreed upon interval (one month during infancy, two months in second year of life and three months thereafter) to measure the growth of young children with a view to detect any deviation at the earliest from the normal path of growth and ensure prompt action.

The growth monitoring is a preventive and promotive strategy. Ideally, it prevents malnutrition and promotes healthy growth. *It makes invisible malnutrition visible.*

Growth monitoring detects the malnutrition at the earliest much before the clinical signs of malnutrition appear.[1–5]

Uses of Growth Monitoring

Growth monitoring is a preventive strategy. There are several uses of growth monitoring:

a. To detect the malnutrition at the earliest and correct it by means of suitable intervention or action at home.
b. To monitor the growth pattern of young children over a period of time (from birth to infancy or in second or third year of life).
c. To assess the nutritional status of young children at a given point of time or period.
d. To assess the weight gain pattern in different ages.
e. To select beneficiaries for supplementary and therapeutic nutrition. It is useful epidemiological tool to study the child on longitudinal basis for prospective studies or cohort studies on growth, morbidity and mortality.
f. Useful tool for effective communication for behaviour change (dietary practices).
g. To demonstrate and observe effectiveness of an intervention or action (supplementary feeding, therapeutic feeding and IFA supplementation and prompt response to illness (diarrhoea, measles, ARI, fever, etc.).
h. To promote integrated maternal and child health interventions.
i. In the long-run growth, monitoring can be used as a tool for nutrition surveillance.
j. It helps to identify various risk factors for growth faltering in population and above all it is a mean to establish contact with home, mothers, parents and families.

Periodicity

Growth monitoring (GM) should begin immediately after birth. All births should be weighed, to help families and mothers, for their survival and growth. Immediately after delivery in hospital, all births should be weighed. In home delivery situation, it is to be ensured on the day of birth by home visit. However, postnatal care after delivery is the weakest component. Traditional birth attendants have been provided with colour coded spring balances for weighing of newborn but these are seldom used. Anganwadi workers have been made responsible for weighing of all births but in practice, coverage is very low. Since Anganwadi workers are locally resident workers, it is feasible to weigh all births and ensure appropriate action.

In family—parents and mothers usually do not allow weighing on cultural reasons, but by motivating and preparing families and pregnant women during antenatal care this barrier can be crossed.

Ideally, during first year of life, the infant should be weighed every month and in the second year of life after every 2 months and thereafter once in every 3 months, up to 5 years of age. Severely malnourished children should be weighed every month irrespective of age. Sick children and severely malnourished children should be weighed more frequently. In ICDS Children below 3 years are being weighed once a month and children between 3 and 5 years weighed every three months.

Integrated Approach

Growth monitoring has been integrated into mother and child protection card (MCPC) activities. Growth monitoring can be a rewarding experience when it is integrated with primary health care and combined with outreach session of immunization at subcentre or at Anganwadi. All pregnant women should also be weighed. Mothers themselves can weigh their children or participate actively in growth monitoring process to ensure all actions for adequate growth. Anganwadi workers must encourage all mothers to weigh their children and see the result of growth on the charts and scale. Ideally, growth monitoring should be handed over to mothers. It has been integrated with integrated management of neonatal and childhood illness (IMCI) and monitoring of developmental mile stones to detect development delay at the earliest.

Custodian of Growth Charts

Growth charts have been designed for mothers and families. It should be with mother and she should be the custodian. Mothers must understand and they should be educated and helped by Anganwadi workers. In practice, the growth charts are kept in a book form safely with Anganwadi workers and seldom shown to mothers. During the training of workers, it should be stressed that growth charts belong to child and mother and it should be at home, valued as home-based record.[2–6]

Tool for Communication

Growth charts are means of communication with mother and family and all workers should use this tool to educate mothers and build upon her all preventive and promotive practices, such as spacing between births, exclusive breastfeeding, adequate feeding at right age, clean eating, continue breastfeeding and feeding during illness and early and prompt response to diarrhoea and other illnesses and prevention of illness by accepting immunization. Visible growth on the chart can be demonstrated to mothers or still better is to show the well-nourished and adequately growing children to mothers and convince them the value of adequate feeding. On several occasions Anganwadi workers have shown and demonstrated effectively to mothers the growth of same age group children, eating well, eating enough and growing well and some who do not eat enough and do not grow well. How effectively this tool is used depends on how well the workers have been trained and supported by the supervisors on their job functions.

Caution

Growth monitoring should not begin and end up with data collection and report preparation or just as a medical encounter, it is an opportunity for contact and education of both worker and mother and is an effective means of communication. This opportunity should never be missed. Messages on feeding and growth can be effectively communicated at right time to the precise need of mother and child.

System of Growth Monitoring

The largest outreach programme for mothers and children, the integrated child development services (ICDS) has been made responsible for growth monitoring of young children. The key person who does growth monitoring is Anganwadi worker who has been trained for 3 months and is being imparted regular on the job training and continuing education. The health system supports the efforts of Anganwadi workers.

Growth Charts (Mother and Child Protection Card)

Prevalence of *underweight, stunting* and *wasting* among under-five childern is estimated by comparing actual measurement to an international standard reference population. In April 2006, the World Health Organization released the 'WHO Child Growth Standard' to replace the widely used National Centre for Health Statistics/WHO reference population which was based on a limited sample of childern from United States, receving bottle and mixed feeding.

The new "WHO Child Growth Standards" globally used have unique features as they *provide how children should grow*—how *every child has right to grow and develop,* with her or his basic needs being met in a nurturing environment. They establish breastfed infants as the *normative growth model* and demonstrate for the first time ever that children born in different regions of the world and given the optimum start in life, have the potential to grow and develop to within the same range of height- and weight-for-age. They also provide reference values for assessing childern obesity and also a unique link between physical growth and motor development. These standards are available for both, girls and boys, below five years for weight-for-age, height-for-age, weight-for-height, BMI for age, and six motor development indicators. With these new standards, parents, communities, child care workers, programme managers, health and child care advocates will know when the nutrition and care needs of children are being compromised. The use of this tool enables them to take timely corrective actions at different levels.

In fact in the new growth charts the cut-off line which demarcates underweight has been shifted downwards and the line which demarcates severely underweight children has been shifted upwards. The implications of new growth charts are:

i Increase in total number of normal weight children.
ii Increase in severely underweight children.
iii Increase in underweight children (moderate and severe) in age group 0–6 months.

The requirement of funds for SNP, Centre and State Contribution would almost double. The new charts would now help in comparing growth of Indian Children within project, districts, states and also other countries.

The Ministry of Women and Child Development in ICDS has adopted 'New WHO Child Growth Standards' and has revised growth monitoring charts as mother and child protection card (MCPC) which describes how children should grow. In the new charts emphasis is on *growth* rather then grades of nutrition (Figs 6.1a and b).

On each growth chart there are three printed growth curves. These are called reference lines or Z scores lines and are used to compare and interpret the growth pattern of child and assess her/his nutritional status. The top curve on the growth chart is the *median*, the second curve is minus two standard deviations of the median and the third curve is minus three standard deviations of the median.

The new growth chart has three coloured tracks rather than earlier classification lines of normal, Grade I, Grade II, Grade III and Grade IV. The children in green track (above–2SD) are normal children. In the new chart Grade I and Grade II have been merged and shown as *yellow track* and children who are plotted in this track would be termed moderately underweight (below –2SD to –3SD). *Below yellow track* there is *orange track* which comprises grade III and grade IV and they will now be termed severely underweight (below–3SD of reference median). The weight of a girl and a boy of a same age differs slightly, therefore separate growth charts for boys (Light blue) and girls (Pink) have been introduced in ICDS.

Process

The correct age of the child is determined—accurate to the nearest month of birth, by use of local events calendar or from birth records. Anganwadi workers must register all births and record date of birth of every child this helps to determine the correct age.

Weighing of children should be done with minimum clothing. The weighing scales used: Salter weighing scale or Beam balance, should be standardised and its accuracy should be checked against a standard weight.

After weighing, the weight should be plotted at a point where weight and age of that child meet. This step can be learned during training and practice.

Interpretation after plotting of weight is important. Child growth curve should be drawn and interpreted along with mother to ensure prompt action.

Growth

Growth is more important than a single weight of a child at a particular point of time. From a single weight and single point, it is not safe to draw conclusions.

The direction of growth is of prime importance. The growth curve can have three directions:[3]

1 Upward — Good
2 Horizontal — Dangerous
3 Downward — Very dangerous

- If the child's growth curve is climbing upwards and follows the direction of reference curve the child growth is good and mothers should be congratulated to keep the child feeding adequately (breastfeeding or supplementary feeding).
- If the growth curve becomes horizontal, it means the child is not growing and growth has faltered. This is dangerous. The reasons for this growth faltering should be discovered and corrective actions by mother and family should be ensured promptly.
- If the growth curve is moving downwards, it means that the child is losing weight. This should be viewed as very dangerous and child should be helped immediately. The downward curve could be due to acute diarrhoea, withholding of foods and fluids, these must be corrected by prompt rehydration by home available fluids or ORS and breastfeeding and feeding according to liking and choice of mothers. If the downward curve is restored upwards, it means that the action taken was successful. Thus, the direction of the curve is helpful to assess the effectiveness of an action.

Position of Growth Curve

The direction of growth curve matters most than the position of the curve in relation to reference line. Each child grows in his/her own channel or trajectory. If the child is growing below the reference line, is healthy and active and there is no illness then there is no cause of worry and health workers must reassure mothers. Only children whose growth curves are well below the lower curve below

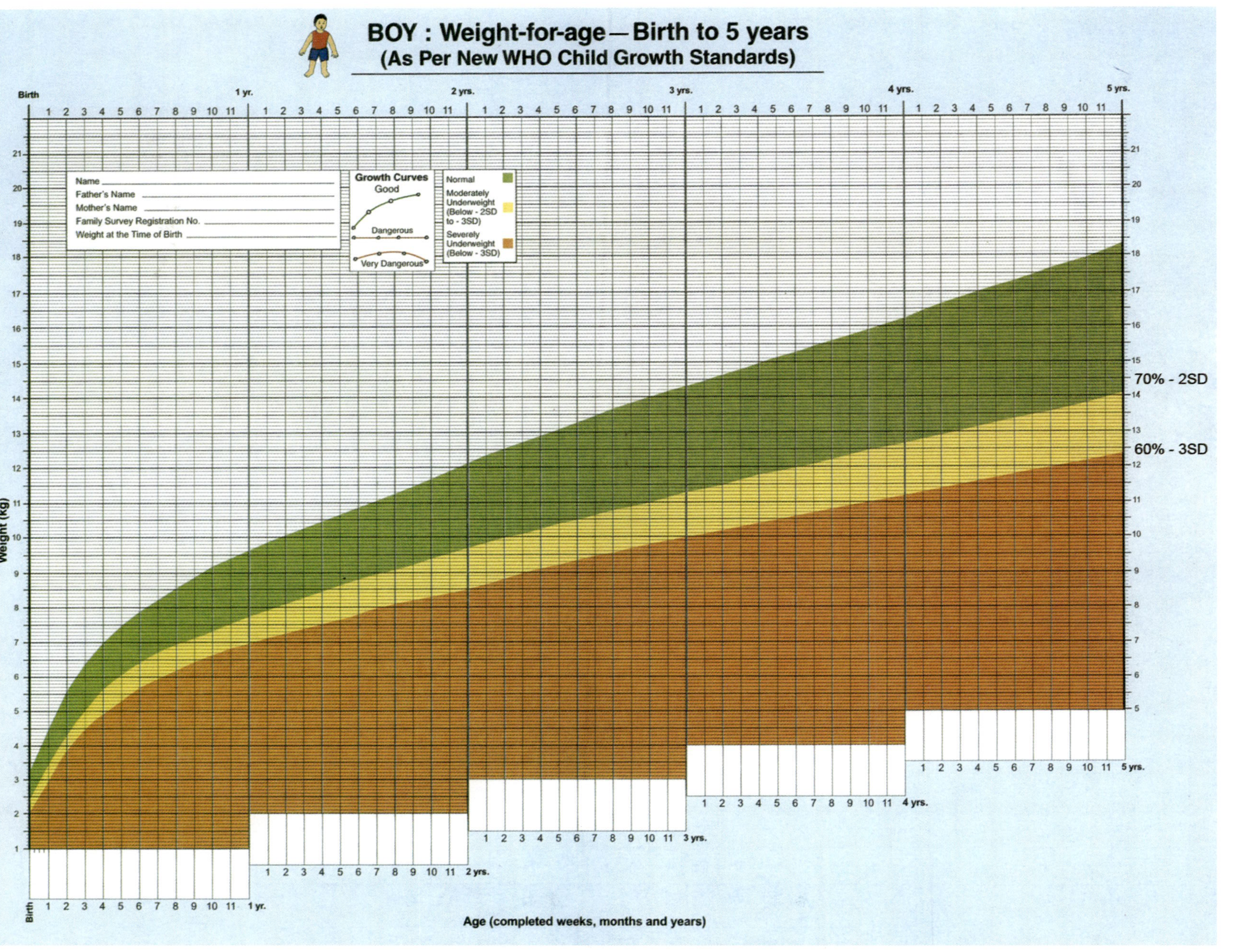

Fig. 6.1a: Growth chart used in ICDS programme

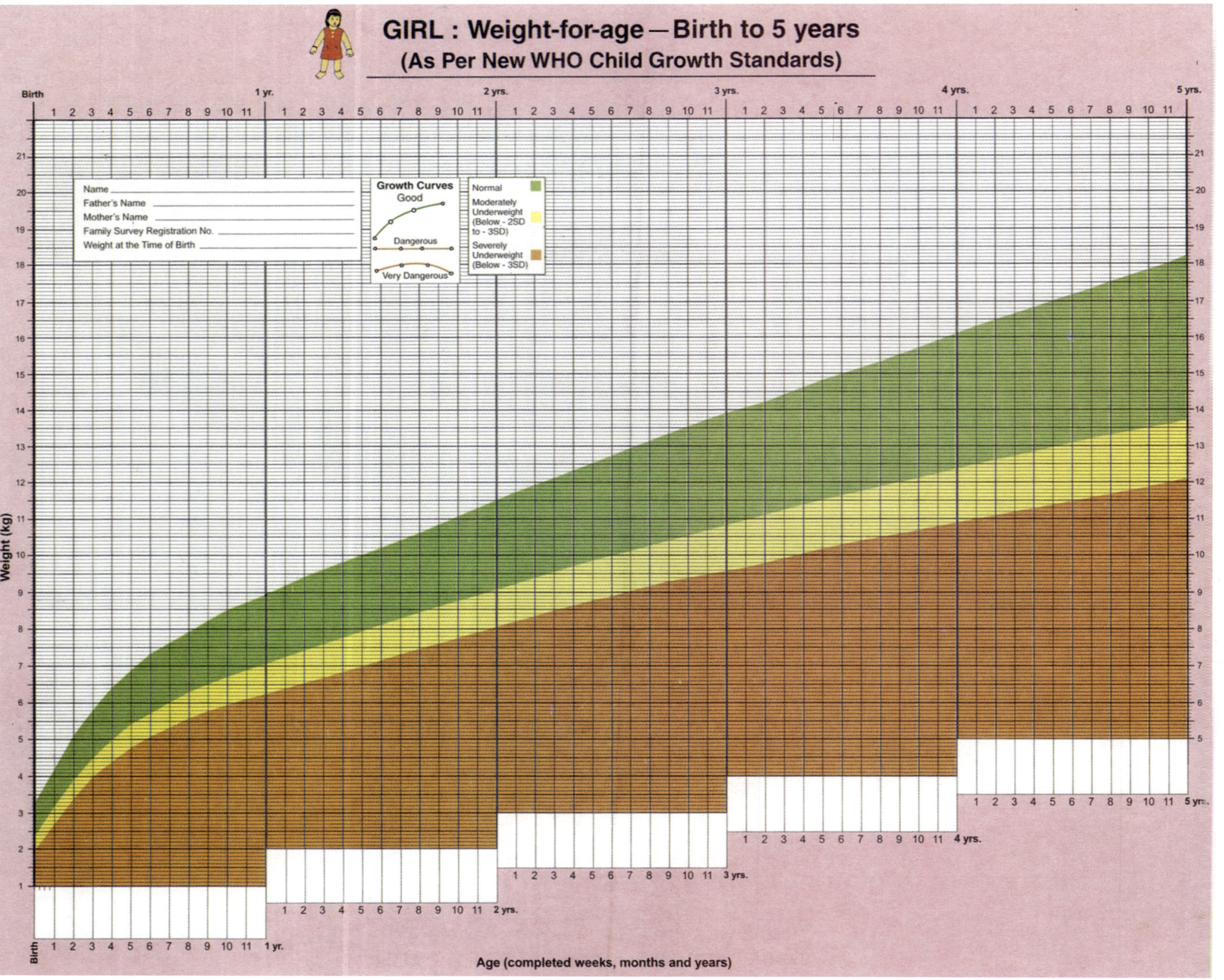

Fig. 6.1b: Growth chart used in ICDS programme

6

3SD should be reassessed and examined and referred to health facility. These children may have chronic illness. The position of the child's growth curve on the chart alone is not sufficient to feel happy about. If the curve becomes flat or moves downward prompt action should be ensured after rapid investigation. Children who are small at birth will grow in lower trajectory or channel if ensured adequate nutrition and care.

Training of Workers and Logistics[7]

Workers need to be trained. Team training of health workers and AWW is always better. Good weighing machines must be in position as also growth charts. Growth monitoring is time consuming process and its quality depends upon good training and experience. Objectives of growth monitoring must be made clear to the workers, and to mothers. Feedback to mothers and actions are more important than preparing reports or updating of records.[7] Regular growth monitoring programme with high quality can become a very useful tool for national nutrition surveillance programme, which is being done by periodical surveys undertaken by NNMB and results are not area specific and much delayed. On the other hand, growth monitoring is local and ensures local action promptly.

Growth monitoring in ICDS needs to be made more realistic and practical. Focus and priority should be on first two or three years at the most. Weighing at birth should be encouraged that will improve the component of postnatal care as well which is quite deficient at the moment. Apart from that, it will improve the birth registration for appropriate action.

Nutrition Surveillance System

Nutrition surveillance means data collection relevant to nutrition for prompt and appropriate action. This involves setting up of a system in the country/state/district/block to continuously collect data at regular interval or periodicity, compile and analyse data and develop information for action and feedback at various levels.

Such a system can help to give warning signal of occurrence of undernutrition well in advance to prepare the system for action in advance. Nutritional surveillance can also be useful for knowing the trend of undernutrition or overnutrition over a long period of time.

Nutritional surveillance also helps in evaluation of impact of various nutritional interventions, it also can identify factors and conditions for good or bad nutrition in a geographical area.

Indicators for Nutrition Surveillance

Wide ranging and common indicators used or collected and analysed at regular intervals are as under, however, it is advisable to collect only limited and essential indicators which are feasible and available through routine records. Special surveys or rapid surveys are needed to collect some special indicators as shown in Table 6.18.

Indicators from Social, Economic and Agriculture Data

These are essential indicators as these determine the adequate production of foods so essential for adequate nutrition.

Rainfall pattern, crop area, crop yield, food production, household food storage, buffer stocks, crop pests and

Table 6.18: Nutrition surveillance indicators[1]

Measurements	*Cut-off level*	*Indicator*	*Agency responsible*
• Birth weight	Less than 2500 g	% less than 2500 g	Health and ICDS
• Weight-for-age	Below – 2SD to – 3SD	% below or above cut-off	ICDS—regularly and NFHS at 5 years intervals
• Height-for-age	Below – 2SD	% above or below the cut-off	NFHS, NNMB
• Weight-for-height	Below – 2SD	% above or below cut-off	--do--
• Exlusive breastfeeding rate	up to six months	% of practice	Health
• Complementary feeding rate	–	% of practice	--do--
• Bottle feeding rate	–	--do--	--do--
• Breastfeeding continuation rate	–		--do-- --do--
• Mild upper arm circumference	13.5 cm	Above or below cut-off level	ICDS and Health
• Bitot's spots	0.5%	--do--	--do--
• Haemoglobin level	WHO reference	Above or below acceptable level	
• Use of iodised salt	100% of households using iodised salt	Percentage of households using iodised salt	Health
• Grades of goiter	TGR < 5%	Percentage of TGR	Health
• Other biochemical levels, such as serum vitamin A, serum cholesterol, fasting triglycerides, etc.	–	–	–

6

animal diseases, live stock and its productivity, cost of food, level of unemployment and below poverty line people are some indicators which are helpful in nutritional surveillance.

Nutrition Surveillance in India

- Nutritional surveillance has been entrusted to ICMR. National Nutrition Monitoring Bureau at NIN, Hyderabad, conducts periodic surveys in Southern states mostly and results are fed back to the system.
- Similarly, food and nutrition board have conducted surveys and available data has been used for effective planning.
- System of integrated child development services (ICDS) collects data on nutritional status of young children on regular basis, which helps state, districts and blocks to take appropriate action to improve the nutritional status. From 1975 to 1995, inputs of regular annual surveys done by consultants of ICDS provided useful data on nutritional surveillance of young children. During 12th plan period, it is proposed to strengthen the system of ICDS further to get quality data for action.
- Recently national family health surveys (NFHS) conducted at five years interval has provided wide ranging data on nutritional status of children, pregnant women and feeding practices, but five years for surveillance is too long a period and it only provides information at state level.[8]
- National Sample Survey Organization (NSSO) undertakes economic survey after every five years and it provides information on expenditure on food at family level.

Nutrition surveillance system as of now has to depend upon ICDS system and NNMB surveys: these must be strengthened so as to provide regular data-based information for action.

REFERENCES

1 WHO. The Health Aspects of Food and Nutrition. Manual for Developing Countries in the Western Pacific Region of the WHO. 3rd edn., Manila: WHO; 1979.
2 Rohde JE. Promoting Healthy Child Growth. NIPHC document; 16. New Delhi.
3 WHO. The Growth Chart: A tool for use in infant and child health care. Geneva: WHO; 1986.
4 Gopalan C. Growth charts in Primary Health Care – Time for Reassessment. NFI Bulletin 1992;13(2).
5 Ghosh S. Nutrition and Child Care – A practical guide. 1st edn., Jaypee Brothers; New Delhi: 1997.
6 Gopalan C, Chatterjee M. Use of growth charts for promoting child nutrition. NFI Special Publication Series 2.
7 NIPCCD. Growth Monitoring Manual. 1st edn., Deptt. of Women and Child Development. Ministry of HRD: 1988.
8 IIPS 2005–06 NFHS-3, Mumbai, India.

MALNUTRITION IN ADOLESCENTS (10–19 YEARS)

Adolescents represent about one-fifth of India's population. Adolescence is a period of second decade of life (10–19 years). During this phase of life, significant physical, physiological, psychological and emotional changes occur; which have bearing on the individual, community and the nation. Adolescence marks the beginning of menstrual cycle or reproduction. Healthy adolescence is a goal. Adolescents gain 50% of their adult weight and more than 20% of their adult height in age group 10–19 years, which we call as growth spurt. For healthy growth and development of adolescents, adequate diet is essential. Dietary requirements for adolescents are shown in Table 6.19.

The RDA for adolescents are seldom met with and consequently there is widespread problem of undernutrition amongst adolescents, particularly teenage girls.

Problem

Undernutrition in teenage girls and boys is the cause of concern in India. Girls do not grow as per norms and their growth potentials are not fully realized.

One-third of boys and girls had adequate weight and two-thirds were underweight (Table 6.20). Around 40% of adolescents were severely underweight for age in rural area.

The situation has not much changed over the years in rural areas. During 2005–06, 11.7% of teenaged married and unmarried girls had height less than 145 cm, and around 46.8% had body mass index (BMI) below 18.5 indicating that two-fifths of them were undernourished and suffer from the effect of chronic energy deficiency. It

Table 6.19: RDA for adolescents (2010) ICMR

	Years	*Body weight*	*Kcal/d*	*Protein g/d*	*Visible fat g/d*	*Calcium mg/d*	*Iron mg/d*	*Vit. A µg/d*	*β-carotene µg/d*
Boys	10–12	34.3	2190	39.9	35	800	21	600	4800
Girls	10–12	35.0	2010	40.4	35	800	27	600	4800
Boys	13–15	47.6	2750	54.3	45	800	32	600	4800
Girls	13–15	46.6	2330	51.9	40	800	27	600	4800
Boys	16–17	55.4	3020	61.5	50	800	28	600	4800
Girls	16–17	52.1	2440	55.5	35	800	26	600	4800

Table 6.20: Nutritional status (Gomez's criteria) of adolescent boys and girls 1990–91* (rural area)

Sex	Nutritional grades (%)				
	Normal	Gr. I	Gr. II	Gr. III	Gr. IV
Boys n = 8196	35.5	14.5	9.9	21.8	18.3
Girls n = 7584	34.4	15.0	11.8	22.5	16.3

*ICDS

indicates high prevalence of nutritional deficiency. In India, this is significant as 30% of adolescent girls get married below the age of 18 years and thus teenage marriages result into high-risk pregnancy and consequently outcome are low birth weight babies and high morbidity and high maternal mortality.

Problem of Anaemia in Adolescents

During the year 2001, overall prevalence of anaemia (haemoglobin < 12 g%) among adolescent girls was quite high. Over 90% of them were anaemic; over 50% had moderate anaemia (Hb 7–10 g%), 32% had mild anaemia (Hb 10–11.9 g%) and 7% had severe anaemia (Hb less than 7 g). High prevalence of anaemia among adolescent girls reflects their poor status of nutrition, and they tend to grow as risky women as their body size and pre-pregnancy weights are low with small size of pelvic bones. Due to chronic deprivation of food particularly during the period of growth and development leads to short stature of girls. Body weights of many girls tend to be less than 45 kg against standard weight of 55 kg.

Malnutrition is a problem that seriously impairs the health of adolescent and adult women and has its roots in early childhood. The causal relationship between anaemia and low birth weight, prematurity, perinatal mortality and maternal mortality has been extensively studied and established. Improvement in health and nutritional status of adolescent girls has an intergenerational impact.

Plan of Action

Adolescent's reproductive health and nutrition has been identified as underserved area under reproductive and child health (RCH) programme, and under National Population Policy, 2000.

1. Out of school adolescent girls belonging to economical weaker sections of society have been covered in ICDS programme for supplementary nutrition services besides vocational training. *Kishori Shakti Yojna* takes care of health, nutrition and development of adolescent girls in the age bracket of 11–18 years.
2. Under national nutritional anaemia control programme, and RMNCH + A, adolescent boys and girls have been covered for IFA supplements.
3. Adolescent girls will be reached through effective school health and nutrition programme. Adolescent to adolescent programme in school can be most effective for peer group education on nutrition and health.
4. **Legal framework:** Enforcing the Child Marriage Restraint Act of 1976 to reduce the incidence of teenage pregnancies. Preventing the marriage of girls below the legally permissible age of 18 should become a national concern. Let all girls first attain womenhood, and cross 18 years of life and attain full physical maturation so that their body size and pelvis and reproductive organs are fully developed.

EMERGING EPIDEMIC OF OBESITY IN URBAN AREAS

Among urban adolescents because of changed lifestyles and changed dietary practices problem of obesity is emerging as an epidemic. One in ten adolescents and young adults is clinically obese. The time trends data of NNMB indicate increase in body weight, height and triceps skin fold thickness of adolescents and it is suggestive that obesity is emerging in adolescents and adult women. Among the middle and high income, schools of Delhi about 30% of adolescents were overweight. NFHS data also indicate around 25% well to do urban women in India have BMI of 25 or more and 6–7% have BMI of 30 or more, which include adolescent girls also. Similarly, NNMB data in adult women indicates overweight of 7–12%. In Delhi and Punjab, more than 30% of adult women have BMI more than 25 (*see* Chapter 13).

The reasons for obesity in adolescents are current dietary trends and physical inactivity. Obesity is also being observed in younger school children, which is a sign of warning for the future (*see* Chapter 13).

MALNUTRITION IN ADULTS CHRONIC ENERGY DEFICIENCY (CED)

Chronic energy deficiency in adults can be measured by body mass index (BMI); which is defined as weight in kg divided by height in square metre (kg/m^2). The BMI of 18.5 in adult men and women is considered to be normal (Table 6.21). The normal BMI ranges are 18.5–25. BMI

Table 6.21: The International classification of adult underweight according to BMI

Classification	BMI kg/m^2 principal cut-off points	Additional cut-off points
Underweight	**< 18.50**	**< 18.50**
Severe thinness	< 16.00	< 16.00
Moderate thinness	16.00–16.99	16.00–16.99
Mild thinness	17.00–18.49	17.00–18.49
Normal range*	**18.50–24.99**	**18.50–22.99** **23.00–24.99**

Source: Adapted from WHO 1995, WHO 2000 and WHO 2004.
*NIN in India recommend normal range of BMI 18.5–23

of less than 18.5 is classified as underweight, < 16.00 is severe, ranges from 16.00 to 16.99 moderate, and from 17.00 to 18.49 is considered as mild chronic energy malnutrition (thinness) respectively.

One-third of adult population (33.7%) were having various grades of chronic energy deficiency while 56.6% were normal, over 9.7% constituted obese grade of BMI (Table 6.22). The effects of undernutrition of childhood are carried over to adolescents, adults and the adult population manifests chronic energy deficiency. Work capacity of adult goes down due to chronic malnutrition of long-standing.

Table 6.22: Prevalence of CED in adults (India nutrition profile 1998 and NFHS-3)*

BMI value	*1998 (Female)*	*NFHS-3 2006 (Both sexes)*
CED < 16–18.5	32.9	33.7
Normal 18.5–25	62.5	56.6
Obese I 25–30	3.8	8.4
Obese II > 30	0.7	1.3
Obese (Total) > 25	4.5	9.7

* All values in percentages

The chronic energy malnutrition in adult women is on the decline; from a high level of 51.8% in 1975–79, it has been reduced to 35.6%. The obesity shows a rising trend from 3.4% in 1975–79 to 12.6% in 2006 even in slum areas, indicating signs of prosperity even in urban slums (Table 6.23).

Table 6.23: Trends in body mass index in adult women (values in %)

BMI value	*NNMB 1975–79 n=6428*	*NNMB 1988–90 n=13422*	*NNMB 1994 n=1832*	*NNMB 1993–94 n=1319 Slums*	*NFHS-3 2006*
< 16 grade III	12.7	11.3	10.4	9.5	15.8
16–17 grade II	13.2	12.9	11.2	9.2	
17–18.5 grade I	25.9	25.1	25.5	18.0	19.7
All < 18.5	**51.8**	**49.3**	**47.1**	**36.7**	**35.6**
Normal 18.5–25	44.8	46.6	46.3	51.7	51.8
Obese > 25	3.4	4.1	6.6	11.6	12.6

Source: HPS Sachdev Bull NFI 1997, 18(2) and NFHS-3

Prevalence

On the basis of current information, 36% of adult women have chronic energy deficiency and 15.8% of adult women have severe chronic energy deficiency. The relationship of LBW with chronic energy malnutrition has been well established. Overall, incidence of LBW in 1991 was 30.5% while in severe CED mothers the incidence of LBW was 53%. In well-nourished mothers (obese grade I) it was around 15%.

MICRONUTRIENTS DEFICIENCY DISORDERS

Nutritional Anaemia

Iron deficiency anaemia is a problem of serious public health significance. Nutritional anaemia (iron deficiency) is the most common micronutrient deficiency in the world affecting more than 700 million persons. Nutritional anaemias are most common in pregnant and lactating mothers, infants, preschool children and adolescent girls.

Causes

Predominant cause is inadequate food intake. Dietary iron intake may be inadequate or insufficient iron is absorbed to meet body requirements or reduced bioavailability of dietary iron or needs for iron get increased or due to chronic blood loss. Iron deficiency is by far the commonest cause of nutritional anaemia. Malaria, hookworm disease (ankylostomiasis or necatoriasis),[1] schistosomiasis and other infections play an important role in tropical climates. Conditions which initiate and perpetuate anaemia will be discussed subsequently.[2]

At Risk Groups

Infants, preschool children, adolescents, women in child-bearing age, particularly pregnant women and lactating mothers are at greatest risk of developing iron deficiency anaemia. Adult males may also be at risk where there is chronic energy malnutrition due to inadequate food intake or frequent parasitic infection.

Definition of Anaemia

Anaemia is defined as reduction of haemoglobin level in circulation. WHO in 2001 has suggested cut-off values for different groups of population as shown in Table 6.24.[3, 4]

Severity of anaemia: Depending upon the level of haemoglobin, the degree of anaemia can be classified as mild, moderate and severe as shown in Table 6.25. The classification helps to determine priorities and launching of intervention and allocation of scarce resource.[4] Health workers track severely anaemics.

Table 6.24: Haemoglobin levels below which anaemia is present in population

Age or gender group	*Haemoglobin g%*
Children 6–59 months	11
Children 5–11 years	11.5
Children 12–14 years	12
Non-pregnant women (above 15 years of age)	12
Pregnant women	11
Men above 15 years of age	13

Table 6.25: Classification of anaemia in pregnancy	
Degree of anaemia	*Level of Hb g%*
Mild	10–10.9
Moderate	7–10
Severe	< 7

Requirements of Iron

The types of diet consumed normally in India should contain 20–30 mg iron to meet the iron requirement of adult. The iron requirements are substantially increased during the special physiological conditions like pregnancy and rapid growth during early childhood period (infancy and preschool period). Similarly, in adolescent girls and boys, the iron requirements are more. The RDA for special age and gender group are as shown in Table 6.26.[5]

Table 6.26: RDA of iron for Indians (ICMR 2010)	
Groups	*Requirement*
Pregnant women	35 mg
Lactating mothers	21 mg
Children 6–12 months	5 mg
Children 1–3 years	9 mg
4–6 years	13 mg
7–9 years	16 mg
Boys 10–12 years	21 mg
Girls 10–12 years	27 mg
Boys 13–15 years	32 mg
Girls 13–15 years	27 mg
Boys 16–17 years	28 mg
Girls 16–17 years	26 mg

Magnitude of Problem of Anaemia

Nutritional anaemia during pregnancy is widespread in India (Table 6.27). As many as 50–87% of pregnant women have haemoglobin level below 11 g% which is unacceptably high prevalence. Of these, 13% are severely anaemic (haemoglobin levels below 7 g%). The prevalence of anaemia in pregnancy over the years has not much changed as per studies of ICMR, it was around 87.5% in 1989 and 85% in the year 2001. It means that all the interventions and programmes against anaemia have not much succeeded, anaemia problem remains where it was.[4,6–10] This further signifies that much remains to be done to reduce the morbidity due to anaemia.

- One in five of all maternal deaths are attributable to anaemia during pregnancy.
- Nearly 70 million, i.e. 60–70% of all children below 6 years suffer from varying degrees of anaemia in our country (NFHS-3 figures for anaemia was 79%).
- More than half 50–90% adolescent girls are anaemic.

Goal: It was envisaged under National Nutritional Policy of India and re-emphasized in 10th plan period to reduce prevalence of anaemia by 25% and severe anaemia by 50% in children, pregnant women, lactating mothers and adolescents.[10, 11] Eleventh plan goal was to reduce anaemia among women and girls by 50% by the end of 11th plan (2012), and 12th plan repeats the same.

Public Health Consequences of Anaemia in Pregnant Women

In Pregnant Women: Anaemia is Killer

Anaemia in pregnant women is reflection of insufficient food intake by pregnant women. This leads to serious consequences. Anaemia during pregnancy is responsible for 19% of all maternal deaths. Anaemia is also a contributory factor of maternal deaths due to haemorrhages, septicaemia and eclampsia. While a healthy woman may tolerate a blood loss up to one litre or more during childbirth, for anaemic women even a normal blood loss of 250 ml can be fatal.

Infection

Since anaemic women have lower resistance to infection and their general health condition is low, they are at higher risk of complications, such as sepsis after delivery (post-puerperal sepsis) which is responsible for 16% of maternal mortality.

Anaemic mothers are more prone to haemorrhages after delivery and are at risk of maternal mortality. Haemorrhages account for 29% of maternal mortality.

Low Birth Weight Babies

Anaemic mothers give birth to low birth weight babies (less than 2.5 kg) and around 28% of births are low birth weight babies in India. Anaemia in pregnancy is one of the significant cause of low birth weight. Anaemic mothers

Table 6.27: Prevalence of anaemia in India[4,6–10] (Figures in %)

At risk groups	*Agency and year of study*				
	ICMR 1989	*Task force*	*NFHS-2*	*ICMR 2001*	*NFHS-3*
Pregnant women	87.5	47–95	49.7	84.9	57.9
Lactating mothers	–	77–95	56.4	–	–
Adolescent girls	–	–	61.0*	90.1	–
Preschool children	–	30-95	74.3	–	79.2

*Seshadri 1998, Rural, Gujarat

have three times greater risk of premature delivery and low birth weight babies, nine times higher risk of perinatal mortality and higher risk of irreversible brain damage in infants born to severely anaemic mothers. Work capacity of women is reduced, they become lethargic, breathless and get tired easily even after normal work. Anaemia incapacitates women and reduces their physical work capacity and productivity.

In Young Children

Anaemia retards physical growth and mental development of child, reduces scholastic performance, decreases attention span, memory and concentration.

In Adolescents

Anaemia may lead to delayed menstrual cycle, poor growth, reduced work capacity and poor reproductive outcome. It reduces their concentration and school performance.

Factors and Conditions Responsible for Anaemia

- In India, prime factor being lack of sufficient intake of food and particularly lack of intake of iron rich foods and poor absorption of iron from food into the body. On the whole bioavailability of vegetarian sources of iron is low. In vegetarian diets based on staple cereals (millets, wheat, rice and vegetables), the iron absorption ranges from 2 to 5%. The iron absorption on an average for mixed cereal diets is 3%. Phytates of cereals, tannins and polyphenol of vegetables inhibit iron absorption. Haem iron is better absorbed. Bioavailability of haem iron is high and absorption ranges from 10 to 20%. It is available from animal sources (meat, fish, poultry and blood products).
- Presence of persistent diarrhoea and worm infestations prevents absorption of iron.
- Once absorbed chronic diseases like malaria, which causes damage to the red blood cells produces anaemia in endemic areas of malaria.
- Increased demand of iron during pregnancy also causes anaemia, repeated pregnancies and short birth interval cause anaemia among women.
- Hookworm disease is another important factor in causation of anaemia due to chronic blood loss.
- Non-haem iron is mainly found in cereals, vegetables and pulses, bioavailability is poor.
- ***Contamination iron:*** From soil dust, water, iron pots, bioavailability is low.
- ***Fortification iron:*** Varied bioavailability depends on composition of food.

Social Factors

Heavy workload and long hours of work combined with inadequate food intake leads to chronic malnutrition including anaemia. Traditional social values requiring women to eat last in the family and observing rituals like fasts during pregnancy and avoidance of certain foods thought to be hot or abortifacient (sugar, jaggeries and even iron and folic acid tablets), seem to be important social factors contributing to anaemia.

Poverty and reproduction behaviour of having too many children and repeated pregnancies deplete iron stores of women. Low status of women and illiteracy are other important social factors.

Poor acceptance: Only 22.3% of mothers consumed IFA tablets for 90 days or more (NFHS-3).

Factors and Causes in Children

In children, iron deficiency in first 6 months is dependent upon the iron reserves acquired from the mother during fetal life. If women are anaemic children born to them will have less iron reserve.

The major factor is delayed weaning and insufficient semisolid and solid food intake by young children. Cereals, pulses and green leafy vegetables are deliberately withheld from the diets of young children because of many wrong beliefs.

Apart from inadequate dietary iron intake, impaired absorption due to persistent diarrhoea and other chronic infections are other factors. Iron supplements are seldom accepted by families.

Adolescent

Adolescent girls are more vulnerable due to poor eating, insufficient foods, onset of menstruation and consequent blood loss and avoidance of IFA tablets.

STRATEGIES FOR PREVENTION OF NUTRITIONAL ANAEMIA[12-16]

Adequate Food and Iron Rich Food

Ensuring adequate food consumption and iron rich food consumption during pregnancy, lactation, early childhood period, adolescent girls, and boys. 50 g of green leafy vegetables consumption per day can provide adequate quantity of iron in diet, besides providing calcium, beta-carotene and vitamin 'C' however, green leafy vegetable consumption per consumption unit is quite low in India (15 g per day). Along with green leafy vegetables, adequate consumption of cereals, rice, wheat, ragi, jowar and bajra, sprouted pulses and jaggery can provide enough of iron in usual diets.

Bajra is good source of iron. Milk is poor source of iron. Bajra has 8.0 mg of iron per 100 g. Wheat contains 5.3 mg, Bengal gram 4.5 mg per 100 g. Amaranth and Bengal gram leaves has 23 mg of iron per 100 g.

Feeding Young Children

Exclusive breastfeeding for 6 months and including green leafy vegetables in the weaning foods of infants after 6 months by mothers and families. Timely weaning and enough food for young child is essential to prevent anaemia.

Promoters

Vitamin C promotes absorption of iron. Vitamin C rich foods are lemon, orange, guava, amla and tomatoes.

Deworming

Deworming pregnant women and children periodically to get rid of worms and promote iron absorption.

Malaria Prophylaxis

Personal protection and prophylaxis by use of insecticide treated bednets should be promoted.

Environmental Sanitation

Promotion of sanitary latrines to avoid contamination of soil with faecal matter and thereby prevention of worm infestation (hookworms). Promoting personal hygiene (handwashing) and wearing of shoes will prevent infection.

Contraception

Contraception and limiting family size to one or two children can prevent anaemia in women.

Supplementary Food and Iron and Folic Acid

Supplementary feeding through ICDS programme for pregnant women, lactating mothers and young children as also distribution of IFA supplements to women, adolescent girls and children have not met with much success.

Food Fortification (Double Fortified Salt)

Technology of salt fortification exists in the country. Salt iodation (iodized salt) is already being done in the country. Technology of double fortification of salt (adding iodate and iron) was developed in India at NIN, Hyderabad. Since iodine was found to be highly unstable in the iron fortified salt developed earlier; an alternative technology was developed by use of sodium hexametaphosphate as the stabilizer along with ferrous sulphate to enhance iron stability and bioavailability. Sodium hexametaphosphate helps to chelate iron, keep it in a soluble form and prevents its interaction with iodine. This has been pilot tested in limited area. However, iron fortified or double fortified salt has not as yet become part of public health programmes to combat anaemia, though feasible and effective. Currently attempts are being made to manufacture and distribute iron fortified salt in Tamil Nadu. Hopefully this will be extended to other parts of the country.

Consumption of locally grown leafy vegetables in home kitchen garden and in farms along with adequate staple foods (cereals and pulses) remain the sheet anchor to prevent malnutrition and anaemia.

POLICY ON CONTROL OF NUTRITIONAL ANAEMIA

Nutritional anaemia is a serious public health problem. To respond to this problem, the Government of India launched National Nutritional Anaemia Prophylaxis Programme (NNAPP) way back in 1970 as part of National Family Planning Programme.

Target Beneficiaries Under NNAPP

Expectant and nursing mothers/acceptors of family planning methods like IUCD, tubectomized women and preschool children were identified as beneficiaries.

Before enrolling them on prophylaxis programme, an estimate of the level of Hb was to be done preferably by Sahli's method. In situations like rural subcentres, where this may not be possible at least the estimation by a Tallqvist Hb scale should be done. Women showing Hb level less than 10 g% and preschool children Hb level less than 8 g% should be put on active anti-anaemia treatment straightway. Those women having Hb level of 10 g and above and children showing Hb level of 8 g and above can be put on prophylaxis programme. All institutions rendering family planning and MCH services like PHCs, SCs and MCH centres and hospitals, urban family welfare centres should implement the programme.

Dosage

Daily recommended dose was one tablet containing 60 mg of ferrous sulphate and 0.1 mg of folic acid for children. Pregnant, nursing mothers and family planning acceptors received 180 mg of ferrous sulphate and 0.5 mg of folic acid daily. The daily administration of tablets should be continued till the level of Hb is attained and maintained at a satisfactory level. Each beneficiary was given one tablet daily for 100 days once in a year. Iron syrup was also introduced for young children. It is necessary that the Hb is repeated at 3–4 months intervals. It is estimated that on an average each beneficiary may require administration of tablets for a period of 6 months. The exact period will depend upon the progress of individual beneficiary.[14,15]

Drug Delivery

For the sake of convenience, the drugs may be issued for fortnight or for a month at a time. The auxiliary nurse midwife/lady health visitor/FP assistant should check on the actual use of tablets by mothers and children during their routine home visits.

Supply of Drugs

The tablets were supplied in two types and two packings:

i Orange coloured small tablets containing 60 mg of ferrous sulphate and 0.1 mg folic acid packed in tin of 1000 and 5000 tablets.

ii A large grey coloured tablet containing 180 mg of ferrous sulphate and 0.5 mg folic acid packed in tin of 1000 and 5000 tablets. The tablets are sugarcoated and therefore are to be preserved in dry cool place to avoid absorption of moisture.

Records and Reports

Records and reports were maintained at above mentioned facilities for monitoring and coverage of beneficiaries. Report format was quite cumbersome.

Drawbacks

The whole concern of programme was to distribute tablets, no nutrition education or dietary improvement component was built into the programme. It was a mechanical programme; supplies ran short, quality of packing and tablets was poor and at many places these were unused. High coverage was only on paper and real ground situation was contrary to the inflated reports of coverage.

Evaluation

An evaluation by Indian Council of Medical Research of the 20 years old national programme for prevention of nutritional anaemia (involving distribution of iron and folic acid tablets 100 days in a year), has shown that prevalence of anaemia among pregnant women has not diminished and continued to be staggering 87.6%. More significantly there was little difference observed in the prevalence of anaemia among pregnant women who were supplied with iron tablets (88.1%) when compared to those who did not get iron supplements (87.6%). It could be inferred that possibly the supplement given was not adequate, the compliance was low and/or quality of tablets was poor.[8,9]

Therefore, the programme was revised and policy on control of nutritional anaemia was revised by MOH and FW, Government of India in 1991 and the name of the programme was changed to "National Nutritional Anaemia Control Programme".[16]

NATIONAL NUTRITIONAL ANAEMIA CONTROL PROGRAMME (NNACP)

Objective

The NNACP aims at significantly decreasing the prevalence and incidence of anaemia in women in reproductive age group, especially pregnant and lactating women and preschool children. Adolescent girls were also included in the programme under RCH programme. The programme focuses on the following strategies:

Strategies

1 Promotion of regular consumption of foods rich in iron.
2 Provision of iron and folate supplements in the form of tablets (folifer tablets) to the high-risk groups.
3 Identification and treatment of severely anaemic cases.
4 Deworming programme.

Implementation: The programme is being implemented through primary health care set-up (PHC and SC). The multipurpose health worker female and male are responsible for distribution of iron tablets (adult and paediatric doses) to pregnant, lactating women, IUD users and children aged 6 months to 5 years, 6–10 years and also to adolescents (10–19 years).[17]

ICDS equal partner: The functionaries of ICDS programme under the department of women and child development are equal partners who help and assist in the distribution of iron tablets in ICDS programme to enhance the coverage of beneficiaries. Anganwadi workers (AWWs) also impart nutrition education to mothers to promote consumption of iron rich foods in the family. Other sectors can be involved to enhance the programme.

The ***Vande Mataram scheme*** has been launched on 9th February 2004 in all the districts of the country with the active collaboration of professional bodies, viz. Federation of Obstetrics and Gynaecological Society of India (FOGSI) and Indian Medical Association (IMA). The aim of the scheme is to reduce the maternal mortality and morbidity of the pregnant and lactating mothers by involving and utilizing the vast resources of specialists/trained workforce available in the private sector. The scheme intends to provide free antenatal and postnatal check-ups, counselling on nutrition, breastfeeding, spacing of birth and distribution of iron and folic acid tablets, etc. through public–private partnership.[17,18]

PREVENTION OF NUTRITIONAL ANAEMIA

Promoting Consumption of Iron Rich Foods

- Regular dietary intake of iron and folic acid rich foods by pregnant and lactating mothers, adolescent girls and children under 5 years must be promoted.
- Regular consumption of iron rich foods, such as green leafy vegetables (mustard leaves), Amaranth (Cholai sag), Colocasia leaves, Knol and Knol leaves *(ganth gobi ka sag)*, Bengal gram leaves, turnip green leaves and cereals, such as wheat, ragi, jowar and bajra, pulses (especially sprouted pulses and gur (Jaggery) must be promoted widely. In addition, whatever culturally and economically feasible, such as consumption of animal flesh foods—meat, liver, etc. must be encouraged.
- Ensure incorporation of iron rich foods as green leafy vegetables in the weaning foods of infants.
- Vitamin C (ascorbic acid) promotes absorption of iron. Regular consumption of vitamin C rich foods, such as lemon, orange, guava, amla, green mango along with iron rich food must be encouraged.
- For increasing availability of iron rich foods, growing of iron rich foods in home gardens, kitchen garden, farms and fields and consumption of these must be promoted (Applied Nutrition Programme).

6

- Tea inhibits absorption of iron in the body. Advise reduced consumption of tea, specially during pregnancy for improving absorption of iron and prevention of anaemia.

To manage the widespread prevalence of anaemia in the country the policy has been revised and **National Iron Plus Initiative** has been launched

National Iron + Initiative, New Strategies Under Reproductive Maternal, Newborn, Child and Adolescent Health (RMNCH + A)

This initiative brings together existing programmes for IFA supplementation among pregnant and lactating women, adolescents and children. The initiative aims to ensure provision of IFA supplements and therapeutic management of mild, moderate and severe anaemia in the most vulnerable groups viz. Children (6 months to 10 years), adolescents (10–19 years) both in and out of school, pregnant and lactating women and women in reproductive age group (15–45 years). This initiative includes:

- Screening and tracking undernutrition and anaemia in homes, schools and anganwadis;
- **Preschool children 6 months to 5 years:** Bi-weekly iron supplementation in home setting under direct observation of ASHA, one tablet of 20 mg elemental iron + 100 mcg folic acid.
- **School children 5–10 years:** 45 mg elemental iron + 400 mcg folic acid weekly throughout the entire period of 5–10 years in government and government aided schools and municipal schools plus deworming.
- **Out of school children 5–10 years:** At Anganwadi Centre weekly IFA supplementation.
- **Adolescent 10–19 years:** Weekly IFA supplementation (WIFS) programme covers adolescents enrolled in class VI–XII (10–19 years) in schools and out of school. IFA tablet of 100 mg elemental iron + 500 mcg folic acid for adolescents is coloured blue (iron ki nili goli). The programme covers adolescents of government, government aided and municipal schools as well as out of school girls.

The Programme Envisages

- Supervised administration of weekly IFA supplement
- Screening of target groups for moderate and severe anaemia and referral to appropriate health facility.
- Bi-annual deworming (Albendazole 400 mg).
- Information and counseling to improve dietary intake and preventive actions for intestinal worm infestation.
- **Pregnant women:** One red tablet containing 100 mg elemental iron + 500 mcg folic acid prophylactically daily, starting after first trimester at 14–16 weeks of gestation for 100 days. If clinically anaemic two such tablets to be given daily for 100 days.
- Nursing mothers and acceptors of family planning: One red tablet containing 100 mg elemental iron + 500 mcg folic acid daily for 100 days.
- **Women in reproductive age group:** One tablet containing 100 mg elemental iron + 500 mcg folic acid weekly throughout reproductive period (15–45 years).
- Use of folic acid is promoted in planned pregnancies during the periconception stage (three months before and three months after conception) for prevention of neural tube defects and other congenital anomalies.

Treatment of Severe Anaemia

Women with Hb level below 7 g% are considered to be severely anaemic. Testing of blood for Hb concentration at field level is neither considered safe nor practical. Therefore, as far as possible, severely anaemic cases should be identified on the basis of clinical signs. All health workers should be trained to identify such anaemic cases.

Recommended therapeutic dose for women in reproductive age group is one tablet (large) of folifer twice daily for a minimum of 100 days. This will provide equivalent to 200 mg elemental iron and 1000 ug of folic acid per day. Further cases of severe anaemia should be referred to PHC medical officers for diagnosis of causative factor and treatment. Tracking system of severely anaemic mothere has been introduced now.

Distribution

These tablets can be distributed during outreach immunization sessions or on the day of antenatal clinic along with Tetanus toxiod immunization or at Anganwadi to children 1–5 years of age. It is important to understand that intake of folifer tablets may cause change in the consistency of stool, i.e. stool may either become loose or hard. The colour of stool may also turn black. There is no cause to get worried with such mild symptoms and one must continue taking folifer tablets. IFA (large) and IFA (small) are distributed free of cost at government health centres. To prevent deterioration of quality of the tablets, it is now supplied in strip of 10 tablets in bubble packs. It is important that drinking tea should be avoided within an hour of taking iron tablets.

Since these tablets are sugar coated, young children may consume excess of iron and toxic effects may occur, at times fatal outcome/accidents have been reported hence the safety should be ensured by family and parents and health workers must educate parents. These tablets should not be accessible to young children in homes.

Goal of 12th Plan

Reduce anaemia among women and girls by 50% by the end of the 12th plan.[19]

REFERENCES

1. WHO. Pawlowski ZS, School GA, Stott GJ. Hookworm infection and anaemia. Approaches to prevention and control. 1991, WHO, Geneva.
2. World Bank. Direction in development: Wasting away—The crisis of Malnutrition in India, 1999. The International Bank for Reconstruction and Development: The World Bank; 1999.
3. WHO. Iron deficiency anaemia, assessment, prevention and control—A guide for programme managers. UNICEF, United Nations, WHO; 2001.
4. ICMR. Micronutrient deficiency disorders in sixteen districts of India. New Delhi: ICMR; 2001.
5. ICMR. Nutrient requirement and recommended dietary allowances for Indians—Report of expert group of ICMR. NIN, Hyderabad: ICMR; 1992.
6. GOI and UNICEF. Report of meeting on prevention and control of nutritional anaemia. New Delhi: GOI, UNICEF; 1989.
7. WHO. Preventing and controlling iron deficiency anaemia through primary health care—A guide for health administrators and programme managers. Geneva: WHO; 1989.
8. IIPS. National Family Health Survey -2, 1998–99. Mumbai: IIPS; 2002, and NFHS-3,2005–06.
9. UNICEF. Children and women in India—A situation analysis. New Delhi: UNICEF; 1990.
10. UNICEF. Rights and opportunities—The situation of children and women in India. India Country Office, New Delhi: UNICEF; 1998.
11. GOI. National plan of action on nutrition. New Delhi: Food and Nutrition Board Department of Women and Child Development; 1995.
12. Planning Commission (GOI). Tenth Five-Year Plan. New Delhi: GOI; 2002–2007.
13. Proceedings of National Workshop on methodologies for assessment of vitamin A deficiency, iron deficiency anaemia and iodine deficiency disorders. 2004 Sep. 13–15; AIIMS, New Delhi.
14. GOI. Policy on control of nutritional anaemia. New Delhi: MOH and FW (GOI); 1994.
15. GOI. National Child Survival and Safe Motherhood Programme. New Delhi: MOH and FW (GOI); 1994.
16. GOI. Basic guide to reproductive and child health programme—for use by NGOs training institutes and health functionaries. New Delhi: MOH and FW (GOI); 1998.
17. GOI. Annual Report 2008–09. New Delhi: GOI; 2009.
18. GOI. Reproductive and Child Health News Letter vol 6: (4) Jan-Mar 2004, MOH and FW, GOI: New Delhi.
19. GOI Towards Faster and more Inclusive Growth. An Approach to the 12th Five-Year Plan: GOI Planning Commission. Yojna Bhavan, New Delhi, Feb 2012.

VITAMIN A DEFICIENCY (VAD)

Vitamin A is essential for normal vision. It also maintains integrity of epithelial cells and is essential for many metabolic functions. It is a fat soluble vitamin and can be stored in liver for a longer time. Vitamin A deficiency (VAD) is common in underprivileged population. Severe forms of VAD (like keratomalacia) has declined considerably, however, it remains a public health problem in many parts of the world including India. The risk of deficiency is greater in preschool children as also in pregnant and lactating women; as their requirements are higher owing to physiological reasons, i.e. rapid growth in children, growing foetus draws its nutrients from pregnant mother and lactating mothers have to produce milk around 700 ml per day.

Requirement of Vitamin A (Retinol)

Groups		*Retinol mcg/day*	*β-carotene**
Infants	0–6 months	350	2800
	6–12 months	350	2800
Children	1–3 years	400	3200
	4–6 years	400	3200
	7–9 years	600	4800
Adolescents	10–17 years	600	4800
Pregnant woman		800	6400
Lactating mother		950	7600

*A conversion ratio of 1:8 is used

For non-pregnant and non-lactating women (NPNL), the recommended dietary allowance (RDA) is 600 mcg/day.

Pregnant and Lactating Mothers

For pregnant women 800 mcg per day of retinol is considered to be adequate. For lactating mothers who secrete 700 ml of breast milk per day require 950 mcg of retinol per day. Additional intake of 350 mcg for lactating mothers is in keeping with the intake of infants below 6 months.

Dietary Intakes

It has been observed that over the years the dietary intake of vitamin A has not improved in India, intake of vitamin A remains much below the RDA for young children as also for pregnant and lactating mothers (Table 6.28).

Dietary Sources of Vitamin A

Rich sources of vitamin A of animal origin are milk, liver and egg where it is available as preformed vitamin A (retinol).

The vegetable rich sources are green leafy vegetables, carrots and yellow fruits (mango, papaya and pumpkins)

Table 6.28: Consumption of food stuffs and nutrient intake (g/Cu/day) and trends in Bitot's spots NNMB—data 1996–97

	1975–79	*1988–90*	*1996–97*
Green leafy vegetables (g)	8	9	15
Vitamin A (mcg)	246	282	300
Bitot's spots (%)	1.8	0.7	0.7

where it is available in the form of β-carotene which can be converted in the body into vitamin A (Retinol). Conversion ratio for β-carotene to vitamin A is 8:1. In India, major dietary sources of vitamin A are green leafy vegetables and milk (Tables 6.29 and 6.30).

Table 6.29: Vitamin A content in food stuffs of animal sources

Items	*Vitamin A mcg per 100 g*
Egg	360 mcg of vitamin A
Liver	6690 mcg of vitamin A
Milk	160–170 mcg of vitamin A
Human milk	137 mcg of vitamin A

Table 6.30: β-carotene content in common food stuffs

Green leafy vegetables and fruits	*β-carotene (mcg) per 100 gm*
Amaranth tender	5520
Bathua leaves	1740
Beet greens	5862
Bengal gram leaves	978
Carrot leaves	5700
Colocacia leaves (black)	12000
Colocacia leaves (green)	10278
Coriander leaves	6918
Curry leaves	7560
Drumstick leaves	6780
Fenugreek leaves	2340
Fetid, cassia	10152
Mint	1620
Spinach leaves	5580
Reddish leaves	5295
Rajagira leaves	14190
Turnip leaves	9396

VAD as Public Health Problem

VAD is considered to be public health problem in many countries including India. According to WHO, if prevalence of any one indicator, such as: Bitot's spot more than 0.5% and corneal xerosis in excess of 0.01% and keratomalacia more than 0.0% and corneal opacity more than 1.0% in young children then it is considered as significant public health problem necessitating urgent response and action.

PROBLEM OF VAD IN INDIA

In India, the level of Bitot's spots which was 2% in 1979 has declined to 0.7% in 2001, indicates that it is still a public health problem. There are considerable interstate variation of prevalence (Table 6.31).

Table 6.31: Problem has been sized up by various surveys[1]

Surveys	*Bitot's spots%*
NIN-1997	0.70
India nutrition profile 1998	0.21
District survey-2001 (ICMR)	0.70
NNMB survey 2011–12	0.2*
Target	< 0.5

* Polled data of seven states (Kerala, Tamil Nadu, Karnataka, AP, Maharashtra, Gujrat and Odisha)

Vulnerability

Young children below the age of 3 years, pregnant and lactating women are most vulnerable to vitamin A deficiency. Young children in age group 9 months to 3 years are most susceptible. Protein energy malnutrition is also common in this age bracket.

Sex: Prevalence is more in male children as compared to female children but it may vary.

Geographical distribution in India: The prevalence of VAD is more pronounced in Rajasthan, Bihar, Madhya Pradesh, Odisha, UP, Tamil Nadu, Karnataka and Andhra Pradesh. There may be pockets with high prevalence of VAD within the state or the district.

Social Significance

VAD may produce blindness; a permanent disability. Around 40,000 children used to become blind due to VAD way back in 1970s, per year.

Famines and Droughts (Monsoon Failure)

Droughts lead to failure of crops and vegetables as also poor yield of milk by animals because of lack of fodder. Children are most vulnerable to droughts and famines and suffer from the effect of malnutrition including vitamin A. Special attention has to be focused on young children during droughts and famines. Vitamin A is more stable than carotene. Light, particularly ultraviolet rays and air have destructive influence on vitamin A. However, ordinary cooking of vegetables causes negligible losses in the carotene content. Fresh green leafy vegetables contain more carotene than do stale ones.

Serum Plasma Level

Serum/plasma vitamin A/retinol concentration of 20 mcg/dl or above is considered to be normal in children. If it is less than that it indicates subclinical deficiency.

Deficiency

Vitamin A deficiency does not occur is isolation. It is a reflection of undernutrition or PEM. Vitamin A deficiency produces night blindness, delayed dark adaptation, and lowers the resistance to infections. Common infections (measles, acute respiratory infections, diarrhoea and worm infestation) increase the demand of vitamin A and produce vitamin A deficiency in young children or precipitate subclinical vitamin A deficiency to clinical deficiency. These infections are quite common in young children and these occur repeatedly and it is not uncommon for young children to have prolonged period of sickness. Consequences of these infections are widespread malnutrition, as half of children below 6 years of age suffer from malnutrition. These infections interfere with the absorption of vitamin A. These infections particularly the measles, lower the vitamin A status of the young children and lead to increased risk of nutritional blindness.

Food Intake

Pregnant women in India are malnourished and during pregnancy food intake including vitamin A are much lower than RDA. This leads to poor vitamin A reserves of liver of neonates, who are born as low birth weight babies. Consequently after delivery these babies get less vitamin A through breast milk as breast milk of poorly nourished women is low in vitamin A content. Further the young children who are often given inadequate quantities of supplementary food (less of milk and less of green vegetables) are susceptible to the effect of VAD. Therefore, VAD is a nutritional deficiency in its origin. Logically, the adequate diets during pregnancy and lactation period with food rich in vitamin A should be encouraged to mitigate VAD.

PREVENTION STRATEGIES

Food-based Approach

Apart from adequate diet, regular consumption of dark green leafy vegetables or yellow fruits and other diets rich in vitamin A during pregnancy, lactation and childhood period prevents vitamin A deficiency.

Infants

Immediately after birth "colostrum feeding" to young babies provides best of vitamin A as colostrum is rich in vitamin A.

Encourage: Exclusive breastfeeding till 6 months of age.

- Adequate quantity of supplementary feeding beyond 6 months of age; add vitamin A rich foods like egg yolk, green leafy vegetables and milk besides staples.
- ***Control infection:*** Early recognition and prompt treatment of diarrhoea, acute respiratory infections and deworming for parasite infection will improve the status of vitamin A.
- Immunization against measles and giving vitamin A 1,00,000 units at 9 months of age.
- ***1–5 years children:*** Adequate diet and vitamin A rich foods and prompt treatment of infection. Vitamin A megadose 2,00,000 IU at 16, 24, 30, 36, 42, 48, 54 and 60 months of age.

Measles, Severe Malnutrition and Vitamin A

- All children suffering from measles should be given one dose of vitamin A, if the child has not received it within the previous one month. Vitamin A reduces measles mortality and associated complications of the respiratory and gastrointestinal tract and hence beneficial (*see* Chapter 12 Measles).
- All cases of severe protein energy malnutrition should be given one additional dose of vitamin A.
- All children with xerophthalmia should be given 2 doses of synthetic vitamin A as per present schedule of Government of India under RCH programme.
- No additional dose of vitamin A is required for children suffering from diarrhoea and respiratory infection.
- No vitamin A mega dose for pregnant or lactating mother recommended under the programme.

Improving diets and dietary intakes of vitamin A holds key in the long run. Growing vitamin A rich foods in the kitchen garden or in farms and fields and consumption of these foods by children, pregnant and lactating women can go a long way. Administration of synthetic vitamin A is a short-term measure and it cannot substitute the adequate intake of vitamin A through food rich in vitamin A and culturally acceptable foods.

Bad Practices and Beliefs

Bad practices and beliefs are discarding of colostrum, delaying supplementation of food, feeding less quantities of food to young children, belief that green leafy vegetables cannot be digested by young children. Many families consider that mango and papaya are 'hot' foods and are harmful for children and pregnant women; hence discouraged. Lack of information to families and community has been a stumbling block.

NATIONAL PROGRAMME FOR VAD (CONTROL OF BLINDNESS)

VAD was recognized as a major public health problem in India in 1970 and in late 1970s it was estimated that 30–40,000 children could lose their eyesight due to VAD in India. The prevalence of eye signs of VAD was as high as 30–50% in some states in 1960. The national prophylaxis programme against blindness due to VAD was launched in 1970 and by 1975 the whole country was covered.

Objective

To prevent nutritional blindness due to VAD, leading to keratomalacia in children under 5 years of age. There were two strategies—short-term and long-term.

Short-term strategy: To administer synthetic vitamin A to young children of 9 months to 5 years of age with the objective of decreasing the prevalence of VAD to below 0.5%.

Long-term strategy: Ultimate solution for prevention of vitamin A deficiency is regular consumption of vitamin A rich foods which are cheap and locally available (food based approach).

Target—short-term strategy: Preschool children in age group 9 months to 5 years were targeted for the programme.

One dose of 2,00,000 IU of vitamin A orally every 6 months. In all, it was intended to administer 9 oral doses from 9 months to 5 years at the interval of 6 months.

Subsequently in 1992 when child survival and safe motherhood programme (CSSM) started, the vitamin A prophylaxis was integrated with universal programme (UIP) of immunization. Children in age group 9 months to 3 years were targeted under CSSM programme for vitamin A prophylaxis. First dose of vitamin A prophylaxis was given along with measles vaccines at age 9 to 12 months (1,00,000 IU units). Now the CSSM programme has been merged with reproductive and child health (RCH) programme.

STRATEGY UNDER CSSM AND RCH PROGRAMME

- To provide vitamin A supplements to children in age group 9 months to 3 years at 6 months intervals.[2]
- Promote exclusive breastfeeding and feeding of colostrum.
- Promote intake of balanced food including green leafy vegetables and yellow fruits.
- Increase coverage with measles vaccine.
- Provide additional attention and monitor areas with identified cases of night blindness in children and areas where measles outbreaks have occurred, since infections deplete vitamin A reserves and increases mortality rate in measles. All children with measles and night blindness need vitamin A.

Vitamin A Prophylaxis Current Strategy

Prevalence of vitamin A deficiency; is maximum in age group 6 months to 3 years. In addition to the risk of blindness, the children with vitamin A deficiency are at a risk of dying due to infections. It is, therefore, imperative that all children in this age group be given vitamin A prophylaxis.

- Every child in age group 9 months–5 years be given 9 doses of vitamin A.
- The first dose of 100,000 IU or 1 ml solution of vitamin A will be given at nine months preferably along with measles immunization.
- The second dose of 200,000 IU will be given at 16 months with booster dose of DPT/OPV.
- Seven more doses of 200,000 IU will be given at 6 months interval thereafter.

Vitamin A Deficiency

In children who have vitamin A deficiency, the surface of cornea becomes dry and rough and may ultimately breakdown partially or completely. This may lead to ulceration and permanent scarring or irreversible damage and permanent loss of eyesight. Ocular signs which are associated with vitamin A deficiency are: night blindness, xerophthalmia, Bitot's spots, corneal xerosis/ulceration, keratomalacia, corneal scars and fundal xerophthalmia. In a child with symptoms of night blindness, therapeutic doses of vitamin A should be given.

- Give 200,000 IU of vitamin A immediately after diagnosis.
- Give one more dose of 200,000 IU four weeks after (dose in infant is 100,000 IU). Children who have an eye lesion must be given the first therapeutic dose of vitamin A and referred urgently for specialist care.

Delivery System

Vitamin A solution is provided to subcentres as part of drug kit A. 12 bottles (1200 ml) per annum are provided in the kit at subcentre.

Multipurpose health worker female (MPHWF) provides vitamin A prophylaxis to children and maintains records and submits reports to primary health centre. She assesses the needs of vitamin A prophylaxis as part of community need assessment under RCH programme.

Similarly, under integrated child development services (ICDS), the Anganwadi workers also help administer vitamin A solution to children in age group 9 months to 5 years. This helps to increase the coverage of vitamin A prophylaxis.

Integration: Administration of vitamin A has been integrated with universal immunization programme to reduce the number of visits of mothers to subcentre or Anganwadi. At least two doses will be ensured—one with measles immunization and one with booster DPT/OPV.

Coverage

Vitamin A prophylaxis coverage level has been low. Overall coverage for first dose as revealed through coverage evaluation survey (2009) in India was around 64%. NFHS-3 indicated that 21% of children in age group 12 to 35 months received a vitamin A dose in the last 6 months. It is linked with coverage of measles immunization which is around 74%. Coverage of second and third doses of vitamin A prophylaxis was dismally low at 3% or at the most 17%. Tracking of children in age group 1–3 years remains a challenge. Health and ICDS system together can increase the coverage.

Logistic Problems

Problem of shortages of supplies and frequent stock outs and delay in supply are the major bottlenecks which interrupt the programme, available infrastructure on the ground needs to ensure adequate coverage.

Vitamin A with national immunization days (NIDs) along with pulse polio immunization (PPI): This strategy was promoted by WHO and UNICEF in UP and Odisha state in October 1999 and March 2000. High level of coverage was ensured in Odisha state but in UP variable coverage was reported. This massive drive ensured the increase in coverage but it was not favoured as a regular strategy in the country.[3]

Pregnant and Lactating Mothers

It is neither possible nor necessary to give vitamin A supplements to all pregnant and lactating mothers in the country. As part of comprehensive antenatal and postnatal care, women should be screened for night blindness. If pregnant/lactating women have night blindness, they should be referred to physician in the nearby primary health centre or any other health facility for appropriate management. In view of the potential toxic and *teratogenic* effects of high doses of vitamin A, pregnant and lactating women with symptoms of night blindness should be treated with vitamin A in dosage not exceeding 10,000 IU per day. They can be given vitamin A till symptoms of night blindness disappear.

Fortified Foods

In several countries including India under the micronutrient initiative programme, attempt has been made to fortify common food items (sugar, wheat flour, candy, etc.) with vitamin A concentrate, however, this has not been favoured as a strategy. Food-based approach holds the key to improve the dietary intake of vitamin A.

Ultimate Solution—Food-based Solution

The ultimate sustainable solution for the prevention of vitamin A deficiency is regular consumption of vitamin A rich foods which are cheap and locally available. Vitamin A consumption must be ensured from birth itself. Breast-feeding, including feeding of colostrum, will protect children from vitamin A deficiency during the first 6 months. From the age of 6 months, it is crucial to introduce complementary (semisolids) food containing rich sources of vitamin A, such as dark green leafy vegetables, yellow vegetables and fruits (carrots, capsicum, yam, pumpkin, papaya, mango). Most leafy vegetables contain more than the recommended dietary allowance (RDA) of vitamin A, for Indian children in about 100 g of edible portion. This quantity on cooking, is reduced to two tablespoons. A child can easily consume this amount with other food items, thereby meeting its total daily requirement.[4–9]

In addition to green leafy vegetables as far as possible, incorporation of other vitamin A rich foods, such as dairy products (milk, cheese, curd, butter) liver, eggs, oil and fat should be encouraged in the daily diet of preschool children who are prone to develop vitamin A deficiency. Such food practices will prevent vitamin A deficiency. Daily consumption of dark green leafy vegetables and other vitamin A rich foods are also recommended during pregnancy and lactation. Mother's vitamin A status influences the vitamin A content of mother's milk and the health status of her children. Adequate intake of vitamin A rich food during pregnancy and lactation will prevent vitamin A deficiency both in mother and child.

Nutrition education, an integral component of primary health care and ICDS programmes, must emphasize on promotion production and consumption of foods rich in vitamin A.

Future strategies: Targeted intervention in areas showing vitamin A deficiency, such as Odisha, MP, Rajasthan, UP and other pockets may be overriding priority.

REFERENCES

1 Indian Council of Medical Research. Micronutrient Deficiency Disorders in 16 districts of India. Part I report of an ICMR task force study—District Nutrition Project ICMR, New Delhi; 2001 and NNMB surveys 1975–2012.

2 Govt. of India. Prevention and treatment of vitamin A deficiency. MOH and FW. GOI, New Delhi; 1991.

3 Kapil U, Srivastava VK. Benefits and safety of administration of vitamin A to preschool children, pregnant and lactating women. A report MOH and FW and AIIMS, New Delhi; Sept. 2000.

4 Gopalan C. Combating vitamin A deficiency—Need for a revised strategy. "Recent trends in Nutrition". The proceedings of First International Symposiums of the Nutrition Foundation of India. Oxford University Press; Dec. 1990.

5 Govt. of India. National Child Survival and Safe Motherhood Programme—Programme Interventions MCH Division, MOH and FW GOI, New Delhi; June 1994.

6 Prahlad Rao N, Reddy V. Textbook of Human Nutrition. Oxford and IBH Publishing company Private Limited. New Delhi and Calcutta; 1996, 287–97.

7 GOI. Basic Guide to Reproductive and Child Health Programme. Deptt. of Family Welfare GOI, New Delhi; 1997.

8 Umesh Kapil. Invited Commentary. Time to stop giving indiscriminate massive doses of synthetic Vitamin 'A' to Indian children. Public Health Nutrition: 12 (2), 285 Feb. 2009.

9 A 2 Z. The USAID Micronutrient and Child Blindness Project—India, 2006–2008.

IODINE DEFICIENCY DISORDERS (IDDs)

Iodine deficiency disorders are prevalent worldwide. Iodine is an essential micronutrient and element and it is necessary for synthesis of the thyroid hormone, i.e. thyroxin (T_4) and tri-iodothyronine (T_3). Thyroid hormone regulates wide variety of vital physiological processes, such as early growth and development of the brain and body in man. Scientific studies in India and abroad have evidence that nutritional iodine deficiency causes deficiency of thyroid hormone during fetal life and childhood.

Why Iodine Deficiency?

Iodine is only present in soil, hence IDDs are environmental problem. Iodine deficiency results from geological rather than socioeconomic conditions. The problem is aggravated by environmental factors, such as accelerated deforestation and soil erosion. Iodine is present in the top crust of soil, frequent floods cause washing of iodine from soil crust and same happens when glaciers slide down mountains. Unlike nutrient, such as iron, calcium or the vitamins, iodine does not occur naturally in specific foods, rather it is present in the soil and is imbibed through food grown on that soil. The ideal situation is where the daily needs of iodine are met from natural foods grown in iodine rich soils.

Foods grown in iodine deficient region can never provide enough iodine to the population and livestock living in such areas. Then, if an area is iodine deficient, IDD cannot be eliminated by changing dietary habits or eating certain kinds of foods grown in that area. The correction has to be achieved by supplying iodine through the external source. This can be done by *fortifying* a commonly consumed food with iodine.

Solution

Iodation of salt is a long-term and sustainable low-cost solution, which will ensure that iodine reaches the entire population and is ingested on regular basis. *Fortification* of salt with iodine has been extremely successful in eliminating iodine deficiency all the world over.

Requirement of Iodine

Iodine is an essential micronutrient. Normal daily requirement of iodine is 100–150 mcg which is absolutely safe for normal growth and development (Table 6.32). Iodine deficiency produces wide-spectrum of disorders and these disorders caused due to deficiency of iodine are called iodine deficiency disorders (IDDs).

Upper Limit of Iodine Intake

Excess of iodine ingestion can be harmful, which may inhibit the synthesis of thyroid hormones. The iodine induced hypothyroidism known as "Wolff Chaikoff" effect.

Table 6.32: Revised Recommended daily iodine intake (WHO/UNICEF/ ICC IDD)[1,2] 2007

Age group	*Requirement (mcg)*
Infant (0–11 months)	90
Children (12–59 months)	90
Children (6–12 years)	120
Adolescents and adults (above 13 years)	150
Pregnant and lactating women	250

Spectrum of IDDs

Lack of iodine in the environment has serious consequences for both human beings and animals. Goitre is only the tip of the iceberg or just one manifestation of spectrum of IDD.

A less obvious but more serious condition affecting million of iodine deficient children include impaired mental functions, poor intellectual performance, lowered IQ, muscular disorders and impaired coordination and sluggishness. In pregnancy, iodine deficiency causes spontaneous abortions, stillbirth, and infant deaths.

Deficiency of iodine in pregnant women interferes with the brain development of foetus and results in birth of iodine deficient babies who may be cretins characterized by mental deficiency, hearing defects, squint and stunted growth. Children born to iodine deficient women can develop, neonatal chemical hypothyroidism (NCH) and develop total brain damage which is permanent and irreversible and limits intellectual growth in later years.

The world's single most significant cause of preventable brain damage and mental retardation is deficiency of iodine. Iodine deficiency is the leading cause of preventable mental retardation in the world. Current research indicates that iodine deficiency results in lowering the average intelligence of the entire school age population by as much as 10–15 IQ points. 40 million school children in endemic areas may lose 400 million IQ points.[3,4]

Effect of Iodine Deficiency in Humans and Animals—Spectrum of IDD in Human Beings[4]

Foetus: Abortions, stillbirth, congenital abnormalities, increased perinatal mortality, increased infant mortality. Neurological cretinism: mental deficiency and deaf-mutism, spastic diplegia, squint. Myxomatous cretinism: dwarfism, mental deficiency and psychomotor defects.

Neonate: Neonatal goitre, neonatal hypothyroidism.

Child and adolescent: Goitre, juvenile hypothyroidism, impaired mental function, retarded physical development.

Adult: Goitre with its complications, hypothyroidism, impaired mental function.

In animals: IDD leads to reduced yield of milk, eggs, meat and wool and reproductive failure.[2]

Epidemiological Criteria for Assessing Severity of IDD and Elimination of IDD

WHO has fixed criteria for classifying IDDs as significant public health problem by following indicators (Table 6.33):

- TGR—total goitre rate (Grade I plus garde II goitre)
- Median urinary iodine excretion.
- Thydroid volume by ultrasound
- Salt iodine content.

For sustainable **elimination** of IDDs, the following three criteria should be met.

1. Ensure 15 ppm of iodine in salt at consumer level and 30 ppm at production level.
2. Median urinary iodine exertion should be 100 µg/L.
3. TGR (percentage of children aged 6–12 with palpable and visible goitre) should be less than 5% (WHO).

Magnitude of Problem

IDDs is a global problem. In 1994, it was estimated that around 1500 million people were at risk of IDD and 225 million had goitre, 0.6 million were cretins and 20 million had mild neurological disorders. Many babies are born as cretins who are mentally retarded, physically stunted, deaf, mute or paralysed. Similarly, many are stillborn. Many more have IQ at least 10 point below their potential.

Magnitude of IDD in India

IDDs have been recognized as a public health problem in India since 1920. Unlike other micronutrient deficiencies, iodine deficiency disorders are due to deficiency of iodine in water, soil and foodstuffs and affect all socioeconomic groups living in a defined geographical area. Initially IDD was thought to be problem in sub-Himalayan region, however surveys carried out subsequently showed that no state in the country is completely free from IDD.

At risk population: The general notion that goitre is confined to endemic area/belt is wrong, it has widespread prevalence. In our country, whole of population is at risk but 200 million people are at serious risk of IDD while the number of persons suffering from goitre and other IDDs is above 71 million (Fig. 6.2). Surveys conducted in the country indicate that no state/union territory is free from problem of IDDs.[5–7] Out of 386 districts surveyed so far, 335 districts are IDD endemic where prevalence of TGR (palpable and visible goitre) is above 5%. There is significant reduction in visible goitre in the country.

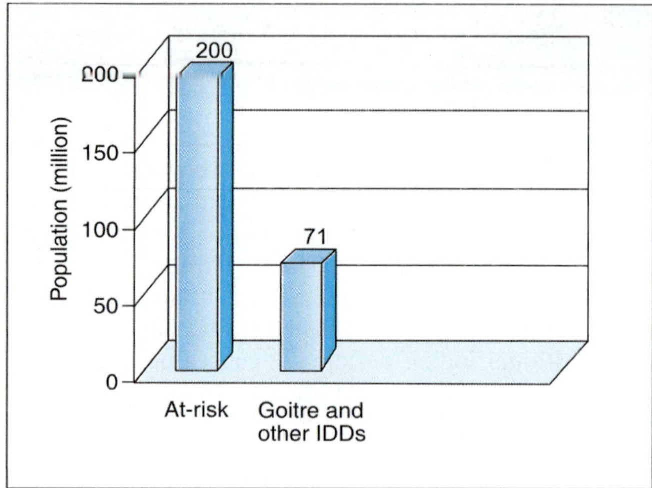

Fig. 6.2: Problem of IDDs in India

Endemic district: The district is declared as endemic district if the total goitre rate is above 5% in the children of age group 6–12 years surveyed.

Prevention

IDDs are preventable. Daily consumption of iodized salt prevents the spectrum of disorders caused due to iodine deficiency. Consumption of iodized salt is safe. Iodation of salt is a low-cost highly effective means of prevention. The cost of iodation is ₹ 2–3 per person per month. The average consumption of iodated salt per person per day is 10 g. The supply of iodated salt must ensure that availability is not less than 150 mcg of iodine per day at consumer level.

NATIONAL IDD CONTROL PROGRAMME (NIDDCP)

Following the successful trial of iodized salt in Kangra valley, Himachal Pradesh, a National Goitre Control Programme (NGCP) was launched in 1962.[8] Initially, the programme aimed at providing iodized salt to well recognized sub-Himalayan "goitre" belt. However, there was no substantial reduction of iodine deficiency disorders

Table 6.33: Epidemiological criteria for assessing the severity of IDD

Indicator	*Target population*	*Severity of public health problem (prevalence)*		
		Mild	Moderate	Severe
Goiter grade > 0	School aged children (6–12)	5–19.9%	20–29.9%	≥ 30%
Median UIE (µg/l)	SAC	50–99	20–49	< 20
Thyroid volume > 97th centile by ultrasound	SAC	5–19.9%	20–29.9%	≥ 30%
TSH > 5 mU/l	Neonates	10–19.9%	20–39.9%	≥ 40%
Median Tg ng/ml serum	C/A	10–19.9%	20–39.9%	≥ 40%

Target population is school aged children (SAC); C/A = Children and adults UIE: urinary iodine excretion due to erratic availability of salt, use of cheaper non-iodized salt and lack of awareness of use of iodized salt.[8,9] In view of the fact that no state was free from IDD, a decision was taken for universal iodation of salt for human consumption, which was implemented in phased manner from 1986. The progress of implementation of this programme was tardy as the production and availability of iodised salt was a fraction of what was required.

Realizing magnitude of the problem, the Government of India launched a 100% centrally assisted National Goitre Control Programme (NGCP) in 1962. In August 1992, the NGCP was renamed as National Iodine Deficiency Disorders Control Programme (NIDDCP) taking into its ambit the control of wide-spectrum of IDDs like mental and physical retardation, deaf mutism, cretinism, stillbirth, abortion, etc. In 1984 policy decision to universal iodization of edible salt was taken by the Government.

Objectives of NIDDCP

The goal of NIDDCP is to reduce the prevalence of IDDs (Iodine deficiency disorders) below 10% in adults by 2015.

The important objectives and components of NIDDCP are as follows:

- Universal iodization of salt and supply of iodated salt all over country in place of common salt.
- Surveys to assess the magnitude of the IDDs.
- Resurvey after every 5 years to assess the extent of IDDs and impact of iodated salt.
- Laboratory monitoring of iodated salt and urinary iodine excretion (UIE).
- Health education and publicity.

Goal of NIDDCP

The goal of NIDDCP is to reduce the prevalence of IDDs below 10% in entire country by 2015.

- Achieve universal access to iodized salt by iodization of 50 lakh MT of edible salt.
- Generate district-wise data on iodized salt consumption.[10]

Strategies[11,12]

1. *Universal salt iodization* (USI) to eliminate IDDs. It is essential to ensure that only iodized salt is made available for human consumption in order to enable children of 21st century to attain their full intellectual potential and take their rightful place in a knowledge-based society. The Government of India took a policy decision to iodate the entire edible salt in the country by 1992. The programme of iodation commenced in 1986, in phased manner. Since then the approach has been to enhance the production, demand and supply of iodated salt. All states and cities have been advised to ban sale of non-iodized salt under prevention of Food Adulteration Act (Now Food Safety and Standards Act, 2006). Ban was imposed by most states. Most states banned non-iodized salt. The ban, however, was lifted in the year 2000 by Central Govt, which was a set back indeed. The central Government again issued the notification banning the sale of non-iodated salt for direct human consumption in the entire country with effect from 17th May, 2006 under the Prevention of Food Adulteration Act, 1954.
2. *Improve the quality of iodized salt by:*
   - Mandatory certification of adequacy of iodization as a prerequisite for getting priority for the transportation of salt.
   - Ensuring that salt is packed in half or one kg consumer poly-packs at production site itself to prevent deterioration in quality during transportation and storage.
   - Periodic checking of iodine content of salts available at wholesale/retail outlets.
   - Quality check at the household level through health workers, ASHA, Anganwadi/school-based testing—using spot testing kits (STK).
3. *Information education and communication (IEC):* To increase the demand for good quality iodized salt providing ready access to iodized salt through targeted public distribution system.
4. *Monitoring:* Monitoring of production and distribution of quality of salt at various levels:
   - Monitoring of prevalence of goitre in 6–12 years age group in schools, urinary excretion of iodine, neonatal thyroid status by appropriate screening techniques may be used to assess the impact on reduction of IDDs.[6,13,14]
   - Monitoring of iodine content of salt at production, distribution and consumer level. The goal of USI is > 90% households should be consuming iodized salt.

Iodization of Salt

Salt is universally consumed by all households. Hence, this has been used as carrier of iodine to mitigate the problem of IDD.

On an average, 10 g of salt is consumed per day per person. To meet daily requirement of 150 mcg of iodine from 10 g of salt we need to ensure 15 parts per million (ppm) or 15 mg of iodine per kg of salt, at consumer level. It is a common knowledge that salt from production centre to consumer takes a long journey and time and is exposed to heat, sunlight, moisture and cooking. Therefore, to ensure iodine content of 15 ppm at consumer level, it is necessary to ensure 30 ppm of iodine at production level so that when salt reaches at household level it retains at least 15 ppm of iodine.[15]

Policy and Standards

The Government of India as per policy has set the minimum iodine content of salt at 15 ppm at the consumer level and 30 ppm of iodine at production level.

Chemicals for Iodization

Salt can be iodized with potassium iodide (KI) or potassium iodate (KIO_3). In India, potassium iodate, which is more stable in Indian weather conditions, has been chosen for iodation of salt. Potassium iodate of 50 ppm (equivalent to 30 ppm of iodine) is added at production level. Since losses are imminent because of transportation, storage and weather conditions (moisture and heat) and cooking it is expected that 50 ppm of iodate at production level will ensure at least 25 ppm of iodate (equivalent to 15 ppm of iodine) at consumer level.

Mixing Process

Potassium iodate is mixed with common salt at production level by spray mixing process, submersion process, the drip feed process, or by dry mixing process. The plants for iodation have been standardized. 96% of salt of the country is produced in three states Gujarat (68%), Tamil Nadu (16%), Rajasthan (12%) and remaining 4% is by other states. 930 private units have been licensed by salt commissioner to produce iodized salt.

Legal Aspects

Salt comes under the preview of "Food Adulteration Act, 1954" (Now Food Safety and Standards Act, 2006). It is mandatory that manufacturers and distribution channels ensure iodine content as 30 and 15 ppm at production and consumer level respectively and salt must confirm other specified standards. Samples of salts are lifted from manufacturers and from retail shops to test the quality of salt for its iodine content. The samples are lifted by food inspectors. It is mandatory to collect 50 salt samples/month/district, 10 samples to be collected from retail shops and 40 at household/consumption level for testing of iodine content in the laboratory.

Testing of Iodine Contents of Salt

Spot testing kit (STK): Iodine content of the salt can be tested at consumer level by spot testing kit (STK). This is a qualitative and rapid test at the field level and at the consumer level. When kit reagent indicator solution is dripped on salt sample spread in a plate or any container a blue colour develops if the salt contains iodine. The intensity of colour can be matched with the colour codes depicted over the kit to judge qualitatively iodine content of sample as: 30 ppm (deep blue), 15 ppm (light blue) 7 ppm (lightest blue), 0 (no colour). Do not jump to conclusion if there is no colour change of salt. This may be due to high alkalinity. Take another sample and spread it on a surface and add sulfuric acid and then add indicator solution on the same spot where sulfuric acid was added and observe the colour change and match it with the colour coded scale.[16] STKs have been supplied to ASHA and health workers.

6

Iodometric Titration

Analysis of iodine content of iodated salt on quantitative basis can be done by iodometric titration, at the district level or state level laboratory. Sample of salt is treated with concentrated sulfuric acid which liberates iodine. The free iodine is titrated with sodium thiosulphate; using starch as an indicator.

Urinary Iodine Excretion (UIE)

If the intake of iodine is optimal the median urinary iodine excretion (UIE) should be not less than 100 mcg per litre and it should range from 100 to 200 mcg/L. This is most important indicator for assessment of impact in salt iodization programme and assessment of intake of iodized salt.

Present Status of Programme

Accessibility of iodized salt: During the year 2015 nearly 74% of the population was consuming iodated salt. District level household survey of 2002–04 indicates that about 30% of households used cooking salt that is iodized at the recommended level of 15 PPM or above, whereas 44% of households used salts that were not iodized at all and another 24% used salt which was inadequately iodized.[17] As per NFHS-3, nearly 51% used adequately iodized salt (iodine content not less than 15 ppm), 24% used non-iodized salt. This much population is yet to be covered under universal iodation programme. The goal of USI is > 90% of households to consume iodized salt.

In India, the target was to reduce prevalence of IDDs below 10% by 2012. ICMR study carried out in year 2001 indicated average prevalence of TGR (grade I plus grade II) of 4.78% in 6–12 years children. The highest prevalence of 31.02% was observed in Dehradun district, 12.5% in Mehboob Nagar district, 8.86% in Bikaner and 8.56% in Dibrugarh district.[18] In India, 303 districts are endemic.

Organization and Implementation of NIDDCP in India

1. The Ministry of Health and Family Welfare is the nodal ministry for policy decision.
2. The central nutrition and iodine deficiency disorders cell at DGHS is responsible for implementation of NIDDCP. The main functions of DGHS are technical guidance, coordination between various sectors and states, monitoring quality of iodated salt, undertaking sample surveys on prevalence and monitoring of programme; and managing finances.
3. Salt commissioner office at Jaipur under Ministry of Industry is responsible for licensing, production, and distribution of iodated salt to states and UTs. This office is also responsible for monitoring the quality of iodated salt from production level and arranges movement of

iodated salt from production centres to the state, through railways.

State/Union Territory IDD cell

Each state has an IDD control cell for implementation of programme in the state. Its functions are to conduct prevalence surveys, to monitor quality of iodated salt, to issue notification–banning the entry and sale of non-iodated salt under Prevention of Food Adulteration Act (1954) conducting training and reporting to DGHS Government of India.

Achievements

The annual production of iodated salt was raised from 5 lakh MT in 1985–86 to 55.08 MT in 2014.

Movement of iodized salt is a priority second to that of defence.

To ensure use of only iodated salt, sale of non-iodized salt has been banned completely in 29 states and all UTs with effect from 17th May 2006 under the PFA Act, 1954.

Standards for iodized salt have been laid down under the prevention of Food Adulteration Act, 1954 (Now Food Safety Standards Act, 2006). These stipulate that iodine content of salt at production and consumption level be at least 30 and 15 ppm respectively.

Realising the importance of IDD in relation with human resource development NIDDCP has been included in the 20 point programme of the Prime Minister.

A national reference laboratory for monitoring of IDD has been set-up at the Biochemistry division in National Institute of Communicable Diseases, Delhi for training medical and paramedical personnel and monitoring the iodine content of salt and urine.

State level IDD monitoring laboratories for the monitoring of iodine content of salt and urinary iodine excretion have been set up.

Guidelines for District IDD Goitre Survey

Purpose is to study the prevalence of IDD with a view to know the magnitude of problem and to assess the impact of interventions.

Focus: School-aged children (SAC) 6–12 years, and general population.

Guidelines for District IDD Survey

Survey Method

The IDD survey at the district may be conducted by using the method of population proportionate to size (PPS) sampling in the age agroup of 6–12 years children. A sample of 30 villages/wards or schools are selected from the district by cluster sampling technique.

Sample

- A sample of 90 children (45 boys and 45 girls) of age group of 6–12 years from the school and out of school/ households of selected village/ward has to be selected as explained below.

Suppose in the selected village the enrolment rates are Boys = 40% and Girls = 30%.

Then, the allocation of samples of 45 boys and 45 girls to be selected from school and out of school would be as under:

	Boys	*Girls*
School	18 (40%)	13 (30%)
Out of school	27 (60%)	32 (70%)
Total	45 (100%)	45 (100%)

For selection of 18 boys from primary school classes, if the number of classes are 5 then the sample would comprise selecting 3 children each from class 1st and 2nd, 4 children each from classes 3, 4 and 5 by random method from attendance register. Similarly, sample of 27 out of school children from the village/ward has to be selected. This has to be allocated into various age groups approximately equal. In the present case, it would be 5 children in each age groups 6, 7, 8 and 12 children from the remaining age groups by random selection. Register of Anganwadi workers can be used for the purpose to locate households/families.

Salt Samples

Every 5th child selected in the earlier steps for goitre survey be covered for collection of salt samples by visiting the corresponding houses.

Sample for Urinary Iodine Excretion

For UIE, every alternate child out of those selected earlier step for salt samples has to be taken for collection of urine sample.

If the school enrolment rate in the village is 90% then the sample may be restricted to school mainly. Alternative if the enrolment rate is as low as 10% then the household approach may only be used.

Monitoring

Fifty samples of salt per month per district, 25 from rural households, 15 from urban households, 7 from rural retailers and 3 from urban retailers are to be collected. 25 samples per district per month for Urinary Iodine Excretion (UIE) should be collected.

Techniques of Examination

From the clinical point of view, the diagnosis of goitre is based entirely on inspection and palpation of the neck. The position taken by the examiner in relation to the person being examined is a matter of personal choice.

Some workers face the subject and usually palpate the isthmus and lobes with two thumbs, the fingers of both hands being spread around the lateral side of the neck. Other workers stand at one side of the subject, the side depending on whether they are right-handed or left handed. The palpation is done with the first or the first and second fingers. The examiner should be so positioned that his eyes are approximately at the level of the subject's neck. This means that in case of young children, the examiner must be seated. When assessing the visibility of an enlarged gland it is important that the subject keeps the head steady so that the eyes and the external aural meatus are on a plane.

To assist in palpation, it is frequently desirable to depress the subject's chin to relax the neck muscles. At the commencement of palpation, the isthmus should first be located and then the thumbs and fingers should move laterally to identify the lobes and assess their size.

In people with a short neck, the sternum may hide a part or the whole thyroid gland; this occasionally makes diagnosis difficult.

Nodules should be noted and recorded separately.

Classification of Goitre

Most classifications distinguish between different grades of goitre and broadly between visible and palpable goitres and record the presence or absence of nodules. Visible goitres, as a general rule, indicate a moderate to severe deficiency of iodine of a relatively long duration and thus tends to be more common among older people. Their presence in children suggests a severe deficiency of iodine. Similarly, nodules are likely to be present to a significant degree only in areas of marked deficiency of iodine for a very long period. Palpable goitres have a special significance in the assessment of the control programme, e.g. salt iodization programme.

As per a recent WHO publication (1994), the previous five grades of goitre namely grade 0, IA, IB, grade II and grade III have been classified into three grades as grade 0, grade I, and grade II. The detailed description of each grade is given below:[6]

Grade Description

- *Grade 0:* No palpable or visible goitre/**no goitre**.
- *Grade I:* A mass in the neck that is consistent with an enlarged thyroid, that is palpable but not visible, when the neck is in normal position. It moves upward in the neck as the subject swallows. Nodular alteration(s) can occur even when the thyroid is not enlarged/**goitre palpable but not visible**.
- *Grade II:* A swelling in the neck that is visible when the neck is in a normal position and is consistent with an enlarged thyroid when the neck is palpated/**goitre visible and palpable**.

Salt Consumption Pattern and Practices

Salt consumption pattern and practices were studied by ICMR in year 1987. It was observed that in rural areas crystal salt was preferred and purchased in bulk by 20% of the households for 3–6 months for human and animal consumption. Most households procure loose salt and store it in earthen pots. Storage practices were bad and most salts were exposed to light and moisture. Over 80% of households preferred loose crystal salt because of being cheaper. Washing of crystal salt was observed in 20% of families.

Cooking in open pan/utensil was common. Pressure-cooker was used by a few households. Iodine losses due to cooking practices could be as high as 20–40%. Most of the families added salt before cooking. Average consumption of salt per person per day was around 10 g.[19–21]

Sustainable elimination of IDDs is possible by daily consumption of iodated salt by all (MDG, 2015).

REFERENCES

1 Partnership-key to success and sustainability. A development sector experience. Bharat Scouts and Guides and ICC IDD Secretariat, AIIMS, New Delhi; 2004.

2 Ranganathan S, Reddy V. Human requirements of iodine and safe use of iodized salt. Indian J Med Res 1995;102: 227–32.

3 UNICEF. Universalization of access to iodized salt – A mid decade goal. Produced by the salt department. Ministry of Industry with Support of UNICEF; 1994.

4 Pandav CS, Kochupillai N. Endemic goitre in India: Prevalence, etiology, attendant disabilities and control measures. Indian J Pediatr 1982;50:259–71.

5 Govt. of India. Policy guidelines on NIDDCP, IDD and Nutrition cell, DGHS, MOH and FW, GOI, New Delhi; 1998.

6 Govt. of India. Policy guidelines on National Iodine Deficiency Disorders Control Programme. IDD and Nutrition cell DGHS, MOH and FW, Govt. of India, New Delhi; 2003.

7 National workshop on Methodologies for assessment of vitamin A deficiency, iron deficiency anaemia and IDD. Jointly organized by Human Nutrition Unit, AIIMS, IAPSM, NFI (Delhi Chapter) and IAP (Nutrition Chapter), AIIMS, New Delhi; 13–15 Sept. 2004.

8 NFI. The National Goitre Control Programme. A blue print for its Intensification. Nutrition Foundation of India, Scientific Report (1); 1983.

9 ICMR. From endemic goitre to iodine deficiency disorders ICMR Bulletin; 13(2); adapted from lead article in lancet November 1983: 1121.

10 Govt. of India. Sectoral Policies and Programmes. Food and Nutrition Security. 10th Five-Year Plan (2002–2007) Vol. II. 2002; 350–52.

11 WHO. Iodine and health. Eliminating iodine deficiency disorders safely through salt iodization. A statement by WHO, Geneva; 1994.

12 Sustaining elimination of iodine deficiency disorders. The National Med. J. India. 1995; 8(2): 49–50.

13 WHO. Universal salt iodization works. Quality Control and Monitoring are critical elements for success. Press release WHO 152, Geneva; 1996.

14 WHO. Recommended iodine levels in salt and guidelines for monitoring their adequacy and effectiveness. Joint WHO/UNICEF/ICCIDD Consultation. WHO, Geneva; 1996.

15 Government of India. National Consultation on Benefits and Safety of Iodized salt. Salt department. Govt. of India, Jaipur 1999.

16 AIIMS. Utility of spot testing kit in the assessment of iodine content of salt. A multicentric study. Department of Human Nutrition AIIMS, New Delhi; 1999.

17 GOI. District Level Household Survey 2002–04, IIPS, Mumbai, MOH and FW, GOI; New Delhi.

18 ICMR. Micronutrient deficiency disorders in 16 districts of India. ICMR, New Delhi; 2001.

19 ICMR. Salt consumption pattern in India. An ICMR Task force study. ICMR, New Delhi; 1987.

20 GOI. CD Alert Monthly Newsletter of NICD, DGHS, June 2005 Vol. 9: (6). GOI.

21 GOI. Revised Policy Guidelines on National Iodine Deficiency Disorders Control Programme. IDD and Nutrition cell. DGHS, MOH and FW GOI, New Delhi. October 2006.

ZINC NUTRITION

Zinc is a trace element or micronutrient. Deficiency of micronutrients like iron and iodine is widespread but zinc deficiency is not that common.

Functions

Zinc is a cofactor for over 200 metal enzymes regulating various cellular functions of the body.

Zinc is associated with wide range of body functions like cell division and growth, membrane function, provides protection against free radical damage, helps in gonadal functions, helps in immune functions, foetal development, brain development and influences metabolism of vitamin A.

Requirements (Table 6.34)

The daily requirement is 5 mg for infants, children up to 10 years 8 mg, and for adults 10–12 mg per day.

Severe Zinc Deficiency

Severe zinc deficiency leads to neuropsychiatric changes, dermal lesions, diarrhoea and loss of hair.

Table 6.34: RDA requirement of zinc (mg per day)

Men	Women	1–3 yrs	4–6	7–9	10–12	13–15
12	10–12	5	7	8	9	11

Acrodermatitis enteropathica: It is an autosomal recessive genetic disorder which leads to intestinal zinc malabsorption. This condition interferes with zinc uptake by the intestinal epithelium. The manifestation of deficiency appears around 6 months of age in the form of severe skin lesions, alopecia, failure to thrive and diarrhoea. Plasma zinc levels are very low in these cases.

Acquired zinc deficiency syndrome: This was described from Egypt in 1960. The syndrome produced dwarfism, hypogonadism, geophagia, anaemia and hepatomegaly. Response to zinc therapy was quite dramatic in these children. Zinc deficiency occurs due to wide ranging pathological disorders, such as chronic alcoholic liver disease, sickle cell anaemia, in severe protein energy malnutrition, chronic malabsorption syndrome.

Zinc deficiency does not occur in isolation. Sometime, back zinc as nutrient was widely recommended to pregnant women, to low birth weight babies and in acute diarrhoeal diseases to promote growth of babies and early recovery from disease process. The widespread use as therapeutic agent or for prevention is hardly justified. Studies done at NIN, Hyderabad, indicated that zinc deficiency is not a significant problem and routine zinc supplements to pregnant women, newborn or to breastfed infants are not necessary.[1,2]

Zinc as adjunct to ORS. Govt. Policy (*see* under diarrhoea Control and ICDS Programme).

Other nutritional deficiency diseases: Vitamin B complex deficiency particularly riboflavin deficiency leading to angular stomatitis, glossitis and cheilosis. Pellagra, which is primarily due to nicotinic acid deficiency, is reported to be caused by excess leucine in the staple jowar leading to amino acid imbalance and decreasing conversion of tryptophan to niacin.

REFERENCES

1 Bhaskaram P, Hemlatha P. Is Zinc deficiency in children a nutritional problem. Nutrition News, NIN 1994 April; 15(2).

2 ICMR. Zinc Status of Indian Children. ICMR Bulletin 1995 Feb.; 25(2).

DIETARY (FOOD CONSUMPTION) SURVEYS

The dietary surveys mean what people eat and how much they eat, what are their likes and dislikes and dietary beliefs as also dietary practices.

Purpose and uses

The primary purpose of dietary survey is:

1 To ascertain dietary intake of most vulnerables.
2 To improve the diets of people at household level particularly to improve the diets or feeding of young children, pregnant and lactating women.

3 For planning of national food strategies, data on dietary consumption is essential.
4 Dietary surveys are also done to assess the effect of nutrition education programme.
5 Periodic dietary surveys done at time intervals provide information on trends of consumption.
6 These surveys also help to know the special preference for a food and foods avoided or disliked and alternate foods consumed during the special conditions like droughts and in tribal areas.
7 When designing specific programme on nutrition, dietary surveys are needed to have evidence-based data.

Dietary surveys in medical profession are not new, however, the only part of "dietary survey" most often known to a medical student/doctor is dietary history, vegetarian or non-vegetarian and it begins and ends there only. No details or dietary intake/assessment are made.

Limitation of Dietary Surveys

These are time consuming and expensive and requires training of workers. The data collected may have limitation and may not be representative of total population.

Types of Dietary Surveys

There are two types of dietary surveys:

1 Qualitative food intake
2 Quantitative intake of food.

Qualitative Survey

The qualitative food intake means food items consumed, their frequency of consumption, daily, weekly or once a while/occasionally, food preferred and food avoided. We can also assess the dietary beliefs and practices of interest. This is rapid method of assessment. Qualitative methods can have focussed attention on dietary practices during infancy, young children, pregnancy and lactational period.[1]

Quantitative Survey

The quantitative dietary survey makes assessment of amount or quantities of food items consumed, are recorded and nutrient composition are determined from tables of food consumption.

Methods of Dietary Surveys

Several methods for dietary surveys have been used at national and international level. These are:[1,2]

1 Food balance sheet (FBS)
2 24 hours recall method
3 Weighment method
4 Inventory method list
5 Expenditure pattern method
6 Diet history
7 Duplicate samples
8 Recording methods.

Before the surveys are conducted, we should list all the family members who partook the meals yesterday, their ages in completed years for adults and completed months for infants and young children, their physiological status (pregnancy and lactation) and occupation (sedentary, moderate, heavy and very heavy worker) as also economic status. This step helps to arrive at adult consumption units.

1. Food Balance Sheet (FBS)

Each country maintains food balance sheet, which indicates total food available or produced in the country as also the available buffer stocks. At the international level, Food and Agricultural Organization (FAO) monitors the food available in each country. India produces 264 million tonnes of food grains every year and there are buffer stocks of 60 million tonnes. It gives an estimate of food available in the country per person per year or per day.[3] It is no guarantee that this much is consumed by each person. This information helps national planners for adequacy or inadequacy of available food. Per person availability of food is determined by:

$$\text{Per person per day of food availability} = \frac{\left(\text{Beginning of the year stock (boys) + total food produced + imports}\right) - \left(\text{Stocks at the end of the year + exports + seeds + cattle/poultry feeds + wastages}\right)}{\text{Total mid-year population} \times 365 \text{ days}}$$

During the year 2013–14 record food grain production of 264 million metric tonnes was achieved in India.

Per capita availability of cereals in India in 2014 per person per day was 474 besides 29 g pulses.[3]

2. 24 Hours Recall Method

This is most popular method, most practical and easy low-cost method to make assessment of quantitative dietary intake. The housewife or individual is asked, which food and what amounts; were consumed on previous day or yesterday. Avoid, festival, fast and feast days.

Information on type of food preparation, ingredients used, raw amount of ingredients used for each preparation and total cooked amount (g/ml) from morning to night are collected on the performa (Table 6.35). Cooked amount in g/ml consumed by individual is obtained/calculated. Equivalent raw amount is arrived at in g/ml.

Gathering this information takes not much time but the conversion of household measures to g/ml can be laborious process. Common household measures are standardized and shown to individual or housewife to get approximate consumption of cooked food and thereafter the equivalent raw amount intake by individual

Table 6.35: Dietary information by 24 hours recall method

Meal pattern	Previous day's intake of family				Individual Intake	
	Type of preparation	Ingredients used	Raw amount used (g/ml)	Total cooked amount (g/ml)	Cooked amount (g/ml)	Equivalent raw amount (g/ml)
(a)	(b)	(c)	(d)	(e)	(f)	(g)
• Morning tea and snacks						
• Breakfast						
• Lunch						
• Evening tea and snacks						
• Dinner						

is arrived at. Much depends upon the cooperation of family and response of individual and the type of investigator. Since practice of cooking of rice is universal; the cooked rice is filled in standardized cups, which are serially numbered and conversion factor is applied to get amount of raw rice consumed (Table 6.36).

To assess the total cooked amount, for the preparation like tea/coffee/milk or any other beverage or soft drink or dal/sambar/curries use the volume of standardised cups and measures. Under field conditions, volumes and weights have to be considered as one and the same. Total cooked amount of rice in the family need not to be assessed since each cup is standardized for its raw amount equivalent. Preparations like chapatis may be assessed in numbers. Assess the individual intake in terms of cooked amount with the help of standardized cups both for rice and for other preparations. Calculate the individual intake in terms of raw amounts in the following way.

$$\text{Individual intake in terms of raw amount (g/ml)} = \frac{\text{Total raw amount of each ingredient used in preparation by the family (g/ml)}}{\text{Total cooked amount of each preparation}} \times \text{Subject intake of cooked amount (ml)}$$

3. Weighment Method

Weighing of raw food and cooked food offers advantage over questionnaire method or 24 hours recall method of dietary survey, as it is more accurate. The family may not allow to weigh the foods. Weighing of cooked food in institutions or hostels is favoured. Usually in field and community survey, raw foods are weighed for consecutive one week. This necessitates presence of investigator each time a preparation is made, hence it is quite difficult and least practical method. Weighing for one day could be considered sufficient in view of practical difficulties involved.

Only edible portions of raw food are weighed before cooking. The results of raw food consumption are expressed as intake of foods in g per consumption unit (CU) or per person as follows:

$$\text{Intake per Cu per day (g/ml)} = \frac{\text{Raw amount of each food (g/ml)}}{\text{Total Cu} \times \text{No. of days of survey}}$$

$$\text{Intake per person per day (g/ml)} = \frac{\text{Raw amounts of each food (g)}}{\text{No. of persons} \times \text{No. of days of survey}}$$

4. Inventory Method List (Logbook Method)

This method is applicable in hostels, orphanage, hospital and other institutions.

In this method, actual amount of foodstuffs issued by the incharge of the institute are taken into account for consumption. If the housewife is able to maintain a log-book of amounts of foodstuff purchased and consumed in a week time then this method can be used for food-consumption at household levels. The average intake of food per person per day is calculated as follows:

$$\frac{\text{Stock at the beginning of week} - \text{Stocks of the end of the week}}{\text{Total number of inmates partaking the meal} \times \text{No. of days of survey}}$$

Table 6.36: Standardization of cups for raw rice equivalents

Take 200 g of raw rice and cook with known amount of water subtract the weight of vessel and calculate the conversion factor

Raw rice (g)	Water used (ml)	Total cooked amount with vessel (g)	Weight of empty vessel (g)	Net weight of cooked amount (g)	Conversion factor (CF) Raw/cooked
200	400	800	200	600	200/600 = 0.33

Note: If individual has eaten 50 g of cooked rice, raw amount is 50 g × 0.33 = 17 g

5. Expenditure Pattern Method

We determine the money spent on food and non-food items by questionnaire. The reference period is fixed and indirectly the amount of food items consumed during a period is arrived at and amount of food items consumed per consumption unit or per person is arrived at. If the instructions are correct and family is cooperative, this method is good proxy method for weighment method.

6. Diet History

This method assesses the qualitative intake of food items and their frequency of intake as discussed in the beginning.

7. Duplicate Samples

What is consumed in the family, the same amount of each food item is kept separately per day as duplicate sample. These samples can be weighed or samples can be sent to laboratory for analysis. Laboratory analysis of nutrients is most accurate method.

8. Recording Method

A record of all items of food eaten is maintained by family or individual for a specified period of time, by actual weighing of the quantities eaten. The cooperative and literate families can provide this information, however it needs validation.

Evaluation of Adequacy of Diet

The adequacy of diet is measured by comparing the actual intake of nutrients to the recommended dietary allowances (RDA) for each nutrients.

$$\text{Percent adequacy of intake} = \frac{\text{Nutrient consumed per day}}{\text{Recommended dietary intake}} \times 100$$

Dietary survey data has to be combined with nutritional assessment survey. Further, we are particularly interested in dietary consumption of preschool, adolescents, pregnant and lactating mothers, as also their nutritional assessment to corroborate the association between intake and nutritional status. Dietary surveys in India are undertaken on sample basis periodically by NNMB, Hyderabad.

REFERENCES

1 World Health Organization (WHO). The Health aspects of food and nutrition. A manual for developing countries in the Western and Pacific Region of WHO. 3rd edn., Manila; 1979.

2 Thimmayamma BVS, Rau P. Textbook of Human Nutrition. Dietary Assessment as part of nutritional status. In: Bamji MS, Rao NP, Reddy V (editors). Textbook of Human Nutrition. New Delhi: Oxford and IBP Publishing Co. Pvt. Ltd., 1996.

3 Govt. of India (GOI). National Health Profile 2008. New Delhi: Central Bureau of Health Intelligence, DGHS, MOH and FW; New Delhi, 2008.

NUTRITION INTERVENTION PROGRAMMES

Some of the direct nutrition intervention programmes which are operative in the country to improve the nutritional status of vulnerables were as under. These broadly fall into two categories.[1,2]

1 Food supply and supplementary nutrition programmes:
   - a Supplementary nutrition programmes for preschool children.
   - b Mid-day meal programme for school children.
   - c Food for work programme—for below poverty line and economically weaker section adults.
   - d Subsidized food through targeted public distribution system (TPDS), to below poverty line families.

2 Specific nutrient supplementation:
   - a Vitamin A prophylaxis for prevention of nutritional blindness.
   - b Iron and folic acid for national nutritional anaemia control programme.
   - c Iodized salt for national iodine deficiency disorders control programme.

SUPPLEMENTARY NUTRITION PROGRAMMES FOR PRESCHOOL CHILDREN (0–6 YEARS)

Logic: Dietary surveys indicated that preschool children diet in the country was inadequate and there was 'food gap' of 300–400 calories and consequently there was wide-spread protein energy malnutrition (undernutrition and severe undernutrition) among preschool children in the country.

To bridge this food gap, supplementary nutrition programmes were started in the country.

Since pregnant women and lactating mothers were also vulnerable groups, they were included in the programme subsequently.

NATIONAL MID-DAY MEAL PROGRAMME (NMDM)

Mid-day meal in Tamil Nadu started way back in 1925–26 by the corporation of Chennai. In July 1956, the school lunch programme was launched as people's movement for organized charity as part of the school improvement efforts. The state achieved another milestone in 1982 with the launch of nutritious meal programme for school children in classes 1st to Xth. During 2001–02 around 5.80 million children were enrolled for the mid-day meal scheme.

The Government of India initiated mid-day meals for primary school children in 1962–63 as a follow-up measure of school health committee report in 1961–62. The supplies for mid-day meals were donated by the cooperative

American relief everywhere (CARE) which were valued as ₹ 40/– per child per year. During the period of droughts in 1966–67, the mid-day meal programme was extended in many areas to cover preschool children, pregnant and lactating mothers, mostly through the CARE programme. Under the scheme, food supplements were to be provided to children of age 6–11 years to meet at least one-third of calories and half of protein requirements for the day. The implementation of programme rests with the education department. The programme coverage was limited and variable.

The national programme of nutritional support to primary education known as national mid-day meal programme (NMMP) was launched in 1995. The honour of starting NMMP goes to Tamil Nadu. The programme took a national shape in 2002. The central government now provides 100 g of grains per child per day as hot cooked meal which provides 300 calories and 10–12 g protein per day for 200 days in a year. Two rupees per child per day are allocated for cooking cost of which one rupee should come from the state government, food grains are provided by the central government free of cost.

Objectives

The objectives of this programme were:

1 To promote universal primary education by increasing enrolment, retention, attendance and continuation rate in primary classes.

2 To improve the nutritional status of students in primary classes as also their learning or scholastic achievements.

Under the scheme, 100 g of wheat or rice per student per school day is provided for 10 academic months. The mandate is to provide cooked food but in practice 3 kg of cereals (wheat or rice) is given as take home grains at the end of each month to each child. Beneficiary has to attend school for 20 days in a month. In Delhi, ready to eat foods are being provided. Lifting of food grains is an important operational problem. Cooked meal is not provided. Take home ration is no surety that it will be consumed by the child. Subsequent to the directive of Supreme Court cooked meal is being provided now.

This programme has enhanced the school enrolment and attendance, particularly in weaker sections of community. It is one of the largest programme for feeding. Improvement of nutritional status by this much ration appears to be doubtful.[3] School health programmes must be revived and converged with NMMP and NMMP itself merged with SSA (*Sarva Shiksha Abhiyan*).[4]

SUPPLEMENTARY NUTRITION PROGRAMME (SNP) THROUGH ICDS

ICDS is the world's largest outreach programme. It is now universal programme in India.[5]

Focus

For supplementary nutrition, the focus is on young children from 0 to 6 years of age, pregnant and lactating mothers as also adolescent girls. ICDS programme started in 1975. ICDS is now universal in India and 7067 projects were operational in the country against 7075 sanctioned.

It is an integrated programme of nutrition, health and education with the objective of overall development of young children by good nutrition, reduced morbidity and mortality and empowerment of mothers and women. It is also a programme of enhancing school enrolment. Adolescent girls are also the beneficiaries of supplementary feeding.

Indira Gandhi Matritva Sahyog Yojna (IGMSY)—a Conditional Maternity Benefit Scheme: The Ministry of Women and Child Development provides cash incentive of ₹ 4000 to pregnant and lactating women of 19 years of age and above, for the first two live births. Cash incentive is provided in three installments. If the conditions are fulfilled. Anganwadi worker and helper receives an incentive of ₹ 200 and ₹ 100 respectively per pregnant and lactating woman.

APPLIED NUTRITION PROGRAMME

Objective

The objective of this programme was to raise the level of nutrition and standard of living of the vulnerable population; preschool children, pregnant and lactating mothers through education in nutrition and to increase production and consumption of protective foods by the above mentioned vulnerable groups.

- The applied nutrition programme (ANP) was one of the nutrition intervention programme extended to entire country in 1963 with the help of UNICEF, FAO and WHO.
- ***Areas:*** It was meant for rural areas. The Ministry of Rural Development exercised administrative control over the programme. Block development officer (BDO) was incharge of the programme at the block level.
- ***Food production:*** Emphasis was local production of protective foods (through poultries, fisheries, community and school kitchen gardens and community dairies, etc.).

Trained officials and non-officials at block and village level were to organize local committees for supervision and implementation of the programme which was undertaken by village Panchayats, schools and *Mahila Mandals* who organized cooking demonstration and feeding programmes for vulnerables. An amount of ₹ 30,000/- per block per annum was provided from central and state funds. During fourth plan, central assistance was raised to 100%. This amount was utilized for digging tube wells, fencing school gardens, establishing community and school gardens and poultry. UNICEF provided vehicles, equipment, supplies and technical experts. The programme failed to generate desired awareness for improved diets and failed to make an impact on production and consumption. The radiating effect of the programme through demonstration was not achieved.

However, the concept of ANP is valid even today, ultimate solution of undernutrition lies in self-reliance and adequate food at home level and that much food for young child is always there. Best of food and nutrition is available in the farm and the home.

TARGETED PUBLIC DISTRIBUTION SYSTEM (TPDS)

While at present, India has in reserve 65 million tonnes of food grains, with heavy post harvest losses. It is now well recognized that the availability of food grains is not a sufficient condition to ensure food security to the poor. It is also necessary that poor have sufficient means to purchase food. The capacity of the poor to purchase food can be ensured in two ways—by raising the incomes or supplying food grains at subsidized prices. While employment generation programmes attempts the first solution, the targeted PDS is a mechanism for the second option.

With a network of 4.62 lakh fair price shops (FPS) for distributing food at subsidized rates, the PDS in India is perhaps the largest distribution network of its kind in the world. It ensures availability of food to the poor.

TPDS now provides 20 kg of grains per month at 50% of economic cost from 1.4.2000 to below poverty line families. In addition, 35 kg of food grains was to be provided to the poorest of the poor families under the *Antyodya Anna Yojna* at a highly subsidized rate of ₹ 2/- per kg for wheat and ₹ 3/- per kg for rice. TPDS ensures household food and nutrition security to the poor.[6]

POVERTY ALLEVIATION IN RURAL INDIA

At the beginning of new millennium, 260 million (27%) people in India did not have incomes to access a consumption basket which defines the poverty line, the estimates for which have been revised to the level of 38% (2009).

Mahatma Gandhi National Rural Employment Guarantee Act and Schemes: It is successor to many employment guarantee schemes of the past. As per the Act any adult who applies for work is entitled to being employed on Public works within 15 days. The work guarantee is limited to 100 days per household per year in rural areas. The Act contains 30% reservations for women.

FOOD FOR WORK PROGRAMME

The food for work programme has been in existence since long. Food grains are given as part of wages to the poor. Food for work (FFW) is now component of employment assurance scheme and is operative in eight drought affected states of Odisha, Bihar, Madhya Pradesh, Chhattisgarh, Gujarat, Rajasthan, Maharashtra and Uttarakhand. The programme aims at augmenting food security through wage employment. Food grains are supplied to states free of cost. However, lifting of foodgrains from Food Corporation of India (FCI) godowns has been slow. All the employment generation schemes now operate under the banner of *Sampoorna Gramin Rozgar Yojna* with the basic aim of provision of food and nutrition security to the poor. Payment of wages is done partly in cash and partly in kind (5 kg of food grains and the balance in cash). The centre and state share the cost of cash component of the scheme in the ratio of 75:25. Renewed thrust has been given to food for work programme in 150 backward districts; the programme will provide 100 days employment to all able bodied rural persons. This will be a step towards national employment guarantee scheme.

The micronutrient supplementary programmes have been discussed earlier in this chapter.

Conclusion

Targeted supplementary nutrition programmes to poorest have beneficial effect to improve the severe malnutrition (PEM) while national mid-day meal programme has a role to improve the universal elementary education but not the nutritional status. On the whole, the supplementary nutrition programmes as a strategy to improve child nutrition have not met much success, it acts as a spring board to develop other activities, such as washing hands, eating clean food, and brushing of teeth, etc.

REFERENCES

1 UNICEF. Study on young child. "Indian case study" New Delhi: UNICEF; 1976.

2 Rao PN. Nutrition intervention programme in India and in neighbouring countries. In: Bamji MS, Rao PN, Reddy V (editors). Textbook of Human Nutrition. 3rd edn, New Delhi Oxford and IBH Publishing Co. Pvt. Ltd.; 1996. p. 467–82.

3 GOI. Planning Commission Strategic Initiatives for Inclusive Development XIth Five-Year Plan: Yojna Bhavan; New Delhi, 2006.

4 NIN. Status of Mid-day meal programme in six states. Nutrition News 1995 Oct; 16(4).

5 NIPCCD. Manual on integrated child development services. New Delhi: NIPCCD; 1984.

6 GOI. Tenth Five-Year Plan (2002–2007), Vol II; New Delhi: GOI; 2002.

NATIONAL NUTRITION POLICY

The National Nutrition Policy adopted in 1993 advocates a comprehensive intersectoral strategy for alleviating the multifaceted problem of malnutrition and achieving an optimal state of nutrition for all sections of the society.

The policy seeks to strike a balance between the short-term measures like direct nutrition intervention and the long-term measures like institutional/structural changes and thus creates an enabling environment and necessary conditions for improving nutritional and health status.

The national nutrition goals which were to be reached by 2000 AD were as under:

- Reduction in moderate and severe malnutrition among preschool children by half.
- Reduction in chronic undernutrition and stunted growth in children.
- Reduction in incidence of low birth weight to less than 10%.
- Eliminate blindness due to vitamin 'A' deficiency.
- Reduction in iron deficiency anaemia among pregnant women by 25%.
- Universal iodization of salt for reduction of iodine deficiency disorders to 10%.
- Giving due emphasis to geriatric nutrition.
- Production of 250 million tonnes of food grains per year.
- Improving household food security through poverty alleviation programmes.
- Promoting appropriate diets and healthy lifestyles.

The overall strategy comprises increased awareness of energy and micronutrient deficiencies and empowering household and communities to tackle these through existing resources. Emphasis is laid on providing sustained support and guidance for better utilization of services and appropriate behavioural actions at community level for improving diets and promoting healthy lifestyle. Advocacy, communication, training and social mobilization play a crucial role in operationalising this plan of action on nutrition.

The policy has identified key areas for action in various spheres like food production, food supply, education, information, health care, rural development, women and child development, people with special needs, and monitoring and surveillance. The policy requires a series of actions to be undertaken by various concerned departments/ministries of the government. Some of the direct interventions enshrined in the policy are as follows.

Direct short-term interventions	***Indirect long-term interventions***
• Expanding the nutrition intervention net (ICDS, UIP, ORT) • Empowering mothers with nutrition and health education • Reaching the adolescent girls • Ensuring better coverage of expectant women • Controlling micronutrient deficiencies • Fortifying essential foods with nutrients	• Food security • Improving dietary pattern • Purchasing power • Public distribution system • Land reforms • Health and family welfare • Nutrition and health education • Education and literacy • Nutrition surveillance • Information and communication • Community participation

SECTORAL PLANS OF ACTION

National development policies and strategies can have an important bearing on the nutritional status of the population. Since many of the basic causes of malnutrition lie outside the immediate field of nutrition, the most effective governmental strategies to reduce malnutrition on a national scale can be those that focus on incorporating nutritional considerations in all development policies and programmes including even the non-nutrition interventions. Maximizing the positive nutritional impacts of development policies both at the national level and in different sectors can significantly contribute to improving nutritional status. At the same time, to ensure an adequate impact from specific nutritional interventions, a favourable environment in terms of both overall development policies and sectoral policies is required.

The sectoral plans, thus, represent a starting point in their process of analysis, articulation, planning, reinforcing and monitoring each sector's contributions for reducing malnutrition in the country. The clear statement of nutritional objectives, review and analysis of existing policies and programme, development of strategies and action plans will help integrate and institutionalize these processes into sectoral planning as well as contribute to strengthening national development planning.

The sectoral plans define the general objectives, specific objectives and activities for the sector which can contribute to nutrition improvement through their respective programmes. These sectors are agriculture, civil supplies, education, food, mother and child health, women and child development, health, environment and forest, rural development and information and broadcasting.

There are certain other sectors like welfare, labour, food processing, industrial, etc., which can make significant contributions to nutrition promotion. These sectors have also been co-opted for integrating nutritional objectives in their sectoral strategies and plans for contributing towards nutritional improvement.

IMPLEMENTATION OF NUTRITION POLICY

The nodal department is department of women and child development which manages ICDS programme is responsible for monitoring of achieving the set goals. The implementation is weak; because of lack of coordination.

- We have achieved self-sufficiency in food grains production (over 264 million tonnes per annum) and targeted public distribution system (TPDS) which ensures food security at household level.
- Purchasing capacity is being increased through employment generation programmes to reduce the level of poverty in India. The current level of poverty (2014) in India is 21.8%. India defines "*poverty line*" in nutritional terms. It is consumption expenditure level below which is a household (of 5.5 persons on an average) cannot meet the recommended intake of 2400 calories per adult in rural areas or 2100 calories in urban area.

Sectoral commitments under National Plan of Action on Nutrition (NPAN)

	Sector	Sectoral commitments in the NPAN
1	Agriculture	To ensure national level food security including buffer stocks and nutritional considerations in agricultural policy.
2	Civil supplies and public distribution	To ensure food security at the household level by making the essential foods available through the public distribution system to the people particularly to the disadvantaged sections.
3	Education	To provide convergent services under education sector to enhance the nutritional and health status of the community with special emphasis on girls' education and improved status of women.
4	Forestry	To popularize the growing of plants/trees supplying food stuffs/fruits with special emphasis on beta carotene (vitamin A) rich species in the social forestry programmes with a view to create nutritional awareness and promote the consumption of nutritious foods.
5	Health	Achieving health for all by 2000 AD through prevention and control of various forms of malnutrition, diseases related to inappropriate diets, creating health awareness among the people and ensuring adequate primary health care for all.
6	Family welfare	Improving the nutritional status of women and children through nutrition prophylaxis programmes, health and nutrition education and public health measures, besides achieving a small family norm.
7	Food	To ensure food security in the country.
8	Food processing industries	To meet the nutritional needs of the people by giving nutrition orientation to the projects in food processing sector.
9	Information and broadcasting	To create a climate of awareness in the country about the importance of nutrition for the well-being of the people and ways and means of preventing various forms of malnutrition through its different units.
10	Labour	To protect and promote the nutrition of various types of labour—agricultural, construction, industrial, etc. with special emphasis on children and women at work, through formulation and enforcement of appropriate labour laws.
11	Rural development	To improve purchasing power of the people in rural areas through employment generation and poverty alleviation programmes with a view to improve food security at the household level.
12	Urban development	To ensure access to social services relating to health care, nutrition, women and child development, preschool and non-formal education and physical amenities like potable water supply, sanitation, sewerage, drainage, etc., with a view to improve the nutritional level of the urban poor.
13	Welfare	To improve nutrition of the disadvantaged sections of society by ensuring implementation of nutritional components of various welfare programme.
14	Women and child	To ensure appropriate development of human resources both through direct nutrition development interventions for special/vulnerable groups as well as through various development policy instruments for improved nutrition as laid down in the National Nutritional Policy. Improving nutrition and health of women and children through strengthening and extension of ICDS programme and setting up of appropriate systems for monitoring the follow-up actions under National Plan of Action for Children.

Source: National Plan of Action on Nutrition (NPAN), Deptt. of Women and Child Development, Govt. of India, New Delhi, 1995.

The other definition of poverty is per capita income less than US$ 1.5 per day. Poverty and unemployment is widespread in India and it indicates need of focussed attention and targeting poor persons for health-nutrition and food for work and employment.

- Dietary intakes of young children and pregnant women are much lower than recommended dietary allowance (RDA) hence there is widespread malnutrition.
- Low intakes of diet in young children, women and adolescent girls are due to wrong beliefs and practices and differential care of girls and boys in terms of feeding.
- Widespread infections like diarrhoeal diseases, worm infestations, acute respiratory infections and measles lower the nutritional status of young children.
- High fertility (repeated pregnancies and short birth interval) and 16.5% of girls getting married below 18 years of age, 90% of them are anaemic.
- National Nutrition Policy has addressed these problems in the policy. Direct nutrition intervention may yield limited results. More emphasis needs to be laid on adequate eating at home and control of infection, fertility, providing safe water supplies, safe-excreta disposal, besides deworming operations and contraception.

In view of emerging epidemic of obesity, diabetes and cardiovascular diseases there is imperative need to revise National Nutrition Policy.

National Nutrition Mission on Anvil

Mapping nutritional levels and monitoring of food distribution through Anganwadis is the basic objective. A GPS tablet of GPS enabled weighing machine will be used to check the weight of every child once a fortnight and monitor the beneficiaries.

PREVENTION OF FOOD ADULTERATION (PFA) ACT

Ministry of Health and Family Welfare is responsible for ensuring availability of safe wholesome and healthy food to the consumers. This is done through "Prevention of Food Adulteration (PFA) Act, 1954". The subject of PFA is in the concurrent list of the constitution. The enforcement of the Act is done by the states.[1]

World Health Day 2015

"From farm to plate make food safe"

New threats to food safety are emerging: Changes in food production, distribution and consumption, changes in the environments, new and emerging pathogens, antimicrobial resistance—all these pose challenges to national food safety system.

THE FOOD SAFETY AND STANDARDS ACT (FSSA)-2006

This Act has been enacted by parliament. The responsibility to implement this Act has been entrusted to Ministry of Health and Family Welfare. FSSA-2006 has come into force with effect from 5th August 2011. PFA 1955, fruit product order 1955, solvent extracted oil order 1967, and other food orders stand repealed.

This Act was enacted to consolidate the laws relating to food being administered by different Ministries/ Departments and to establish the Food Safety and Standards Authority of India (FSSAI) for laying down science based standards for articles of food and to regulate their manufacture, storage, distribution, sale and import, to ensure availability of safe and wholesome food for human consumption.

Pure food is essential for maintenance of health. The food available to consumer should be nutritious, wholesome and pure. It is observed that the evil of food adulteration prevails in the country on large scale.

For the first time a limit of 1 ppb (part per billion) for each pesticide has been fixed in carbonated water (like cola drinks) by notification in june 2009. The govt. has reduced the maximum limit of caffeine from 200 ppm to 140 ppm in june 2009.

REASONS FOR ADULTERATION

Reasons are molstly socioeconomic and to get rich quickly by adopting unscrupulous practices. It is also because of processing or preservation of food items to increase the acceptability, appearance and shelf life of food. The manufacturers or food processors use food additives which may be harmful to the health.

Objectives of PFA

i The PFA has been enacted to ensure protection of health of the consumers.

ii To prevent gross food adulteration, to control over contaminants and additives and to control over dumping of substandard foods.

iii To improve the nutritional status of population by ensuring wholesome food.

iv To earn foreign exchange by supply and sale of quality food items (exporting of food).

v Banning the entry and sale of non-iodated salt.

Implementation

The food samples are collected from the grocer's shops, fair price shops, milk sellers, dairy development and cooperative and from traders by the designated food inspectors or even consumer can collect the sample by observing proper instructions. The food samples are sent to designated laboratory. There are 72 food laboratories under the administrative control of various states/union territory Governments and local bodies. In addition, there are four central food laboratories at Mysore, Kolkata, Ghaziabad and Pune. Three food samples are collected, one is sent to the designated laboratory, the second one is left with the retailer and the third is kept with the food authority at district level.

Common Adulterants in Food

1 Colouring agents—non-permitted coal tar dyes and colours, excessive lead and lead chromate. Most pulses are coloured with coal tar dyes.

2 Artificial sweeteners like dulcin, saccharin.

3 Starches.

4 Citric acid, saw dust.

5 Non-permitted flavours and preservatives, non-permitted acids.

6 Mixing of cheaper edible oils in pure ghee, animal fat, rancid stuff, mineral oils, argemone oil, argemone seeds, excess sand dirt and grit.

7 Fats abstraction and addition of water and starches in milk besides urea mixing in milk to prevent curdling.

8 Ripening agents like calcium carbide for ripening of bananas and mangoes.

Synthetic milk is deadly mixture of caustic soda, detergent, urea, vegetable oil white paint and paper pulp.

9 Formalin—a toxic and carcinogen chemical is used to make fish look fresh.

In addition, the food may be sold as misbranded and wrong label or without label or with excessive moisture. Varieties of foreign seeds/matters may be added.

The prevalence of adulteration has declined from 14.2 to 7% but still one out of 14 food items is adulterated and this is unacceptably very high (Table 6.37).[2]

During the year 2008, Chhattisgarh topped the list where 23% of all food items were found adulterated. The

Table 6.37: Trends of food adulteration in India

Year	No. of samples examined	No. of samples found adulterated	% of adulteration
1981	133242	19050	14.2
1982	129595	16765	12.9
1983	129062	17965	13.9
1984	122296	14990	12.2
1985	128511	14677	11.4
1986	121969	13730	11.2
1987	131391	14091	10.7
1988	130390	15365	11.8
1989	122599	11549	9.4
1990	118580	11124	9.3
1991	115554	12841	11.1
1992	111591	11853	10.6
1993	99278	8562	8.6
1994	107360	10370	9.7
1995	103638	9424	9.1
1996	106229	11221	10.5
1997	95110	9315	9.8
1998	96479	7834	8.1
1999	88929	8197	9.2
2000	82701	8877	10.7
2008	63035	4096	7.0
2012–13	72200	58429	81.3

corresponding figures for rest of the states in India were: Himachal 20%, Punjab 19%, Jharkhand 18%, Jammu and Kashmir 15%, Uttarakhand 13% and Chandigarh 9%. Lowest food impurity levels were found in Arunachal 1%, Kerala 2.58% and Nagaland 3.25%. Most worrisome is the laxity of state governments on prosecution front as proceedings against 51% of cases/adulterators have not been launched.[3]

During 2012–13 out of 72200 food samples 13571 cleared the laboratory test, this means 81.3% of the samples failed the test for food safety. In 2011–12 only 8247 samples out of 64593 met food safety standards. This amounts to adulteration evidence in 85.3% of samples. Similarly in 2014–15 nearly 20% of food samples were adulterated or misbranded against the WHO norms of 5%

National Survey on Milk Adulteration

Milk and milk products are the most commonly adulterated items, followed by beverages and edible oils, fats and vanaspati ghee (Table 6.38).[4] National Survey on Milk Adulteration (2011) found that 68.4% of milk samples were found adulterated in India (FSSAI-2011). Adulteration in urban areas was higher than rural areas and more so in loose milk samples.[5]

Table 6.38: Percentage of food articles found adulterated in India (1998–2008)

	Name of food	Percentage adulterated 1998	2000	2006–08
1	Milk	26.33	19.36	7.43
2	Non-alcoholic and alcoholic beverages	11.86	12.6	
3	Milk products, butter, ghee, ice cream	14.92	30.4	
4	Spices and condiments	5.59	7.84	
5	Cereals and pulses	6.18	7.47	
6	Tea, coffee, cocoa and chikory	1.4	2.56	
7	Fruit products	7.93	2.91	
8	Edible oil, fats and vanaspati	8.41	10.39	7.43
9	Sweetening agents	6.56	11.70	
10	All foods	8.1	10.7	7.0

Food Additives

Food additives are substances which are added to food in controlled amount to process the food, preserve or improve its outlook and acceptability or to improve keeping qualities of food items or to enhance palatability. Monosodium Glutamate (MSG) is a common food additive as flavour enhancer.

The type and amount of most additives are controlled by law in most countries and only those substances, "generally recognized as safe" are allowed in the minimum amounts (permissible limits). Food additives are non-nutritious substances.

Commonly food additives which are added in the home or factory to preserve and process food; include: food preservatives, colouring agents, flavouring agents, ripening agent, sweeteners and antibiotics, etc.

Commonly used additives include nitrates used to preserve flavour and texture of meat products, to enhance the colour and to protect from *Clostridium botulinum* (which forms the fatal toxins). Nitrates can be converted to nitrites which in turn can interact with amines and amides in the meat or body to form nitrosomines which are carcinogenic. It is, therefore, important that the amount of nitrate and nitrite, is carefully controlled and the risks of cancer be weighed against the risk of botulinum poisoning.

Unpermitted artificial sweeteners, i.e. dulcin in soft-drinks and confectionary and other foods, excessive amounts of preservatives, antioxidants and other additives or unpermitted colours or excess amount of coal tar colours can be carcinogenic. Similarly, use of *pesticides* and *insecticides* in foodgrains and vegetables, fruits can be injurious to health.

The FSSI has approved 12000 standards for additives and ingredients.

Punishment under PFA

When the adulterated food is likely to cause death or injury to the body or amounts to grievous hurt it can be punished according to section 320 of Indian Penal Code. There is an imprisonment of not less than 7 years extendable up to life term and with a fine not less than ₹ 10 Lakh.[1]

Six year jail and 5 lakh for grievous harm caused by unsafe food intake and one year jail and 3 lakh fine for non grievous harm. Even for misbranding a seller could face 6 months jail and ₹ 1 lakh fine.

The food adulteration Act is a partial solution. The problem of adulteration needs to be mitigated by strong component of education of people, voluntary organizations, manufacturers and retailers.

Codex

The issue of international trade in food has become very important. Food standards at the international level are set by Codex Alimentarius Commission established by UN and WHO. India has participated in the meeting of the commission and has effectively advocated the stand of developing countries regarding the process of standard settings so that their interests are kept in view. An attempt is being made to harmonize to the extent possible the standards under the PFA rules with Codex.

Agmark and ISI

These are two other agencies which set standards for food. The work on standardization being highly specialized activity, these two organizations have developed the elaborate capacity and these agencies extend their laboratory services for testing of foods to the private industry, trade and consumers at nominal cost. Many food items bear ISI or Agmark as a mark of standard.[3]

FOOD FORTIFICATION

Food fortification means the addition of nutrients to a food so that the quality is maintained or improved without the quantity being significantly increased.

Food fortification can be important part of nutrition intervention strategy as a means of delivering nutrient to population. Micronutrient deficiency, such as iodine, vitamin A and iron is widespread in India. To deliver these nutrients to the community, the programme of fortification has been launched. The best example of fortification is iodation of common salt with potassium iodate to deliver nutrient-iodine, 15 PPM in salt at the consumer level, to eliminate Iodine Deficiency Disorders (IDDs). Similarly, delivery of iron through common salt was launched by National Institute of Nutrition (NIN) on experimental basis to mitigate the problem of anaemia.

Definition

Nutrient added to a food or an article of diet to improve the quality of diet of a group, community or population (WHO).

Improving Quality of Food

Examples: Wheat proteins are deficient in lysine and it can be improved by addition of lysine in wheat flour. Maize protein is deficient in lysine as well as tryptophan and we can add these amino acids to improve the quality of maize proteins.

Similarly, highly milled and polished rice are deficient in B-group of vitamins (thiamine) we can add vitamin B to enrich the polished rice.

To improve the quality of vanaspati ghee (hydrogenated oils), we used to fortify all hydrogenated oils with vitamin A—700 IU and vitamin D—50 IU per ounce as per regulations but now it is optional.

Enrichment of Food

Enrichment is another term for fortification. It is a process to add back a nutrient to food lost due to processing of that food. It is also called restoration of food quality. During the process of milling and polishing of rice, vitamins of B group are lost as also threonine (protein). Similarly, preparing of fruit juices causes loss of vitamin C. Hydrogenation of vegetable oils causes loss of essential fatty acids (EFA). During the process of baking of bread lysine is lost. Adding lost nutrients like vitamin C, EFA and vitamin B to above-mentioned foods is known as enrichment or restoration process.

Fortification as Tool to Deliver a Nutrient

The examples have been already given. To deliver iodine to population by universal salt iodation and to deliver iron by fortification of salt (double fortification with iron and iodate). Similarly, delivering vitamin. A through the vehicle of monosodium glutamate (MSG) to mitigate the problem of vitamin A deficiency.

Fortification of common salt has been a successful intervention to reduce the prevalence of iodine deficiency disorders in India. However, fortification rarely solves all the nutritional problems of a country.

Justification and Criteria for Fortification

1 The deficiency of nutrient should be widespread.
2 The vehicle food must be consumed by the target group, e.g. salt consumption is universal in India on an average 10 g of salt is consumed per day per person. This is an ideal food for iodate fortification. Similarly, sugar is also consumed in every household.
3 The high consumption of fortified food will not lead to toxicity.
4 The addition of micronutrient should not change the taste, colour, flavour, texture and shelf-life of the food item.
5 The item of food should be centrally controlled and monitored.
6 The cost of fortification should be affordable.

NEUROLATHYRISM

In India, neurolathyrism has almost disappeared and now sporadic cases may be there. Diets which were predominately based on the pulse *lathyrus sativus* (Khesari Dal) led to spastic paraplegia. The toxic factor in the pulse which led to spastic paralysis was identified as BOAA (β-oxalyl aminoalanine). The disease used to occur in epidemic proportion in central India and epidemics continued from 1844 to 1974. Since 1974, the epidemics have stopped; however, sporadic cases do occur from time to time but the disease has virtually disappeared by late 1980. Cultivation of Khesari dal was banned. Now the Government is considering to allow cultivation of three new varieties (Ratan, Parteek and Mahateara) which are safe for human consumption.

Measures which Succeeded

- Labourers avoided using *Lathyrus sativus* as the sole staple diet and instead used small quantities.
- Soaking of lathyrus sativus for 15 minutes in water before cooking or parboiling of pulse could remove the toxin.
- Banning payment of wages in the shape of lathyrus sativus to farm labourers with effect from 1983.
- This pulse became costlier item and landlords could not afford to distribute this item to poor labourers from 1980 onwards.

EPIDEMIC DROPSY

Argemone mexicana (Prickly Poppy) seeds grow as wild weeds in the field. The seeds of this plant resemble mustard seeds. The argemone seeds contain two toxic alkaloids: Sanguinarine and dihydrosanguinarine. The other minor alkaloids present are berberine propionate, cheletrythrine and coptisine which are less toxic.

The consumption of adulterated mustard oil with *Argemone mexicana* seeds leads to epidemic dropsy. In the recent past, Delhi and neighbouring states experienced outbreak of epidemic dropsy which affected 2000 people and caused 50 deaths.

The symptoms of poisoning appear within 5–20 days of consumption of adulterated oil containing 2–10% argemone oil.

Effects

The symptoms include vomiting, diarrhoea, abdominal pain, oedema of feet and legs. The patients may complain of lethargy, low grade fever and dyspnoea. Liver enlargement may occur without jaundice.

The cardiovascular manifestations include tachycardia and precardial pain. The ocular manifestations include itching and burning of eyes with superficial retinal haemorrhages, disc oedema and glaucoma in some cases. Death occurs due to cardiac arrest

Tests for detection of argemone oil: The permissible level of argemone oil in edible oil is 0.01%.

Concentrated nitric acid test is nonspecific test. Ferric chloride test can detect 0.25% of argemone oil.

Cupric acetate test can detect 0.5% of argemone oil.

Hydrochloric acid test is most sensitive and specific test and can detect argemone oil up to 0.001% in edible oil.

Thin layer chromatography (TLC) is done for biological samples.

Prevention

- Use of unsealed oil is not advisable.
- Enforcement of Food Adulteration Act.
- Education of people about early signs.

FOOD POISONING

Worldwide unsafe food is linked to the deaths of estimated 2 million people mostly children. Food contamination with bacteria or their toxins is a common feature in India because of poor hygienic conditions. Contamination is more common during mass cooking, feasts and festivals. Food contamination can occur during preparation, processing, cooking, storage or serving of foods.

Food-borne Infection

These infections are caused by consuming foods or liquids contaminated with bacteria, viruses and parasites. These pathogens cause infection by:

- Invading and multiplication in the lining of intestine and/or other tissues.
- Invading and multiplication in the intestinal tract and releasing toxin (bacteria only).

Food-borne intoxication—caused by consuming foods or beverages already contaminated with a toxin. Sources of toxins are as follows:

- Certain bacteria (preformed toxins)
- Poisonous chemicals—malathion, parathion and toxic metals
- Natural toxins found in animals, plants and fungi.

Occurrence

This may be sporadic and effect is limited to number of persons in household. Many a times outbreaks and particularly explosive outbreaks occur due to *Staphylococcus enterotoxin*.

Food borne disease outbreaks are defined as the "Occurrence of two or more cases of a similar illness resulting from ingestion of a common food or when observed number of cases exceeds the expected number. These can be confirmed (when at least 1 causal agent is identified) or suspected (based on clinical and epidemiological information)".

Common Features

Staphylococcal and Bacillus cereus

Food poisoning

Enterotoxins A, B, C, D and E of *Staphylococcus aureus* from food handlers, skin lesions, and nose. The symptoms appear within 1–6 hours. Common symptoms include nausea, vomiting, abdominal cramps and diarrhoea but no fever.

Salmonella sp, Campylobacter jejuni

These organisms from faeces of infected humans and animals can contaminate food items and produce inflammatory diarrhoea. Signs and symptoms appear in 18–36 hours. Manifestations are abdominal pain, fever and chills, nausea and vomiting.

Vibrio Cholerae, Enterotoxigenic E. coli

Incubation period varies from 6 hours to 5 days. These organisms produce watery diarrhoea. Enterohaemorrhagic *E. coli* produce bloody diarrhoea.

Botulism

Enteroneurotoxins A, B, E, and F of *Clostridium botulinum*. Spores are found in soil and animal intestine. The signs and symptoms of poisoning appear within 18–36 hours which include gastrointestinal symptoms and neurological symptoms.

Clostridium Perfringens and B. cereus Gastroenteritis

Enterotoxin of *C. perfringens* and *B. cereus* produce abdominal cramps and diarrhoea within 8–16 hours.

Epidemiological Investigations

Epidemiological investigations of food poisoning outbreak is an important exercise.

Food items can be pinpointed by thorough investigations. Attack rate can be determined in persons who consumed that food, and similarly attack rate can be determined in those who did not consume that food item and finally odds ratio can be worked out to arrive at incidence in exposed and non-exposed persons.

Stool samples, vomitus, gastric aspirate and food items for isolation of organisms and toxins can be collected as soon as possible after onset of illness. Government has approved for the first time for carrying out standard bacteriological tests for items like milk and milk products like cheese, curd, ice cream, etc.

Treatment: Correct dehydration by oral rehydration therapy or by IV fluids. Specific treatment in case of pesticide poisoning with chelating agents may be done under medical supervision.

Prevention: Hazard Analysis and Critical Control Point (HACCP) is a systematic preventive approach to food safety that addresses physical, chemical and biological hazard as a means of prevention rather than finished product inspection.

Five keys for safer food:

1 Wash your hands before handling food and food preparation.
2 Separate raw and cooked food.
3 Cook thoroughly.
4 Keep food at safe temperature.
5 Use safe water and raw material.

World health Day 2015 is an opportunity to alert people working in different government sectors, farmers, manufacturers, retailers, health practitioners as well as consumers about the importance of food safety.

GENETICALLY MODIFIED (GM) CROPS

GM crops being promoted by foreign multinational biotech. Companies are proving to be serious hazards for both environments and human and livestock health. GM will not solve the world food problem. GM crops lead to reduction of soil fertility. Increased use of toxic, carcinogenic and mutagenic agriculture chemicals lead to water, air and soil pollution and increased incidence of cancer, birth defects and other diseases.

REFERENCES

1 Chadha DS. National Programme on Prevention of Food Adulteration, New Delhi: NIHFW; 1988.
2 CBHI. Health Information of India 2000–01. New Delhi: DGHS, MOH and FW, GOI; 2001.
3 The Sunday Tribune, Haryana Edition–Adulteration: Northern region takes the cake – Vol 130, No 71 March 14, 2010 by Aditi Tandon.
4 GOI. Annual Report 2003–04. New Delhi: MOH and FW GOI; 2004.
5 FSSAI-National Survey on Milk Adulteration, 2011.

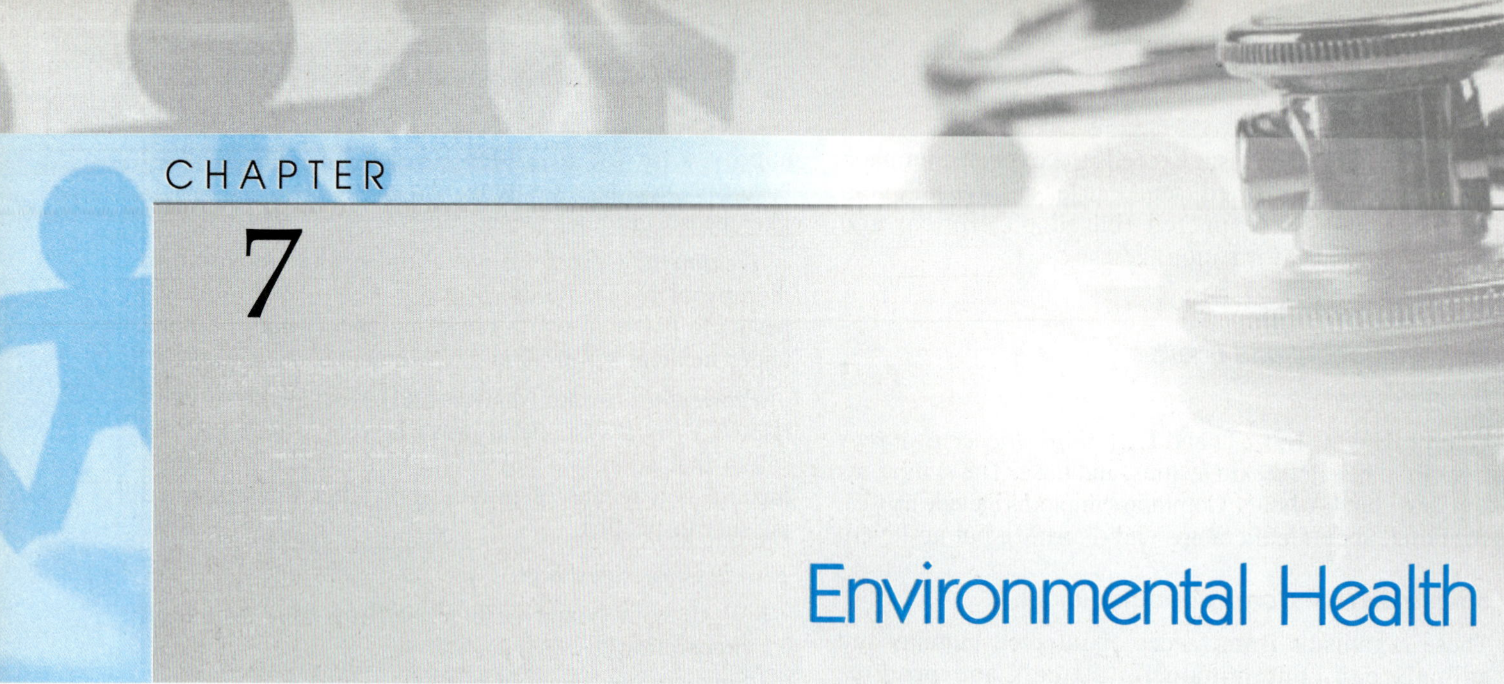

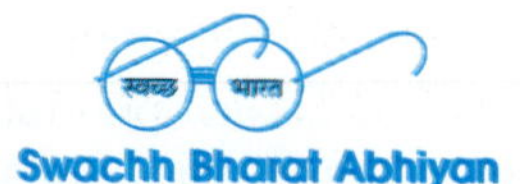

SAFE WATER

Environment is most important *determinant* of health—"Achieve universal and equitable access to safe drinking water and sanitation and hygiene for all and end open defecation by 2030". It is one of the goal of UNs Sustainable Development.

Water is literally, the source of life on our planet (Earth). The human body is 70% water. Close to 6% of DALYs lost in developing countries are attributed to unsafe water, sanitation and hygiene.[1] Water is essential for all metabolic functions of life. The availability of fresh and safe water is a challenge in view of increasing population, industrial and agricultural activities. Further, the fresh water is a finite source and pollution is a widespread phenomenon.

"Water is fundamental for life and health. The human right to water is indispensable for leading a healthy life and human dignity. It is prerequisite to the realization of all other human rights". Everyone should have access to safe water and secure drinking water and sanitation facilities.[2]

The framework for safe drinking water and recommended approach for regulations, policies and programmes are based on Stockholm Framework (1999).

As indicated in Chapter 18 of "Agenda 21" of United Nations Conference on Environment and Development (UNCED), "…. An estimated 80% of all diseases and over one-third of deaths in developing countries are caused by the consumption of contaminated water and on an average as much as one-tenth of each person's productive time is sacrificed to water related diseases".[3,4]

In view of the International Conference on Primary Health Care, jointly organized by WHO and UNICEF in Alma-Ata USSR in September 1978, it was enunciated that "Adequate supply of safe water and basic sanitation" would be one of the essential components of primary health care to attain minimum level of health for all citizens of the world by 2000 AD.

Daily Requirement for Drinking Purposes

Average daily consumption for drinking water varies in view of variations in climate, temperature and physical activity. On an average, two litres of water are required per day per adult person for drinking purposes alone, and child requires one litre per day.

Water Requirement Norms for Rural Areas

Different norms/standards have been adopted by developing and developed countries. In India, standard of 40 lpcd (litres per capita per day) has been adopted and considered to be necessary minimum to meet the needs of drinking and sanitation. The stipulated norms of supply of 40 lpcd of safe water within a walking distance of 1.6 km or elevation differences of 100 metres in hilly areas, can be relaxed as per field conditions applicable to arid, semi-arid and hilly areas.[5]

At least one hand pump/spot source for every 250 persons and additional water of 30 litres in desert development programme (DDP) for cattle, based on the cattle population is to be provided. The water requirements for cattle need not necessarily be met through piped water supply and could be made through rainwater harvesting structure/spot sources.

In the states, where 40 lpcd has been achieved in all habitations, the next step is to raise the level of availability to 55 lpcd. Population/distance/elevation norms may also be liberalized for states which have achieved full coverage as per existing norms subject to the cost sharing by the beneficiaries.

Norms of Water Supply for Urban Areas

The manual on water supply and treatment published in May 1999 by Central Public Health Environmental Engineering Organization (CPHEEO), Ministry of Urban Development and poverty alleviation specifies the norms and standards of municipal water supply for domestic and non-domestic needs such as institutional, commercial, fire-fighting and industrial requirements. The requirements/ norms are as under:[5]

1 Towns with piped water supply but without sewerage system: 70 litres per capita per day (lpcd).
2 Cities with piped water supply and existing or planned sewerage system: 135 lpcd.
3 Metropolitan and megacities with piped water supply and sewerage: 150 lpcd.
4 Public stand post–40 lpcd.

The above figures exclude unaccounted for water (UFW), which should be limited to 15%.

With the level and scale of development of an area, the norms will be scaled up and periodically these norms are reviewed. These norms have hardly been met in most cities though these norms are the bare minimum and not the ceiling or limit fixed. The eighth plan specified one source for 150 persons with maximum walking distance of 100 metres.[5]

Millennium Development Goals: Halve by 2015 the proportion of people without sustainable access to safe drinking water and basic sanitation.

Fresh Water Availability and Use

Only 3% of all water on earth is fresh water and rest 97% is in oceans. Most of the fresh water is locked away in icecaps and glaciers or deep underground aquifers and only 1% is considered easily accessible through lakes, rivers and shallow aquifers (underground levels shallow enough to be tapped by an affordable cost). Only this amount is regularly renewed by rain and snowfall and thus available on sustainable basis.[6]

Usage

The major use of fresh water is in the area of agriculture (production of food and rearing of animals). Worldwide over 69% of all annual water withdrawal is for agriculture, 23% for industry and 8% for domestic use. India uses 90% of all water for agriculture purposes with just 7% for industry and 3% for domestic use.[6]

SOURCES OF WATER

Drinking water comes from various sources such as groundwater, surface water (lakes, ponds, rivers, etc.) and rainwater.

Groundwater

Groundwater is available in different layers of earth. Aquifer is a layer or section of earth or rock that contains fresh water known as groundwater (any water that is stored naturally underground or that flows through rock or soil supplying springs and wells). Groundwater is dependable source of water supply. Groundwater in aquifers if recharged periodically by adequate rainfall or from river-beds is called a *renewable* water resource. Water in aquifers and other natural reservoirs that is not recharged by the hydrological cycle or is recharged so slowly that significant withdrawal for human use causes depletion are thus *nonrenewable* water sources.

Qualities

Groundwater is somewhat dependable source of water supply.

In most situations, it is available at affordable cost but in rocky areas access is difficult.

It is less liable to be polluted if source is adequately protected.

Disadvantages

It is highly mineralized and hardness varies from place to place. Sometimes, groundwater may contain excess of fluorides and arsenic which are harmful for human beings. Excess of iron causes taste problem.

Groundwater is susceptible to pollution through industrial chemical wastes and agriculture pesticides and insecticides. Excessive withdrawal of groundwater by everincreasing population poses several problems.

Shallow Open Wells

These wells draw water from superficial water table above the impervious layer. These wells are located intentionally near the ponds or canals or river beds from where these are charged continuously and provide sweet water of acceptable taste. Rural population depends on such wells. These wells over the times have dried up and are no longer dependable source of water supply.

- Often these wells are contaminated by human activities as also through seepage and poor maintenance of parapet around the well. Unclean buckets and washings often pollute these wells.
- People love the taste of well water and are adapted to it. Moreover, they believe that it is good for abdominal ailments, it quenches their thirst easily and is readily available. People prefer well water to piped water.

Deep Wells

These wells draw water from deep water table and water available between two aquifers. It is more dependable source and less liable to pollution but much depends upon the integrity of aquifer. If it is friable and broken there are more chances of contamination from surface water, industrial and agricultural activity. Deep wells have high mineral contents and the water is often hard.

Tube Wells

Water is drawn from the superficial or deep water table underground by boring into the ground. Accordingly, the tube wells are categorized as shallow and deep tube wells. With appropriate local technology, the hand pumps are widely used in rural areas. India mark II and mark III hand pumps are classical example of development of appropriate technology to draw under groundwater from rocky areas, and training local women and men for maintenance and upkeep of these pumps. Training of Rural Youth for Self-Employment (TRYSEM) Scheme was exploited for hand pump maintenance at local level and participation of youth was quite encouraging. UNICEF played pivotal role in advancement and popularization of India mark II and mark III hand pumps. Around 8.9% of urban and 8.3% of rural households use tube wells/borewells.

Surface Water

Surface water is available to us through lakes, rivers, and ponds. Around 11.6% of families in West Bengal in rural settings use ponds (Dobas) for drinking purposes. Ponds are heavily contaminated due to human activities such as ablution and washing of dirty linens as also animal bathing. These are unsafe sources of drinking water; but only means of drinking water to some families.

Rivers are the mainstay of surface water to urban areas. All big cities depend considerably on rivers for drinking water, therefore, it is necessary to keep the rivers clean. Unfortunately, all the 14 major rivers in India are heavily polluted because of discharge of raw sewage of municipality towns, industrial effluents and agriculture activities. Central and state pollution control boards are there to regulate river cleanliness, but these bodies are not effective to deal with the menace of river pollution.

Census 2011 data indicated that 43.5% of households in India used piped drinking water, while 33.5% drink water from hand pumps, 11% used well water, 8.5% drink from tube well/borewell and remaining 3.4% used surface water and other sources. In rural areas 43.6% of households drink water from hand pumps, 30.8% depend on tap water (piped water supply), 13.3% use wells, 8.3% use tube wells/borewells and remaining 4% use surface water or other sources. Piped water supply is available to 70.6% urban households against 30.8% in rural households. Only 41% of families have source of water (tap, well, etc.) within the premises.

Water Pollution Problem

Agriculture is the biggest polluter, even more so than industries and municipalities. Widespread use of insecticides and pesticides indiscriminately have led to contamination of groundwater aquifers and surface water. The water that goes back into rivers and streams after being used for irrigation is often severely degraded by excess nutrients, salinity and pathogens that render it unfit for any further use. India which depends on irrigated agriculture for food supplies, more than 4 million hectares of high quality land have been abandoned because of salinization and water logging caused by too much irrigation.[6]

Pollution through Industrial Activities

While agriculture remains the biggest source of water pollution, wastes from industries have increased tremendously in recent years. Industrial wastes generate between 200 and 400 major chemicals, which are directly dumped into waterways. Moreover, pollutants such as sulfur dioxide and oxides of nitrogen which combine in the atmosphere to form acid rain, have pervasive effects on both fresh water and land ecosystems. In the soil, acid can release heavy metals such as lead, mercury, and cadmium that can percolate into waterways. Further synthetic chemicals particularly persistent organic pollutants (POPs), which include hydrogenated hydrocarbons, dioxins, and organochlorides such as DDT are long-lived and highly toxic in the environments. These do not breakdown easily under natural processes and thus tend to accumulate up the biological food chain until they pose risk to human health. Industrial chemicals have led to pollution of groundwater with arsenic (in West Bengal and Bangladesh) and consequently produced ill effects on human health in the form of melanosis, keratosis and skin cancers.

Industrial fluorosis in population living near industries, which release fluorides into water channels, is yet another example of toxicity through polluted groundwater. Near Agra, Yamuna river water is red due to heavy pollution with industrial dyes and chemicals. Total dissolved solids (TDS) in water exceed many many times than the prescribed limit of 800 ppm.

Municipal Pollutants

Human and animal wastes are let into waterways. Raw sewage of towns and megacities finds its way into rivers. All of India's 14 major rivers are badly polluted. Together they transport 50 million cubic meters of untreated sewage into India's coastal waters every year. The city of New Delhi dumps 200 million litres of raw sewage and 20 million litres of industrial wastes into Yamuna river everyday as the river passes through the city on its way to Ganges. Many water-borne outbreaks and epidemics have occurred on this account in the past in the city of Delhi. Outbreaks of viral hepatitis (hepatitis A and E) have become perpetual affair. During 1958, outbreak in Delhi 30,000 cases of viral hepatitis were reported; due to heavy pollution of River Yamuna with sewage near Wazirabad water works.

Health Dimensions of Water Pollution

About 2.3 billion people in the world suffer from diseases that are linked to water. In Bangladesh, e.g. an estimated 75% of all diseases are related to unsafe water and inadequate sanitation facilities. In Pakistan, one quarter of all people attending hospitals are ill from water-related diseases. In India, too very high proportion of illnesses are water-related, about 1.5 million infants die of diarrhoeal diseases every year.[6–8]

Providing clean supplies of water and ensuring proper sanitation facilities can save million of lives by reducing the prevalence of water-related diseases.

Water-borne Diseases (WBD)

WBDs are dirty water diseases; those caused by water that has been contaminated by human, animal and chemical wastes. Water-borne diseases include diarrhoeal diseases, cholera, typhoid, dysentery, polio, hepatitis A and E. Diarrhoeal diseases kill over a million of young children in India and produce malnutrition and disabilities in survivors. Improved water supply reduces diarrhoea morbidity by 6–25%.

Water-based Diseases

Snails and cyclops live in water and act as intermediate hosts. Schistosomiasis is transmitted through snails. Infected faeces reach water, schistosome eggs hatch, embryo penetrate the snail where infective larvae develop, larvae leave snail and enter into water, when man comes in contact with such water these larvae penetrate through the skin of human body and cause schistosomiasis.[6]

Infected cyclops when ingested produce guinea worm disease in man. Thus, cyclops act as intermediate host for guinea worm disease (dracunculiasis). Guinea worm disease has been successfully eradicated from India.

Water-related Vector-borne Diseases

Mosquitoes and tsetse flies that breed and live in or near both polluted and unpolluted water can transmit diseases like malaria, yellow fever, dengue fever, dengue haemorrhagic fever, sleeping sickness, filariasis and Japanese encephalitis.[6]

Water Scarce Diseases (Water-washed Diseases)

Many diseases including trachoma, scabies, skin sepsis, lice infestation, conjunctivitis, bacillary and amoebic dysentery, salmonellosis and worm infestations are due to lack of water and personal hygiene. These diseases are also called "water-washed" diseases. These diseases thrive because of scarcity of water and consequently poor hygienic practices.

***The Swachh Bharat Abhiyan*:** Clean India drive has been launched in 2014 to reduce water and vector-borne diseases and improved solid waste management.

WATER PURIFICATION

The aim of water purification is to make water safe, i.e. free from pathogens or disease producing organisms.

Safe water is one that is free from pathogenic organisms, harmful chemical substances, excessive amounts of minerals which could produce undesirable physiological effects. It does not harm the consumer when consumed over prolonged period.

***Potable/wholesome water*:** It is safe water which is pleasant to taste, odourless, cool and colourless and does not stain clothes or utensils.

Water can be made safe and potable through time tested technologies and natural process to diminish organic and inorganic suspended particles.

NATURAL METHODS

A. Dilution

Controlling pollution by dilution is a natural way in rivers and stream water. Small amount of sewage or polluting matter, which enters river or stream gets diluted so much that it loses its bad effect on human health. Dilution is an important means of purification.

B. Sedimentation

If water is allowed to stand or stored in a reservoir or tank, it is exposed to natural sunlight and air which leads to aeration and adds oxygen to water and oxidizes organic matter to a large extent.

Ultraviolet rays help to destroy the harmful organisms. The suspended organic matter (bacteria, protozoa) and inorganic matter settles down at the bottom, if the water is allowed to stand in reservoir tank for 24 hours or longer. This is the common method used in water purification for piped water supply system. Aquatic plants, which grow at the bottom of tank over a time period help oxidize the organic matter and trap harmful microorganisms. Over 90% of suspended impurities settle down in 24 hours of sedimentation process. The raw water drawn from a source of canal/river is quite turbid because of suspended impurities. During the process of sedimentation, the turbidity gets reduced and water becomes clearer and most of suspended matter settles down at the bottom. The storage and sedimentation therefore are natural purifiers of water and form the preliminary stage in purification of water in slow sand filters. Over the period after sedimentation, sludge accumulates at the bottom of the tank which has to be removed periodically.

PURIFICATION BY ARTIFICIAL MEANS

C. Filtration

The objective of filtration is to make water safe by removing pathogenic organisms. Over 98–99% of bacteria get removed by the process of filtration.

Slow Sand Filters

These filter beds are made with filter media:

- The surface layer or top layer consists of fine sand graded particles. The thickness this layer varies from 3′ to 5′.
- The second layer is of coarse sand 6″–12″ in thickness.
- The third layer is graded gravels or stones 6″–12″.
- Bottom layer is two layers of bricks arranged in the form of drain over perforated pipes.

- The total depth of slow sand filter is 9′–12′.
- The sizes of the slow sand filters vary depending upon the size of community to be served.

Function of Slow Sand Filter

- It acts as sedimentation tank as well as removes suspended organic and inorganic matters.
- It acts as strainer and removes suspended matter.
- Slimy layer develops on the top surface of the filter bed. It is vital layer of the filter which is called *zoogleal* or *biological layer*. It is also called schmutzdecke or dirty skin. It adsorbs the colloidal particles and bacteria. Real biological action is done by this layer and the process of nitrification also occurs at this layer.
- There occurs oxidation of organic matter in filter bed pores.

Limitations

- The filter occupies large space/land area.
- Rate of filtrations is low. It gets chocked frequently.

Efficiency

The efficiency of slow sand filter is maximum as it holds back 99% of bacteria.

Rapid Sand Filter (Mechanical Filter)

Mechanical or rapid sand filters have replaced slow sand filters. Speed or rate of filtration is quite rapid and these filters occupy less space. These filters are of two types:

1. Gravity type rapid filter
2. Pressure type rapid sand filter.

Gravity Type Rapid Filter

It is a water tight chamber containing 33" of sand and about 18" graded gravel underneath.

In this filter, the vital layer is artificially made by producing flocculent precipitate with which the colloidal silt settles on the surface of the sand. Aluminium hydroxide or "alum floc" forms slimy layer over the sand bed of filter, which performs the functions of adsorbing bacteria from water. Oxidation of ammonia also occurs in the vital layer.

Coagulation: Process of coagulation is essential step for rapid sand filtration. Coagulation is done by mixing aluminium hydroxide 5–40 mg/L or adjusted according to turbidity level of water. When alum is added to water it results into formation of white flocculent precipitate of aluminium hydroxide, which is allowed to settle in sedimentation tank. Clear water is then allowed to pass through filter bed.

Back washing: Rapid sand filter gets clogged with excess of floccules of aluminium hydroxide and has to be washed by pressure periodically, it is called back washing or backflushing.

Efficiency: Bacterial removing efficiency is to the extent of 90–95%.

Rapid Sand Filter (Pressure Type)

The filter media is placed in an entirely closed steel tank and operates under pressure higher than atmosphere pressure. The filter bed is same as that of rapid sand gravity filter. Strainers are provided at the bottom instead of perforated pipes. Raw water dosed with aluminium hydroxide passes on the top of the sand and forms a gelatinous film without previous mixing. Consequently, the quality of effluent is inferior to that of gravity type filter. These filters are suitable for small installations.

Domestic Filters (Household Level)

Their action is purely mechanical. An effective domestic filter must keep back all germs and raw substances.

Usually, the filter media we use is infusorial earth, clay, porcelain or patent combination of porcelain or clay or animal charcoal.

Some of the Common Domestic Filters

i. *Pasteur-Chamberland filter:* This consists of porous tubes or bougies of unglazed porcelain. These tubes can be screwed onto a tap. The action is purely mechanical. It can separate the suspended particles including bacteria. It is reliable filter but action is slow.
ii. *The Berkefeld filter:* This consists of cylinder made of infusorial earth.

Domestic filters need frequent cleansing. Filtered water is not always above suspicion, sometimes these filters give us a false sense of security as they very often get clogged.

Meta Filters and Stellar Filters

These were extensively used in World War II. These are pressure filters of domestic use taking water directly from the tap. The actual filter bed consists Kieselgurh coated with silver and intermixed with aluminum hydrate, forms a layer over the metallic filter pack.

Modern techniques: Online Filters, Aquaguard, Kent, Pureit, Philips-389 filters are available in the market. Besides mechanical filtration, the function of reverse osmosis and UV rays are built in these filters. Such systems help in removing bacteria, hardness, and excess of fluorides and arsenic.

D. Disinfection of Water

All water supplies need to be disinfected before consumption of water. Various methods of disinfection are as follows.

Boiling

Boiling is the best method to destroy all organisms and it makes the water sterile but this method is not practical. It can be practiced at individual, households and for high-risk individuals.

Ozone

It is a powerful sterilising and oxidizing agent. It inactivates viruses very quickly. Ozonized air when brought into contact with water destroys the germs. 0.2–1.5 mg of ozone is required to purify one litre of water. It is somewhat expensive. There is no residual effect of ozone as it decomposes and disappears within a short time. A minimal dose of chlorine if added to ozonized water before distribution ensures residual free chlorine in water.

Ozonation is practiced in advanced countries.

Ultraviolet Rays

Sterilization of water can be done by ultraviolet rays. It is being used in developed countries; and in domestic filters: Like Aquagard. Bacteria and viruses are killed by UV rays.

Chemical Methods

Terminal disinfection is essential for surface water treatment and for protected groundwater sources when *E. coli* or thermotolerant (faecal) coliforms are detected. For effective disinfection, there should be a residual concentration of free chlorine of $> = 0.5$ mg/L after at least 30 minutes. Contact time at pH < 8.0. A chlorine residual should be maintained throughout the distribution system. At the point of delivery, the minimum residual concentration of free chlorine should be 0.2 mg/L. In emergencies, e.g. in refugee camps, during outbreak of potentially water-borne disease, or when fecal contamination of water supply is detected, the concentration of free chlorine should be increased to greater than 0.5 mg/L throughout the system.

Chlorine has been the mainstay of disinfection of water and is the most commonly used disinfectant worldwide. When chlorine is added to water it forms hydrochloric acid and hypochlorous acid.

$$Cl_2 + H_2O = HCl + HOCl$$

The hypochlorous acid (HOCl) further ionizes to $H^+ + OCl^-$ (hypochlorite ion). The disinfection action of chlorine is mainly due to hypochlorous acid and partly by hypochlorite ions. Best action of chlorine is achieved when pH is around 7.0.

Limitation

Normal doses of chlorine do not destroy hepatitis virus, protozoal cysts, spores, and helminth eggs. Higher doses or superchlorination is required to destroy these forms of pathogens. At least 0.5 mg/L of free residual chlorine throughout the system is required to kill these organisms.[3] Chemical disinfection of drinking water supply that is faecally contaminated will reduce the overall risk of diseases but may not necessarily make the supply safe. Chlorine disinfection has limitation against the pathogens—in particular cryptosporidium and some viruses.

Methods of Chlorine Application

Chlorine gas: In big water purification plants, chlorine is used in gaseous form with the help of mechanical injector called 'chloronomes'. The compressed gas is cheaper and easier for application. The dosing machine carries out chlorination automatically to ensure 0.2 PPM of residual chlorine at consumer's end or household level. At the plant, itself the free chlorine of 0.5 PPM is ensured.

Water purification process is shown in Fig. 7.1.

Chloramination: Chloramine is produced by interaction of ammonia and chlorine. It imparts less chlorinous taste in water and ensures persistent type of residual chlorine, however, chloroamines are slower in action. Chloramination could be useful in large urban areas when water is to make very long journey through pipes.

Bleaching powder: It is also known as chlorinated lime. Bleaching powder decomposes in water into calcium hypochlorite and calcium chloride.

$$CaO + 2Cl = CaOCl_2 \text{ (bleaching powder)}$$

$$2CaOCl_2 + H_2O = Ca(OCl)_2 + CaCl_2 + H_2O$$

Bleaching powder of good quality should contain 33% of available chlorine. It is white amorphous powder, unstable with pungent smell. Moisture, light, air and CO_2 reduce the available chlorine content of bleaching powder.

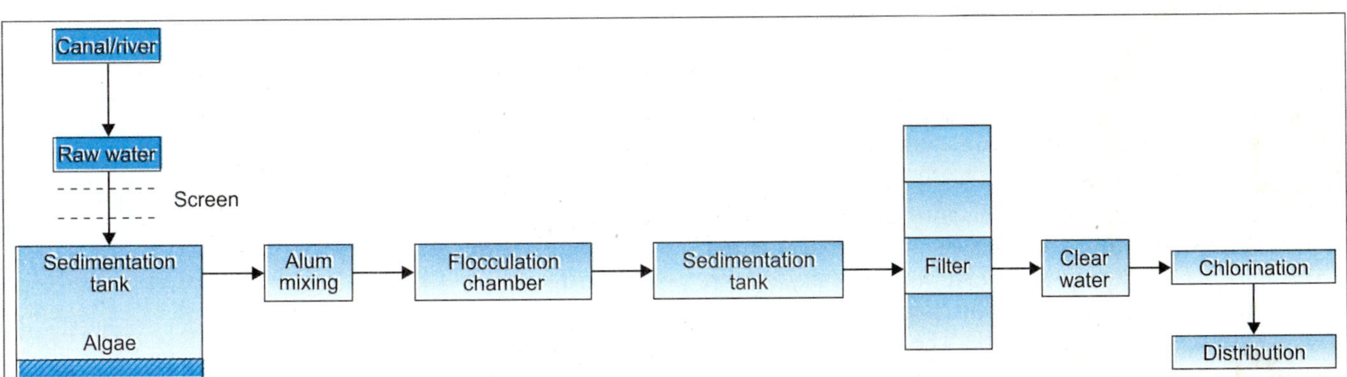

Fig. 7.1: Water purification process

Bleaching powder is by far the most used disinfectant for water supplies and ideally suited for small water supplies in rural areas. The potency of unstable bleaching powder lasts for 3 months with chlorine content of 25–30%. It should be stored in cool dry and dark place, once opened should be used on the same day so it is advisable to store in small containers.

Under proper and optimal storage conditions chlorine content of bleaching powder is expected to fall below 20% in the course of one year.

Stabilized bleach: The stabilized bleaching powder has higher chlorine content 50–70%. The life of stabilized bleaching powder is normally taken as one year for which period it retains its chlorine contents.

Water sterilizing powder: Keeping qualities of bleaching powder can be considerably improved by addition of quick lime in the proportion of 80:20, when it is called as water sterilizing powder (WSP). The available chlorine in WSP is 25%. WSP is soluble in about twenty times its weight in water. Chlorine solution can maintain its strength for weeks if stored properly. For preparing stock solution of chlorine see guidelines of chapter on cholera control. To prepare 1% of solution we add 33 g of bleaching powder in one litre of water.

Chlorine Demand

"Chlorine demand is the amount of chlorine required to kill bacteria and to oxidize the organic matter and ammoniacal substances present in the water".

Dose of chlorine is chlorine demand plus the free residual chlorine of at least 0.5 ppm, is the correct dose of chlorine.

Contact time: Minimum contact time of 30 minutes of bleaching powder with water is required for disinfection. This can be determined by orthotoluidine test. If chlorinated water shows positive orthotoluidine test after half an hour it means residual chlorine of 0.5 ppm is present in that water.

Determination of Demands of Chlorine

The demand of chlorine and dose of bleaching powder is determined by Horrock's apparatus. The Horrock's outfit consists of six white cups of 200 ml capacity each and one black cup of 240 ml capacity, two metal scoops each capable of holding 2 g of bleaching powder/WSP when filled level with brim, a bottle of cadmium iodide starch solution, glass stirring rods and pipettes.

1. Prepare stock solution of bleaching powder or WSP. One level scoopful of fresh bleaching powder is put up into the black cup and made into thin paste with minimum quantity of water and thereafter more water is added up to the white mark. The mixture is stirred with glass rod. This is the stock solution.
2. Fill 6 white cups with clear water.
3. Drops of stock solution are added with pipette in each glass, 1 drop to first glass, 2 in second, 3 in third, 4 drops in fourth, 5 in fifth and 6 drops in the sixth cup. One drop represents 1 ppm (parts per million), i.e. one part of chlorine in a million parts of water.
4. Contents of each cup are stirred with glass rod and contact time of half an hour is allowed.
5. After contact time of half an hour, three drops of indicator (cadmium starch solution) are added to each cup.
6. Serial number of first of the cup showing blue colour indicates number of scoopful of bleaching powder required to sterilize 500 litres of water with 1 ppm of residual chlorine after half an hour. If second cup shows blue colour, it means 4 g of bleaching powder is the demand and this much should be added in 500 litres of water.

If superchlorination is advised, one more scoopful of 2 g of bleaching powder in 500 litres of water is required to be added. This will give 2 ppm of free chlorine in water after 15 minutes of contact time.

Pot Chlorination

Chlorine tablets are available for pot chlorination at home. A safe dose of 2–3 mg/L of water is suggested this is equivalent to 1–2 drops of bleaching powder liquor with 3% available chlorine for each litre of water.[9]

Chlorination in Practice

In rural settings, well chlorination and at small water works supplies the chlorination is not a routine or regular affair. It tends to be irregular or symbolic and resorted during outbreak or epidemic of water-borne diseases or if death due to water-borne diseases is reported.

DISINFECTION OF OPEN WELLS

Around 11% of Indian rural households depend on wells to meet their need of drinking water. Well chlorination therefore deserves special attention. Chlorine demand and dose is determined by simple formula-5 D^2H, where D denotes the diameter of well in feet; H indicates the depth of water column in feet. The quantity of water is estimated in gallons (1 gallon = 4.55 litres). 2.5 g of fresh bleaching powder per 1000 litres of water is the rough estimate of demand of chlorine. Half an hour after adding bleaching powder; the well water is tested for residual free chlorine by orthotoluidine test and if the test is positive it indicates successful chlorination. The health worker male keeps records of all wells in his area and ensures their chlorination, usually on demand basis.

Method

The calculated amount of bleaching powder is mixed with a small quantity of water in a bucket to make a thin paste; more water is added to get an even solution of chlorine. The sediments are discarded by pouring supernatant in another clean bucket. The bucket containing chlorine solution is lowered about two-feet below the water level and mixing it by giving rotatory movements to the rope tied to the bucket and drawing it up and down several times below the water surface. The bottom of the well should not be agitated as it disturbs the organic matter and it increases the turbidity of water which can protect the organisms from the effect of disinfection, stimulate the growth of bacteria and gives rise to a significant chlorine demand.

Frequency of Well Chlorination

It is determined by orthotoluidine test. Ideally it should be done daily in the evening by the village volunteers themselves. This ideal is seldom achieved.[9]

Orthotoluidine Test

This test is done at least half an hour after the water has been chlorinated. Objective of the test is to determine the **residual free chlorine** qualitatively and quantitatively. If the test is positive, it is inferred that residual chlorine of at least 0.5 ppm is present in the water.

The reagent consists of analytical grade of orthotoluidine dissolved in 10% solution of hydrochloric acid. A sample of chlorinated water (10 ml) is taken in a test tube and 2–3 drops of orthotoluidine (OT) are added and observe the colour of water. The yellow colour produced immediately after adding OT solution indicates free residual chlorine and a colour appearing after 20 minutes indicates both free and combined chlorine. The residual chlorine content of the water sample can be determined quantitatively with greater accuracy by matching the colour developed in the sample of water with standards contained in the sealed tubes using the chlorine comparator.

It may be noted that even if a trace of residual chlorine is present it gives a characteristic smell and taste. Villagers can smell or taste the water after half an hour to know if chlorine is present in the well water or pot water.

Successful stories of regular chlorination are very few. One experience is, however, worth quoting.

Intensive education to women was given in villages. Women groups took responsibility for home chlorination, inspired by young school children who were trained at school for chlorination. Chlorine tablets/bleaching powder packets were provided free of cost through Anganwadi workers and subcentres. Women had a pride and at least in ten villages they were emphatic and sure that they successfully kept away diarrhoea, drugs and doctors "because of regular pot chlorination; washing hands and improved water storage practices at home". However, civil surgeon of the district was annoyed with us as we were consuming half of the total supply of bleaching powder in just one block only. Demand for bleaching powder and chlorine tablets was generated in many villages but we could not meet this demand or sustain the supplies on regular basis. There was no local source of supply of bleaching powder.

Case study I: Young women of 10 villages were trained on chlorination of well and pot chlorination at home. One of the enthusiastic daughter-in-law of village Sehri carried the stock of chlorine tablets to her in-laws home. She chlorinated the pot. Mother-in-law got suspicious of the activity of her daughter-in-law, she suspected her daughter-in-law of adding poison in the water and consequently the daughter-in-law was beaten severely. The message went like wild fire in that village. A doctor was summoned from nearby primary health centre to testify the poison in the pot. Doctor verified and certified that tablets were not poison, but chlorine tablets meant to purify water. He was brave enough to consume one glass of chlorinated water in the presence of village crowd and stayed there for about half an hour and thus effectively demonstrated that nothing happened to him by consumption of that chlorinated water.[9]

A woman adopted the practice of pot chlorination in her home. For the first three days, she would ask her husband every evening "Are you fit and fine?" Husband retorted back on the third day as to why do you ask me the same silly question every evening? What has happened to you? The wife disclosed that she was serving him the chlorinated water for the past three days and was really worried and feels concerned for his health and less any bad effect of chlorine.

Women, men and children draw water from pot by dipping their soiled hands and glass every time they feel the need of drinking water. Unwashed and dirty hands leave, lot of dirt and dust in pot. This was demonstrated to a group of women. Women were asked to wash their hands in steel bowl and the clean water in the bowl turned muddy (after dipping and rinsing hands in it). Women were asked to drink this water, they refused and appreciated that repeated dipping of dirty hands in pot spoils the drinking water we therefore advocated use of ladles to draw water from pot.

60 ladles were distributed free of cost under *Mahila Swasthya Sangh* group meetings in some villages to help some women to adopt healthy practices for drawal of drinking water from the pot. The left out women kept on waiting for arrival of free ladles and used to ask frequently when you will bring free supply of ladles? Lesson was learnt that free supply did not motivate the left out women to buy their own ladles to keep water clean.

Case study II: We advocated and demonstrated use of clean glass for drinking water, this was our belief and thinking that people would practice use of clean glass. We soon realized our mistake. People in this part of the country are habitual to drink water by cupping of their hand/hands. They draw the water from pot by using a common glass but use their hands to drink water. Explanation and reasoning of this practice was very sound and simple that no one else could use their hands and it is a pure act limited for oneself. Use of glasses for drinking water is restricted to guests only. The focus of education was shifted soon and we promoted the practice of washing hands before drinking water. But, adoption of this practice meant more water and people want to conserve water for drinking.

All along these years the emphasis remained on achieving the target of "coverage of rural population", thrust has been more on quantity of water (40 litres/day/ person). The massive programme of rural water supply adopted "Provider's approach" and quality aspects of water supply and education of people has been neglected to a great extent all these years.

Due to alarming growth of population, there is mounting pressure on "drinking water" which is becoming a scarce resource and widespread contamination due to human excreta and garbage continues. Due to widespread ignorance and illiteracy, the "concept of safe water" eludes the common man. Consequently, the outbreak of water-borne diseases and several endemic diseases remain a great burden on the society.

Our experience and results of several studies reveal that over 80% of rural people in this part of the country depend on well or hand pump water. Well water is preferred and is the first priority whenever this is available. Hand pumps rank second in preference. Barely 20% of rural people use piped water system. Piped water supply is considered to be undependable, unsafe, taste is not liked by many (unpalatable), smell of chlorine is resented and according to many, it does not quench their thirst. Some people associate piped water with common cold and abdominal ailments. Most common and preferred use of piped water in this area consists of bathing, washing of clothes and utensils, cooking and preparing tea. People have experienced that soap works better on piped water and hence this water is good for washing clothes and hair.[9]

Overall acceptance of piped water system tends to be low. Common villagers rate the piped water supply system as much inferior to that of well or hand pump water supply. Village people see their peers using raw water for ablution, lot of mud, dirt, dust and even dead animals and birds present in the storage system or raw water channels. How can I drink someone else's faeces? Is a common question asked by villagers? Concept of filtration and treatment system of waterworks is miles away from their imagination. Seeing is believing and the villagers have never seen the treatment process at waterworks. Women groups were taken to waterworks system and a demonstration was organized for them at the site, they got convinced and on return they demonstrated to fellow women and convinced other women in their village of the benefit of safe water supply.

7

The practice of chlorination and ensuring quality of water supply in rural setting more often than not, becomes a "crisis response". The practice of chlorination and subjecting the water to laboratory testing assumes significance during outbreaks only or at best chlorination happens to be a seasonal activity. Routine and regular chlorination and testing of water samples are conspicuous by their absence. Chlorination of well water is resorted to as compliance to an order from higher formation and workers tend to adopt a line of "all-or-none law" that is heavy chlorination of wells beyond the acceptable limits, forcing people to leave the regular source and switch over to alternate unsafe sources of water supply. They (workers) do this deliberately to show their presence to authorities. Further, the task of regular chlorination of sources is beyond the capacities of health workers. People must participate and take responsibility of chlorination and maintenance of water sources. Some of the operational research studies undertaken in field practice areas of Medical Colleges, Rohtak, paid rich dividends. School teachers undertook the responsibility of chlorinating the supply system in their schools, school children promoted the pot chlorination in their homes, women groups influenced women and built the practice of pot chlorination and took the responsibility of chlorination of village wells, they thus became self-reliant.

At home level, the storage practices and drawing water from the pot are deplorable. Water is stored in pitcher or metallic pots. Everyone dips hands to draw water from the pot, so water is liable to be contaminated. Storage of water in narrow mouthed pots (SURAHI) can prevent contamination of water at home. Use of ladles to draw water from pot is a rare practice. People are habitual to drink water by cupping of their hand/hands and use of glass for drinking is reserved for guests only. Repeated demonstrations of clean water and unclean water were organized in schools and with women groups in the villages to inculcate practice of regular hand washing and use of ladles to draw water. The success of inculcating the practice of hand washing in preschool children and school children was quite high and sustainable, but it meant more water and more burden on women.

E. Quality and Standard of Water

WHO has developed guidelines for drinking water quality. The latest guidelines (published in the year 2011) are being reproduced in Table 7.1.

Microbiological Aspects

Indicator Organisms

Ideally drinking water should not contain any micro-organism known to be pathogenic, capable of causing disease or any bacteria indicative of faecal pollution. The detection of *Escherichia coli* provides definite evidence of faecal contamination; in practice, the detection of thermotolerant coliform bacteria is an acceptable alternative.

Table 7.1: Guideline values for verification of microbial quality[a] WHO 2011

Organisms	*Guideline value*
All water directly intended for drinking	
E. coli or thermotolerant coliform bacteria[b,c]	Must not be detectable in any 100 ml sample
Treated water entering the distribution system	
E. coli or thermotolerant coliform bacteria[b]	Must not be detectable in any 100 ml sample
Treated water in the distribution system	
E. coli or thermotolerant coliform bacteria[b]	Must not be detectable in any 100 ml sample

[a] Immediate investigative action must be taken if *E. coli* are detected.
[b] Although *E. coli* is the more precise indicator of faecal pollution, the count of thermotolerant coliform bacteria is an acceptable alternative. If necessary, proper confirmatory tests must be carried out. Total coliform bacteria are not acceptable indicators of the sanitary quality of water supplies, particularly in tropical areas where many bacteria of no sanitary significance occur in almost all untreated supplies.
[c] It is recognized that, in the great majority of rural water supplies in developing countries, faecal contamination is widespread. Under these conditions, the national surveillance agency should set medium-term targets for the progressive improvement of water supplies.

Escherichia coli is abundant in human and animal faeces, in fresh faeces it may attain concentration of 10^9 per gram. It is found in sewage, treated effluents and all natural water and soils recently contaminated with faecal matter. *E. coli* count should be zero and not detectable in any water sample meant for drinking purposes.[3,10,11]

Characters: *Escherichia coli* (*E. coli*) possesses enzymes β-galactosidase and β-glucuronidase. It grows at 44 to 45°C on complex media, ferments lactose and mannitol with production of acid and gas and produces indole and tryptophan.

However, increased attention has focused on the shortcomings of traditional indicators such as *E. coli*, as indicator organisms for enteric viruses and protozoa. Viruses and protozoa are more resistant to conventional environmental conditions or treatment technologies, including filtration and disinfection, may be present in treated drinking water in the absence of *E. coli*. Retrospective studies of water-borne diseases outbreaks have shown that complete reliance on assumptions surrounding the absence or presence of *E. coli* may not ensure safety. More resistant organisms such as bacteriophages and/or bacterial spores may be included as indicators of persistent microbial hazards under certain circumstances.

Thermotolerant Coliform Bacteria

These are coliform organisms that are able to ferment lactose at 44–45°C; the group includes the genus *Escherichia* and some species of *Klebsiella, Enterobacter* and *Citrobacter*. Thermotolerant coliform other than *E. coli* may also originate from industrial effluents or from decaying plant materials and soils. For this reason the term "faecal" coliform though frequently employed, is not correct and its use should be discontinued.

Virological Aspects—Residual Chlorine

At least 0.5 mg/L free residual chlorine after a minimum contact of 30 minutes at a pH less than 8.0 is sufficient to inactivate enteric viruses. This level of free residual chlorine is to be insisted upon in all disinfected supplies in areas suspected of endemicity of infectious hepatitis. For emergency and outbreak situation, the level of chlorine should be increased to greater than 0.5 mg/L throughout the system. For other areas, free residual chlorine of 0.5 mg/L throughout the system is desirable. High level of turbidity can protect microorganisms from the effect of disinfection hence the turbidity should always be less than 5 NTU (nephelometric turbidity unit).

Major indicators of quality of drinking water are

i Residual chlorine mg/L
ii *E. coli* or thermotolerant coliform bacteria count: It should be zero.
iii Turbidity NTU—It should be less than 5 NTU: Ideally should be below 1 NTU.
iv pH less than 8.0.

Further the drinking water should be colourless, tasteless, odourless and cool.

SAMPLING OF WATER

These are collected for:

- Physical and chemical examination.
- Bacteriological examination.

Physical examination consists of colour, turbidity, pH.

Chemical examination consists of determining the level of various chemicals (Table 7.2).

Bacteriological examination: Water should be collected in sterilized or boiled bottles obtained from laboratory. People and health workers themselves can collect these samples. 200–250 ml of water is collected and labelled properly depicting date, time, source and place. These water samples should be transported in cold chain system or on ice to microbiological laboratory.

Frequency of Collection of Samples

In case of outbreaks, the bacteriological examination is to be done daily. Samples should be collected from different areas of distribution system.[12] Periodicity of sampling depend on size of population.

Table 7.2: Chemicals of health significance in drinking water

Inorganic constituents	*Guideline value (mg/L)*	*Organic Industrial constituents*	*Levels (µg/L)*		*Levels mg/L*
• Antimony	0.02	*Chlorinated alkanes*		• Atrazine	100
• Arsenic	0.01 (A, T)	• Carbon tetrachloride	4	• Bentazone	30
• Barium	0.7	Dichloromethane	20	• Carbofuran	7
• Benzo (a) pyrene	0.0007[a]	• 1,2-dichloroethane	30[a]	• Chlordane	0.2
• Boron	2.4	• 1,2-dichloroethene	50	• Chlorotoluron	30
• Cadmium	0.003	Trichloroethene	20 (P)	• Lindane	2
• Chromium	0.05 (P)	• Tetrachloroethene	40	• Methoxychlor	20
• Vinyl chloride	0.0003[a]	1, 4-*Dichlorobenzenes*	300 (C)	• Metolachlor	10
• Fluoride	1.5	• 1, 2-Dichlorobenzene	1000 (C)	• Molinate	6
• Lead	0.01 (A, T)	*Xylenes*	500 (C)	• Pendimethalin	20
• Mercury (inorganic)	0.006	• Toluene	700 (C)	**Radioactive constituents of drinking water**	
• Nickel	0.07	• di(2-ethylhexyl)phthalate	8	• Uranium 238	10 Bq/L
• Nitrate (as NO_3^-)	50	• Benzene	10[a]	• Uranium 234	1 Bq/L
• Nitrite (as NO_2^-)	3 (P)			• Thorium 230	1 Bq/L
• Selenium	0.04 (P)	**Pesticides used in agriculture**	**Levels (µg/L)**	• Radium 226	1 Bq/L
• Uranium (chemical aspects)	0.03 (P)			• Plutonium 239	1 Bq/L
		• Alachlor	20[a]		
		• Aldicarb	10		
		• Aldrin/dieldrin	0.03		

A, provisional guideline value because calculated guideline value is below the achievable quantification level; C, concentration of the substance at or below the health-based guideline value may affect the appearance, taste or odour of the water, leading to consumer complaints: P, provisional guideline value because disinfection is likely to result in the guideline value being exceeded; P, provisional guideline value because of uncertainties in the health database; T, provisional guideline value because calculated guideline value is below the level that can be achieved through practical treatment methods source protection, etc. [a]For substances that are considered to be carcionogenic the guideline value is the concentration in drinking-water associated with an upper-bound excess lifetime cancer risk of 10^5 (one additional case of cancer per 1,00,000 of the population ingesting drinking-water containing the substance at the guideline value for 70 years). Concentration associated with estimated upper-bound excess lifetime cancer risks of 10^4 and 10^6 can be calculated by multiplying and dividing, respectively, the guideline value by 10.

Table 7.3: Categorization of drinking water systems on the basis of population size and quality rating in order to prioritize actions (*see* also Table 7.1)

	Proportion (%) of samples negative for E. coli		
Quality of drinking water system[a]	*<5000 population*	*5000–1,00,000 population*	*>1,00,000 population*
A	90	95	99
B	80	90	95
C	70	85	90
D	60	80	85

[a]Quality decreases A to D

Example of assessment of priority of remedial actions of community drinking water supplies based on a grading system of microbial quality and sanitary inspection rating or score[a]

		Sanitary inspection risk score (susceptibility of supply to contamination from—human and animal faeces)			
		0–2	*3–5*	*6–8*	*9–10*
E. coli classification[b]	A				
	B				
	C				
	D				
		Low-risk: No action required	Intermediate risk: Low action priority		High-risk: Higher action priority

[a]Where there is a potential discrepancy between results of the microbial water quality assessment and the sanitary inspection, further follow-up or investigation is required.

[b]Classifications based on those shown in Table 7.3. Quality decreases from A to D. Source: Adapted from Lloyd and Betram (1991).

Water Quality Control (WQC)

WQC is primarily responsibility of water supplying agency and it is aimed at meeting the water quality standards by regulatory authority. WQC can provide the water supplying agency valuable information:

- It indicates quality of source of water.
- It helps to assess efficiency of treatment and also indicates whether the water quality variables are within acceptable limits.
- It provides useful information on natural and seasonal variations.
- It identifies need for taking remedial action.

Operating Practices

The supplying agency should ensure suitable preventive maintenance, and exercise strict day-to-day control on water quality; collect routine water samples and test at various points including the source of water, conveyance, treatment and distribution, supplemented by sanitary inspection.

Water Quality Surveillance (WQS)

WQS is done by independent agency. Objective is to ensure safe water supply to community. This system investigates the activity and identifies the corrective or preventive measures and gives feedback to water supplying agency. Responsibility of WQS is entrusted to health department. Following must be ensured for effective surveillance:

- Regular testing of residual chlorine at consumer level.
- Regular collection of water samples and testing of water samples for *E. coli* or thermotolerant coliform bacteria.
- Regular interaction with supplying agency.
- Monitor and surveillance of water-borne, water-related and water-associated diseases for early warning as part of integrated disease surveillance programme.
- Monitor outbreaks of water-borne diseases.
- Carry out sanitary inspection of water sources.
- Preparing and distribution of educational material to people on water management.
- Training of community members and Panchayati Raj Institutions (PRIs) for home and well chlorination besides education on safe water.
- Continuing education of health teams.
- Intersectoral coordination with ICDS, rural development and education, PRIs and non-Governmental organizations.[12–15]
- Combined analysis of sanitary inspection and water quality data can be used to identify the most important causes of and control measures for contamination.

Field Test Kits for Potable Water Quality Assurance

These kits have been developed for rapid surveillance of quality of drinking water. These can be carried to the field and can run on alternate source of power. These kits can test, essential physical, chemical and bacteriological parameters on the spot and during emergencies. These kits have been developed by:

- Defence Research Laboratory, Jodhpur
- National Environmental Engineering Research Institute (NEERI), Nagpur
- Industrial Toxicology Research Centre, Lucknow
- All India Institute of Hygiene and Public Health, Calcutta
- Central Scientific Instrument Organization, Chandigarh
- Other private organizations/entrepreneurs of national and international level.
- H_2S strip test for drinking water: This is used as rapid screening test for testing the microbiological quality of water. Cost is very low. Dry and sterile media are provided in screw capped bottle. Fill the water to be tested up to upper level of the label. Shake the bottle gently for 5 minutes. Keep the bottle at room temperature of 30–35°C or in incubator at 37°C for 18 hours. If none is available it can be kept in the pocket while sleeping in the night. If the medium turns black the water is considered to be unfit (KS Manja). This is purely a qualitative test. These kits have been supplied to Health Workers under NRHM.

ARSENIC CONTAMINATION

Problem

West Bengal, Bihar, UP, Assam and 6 districts each in Haryana and Punjab are major states where arsenic contamination is prevalent in groundwater. Around 16 million people are at risk of arsenicosis (keratosis and melanosis). The number of habitations affected with arsenic in rural areas has increased from 7067 in six states to 10,004 in 14 states in 2009.

Arsenic contaminated habitations have been identified in eight districts of West Bengal (North and South 24 Parganas, Murshidabad, Malda, Nadia, Howrah, Hugli and Bardhman). Arsenic is released through industrial activities such as coal burning, copper smelters and industrial effluents which contaminate the groundwater and when waste from coal mines is dumped along river bed. Industries such as metallurgical industries, glassware, ceramic, dye and pesticide manufacturing units, petroleum refineries use arsenic in many of the processes.

Because of large scale overuse of groundwater due to rise in population and industrial activities led to ground water pollution.

Permissible arsenic limit in drinking water by WHO standard is 0.01 mg/L.[10] The range of arsenic content in drinking water in eight districts of West Bengal is 0.055–3.20 mg/L.[16,17]

Health Effects

Excess of arsenic in water produces arsenicosis. Skin pigmentation, arsenical dermatosis, mellanosis, excessive keratosis of skin and cancer of skin, hepatomegaly are the visible bad effects of arsenicosis.

Solutions

Providing safe water with arsenic level of acceptable limits. The Government of India introduced an arsenic submission in 1994 under the Rajiv Gandhi National Drinking Water Mission to tackle the arsenic problem in West Bengal on 75:25 cost sharing basis.[18]

Measures

1 Utilization of surface water from rivers, lakes, ponds, which are normally free from arsenic contamination.

2 Sanitary protected ring wells tapping shallow aquifers.
3 Tapping of deeper third layer beyond 100–150 metres below ground level, which is found to be arsenic free.
4 Adopting arsenic removal techniques through domestic filters, attached with hand pumps and arsenic removal plants in piped water schemes (by oxidation followed by coagulation and filtration, adsorption, osmosis, reverse osmosis and ion exchange).

ENDEMIC FLUOROSIS

Excess of fluoride in drinking water leads to endemic fluorosis. Fluorosis is endemic in 20 states of India.[19,20]

Permissible Level of Fluoride in Water

The World Health Organization (WHO) has set the standard of fluoride in drinking water at 1.5 mg/L to be adopted by nations. WHO guidelines further state that climatic conditions, volume of water consumed and intake from other sources be considered while setting national standards. Because of widespread problem of fluorosis in India, the Bureau of Indian Standards (BIS) has fixed the upper limit of fluoride in drinking water at one mg/L. WHO guidelines are under review and levels of 0.5 mg/L has been favoured in 2000 AD by International Workshop held in Chiang Mai, Thailand.[19]

Geographical Distribution and Population Affected

In India, fluorosis is endemic in 275 districts of 20 states. Over 70–100% of districts are affected in the state of Rajasthan, Gujarat and Andhra Pradesh, where the problem is very severe. These are the states where drinking water problem is also very serious, people depend and draw underground water and suffer silently from fluorosis.

- 40–70% of districts are endemic in the state of Punjab, Haryana, Delhi, UP, Bihar, MP, Maharashtra, Karnataka and Tamil Nadu.
- 10–40% of districts are endemic in J&K, Assam, West Bengal, Odisha and Kerala. For the remaining states, the endemicity is not known precisely.[20–22]

Recently fluoride mapping in the country has been done by Dental Council of India (2004). The evidence indicates that about 27% of households in India use water with fluoride levels of 1.5 ppm or more (Fig. 7.2).

While 40–50% of households in Gujarat, Maharashtra, Karnataka, Kerala, Tamil Nadu and Haryana had used drinking water with fluoride level of 1.5 or more ppm. Fluoride content of water in Delhi, Puducherry and Chandigarh is low.[22]

Magnitude of fluorosis determined by UNICEF indicates that 25 million people are actually affected by fluorosis and over 66 million stand exposed to the risk of fluorosis. Thus, fluorosis is a widespread problem in India. Number of fluoride affected habitations in the rural areas has increased from 29,030 in 17 states in 2006 to 33,071 in 19 states in 2009.

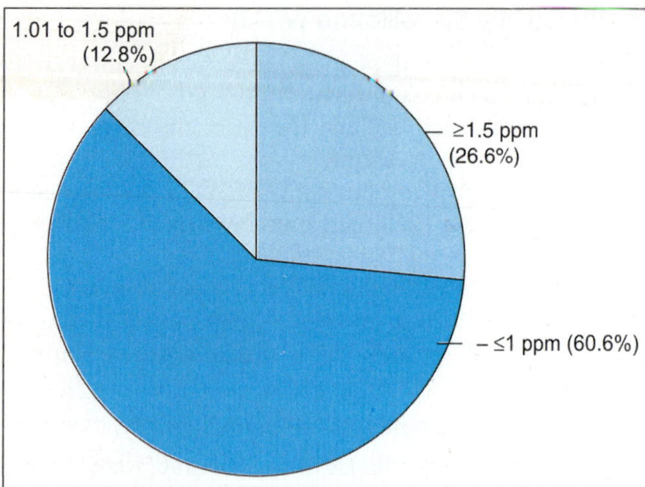

Fig. 7.2: Fluoride content of drinking water in India (households %)

Social and Economic Implications

Social and economic implications due to fluorosis in India are enormous because of widespread crippling effects, disability, dependence and decreased work capacity. Discoloration of teeth leads to social problems in children.

Rural Urban Distribution

It is more in rural areas but in some parts, it is equally prevalent because of excess of fluoride in water.

Risk Factors

- A dramatic increase in population and industrialization and perpetual shortages of drinking water supply.
- Groundwater supply having excess of fluoride content.
- Lack of awareness.
- Undernutrition.
- Use of toothpastes having fluorides.
- Food habits of consumption of excess of black tea, supari, tobacco and black salt.
- Children and pregnant women and lactating mothers are most vulnerable.

Exposure Time

The prolonged consumption of water having excess of fluoride leads to fluorosis. Excess of fluoride in water does not change the colour of water or alters its taste, thus the consumer will not know unless frank stage of fluorosis is produced either in teeth or in bones.

Types of Fluorosis

Excess of fluorides affect all parts of body predominantly it affects skeletal system (skeletal fluorosis) and teeth (dental fluorosis). Skeletal and dental fluorosis are irreversible conditions and not curable by any drug or medicine. Further skeletal and dental fluorosis produce crippling effects, permanent disability, loss of teeth and permanent discoloration of teeth.

Non-skeletal Fluorosis

Non-skeletal fluorosis affects soft tissues, red blood cells, muscles, ligaments, gastrointestinal system and it leads to development of vague signs and symptoms.

Dental Fluorosis

Dental fluorosis is an indicator of prevalence of fluorosis in the community, hence rapid survey of school children of 6–12 years of age can measure the extent of fluorosis in the community.

Mottling of teeth is one of the earliest and most easily recognizable sign of fluorosis. Dental fluorosis is not just a cosmetic problem, as generally perceived but also a window to what might happen to some of the vital organs of body. In mottled teeth, the enamel loses its lustre and becomes rough, opaque and chalky white. A yellow white discoloration appears which turns brown and presents itself in horizontal streaks. In late stages, the teeth become black, get pitted and perforated and may even get chipped off. There occurs premature loss of teeth. Dental fluorosis is irreversible and incurable. Children under 10 are most vulnerable.

Skeletal Fluorosis

Early symptoms of fluorosis include pain and stiffness in the neck, back and major joints. Entire spine may become one column of bone in late stage, manifesting a condition called "pokers back". Finally, various ligaments of the spine become ossified. This spreads to other joints as well and produces deformities of hip, knee and other joints. Skeletal fluorosis leads to crippling in high endemic areas.

Hydrofluorosis

Water-borne fluorosis due to excess of fluoride in water is called hydrofluorosis and if food chain contains high fluoride, it results into food-borne fluorosis. It is well-established fact that consumption of fluoride contaminated water and/or food for a period of 6 months to one year is sufficient to have the ill effects on health.

Industrial Fluorosis

Industries which use fluoride in the manufacturing process produce lot of dust and fumes which pollute the environments, inhaling dust and fumes is as dangerous as fluoride containing food or contaminated water with fluoride. The industrial workers and population nearby are the victims of fluoride toxicity or fluorosis. Such fluorosis is known as industrial fluorosis. The industries that use fluoride are: Aluminium, steel, enamel, pottery, glass and ceramics, bricks, phosphate, fertilizer, welding, refrigeration, rust removal, oil refinery, plastic, pharmaceutical, toothpaste, chemical industries and automobile industries, etc. Monitoring of levels of fluoride in such industries is essential to control the level of fluoride at the source.

Neighbourhood Fluorosis

Industries listed above may discharge the effluents into streams or rivers and pollute the groundwater or surface water. The people living nearby these industries who depend on groundwater may suffer the ill effects of fluorosis. Such fluorosis is known as neighbourhood fluorosis. Industrial town of Faridabad in Haryana bears the testimony. Underground water table of this town shows unacceptable high level of fluorides ranging from 5 to 20 mg/L.

NATIONAL PROGRAMME FOR PREVENTION AND CONTROL OF FLUOROSIS (NPPCF)

Since there is no cure of skeletal and dental fluorosis, prevention is the only means to tackle the problem of fluorosis. Fluoride once impregnated in tooth and bone stays there for life time. Government of India initiated preventive measures against fluorosis as a part of safe water supply.

Rajiv Gandhi National Drinking Water Mission (RGNDWM)[18]

Guidelines for Fluoride Control

Fluoride control was taken up as sub-mission of RGNDWM. Major guidelines are:

- i To identify and label any potable source SAFE and educate the population to conserve/use the source for drinking and cooking only.
- ii To tap safe low fluoride aquifers.
- iii To arrange for blending of water from different sources to obtain adequate quantities of safe water, and to supply this potable, "mixture" through designated "safe" standposts.
- iv To provide piped water supply schemes through distant sources.
- v Rainwater harvesting techniques have been used to mitigate fluorosis.
- vi To provide community treatment plants to remove excess of fluoride.

A 100% centrally sponsored new health initiative entitled "National Programme for Prevention and Control of Fluorosis" was taken during the XIth Five-Year Plan in the year 2008 with a goal to prevent and control fluorosis in the country with the following objectives:

- i To assess and use the base line survey data on fluorosis of Ministry of Drinking Water and Sanitation.
- ii Comprehensive management of fluorosis in selected areas.

iii Capacity building for prevention, diagnosis and management of fluorosis cases.

Strategies

1. Surveillance of fluorosis in the community
2. Training to health personnel for preventive, health promotion, early diagnosis and prompt treatment/ intervention, deformity correction, and rehabilitation, capacity building of district and medical college hospital for reconstructive surgery and rehabilitation.
3. Health education for prevention and control
4. Establishment of diagnostic facilities at district level. NPPCF has already been initiated in 6 districts, namely Nellore, Jamnagar, Ujjain, Nayagarh, Nagaur and Dharmapur in 2008–09. The programme has been expanded to cover 100 districts of the country in phased manner. The programme is being implemented in 111 districts. The 12th plan intends to cover 84 new districts in phased manner.

Defluoridation of Water

Defluoridation is the removal of excess fluoride from water. It should be considered only if none of the above solutions work.

Defluoridation methods: Precipitation and adsorption/ ion exchange.[23]

Precipitation Method

These methods involve the addition of soluble chemical to water, which leads to precipitation and/or adsorption of fluoride on the precipitate formed.

1. *Lime treatment:* By adding lime excess of fluoride can be removed from water. This method is effective only for waters with a fluoride concentration in the range of 3–4 mg/L.
2. *Alum coagulation:* The addition of high doses of alum results in removal of fluoride from water. Large alum doses, however, can lead to the presence of high residual aluminium in the treated water.
3. *Nalgonda technique:* This method was developed in India in 1975 by the National Environmental Engineering Research Institute (NEERI) at Nagpur. It involves the addition in sequence, of lime, bleaching powder (optimal) and filter alum in fluoride rich water and rapid mixing, which results in the formation of alum flocs (coagulation). These flocs are allowed to settle (sedimentation) and the supernatant water which is free of excess fluoride is filtered. Fluoride removal is probably due to formation of polyhydroxy aluminium complexes with fluoride and their adsorption into polymeric aluminium hydroxides. Technology is simple and economical (cost of filter is ₹ 700 only) and is very popular in India. The dose of alum and lime varies from source to source depending upon alkalinity and fluoride level in raw water.

Adsorption/Ion Exchange Method

Activated Alumina

Defluoridation of drinking water by activated alumina (AA) is the method of choice in developed countries. The Indian Institute of Technology (IIT), Kanpur has developed defluoridation systems based on activated alumina technology including domestic defluoridation filter and a hand pump attachable defluoridation plant. Domestic filters using activated alumina have been accepted by users. Use of proper grade of AA is a must to obtain satisfactory result. Exhausted AA has to be regenerated after 4–5 months.

In India, Nalgonda technique has been used extensively in large scale water treatment but it appears to be cosmetic effect and cannot meet the requirements of affected community. Maintenance of plants has been a perpetual problem. At household level, both Nalgonda and AA-based domestic defluoridation units are in use.

Domestic Defluoridation by Nalgonda Technology

Defluoridation of water can be carried out at home level after training local women.

Example: 40 litres of raw water (3 ppm fluoride content and alkalinity 200 ppm is reduced to fluoride content of 1 ppm) when mixed with 6 ml of lime solution (10 g of quick lime in one litre of water), 120 mg of bleaching powder mixed well and then 120 ml of alum solution (100 g of alum dissolved in one litre of water) is added and stirred slowly for 20 minutes and allowed settling for nearly one hour. The supernatant, which contains permissible amount of fluoride, is withdrawn for consumption. The settled sludge is discarded.

Nutritional Intervention

Non-skeletal fluorosis can be reversed by promoting intake of vitamins C, E, calcium and antioxidants. These help in the prevention and control of skeletal and non-skeletal fluorosis. In terms of diets promoting vitamin C rich foods such as amla, lemon, oranges, tomato, green leafy vegetables, carrots and salads help in reduction of fluoride levels.

Similarly, milk, green leafy vegetables and cereals are rich sources of calcium in diet.

Antioxidant foods such as garlic, turmeric, ginger, carrot, onion, green leafy vegetables, papaya and pumpkin should be encouraged.

Community Participation

Information education and communication on all aspects of fluorosis is vital to mitigate fluorosis problem. People in endemic and high endemic areas should be empowered for self-help to use safe and alternate sources of water in their village. Government alone cannot solve this problem. Fluorosis mitigation should be the concern of development agencies. Voluntary agencies and Non-Governmental Organizations should take the lead.

International Organizations

UNICEF and DANIDA are working closely with Government of India and helping to strengthen the district water quality laboratories, development of activated alumina (AA) based domestic defluoridation by IIT Kanpur, as also educational material and support to non-Governmental organization. DANIDA is supporting Rural Drinking Water Supply and Sanitation Project (RDWSSP) in Karnataka.

NATIONAL RURAL DRINKING WATER SUPPLY AND SANITATION PROGRAMME

RAJIV GANDHI NATIONAL DRINKING WATER MISSION (RGNDWM)

Provision of safe drinking water in rural areas is the responsibility of states and funds have been provided in the budgets of the states right from the commencement of First Five-Year Plan. A national water supply and sanitation programme was started in the social welfare sector in the year 1954.

Taking into account the magnitude of the *problem villages*, the central Government introduced the accelerated rural water supply programme (ARWSP) in 1972–73 to assist the states and union territories with 100% grants in aid to implement the scheme in such villages (problem villages).[5]

Focus

The focus remained on problem villages. The programme of rural water supply in the country is based on identification of problem villages/habitations through surveys conducted in 1972, 80, 85 and 1991–94. India is a signatory to 1977 UN General Assembly Resolution on International Drinking Water Supply and Sanitation Decade (IDWSSD) (1981–90). Goal during the decade (1981–90) was to provide safe drinking water and adequate sanitation to all its citizens. Target was to cover 100% of rural and urban areas with safe water, i.e. *water for all.*

Problem Village/Habitations

- Water scarcity was the first consideration. Any village/hasbitation which do not have a safe source within 1.6 km with 15 meters depth in the plains and 100 meters elevation difference in the hills is called a problem village. The drinking water is considered *safe* if it is free from chemical contaminants (excess fluoride, arsenic, brackishness, iron and other toxic elements) or biological contamination (leading to diarrhoea, cholera, typhoid, hepatitis and worm infestations).
- Villages where cholera and dracunculiasis were endemic.
- Villages having excess of fluoride, iron and brackishness and excess of arsenic.

National Technology Mission on Drinking Water

New push: "Water for all"

In 1986, the entire programme was given a mission approach to make intensive efforts to cover problem villages. The programme was named as Rajiv Gandhi National Drinking Water Mission (RGNDWM). Out of 5.75 lakh villages, 2.27 lakh (39%) were identified as problem villages' for water in 1987. The mission specific objectives were:

- Cover 2.27 lakh residual problem villages by 1990, i.e. 39% of total villages.
- Supply potable water of 40 litres per capita/day (lpcd).
- Supply water in desert area at the rate of 40 lpcd for human beings and 30 lpcd for cattle.
- Evolve cost-effective technology mix to achieve above objectives.
- Take adequate measures for sustained water supply.

Major Objectives of Technology Mission[5]

- Identify water sources in uncovered villages.
- Use appropriate technologies to ensure that potable water is made available to the population
- Monitor quality of water supply
- Ensure that quantity and quality of water supply is sustained on a long-term basis.

Prior to launching of mission in 1986, the emphasis was on coverage of problem villages with safe water sources. The mission since inception paid attention to water quality issue by:

- Adoption of quality standards.
- Establishing district level water testing laboratories.
- Establishing regional centres to network with state Government agencies to promote water quality monitoring programme.

The identified problem villages were provided safe drinking water facilities based on groundwater and surface water schemes like hand pumps, piped water supply schemes, sanitary wells and rain harvesting structures.

Sub-missions of Technology Mission[5,18]

Under the mission five sub-missions were set-up:

i ***Sub-mission on control of brackishness:*** To tackle the problem of excessive salinity by setting up 130 desalination plants in areas having problem of excessive salinity.

7

ii ***Sub-mission on removal of excess of iron:*** Excess iron imparts colour and unacceptable taste to drinking water. Such water supplies impart stains to clothes and utensils. Sub-mission has set up plants to remove excess of iron with the help of NEERI, Nagpur.

iii ***Sub-mission for control of fluorosis:*** Excess of fluoride is problem of considerable magnitude, as 66 million population is exposed to the risk of fluorosis and 25 million people are actually affected with endemic fluorosis. Mission has provided alternate sources of safe drinking water apart from defluoridation plants in endemic areas.

iv ***Sub-mission to deal with arsenic contamination:*** This sub-mission was set up in 1994 to deal with the problem of excess of arsenic in drinking water in eight districts of West Bengal.

v ***Sub-mission on guinea worm control and eradication:*** Guinea worm has been successfully eradicated in India (2000) by concerted action of technology mission.

Coverage Levels/Achievements

While nearly 96% of rural population has access to safe water (census 2011). Around 52% of rural households were being served by tube wells/hand pumps/borehole, 13% by wells and 30.8% by taps (piped water supply). Only 31% of households reported having their source of water within their premises. Only about 60% have access to 40 litres per person per day. Over the coming years, priority needs to be given to ensure access to at least the minimum quantity for the entire rural population. Census 2011 reported that 68.2% of households in India have access to safe drinking water. According to other estimates 94% of rural population and 91% of people living in urban areas have access to safe drinking water (Water Aid India–2008).[24] Government has provided a water connection and a 200 litres tank free of cost to scheduled caste families.

Priorities in 10th, 11th and 12th Plan[5]

1 Highest priority is to be given to 'not covered' habitations for supply of drinking water of 40 lpcd within a horizontal walking distance of 1.6 km in plains or elevation difference of 100 metres in hilly areas.

2 All partially covered habitations having a supply level of less than 10 litres per capita per day (lpcd) and those habitations facing a severe water quality problem are to be 'fully covered' with safe drinking water.

3 Thereafter other 'partially covered' and quality affected habitations are to be covered.

4 Once the supply of drinking water to all rural habitations by 2004 is achieved, the remaining part of 10th plan was utilized for consolidation. This involved covering newly emerged habitations and those which have slipped back to 'partially covered' or 'not covered' status due to any reason.

5 Identify and cover habitations where water quality problems have emerged recently.

6 Cover scheduled caste/scheduled tribe and other poor and weaker sections on priority basis.

11th Plan Targets: MOH and FW will take up programme for Prevention and Control of water-borne diseases as part of *Sarva Swasthya Abhiyan* (SSA) with the objective of:

1 To reduce the burden of water-borne diseases to 75% of the present level by 2010 and by 2015 to reduce the burden to 50% of the present level. In order to achieve 100% coverage of clean water and sanitation, Eleventh Five-Year Plan strategies include:
   - Convergence of health care, hygiene, sanitation, and drinking water at the village level through village health sanitation and nutrition committees (VHSNCs) under NRHM.
   - Renewed efforts under NUHM to cover primary health care, safe drinking water, and sanitation in urban areas.

2 Provide clean drinking water for all by 2009 and ensure that there are no slip backs. The 10th plan target of providing potable drinking water to all villages has not been achieved. Under *Bharat Nirman* now it is planned to cover 55,067 uncovered habitations in 7 years (2005–12). Though more than 95% coverage was achieved prior to *Bharat Nirman*, 2.8 lakh out of 14.22 lakh habitations in the country have, slipped back to from fully covered to partially covered status. Another 2.17 lakh habitations have problem with the quality of water, about 6000 habitations face serious problems of salinity or arsenic and fluoride contamination. These habitations will be taken up under *Bharat Nirman*,[25] which includes components of irrigation, drinking water, electrification, telephone connectivity, housing and roads, which is a flagship programme of Govt. of India for rural development launched in 2005.

Targets in 12th Plan, 2012–17

- In the states, where 40 lpcd have been achieved the next step is to raise the level of availability to 55 litres.
- By 2017, at least 50% of rural population in the country (as against 35% today will have access to 40 Ipcd piped water supply within their household premises or within 100 meters radius (and within 10 meters elevation in hilly areas) from their household.
- By 2017, at least 35% rusal population will have individual household connections as against 13% currently.[26]

Decentralization of Rural Water Supply

Panchayati Raj Institutions (PRIs): Currently planning of rural water supply is made at the central and state levels. Water supply projects are designed and executed by implementing departments and handed over to the end users. The system is supply driven, people and PRIs are not involved. The installed supply system fails because of lack of maintenance. PRIs are unwilling to take responsibility for maintenance of rural water supplies.

People First

A paradigm shift from "Government oriented supply driven approach" to "People-oriented demand responsive approach" was adopted in 1999.

People and PRIs should be involved and consulted as to what system of supply suits them. Cost sharing by users and PRIs is essential. Presently large number of private organizations in rural areas are operating and have given water connections to household level and charge at the rate of ₹ 100–200 per household per month and people pay willingly to private operators. These private organizations use source of groundwater, shallow or deep tube wells. Reverse osmosis plants in Punjab with the assistance of Govt of India have been set up in many villages and safe water is being provided to rural people at subsidized/affordable rate (₹ one per ten litre). Government piped water supply system in these villages is not accepted. Piped water is used for everything except for drinking (bathing, washing clothes, utensils and preparation of tea as it is soft water, soap, works well on it and milk in tea pot does not curdle). Consumer consultation is essential to decide the kind of supply they want. PRIs should be empowered for devolution of powers and responsibility and to meet out part of cost of water supply. PRIs should be strengthened and entrusted with all activities relating to water supplies, sanitation, hygiene and nutrition. The participatory approach has become a necessity to share project cost but major source of funding for rural water supply schemes has to be from budget of the State and Central Government.

INTEGRATED WATER MANAGEMENT IN RURAL AREAS

The three major and widely prevalent problems in sustainable supply of drinking water—scarcity, brackishness and excess fluoride content are manifested in low rainfall and high potential evaporation areas. This calls for integrated water and sanitation programme with emphasis on conservation of water, rain water harvesting and groundwater recharging, storing of rainwater for harvesting and drinking—exploiting traditional sources of water and changing cropping pattern in drought hit areas.

Operation Maintenance

As more than 3.5 million hand pumps and over 1,00,000 piped water schemes have been installed in the country under the rural water supply programme. The total maintenance cost would be around 2000 crores per year (10–15% of capital cost). A majority of schemes remain non-functional and many other become permanently defunct due to lack of proper maintenance and repairs for want of funds. Funds of minimum needs programme (MNP) and the accelerated rural water supply programme (ARWSP) are already available to meet some of the operational and maintenance cost. Community should share the responsibility of maintenance cost.

Water Quality Monitoring and Surveillance

This is minimal in rural water supply system. Regular monitoring of quality and surveillance though most desirable is lacking. It operates only during "crisis" situations, such as outbreaks and epidemics. People only demand chlorination when they observe large number of mosquitoes larvae in the water supply of wells or during outbreak situation. Monitoring and surveillance system needs to be strengthened to a great extent by developing district laboratories and local capacity to test minimum parameters, such as residual chlorine, coliform count and *E. coli* count. The Government of India launched *National Rural Drinking Water Quality Monitoring and Surveillance Programme in February 2006*. This seeks to ensure community participation for monitoring and surveillance of drinking water sources at the grass root level by village panchayats and village water and sanitation committees with support of district laboratories.

URBAN WATER SUPPLY SYSTEM

Responsibility

Around 31% of population of India is urban and this proportion is going to rise in coming years. Municipal bodies have the responsibility of providing civic amenities including drinking water. Department of drinking water and sanitation has been upgraded as Ministry of Drinking Water and Sanitation.

Goal

Eleventh Five-Year Plan envisaged 100% coverage of urban and rural population with safe drinking water and sanitation as per stipulated norms and standards.

Norms of Water Supply in Urban Areas

Towns with piped water supply but without sewerage; 70 lpcd and cities with existing or planned sewerage systems; 135 lpcd, metropolitan towns and megacities with piped water supply and sewerage; 150 lpcd and public standpost; 40 lpcd.

Present Status

Improved drinking water sources include: Piped water supply at household, plot or public tap and protected tube wells, bore wells springs and rainwater harvested from roof and ground catchment and stored in containers.

Over 96% of rural households and 98% of urban households have access to improved drinking water source (2011). According to 54th round of national sample survey (NSS), and census 2011, an estimated 70% of urban households are being served by taps, 20% by tube wells or hand pumps. Sixty per cent of households had drinking source within their premises, while 32% had it within 0.2 km; and 59% shared the public post. Fifteen per cent of households did not get sufficient water from their principal source.

Coverage figures do not reveal many things. Sufficient quantities as per norms are available to 60% of households, quality of water supplies in urban areas is very difficult to ensure. Pressure of growing population and habitations is mounting and supplies always run short. Condition in urban slums are deteriorating fast because of large influx of migration of population to towns and industrial development. Widespread insanitary conditions hold perpetual threat of water contamination and consequently outbreaks of diseases and high incidence of water-borne diseases.[24]

Water Post

One post or source for 150 persons at a distance of 100 metres.

Finances

The financial health of municipal bodies is poor and amount of user charges collected in urban area is insufficient to meet the norms and augment and maintain water supplies. State government and municipal bodies share the cost of urban water supply. The central Government only provides assistance through central sponsored schemes of accelerated urban water supply (AUWS) programme.

Centrally Sponsored Accelerated Urban Water Supply Programme (AUWSP)

This was launched in 1993–94 to provide water supply in towns with population of less than 20,000 as many as 2151 towns qualified for this scheme. The project funding is shared equally between central and state governments with 5% contribution from beneficiary. The centre meets the entire cost in union territories. Priority is given to towns with special problems such as very low per capita supply, very distant and deep water source, drought prone area, excessive salinity, fluoride and iron content in water source and high incidence of water-borne diseases. The per capita cost is normally limited to ₹ 1000.

Sources

Urban area water supply depends upon surface water (canals) or underground water. The raw water undergoes through all processes of cleaning and making it safe for consumption. The raw water passes through sieving → storage tanks → sedimentation → coagulation → clarification → chlorination → distribution. Usually rapid sand filter system operates in urban areas (*see* Fig. 7.1). All said and done the quality and quantity of water supply in urban area is poor and water supply system is under pressure of everincreasing population and outbreaks of water-borne diseases are perpetual phenomenon. Viral hepatitis and other water-borne diseases have become endemic in many urban areas.

REFERENCES

1 World Health Organization (WHO). Statistics and maps, Geneva: WHO; World Health Report, 2002.

2 World Health Organization (WHO). Water for Health enshrined as human right WHO/91. Press release 27 Nov. 2002.

3 World Health Organization. Guidelines for drinking water quality. 4th Edition. Geneva: WHO; 2011.

4 WHO. Alma-Ata 1978: Primary health care. Geneva: WHO; 1978.

5 Planning Commission GOI. 10th Five-Year Plan, 2002–07. New Delhi: GOI; 2002.

6 School of hygiene and Public Health (USA) Population reports—solutions for a water shortage world. Dr. Jain Clinic, New Delhi 1999; 26(14).

7 Indian Institute of Population Sciences (IIPS) and ORC macro. National Family Health Survey (NFHS-2). India (Mumbai): IIPS; 2002.

8 School of Hygiene and Public Health (USA). Population reports—population and the environment—the global challenge. Dr. Jain Clinic. New Delhi Feb 2001; 28(3).

9 United National International Children Emergency Fund (UNICEF/MNIO). Training Modules on sanitation. New Delhi: UNICEF.

10 World Health Organization. Guidelines for drinking water quality. Second Edition. Geneva: WHO; 1993.

11 World Health Organization. Guidelines for drinking water quality. Health Criteria and other supporting information. Geneva: WHO; 1984.

12 Ministry of Rural Areas and Employment/WHO/UNICEF. Technical papers—national workshop on water quality monitoring and surveillance in rural areas. New Delhi: Ministry of Rural Area and Employment; 1997.

13 World Health Organization (WHO). Action plan for the development of national drinking water quality surveillance. Proceedings of regional consultations on planning and developing drinking water quality surveillance and control programme; Sept 1996. 16–19; Kathmandu, Nepal.

14 Government of India (GOI). Monograph on Intregrated Training on National Programmes for mother and child development. First edition, New Delhi: Central Technical Committee on Health and Nutrition, Deptt. of Women and Child Development, 1990.

15 Oxford University. World Development Report 1993, Investing in Health. New York: Oxford University Press; 1993.

16 Sushila AK. Arsenic in drinking water—a public health hazard. Bulletin of Nutrition Foundation of India, October 1998; 19(4).

17 GOI. Annual Report 2006–2007, Ministry of Health and Family Welfare. GOI, NRHM, New Delhi.
18 Government of India. Annual Report. New Delhi; Ministry of Health and Family Welfare. GOI; 2003.
19 Susheela AK. Excess fluoride in Drinking Water and Fluorosis Mitigation. New Delhi; Fluorosis research and rural development foundation; 2003.
20 Susheela AK. A treatise on fluorosis (2001). Fluorosis Research and Rural Development Foundation C-103-SARANSH. I.P. extension, Delhi, India.
21 National Technology Mission on Drinking Water. Prevention and Control of Fluorosis. Water Mission-Sub-mission on Control of Fluorosis, 1991.
22 National Oral Health Survey and Fluoride Mapping-2002–03 (India). Dental Council of India, New Delhi, 2004.
23 NICD. CD Alert. Fluorosis prevention and control. May–June 2002; 6(5).
24 Water Aid Drinking water quality in rural India: Issues and approaches background paper-2008 by Indira Khurana and Romit Sen, Water Aid.
25 GOI Towards Faster and More Inclusive Growth. An Approach to the 11th Five-Year Plan. GOI Planning *Commission Yojna Bhawan*, New Delhi, Dec 2006.
26 Planning Commission. Rural Drinking water and Sonitation in Twelfth Five Year Plan 2012–17, Vol. II, New Delhi.

RURAL AND URBAN SANITATION

The WHO/UNICEF estimates that 2.5 billion people—40% of the world's population lack access to even basic sanitation. It stands as the most neglected Millennium Development Goal.[1]

World Bank water and sanitation programme study reported that poor sanitation cost India \$54 billion or 6.4% of GDP in 2006. There are losses in terms of education, productivity, time and tourism. Around 3.5 lakh children aged below 5, die of diarrhoea alone in India every year.

India tops the list of countries where people defecate in open, exposing them to soil and water borne infections.

'Sanitation is a way of life', it should be people's programme. Definition: 'Sanitation' is collection, transport, treatment and disposal or reuse of human excreta, domestic waste water and solid waste, and associated hygiene promotion'. The insanitary conditions are appalling in India. Sanitary conditions have not much changed in rural India. Only 33% of rural households were using latrines and the rest 67% defecated in open, as revealed by census 2011 data; against 87.4% of urban households, while the national average being 50%. It means 12.6% of urban population defecte in open. The rural sanitation programme till 1995 was restricted to construction of latrines only. Relative to the attention given to safe water, sanitation programme has had a very late start. There is now a distinct change in the strategy of "promoting sanitation" by the Government. The *central rural sanitation programme* now promotes sanitation as a seven component package.[1, 2]

1 Safe handling of drinking water.
2 Scientific disposal of waste water.
3 Safe disposal of human excreta including child excreta.
4 Disposal of garbage and animal excreta.
5 Home sanitation and food hygiene.
6 Improved personal hygiene.
7 Village sanitation.

Now the Government intends to promote rural sanitation as a package as stated above.

The priorities for rural sanitation have been fixed as:

i Preference will be given to the twin pit model of water seal latrine. The successful model of Midnapur single pit latrine may also be adopted.
ii School sanitation (providing toilets) should be given highest priority to inculcate safe hygiene habits among school children.
iii Village Panchayats should adopt building by-laws where dry latrines are not permissible only water seal type latrines are to be constructed.
iv The State Council proposed for urban sanitation sector should also have the mandate for rural sanitation.
v Subsidy for low cost household toilets should only be given to rural below poverty line (BPL) families and it should be at par with subsidy for urban households. For the success of the scheme, a subsidy of 50% of the cost of unit inclusive of sub- and superstructures for the basic twin pit pour flush system appears to be necessary.
vi In order to mobilize funds for rural sanitation, financial institutions/banks including HUDCO and the National Bank of Agriculture and Rural Development (NABARD) should extend loan to states at lower rates of interest for provision of sanitation facilities.
vii Private sector should be encouraged in setting up of building centres and sanitary marts in rural areas to provide cost-effective sanitation technology.
viii The recommendations made for urban low cost sanitation should also apply to rural areas as well.
ix Sanitation is a way of life. To change behaviour and adoption of sanitary practices, intensive, communication, education and appropriate information is necessary to be disseminated to women groups, PRIs and Village Health and Sanitation Committee through multiple channels. Participation of non-governmental organizations like Safai Vidayala, Ahmedabad, has made a real difference.

Social Factors Related to Excreta Disposal: "Easing for Diseases"

Seventy to eighty per cent of illnesses are related to water contamination and poor sanitation. Because of age-old practice of indiscriminate open field defecation, widespread soil pollution occurs in villages as also in urban slums.

7

1 Human excreta which contains pathogenic organisms pollutes soil and drinking water by way of contamination because of human behaviour such as ablution, washing of dirty linen, hands and utensils at the source or nearby source. Soil in and around house get contaminated repeatedly because of human behaviour.
2 Excreta of children is considered to be harmless which is a wrong perception. Because of this perception children are allowed to defecate in and around home which leads to contamination of soil, food and drinking water at home; because children and adults may handle drinking water with soiled hands and fingers.
3 Open defecation is generally not seen as a health hazard by the community. Women folk defecate during dusk and dawn not very far from their dwellings, around village periphery near cow dung cake stores/heaps, in groups. Because of population explosion the defecating grounds are shrinking.
4 Men folk choose to defecate a bit away from village (about ½–1 km). They combine the act of defecation with morning walk and smoking with a firm belief that smoking helps the act of defecation, which has no scientific base.
5 Hands are used for the act of ablution and washing of hands after defecation is done with plain water or water and mud. Soap is seldom used.
6 People draw drinking water from pitcher/container by dipping their fingers and hands which are quite often soiled/unclean, this practice contaminates the stored water in the pitcher/containers and may act as risk factor for water-borne diseases.
7 Latrines are considered to be dirty places and nuisance of odour and flies.
8 Toilet built by the Government or with subsidies of Government are seldom used by people as these are considered as "*Sarkari* toilets" and often used as storage bins.

While improved quality of water resulted in one-sixth reduction in diarrhoea, however, improved excreta disposal resulted in one-third reduction in diarrhoea. By adopting a practice of excreta disposal to pit latrine or similar faecal disposal system along with improved water supply could reduce prevalence of diarrhoea to the extent of 44%. The highest rates of diarrhoea are found among slum children whose families did not have latrines.

Learning Personal Hygiene—Washing Hands

Practice of handwashing with soap before handling food, and water and after defecation can reduce the incidence of diarrhoeal diseases and worm infestation. This is a lifestyle and most important habit; must be developed in young children and should be practiced by every one to avoid diseases.

Recent studies have shown that personal hygiene practices like washing one's hands with soap and water after defecation and before eating could reduce diarrhoeal disease incidence and worm infestation by 43%.[1] Practice of handwashing amongst young children should be inculcated by parents and family members, by Anganwadi workers in the Anganwadis before serving supplementary food, the young children should wash their hands. Large majority of Anganwadi workers have done it successfully. In our experience, once the young children develop the habit of washing their hands at Anganwadi centre, these children insist their parents to wash their hands before eating and some of the parents/mothers complained to Anganwadi workers that they have to bring now extra water to wash the hands of their children; and their water consumption has gone high.

School teachers should also inculcate habit of handwashing among school children by demonstration and becoming a good role model. Learning hygiene at school should be part of education and lifestyle. School sanitation programme has been chosen as priority area of rural sanitation programme as a part of seven component package as also component of TSC.[3]

Learning trimming of nails and cleaning nailbeds prevents diseases. Similarly, eating clean food with clean hands and using clean utensils and clean water prevents water-borne diseases. These measures are measures of personal hygiene practices acquired in the family, at Anganwadi at school or at workplace.

Water Storage Practices

Storing clean water in clean utensil and keeping the water container covered was adopted by most families in rural areas but positive effect of this practice were negated when people dipped their fingers and hands, while retrieving and using the water from pitcher/container. Storage of water in narrow mouthed pot (SURAHI) prevents contamination.

SAFE DISPOSAL OF HUMAN EXCRETA

Human excreta contains disease producing organisms and is the chief source of many diseases. Human excreta comes back to human mouth by contaminated water, dirty hands, flies, insects and eating raw and unwashed vegetables. Therefore human excreta must be disposed off safely.

METHODS OF HUMAN EXCRETA DISPOSAL

Methods of human excreta disposal by use of sanitary latrines: Sanitary latrines should be acceptable, affordable and accessible. A sanitary latrine is one which does not contaminate the source of water, where excreta is out of bounds to flies and it does not produce objectionable odour and it is kept clean and acceptable to people. Some of the commonly used latrines in rural areas are as under.

Borehole Latrine

Digging a hole of 12" to 16" diameter with special instrument called 'auger' up to a depth of 10'–20' underground.

The concrete squatting plate with central hole is placed on the borehole. The excreta and ablution water directly falls into the hole and undergoes anaerobic digestion. The hole gets filled up in 1–2 years time. The hole can be lined with appropriate affordable material such as earthen rings, bamboo matting, etc.

Pit Latrine

Pit latrines are used where the water is scarce and solid materials or minimum quantity of water are used for anal cleaning. This latrine is very simple to construct and cost is very low. A pit of 0.75 × 0.85 × 2.50 meters is dug and covered with a squatting slab having an opening. Excreta goes into the pit directly. The excreta may be covered with earth after defecation. The disadvantage of this type of latrine is that flies can come in direct contact with the excreta and moreover objectionable odour is a problem. Decomposition of excreta occurs by soil bacteria. Life of this latrine depends upon size of pit and number of users (Fig. 7.3).[4,5] Pit can have water seal hand flush system (Midnapore design) to avoid fly breeding and bad smell.

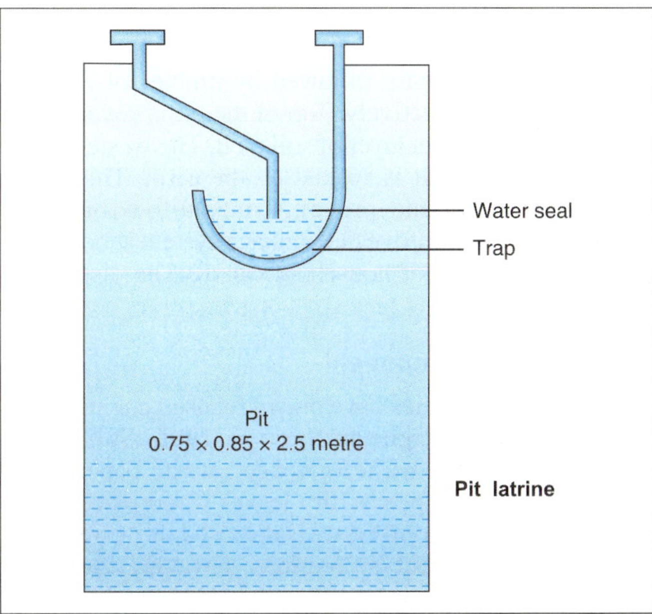

Fig. 7.3: Low cost hand flush single pit sanitary latrine (Midnapore design) for rural area

After the outstanding action research contribution of The Planning and Research Action Institute (PRAI), Lucknow and Research-cum-Action (RCA) Project of ICMR and All India Institute of Hygiene and Public Health, Calcutta, RCA latrine (single pit or twin pit) design has been accepted and being promoted under Total Sanitation Campaign (TSC) in rural India. Over 9% of Indians use pit latrines.

Flush Type Water Seal Latrine (Twin Pit Water Seal Latrine)

This type of latrine requires water for flushing usually hand flushed, requiring at least 2 litres of water per user. The essential feature of flush type is the "water seal"—this is

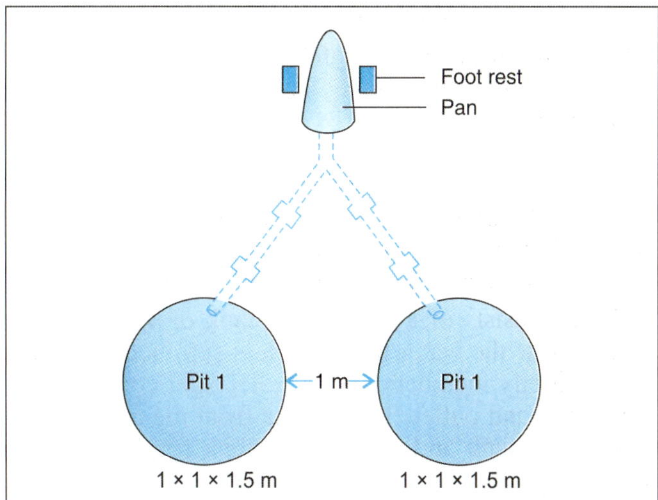

Fig. 7.4: Two pits water seal latrine for rural area for safe disposal of human excreta

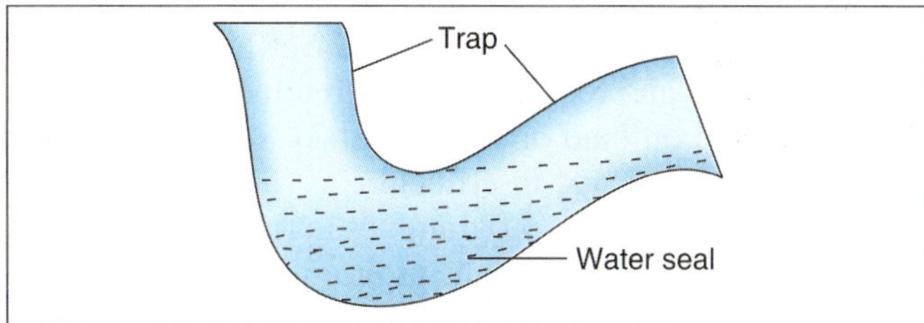

Fig. 7.5: Trap with water seal

the amount of water which remains in the trap and prevents entry of flies/fly breeding and bad odour coming out of the pit (Figs 7.4 and 7.5).

Latrine pan/seat is connected to two pits by Y-shaped drain. Two pits of 1.5 meter deep and one meter diameter (circular or rectangular) are dug and connected through pipes to pan. One pit is put to use at a time. One pit can last for 3 years for 5 persons.[4,5]

Once the first pit is filled up in about three years, the second pit is then used. The excreta in first pit is left undisturbed for a period of 2 years. After this much period the excreta gets self-digested by soil bacteria anaerobically and is rendered harmless. The contents of the pit can be removed/emptied safely and used as good manure, which is quite harmless. Hence, two pits are used alternately.

If only one pit is used to reduce the cost and space, it can be located directly under the slab incorporating the water seal unit. When the pit is filled up, the contents have to be removed to second pit specially dug for this purpose, which is then covered with earth and left undisturbed for two years for decomposition of excreta. Alternately a new latrine can be constructed.

Ventilated Improved Pit Latrine (VIPL)

When a vent pipe is added to the pit to help escape of gases it helps in removing the bad smell. Fly screen is fitted at the top of vent pipe to act as trap for flies.[6,7]

Location of Latrine

The flush latrine can be safely located 10 meters away from drinking water source; however, the safest distance is 15 meters.

Septic Tank

Septic tanks are in use in urban areas mainly and by some well to do households in rural areas. 22% of urban, 14.7% of rural households are using septic tank latrines.

This consists of a rectangular tank of $4^1/_2' \times 3' \times 3'$ deep below the water line, which is sufficient for a unit of six family members. It is a water tight compartment, with inlet and outlet. The excreta from the pan and trap flows into tank and stays in the tank for considerable time. The excreta undergoes anaerobic decomposition in the tank.

The digested sludge at the bottom of the tank has to be removed periodically say once a year, which can be used for horticulture or agriculture purposes or manure. The effluent is usually let into drains but the effluent is as strong as city sewage and requires further treatment before it can be discharged on land or water courses. Large number of helminths eggs escape in effluent.

Promotion of latrine programmes in rural areas through the community development programmes initiated way back in 1952, through education department in schools and through Anganwadi workers in ICDS programme has not achieved much success.[8] In some states like Gujarat, this programme has achieved some success. In some rural areas of Haryana (Distt. Sirsa), dug well latrine, is almost a universal practice in each home for women and children for security and privacy and it is their felt need for that purpose. These latrines can be constructed with local technology and local resources with minimum cost. The cost was subsidized by the Government for economically weaker sections and below poverty line families. One of the stated function of the primary health centre was 'environmental sanitation'. One sanitary inspector was made available at each primary health centre to promote environmental sanitation including latrine promotion programme as also ensuring regular chlorination of wells. Most of the tasks related to environmental sanitation have remained unaccomplished and it is too big a function to be performed by health centre. Seven components of rural sanitation as package need to be implemented through integrated efforts involving village Panchayats, VHSC, development functionaries, health; education and ICDS sector, women organization, voluntary and Non-Governmental Organizations.

Case Study of a Dug Well Latrine

One of the police station in district Sirsa in Haryana had a dug well latrine which was used infrequently. In the past 6 months, the latrine was used only on a few occasions. One fine morning a police man had to use this latrine. Being a chronic smoker, he was habitual to smoke before the act of defecation. Most men in this part smoke before defecation with a firm belief that smoking facilitates the act of defecation. While squatting on the seat, this gentleman lighted a cigarette and burning matchstick was thrown in the pit of dug well latrine. Amazingly all of a sudden fire erupted in that pit and it caused perineal burns, before this man could escape from the site of latrine. Thus, the man was penalised for smoking by nature. Fire erupted because of accumulation of methane gas under the scum of human excreta which acted as partial seal. During the act of defecation on that day, the seal got disturbed and gave way to methane and burning matchstick led to fire flame in the pit.

Disposal of Waste Water at Household Level

Soakage pit can be constructed to dispose waste water or waste water can be discharged to kitchen garden. A soakage pit is a pit of 1×1×1 meter dug and filled with stones or rubbles, broken bricks and pebbles and the top of the pit is covered with layer of soil. Usually 10–15 cm rubbles or broken bricks are placed at the bottom of pit to fill up to one-third of the depth, followed by rubbles of 5–10 cm and 1 cm size respectively. Top of the pit is covered with gunny bag with 5 cm layer of soil on it. The waste water is led to this pit and it is soaked by the earth. This avoids water collection and prevents mosquitoes breeding. Community can improve the drainage system at household level. Waste water of household can also be disposed in kitchen garden.

Solid Waste Management

Towns and mega cities have drawn focused attention after the outbreak of plague in Surat in 1995. Solid waste consists of kitchen waste (garbage), waste papers, rags, glass pieces, metal pieces, dry leaves wood pieces, brick bats, plastics, etc. Solid waste is disposed of by trenching, sanitary land fill and by biomass. Growing towns and slums, implementation of urban development and rise in population; pose serious problem to manage solid waste disposal. Plastic era has added to the problem of blocked sewers and non-biodegradable qualities of plastic material inhibit process of composting. Proper management of biomedical waste management is another problem.

Disposal of Garbage and Animal Excreta (Composting)

Garbage is wet refuse (kitchen waste, vegetable and fruit peelings, left out vegetables, left out food) and if it is disposed indiscriminately or heaped up around houses is a breeding ground for flies which can carry disease organisms and contaminate the food. Similarly, animal excreta is rich in organic matter, hence is most suitable for fly breeding. Garbage disposal and animal excreta disposal can be done in manure pits. Location of manure pits should be away from home. Every week a layer of soil 2" thick is laid over levelled garbage to prevent fly breeding when the pit is filled it is covered with layer of firm soil and left undistributed. After 3 months, the contents of pit become good manure. A compact earth bank of 4" is raised around the pit to prevent flow of rain water into pit. *Bangalore* method of composting night soil plus refuse in alternate layers by anaerobic method is quite simple and most popular method. *Indore* method of composting refuse and night soil by aerobic method is yet another method of safe disposal of refuse and night soil.

Gobar gas plant is an appropriate technology, which can be used for safe disposal of animal excreta. Minimum quantity of 40–50 kg of Gobar (cow dung) per day is essential to feed the plant. This technology yields methane gas which can be used for cooking and the slurry or sludge formed after the process can be used as good manure. This requires keeping of 3–4 cattle and the cost may be unaffordable by below poverty line families, the maintenance of plant poses several problems, but these can be obviated by good training and upkeep of the plant.

Smokeless Chullah (Earthenware Stove)

Over 80% of houses in rural areas in India use unprocessed biomass fuel (firewood, crop wastes and cow dung cakes) which generate lot of smoke in the kitchen.[8–9] More often than not the kitchens are ill-ventilated and the smoke generated by the fuel enters the respiratory system of women and children who are most susceptible. Indoor air pollution in rural homes is thus a widespread phenomenon. Its ill effects are acute as well as chronic respiratory diseases and also associated with long-term cardiovascular effects and increased risk to lung cancer in women and children. These ill effects can be avoided by improving the ventilation in the kitchen and by using smokeless chullahs. District rural development agencies are promoting the use of these chullahs and village women themselves can install such chullahs in their kitchen by use of local technology. In addition, such chullahs offer the additional advantage of saving the fuel as these are fuel efficient, thus saving the energy and workload of women. *Mahila Mandals* have come forward to popularize these chullahs. In nutshell, these chullahs are user-friendly and prevent indoor air pollution.

Use of Solar Cookers

It is yet another technological advance and user-friendly device of non-conventional source of energy. Use of solar cookers in rural areas is becoming popular as it saves work-load of women and it is environment-friendly, acceptable and affordable device.

Total Sanitation Campaign (TSC)

As per census 2011 data, nearly 50% of households use toilets. This percentage is lower in villages where only 33% use toilet. Total sanitation campaign is a sound beginning. Its objectives are to bring about improvement in general quality of life in rural areas, accelerate sanitation coverage and generate demand for toilets in all schools and Anganwadis in rural areas through awareness and education. TSC is presently being implemented in 572 districts. Components of TSC include IEC activities, rural sanitary marts, individual household toilets, women sanitary complex school sanitation programme and Anganwadi sanitation.[9–11] *Nirmal Gram Puruskar*, a National Award under TSC has been launched in February 2005 by the Government. Goal is to achieve open defecation free India by the year 2019 Under *Swachh Bharat Abhiyan*. The 7th World Toilet Summit was held at India in Delhi in November 2007 wherein 40 countries participated, with focus on to meet the sanitation needs of people worldwide. The UN (United Nations) has declared 2008 as the International Year of Sanitation with an objective of providing toilet for all by 2030.

Sustainable Development Goal 6 of UN: Universal and equitable access to safe and affordable drinking water and sanitation for all by 2030 and end open defection paying special attention to the needs of women. United Nations has adopted a landmark resolution recognising the human right to "Sanitation" along with the right to safe drinking water.

URBAN SANITATION

Problem

Census 2011 reported that 12.6% of households reported using no latrine, 38.2% reported using septic tank and 32.7% reported using sewerage system. This indicates that as many as 12.6% of households in urban areas had either no latrines or no connection to septic tank or sewerage and practice open field defecation. Overall 87.4% of urban households have latrine facility within the premises.

Out of 300 class I cities, about 70 have partially sewerage system and sewage treatment facilities. Levels of sewage treatment are reported to be very low. Nearly 90% of the liquid sewage generated daily by Indian cities flows into streams, rivers and sea untreated (Central Pollution Control Board). Cities produce around 38, 254 million litres of waste water each day and India presently has the capacity to treat 11,500 million litres of waste water everyday (31%) but just 39% of treated waste meets the environment norms. Thus, the untreated and partially treated municipal waste water finds its way into water resources such as rivers, lakes and groundwater, causing water pollution. On the other hand, programme of low cost sanitation which offers an affordable alternative technology has made very little progress despite being linked to social problem of manual scavenging which is prohibited by law.

The poor sanitary conditions in urban slums are linked to outbreaks of cholera and gastroenteritis. Water-borne diseases are a major cause of mortality throughout India and impose a huge burden in terms of loss of lives and productivity.

Low-cost Sanitation (LCS)

The centrally sponsored scheme of urban low-cost sanitation for liberation of the scavengers started from 1980–81, initially through the Ministry of Home Affairs and later through Ministry of Welfare. From 1989–90 it came under the Ministry of Urban Development.

Objective

The main objective of LCS is to convert dry latrines into low cost pour flush latrines and provide alternate employment to the liberated scavengers.

Coverage

The scheme covers all the households which have dry latrines and households having no sanitation facilities including households in slums and squatter colonies.

Loan Assistance

Under the scheme, loan and central subsidy are extended simultaneously by HUDCO. Subsidy is graded according to economic status, being set at 45% for economically weaker sections (EWS) and 25% for low income group (LIG) and nil subsidy for middle and high income groups. Loan ranging from 50 to 75% of the cost is given at 10% interest repayable over 15 years. Loan is also given for construction of community latrines on "pay and use" principle, shared latrines in slums and housing chawls. Subsidy is limited to the cost of sub-structure but HUDCO loan can also be used for superstructure.

Number of households that need LCS or community toilet facilities may be as high as 15 million at least, may be more. LCS is not a programme solely of urban poor or slum population, it has to be propagated as appropriate solution wherever the costly option of drainage is not feasible. In this sense, there is need to offer more options to households that desire sanitation facilities, which while being based on the 'twin pit pour flush' model, is in keeping with their needs and capacity to invest. LCS intends to have integrated approach: water supply plus sanitation together.

NGO's Role: NGO Like Sulabh International

NGO's role: NGO like Sulabh International has played key role in the construction and maintenance of "pay and use" toilets for floating population or places such as bus stands, markets, parks and other places where people congregate.

Community Toilets

The scheme of LCS also includes community toilets. However, the experience of upkeep and maintenance of community toilets by municipality has been quite dismal, with the conditions turning so insanitary that the people prefer open air defecation to using public toilets. Public latrine are used by 3.2 percent of people.

Treatment of Urban Waste Water

Three-fourths of surface water resources are polluted and 80% of the pollution is due to sewage alone. Sewage is rich manure apart from economic source of methane gas. Waste water or sewage treatment facilities are missing in most towns. Sewerage system is the answer for the problem but sewage treatment facilities needs to be geared up.

Scheme to Provide Sewerage for River Bank Towns

Urban waste both solids and liquids of towns located on the banks of river finds its way directly to river. The Ministry of Environment and Forest is implementing a massive programme of cleaning of rivers and lakes in the country. The programme which was started with Ganga Action Plan (GAP) in 1985 now extends to the polluted stretches of 27 major rivers with sewerage system works spread over to 149 towns in 16 states.

Sewage (Human Excreta) Treatment Processes

Sewage: It is human excreta, wash water and liquid waste. Sewage consists of more than 99% of waste water and solid content is less than 1%.

Sewage treatment facilities are available in metropolitan and mega cities only and missing in most other cities. Raw sewage or untreated sewage is used for agriculture and horticulture proposes (mainly as organic manure), this is risky practice and waste may come back to human beings through flies and raw vegetables and this pollutes the water sources of the city, if it is let into the river.

- Primary treatment of sewage consists of—screening → grit removal → primary sedimentation → sludge digestion.
- Secondary treatment consists of—biological treatment by → aeration, addition of activated sludge → final sedimentation followed by chlorination of effluent and sludge digestion → sludge drying (Fig. 7.6).

The biological process consists conventional techniques such as trickling filters, activated sludge process, extended aeration, aerated lagoons, oxidation ditches, up-flow anaerobic sludge blanket reactor, contact biological disk reactors, etc.

In most of the towns, only the primary treatment is done and secondary treatment facilities are not made available because of cost factor. Thus, most of sewage is partially treated and is not free from health risks.

Screening

Sewage is passed through a coarse screen or iron bars, this process holds back the floating objects in the sewage.

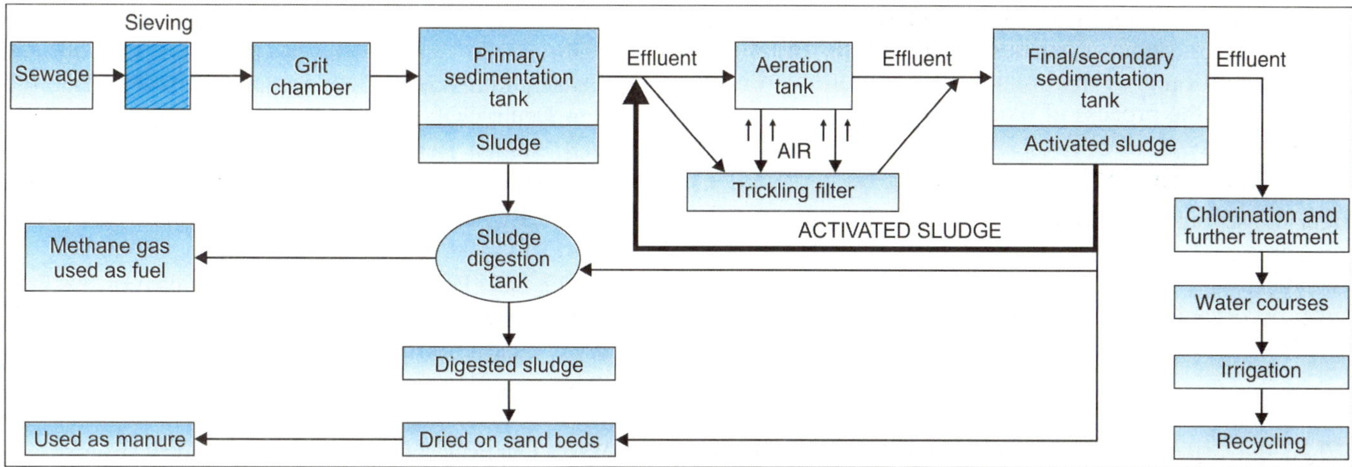

Fig. 7.6: Sewage treatment process

Grit Chamber or Detritus Tank

After screening when sewage is collected in small tanks, the heavy suspended material such as gravel, sand debris and ashes (inorganic material) settle down in this chamber.

Sedimentation

Sewage is allowed to stand for some period say half an hour to three hours in tanks, the suspended organic matter will settle down at the bottom is called "sludge" when the process of sedimentation is applied to new sewage it is called as primary sedimentation.

Screening, grit removal and primary sedimentation and sludge digestion process is called primary treatment of sewage.

Secondary Treatment

The secondary treatment of sewage consists of oxidation and aeration of sewage, percolation through trickling filter activated sludge mixing, oxidation ponds and oxidation lagoons.

Percolation or Trickling Filter

The effluent (liquid part of sewage) from primary sedimentation tank is sprinkled in spray form by perforated rotating pipes, over filter bed similar to slow sand filter described for water purification. The effluent trickles through filter and comes in contact with topmost vital layer or "Zoogleal layer" which removes bacteria, fungi and it is oxidized by atmospheric oxygen and the effluent after passing through filter bed gets clarified and it loses much of its venom. An efficient trickling filter would reduce the biochemical oxygen demand (BOD) of sewage to the extent of 85–95%.

Final Sedimentation or Secondary Sedimentation Process

The effluent from bottom of trickling filter is allowed to stay in secondary sedimentation tank. Aerated sludge or activated sludge settles at the bottom of the secondary sedimentation tank. The sludge is allowed to dry upon the drying beds of the ground and can be removed after drying and can be used as manure or mixed with soil as soil conditioner.

Activated Sludge Process

Part of the activated sludge from secondary sedimentation tank which contains the active aerobic bacteria is recirculated and allowed to mix with effluent coming out of primary sedimentation tank, as also mixed with sludge of primary sedimentation tank. The sludge from primary sedimentation tank and active sludge is further aerated by diffusion of air in *aeration tank*. This process reduces the biochemical demand of oxygen and it reduces load on the system and improves the efficiency of the process. Oxidation of ammonia to nitrates and nitrites also gets faster with this process. This process is called biological treatment of sewage.

SLUDGE DIGESTION

Sludge which settles at the bottom of primary sedimentation tank and secondary sedimentation tank is led to sludge digestion tank, which is a closed tank. Here anaerobic digestion of sludge takes place and this process produces lot of methane gas and carbon dioxide. The methane thus generated can be used as fuel and power for various processes of sewage treatment. The digested sludge is removed from the digestion tank and dried on sand beds or taken to lagoon and allowed to dry up or else it is dried up by pressure filter process. The dried sludge serves as good manure.

OXIDATION POND

Here the sewage is exposed to sunshine and air in leak proof tanks, after the sedimentation (primary and secondary sedimentation). This process converts the organic matter of the sewage into harmless sludge which can be removed periodically or subjected to digestion by anaerobic or aerobic processes as described. The algae protozoa and fungi at the bottom of oxidation pond help and enhance the process of oxidation.

Oxidation Ditch/Aerated Lagoon

Here the sewage is mechanically aerated. It occupies less land area and efficiently oxidizes the suspended matter and dissolved organic matter by aerobic bacteria. The coliform organisms in sewage can be reduced by 90–95% by biological oxidation.

Tertiary Treatment of Sewage

When the water is scarce and the waste water is to be recycled for drinking purposes or recreational and industrial use, the effluent is further subjected to final treatment to make it absolutely harmless. Filtration and coagulation processes make the effluent more safe. Ozonization is most efficient method to destroy all sorts of pathogens, but it is quite costly. Superchlorination is another alternative to make effluent safe.

Disposal of Effluent

- The effluent after treatment (chlorination) is used for irrigation purposes. Sewage farming is common in many areas.
- The treated effluent can be disposed of in water courses such as rivers, streams, lakes, sea, ponds and canals. This is known as disposal by dilution (Fig. 7.6).

Biochemical Oxygen Demand (BOD)

It is the amount of oxygen absorbed by the specified amount of sewage (one liter) at particular temperature (20°C) for specified period (5 days) for aerobic digestion of sewage. It measures the efficiency of treatment process as also the extent of strength of sewage. BOD of 300 mg/L (300 ppm) or above is called strong while that of 100 mg/L (100 ppm) is called weak.

The standard for biochemical oxygen demand (BOD), which represents the extent of organic pollution in a water body, is fixed at 30 mg/L in the country. This means any industry or infrastructure project or municipality has to treat sewage or effluent to a level of 30 mg/L prior to discharging the same to a water body. The standards in the developed countries are being revised and are now being based on the total maximum daily load (TMDL) calculation rather than a source based limit. In India, the level of BOD in source of drinking water has been fixed as BOD 2 mg/L or less.

REFERENCES

1. Water Aid Report July 2008. Tackling the silent killer. The case for sanitation 47–49 Durham street, London, Oliver Cumming.
2. UNICEF. State of World's children. New Delhi: UNICEF; 1998.
3. Planning Commission GOI. Tenth Five-Year Plan 2002–07. New Delhi: GOI; 2002.
4. GOI. School Health Committee Report-I. New Delhi: Ministry of Health, School Health Committee, CHEB; 1961.
5. UNICEF. Training modules on sanitation. New Delhi: UNICEF; 1988.
6. Patel I. Sasti Pariyavaran Swachhta Suvidhayen. 3rd Edn., Ahmedabad: Pariyavaran Swachhta Sansthan; 1998.
7. WHO. Guidelines for Cholera control. WHO; Geneva, 1993.
8. Bhaskaran RR, Sampathkumaran MA (ICMR). Review of Work Done on rural Latrines in India; 1966 Report No. 54.
9. WHO. Our planet our health—Report of WHO Commission on Health and Environment. Geneva: WHO; 1992.
10. Govt. of India. National Rural Health Mission (2005–2012). Mission Document, MOH and FW; Govt. of India, New Delhi.
11. GOI. Central Rural Sanitation Programme (Total Sanitation Campaign). Department of drinking water supply, MORD, GOI; May 2002.
12. Nirmal Gram Puraskar. Hindustan Times, New Delhi. Friday, May 4, 2007.

SOIL POLLUTION

Soil—*Dharti Ma* (Mother Earth) in India is respected and worshipped, but because of compulsive life and exploding population this respect is diminishing fast. Soils are formed by the disintegration and decomposition of rocks, vegetation and animal fossils embedded in them. Decomposition and disintegration is brought about by action of rain water, running streams, glaciers, wind, high and low temperatures, storms, volcanic activity, apart from action of soil organisms such as many soil bacteria, fungi, protozoa, earthworms, etc. and interaction of various chemicals. Soil structure and composition varies from region to region, district to district and state to state. It could be categorized as sandy soil, clay soil and loamy soil or alluvial, black, red, laterite, arid and desert, mountain and hilly, saline and alkaline, peaty and other organic soil.

Humus

Humus is decomposed vegetable matter dead roots, fruits, flowers, trunks, branches and leaves. It forms dark coloured surface layer on the ground. It is rich in nitrogen and can absorb lot of water. Humus is used for conditioning of soil, if it is added to sandy soil to improve its quality. Humus is an important seat for bacterial activity. Soil organisms and bacteria help decomposition of organic matter in the soil including human excreta. Pit latrines and trench latrine excreta gets decomposed by soil bacteria and organisms and over a period of time it gets converted to good manure for use in agriculture. Soil contains varieties of bacteria like nitrifying bacteria, nitrogen fixing bacteria, ammonifying bacteria, and sulphur bacteria. Lot of fungi and algae also help in decomposition of organic matter.

Human Population (Easing for Diseases)

Growing population and human excreta is enormous problem. Management of human excreta is uphill task in itself. No more than 33% of villagers use sanitary latrines, while 67% defecate in open field. Similarly, 12.6% of urban slum dwellers have no facility of latrine and use all sorts of available grounds, open areas, railway tracks for indiscriminate defecation. Almost every big city has enormous problem of human faecal matter. Scene and obnoxious smell of excreta along railway tracks is awful in capital city of Delhi and other big cities.[1]

Indiscriminate defecation by people in urban and rural areas leads to widespread soil pollution in India.

Sewage and Sludge

Sewage: It is raw water or waste water or human or animal excreta plus water.

Sewer: It means network of pipes laid underground to carry sewage.

Very few towns in India have complete facility of sewage treatment, sewage is collected through sewer system and disposed off untreated or partially treated outside town or led into water courses. Towns and cities along the river bank dispose off their raw sewage into rivers thus polluting drinking water sources. The sanitary disposal of night soil with effective control of foul smell and fly nuisance is therefore a serious problem all over the country.

Raw sewage and partially treated sewage as also sludge are used in farms, which is called *sewage farming*. This practice is hazardous. Vegetables grown on soil manured with untreated sewage and sludge is real danger to health. Human excreta comes back to human beings through vegetables and fruits (vegetables grown on such soils and consumed by human beings as unwashed, partially washed or uncooked). Taenia eggs can survive for long in soil and can survive many sewage treatment processes.

Garbage and Refuse

Garbage and refuse collection and disposal in cities and rural areas leaves much to be desired. Quite often it is just heaped up on the outskirts of city and is not subjected to composting. Manure pits or trenches are seldom dug by municipal authorities. Garbage and refuse which is just dumped at outskirts of city poses several health problems. Biodegradable and non-biodegradable waste is dumped up together and no effort is made to segregate the waste. Plastic bags and plastic material hinders the process of composting. Rag pickers bring back the dirt to; market and town population. Indiscriminate disposal of garbage and refuse produces soil contamination and health hazards of several kinds (fly breeding apart from contamination of soil with plastic). Spores of *B. anthracis* remain viable in contaminated soil for many years. Rodents and cattle excrete large number of leptospires organisms in their urine and are thus responsible for the contamination of soil. The salinity of soil provides favourable environments for survival of leptospires.

Industrial Effluents and Soil Pollution

Urbanization and industrialization are inevitable for economic development, but uncontrolled industrialization has its own drawbacks. Many polluting and hazardous units are located in non-confirming areas (within the residential complexes). Dangerous and hazardous industrial wastes and effluents are dumped into the soil which leads to widespread soil pollution and air pollution. Most toxic wastes come from chemical industry but others including the metal, petroleum, transport electrical equipment, and leather tanning industries also produce significant quantities of hazardous waste. Sewage; sludge and hospital wastes are also hazardous. Indiscriminate disposal and dumping of industrial wastes have resulted in widespread soil pollution and underground water pollution, besides air pollution. The discharge of methyl mercury contaminated waste into river, resulting in hundreds of deaths and thousands of cases of disablement at Minamata Bay in Japan (Minamata disease). Mercury contamination produced serious problems in many North American water bodies and has been noted in Alexandria, Bangkok, Bombay, Cartagena, Managua Perai and various Chinese cities. Significant build ups of mercury lead, arsenic, fluoride, cadmium, copper and chromium have been reported in recent years in almost every industrialized country in South East Asia. The Kalu river, which runs through two of Bombay's industrial suburbs received liquid effluents containing heavy metals from over 150 industrial units. This causes heavy levels of mercury and lead in the water of nearby villages. Heavy metals enter the food chain through cattle browsing on river bank vegetation. When contaminated water from industries is used for irrigation the heavy metals enter the food chain through vegetations and plants grown on such fields and when consumed by local population over long time produce toxic effects. These heavy metals become stock pollutant of the agriculture land.[2] Radioactive substances from laboratories and industries, or atmospheric fall out from nuclear explosion can pollute soil and may enter the food chain through vegetation and plants.

Agriculture and Soil Pollution

Human exposure to persistent organic pollutants (POPs) occurs as pesticide residue. Indiscriminate use of pesticides on crops pollute soil. POPs are organic compounds and have long life in environment and undergo physical, chemical and biological changes over time. Through crops and foods, these pesticides climb the food chain and accumulate in tissues of animals and man and produce untowards hormonal effects in the long run. POPs can travel great distance in air or water.[2]

Health Hazards of Soil Pollution

Soil-transmitted helminths like *Ascaris lumbricoides* (roundworm), *Trichuris trichiura* and *Ancylostoma duodenale* (hookworm) are very common in India. High prevalence of soil transmitted helminthic (STH) infection in population has been observed, where open field defecation is practiced, due to soil pollution with human excreta. Excreta comes back to human from contaminated soil through dirty hands, by flies and contaminated water. Person with bare feet who walks or works on such soil or 241 million children who play on such soil are at risk of contracting helminthic infection and diarrhoeal diseases. DALYs lost due to STH have been estimated around 39 million against 34.1 million due to measles, 35.7 million due to malaria and 46.5 million due to tuberculosis.[3,4]

Heavy metal poisoning (lead, mercury, arsenic) due to indiscriminate disposal of industrial wastes and carcinogenic effects of radioactive waste/material have been reported in many parts of the world. These substances either pollute groundwater or atmosphere and affect human beings.

Tetanus is transmitted through soil, which is contaminated by animal excreta. Tetanus spores are present in superficial layer of earth mostly in humus. Due to infection of wound by the spores of tetanus bacilli from polluted soil, street dust or dusty air, the danger of tetanus neonatorum and tetanus in adults persist in rural and urban slum areas. Road side accidents which contaminate the wound with dirt and dust can be risk factor for occurrence of tetanus.

Diarrhoeal disease, cholera, amoebic dysentery, typhoid fever, infective hepatitis may occur from infected or polluted soil indirectly through contaminated water, dust and flies. Outbreaks of diarrhoeal diseases, cholera and infective hepatitis may occur when large scale contamination occurs by rains, flood or sewage. Anthrax spores have been found in fields where infected animals are allowed to graze.[5]

Prevention and Control of Soil Pollution

Good environmental health is a necessary prerequisite for health of mankind. All efforts must be directed to prevent environmental pollution/soil pollution by:

- Controlling population.
- Promoting safe disposal of human excreta by sanitary latrines, sewerage system and treatment of sewage.
- Safe disposal of garbage and refuse, by composting in trenches or manure pits.
- Safe disposal of industrial wastes and effluents by adequate planning and enforcing the laws and by-laws for polluting units.

7

Health Education

Improving Habits and Practices

The social attitudes are at the heart of environmental concern. Much of personal hygiene like washing hands, wearing of shoes and storing water clean at household level and open defection are the mindsets of individual—families and community, these must be inculcated at all levels to prevent diseases, especially transmitted through soil pollution and water pollution. Families and schools as transmitter of values to next generation become central and so too does media in its role of shaping what is acceptable social behaviour.

REFERENCES

1. UNICEF. Right and opportunities: The situation of children and women in India. New Delhi: UNICEF; 1998.
2. WHO. Our planet our health—report of WHO commission on health and environment. Geneva: WHO; 1992.
3. NICD. Proceedings National workshop to develop National Plan of action for prevention and control of Soil Transmitted Helminths (STH) in India, 2004 Jan. 15–16; NICD: New Delhi.
4. WHO. Hookwarm Infection and anaemia approaches to prevention and control. Pawlowski ZS, Schad GA, Stott GJ. World Health Organization; Geneva, 1992.
5. Population Report. Population and the environment. The Global Challenge Feb. 2001; Series M(15): 1–30.

AIR POLLUTION

Air, water and soil contamination has drawn the attention of all Governments. Epidemiologists are deeply concerned with deteriorating environments, as these determine the health status of individual, family and community. Air pollution is widespread in developed and developing countries, affecting urban and rural areas. The main source of air pollution is combustion of solid fuels (coal, lignite, wood) and liquid fuel (from petroleum source). Due to population explosion, the need for more electricity has led to steep rise in power generation through coal as India has limited reserves of natural gas. Increased urbanization and economic activities have increased vehicular traffic using diesel and petrol both of which add to NOx and SOx emissions in cities. Heavy vehicles which use diesel as fuel, emit large quantities of RPM (respirable suspended particulate matter). Shortage of electric power has led to increased use of diesel generator sets in the commercial, household and agriculture sector. Air pollution kills an estimated 7 million people every year—about 12.5% of all deaths annually. 9 out of 10 deaths due to air pollution take place in the developing world where 82% of all people live. About 2.5 billion people almost all in developing countries suffer from high level of indoor air pollution. Indoor air pollution is due to burning wood, animal dung, crop residues and coal for cooking and heating. Most of the victims of indoor air pollution are women and girls who have the primary responsibility for cooking and tending the house. Outdoor air pollution harms more than 1.1 billion people mostly in cities. WHO estimates that about 7,00,000 deaths annually could be prevented in developing countries, if three major atmospheric pollutants—carbon monoxide, suspended particulate matter and lead were brought down to safer levels.[1]

Composition of Air

It is composed of oxygen (20.94%), nitrogen (78.09%), carbon dioxide (0.03%), argon (0.93%), water vapour, ozone, krypton and other gases. In addition, the natural electrical discharge during thunder storms produces oxides of nitrogen, volcanic disturbances produce sulphur dioxide, hydrogen fluoride and hydrogen chloride, hydrogen sulphide and ozone formed photochemically. Dust and aerosols of natural origin present in atmosphere consist of salt particles from sea water, various types of condensation nuclei, air-borne particles from coal and vegetation, dust of meteorite origin, bacterial spores and pollens. Adult person breathes 500 ml of air per breath or 6 litres per minute.

OUTDOOR AIR POLLUTION (AMBIENT AIR POLLUTION)

The air of large/mega cities is often polluted and unhealthy. Cities such as Mumbai (Bombay), Kolkata, Delhi, Chennai (Madras), Kanpur, Ahmedabad, Nagpur have severe air pollution problems with the annual levels of total suspended particles (TSPs) at least three times as high as the WHO standards.[2]

Major Air Pollutants

The air pollutants are classified into two major categories:

1. Particulate
2. Gaseous

Particulate: The particulate includes substances which may exist as solid or liquid at normal temperature and pressure. Depending upon the size, the particulate may remain suspended in air or settle down. Generally, particulates below 5×10^6 Å diameter remain suspended in air and are referred as suspended particulate matter (SPM). The particulate pollutants include dust, fumes, mist, spray and smoke.

Gaseous: The gaseous pollutants include sulphur dioxide (SO_2), carbon monoxide (CO), nitrogen dioxide (NO_2), hydrocarbon (HC) and photochemical oxidants (OX).

Sources of Air Pollution

Fossil fuels (coal and petroleum products including diesel) are the largest sources of air and atmospheric pollution. Most industries, power plants and automobiles depend on fossil fuel. Fossil fuels account for nearly 90% of the world's commercial energy production. While complete combustion of fossil fuels produces carbon dioxide and water together with some oxides of nitrogen generated by fixation of atmosphere nitrogen at high temperature. Post-harvesting burning stubble of paddy and wheat crops also leads to outdoor air pollution. It is widespread practice in Punjab, Haryana, UP and MP.

Suspended Particulate Matter (SPM)

The incomplete combustion of fossil fuels leads to black smoke which consists of finely divided particles of carbon or complex hydrocarbons. These particles of varying sizes constitute suspended particulate matter (SPM)—small particles floating in the air or atmosphere. The fine suspended particulate matters are called aerosols, which can enter the tracheobronchial tree. Finest particles can reach the alveoli of lung and remain suspended in the air for longer time. Sulfur and nitrogen oxides emitted from fossil fuels in the atmosphere are converted to acids and eventually fall to the ground as acid rain or snow. Acid rain destroys many flora, fauna on earth apart from contaminating drinking water. WHO guidelines have fixed the level of suspended particulate matter which ranges from 60 to 90 micrograms per cubic meter and in many of the mega cities these levels range from 100 to 400 μg (micrograms) per cubic meter of air.

Sulfur Dioxide and Metals

Most of the sulfur present in the fossil fuels is emitted as sulfur dioxide and metals are emitted as vapour or present in ash or emitted in gases.

Ozone

At ground level ozone is powerful secondary pollutant formed due to photosynthesis of nitrous oxide gas released mostly from automobiles exhaust, industrial effluents, mass fuel burners, ultraviolet radiation from sun, thunderstorm and lightning discharge, photocopier machines, arc welding, and decay of potassium nitrate in agricultural fields during post-harvesting season. The ozone is major secondary pollutant formed within photochemical smog seen in big cities with mounting population of motor vehicles and automobiles. The problem was first recognized in Los Angeles as "Los Angeles Smog", now it is widespread in many cities.[3] Ozone is main component of smog. Another powerful secondary pollutant is acid rain, formed when SO_2 and oxides of nitrogen combine with water vapour of oxygen in the presence of sunlight to form a diluted "soup" of sulfuric and nitric acids. They can fall as both wet (acid rain) or dry deposition.

Lead

Lead is used as an additive in petrol. Air-borne lead from vehicles remains a big problem, further the lead is retained on the surface layer of soil and poses threat to human health and more severe effects are visible in young children.

Problem of Air Pollution—Choked Cities

In Latin America, cities such as Sao Paulo and Santiago have recorded suspended particulate matter that averages 100–400 micrograms per cubic meter of air. Many Asian cities face similar problems. In 1991, following Asian cities exceeded WHO thresholds for suspended particulate matter of sulfur dioxide for much of the year. Beijing 272 days, Jakarta 173 days, Mumbai 100 days; and New Delhi 294 days.[4] The situation has become worse since then, as the population of these cities have grown rapidly over the past decades. With more people, the cities have more industry, more households, more fuel use, and more motor vehicles and thus more air pollution. In New Delhi, India, vehicle exhausts account for 70% of air pollution, according to 2000 estimate. City of Delhi is often entombed with pall of pollution from trucks, cars and uncontrolled industrial emissions. With the use of CNG fuel the levels of pollution in Delhi have come down substantially. In US, many cities had suspended particulate matter levels ranging from 20–30 micrograms per cubic meter of air, while the national standard is no more than 15 micrograms per cubic meter (of fine particles less than 2.5 micrometers in diameter).

Mumbai is one of the most populous cities in the world. It is also one of the most polluted city. Mumbai reports average level of suspended particulate matter in the air nearly 240 micrograms far exceeding WHO standard of 60–90 micrograms per cubic meter. The Mahim Nature Park Project has effectively demonstrated the effect of green spaces to clean-up Mumbai and decreasing pollution levels.[4]

Death by Breath

Worldwide WHO estimates that 1.5 billion urban dwellers face levels of outdoor air pollution that are above the maximum recommended levels and hence are exposed to health risk of air pollution. About 3.7 million death each year can be attributed just to particulate matter and sulfur dioxide in outdoor air. Outdoor air pollution is usually considered a problem of developed countries, as a consequence of their high level of industrial activity and vehicle use. More than 88% deaths due to outdoor air pollution occur in the developing world, however, because population is larger and pollution standards often are less strict than in the more developed world. In Asia, with half of the world's urban population, more than 1.5 million people die every year from diseases related to air pollution. In India, alone air pollution causes an estimated 84,000 premature deaths each year (Table 7.4). WHO analysis on

Table 7.4: Death by breath—estimates of deaths due to air pollution by regions, 2012 (WHO)

Region or country	*Deaths from indoor pollution*	*Deaths from outdoor pollution*
South East Asia	16,91,600	9,36,000
Western Pacific	16,20,100	17,37,000
India	14,00,000	84,000
America	81300	1,52,000
Europian countries	1,17,200	4,82,000
Africa	5,81,300	1,76,000
Eastern Mediterranian	2,00,800	2,50,000
Grand total	**42,92,300**	**37,33,000**

Source: WHO, 2014 India data not included in total

Outdoor air pollution deaths—breakdown by diseases: Ishaemic heart disease 40%, strokes 40%, chronic obstructive pulmonary disease (COPD) 11%, lung cancer 6% and acute lower respiratory infections in children 3%.

In the US, nearly half of all urban residents are exposed to harmful levels of ozone. A recent study estimated that particulate pollution, mostly from vehicle emissions, causes up to one-fifth of all lung cancers in the US. Researchers found an 8% increased risk of lung cancer for every increase of 10 micrograms of particulates per cubic meter of air. In the United Kingdom, suspended particulate kill an estimated 482000 people each year.[4]

INDOOR AIR POLLUTION (HOUSEHOLD AIR POLLUTION)

About 2.5 billion people, almost all in developing countries suffer from high levels of indoor air pollution. Indoor air pollution is common in rural areas as also poor people in urban slums. Some estimates suggest that worldwide urban and rural indoor air pollution kills prematurely about 4.3 million people annually. Indoor air pollution is a major health problem because worldwide almost 3 billion people rely on unprocessed biomass fuels—mostly fire wood, charcoal, animal dung, logging wastes and saw dust, grass leaves, crop residues for household cooking and heating. WHO estimates that biomass fuels are used to meet the energy needs of nearly half of world's population. These are often burnt in open fires or inefficient stoves and poorly ventilated houses.

In China, India and sub-Saharan Africa more than 86.5% of rural and 26.1% urban households use biomass fuel for cooking.[5–7] These fuels do not burn cleanly and emit large amount of smoke, often directly inside dwellings with inadequate ventilation. The combustion of raw biomass fuels produce hundreds of chemical compounds including suspended particulate matter, carbon monoxide, oxides of nitrogen and sulfur, hydrocarbons, aldehydes, benzene, denol, cresol, toluene and more complex hydrocarbon compounds including polyaromatic hydrocarbons. Use of improved stoves with ventilation and exhaust chimneys can reduce the emission of suspended particulate matter by up to 60%; of carbon monoxide by up to 86%. While rural areas may lack access to modern stoves or clean fuels, the urban poor often cannot afford cleaner fuels such as kerosene, natural gas, or electricity. They have no choice but to use biomass fuels. Women and children suffer most from indoor air pollution because they spend many hours each day in their homes, where often the air is polluted.

Similarly, fossil fuels are widely used for space or water heating in the home or for cooking in many countries. Because of poor combustion conditions, coal fumes become major source of air pollution in homes. The production of sulfur dioxide from coal is inevitable besides carbon monoxide, which can reach lethal concentrations at times. The risk from oxides of nitrogen also remain because of poor combustion.

Effects on Health

Adverse health effects have been associated with:

i Sulfur dioxide and particulate suspended matter (soot, ash, dust, smoke fumes, mist and spray) from fossil fuels and poor combustion of biomass fuel.

ii Photochemical oxidants (secondary pollutants like ozone) due to heavy emission of oxide of nitrogen from road vehicles, which combine with atmospheric oxygen in the presence of sunlight.

iii Pollutants from inorganic metals such as arsenic, asbestos, beryllium, cadmium, hydrogen sulfide, lead and mercury.

Respiratory System

Air pollution is a potential risk and has led to an increase in respiratory problems/diseases in cities.

The most serious health risks of indoor air pollution are burns and smoke inhalation. Exposure to pollutants is 60 times higher in indoor environments in the rural area of developing countries than in urban areas of developed countries. The principal adverse effects on health are respiratory and CO poisoning. Women working indoor on stoves have higher risks of inhaling total suspended particulate and benzo(a) pyrene. This creates risk of respiratory cancer. Chronic effects include inflammation of the respiratory tract caused by continued exposure to irritant gases and fumes. These may lead to development of emphysema and chronic obstructive pulmonary disease (COPD) and cor pulmonale. As women and girls tend the fires and do the cooking inhaling large concentration of pollutants over longer period and thereby increasing prevalence of chronic bronchitis by 100% in those chronically exposed to biomass fuels. Similarly, infants and children may be heavily exposed because they remain with their mother while fires are tended and cooking is done. In many cities, the concentration of air pollutants are already high enough to cause morbidity in susceptible individuals and premature mortality in aged, particularly those with respiratory infection.

Reduced lung function in school children have been reported due to air pollution. Similarly, acute respiratory illness like acute bronchitis and pneumonia in adults have been incriminated due to air pollution.

WHO analysis on indoor air pollution death—breakdown by diseases: Strokes 34%, ischaemic heart disease 26%, COPD 22%, acute lower respiratory tract infections in children 12% and lung cancer 6%.

Chronic Lung Diseases

According to World Health Report 2002, analysis based on particulate matter estimates report that ambient air pollution causes about 5% of trachea, bronchus and lung cancer, 2% cardiorespiratory mortality and about 1% of respiratory infections mortality globally. This amounts to about 1.4% (0.8 million) deaths and 0.8% (7.9 million) of disability adjusted life years. The adverse effects of air pollution are more pronounced in developing countries.[8]

Air pollution leads to worsening of or exacerbation of chronic lung diseases due to high concentration of smoke and sulfur dioxide. The persons already having chronic lung disease are extremely susceptible to air pollution.

A protective layer of ozone is present in the region of 16–30 km above the earth's surface at a concentration of 1–10 parts per million (ppm). This is referred to as stratosphere that performs indispensable function of absorbing harmful ultraviolet radiation to shield the biosphere.

Every year due to depletion of ozone layer, more and more people are being exposed to ultraviolet (UV) radiation from the sun thus causing 2–3 million new cases of nonmalignant melanomas and more than 1,30,000 new melanoma skin cases worldwide. An estimated 66,000 deaths occur annually from melanoma and other skin cancers. The new educational materials were launched on the occasion of International day for the preservation of the ozone layer, which held its theme in 2003 as "Save O_3ur sky: There is a hole lot more to do for our children".[9]

Air Pollution and Sensory Irritation

The odour of air-borne substances and irritation to the eyes, nose, skin and throat are most common and annoying aspects of air pollution. Ozone the component of photochemical smog directly irritates the eyes, pharynx and trachea, causing a burning sensation in chest, chest discomfort, headache and various other symptoms in school children playing outdoor on "Smog alert" days. Ozone can inflame and damage lung cells besides aggravating chronic lung diseases. Safe level of ozone is 64 parts per billion (ppb).

Carbon monoxide can alter human performance as well as cardiac function. Inhalation of lead can cause neurogenic disturbances and can adversely affect the central nervous system. Children are most susceptible to lead toxicity.

The stratospheric ozone layer is being damaged by the release into the atmosphere of various chemicals including chlorofluorocarbons used in refrigerant, aerosols, plastic foam blowers and other equipment, halogens used by fire fighting services and various organic solvents. Depletion of ozone layer leads to higher levels of active ultraviolet radiation at the earth's surface. UV radiation increases the incidence of skin cancer and cataract in humans.

Greenhouse Gases (Global Warming)

Air pollution can build up greenhouse gases (CO_2, methane, nitrogen, oxide) in the atmosphere which is likely to lead to global warming and rise in sea level by melting of ice caps. Carbon dioxide and chlorofluorocarbons are mainly responsible for global warming effect.

Global warming has resulted in increase of mean surface temperature by 0.4 to 0.8°C during the last 100 years.

Heat strokes and heat stress because of global warming can affect human population particularly old and young people. It may also lead to changes in rainfall, droughts, floods, desertification and agriculture may be affected seriously. There has been significant decrease in sunshine hours.

PREVENTION AND CONTROL OF AIR POLLUTION

Outdoor Air Pollution

Outdoor air pollution can be controlled and prevented by:

- Efficient public transport system and reduction of population of private vehicles.
- Use of lead free petrol.
- Reducing air pollution from fossil fuels use by appropriate technologies such as use of catalytic converters which can reduce the emission of oxides of nitrogen, carbon monoxide and volatile organic compounds from motor vehicles fuelled with lead-free petrol.
- Alternate fuel such as CNG (compressed natural gas) for automobiles instead of petrol and diesel. The landmark ruling of Honourable Supreme Court came on 5th April 2002, declaring that all public transport in Delhi will run on CNG. Similarly, it was mentioned that cities such as Lucknow, Pune and Jodhpur will also switch over to CNG for running their public transport. With this proclamation, the level of air pollution in Delhi has come down to a significant level.
- Green belts, plantation of trees to create a buffer zone between residential areas and industrial estates. These absorb CO_2 of the air. Hence, massive afforestation drives can improve earth's lung capacity.
- Plan industries away from residential areas and ensure regulation.
- Controlling emissions at source level in industrial set-up by use of electrostatic precipitators and bag filters can trap large amount of particulates (dust, ash and soot) in factories or power plant exhaust gases.
- Fitting power station with scrubbers can reduce sulfur dioxide emission by up to 95% and equipping them with catalytic converters can significantly reduce emissions of oxides of nitrogen.
- **Legislation to control air pollution:** The Air (prevention and control of pollution) Act, 1981 and Environment Act, 1986 forms the basis of monitoring and controlling air pollution in the country especially after Bhopal gas tragedy in 1984. Implement ban on burning of straw and other organic waste. Curtail the use of polythene.
- Development of alternate sources of energy such as biodiesel which is renewable energy source with properties of decreasing the emission of CO_2 and SO_2 and unburnt hydrocarbons during the combustion process is most welcome. Such a fuel could substitute fossil fuels.
- **Central Pollution Control Board (CPCB)** has established a national air quality monitoring network covering 290 stations spread over in 90 cities and towns. The measures taken to control air pollution are:
  - Setting up of ambient air quality standard (AAQS) for short-term (24 hours) and annual for industrial, residential, rural and other areas with respect to various pollutants like SO_2, NO_2, RPM, Pb and CO.
  - Monitoring of air quality is done with regard to SO_2, NO_2 and SPM and in selected stations, ammonia, hydrogen sulphide, RPM (respirable suspended particulate matter) and polycyclic aromatic hydrocarbons are also monitored.
  - To reduce vehicular pollution, emission standards for petrol and diesel driven vehicles were introduced in 1990, further modified in 1996 and 2000.
  - The fitting of catalytic converters in petrol driven vehicles have been made compulsory in the four metro cities. Specifications of diesel and gasoline have been revised further to reduce sulphur, aromatics and lead content. Lead in gasoline has been phased out since 2000.
  - Guidelines have been laid down for setting up of industries. A project for district wise zoning atlas has been taken up that would guide suitable location of industry.
  - Submission of environment statement by polluting units has been made mandatory since 1992.
  - Environment impact assessment has been made mandatory for 29 categories of projects since 1994 and public hearings have been prescribed since 1997.

Indoor Air Pollution

Indoor air pollution can be controlled and prevented by:

- Improved ventilation: Can reduce the levels of SO_2 and particulate matter.

- Use of improved and efficient stoves with exhaust chimneys. Fuel efficient stoves save lot of fuel and are better accepted by people.
- Use of modern fuels—like kerosene oil, electricity and LPG (liquefied petroleum gas).
- Use of non-conventional source of energy such as solar cookers, wind energy, biogas plants—these are user-friendly and environmental friendly source of energy and produce no air pollution or least air pollution.
- ***Local innovation:*** Use of biomass fuel (animal dung) in improvised device called "Hara" in local language, is self-regulated device of burning animal dung outside kitchen, for heating milk, water and cooking purposes; keeps away smoke and unburnt particles, but it leads to outdoor air pollution.

Monitoring Indicators of Air Pollution

Following indicators and measurements can provide index of health risks:

- Sulfur dioxide levels
- SPM in air
- Smoke index
- Dust fall
- Air content of CO, nitrogen oxide, lead and various oxidants.

At global level—global environmental monitoring system (GEMS) of WHO conducts regular periodical monitoring of air quality and it has laid down acceptable standards. At national level, National Environmental Engineering Research Institute (NEERI) at Nagpur monitors the quality of air.

Goal: Attain WHO standards of air quality in all major cities by 2011–12.[10]

REFERENCES

1 Population and the environment—the global challenges. Population Report June 2003; M(15).

2 Patel TS. Air pollution—problem and perspectives. ICMR Bulletin June 1997; 27(6).

3 WHO. Our planet our health—report of WHO commission on health and environment. Geneva: WHO; 1992.

4 Meeting the urban challenge. Population report May–June 2003; M(16).

5 WHO. News release 25th march 2014 march 2014/Geneva.

6 IIPS and ORC Macro. National Family Health Survey-2 and 3 1998–99. Mumbai: IIPS; 2002 and 2005–06.

7 UNICEF. Facts for life—a communication challenge. Indian edition. New Delhi: UNICEF; 1990.

8 World Health Organization. World Health Report 2002, WHO: Geneva, 2002.

9 WHO. Children suffer from most effects of ozone depletion. WHO Press Release Sept. 16 2003.

10 GOI. Towards Faster and more Inclusive Growth. An Approach to the 11th Five-Year Plan. GOI. Planning Commission, Yojna Bhavan, New Delhi, Dec 2006.

NOISE POLLUTION

Noise is undesirable and annoying level of sound which affects human beings. Noise like any sound is defined in terms of its duration, frequency spectrum (measured in Hz) and intensity measured in sound pressure level (SPL) and expressed in decibels (dB). Noise may be continuous, intermittent, impulsive or explosive. Noise has been notified as pollutant under the Air (prevention and control of pollution) Act, 1981.[1]

The unit of measurement: The unit of measurement of noise is decibel (dB) on A-weighted scale.[2]

SAFE LIMIT

The international organization for standardization (ISO) has considered the safe limit of exposure to noise as 90 dB. In India, ISO standards are followed. Noise induced hearing loss has been incorporated in the Factories Act, 1948 amended in 1976, as a notifiable disease and also made compensable.[1] Way back, in UK in 1972 maximum level of noise exposure (equivalent continuous noise level—Leq) for an 8-hour working day were fixed at 90 dB.

Noise Level in Industries

Sound pressure levels (SPLs) in many of the industries may be very high and beyond the acceptable limit of 90 dB. The example of industrial operations which produce lot of noise induced damages include:

- Blasting, drilling and loading operations, boiler makers and iron foundries.
- Air compressors, motors, blowers, generators, pumps and steam turbines.
- Sawing operation

Noise pollution in industries is an occupational hazard and workers who are exposed to the risk of high noise may suffer from various grades of hearing loss after prolonged exposure.

Community Exposure

The noise appears to be endemic in urban areas. The main causes in cities are traffic noise due to motors, trucks, buses and motor cycles and exhaust system of automobiles.

Railways, horns, whistles, aircraft, public address system, high-pitched pop music and personal cassette players and radio for entertainment are common sources of noise. Crackers on the eve of festival, produce intolerable noise and acute traumatic effect on eardrum besides air pollution. Otitic blast injuries are produced due to sudden explosive forces in bombs.[3, 4]

Effects on Health

Hearing Loss

The most intense and continued exposure to noise occurs at work place, especially in industry. Workers manifest varying degree of noise induced hearing loss. Persistent exposure to high levels of noise can lead to hearing loss that is initially temporary, but can later become permanent.[2]

- Industrial accidents on account of hearing impairment may result because of poor communication and disturbance of sound.
- Fatigue and tiredness may set early.

People who are exposed to the risk of surface rail noise, underground rail noise, road traffic noise and aircraft noise run a risk of hearing loss, which may be temporary or permanent.[3,4]

Non-auditory Effects

Behavioural effects are more than auditory effects. It creates annoyance, disturbed sleep (insomnia) and fatigueness and decreases intellectual and work performance. Cognitive and psychomotor functions are altered and noise can alter neurosensory coordination, psychological reactions and psychological responses.

PREVENTION AND CONTROL

Engineering Control Mechanisms

Using efficient machinery and soundproofing and isolation of noisy machinery in industrial set-up has been adopted to reduce the noise.

Legislation

Enforcing legislation, i.e. implementation of Factory Act (1976 modified) in industrial set-up. Regular monitoring of noise is essential.

Personal Protection

Use of hearing protectors (earmuffs and headphones and helmets) and periodic audiometric monitoring by periodic health check-up of exposed workers to ensure that damage is reduced to minimum.

- See also National Programme for Prevention and Control of Deafness.

REFERENCES

1 ICMR. Studies on Noise Pollution. ICMR Bulletin 1996; 26(8).

2 Alberti PW. Noise and the ear. In: Booth JB (ed). Scott Brown's Otolaryngology, Sixth Edition. Adult audiology Vol. 2/11/1. Bath: Bath Press, 2002.

3 Centre for occupational and environmental health. Bulletin of occupational and environmental health Jan–June 2002; 1(3), MAMC—New Delhi.

4 WHO. Our planet our health—Report of WHO Commission on health and environment. Geneva: WHO; 1992.

7

CHAPTER

8

Epidemiology and its Applications in Prevention and Control of Diseases and Epidemics

CONCEPT OF EPIDEMIOLOGY AND EPIDEMIOLOGY OF DISEASES

EPIDEMIOLOGY

"Think epidemiologically and act socially" holds true in all situations. Teachers should strive to develop epidemiological and analytical thinking amongst the students.

"Epidemiology is defined as the study of the distribution and determinants of health-related states or events in specified populations and the application of this study to control the health problems" (Last 1988).

Distribution: It means distribution of health events/states by *time*, *place* and *person* (TPP), *when* and *where* the health event occurred and *who* were affected most? TPP distribution is the function of *descriptive* epidemiology.

Determinants: Determinants mean causes or risk factors of health events and states. *Why* did the event occur? Or *what* causes the event to occur is a function of *analytical* epidemiology which is concerned with the search of causes and risk factors.

How the health event can be controlled and prevented is the function of *experimental* or *intervention* epidemiology.

The science of epidemiology focuses on "human population". There are 5 Ws in epidemiology. *What* is the problem, *who* suffers most, *where* does it occur, *when* does it occur and *why* does it occur (causes) and *how* to control it?

APPLICATION OF EPIDEMIOLOGY

The epidemiology is useful in:

1. Search of cause/causes of disease/diseases.
2. Helps to describe the health status of population or groups.
3. Helps to discover and bridge gaps in natural history of diseases.
4. Helps in controlling the diseases to break the weakest link in chain of transmission of communicable and non-communicable diseases.
5. Helps in planning of health programmes on evidence basis and setting up of health priorities.
6. Helps to evaluate health programmes and interventions.
7. Helps to determine the chances or probability of occurrence of disease/deaths and disability.
8. Helps in better management of health services and hospital services.
9. Helps to set-up cut-off levels between normal and abnormal population and establishes trigger levels for action or intervention.

EPIDEMIOLOGY OF COMMUNICABLE DISEASES (CCD)

The objective of understanding epidemiology of CCD is to reduce the incidence and prevalence of these diseases and it may help to eradicate a disease or eliminate a disease from the globe or geographical area, e.g. India.[1]

DEFINITION

A communicable or infectious disease is an illness caused by transmission of a specific infectious agent or its toxic products from an infected person or an animal to a susceptible host, either directly or indirectly through an intermediate, animal host, vector or inanimate environment (Last 1995) (Fig. 8.1).[1]

Disease burden due to communicable diseases is colossal and these diseases cause heavy mortality, disability and economic loss to the country. CCD burden in India accounts for 44% of *DALYs* losses. CCD continue to present the most important *acute health problems* in all the countries in the form of outbreaks and epidemics.

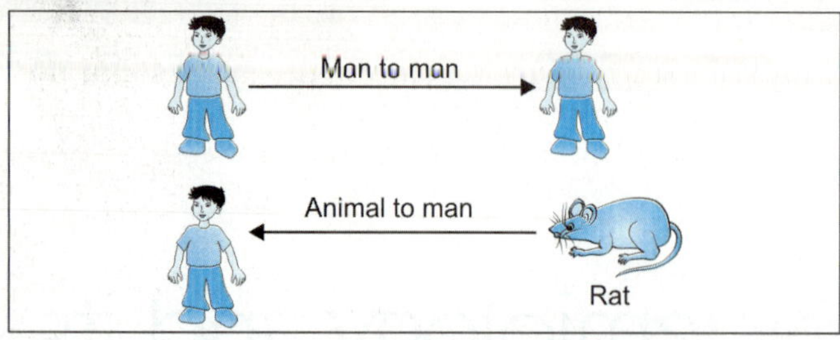

Fig. 8.1: Disease transmission

CHANGING PATTERN OF INFECTIOUS/ COMMUNICABLE DISEASES IN INDIA

- While smallpox, Guinea worm, have been eradicated, leprosy has been eliminated, maternal and neonatal tetanus eliminated and WHO has certified India as polio-free since 2014.
- The incidence of measles, hepatitis B and rheumatic fever has been significantly reduced.
- Diarrhoeal diseases, acute respiratory infections, tuberculosis and malaria incidence remain high with reduced mortality.
- Some infectious diseases like hepatitis B and C as also, HIV, HPV and JE have long-term consequences like chronic hepatitis, cancer and mental health.
- The emerging and re-emerging infectious diseases are global phenomena and most of these diseases result in widespread epidemics, with high mortality and morbidity. In addition to the immense suffering to the mankind these diseases, especially the epidemics, disturb international trade and economic development.

Emerging Infectious Diseases (IDs)[2, 3]—New IDs

Emerging infectious diseases are newly identified and previously unknown infections, or those spreading to new geographical areas, which cause public health problems either nationally or internationally. These include:

- HIV/AIDS burden: 2.11 million in India (2015).
- Severe acute respiratory syndrome (SARS).
- Middle East respiratory syndrome (MERS).
- Bird flu or avian influenza (H5N1 virus).
- Pandemic influenza (H1N1), 2009.
- Multidrug resistant tuberculosis (MDR/XDR).
- Hepatitis C, B and E.
- Japanese encephalitis.
- A new form of cholera—*Vibrio cholerae* 0139.
- Leptospirosis.
- *Nipah virus disease:* A recently emerged, zoonotic paramyxovirus was implicated as the cause of a highly fatal febrile human encephalitis in Malaysia and Singapore in 1991, Bangladesh in 2001–2004. Outbreaks from India have been reported from West Bengal in 2001 and recently in 2007.
- A variant of Creutzfeldt-Jakob disease: A disease of central nervous system.
- Zika virus infection is linked to microcephaly in newborn.
- Haemolytic uraemia syndrome caused by *E.coli* 0157: H7.
- Ebola viral disease or Ebola haemorrhagic fever.
- Hantavirus: Haemorrhagic fever with renal syndrome.
- A highly fatal respiratory disease caused by virus called Sin Nombre virus.
- Lassa fever.
- Crimean-congo haemorrhagic fever (CCHF).

Re-emerging Infectious Diseases[2, 3]

Re-emerging infectious diseases are known infections which had ceased to be major public health problems and now reappearing, often in epidemic proportions. These include:

- Tuberculosis due to its close association with HIV infection, a leading killer of adults in India, accounts for one-fifth of global incidence. Around 2.5 million is disease burden of which about 1 million are bacillary cases.
- Cholera: Occurs in epidemics.
- Dengue: Dengue haemorrhagic fever and dengue shock syndrome.
- Malaria: Drug resistance and rising incidence of Pf malaria.
- Chikungunya: Occurs in outbreaks.
- Plague: Outbreak was reported in India in 1994.
- Kala-azar: Endemic in four states of India.
- Meningococcal meningitis: Outbreaks.
- Diphtheria: Outbreaks.

Major Reasons for Emergence of Infectious Diseases

- High population growth, and density, uncontrolled and unplanned urbanization.
- Poor environmental sanitation.
- Migration of population.
- Natural disasters.
- Growing international trade, tourism and rapid travel.
- Alterations in microorganisms.
- Resistance to antimicrobials/antibiotics misuse.
- Insecticide resistance.
- Weak public health system and dysfunctional governments.
- Illiteracy and ignorance.

The World Health Day on 7th April 1997 chose a theme "Emerging infectious diseases—global response—global alert".

Emergence and re-emergence of many infectious diseases has resulted in more serious health problems in India as compared to many other developing nations. These diseases are responsible for significant number of deaths and illnesses and have caused massive disruption in the national economy.

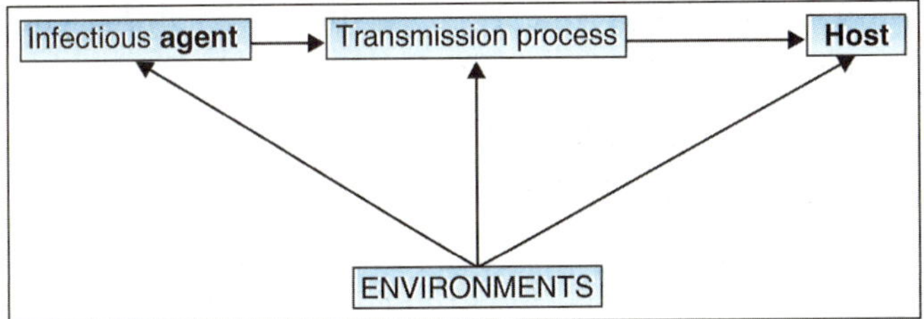

Components of chain of infection in CCD (epidemiological triad)

CHAIN OF INFECTION OR MODES OF TRANSMISSION

The communicable disease occurs as a result of the interaction of infectious *agent*, the transmission process, the *host* and *environments*.

Epidemiological Triad or Triangle

The epidemiological triad consists of an external *agent*, a *susceptible host* and an *environment* that bring the host and agent together. The disease results from the interaction between the agent and susceptible host in an environment that supports transmission of agent from source to host.

The *environments* influence all the three components of chain of infection. Knowledge of each component of chain of infection is helpful to understand the natural history of CCD for effective intervention and control of communicable diseases.

(A) INFECTIOUS AGENT

i Large number of agents like microbiological organisms (biological agents) is responsible for infection and occurrence of communicable diseases. These organisms live or develop and multiply in various hosts or in environments. Knowledge of these microorganisms helps to control the infection and CCD. The micro-organisms belong to different categories like bacteria, parasites, viruses, fungi and rickettsial organisms; besides spirochaetes.

ii Other agents—physical—heat, cold, radiation, noise etc.
   - Chemical agents—lead and silica, etc.
   - Lifestyles in noncommunicable diseases.

Pathogenicity

Pathogenicity of an agent is its ability to produce disease which can be measured by the ratio of number of persons developing clinical illness to the numbers exposed to infection.

Virulence

It is a measure of severity of disease, which can vary from high to low.

Infectivity

Infectivity is the ability of an organism to invade and produce infection in the host.

(B) TRANSMISSION PROCESS

This is the second important link in the chain of infection.

Transmission is defined as "spread of infectious agent through the environment, to another person, or from the reservoir and source".

Modes of Transmission

There are two major modes of transmission of an infectious agent:

1 Direct
2 Indirect

Direct Mode of Transmission

Here the method of transmission involves intimate or close contact between the infected person or reservoir of infection with susceptible host. Direct transmission occurs by:

- Touching
- Kissing
- Sexual intercourse
- Childbirth
- Breastfeeding
- Air-borne, short distance via droplets (by coughing, laughing, sneezing, spitting).
- Transfusion of blood and by unsafe injection
- Transplacental from mother to foetus
- Bite by rabid animal
- Organ transplantation
- Soil transmission (hookworm)

Indirect Mode of Transmission

- Vehicle-borne transmission (by contaminated food, water, and blood).
- Vector-borne transmission
- Air-borne transmission
- Fomite transmission
- Unclean hands

Direct Transmission

Here the method of transmission involves direct and intimate contact or close contact between the infected person or reservoir of infection with the healthy susceptible person. The infectious organisms get transferred from an infected person to the healthy person. Best example of contact transmission is by sexual intercourse, when a healthy person with a high-risk behaviour indulges into unsafe sex with multiple sexual partners or with commercial sex workers, who may harbour HIV infection, may acquire HIV infection. Healthy persons get HIV infection from HIV-infected persons like commercial sex workers or other persons known to have HIV infection. In an infected individual, the HIV is present in body fluids and secretions including semen and vaginal secretions. The HIV infection gets transmitted from men to women,

women to men and men to men by unprotected sexual intercourse (heterosexual and homosexual). Over 85.8% of HIV transmission is through unprotected sexual intercourse. People infected with HIV are both infected and infectious for life. Thus, HIV infection in nature is being maintained in human population by direct transmission of virus from person to person. The virus is fragile and cannot survive outside human body for long (Table 8.1).

Table 8.1: Sources of infections

Disease	Source(s)
HIV/AIDS	Blood, semen, vaginal fluids and breast milk
Cholera and hepatitis A and E	Contaminated water and food
Tuberculosis	Sputum
Food poisoning	Contaminated food

All sexually transmitted infections (STIs) like syphilis, gonorrhoea, trichomonal infections, human papillomavirus are transmitted by unprotected sexual intercourse.

Implications

The implication of sexual transmission involves modification of risky sexual behaviour of young people, which is an uphill task. Adolescents and young people account for 40% of all new HIV infections and hence changing their sexual behaviour is a significant strategy in control programme of HIV epidemic, unless that happens the epidemic will continue to spread. HIV/AIDS has no cure.

Nosocomial Transmission

It is cross infection acquired in a hospital. Infections are considered nosocomial if they appear 48 hours or more after hospital admission or within 30 days of discharge. This could be due to lack of practice of universal precautions by providers of health services.

Transfusion of Blood

HIV and AIDS can also be transmitted through unsafe blood transfusion. Other diseases, which can be transmitted by unsafe blood transfusion include malaria, hepatitis B, hepatitis C, syphilis and HIV.

Screen all the blood collected in the blood bank before transfusion and discard those, which are positive for HIV, hepatitis B, hepatitis C, syphilis and malaria.

Transplacental (Vertical) Transmission

HIV can also be transmitted from HIV positive pregnant mother to foetus through placenta and during the birth and after to newborn through vaginal secretions and through breast milk respectively.

Risk of mother to child transmission (MTCT) can be controlled by multidrug ARV prophylaxis to HIV positive pregnant women lifelong period and nevirapine to newborn daily for six weeks. Breastfeeding to baby is not indicated if mother is HIV positive.[4] Syphilis and toxoplasmosis can also be transmitted through placenta.

Transmission in Tuberculosis (Air-borne Transmission)

TB like common cold is an air-borne infection. TB spreads through air from one person to another when a person with tuberculosis of lung (open case) coughs, sneezes, talks or even sings or laughs, the bacteria are sprayed out into the air as infectious droplets. These droplets dry up rapidly and the smallest of them remain suspended in the air for several hours. People nearby (as household or family contacts) may inhale these bacteria and become infected. Exposure to an infectious case of TB is a prerequisite for acquiring TB infection. If there is an open case in the family and he indiscriminately coughs, he can infect others in the family and most susceptibles are **young children** and other contacts in the family. Thus, tuberculosis spreads through close contacts as also the infection can spread to long distances. Droplet nuclei disperse rapidly throughout the air in a room and can be carried wherever air currents take them.

Implications

Preventing infectious cases from producing droplets by covering mouth and nose during coughing is very effective method of reducing the probability of transmission. Collection of sputum and its safe disposal prevents spread of tuberculosis. Person should spit in sputum cups, which contain sputum, can be burnt in a pit at a safe distance from home.

There is no need of isolation of a case of tuberculosis. Similarly, opening windows during and after cough inducing procedures or in hospital wards is one of the most efficient means of reducing probability of exposed persons becoming infected.

Every sputum positive patient can infect 10–15 individuals in a year, if left untreated; hence early treatment and regular treatment with DOTS strategy makes 80% of persons non-infectious within two months of treatment, thus it reduces the pool of infectious cases in the population.[5]

High density of population and overcrowding in urban slums increases the chances of spread of tuberculosis. These populations are risk population for tuberculosis apart from many other diseases.

Similarly, scabies spreads from person to person contacts and rabies by rabid animal bite.

Indirect Transmission

Vehicle-borne Transmission

Drinking unsafe water contaminated with human and animal excreta, by agricultural and industrial activities are common features in India and other developing countries. Polluted and contaminated water becomes major source of disease transmission in urban and rural areas. Human beings are the biggest polluters of water supplies and sources of water. Human beings and animals can act as hosts to bacterial, viral or protozoal organisms that cause many diseases. Indiscriminate defecation is quite common. The city of New Delhi alone dumps 200 million litres of raw sewage and 20 million litres of industrial wastes into Yamuna River everyday as the river passes through the city on its way to the Ganges.

Worldwide 2.3 billion people suffer from diseases that are linked to polluted water problems. Water-related and water-borne diseases kill millions of people each year. Nearly half of the urban residents in Asia suffer from one or more of the main diseases associated with inadequate provision of water and sanitation. Problem of sanitation is acute in rural areas and water-borne diseases include diarrhoeal diseases, cholera, typhoid, dysentery, hepatitis A and E and polio. Diarrhoeal diseases are the major water-borne malady responsible for 90% of the health problems related to water supply and sanitation. An estimated 4 billion cases of diarrhoeal diseases occur every year, causing 3 to 4 million deaths, mostly among children. Other diseases like cholera and hepatitis A and E may occur in epidemics and become endemic when there is poor food hygiene, lack of sanitation or unsafe drinking water. Contaminated food can produce food poisoning and many other diseases.

Implications

The implications of vehicle transmission (transmission through contaminated water and food) are quite serious. The challenge is to provide safe water, free from germs with safe levels of fluorides, heavy metals and other contaminants, to people. "Safe water for all" is the biggest challenge. Every year in India, many areas report occurrence of outbreaks of hepatitis E, A and cholera as also diarrhoeal diseases apart from food poisoning. These occurrences indicate regular and continuous contamination of water supplies.

The problem of safe disposal of human excreta is quite acute. There are no easy solutions because of rising population.

One observes defecation grounds everywhere and anywhere leading to widespread soil pollution and water pollution. Treatment and safe disposal of sewage is complex and costs lot of money and unsafe disposal to watercourses, rivers, or canals or to fields poses problem of water pollution and soil pollution. Faecal matter comes back to us through water and vegetables. Hence, vehicle transmission in epidemiology is a substantial challenge.

Vector-borne Transmission

Diseases, which are spread by insects, are called vector transmission or vector-borne diseases (Table 8.2).

The disease-producing organisms live, multiply, develop and complete the part of their life cycle in a vector. The **infected vector** spreads these organisms to human beings by injecting these to human circulation.

Table 8.2: Important vectors in India

Infected of vector	*Disease transmitted*
Anopheline mosquitoes	Malaria
Aedes aegypti	Dengue haemorrhagic fever and dengue shock syndrome, zika virus and yellow fever (not present in India)
Culex vishnui	Japanese encephalitis
Culex quinquefasciatus	Filaria (Bancroftian)
Sandfly	Kala-azar (Leishmaniasis)
Rat flea (*Xenopsylla* genus)	Bubonic plague
Body louse	Typhus fever

A disease-producing organism may simply multiply in the vector such as dengue virus multiplies in *Aedes aegypti* mosquitoes and *Pasteurella pestis* multiplies in rat flea and these vectors spread these organisms to healthy human beings. This is called *propagative transmission.*

A disease producing organism such as microfilaria undergoes development in the body of *Culex* mosquito but does not multiply in vector. Such a spread is known as *cyclo-developmental transmission.*

A disease producing organism like malaria parasite undergoes development as well as multiplication in the body of Anopheles mosquito and mosquitoes spread the disease from one person to another. We call this transmission as *cyclo-propagative transmission.*

Vector-borne diseases like malaria, filaria, kala-azar, Japanese encephalitis, dengue haemorrhagic fever (DHF), and dengue shock syndrome (DSS) and chikungunya are examples of vector-borne or vector-transmitted diseases. These diseases are significant problems in India and pose constant threat of epidemics and outbreaks leading to high mortality and economic loss. Malaria and filaria are endemic in India.

Houseflies transmit diseases by *mechanically* transporting infected organisms from faecal matter to uncovered food and eatables.

Implications

Vector-borne disease transmission in India is quite rampant. Vector-borne diseases like malaria and filaria are major public health problems in the country. Malaria is endemic in the country and 1.49 million cases were reported in the year 2010. Of these, 0.77 million were due to *Plasmodium falciparum* (Pf). Outbreaks of malaria have come to surface every now and then. In view of significant problem of vector-borne diseases, national vector-borne disease control programme (NVBDCP) has been launched in the year 2003–04 by convergence of ongoing programmes of national anti-malaria programme, filaria, Japanese encephalitis (JE), kala-azar, dengue and dengue haemorrhagic fever (DHF) and chikungunya.

Vector control is the major strategy in all the above mentioned vector-borne diseases. Anti-vector measures include source reduction, i.e. controlling breeding places, anti-larval measures and anti-adult measures besides personal protection measures like use of impregnated bed nets. Integrated vector control measures involve biological control measures as well; which are environment-friendly. The major challenge to control vectors of diseases is to *control the environments*, i.e. waste water management in urban and rural area. Insecticides as weapon against malaria vectors have become blunt due to development of **resistance**. Anti-larval measures are extremely costlier and labour intensive.

Air-borne Transmission

Tuberculosis spreads through fine droplets in those persons who are close by to a case of tuberculosis if the open case does not observe precautions. However, tuberculosis is not as easily transmitted as certain other air-borne infectious diseases. Most TB infections are acquired by continued exposure rather than casual contact, because respiratory defence mechanisms can kill small number of mycobacteria.

TB bacilli can remain viable in wet sputum for months and in dried sputum for weeks. Fine droplets containing viable TB germs can reach through air far away from index case to distant place and affect the people who are not close to the index case. Therefore, it becomes imperative that indiscriminate spitting by open cases should be controlled and sputum disposal should be appropriate and most important is to put the persons on treatment and make them non-infectious to reduce the pool of infection in the community.

Influenza is another example of air-borne transmission.

Parenteral Transmission

Parenteral transmission occurs by use of common needles and syringes or sharing of needle and syringe amongst **injecting drug-users.** This is the common mode of spread of HIV in some of the North-Eastern states of India. Overall 1.7% of HIV infections are transmitted by this way. Apart from HIV, many other dreaded diseases like hepatitis B and hepatitis C are also transmitted by unsafe injections.

Implications

The implications of such a transmission are to control the drug menace, change the behaviour and provide safe needles and syringe services (safe injections).

Fomite Transmission

Fomite transmission means transmission of CCD through contaminated articles—instruments, linen, dressings, beddings, soiled clothes, handkerchiefs, toys, books and utensils. "Contamination" means the presence of infectious agent or matter on human body/animal body or surface. To prevent fomite transmission it is essential to use sterile linen and instruments and disinfect the contaminated articles and observe personal hygiene above all.

Hands

Unclean hands or soiled hands often transmit faeco-oral diseases. Children quite often put their soiled and dirty hands, fingers in their mouth and similarly if adults do not wash their hands after defecation, they are liable to eat with dirty hands and thus ingest dangerous germs and get diseases—most often diarrhoea and worm infestation. Handwashing also reduces the risk of respiratory infection including swine flu and influenza besides Middle East respiratory syndrome. "Namaste" is much better than "Hand-shake" and well accepted in Indian culture.

Implications

Handwashing practice should become universal in children and adults before eating and after defecation. Handwashing itself reduces incidence of diarrhoeal diseases by about one-third.

(C) HOST IN CHAIN OF INFECTION

The host is the third link in the chain of transmission. Host is a person or animal that provides a suitable place for an infectious agent to grow and multiply under natural conditions.

Reservoir and Source of Infection in CCD

The reservoir in CCD is a person or an animal or an insect, plant, soil or substance who harbours the infectious organism of a CCD and acts as a source of infection in the community.[6,7] The disease producing organism lives, multiplies, develops and depends primarily for its survival in the reservoir. The person who harbours disease-producing organism is called host. The reservoir acts as natural habitat of the organism. The natural habitat of an infectious agent is called its "reservoir" and it may be humans, animals and environments.

The "reservoir" is defined as "man, animals, arthropods, plants, soil or inanimate organic matter/substance (or combination of these) in which the infectious agent lives and multiplies, and depends for its survival, reproduces itself in such a manner that it can be transmitted to susceptible host". Man himself is the most frequent reservoir of infectious agents pathogenic for man.

"Source" of infection is the person (living) or object (non-living) from which the host acquires the agent.

or

"Source of infection: The thing, person, object or substance from which an infectious agent passes immediately to a host."

Knowledge of both the reservoir and source is necessary for control measures.

Common reservoirs and sources of infection, some examples:

Disease	Reservoir	Source
Tuberculosis	Man	Sputum
HIV/AIDS	Man	Body fluids and secretions
Malaria	Man and mosquito	Infected mosquito
Rabies	Dog and other animals	Saliva
Measles	Man	Droplets
JE	Pig and birds	Infected mosquitoes
Cholera	Man	Unsafe water and food
Plague	Rodents	Infected flea
Typhoid	Man	Unsafe water and food
Tetanus	Soil	Soil

Significance

If we know the reservoir and source of infection, the chain of infection can be broken and CCD can be effectively controlled. Where man is the reservoir of infection of CCD the attempt is made to treat man to eliminate the infectious organisms or reduce their population to such a low level where they cannot produce disease.

Example: In tuberculosis we treat the reservoir (men/women suffering from tuberculosis) by chemotherapy or DOTS to render the reservoir non-infectious.

Treating malaria in man means controlling infection in the reservoir to make man non-infectious.

If the reservoir and source of infection is an animal or an insect, attempt is made to kill insects with insecticide or not to allow breeding of mosquitoes (source reduction) and control the animals population by various methods (e.g. sterilization of dogs, or vaccination of dogs against rabies or licensing of dogs, and killing of rodents).

Where the source of infection is inanimate reservoir like contaminated water, we treat the water by boiling or by chlorination to destroy the disease-producing organisms in order to prevent the water-borne diseases. Safe water supply to community means prevention of many water-borne diseases.

Host factors are important in distribution and determinants of communicable disease. Host factors include age, sex, marital status, nutritional and immunization status, apart from literacy, occupation and past experience or exposure with infection and risk behaviour. The occurrence and distribution of CCD vary in persons. All are not at equal risk. This can be better understood by some examples. Who is at risk of contracting HIV and tuberculosis? The answers are:

Age and Sex

Young people are disproportionately affected by HIV and AIDS. Around 40% of all new HIV infections are in young people aged 15–24 years, the range in which most people start their sexual life.

High-risk Groups

For HIV and AIDS, high-risk groups are injecting drug-users (IDUs), commercial sex workers and persons who receive repeated blood transfusion, persons having tuberculosis and persons having sexually transmitted diseases and men having sex with men.

Implication

Targeted interventions are focused on high-risk groups under the National AIDS Control Programme.

Presence of STD

There is strong evidence that men and women with genital ulcer disease or urethral discharge are at increased risk of acquiring and transmitting HIV. High prevalence of STD means high prevalence of unprotected sexual intercourse.

Behaviour of Host

Pre-marital sex, extramarital sex and having multiple sexual partners are risk factors in HIV and AIDS. Cultural and behaviour pattern of host-like men having sex with men also contributes to HIV transmission.

Immunity

HIV destroys the immune system. There is no immunity against HIV infection. Host immunity is a mechanism, which protects it from diseases.

Immunity is acquired by having natural infection, e.g. an attack of measles confers lifelong immunity provided the child survives after an attack of measles. Similarly, immunity can be acquired by having measles immunization at the age of 9 months, it provides sufficient immunity against measles. Improved nutritional status also builds to fight infection in a better way. Therefore, unimmunized children are susceptible hosts for occurrence of communicable diseases.

Mechanism of Entry of Infectious Organism in Host

- The infectious organism can enter in the body of host through intact skin and mucous membrane. Hookworm larvae can penetrate intact skin. Rabies virus can enter the body through wound and intact mucous membrane.
- Through oral cavity and gastrointestinal tract, contaminated water and food having infectious organisms enter through mouth and gastrointestinal tract.
- Through respiratory system: *Mycobacterium tuberculosis* enters through respiratory system.
- By insect bite, the disease producing organisms can be injected to bloodstream.

- Parenteral transmission occurs by use of unsafe needles and syringes as also through unsafe blood transfusion and through needle stick injury. Thus, the disease-producing organisms enter human host through several routes specific to each disease.

Host Reactions

Once the infectious organisms enter human host, the host reacts and host defence system comes into action. There are following possibilities (Flowchart 8.1).

Flowchart 8.1: Host reactions

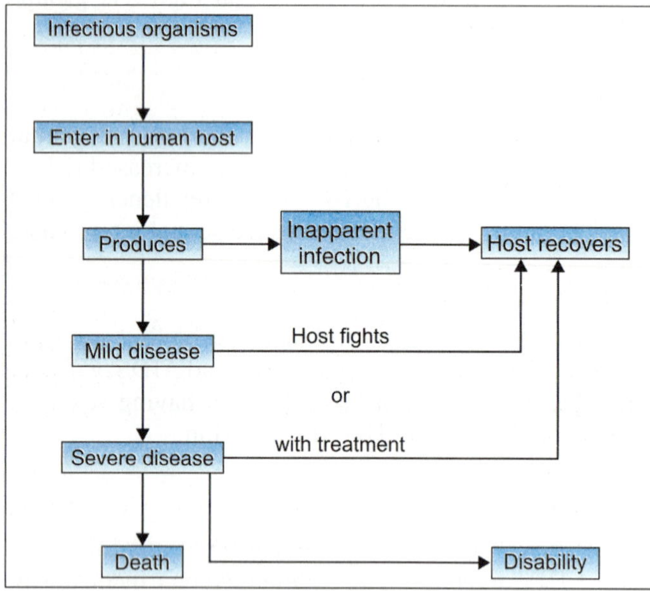

Infection

The infection is not equivalent to disease. Infection means the entry, development or multiplication of an infectious agent in the body of man or animal that may constitute a public health risk. Infection is not synonymous with disease as explained below.

TB Infection

Once a person breathes in, the air that contains droplets contaminated with TB bacilli, most of the larger droplets settle in the nose or throat where they are unlikely to establish infection. However, fine droplets containing as few as 1–3 TB bacilli may reach the alveoli. Within alveoli, the bacilli are ingested by alveolar macrophages and other phagocytes. Live virulent bacilli multiply within macrophages, which get destroyed in the process. The bacilli are subsequently ingested by other tissue macrophages. Bacterial multiplication cannot be stopped within those non-activated macrophages. Within 2–4 weeks after infection, the host mounts a specific cell-mediated immunity that will arrest TB infection in more than 90% of infected individuals.

TB infection means that tubercle bacilli are viable within the body but are not multiplying and causing disease due to body immune system. People who have TB infection but not TB disease are not infectious; in other words, they cannot spread the infection to others. They look and feel quite healthy persons. Infection in a person can be detected by tuberculin test. Prevalence of TB infection in India is about 30%.

TB Disease

Only 10% of TB infected persons have the chances of developing disease in their lifetime; however, if HIV infection occurs to infected people, it enhances the risk of lifetime occurrence of disease to 60%. HIV and TB infection is a deadly combination.[7]

In tuberculosis disease, a person develops pulmonary tuberculosis or brain tuberculosis, bone tuberculosis or tuberculosis of any other organ. The course of disease depends upon treatment and intervention. The severity of disease will depend upon host factors and agent factors.

Carriers

In some situation, the inapparent infection in host leads to carrier state. Carriers are infected persons who are apparently healthy persons, do not shows any clinical signs and symptoms of disease but harbour disease producing organisms and continue to discharge the organisms from their body. Various types of carriers have been described.

Incubatory, Convalescent, and Chronic Carriers

Incubatory carriers are those who shed the disease-producing organisms during the incubation period of disease, convalescent carriers are those who continue to shed the organisms during the recovery stage of the disease.

In some diseases like typhoid fever, the carrier state may persist for a very long time and such persons are called chronic carriers. Chronic carrier state persists in hepatitis B and C.

(D) ENVIRONMENTS IN CHAIN OF INFECTION

Environments (Δ)

It is an aggregate of all the external conditions and factors, which affect the life and development of an organism. Environmental degradation is leading to development of many of the diseases. Protection and promotion of healthy environments is a global concern.

Environment is getting worse because of rapid population growth, and increased pressure on natural resources; threatening public health and development. The most important concern is water shortages, soil exhaustion, loss of forest leading to air and water pollution, besides soil pollution and degradation of coast lines. As the population grows, improving living standards without destroying the environments is a global concern. The environments can be categorized into *physical* environments (water, air, temperature, humidity, radiation, etc.), *biological* environments (all living organisms, plants and animals), *chemical* environments (agriculture and industrial chemicals) and *social* environments (men around men).

Environments are the major *determinant of health* and *disease* in the chain of infection. The environment affect the life and development of infectious organisms or agents of disease, it influences the transmission process and also affects the host. Environments form the *fulcrum* in chain of infection. Environments can tilt the pendulum of chain of infection to favourable or unfavourable side. Over 60–80% of infectious diseases are related to bad physical environments like contaminated water supplies, poor drainage system, widespread filth and insanitary conditions and indiscriminate defecation. This leads to faeco-oral transmission of diseases in epidemic form and many diseases get rooted as endemic diseases. Soil pollution has led to soil transmitted helminthic diseases apart from killer diarrhoeal diseases in children.

Implications

The challenge is to provide safe drinking water, safe disposal of human, and animal excreta, source reduction or control of breeding of insects or vectors of disease transmission. In summary, protection of environments and population control is a global emergency. In controlling communicable diseases treating environments becomes a necessity in addition to treatment of sick people. Hospitals treat patients while an epidemiologist treats both environments and patients and biggest concern is to keep the people healthy-free from disease.

PATTERN OF COMMUNICABLE DISEASES

An illness due to specific infectious agent or its toxic products, which arises through transmission of that agent or its products from the reservoir to a susceptible host, either directly as from an infected person or animal or indirectly through the agency of an intermediate animal host, vector, or the inanimate environment. The communicable disease occurs in various patterns.

1. Sporadic

Sporadic occurrence refers to a disease that occurs infrequently and irregularly.

2. Endemic

It means stable pattern of occurrence of a disease in a given population. It refers to constant presence and/or usual prevalence of a disease or infections agent in a population within a geographical area. It signifies that factors and conditions for survival of infectious agent of that disease are always favourable in that community and regular transmission goes on with some seasonal variation. The prevalence and incidence is maintained at expected level.

Examples: Malaria and tuberculosis are endemic in India and similarly leprosy and filaria are also endemic.

3. Hyper-endemic

Refers to persistent high level of disease occurrence.

Level of Endemicity

The level of endemicity of a disease is not uniform in all the geographical areas, some geographical areas show high level of endemicity or prevalence while other areas may show low level of endemicity. For example, Haryana is low endemic area for leprosy. Some other states like Chhattisgarh, Odisha, Uttar Pradesh, Bihar, Maharashtra have very high prevalence rates, while the states like West Bengal, Andhra Pradesh have high prevalence rates. Level of endemicity can be determined on the basis of prevalence rate or incidence rates (for cholera, malaria and diarrhoeal diseases, etc.). When conditions become favourable or if the number of susceptible persons in the population increase or in conditions like heavy rains, floods and other natural disasters the **endemic disease becomes epidemic** in endemic areas. Outbreaks of cholera, diarrhoea and malaria are quite common in India.

4. Epidemic of CCD

An *epidemic* or outbreak is the occurrence in a community of illnesses of similar nature, clearly in excess of normal expectancy and derived from a common or propagated source.

While an *outbreak* is usually limited to a small focal area, an epidemic covers large geographical area and has more than one focal point.

There is yet another definition of an *outbreak*—"Occurrence of two or more epidemiologically linked cases (occurrence at the same time and same location as other confirmed cases) of a disease of outbreak potential (e.g. measles, cholera, dengue, JE, AFP and plague)".

The number of cases indicating presence of an *epidemic* varies according to the infectious agent, size and type of population exposed, previous experience or lack of exposure to the disease, and time and place of occurrence. Epidemicity is thus relative to usual frequency of the disease in the same area, among the specified population, at the same season of the year.

A single case of wild poliovirus is an epidemic or outbreak, because of its significance and rapid spread and many inapparent infections in the community. If an unknown disease or disease which is absent from an area for quite long time is introduced, even a single case of that disease will constitute an *epidemic* occurrence.

Example: HIV epidemic, hepatitis E and A epidemic and JE epidemic.

EPIDEMIC—PATTERNS OF CCD

Point Common Source Epidemic

In a point source epidemic, the susceptible individuals are exposed more or less simultaneously to one source of infection. This results in very rapid increase in the number of cases often in a few days/hours. The cholera outbreak is an example of point source epidemic. Similarly, hepatitis E and A are point source outbreaks. If the population is exposed over a relatively brief period, so that everyone who becomes ill does so within one incubation period. The resulting **graph** or **epidemic curve** has a steep rise and gradual decline. In some common source outbreaks, cases may have been exposed over a period of days, weeks and longer. In a continuous common source outbreak, the range of exposure and range of incubation period tends to flatten and widen the peaks of epidemic curve.

Contagious Epidemic (Propagated Outbreak)

In this epidemic or outbreak, the disease is passed from one person to other person and the initial rise in the number of cases is slower. The example is measles outbreak. Measles outbreaks are commonly observed in children who have not been immunized against measles. In the urban slum areas having dense population, the children are exposed to more risk of outbreak of measles if they are left over for measles immunization. In propagated outbreaks, increasing number of cases in each generation—should have a series of progressively taller peaks, one incubation apart (10–14 days apart).

Vector-borne Epidemics/Outbreaks

JE produces sporadic cases, one or two cases in a village but these are widespread while DHF and DSS outbreaks produce many cases and affect all persons.

Outbreaks of vector-borne diseases may result from sufficient presence of vectors, sufficient prevalence of infection and human vector interaction.

5. Pandemic

When the epidemic occurs in more than one country or widely spread over the globe it is called pandemic. HIV/AIDS is global in distribution and several countries of the world are in grip of epidemic; hence, HIV pandemic is going on currently. Over seven pandemics of cholera have been witnessed in the world. Influenza spreads like wild fire and it sweeps over different countries very rapidly. Pandemics have been correlated with rapid movements of persons from one country to another by air, sea and land routes. Recently, SARS pandemic was observed in several countries and bird flu pandemic is yet another example besides swine flu pandemic and ebola pandemic.

CONTROL OF COMMUNICABLE DISEASES (CCDs)

Knowledge of the chain of infection helps us to control communicable diseases.

The control of CCD has received priority attention right from independence. Vaccines and effective antibiotics for prevention of CCD were the major factors responsible for steep decline in crude death rates. However, morbidity due to CCD continues to be high. Deteriorating urban sanitation, poor liquid and solid waste management and overcrowding have contributed to increasing incidence of CCD. Emerging antibiotic resistance is a serious problem.

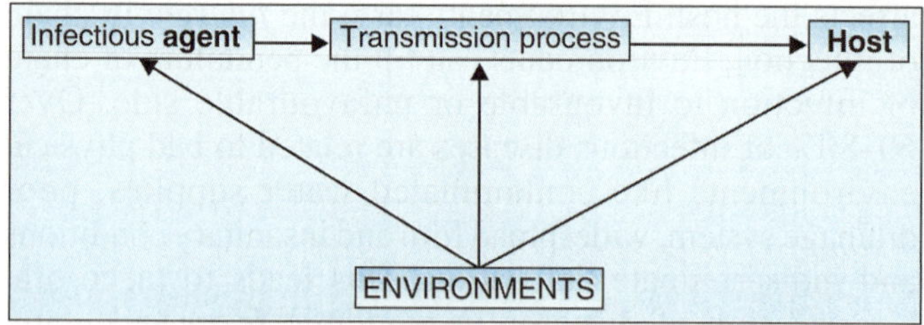

Epidemiological triad (triangle)

Control of Infectious Agents in the Environments

The infectious agent of a disease after exit from host lives, multiplies and develops in environments and gets transmitted through the environment readily to human host. Therefore, control of the infectious organism at source is an important strategy. This means *treating* the *environments* (water and excreta).

1. Controlling Sources of Infection

i Supply of safe drinking water by treatment and chlorination of water, and pasteurization of milk.

ii Safe disposal of human excreta and animal excreta by sewerage system, sanitary latrines, compost pits/manure pits and sewage treatment.

iii Integrated control of vectors of diseases—by source reduction and anti-larval and anti-adult measures.

iv Animals—vaccinate dogs against rabies and animal birth control.

v Rodent control measures—trapping and killing.

vi Hospital waste management.

vii *Disinfection:* The killing of infectious agents outside the body by chemical or physical means is known as disinfection. Concurrent disinfection is the application of disinfectant as soon as possible after the discharge of infectious material from the body of an infected person. All soiled articles with secretion, excretions of infectious patient are treated with suitable chemical, e.g. hypochlorite solution 1% or other suitable chemicals: Phenol, cresol, dettol, cetavlon, savlon, alcohol and iodine. Washing with detergents, bleaching powder solution, steaming, sun drying and autoclaving are common methods of disinfection of soiled articles. If one can afford these can be burnt or incinerated as dangerous waste material.

2. Immunization Against CCD

Massive programmes of immunization for vaccine preventable diseases (VPDs) have been launched in the country to control communicable diseases like polio, measles, whooping cough, diphtheria, tetanus neonatorum and tuberculosis. Hepatitis B vaccine has been launched in India. Newer vaccines against other diseases have been launched. The purpose of immunization is to ensure high level of coverage and to prevent outbreaks as also to reduce the incidence of disease and ultimately to eliminate and eradicate the communicable diseases.

3. Control of Infectious Agent in Host

1 ***Reservoir control:*** To reduce the pool of infected persons and cases of communicable diseases like tuberculosis, leprosy, filaria, malaria, early diagnosis and prompt treatment is the strategy under various national programmes of CCD. Complete and early treatment of disease by standard treatment protocol in man renders the reservoir non-infectious.

4. Practice of Chemoprophylaxis

- In high-risk areas of *P. falciparum* malaria, like Africa, chemoprophylaxis in pregnant women is recommended to prevent morbidity and mortality in pregnant women due to *P. falciparum* malaria as also to reduce the incidence of low birth weight babies. Tablet chloroquine once a week after first trimester has been advocated. Malaria prophylaxis in high-risk areas has been recommended for travellers and army personnels.
- *Use of isoniazid as prophylaxis:* In children who are in contact with sputum positive case, use of chemoprophylaxis is well established. Six months of daily isoniazid alone or 2 months of rifampicin and pyrazinamide are both found to be useful regimens for these children.

  However, infectious case is priority, i.e. treat all sputum positive tuberculosis cases, to reduce reservoir.

5. Surveillance

Surveillance means detection of cases at the earliest and treat them promptly at home or at the facility (Hospital, Health Centre and Sub-centre).

a **Surveillance of CCD:** The purpose of surveillance in CCD *is to collect information for action*. National surveillance programme for malaria control, polio-eradication and control of HIV/AIDS has already been mounted in the country. In addition, all institutions in India are required to report cases and deaths of 20 communicable diseases every month to the next higher level. The state bureau of health intelligence/vital statistical units consolidate this information to transmit to Central Bureau of Health Intelligence (CBHI). The report is published every year.

Malaria programme has one of the best surveillance programme in the country. To promote the principle of convergence the Government of India has approved national vector-borne disease control programme and hopefully surveillance against other diseases like JE, dengue will get strengthened besides malaria, filaria and kala-azar.

National project on integrated disease surveillance programme (IDSP) for communicable and non-communicable diseases has been initiated in the year 2004 to predict and control outbreaks/epidemics.

The basic purpose of surveillance at local level is to initiate prompt action to control outbreaks of diseases and prevent occurrence of epidemics. Epidemiological unit at the level of district plays pivotal role to build local support to all Peripheral Units (PHC and CHCs). National Project 2004 (IDSP) envisages strengthening laboratory services at district level. Routine reporting system at village, subcentre and PHC level is critical for early detection of outbreaks and action at local level by Rapid Response Teams.

b **Entomological surveillance and vector control.**

c **Environmental surveillance:** Isolation of polio-viruses form sewage samples, air samples, water samples, etc. for air and water pollution respectively.

6. Environmental modification and manipulation

7. Notification

Notification of diseases: When reporting is required by law, the diseases or conditions to be reported are known as *notifiable* diseases. Cases and deaths of 20 communicable diseases in India are reported every month by all health facilities. It helps to control the spread of diseases. Cholera, yellow fever and plague are internationally notifiable diseases, besides other public health emergencies of international concern.

8. Quarantine

a *Complete quarantine:* Quarantine means limitation of freedom of movement of such well persons or domestic animals, who have been exposed to communicable disease, for a period of time equal to the longest usual incubation period of the disease, in such a manner as to prevent effective contact with those not so exposed.

b *Modified quarantine:* It is a selective, partial limitation of freedom of movement of persons or domestic animals. Examples are exclusion of children from school, restriction of military population to the post or to quarters.

c *Isolation:* Practice of isolation applies to *cases* of communicable diseases. "Isolation" means separation for the period of communicability of infected persons from other persons, in such places and under such conditions as will prevent the direct or indirect conveyance of the infectious agent from infected persons to persons who are susceptible or who may spread the agent to others. This also applies to animals, affected baggage, containers, goods, etc. Isolation of patients has but a little effect in limiting the spread of many diseases for instance poliomyelitis, and tuberculosis. Practice of isolation is limited. Some states have infectious disease hospitals and others practice isolation in segregated rooms.

9. Education and Behaviour Change

Improving personal hygiene practices like washing hands, eating clean food and drinking clean water, wearing shoes and safe sex will prevent many communicable diseases. Use of impregnated bed nets prevents bite of mosquitoes and prevents vector-borne diseases.

Control of Outbreaks of CCD/Infectious Diseases

Communicable diseases like malaria, JE, DHF and DSS, hepatitis E and A, hepatitis B and diarrhoeal diseases quite often occur in epidemic proportion. Many local and focal outbreaks are being reported quite frequently; hence, control of outbreaks of these diseases is an essential requirement. Local capacity should be built in for rapid response and recognition of outbreaks. Standard protocols have been evolved for control of outbreaks and general guidelines issued by NICD should be followed.

Other Measures

1. *Legislation:* Epidemic disease Act of 1897, and notification helps control of CCD. The Act of 1897 is being replaced by Public Health (prevention, control and management of epidemics, bioterrorism and disasters) Bill of 2005, which is most comprehensive and stringent.
2. *Observe international health regulations (IHRs):* Observe international regulations on notification, immunization and quarantine measures. Internationally notifiable disease, include cholera, plague and yellow fever besides notification of an event/events that may constitute a public health emergency of international concern (WHO, 2005). All nations are required to report these diseases to WHO regularly. The diseases like louse-borne typhus fever, relapsing fever, paralytic polio, malaria and viral influenza are under WHO surveillance. IHR have been revised in 2005 and the scope has been enlarged to cover public health emergencies.
3. *Observing universal practices and precautions:* Prevents occurrence and spread of CCD.
4. Train and employ more epidemiologists and public health experts.
5. Strengthen health systems.

Specific Measures for Control of HIV Epidemic

Massive control programme for HIV and AIDS has been launched ever since 1986. The objective is to reduce the spread of epidemic of HIV and to reduce the disease load in the community. The major strategies include:

i. *Targeted interventions for groups at high-risk:* Provide counselling, condoms and treatment of sexually transmitted infections.
ii. Control of sexually transmitted diseases/infections.
iii. Information education and communication for universal awareness on prevention methods.

Blood Safety

Blood safety and screening of all blood units for HIV, malaria, hepatitis B, syphilis, hepatitis C is mandatory now. This would prevent spread of these diseases.

Injection Safety

Injection safety is essential to prevent the spread of hepatitis B, hepatitis C, malaria and HIV.

Universal Safe Practices/Precautions

Universal precautions and practices should be routinely ensured in all the institutions. Hospitals waste disposal should be ensured after disinfection. These steps would prevent transmission of infections and communicable disease.

As a result of ongoing epidemiological, demographic and lifestyles transition in the country, NCDs have emerged as major cause of morbidity and mortality.

Non-communicable diseases cover wide range of heterogeneous conditions affecting different organs and systems of different age and socioeconomic groups. Over the last two decades, morbidity and mortality due to cardiovascular diseases, mental disorders, cancer and trauma have been rising due to following causes.

Causes

1. Rise in life expectancy and increasing number of senior citizens.
2. *Changing lifestyles:* Faulty diet, use of alcohol, sedentary life—physical inactivity and rising stress-leading to obesity and stress-related problems.
3. Use of tobacco.
4. Exposure to environmental risk factors—air pollution.
5. Increasing population and rise in population of vehicles, automobiles and trauma incidence.

Data from NSSO, 52nd round showed that tobacco use (smoking and smokeless-tobacco) and alcohol use are higher in the poorest 20% of income quintile (Fig. 8.2) and hence, the prevalence of tobacco-related non-communicable diseases is likely to be high in this income group.

Implications

In view of the chronic morbidity and high cost involved in the management of non-communicable diseases attention need to be focussed on prevention, early detection and appropriate management. Further, these diseases cause lot of disability and dependency and disease burden.

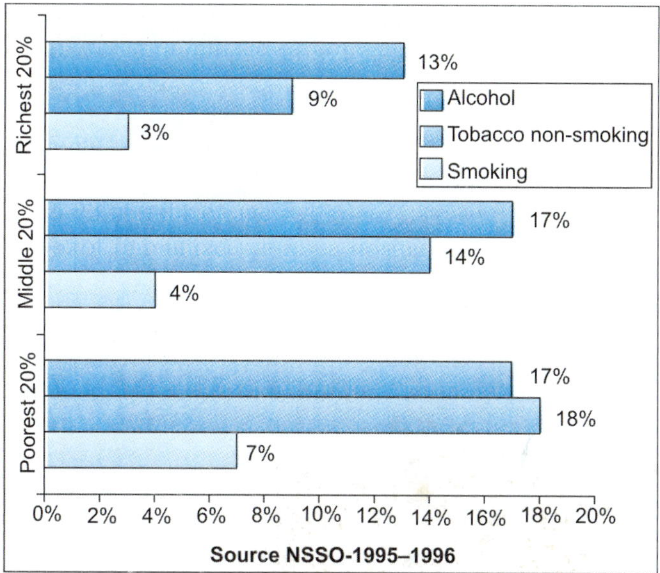

Fig. 8.2: Prevalence of alcohol and tobacco use in India by income quintile

Disease Burden of NCD

There are 2.5 million of cancer cases in the country and load will double over the next two decades. Data on prevalence of cardiovascular diseases is insufficient for national level projection. The reported prevalence of coronary heart disease (CHD) in adults in urban Kerala is 14% (17% in men and 10% in women) and 7% in rural Thiruvananthapuram and 3% in rural parts of North India. 10% of urban and 5% of rural adult population suffer from hypertension. The estimated prevalence of rheumatic heart disease which constitute 20–30% of hospital admissions due to all cardiovascular disease (CVS) in India, is 5–7 per 1000 in the 5–15 years age group. A recent study carried out in six cities in India showed an age-standardized prevalence of diabetes and impaired glucose tolerance in 12.1% and 14.0% respectively with no gender difference. It indicates that NCDs constitute heavy burden of disease and this is going to rise further.[8, 9]

MULTIFACTORIAL ORIGIN

Causes of NCD are multifactorial. Range of lifestyles: Risk taking behaviour, changing dietary pattern, physical inactivity, use of alcohol and tobacco and stress in life have been incriminated.

Future

During the 10th and 11th plan period, efforts were made to improve preventive, promotive, curative and rehabilitative services for non-communicable diseases throughout the country at all levels of care so as to reduce morbidity and mortality. The major thrust was on:[9,10]

1 Well-structured information education and communication for primary and secondary prevention of NCD.

2 Reorientation and skill upgradation of health care providers.

3 Establishment of referral linkages among primary, secondary and tertiary institutions.

4 Production and provision of drugs for NCDs.

5 Development of institution for rehabilitation of disabled persons due to NCDs, teaching persons to live with their disability.

6 Development of hospices for terminally ill people who cannot have home-based care.

7 Creation of epidemiological database of NCD especially, CVDs, strokes and diabetes through survey and surveillance of risk factors in the community.[10]

REFERENCES

1 Beaglehole R, Bonita R, Kjellstrom T. Basic epidemiology. Geneva: WHO; 1993.

2 WHO. "Emerging infectious diseases—Global Response Global Alert". Backgrounder World Health Day, 7th April 1997. WHO, Geneva.

3 NICD. Emerging and Re-emerging and new infections. CD Alert. Monthly Newsletter on Communicable diseases 1997; (1): 1.

4 UNAIDS. HIV Voluntary Counselling and Testing—A gateway to prevention and care. UNAIDS Case Study—June 2002.

5 Narain JP. Tuberculosis epidemiology and control. First Edn., New Delhi: WHO Regional Office for South East Asia; 2002.

6 Benenson S. Control of communicable diseases in man. Thirteenth Edn., New York: American Public Health Association; 1981.

7 Gordon JE. Control of communicable diseases in man. Tenth Edn., New York: American Public Health Association; 1965.

8 GOI. Annual report 2003–04. New Delhi: MOH and FW, GOI; 2004.

9 Planning Commission. Tenth Five-Year Plan 2002–07. New Delhi: Planning Commission, GOI; 2002.

10 GOI. Annual report 2007–08. MOH and FW. Government of India.

CAUSATION IN EPIDEMIOLOGY

One of the major use of epidemiology is to discover or identify the causes of disease and help in prevention and control of disease in population.

Disease occurs because of some external stimulus. Before the disease occurs, there is interplay of external stimuli/stimulus between "environments", disease producing "organism/factors" and the "host", which we call as *epidemiological* triad (Fig. 8.3).

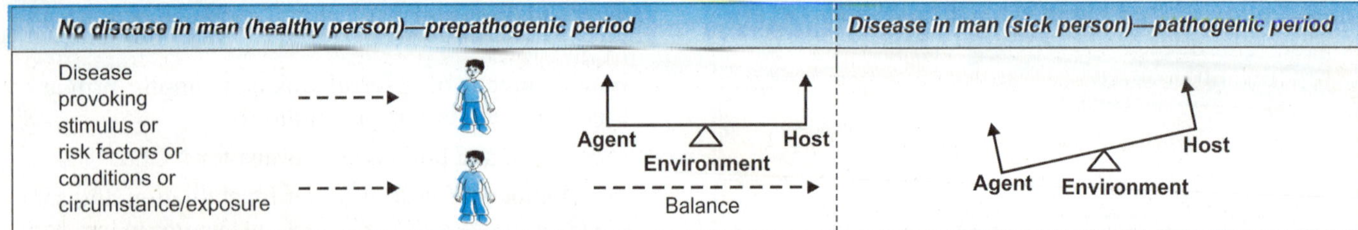

Fig. 8.3: Interplay of external stimuli between agent, host and environments (natural history of disease)

Cause is something, which precedes the occurrence of disease or effect or unfavourable outcome. Logically cause must precede a disease.

Example

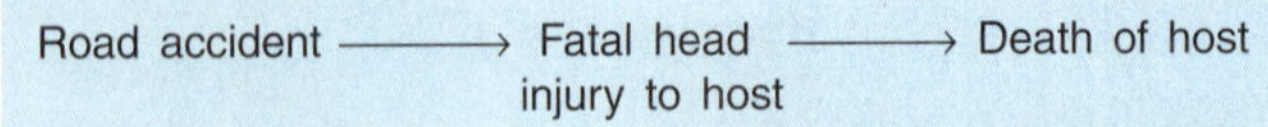

Road accident caused fatal head injury to host and the host died. Here the final outcome or unfavourable outcome or effect was death. Fatal injury precedes death. Therefore, cause of death is road accident and fatal injury. Here the cause is injury, which initiated the train of morbid events leading directly to death.

Definition of Cause

A cause of disease is defined as an event, circumstance, condition, risk factor, exposure, characteristic or a combination of these factors, which result in producing the disease.

Necessary Cause

Vibrio cholerae is a cause of cholera disease. The causation is somewhat better understood in communicable diseases, e.g. *Vibrio cholerae* is a cause of cholera disease. The cholera cannot develop or occur in the absence of *Vibrio cholerae*. In other words, the *Vibrio cholerae* is *essential* for cholera to occur. This is termed as "*necessary cause*" for occurrence of cholera.

In outbreak or epidemic of cholera, not all people who drink contaminated water suffer, some suffer cholera, while many escape despite ingesting *Vibrio cholera*e through contaminated water. It proves that *Vibrio cholerae* is not a *sufficient cause* of cholera, though it is necessary cause. *Sufficient causes* other than necessary cause must exist together for occurrence of cholera.

The sufficient causes for cholera are insanitary conditions, water contamination, adequate dose of *Vibrio cholerae*, survival of organism, host factors (resistance or immunity, nutritional status, and personal hygiene, etc.).

Sufficient Cause

8

"Sufficient cause" or sufficient causes are factors and conditions, which are other than the etiological cause of disease. "Sufficient causes" include factors in the environments, and factors and conditions in the host, which produce a disease provoking stimulus/stimuli for initiating the disease process in the host (Fig. 8.3). Sufficient cause often comprises several components.

Approach

Science of epidemiology helps determining the causes. We may begin with a *disease* problem and then search for its causes or we may begin with *healthy people* and study the effect of an *exposure* on them. Most of the clues and sufficient causes of a disease come through descriptive studies (observational epidemiology). Snow described occurrence of cholera deaths due to contaminated water much earlier (in 1853) than the discovery of disease producing organism in 1883 (*Vibrio cholerae*). Control measures were initiated much before the discovery of *Vibrio cholerae*, on the strength of descriptive epidemiology.

Single and Multiple Causes

In communicable diseases, usually the etiological organisms are responsible for occurrence of diseases in combination with sufficient causes. These organisms can be isolated and proved to be cause of a disease. In the later part of 19th century, most of the disease-producing organisms were discovered and interest concentrated on microorganisms. Koch's laid down postulates or rules for occurrence of disease due to living organism:

a. The organism must be present in every case of disease.
b. One should be able to isolate the organism on culture.
c. The isolated organism when inoculated should be able to produce disease in susceptible animal.
d. The organism must then be recovered from the animal and identified.

Koch's postulates are not wholly true in all circumstances. We may not be able to isolate *Mycobacterium tuberculosis* from all those persons who have the disease, but certainly, the *M. tuberculosis* is necessary cause of tuberculosis.

In communicable diseases, the aetiology of disease is well established but in many of the non-communicable diseases, there are multiple causes.

Multifactorial Diseases

Non-communicable diseases like coronary heart disease, diabetes and cancer have multiple factors for their occurrence and causation. Web of causation in non-communicable diseases is much more complex as no single factor can be pinpointed or incriminated as an aetiological factor.

Coronary heart disease risk factors include high level of saturated fats in diet, physical inactivity, raised serum cholesterol, level of unfavourable lipid concentration, hypertension, smoking and obesity explain at least 75% of new cases of cardiovascular disease in the community. Science of epidemiology through studies like Framingham study and MONICA study, the largest global study ever undertaken on cardiovascular diseases, have proved the role of multiple risk factors as described above, by undertaking longitudinal (cohort) study lasting for several years. Sufficient evidence has accumulated on coronary heart disease prevention which centres around primordial prevention, i.e. adoption of healthy lifestyles by people and adoption of population-based strategies to avoid the emergence of risk factors in population such as controlling tobacco, controlling fats and promoting healthy eating and physical activity.

HOW TO ESTABLISH CAUSE OF DISEASE?

Cause and effect relationship can be established by following epidemiological principles tested over time.

Temporal Relationship

Temporal relationship or time series studies, the cause must precede the effect. If the cause is an exposure or toxic substance in a factory (say lead), the level of exposure must reach to a certain level before it can produce toxic effects on a person; hence, the persons exposed to lead should be observed at various points in time to measure the effect of exposure (lead).

The time to measure the effect could be every 6 months. The exposure to lead can be observed at 6, 12, 18 and 24 months to measure the effect. Repeated measurements of lead exposure at more than one point of time at different locations may provide useful and stronger evidence than only one measurement at one point in time. Cross-sectional studies and case control studies, in which the cause and effect are measured at the same point of time, are not suitable to establish the cause and effect relationship. Thus, **time series studies** and temporal relationship between **cause** and **effect** can provide better evidence to establish cause of an effect.

Strength of Association

Relative risk measures the strength of association between **cause** and **effect.** Relative risk of more than two means the association is causal. If the relative risk is manyfolds say 4 times or 10 times, it is much stronger evidence that the exposure is cause to effect. The size of risk ratio which measures the incidence in exposed and the incidence in non-exposed (I_E/I_{NE}) helps to establish cause to effect relationship.

Dose Response Relationship

If a dose response relationship can be demonstrated, it strengthens the argument for *cause* and *effect*.

Doll and Hill established in 1950s the relationship between cigarette smoking and lung cancer. Relationship between average number of cigarettes smoked per day and annual lung cancer death rates per 1000, measures dose response. With the increase in number of cigarettes per day the mortality effects are increased. This way it could be established that heavy smokers (cause) experienced high rate of cancer lung (effect). Many studies have demonstrated dose response relationship of this kind. Thus, it was concluded that smoking had causal relationship with lung cancer.

Reversible Association

If the exposure or cause is removed, it results in decreased risk of disease, i.e. the association between smoking and lung cancer is reversible if smoking is stopped. It was proved by Doll and Hill that if smoking was stopped the risk of mortality due to lung cancer decreased substantially. These observations establish the *cause* to *effect* relationship.

Consistency

If the results of several studies done in different parts of the country come out with similar results it can be concluded that the evidence of causal relationship exists.

Meta-analysis technique can be adopted and results of various randomized controlled trials done over different parts of the country can be pooled to generate evidence. If the results are consistent or similar in different parts it probably establishes that cause and effect have strong association. Results of BCG trials to establish its efficacy, varied from 0 to 80% over different parts of the World, thus it was concluded that BCG does not reduce the incidence and prevalence of tuberculosis but certainly it prevents serious forms of tuberculosis in children.

Plausibility

It means that cause to effect association should be consistent with knowledge. Knowledge changes with the passage of time and advancement. Effects observed due to a cause should take into the consideration the results of experiments in laboratories done on animals and all other scientific evidences.

Study Design

The study design to establish cause to effect relationship is most important. The randomized controlled trials (RCT) produce best evidence for effect of treatment or an intervention, however, evidence of causation is rarely available from this type of study. Most often, the evidence comes from observational studies; almost all the evidence of most of the water-borne diseases came from observational or descriptive epidemiology. **Cohort studies** provide **strong evidence** for **cause to effect** relationship and similarly **case control studies** when pursued over different points in time produce moderate evidence of cause to effect relationship. However, **cross-sectional** studies which measure the cause and effect at the same point in time provide weak evidence of cause to effect relationship and similarly **ecological studies** provide least satisfactory evidence for *cause* to *effect*.

Weighing the Evidence

The available evidence on cause and effect must be weighed to make valuable judgment. After examining all the available evidences, the judgment of cause can be made but sometimes it may be difficult.

MEASURING HEALTH AND DISEASE

Epidemiology measures occurrence of disease, death, disability and health status in the community with a view to control the disease/diseases and to eliminate and eradicate disease from the globe or a defined territory.

Objectives of Health and Disease Measurement

The objectives are:

1. To determine load of disease in community (incidence and prevalence) and measure trends.
2. To measure the health status of community.
3. To plan, implement and monitor the programme (allocation of funds).
4. To evaluate the intervention or programme we use incidence and prevalence of morbidity.
5. To know the changing pattern of diseases.

MEASUREMENT OF DISEASE OR MORBIDITY

The disease definition should be clear. It means one needs to define a case of disease. Operational definition of a case must be worked out. Some of the examples of case definitions have been given under epidemiological surveillance of diseases. The International Classification of Diseases-10th Rev. (ICD-10) and WHO guidelines on definition of diseases is followed to arrive at uniformity and to achieve the purpose of comparison.[1]

Data on morbidity is generated through subcentres, primary health centres and community health centres. The quality of the data may be poor but it does serve useful purpose at local level.

Secondary and tertiary level of care institutes also generate lot of data on diseases. It should not be mixed with primary health care as each has its distinct significance. Private health sector also generate lot of data on disease.

8

However, in India, reliable information on overall morbidity is not available. In the absence of reliable morbidity and mortality statistics, survey and surveillance data have formed the basis on which policy makers and managers evolved public health programmes and allocated funds. Statistical units involved in morbidity statistics should include:

- Number of sick persons
- Number of illnesses
- Spells or episodes
- Period of sickness or average duration of sickness per spell of sickness
- Proportion of time lost due to sickness (days, months, etc.).

Count

Morbidity measure could be simple counts of a disease or diseased persons.

This is the simplest type of measure of disease or sick person just count the number of events or subjects.

Example: Number of patients seen at a facility per week, per month or per year; number of fever cases and malaria positives detected per month by surveillance programme. Simple count helps to know if disease is increasing or falling. This indicates trends and helps in forecasting the development of outbreaks. WHO weekly epidemiological report relies on simple count of international notifiable diseases (cholera, yellow fever and plague).[2]

Rate

It is a measure of the frequency with which some event occurs. To determine the rate, we require the information on:

- Occurrence of an *event* or disease (numerator)
- *Population* at *risk* (denominator) to that event or disease
- *Defined area*, where the event occurred
- *Time period* of occurrence of event or disease.

The population at risk means the individuals or people, or group of people who are exposed to the risk of that disease or event. Knowledge of population at risk helps to use this figure as denominator for calculation of rates.

In some diseases, total population is at risk, e.g. malaria, while for maternal deaths only women who become pregnant are at risk of maternal deaths and not the whole population. At risk population for HIV/AIDS is sexually active persons in the age of 15–49. For senile cataract, people above the age group of 50 are at risk. Rate allows epidemiologist to compare disease occurrence across different populations and geographical areas.

Ratio

A ratio places in relation two quantities that may be unrelated. It is quotient of two numbers, numerator not necessarily included in the denominator. Examples: Male female ratio in India 1000:940, doctor population ratio and waist hip ratio.

Proportion

It is a special type of ratio expressing a relationship between part and the whole. Here numerator is part of denominator. All proportions are ratios but all ratios are not proportions.

For example, proportion of a disease to total disease load or proportional mortality ratio due to a disease. The other examples of proportion are one-third of births are low birth weight babies, one-fifth are adolescents.

Percentage

A proportion multiplied by 100, e.g. 28% of births in India are low birth weights. Over 80% of pregnant women are anaemic and 69% of people live in rural areas.

Prevalence

The prevalence means the number of existing cases (new and old both) of a disease in a given population in a geographical area at a specified point or period of time.

Uses

- Prevalence measures disease burden/load in population and helps to justify allocation of resources. Some diseases are highly prevalent in India.
  Malnutrition, tuberculosis, blindness, and endemic goitre are highly prevalent and other noncommunicable diseases like cardiovascular diseases, diabetes and hypertension are showing rising prevalence in India due to unhealthy lifestyles and longer survival.
- Prevalence also helps to identify high-risk population and geographical areas affected most.

Incidence

It is the number of new cases, which occur in a given population at a specified point or period of time.

Uses

Incidence measures occurrence of new cases and it is helpful in evaluation of programme as an impact indicator. The purpose of primary prevention is to reduce incidence of disease.

Incidence is usually calculated for acute disease lasting for a short period, e.g. fever incidence, flu, acute watery diarrhoea, injuries, etc.

DIFFICULTIES IN MEASURING MORBIDITY

The disease or sickness has a period and it runs a variable course, some diseases are subclinical, still others are at early stage and not detectable so easily while some diseases manifest signs and symptoms which are quite obvious and visible. Thus, for a single manifesting case there may be many persons who may have inapparent infection of disease.

Further one person may have multiple sicknesses (e.g. old people have multitudes of diseases). Some patients have several other diseases apart from the presenting problem. Sickness also occurs in spells and some sicknesses occur again and again, doctors or a facility cures the person, the person returns to the same environments and gets the disease again and again.

In view of demographic and epidemiological transition the disease pattern is changing and in future the country is likely to face much more problem of non-communicable diseases and some of the lifestyle diseases already are showing their ugly heads (accidents, cardiovascular diseases, cancers, HIV/AIDS, diabetes and hypertension). Right now, we have the problem of double burden of disease: Communicable diseases, maternal and child health problems besides non-communicable diseases.[3]

$$\text{Prevalence rate} = \frac{\text{Total number of cases of a disease (new and old both) at a specified time}}{\text{Population at risk at the specified time}} \times 100$$

Example

i Total population of India in 2000 at risk = 1000 million

ii Total no. of tuberculosis cases in India in the year 2000 = 14 million or prevalence of tuberculosis was 1.4% (14/1000) × 100 = 1.4%.

iii Prevalence of sputum positive cases 0.4%.

Sputum positive cases = 4.0 million (4/1000) × 100 = 0.4%.

With this level of prevalence, it can be stated that tuberculosis is a major public health problem in India because of high prevalence and high burden of disease. Of all tuberculosis cases nearly one-fourth are infectious cases (prevalence rate of sputum positive cases is around 0.4% in population). Because of heavy burden of tuberculosis, high priority has been accorded to control the disease by DOTS strategy.[4]

$$\text{Prevalence of infection due to tuberculosis} = \frac{\text{No. of persons showing tuberculin positive tests}}{\text{No. of tuberculin tests done}} \times 100$$

$$\text{Example} = \frac{400}{1000} \times 100 = 40\%$$

40% of people in India have tuberculous infection. They are infected but not diseased (Fig. 8.4).[5]

Prevalence rate for leprosy[6] in India is 0.84/10,000.

Prevalence of a disease quite often relates to a period prevalence.

Point prevalence means total number of existing cases of a disease (old and new) at one point in time per 100 or per 1000 people at risk at the specified time.

$$\text{Point prevalence} = \frac{\text{Total number of cases of a disease at a point in time}}{\text{Number of people at risk at that point in time}} \times 100$$

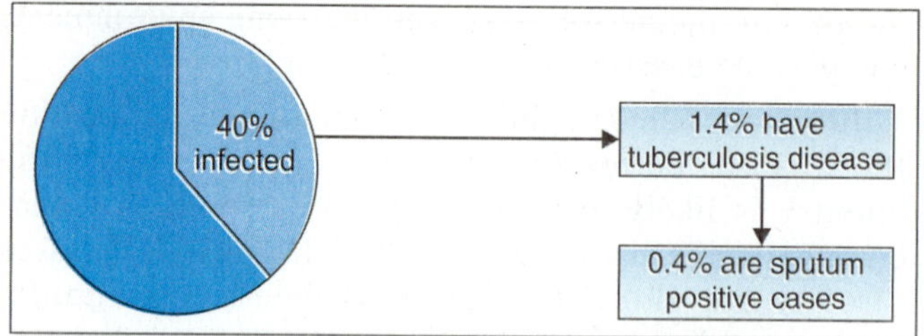

Fig. 8.4: Prevalence of tuberculous infection

Period Prevalence

The period prevalence from 1.1.2004 to 31.12.2004 would be 6 persons (students) which include no. 1, 2, 3, 4, 5 and 6 (Fig. 8.5).

Point Prevalence

Say on 31st Dec 2004, it would be 3 (student no. 1, 2 and 6) as shown in Fig. 8.5.

Incidence

New cases between 1st Jan and 31st Dec 2004 would be 3 (student no. 2, 3 and 6) as shown in Fig. 8.5.

INCIDENCE OF A DISEASE

Definition

Incidence means new cases of a disease that occur in a defined period in population at risk.

$$\text{Incidence} = \frac{\text{Number of new cases of a disease in one year}}{\text{Total population at risk in that year}} \times 100$$

Example

$$\text{Fever incidence} = \frac{\text{100 million fever cases were reported in the year 2000 in India}}{\text{Population at risk was 1000 million in that year}} \times 100$$

$$= 10\% \text{ per annum.}$$

The incidence of fever in community in the year 2000 was 10% per year.

$$\text{Annual parasite incidence (API) of malaria in India in the year 2000} = \frac{\text{2 million cases of malaria in the year 2000 in India}}{\text{Population at risk 1000 million in year 2000}} \times 1000$$

$$= \text{API} = 2$$

The annual parasite incidence for malaria was two in the year 2000 in India. The incidence of malaria can be obtained every fortnightly, every month, or every year under the national malaria control programme. The data are generated by regular surveillance of fever in the community. The population at risk of fever in this example is the total population of the country (1000 million) in the year 2000 because whole population was under surveillance and exposed to the risk of malaria.[6,7]

At risk population usually is seldom available precisely and therefore the mid-year population or total population of area constitutes population at risk in malaria, this may be true for many other situations.

The **incidence** is determined usually by **cohort study,** by longitudinal follow-up of healthy subjects. For example, 20 healthy children between 1 and 2 years of age group were followed for 4 weeks period, of these 4 developed acute watery diarrhoea at the end of 4 weeks of follow-up. We can calculate incidence of diarrhoea by knowing person weeks of follow-up in these 20 children.

Three children were followed for all the 4 weeks and hence they contributed 12 weeks of follow-up, 4 children

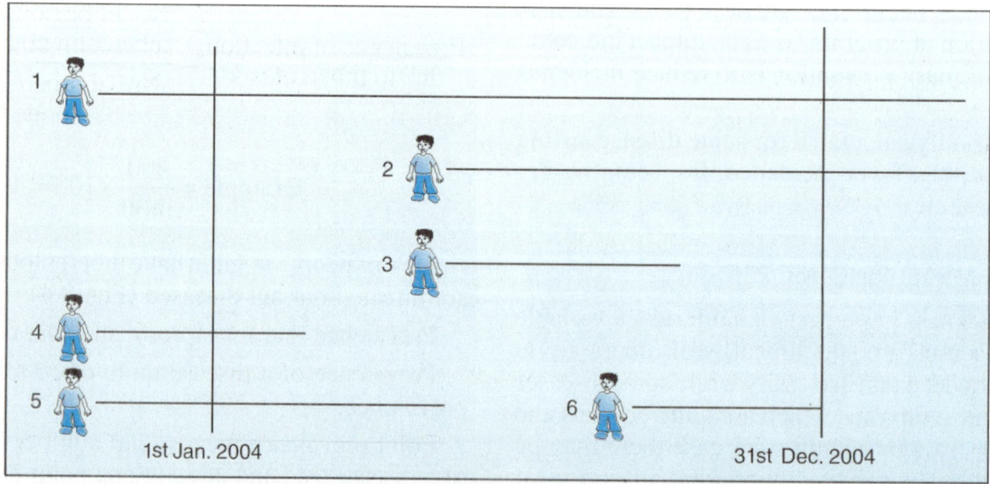

Fig. 8.5: Six students who start their sickness at different point in time

were followed up for 3 weeks, they contributed 12 weeks, 3 children could be followed up for 2 weeks they contributed 6 weeks and 10 children were followed up for one week they contributed 10 weeks of follow-up. Total person weeks of follow-up were 40 weeks (Table 8.3).

Table 8.3: Four weeks follow-up 20 healthy children

No. of weeks of children	*Total follow-up*	*No. of weeks*	*Developed diarrhoea*
3	4	12	1
4	3	12	1
3	2	6	0
10	1	10	2
20	**10**	**40**	**4**

$$\text{Incidence of diarrhoea} = \frac{\text{No. of children who developed diarrhoea}}{\text{Total child weeks of follow-up}} \times 100$$

$$= \frac{4}{40} \times 100 = 10 \text{ per 100 child weeks of follow-up}$$

This method is most appropriate as in this **cohort** of 20 children all could not enter the study at one point in time and further all could not be followed up for all the 4 weeks, some left the study area and were away to relatives. In short, risk time of each child is calculated in terms of weeks or days a child is observed or followed up. The unit of time depends upon the nature of study.

The incidence of this cohort study can be expressed by *cumulative incidence* (CI) rate.

$$\text{CI} = \frac{\text{No. of children who experienced diarrhoea during 4 weeks of follow-up}}{\text{No. of children who were free of diarrhoea at the beginning of the study}} \times 100$$

$$= \frac{4}{20} \times 100 = 20\%$$

It means 20% of children experienced diarrhoea in four weeks of follow-up.

Further, the duration of diarrhoea in 4 children was 14 days. The average duration of disease was 14/4 = 3.5 days or half week.

Inter-relationship of Prevalence and Incidence

The prevalence rate is dependent on both incidence rate and duration of disease provided that the prevalence rate is low and does not alter much with time.

P = Incidence rate × average duration of disease

From the above example of incidence of diarrhoea and average duration of diarrhoea (one episode), the prevalence can be arrived at by:

= 10/100 weeks × half week (3.5 days)

P = 5 cases per 100 children between 1 and 2 years.

Attack Rate

It is also an expression of incidence of a disease. It is special incidence rate when a particular disease occurs in an **epidemic proportion** or outbreak in population we usually calculate attack rate, e.g. in the year 1996 out of 4000 population in a village, 2800 persons were affected with fever from mid-August to mid-September, it was an outbreak of malaria.

$$\text{Attack rate} = \frac{\text{No. of persons who had fever from mid-August to mid-September}}{\text{Total population exposed to risk in the same period}} \times 100$$

$$= \frac{2800}{4000} \times 100 = 70\%$$

It means 70% of people of that village were attacked by fever proved to be malaria.

Secondary Attack Rate

In outbreak situation like measles, cases start occurring one after the other in the family. The primary case in the family spreads infection to other members of the family. The secondary attack rate measures the **contagiousness** of a disease.

Secondary attack rate is defined as number of exposed individuals who develop the disease within the expected range of incubation period of that disease following exposure to primary case.

In the secondary attack rate, the contacts who have not been immunized against measles are at risk of developing measles if they come in contact with a case of measles.

$$\text{Secondary attack rate} = \frac{\text{Number of contact persons who developed the disease within the range of incubation period following exposure}}{\text{Total number of exposed/contacts}} \times 100$$

The contacts can be within the family, in the neighbourhood, or in an extrafamilial institution. Secondary attack rate in measles is very high (90%).

MORTALITY STATISTICS

The mortality rates and ratio are outcome indicators or impact indicators and are used to measure the long-term impact of the programme or an intervention. Traditionally, policy makers have used mortality statistics for identifying major public health problems. In India, reliable age specific mortality data is available through SRS, though there are lacunae in the system to ascertain cause of death.

If mortality rates are collected over a long period, we get the secular trends of mortality. Mortality rates can be compared between various states, regions and districts, at the same point in time or over the different points in time of the same area. Unlike morbidity, the mortality is unambiguous, easy to define and can be collected even by lay persons. Mortality statistics are somewhat easier to collect. Compulsory birth and death registration Act in India is there but its implementation is tardy and consequently the routine registrations of deaths are always incomplete and causes of death are not recorded or are incorrect. Therefore, we rely on alternate system of getting accurate and reliable account of deaths through sample registration system (SRS). The most common mortality rates used in the country are:

Crude Death Rate (CDR) (Incidence of Deaths)

This is the most common measure of mortality available and used for several purposes. It is easiest to compute. In epidemiological terms, crude death rate is speed of death or *incidence measure* during a specified time period, usually a year.

Definition

Crude death rate (CDR) is defined as total number of deaths in population over a period of one year in an area, divided by total population at the middle of the year.

$$\text{CDR} = \frac{\text{Total number of deaths in one year}}{\text{Mid-year population}} \times 1000$$

Limitations

The CDR does not take into account the age and sex composition of the population. It is an established fact that the mortality rate during the first year of life, early childhood period up to 5 years of age and mortality in elderly people are much higher than other age groups. Similarly, death rates among female and during reproductive period tend to be higher. Thus, it is imperative to interpret crude death rates with composition of population. For example, Kashi and Haridwar in India are religious places for Hindus; many of the old people make these towns as home after attaining old age and prefer to die at holy place. The population composition of these towns is likely to change and crude death rates may be much higher.

The SRS provides reliable estimates of crude death rate in the country by statewise, every year. The death rates can be compared between various states and union territories of India. Rural rates are higher in comparison to urban rates. Over the years, India has achieved reduction of death rates from 27.4 in the year 1951 to 7.0 in the year 2013, which is a significant milestone of overall development and quality of life (Table 8.4). Thus, the crude death rate in spite of various limitations is useful to measure the progress of a nation or state.[8,9]

8

Table 8.4: Trends of crude death rates in India

Year	*Crude death rate*
1901–11	42.6
1911–21	47.6
1921–31	36.3
1941–51	27.4
1971	14.9
1981	12.5
1991	9.8
2003	8.0
2006	7.5
2007	7.4
2008	8.0
2009	7.3
2010	7.2
2011	7.1
2012	7.0
2013	7.0

Source: SRS Bulletin—2005, Oct 2006 and Oct. 2007 to 2013

Standardization

Standardization of crude death rates is done to achieve comparability between different populations over the same period. This is done by direct and indirect standardization methods.

Standard million: Population distribution when calculated for each age and sex group in such a manner as to give a total of 1 million persons, preserving the same proportional age and sex distribution as in the total population. This is called "Standard million population".

Direct Method

Age and sex specific death rates of a local population are applied to standard million population of male and female to arrive at adjusted or standard death rate. Age and sex specific deaths rate of local population is very very difficult to obtain.

Indirect Method

Here the specific death rates of standard population are applied to local population to arrive at expected standard death rate in that population. Even age and sex composition of local population may be herculean task to obtain. It can be obtained for a district or state from census data as rough approximate of the population where one is interested to arrive at such rates.

Since crude death rates need to be refined by age and sex specific death rate to get more reliable indicators of measuring health status of the country or an area, the following age specific mortality rates are widely used to measure the health status and quality of life and overall development of a nation.

Infant Mortality Rate (IMR)

It is age specific mortality. It measures speed of death during the first year of life. It is considered to be most sensitive and reliable index of level of health or health status of a community.

$$\text{IMR} = \frac{\text{Number of deaths below one year of age in a geographical area}}{\text{Total number of live births during the same year in a geographical area}} \times 1000$$

Infant mortality is sensitive to health programmes and interventions as also to socioeconomic changes in the country. In calculating IMR, we use live births as denominator since it is difficult to obtain the population of 0–1 year age in the community (Table 8.5).

Table 8.5: Trends of IMR in India

1980	*1985*	*1990*	*2003*	*2006*	*2007*	*2009*	*2012*
114	97	80	60	57	55	50	42

The trend in infant mortality is declining. In the last 22 years, it has been halved (50% reduction). After year 2003, slow decline is obvious. Achieving target of 30 by the year 2015 appears to be difficult. There were wide variations of IMR statewise in India. District level data are not available through SRS.[9]

Under-five Mortality

This is a composite measure of mortality, again a very sensitive and reliable index of human development and health status of the country or an area. This has been explained in the section of childhood mortality.

The other measures of mortality are mortality in age bracket 1–4, maternal mortality rates, which have been explained in respective chapters.

Case Fatality

If the disease is severe, the case fatality is high, e.g. JE (Japanese encephalitis has high case fatality).

This is the proportion of cases of a disease who experience death within a specified period of time.

$$\text{Case fatality} = \frac{\text{No. of deaths from a disease in a specified period}}{\text{Total number of cases diagnosed in the same period}} \times 100$$

Case fatality due to JE in year 2000 was 670/2241 × 100 = 30%. In rabies and AIDS cases, fatality is 100%.

During the year 1996, the outbreak of dengue haemorrhagic fever (DHF) and dengue shock syndrome (DSS), there were about 10,000 cases and 400 deaths.[10] The case fatality due to dengue outbreak was thus 4%.

$$\text{Case fatality due to dengue in National Capital of Delhi} = \frac{\text{Deaths due to DHF and DSS from mid-Aug. to Nov. 1996}}{\text{Total cases of DHF and DSS from mid-Aug. to Nov. 1996}} \times 100$$

$$= \frac{400}{10000} \times 100 = 4\%$$

Proportional Mortality Rate/Ratio (PMR)

This is expressed as:

$$\text{PMR} = \frac{\text{No. of deaths from a specified disease in a specified period}}{\text{Total number of deaths from all causes during that specified period}} \times 100$$

The proportional mortality rate due to diseases of respiratory system was 29.47%. It means in this area over 29% of deaths were due to respiratory diseases including tuberculosis, or else we can say major killers in this area were respiratory diseases followed by digestive disorders and accidents. It is an evidence which diseases should get our attention most in rural areas (Table 8.6).

Proportional mortality due to prematurity in infants (rural area) in 1994 was determined in India. 46.4% of infant mortality in India was due to prematurity. It signifies that to reduce infant mortality, one has to focus on reduction of prematurity (Fig. 8.6).[11]

Table 8.6: Distribution of deaths by major cause group in a rural block—1996–97

Major cause group	*Proportion of death*
Cough (disease of respiratory system)	29.47
Digestive disorders	13.45
Accidents and injuries	12.87
Fevers	10.88
Other clear symptoms	8.54
Causes peculiar to infancy	7.95
Senility	7.13
CNS disorders	4.80
Disorders of circulatory system	4.68
Child birth and pregnancy complication	0.23
Total	**100.00**

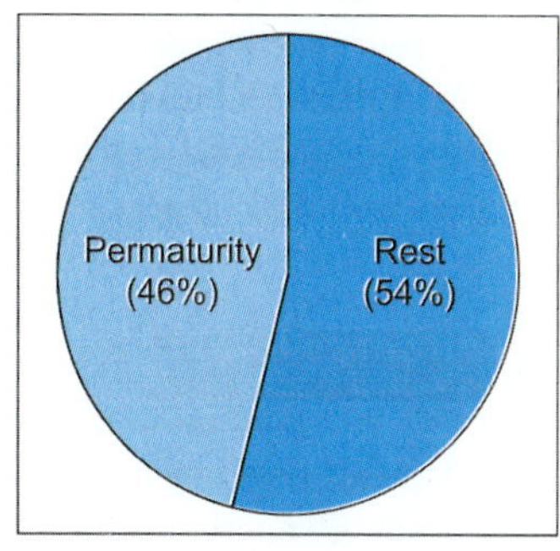

Fig. 8.6: Causes of infant mortality in rural area 1994 (SRS)

8

The proportional mortality rate of different age brackets in a rural block in the year 1996–97 is presented for clear understanding (Table 8.7).

Table 8.7: Proportional mortality rate of rural block—1996–97

Age group (years)	Total deaths	Proportional mortality rate (%)
Below one year	166	19.42
1–4	42	4.91
5–14	32	3.74
15–44	161	18.83
45–59	73	8.54
60 and above	381	44.56
All ages groups	855	100

The proportional mortality rate (ratio) for infants in this block was 19.42%, though the infants constitute 3% of total population but experience almost one-fifth of total deaths. It means the mortality effects are much more in the first year of life. Proportional mortality rate for persons age 60 and above was 44.56%. It means that over 44% of deaths were experienced by persons above the age group 60. Thus, the mortality was highest in extreme of age (highest in first year and above 60 years). This also speaks of vulnerability of infants and aged people who were most vulnerable to mortality. It also raises the question of where to invest? Prevention of infant and child mortality clearly is overriding priority.

Causes of Death Statistics—Million Death Study

The causes of death statistics are essential to capture the leading killers diseases in order to control these diseases. Cause of death till 1994 were being generated by SRS by using lay diagnosis reporting system from rural areas under model registration scheme, however, the scheme was suspended. It has now been revived to capture causes of death by verbal autopsy, since 1999 in urban and rural areas.

Over 75% of the 95 lakh annual deaths in India occur at home and majority of these do not have certified cause. Recognizing the need for better data, the government has undertaken the world's largest study to track the causes of death in the country called the "prospective study of one million deaths in India". The study lasted for 16 years (1998–2014). This is known as "Million Death Study" (MDS) undertaken by sample registration system. The verbal autopsy (VA) called "RHIME" or Representative, Re-sampled, Routine Household Interview of Mortality with Medical Evaluation method to determine the causes of death. Causes of neonatal mortality in India in 2005 as per million death study (MDS) were prematurity and low birth weight 14%, birth asphyxia and birth trauma 8%, neonatal infection 12%, neonatal tetanus 1%, diarrhoea 1% and others 7%. Causes of child mortality—pneumonia 16%, diarrhoeal diseases 13%, other infectious diseases 11% and others 17%.

Cause of death is also obtained from hospital statistics, as these deaths are attended by physicians (doctors) hence the causes are more reliable but unfortunately many of the hospitals do not adhere to ICD-10 classification of diseases and deaths, hence, value of an important source of data get lost.[12, 13]

MEASURING THE BURDEN OF DISEASE

Relative importance of different diseases is based on how many deaths they cause. This convention has certain merits as death is an unambiguous event and many countries collect these statistics routinely.

There are, however, many diseases or conditions which are not fatal but are responsible for great loss of healthy life, e.g. chronic depression and paralysis caused by polio. Therefore, World Bank and WHO jointly undertook an exercise and recommended DALYs as measure of disease burden.

Disability-adjusted life years (DALYs) have been used to assess the disease burden in the community.

One DALY is equal to the loss of one year of healthy life, e.g. a person who lives up to 70 years but suffers an incapacitating stroke at age 65, has lost 5 DALYs.

DALY combines: (a) losses from premature death, which is defined as the difference between actual age at death and life expectancy at that age in a low mortality population, and (b) loss of healthy life resulting from disability. The global burden of disease is measured in units of disability-adjusted life years (DALYs). Worldwide 1.36 billion DALYs were lost in 1990, the equivalent of 42 million deaths of newborn children or of 80 million deaths at age 50.

Premature deaths were responsible for 66% of DALYs losses in developing countries. The comparison of absolute number of DALYs may be misleading because of variation in size of population of a country. India lost 344 DALYs per 1000 population in the year 1990.

The World Bank report 1993 estimated that in India 50.5% of DALYs loss was due to communicable diseases, 40.4% of DALYs loss was due to non-communicable diseases, and 9.1% of DALYs loss was due to injuries and accidents (Fig. 8.6A).[3]

MEASUREMENT OF HEALTH (*see* Chapter 3)

Disability—Measurement[14–16]

Apart from measuring morbidity and mortality, the measurement of disability in population is significant to have an assessment of magnitude of disability (prevalence and incidence). Disability results in dependency, loss of productivity apart from social implications of disability. The measurement of DALYs proposed by WHO and World Bank gives due importance to healthy life lost due to disability.

There is no accurate estimate of the number of disabled persons in the country. Year 1981 was observed as an International Year of Disabled Persons (IYDPs). Of every

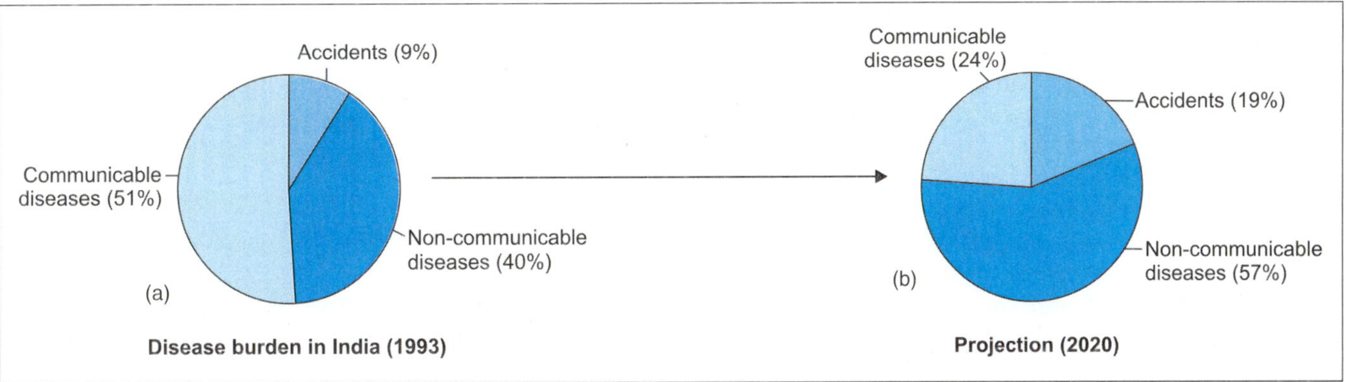

Fig. 8.6(a and b): Disease burden and projection in India (Source: World Bank report (1993)

10 children in the world, one child is born with an impairment or acquires it early in life.

It was estimated in 1981 that in India, there were 2 million mentally retarded, 5 lakh physically disabled, 2 lakhs deaf and 8 lakh blind children. Accidents and injuries produce disability in youth, adults, and is assuming epidemic proportion. Trauma is major cause of morbidity, mortality and disability in adults.

Common Impairments[17]

Census 2011 reveals that 2.14% of our population or approximately 26.8 million people in India suffer from severe disability.

1 ***Physical/locomotor limitation:*** Due to accidents and trauma, poliomyelitis, and leprosy. In 2011, census, locomotor disability was reported in 5,436,604 persons (20.0%).
2 ***Mental retardation:*** Due to iodine deficiency disorders, rubella infection, bacterial and viral infection, asphyxia and trauma during birth, toxoplasmosis, cerebral palsy, and genetic disorders. 1505624 persons had mental disability in 2011 (5.6%).

   Mental illness: 722826 (3%) most likely severe mental illness.
3 ***Blindness and visual impairment:*** Due to vitamin A deficiency, onchocerchiasis, accidents, cataract and glaucoma. 5032463 had visual disability in the year 2011 (19.1%).
4 ***Deafness/hearing impairment:*** Congenital, chronic suppurative otitis media, prolonged exposure to noise and accidents. 5071007 persons had hearing disability in the year 2011 (19.3%).
5 ***Speech:*** Due to consequences of various diseases. 1998535 persons had speech disability in the year 2011 (7.3%).
6 ***Any other:*** 4927011 (18.4%)
7 ***Multiple disabilities:*** 2116487 (8%)

The impairment, disabilities and handicap may result which may be permanent or temporary, progressive or regressive. These terms have been defined by WHO (1980) as follows.

Impairment

"Any loss or abnormality of psychological, physiological or anatomical structure or function".

Example: An abnormality, a temporary or permanent loss such as a missing or defective body part (loss of limb), paralysis after polio, diabetes, mental retardation, and near-sightedness.

Disability

"Any restriction or lack resulting from impairment to perform an activity in the manner or within the range considered normal for a human being".

In other words, it is any restriction of a function considered normal for human beings resulting from an impairment. This would involve difficulty in seeing, hearing, walking, writing or speaking. Now the term disability serves as an umbrella term for impairments, activity limitation and participation restrictions.

Handicap

"A disadvantage for a given individual, resulting from an impairment or disability, that limits or prevents the fulfilment of a role that is normal (depending on age, sex and social and cultural factors) for that individual".

A disability only becomes a handicap, if it is allowed to interfere with doing what is normally expected at a certain age. Now the term handicap has been dropped.

INTERNATIONAL CLASSIFICATION OF FUNCTIONING (ICF), DISABILITY AND HEALTH

The WHO has revised the international classification system of impairment, disability, and handicap (ICIDH), which was first published by WHO in 1980 for trial purposes. WHO recognizes the importance of full participation of persons with disabilities, in the revision of classification of functioning and disability.

The term "handicap" has been dropped entirely and not to use the term "disability" as the name of the component but to keep it as overall umbrella term. The term impairment has been retained.

Now the *international classification of functioning, disability and health* known as ICF is in place. The overall aim of ICF is to produce a unified and standard language and framework for the description of health and health-related states. The domains contained in ICF can, therefore, be seen as *health domains and health-related domains.*[18] These domains are described from the perspective of the body, the individual and society, formulated in two components:

1. Body functions and structures
2. Activities and participation

As a classification, ICF systematically groups different domains for a person in a given health condition (e.g. what a person with a disease or disorder does do or can do).

The old ICIDH terms (impairments, disabilities and handicaps) and their definitions have been replaced by new terms and definitions. ICF also lists environmental factors that interact with all these constructs. In this way, it enables the user to record useful profiles of the individuals functioning, disability and health in various domains.[18]

It is important to stress, moreover, that ICF is not a classification of people at all. It is a classification of people's health characteristics within the context of their individual life situations and environmental impacts. For example, instead of referring to a "mentally handicapped person" the classification uses the phrase "person with problem in learning". The term "differently-abled" persons is used for persons with physical shortcomings.

New terms and definitions

Functioning: It is a generic term for body functions, body structures, activities and participation. It denotes the positive aspects of interaction between an individual (with a health condition) and that individual's contextual factors (environmental and personal)

- Body functions are the physiological functions of body systems (including psychological functions)
- Body structures are anatomical parts of the body such as organs, limbs and their components

Disability is an umbrella term for impairment, activity limitation and participation restrictions. It denotes the negative aspects of interaction between an individual (with a health condition) and that individual's contextual factors (environmental and personal)

- Impairments are problems in body function or structure such as a significant deviation or loss
- Activity is the execution of a task or action by an individual
- Participation is involvement in a life situation
- Activity limitations are difficulties an individual may have in executing activities
- Participation restrictions are problems an individual may experience in involvement in life situations
- Environmental factors make up the physical, social and attitudinal environment in which people live and conduct their lives

An overview of these concepts is given in Table 8.8. ICF classifies health and related states in two parts:

Part 1. Functioning and disability

a. Body functions and structures
b. Activities and participation

Part 2. Contextual factors

a. Environmental factors
b. Personal factors
    - Each component can be expressed in both positive and negative terms.
    - Each component consists of various domains and, within each domain, categories, which are the units of classification. Health and health-related states of an individual may be recorded by selecting the appropriate category code or codes and then adding *qualifiers*, which are numeric codes that specify the extent or magnitude of the functoning or disability in that category, or the extent to which an environmental factor is a facilitator or barrier.

Measurement of Disability

1. Prevalence rate of disability
2. Incidence of disability
3. Disability adjusted life years (DALYs).

Example

Incidence: During the year 1981–82, the annual incidence rate of poliomyelitis per thousand children (0–4 years) in India was measured which were 1.7 and 1.6/1000 children (0–4 years) in rural and urban areas respectively (Table 8.9).

This survey was carried out when EPI programme was still in its infancy when coverage with poliovaccine was negligible. It provided useful estimate of poliomyelitis disability in children (0–4 years).

In census 1981, attempt was made to determine the prevalence of disability in the country.

Prevalence: Similarly, in the year 2001–2002, prevalence of *blindness* above the age of 50 in India was mapped out as 8.5% and estimated prevalence in general population was 1.1%, cataract was the main cause of blindness (62.6%). Prevalence of disability due to leprosy in the year 2004 was 1.4% (deformity grade II).

DALYs: This has been explained in Chapter 2.

CAUSES OF IMPAIRMENTS

- Accidents and injuries.
- Leprosy.
- Vitamin A deficiency and malnutrition in children.
- Malnutrition in mothers during pregnancy.
- Iodine deficiency disorders.
- Congenital rubella and other genetic factors.

Table 8.8: An overview of ICF

	Part 1: Functioning and disability		*Part 2: Contextual factors*	
Components	Body functions and structures	Activities and participation	Environmental factors	Personal factors
Domains	Body functions Body structures	Life areas (tasks, actions)	External influences on functioning and disability	Internal influences on functioning and disability
Constructs	Change in body functions (physiological) Change in body structures (anatomical)	Capacity Executing tasks in a standard environment Performance Executing tasks in the current environment	Facilitating or hindering impact of features of the physical, social and attitudinal world	Impact of attributes of the person
Positive aspect	Functional and structural integrity	Activities participation	Facilitators	Not applicable
	Functioning			
Negative aspect	Impairment	Activity limitation Participation restriction	Barriers/hindrances	Not applicable
	Disability			

- Infectious diseases such as polio (it used to be major cause earlier on now it has been eradicated).
- Misuse of drugs by mothers.
- Environmental pollution (noise pollution in particular) and food adulteration.
- Lack of sanitation, man-made and natural disasters.

Prevention of Impairment

1 By immunization to prevent infectious diseases like measles, mumps, rubella and poliomyelitis. Rubella infection can be prevented by immunization.

Table 8.9: Annual incidence rate of poliomyelitis per 1000 children 0–4 years (based on sample surveys 1981–82)

State/UT	*Incidence rate per 1000 children*	
	Rural	*Urban*
Andhra Pradesh	1.7	1.4
Gujarat	2.5	2.2
Haryana and Punjab	3.1	1.7
Chandigarh	–	–
Karnataka, Goa	1.2	1.2
Madhya Pradesh (Bhopal and Jabalpur division)	1.9	1.7
Odisha	0.8	0.7
Rajasthan (Jaipur division)	3.1	2.5
Uttar Pradesh (Allahabad division)	2.3	1.6
West Bengal	0.8	1.0
Delhi	–	1.6
India	**1.7**	**1.6**

2 By regular consumption of iodized salt.
3 Improved maternal and child nutrition.
4 Vitamin A prophylaxis
5 Prevention of accidents—roadside, home and factories.
6 Avoidance of drugs and radiation during pregnancy.
7 Improved conditions and facilities during delivery.
8 Genetic counselling
9 Elimination of environmental hazards.
10 Proper care and treatment of acute respiratory infections.
11 Reduction of prolonged exposure to high noise.

Apart from primary prevention, the impairment can be controlled by early diagnosis and prompt treatment like provision of glasses for defective vision, cataract surgery, treatment of glaucoma, diabetes, hypertension, leprosy, etc. If the impairment progresses to disability and handicap, the tertiary prevention is applicable to limit disability and to rehabilitate persons who have handicaps. Scheme of setting up of Physical Medicine and Rehabilitation (PMR). Departments in 21 Medical Colleges of the country has been initiated for medical rehabilitation services.

The world summit for children included indicators of disability like disability type specific prevalence. The total number of persons with disability, specifying the number having serious difficulty in seeing, hearing, or speaking, moving, learning or comprehending, or having strange or unusual behaviour or other disability of duration of at least 6 months or of an irreversible nature, in the following age groups: 0–4, 5–14, 15–19 and 20 and over. Child-disability: One in twenty of those aged 14 years or younger live with a moderate or severe disability.

REFERENCES

1 WHO. International Statistical Classification of Diseases and Health-related problems. Tenth revision. Vol. 2. Geneva: WHO; 1993.

2 Aga Khan Foundation. PHC MAP Module 5 Users guide. Geneva: University Research Corporation Centre for Human Services, Aga Khan Foundation.

3 UNDP. World Development Report 1993. Investing in Health: New York: Oxford University Press; 1993.

4 Planning Commission. Tenth Five-Year Plan 2002–07. New Delhi: Planning Commission MOH and FW, GOI; 2002.

5 Narain JP. Tuberculosis epidemiology and control. First Edn., New Delhi: WHO Regional Office for South East Asia; 2002.

6 GOI. Annual Report 2003–04 and 2006–07. New Delhi: MOH and FW, GOI; 2004 and 2007.

7 GOI. Proceedings of the National Conference of Public Private Partnership for up-scaling use of insecticide treated bednets; 2003 May 1–3; Indian Habitat Centre, New Delhi.

8 UNICEF. Rights and opportunities, Situation of children and women. New Delhi: UNICEF India Country Office; 1998.

9 Registrar General India SRS. Sample Registration System Bulletin 2005, April; 39(1) and 2007 October; 42(1).

10 Ranbaxy Science Foundation. Dengue Outbreak in Delhi 1996. Proceedings of Round Table Conference Series 1; 1996 December; New Delhi.

11 Kumar V. Causes of mortality in rural community development block, Lakhanmajra (dissertation), Rohtak Maharshi Dayanand University; 1999.

12 WHO. International Classification of diseases 1975 Revision Vol. 1. Geneva: WHO; 1977.

13 UNICEF. The State of the World's Children 2004. New Delhi: UNICEF Regional Office for South East Asia; 2004.

14 WHO. What you should know about impairments. Proceedings of United Nations Inter Agency meeting on disability-prevention and rehabilitation of disabled; 1978; Geneva.

15 WHO. International Classification of impairments, disabilities and handicap. Geneva: WHO; 1980.

16 UNICEF. Facts about disability. New Delhi: UNICEF Information Office; 1982.

17 National Health Profile 2005. CBHI, DGHS, MOH and FW; New Delhi.

18 WHO. Fifty-fourth World Health Assembly. ICF. (Resolution WHA 54.21).

RISK MEASUREMENT IN EPIDEMIOLOGY

8

It is a common observation that some persons have higher risk, than others, to develop or contract a disease or death, these persons, who stand to higher risk of developing a disease or death are called "high-risk individuals". *Example*—infant born with low birth weight stands to high-risk of infant death as compared to infant born with adequate weight. Thus, low birth weight is a risk factor to high infant mortality in general.

What is Risk?

The dictionary meaning of risk is danger, hazard, or exposure to mischance. Risk or hazard develops before the occurrence of disease.

Risk Factors

Definition: The risk factor is a characteristic or a circumstance of individuals or groups, which is associated with an increased "risk" of developing an untoward or unwanted outcome.[1]

The risk factors can be "causes or signals" of an outcome. The risk factors can be identified and detected before the occurrence of an undesirable event. The risk factors vary with different diseases.

Common Risk Factors

- Diet high in saturated fats is a risk factor for coronary heart disease.
- Tobacco is risk factor for lung and oral cancer and many other diseases heart diseases.
- Chewing tobacco is a risk factor for oral cancer.
- High blood pressure is risk factor for strokes.
- Unprotected or unsafe sex is risk factor for sexually transmitted infections and HIV.
- Physical inactivity is risk factor to obesity and heart diseases.
- Unsafe water is a risk factor for water-borne diseases.

Grading of Risk

The risk can be graded based on objective criteria and experience. According to birth weight, the infants can be graded in following categories:

Grading of risk

Birth weight	*Risk category*
2500 g and above	Who carry very low-risk of death
2000–2499	Low-risk of death
1500–1999	Moderate risk
1000–1499	High-risk
Less than 1000 g	Very high-risk

This is to be observed that no birth is without risk of death, some stand to very high-risk of death such as weighing less than 1000 g and high-risk in births weighing 1000–1499 g. Thus, grading helps to decide the level of management. Infants weighing between 2000 and 2499 g at birth can be managed at home by appropriate neonatal care. While infants, weighing less than 2000 g should be managed at institutional level.

Overall risk of dying within first year of life in India (in the year 2005) was 6%, i.e. out of 100 births 6 will die within first year of life. However, in 100 births with weight less than 2000 g at birth, 18 infants may die within first year of life, then the risk of death is three times if the birth weight is less than 2000 g or else, the chances of survival are much more if the birth weight is more than 2500 g.

Population at Risk

In some situations, the whole population is at risk of developing or contracting a disease, e.g. tuberculosis and malaria.

But in most situations part of the population is exposed to the risk of developing a disease, e.g. carcinoma of cervix occurs commonly in women in age group 30–49 years, therefore the screening programme should focus only on this age bracket or on population at risk.

Application

The knowledge of risk factors helps in prevention of diseases. The primordial prevention aims at prevention of development of risk factors in population/person. If the risk factors are eliminated, the disease will not occur. Primary prevention aims at to prevent the development of disease in persons having risk factors. Attempt is made to modify the risk factors in such persons.

Uses

- Risk factor can predict the occurrence of a disease/ event.
- Helps in prevention and control of disease.
- Helps in allocation of resources and determination of priorities.

Measurement of Risk

The science of epidemiology measures the risk factors and determines the chances of development of unfavourable outcome or an event. There are several measures of risk. Risk can be categorized as:

1 Attributable risk
2 Attributable fraction
3 Population attributable risk
4 Percentage population attributable risk
5 Relative risk

1. Attributable Risk (AR)

In Table 8.10, we have chosen low birth weight (LBW) as a risk factor for infant deaths. There were 2700 births in a rural block, of these 1800 were of adequate weight (2.5 kg or more) and 900 were below 2.5 kg of weight at birth, the incidence of deaths among these infants within one year period was recorded. The incidence of infant death was 40/1000 among infants having birth weight of 2.5 kg or more and higher incidence of 120 infant deaths per 1000 live births was recorded in infants with birth weight less than 2.5 kg. In this situation, the risk of infant death, which can be attributable to low birth weight risk factor is as under:

$$\text{Attributable risk} = \begin{array}{c}\text{Incidence of infant}\\ \text{deaths in babies with}\\ \text{low birth weight}\end{array} (-) \begin{array}{c}\text{Incidence of infant}\\ \text{deaths in babies with}\\ \text{adequate weight}\end{array}$$

or

$$AR = 120 - 40 = 80$$

$$\begin{array}{c}\text{Proportion of low birth}\\ \text{weight babies in the}\\ \text{community}\end{array} = \frac{900}{2700} = \frac{1}{3}$$

Attributable risk is also called "risk difference", i.e. difference of incidence of infant deaths in two categories: One with risk of "low birth weight" and other without risk, i.e. "adequate weight at birth". We can say that there is additional risk of 80 points in high-risk infants born with low birth weight.

Significance

Attributable risk is a useful measure of the extent of mortality caused by the low birth weights in the community. Incidence of 80/1000 infant deaths is attributable to low birth weights.

2. Attributable Fraction

The attributable fraction or aetiological fraction is obtained by dividing the attributable risk or risk difference by the incidence of infant mortality occurring in low birth weight babies.

$$\frac{80}{120} \times 100 = 66\%$$

Significance

Sixty-six percent of mortality in low birth weight babies is attributable to low birth weight. It means that 66% of incidence of mortality in infants of low birth weight could

Table 8.10: Risk of dying within one-year in infants with normal and low birth weight in a rural block

Birth weight	*Total births*	*No. died within one year*	*Incidence per 1000 live births*
>2.5 kg (adequate)	1800	72	40
<2.5 kg (low birth weight)	900	108	120
Total	**2700**	**180**	**67**

8

be reduced if the risk factor of low birth weight in the community is eliminated.

3. Population Attributable Risk

The population attributable risk is a measure of excess of rate of infant deaths in a total study population which is attributable to low birth weight. In the present example: What is the incidence of infant deaths in the population associated with occurrence of low birth weight? The population attributable risk is the product of attributable risk and proportion of low birth weight in the community.

Attributable risk × Proportion of infants with low birth weight babies in community

or

$$80 \times \frac{900}{2700} = 80 \times \frac{1}{3} = 27$$

Significance

It measures the excess rate of incidence of infant deaths in the community that is associated with a risk factor of low birth weight. Population AR is useful to determine the relative significance of low birth weight in the community. Thus the excess annual incidence of avoidable infant deaths in this population is 27 per thousand.

4. Percentage Population Attributable Risk

The fraction of infant deaths occurring in population that is associated with LBW is obtained by dividing the population AR by the total infant mortality rate in the population.

$$\text{Percentage population AR} = \frac{\text{Population attributable risk}}{\text{Total incidence of infant mortality}} \times 100 = \frac{27}{67} \times 100 = 40\%$$

Forty percent of overall or total infant mortality could be prevented in the population if the risk factor of low birth weight is eliminated in the community.

The concept can be applied to disease, death, disability, survival, or any other event like accident, etc.

5. Relative Risk (RR)

One may ask how many times a low birth weight baby experiences mortality relative to baby with adequate birth weight? This can be answered by calculating *relative risk or risk ratio*. This is the ratio of incidence of infant deaths in low birth weight babies and incidence of infant deaths in babies with adequate birth weight. In the present example:

$$\text{Relative risk} = \frac{120}{40} = 3$$

Thus, we can answer that low birth weight babies are likely to experience mortality during infancy three times higher than babies with adequate birth weight.

Significance

The relative risk measures the strength of association between the risk factor and the unfavourable outcome. A relative risk greater than 2 can be considered as strong association between the risk factor and the unwanted outcome. In the present case, RR of three means LBW as a risk factor has strong association with infant mortality.

Summary of Risk Measurement

$$\text{Attributable risk (AR)} = \text{Incidence of an event in persons exposed to risk factor} \; (-) \; \text{Incidence of an event in persons not exposed to risk factor}$$

or

$$= I_E - I_{NE}$$

Population AR = AR × incidence of risk factor in the community

Attributable fraction = AR/incidence of risk in cexposed population

$$\text{Percentage population attributable risk} = \frac{\text{Population AR}}{\text{Total incidence of outcome in the community}} \times 100$$

$$\text{Relative risk (RR)} = \frac{\text{Incidence in person exposed to risk factor } (I_E)}{\text{Incidence in persons not exposed to risk factor } (I_{NE})}$$

SCREENING

Lead Time

Risk factors are present before the undesired outcome occurs. Time taken between presence of risk factors in population/person, and development of disease/event is significant for intervention or action. The time gap between presence of risk factor and development of disease provides useful opportunity for appropriate action. Screening of population or subgroups for detection of risk factor is essential step for prevention of unwanted outcome/disease.

Focus

Screening focuses on apparently healthy persons/groups. Thus, screening is the process by which risk factors or danger signs of unrecognized diseases/defects are identified by tests that can be applied rapidly on a large scale. Screening tests sort-out apparently healthy people from those who have a risk factor or have a chance to develop unfavourable outcome. Screening is not a final diagnosis it usually requires further tests for confirmation. Screening rates remain woefully low in our country.

Criteria for Screening[2]

1 The disease should be highly prevalent and severe enough to necessitate screening, i.e. it affects large number of people and geographically widespread and is important cause of death in the country or region.
2 The gap between exposure and development of disease should be sufficient for intervention or action.
3 Availability of sensitive, specific, reliable, cheap and safe test available for screening.
4 Effective, safe and acceptable interventions are available.
5 Screening without action or intervention is useless.

Example: Screening for cancer cervix, breast cancer, tuberculosis, diabetes, obesity and coronary heart disease, blood for its safety and 4 Ds in RBSK.

Objectives

The screening programme have the following objectives:

i To identify a risk factor.
ii To detect a disease at preclinical stage.
iii To detect syndrome at early stage.

Types of Screening[3]

- ***Whole population or mass screening:*** Whole population is subjected to screening. *Example:* All schoolchildren as they enter in school are examined or given a health check-up to screen out health conditions.
- ***Targeted screening:*** Screening which is directed towards a special group of population or high-risk groups—commercial sex workers, factory workers, pregnant women, infants, etc.
- ***Opportunistic screening:*** Restricting screening to patients who consult a health physician in hospital or clinic.
- ***Multiple or multiphase screening*** using multiple screening tests at the same time, e.g. testing vision, weighing, testing hearing, testing blood, at the same time.

The disease may be either present or absent and similarly the test result may be either positive or negative. There are thus four possible combinations:

1 ***True positive:*** When the disease condition is present and test is positive.
2 ***True negative:*** When the disease condition is absent and the test is negative.
3 ***False positive:*** When the disease condition is absent but the test is positive.
4 ***False negative:*** When the disease condition is present but the test result is negative (Table 8.11).

Sensitivity

Sensitivity means proportion of truly disease persons who are categorized as abnormal by the test.

or

Proportion of true positive persons (who have the disease) and test is positive.

Calculation: It is calculated by a/a + c.

Specificity

Specificity means proportion of truly normal people categorized as normal by the test.

or

Proportion of true negative persons (who do not have the disease) and test is negative.

Calculation: It is calculated by d/b + d.

Positive Predictive Value (PPV)

This is the probability of a disease in a patient with an abnormal test result.

Calculation: It is calculated by a/a + b.

Negative Predictive Value (NPV)

This is the probability of a person not having a disease when the result of a test is negative.

Calculation: It is calculated by d/c + d.

The predictive value depends upon the sensitivity and specificity of a test and most importantly on the prevalence of disease in the community being tested. Predictive value is more important determinant in view of variation in

Table 8.11: Validity of a screening test

		Risk factor/disease		
		(Present) +	*(Absent)* –	*Total*
SCREENING TEST	+ (Positive)	a	b	a + b
	– (Negative)	c	d	c + d
	Total	**a + c**	**b + d**	**a + b + c + d**

a: Indicates number of true positives, i.e. those who have the risk factor or disease condition and test is also positive.
b: Number of false positive, who have no disease but the test is positive.
c: Indicates number of false negative, i.e. number of persons who have the risk factor/disease but the test is negative.
d: True negative—who have no disease and test is negative (Table 8.11).

prevalence of disease from one state to another and from one region to another.

VALIDITY OF TEST

Validity is an expression of the degree to which test is capable of measuring what it intended to measure. In validity, we consider 4 elements, namely: Sensitivity, specificity, positive predictive value and negative predictive value of the measurement or test. All the available tests have their limitations; hence one should use multiple tests to increase the validity.

Typical sensitivity and specificity values for commonly used laboratory tests today for detecting HIV-1 infection (ELISA, rapid and simple test) are at 99%. The first generation ELISA had a sensitivity of 95% and the Western Blot has a specificity of 99.99% (Tables 8.12 and 8.13).

Second generation ELISA tests have high sensitivity and high specificity.

Low rate of false negative is the priority for blood transfusion safety, in contrast, if the objective is case identification, a low rate of false positive is very important.

ELISA is most commonly performed screening test for blood safety. It is easy to perform, it is sensitive and specific and cost-effective and adoptable to large number of samples.

Supplemental Western Blot of all initially ELISA positives is a confirmatory/diagnostic test. Therefore, "total population" for the Western Blot is 5850 (Table 8.13).

Since HIV is life-threatening infection high sensitivity and high specificity is desirable. Both ELISA and Western Blot tests are highly sensitive and have high specificity.

SCREENING IN NON-COMMUNICABLE DISEASES (NCDs)

The following risk factors for non-communicable diseases have been identified.

Behavioural Risk Factors

- Tobacco and harmful alcohol use.
- High saturated fats and inappropriate dietary habits.
- Physical inactivity.

Table 8.12: Validity of ELISA test[4]

		True infection status		
		Infected	Non-infected	Total
ELISA RESULT	+ (Positive)	4900 (A)	950 (B)	5850 (A + B)
	– (Negative)	100 (C)	94,050 (D)	94,150 (C + D)
	Total	5000 (A + C)	95,000 (B + D)	1,00,000 (A + B + C + D)

Persons tested = 1,00,000

Prevalence of HIV infection $= \frac{5000}{100000} \times 100 = 5\%$

A: True positives, *B*: False positives, *C*: False negatives, *D*: True negatives

Sensitivity $= \frac{A}{A+C} = \frac{4900}{5000} \times 100 = 98\%$

Specificity $= \frac{D}{B+D} = \frac{94050}{95000} \times 100 = 99\%$

Positive predictive value $= \frac{A}{A+B} \times 100 = \frac{4900}{5850} \times 100 = 83.8\%$

Negative predictive value $= \frac{D}{C+D} \times 100 = \frac{94050}{94150} \times 100 = 99.9\%$

Table 8.13: Validity of Western Blot test[4]

		True infection status		
		Infected	*Non-infected*	*Total*
WESTERN BLOT	+ (Positive)	4655 (A)	1 (B)	4656 (A + B)
	– (Negative)	245 (C)	949 (D)	1194 (C + D)
	Total	4900 (A + C)	950 (B + D)	5850 (A + B + C + D)

Total population: 5850, *A*: True positives = 4655, *B*: False positives = 1, *C*: False negatives = 245, *D*: True negatives = 949

Sensitivity $= \frac{A}{A+C} = \frac{4655}{4900} \times 100 = 95\%$

Positive predictive value $= \frac{A}{A+B} = \frac{4655}{4656} \times 100 = 99.9\%$

Specificity $= \frac{D}{B+D} = \frac{949}{950} \times 100 = 99.9\%$

Negative predictive value $= \frac{D}{C+D} = \frac{949}{1194} \times 100 = 79.5\%$

Metabolic or Physiological Risk Factors

- High body mass index—obesity
- Raised blood pressure
- Raised blood glucose
- Raised cholestrol

Measurements

- ***Biochemical assessment:*** By blood sugar, and blood cholesterol.
- ***Physical measurements:*** Height, weight, waist circumference, blood pressure, pulse rate.

Strategies of Screening for Non-communicable Diseases (NCDs) Risk Factors[5]

1. Monitor trends of important risk factors of NCD in the community over a period of time.
2. Evolve strategies for interventions of these risk factors so as to reduce the burden of disease due to NCD (these have been explained in the book in Chapter 13 on NCD).
3. Strengthen NCD surveillance at district level.

Integrate NCD risk factors surveillance with IDSP (integrated disease surveillance programme).

Common Screening Tests

Safe Blood

1. Screening blood before transfusion is mandatory for HIV, HBV, malaria and syphilis. Before transfusion, blood is screened for all these infections and we have now introduced screening for HCV as well.
2. *Cancer cervix:* Cervical smears (PAP test) for early detection of asymptomatics, pre-cancerous cervical lesion usually done in married women above 35 years of age. This is the strategy adopted in national cancer control programme.
3. Screening of risk factors for epidemic of cardiovascular diseases. The major risk factors are inappropriate diet and physical inactivity (as expressed through unfavourable lipid concentration, high body mass index and raised blood pressure), together with tobacco use.

Screening for Tuberculosis

First stage: Encourage health workers and Medical Officers to identify pulmonary tuberculosis suspects as early as possible to prevent further spread of infection.

- Every patient who has cough for 2 weeks or more with or without other symptoms should have two sputum samples examined for AFB. Around 2% of adult population in general OPD have cough for 2 weeks or more (Fig. 8.7).

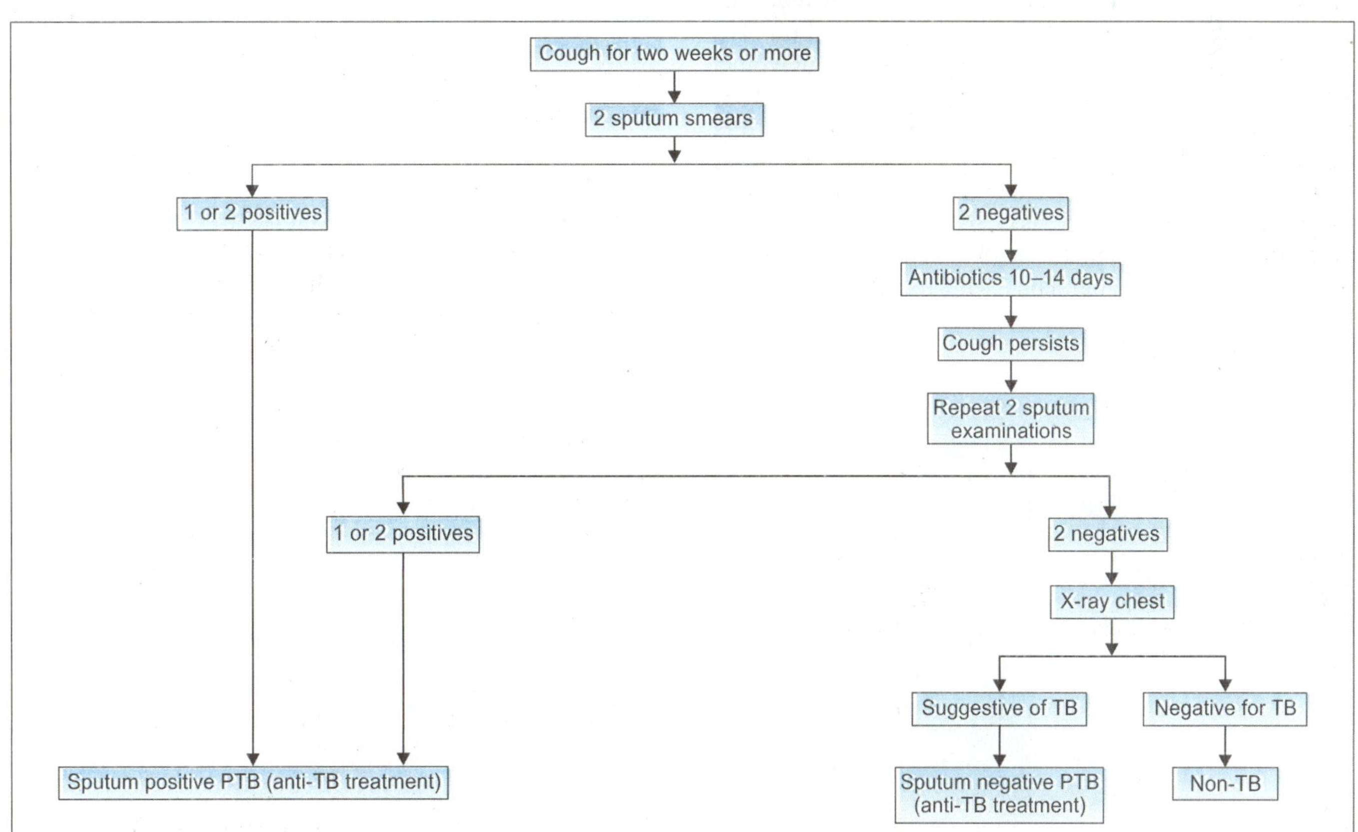

Fig. 8.7: Diagnosis and algorithm for pulmonary TB

- The diagnosis of tuberculosis by X-ray alone is unreliable. Unless the diagnostic algorithm is followed, a large proportion of patients not actually having tuberculosis may be treated for tuberculosis on the basis of abnormal X-ray alone.

X-ray-based evaluation causes over-diagnosis of TB as 40% of cases diagnosed and put on treatment on the basis of X-ray did not actually have tuberculosis. Thus, the patients are subjected to unnecessary expensive and potentially toxic medicines (NIT, Bangalore Ind. J. Tub., 1974).

X-ray chest for diagnosis of TB is not specific, sputum test is specific for pulmonary tuberculosis. X-ray results should be read carefully and should be corroborated with clinical signs and symptoms.[6,7]

Risk Approach in Maternal Health

Much discussion has gone into the formulation of a risk approach for maternal and child care. Epidemiologically, risk approach implies that there are criteria to screen potential danger, identify those in danger and provide special care. In the context of maternity, this would mean that certain conditions have a higher probability of death. Risk factors identified for pregnant women are anaemia, short stature, bad obstetrical history, etc. If these factors are taken into account, over 90% of India's pregnant women are at risk. Therefore, the approach does not have focus action and all women should get essential obstetrical care.[8]

Recent studies related to women who died due to pregnancy and childbirth revealed that 50% of them had one or more risk factors, and 50% of them had no "risk factors". In other words, the probability of pregnant women with any risk factor dying due to pregnancy-related causes is just as much as in women without any risk factor. Further, risk approach for maternal care "conveys" to the health workers the impression that they cannot render any care to pregnant women with risks. Attempts to refer such pregnant women to hospitals lead to increased reliance on the traditional birth attendants with its added problems. This underlines the need to provide essential "obstetrical care for all" (Fig. 8.8).

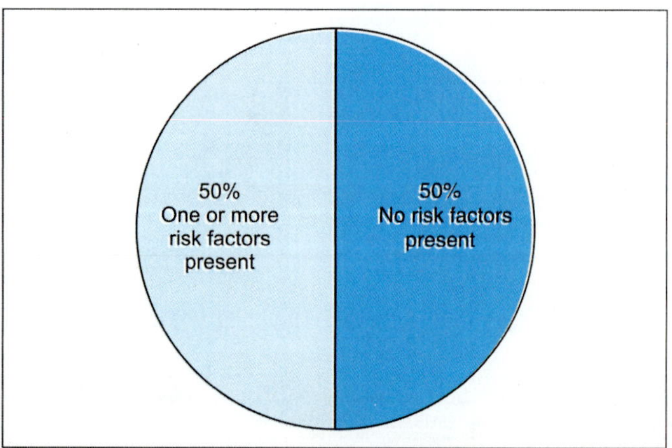

Fig. 8.8: Maternal deaths

REFERENCES

1 IGNOU. School of Health Sciences. Epidemiology in maternal and child health. Preventive MCH, MME-101. New Delhi: IGNOU; 2003.

2 Beaglehole R. Global cardiovascular disease prevention: Time to get serious "viewpoint". Lancet 2001; 358: 661–3.

3 Beaglehole R, Bonita R, Kjellstrom. Basic epidemiology. Geneva: WHO; 1993.

4 NACO. Training manual on sentinel surveillance of HIV/AIDS. New Delhi: NACO: MOH and FW, GOI; 1993.

5 WHO. The World Health Report 2002—Reducing risks, promoting healthy life. Geneva: WHO; 2002.

6 GOI. TB India 2002, RNTCP Status Report. Stop TB Fight poverty. New Delhi: Central TB Division, DGHS, MOH and FW; 2002.

7 GOI. Managing the Revised National Tuberculosis Control Programme in your area. Training Course Module 1–4. New Delhi: Central TB Division, DGHS, MOH and FW; 2004.

8 MOH and FW. National Child Survival and Safe-motherhood Programme. Programme intervention, New Delhi. MOH and FW, GOI; 1992.

PUBLIC HEALTH SURVEILLANCE

What is Surveillance?

Surveillance is information for action. This is the simplest definition of surveillance. Surveillance is a French word meaning, "watch with attention, suspicion and authority".

Centre for disease control (CDC), which defines epidemiological surveillance as "the ongoing and systematic collection, analysis and interpretation of health data essential to planning, implementation and evaluation of public health practice and programmes closely integrated with timely dissemination of these data to those who need to know." The final link in the surveillance chain is the application of the information to prevention and control. A surveillance system includes a functional capacity for data collection, analysis and dissemination linked to public health programmes.[1] Surveillance is not made to "Keep statistics" but to guide decision/action to prevent and control diseases.

or

Surveillance is—"Information for Action"

Objective of Epidemiological Surveillance

The surveillance could have limited or many objectives. Some of the objectives are:

1 To determine incidence of disease.

2 To know the geographical distribution or spread of disease/event.

3 To identify population at risk of that disease/event.
4 To monitor trend of disease over a long-time period.
5 To capture the factors and conditions responsible for occurrence and spread of a disease.
6 To predict the occurrence of epidemic and control epidemic.
7 To evaluate the effectiveness of an intervention or programme.
8 To assess the disease burden in the community or health needs of community.

These are the broad objectives of epidemiological surveillance, however, depending upon the resources and needs, the objectives could be limited to one or two specific areas or these could be expanded. But keep it short and specific (KISS), limited to a few indicators.

Scope

The surveillance is an important epidemiological tool and it limits to a specific disease/diseases which is/are of national significance and has high priority in terms of control/elimination/eradication. Malaria and acute flaccid paralysis surveillance (for eradication of polio) are significant in India. Currently, the vertical national programme of epidemiological surveillance of the following diseases is going on in the country, independently without much coordination.

- Acute flaccid paralysis (AFP) surveillance to eradicate polio.
- HIV/AIDS surveillance
- National vector borne diseases surveillance.
- Vaccine preventable disease (VPD) surveillance.
- Acute respiratory infections in children.
- Diarrhoeal diseases in children.
- Nutrition surveillance
- Sentinel surveillance for blindness control.
- Surveillance of noncommunicable diseases.

ESSENTIAL ELEMENTS OF SURVEILLANCE

A Collection of data
B Compilation and transmission of data
C Analysis and interpretation
D Action
E Feedback

Surveillance Methods for Data Collection

A surveillance system counts the same event consistently everyday. The commonly used surveillance methods for data collection are as under:[2]

1 Community level surveillance.
2 Routine reporting system.
3 Active surveillance and passive surveillance for malaria.
4 Sentinel surveillance.
5 Surveys and special studies.
6 Case and outbreak investigation.
7 Verbal autopsy.
8 Laboratory surveillance.
9 Entomological surveillance.

1. Community Level Surveillance

People themselves (community informants) report births, deaths, outbreaks and unusual events.

- ASHAs, Anganwadi workers, self help groups and village panches/panchayats as also press report unusual events or significant health events. Disease surveillance system at village level is being strengthened under NRHM. Informants at community level need to be contacted on regular basis.

2. Routine Reporting (Institutional Based or Passive Reporting—Provider's Initiated)

In routine reporting, health staff collects information about number of cases of reportable diseases and deaths that occur in their area in relation to all national health programmes.

This system relies on government-established system of subcentres, primary health centres, community health centres and hospitals data. Whosoever comes to these facilities are recorded and reported. This is passive routine reporting system. This is the simplest and most widely prescribed way of collecting information for action.

Medical institutions in India are required to report cases and deaths attended in the outpatients or inpatients which include the enlisted 20 communicable diseases, *every month* to the next higher level. The State Bureau of Health Intelligence/Vital Statistical Unit consolidates the data received from district health officers and transmits it to the Central Bureau of Health Intelligence (CBHI).[2]

Advantages

- Routine reporting system is simplest and least costly or inexpensive.
- It is efficient and quickest method to obtain the information.

Disadvantages

Routine reporting system provides:

- Incomplete information or reporting
- Quality of data highly variable and reliability is also variable
- These systems almost always provide incomplete picture of the total number of cases that occur. Some of the reasons of incomplete reporting are:
  – Not all cases come to health facility for treatment. Some people or most people may go to private

practitioners for treatment, some may not seek any treatment, and some may go to other facilities.

- Some diseases such as neonatal tetanus are more commonly treated at hospitals than health centres.
- Complete and accurate reporting are always problem in PHCs and CHCs.

Nevertheless, routine reporting is the most common method used in surveillance because it is so inexpensive.

3. Active Surveillance

It is usually limited to a specific disease. However good the routine reporting system there will still be cases that will not be recorded under this system. The cases with mild or moderate form of the disease may not seek treatment from the health centre/hospital. They may stay at home or may go to private practitioners or traditional healers. These will not be recorded under the routine reporting or institutional surveillance. It is also possible that patients in severe conditions are taken to large hospital in another district for specialized care and some cases may die within a short period of onset of symptoms.

Active surveillance means actively looking or searching for a particular type or group of diseases, is useful in detecting these unreported cases, it involves active participation of health personnel as well as the community. The degree of *reporting is more complete* than by any other method, especially for the clinically distinct and easily recognizable diseases/syndromes.

i Active surveillance for malaria control/eradication programme has been the time-tested strategy and is still going on strong. Workers have fixed beat programme and fortnightly visit to every home/household to capture all fever cases in assigned population of 5000 in a subcentre area, preparation of blood smears (thick and thin) and full therapeutic treatment for malaria.

ii Active search for smallpox cases was an important strategy for smallpox eradication programme. Photo flash cards were used for easy recognition of disease in the community.

iii In the guinea worm, eradication programme search was conducted twice in a year in the affected area. Photo flash cards were used for easy recognition of case.

iv People themselves, multipurpose health workers, village health guides, Anganwadi workers have played important role in active surveillance of diseases in the community. This type of community surveillance can detect early cases of a possible impending outbreak/epidemic.

v Active search may be called during outbreaks to determine the extent of outbreak and to keep mortality rate low, to check the reports received by rumour registry, active surveillance is also undertaken for acute flaccid paralysis (AFP) as also to confirm the absence of even a single case during pre-certification phase of disease eradication, as "Zero" incidence has to be maintained for a period of 3 years.

Only a few diseases should be selected for active surveillance. These should include those diseases for which control programme is operating and which are epidemic prone such as malaria, polio, diarrhoeal diseases and ARI in children. The channel of flow of community surveillance and institutional surveillance is presented to understand the system of flow of information (Fig. 8.9).

Passive Surveillance

It means collection of data from persons, themselves reporting to a facility (hospital, clinic, subcentre, PHC and CHC, etc.) as elaborated under routine reporting. At times during outbreak investigator may conduct what is sometimes called *stimulated* or *enhanced* passive surveillance by sending a letter describing the situation and asking for reports of similar cases.

4. Sentinel Surveillance

In sentinel systems, a small number of health units are selected to report cases of diseases and deaths that are seen or diagnosed at their facility.

These sentinel sites also collect and report additional information such as age, immunization status and other details. Staff at sentinel sites is given special training and supervised to ensure that reporting is complete and accurate.

Common Sentinel Sites

A hospital (infectious diseases, TB, paediatric hospital), health centre, antenatal clinics, sexually transmitted infection clinic, laboratory or rehabilitation centre, which attends large number of particular type of cases can be considered as a possible sentinel site/centre. Many institutions such as teaching hospitals and national institutes may already be collecting the information desired.

Advantages

- The sentinel sites collect more reliable and accurate data because trained staff and specialists handle the cases.
- Their records are more accurate and timely and these sites provide consistent and quality data/information. They are also relatively inexpensive to set-up and operate.

Disadvantages

A major disadvantage of sentinel system is that they are not representative of entire population at risk. We cannot calculate incidence or prevalence rates, because of lack of denominator; which are important for assessing changes in health status. The information cannot be generalized to estimate the national or state incidence rate. Another disadvantage is that population served by sentinel site may change making the study or trends invalid.

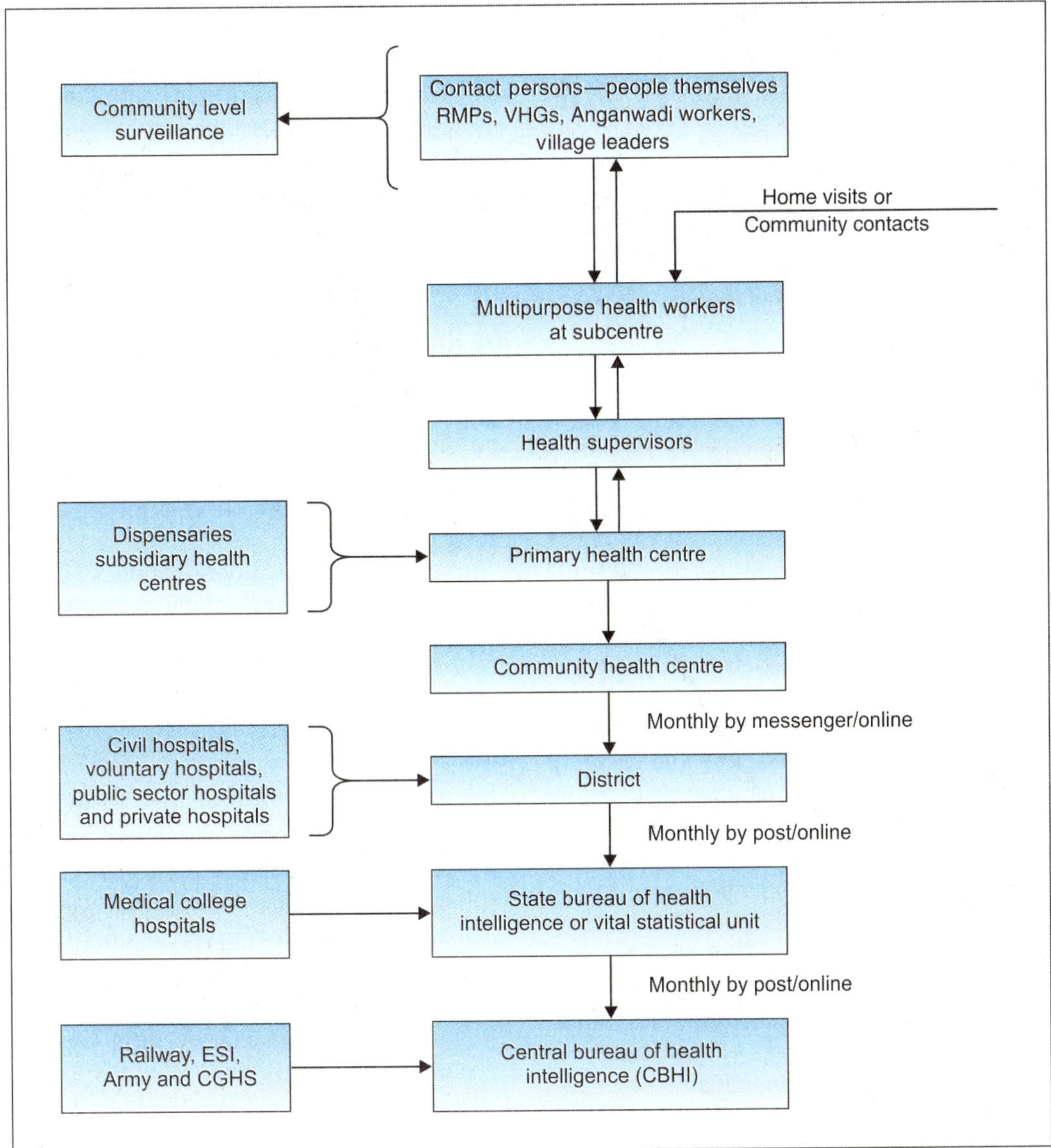

Fig. 8.9: Channel of information flow in community and institutional level surveillance

Criteria

An institution may act as sentinel centre for one or group of diseases depending upon the number and type of cases attended by them. The following minimum criteria need to be observed in selection of centre:

i Large attendance of patients with the particular disease.

ii Diagnosis is reasonable accurate and laboratory support is available.

iii Good recording and reporting facilities available.

iv Willingness to submit regular reports.

Uses

The data collected by sentinel centres can be effectively used both for immediate action in the field as well as for future plans and policy decisions.

- Reporting large number of cases as compared to corresponding period (month or quarter) of previous years serve as an early warning of a potential epidemic. An abnormal increase in the number of cases calls for an immediate investigation and institution of necessary preventive measures by the local health officer.
- The seasonal pattern of disease is clearly established from the reports of the sentinel centres and plans for preventive programmes are made accordingly.
- The sentinel centres can serve as indicator of the impact of the services provided. For example, data can tell whether the children are getting the diseases after completion of immunization. These centres can be efficient "watch dogs" of quality of preventive health services.
- The information may indicate the shifting of disease to higher age groups or clustering of cases in selected

localities. Plans can be modified according to changing pattern of the diseases.

The sentinel surveillance system was used to capture incidence of vaccine preventable diseases.

Annual unlinked anonymous *sentinel surveillance* is being carried out since 1998, to capture HIV/AIDS prevalence in the country and to determine trends, HIV load in the country as also to identify the population at risk and geographical distribution of epidemic of HIV in the country.

5. Surveys and Special Studies

Sample survey or disease survey is an active and efficient method of surveillance, which can complement the other methods. Two surveys done at an interval of several years apart may be able to demonstrate changes in disease incidence. The first survey for collecting reliable baseline epidemiological information and the subsequent one for evaluation of the control programme or intervention. In some selected instances (e.g. poliomyelitis lameness surveys), it may be possible to conduct one survey at one point in time utilizing two different age groups to collect both baseline and current performance data. In planning a national disease control strategy, survey is needed to establish priorities between various diseases.

Survey on blindness at different points in time in India provides information on prevalence of blindness and effect of interventions on blindness.

National oral health survey and fluoride mapping provides useful information on oral health status and problems.

Survey of risk factors for non-communicable diseases is being undertaken at 3–5 years interval under IDSP programme.

Limitations

Surveys are difficult to conduct, relatively expensive and call for highly skilled persons with organizational abilities. The sample size, questionnaires and forms must be well designed to avoid bias and misinterpretation of data. Some diseases require laboratory back-up for accurate diagnosis, which make the surveys even more difficult. House to house surveys require an important investment of organizational efforts; manpower and other resources. It is difficult to justify this investment merely to study one disease. With appropriate multipurpose survey designs, several disease conditions can be studied in the same sample population.

A simple method using cluster-sampling technique (recommended for vaccination coverage evaluation surveys by the World Health Organization) with necessary modifications has been proposed for surveys of various diseases.

6. Case and Outbreak Investigation

The major objective of an epidemiological investigation of a disease outbreak is to help control the spread of disease by indicating the most appropriate preventive measures by identifying where and to whom and how to apply these measures and subsequently by monitoring the progress of control efforts. Outbreak investigations can also provide important supplementary information, not often gained from other surveillance methods. This includes, age specific attack rates, case fatality rates, rate of serious disability and estimates of vaccine efficacy. Measles surveillance in the country is based on "measles outbreak" investigation. It also attempts to identify the causes of death and disease.

They are not alternatives to routine and sentinel systems but are used as the next step in epidemiological investigation.

In general, a "case" investigation is an investigation of a single case of a disease or death; an "outbreak" investigation is an investigation of many cases. However, when the occurrence of a particular disease is very low, polio for example, even one case can be considered as an outbreak.

Purpose

The usual purposes of these investigations are:

1. To confirm diagnosis and determine the causes.
2. Confirm the existence of an outbreak (an increase in the number of cases/deaths than usual frequency).
3. Identify the most appropriate control measures.
4. Identify where and to whom to apply these measures.
5. Determine why the outbreak occurred?
6. Determine what can be done to prevent similar outbreaks in the future?

These investigations are conducted systematically by having a written protocol or plan to identify the underlying cause of the problem.

7. Verbal Autopsy

It is a special technique for investigation of cause of death. Trained worker or investigator conducts an in-depth investigation of the death (maternal or infant death or any other death) through interviews with the mother or any one else who was a witness to the death and the circumstances leading up to it. The investigations are done on a standard designed format or protocol.

Purpose

- The purpose is to ascertain the most probable cause of death.
- Whether the death could have been prevented or avoided by timely and appropriate measures.
- Workers can educate community as to how to prevent deaths as also common causes of death in the community.

8. Laboratory Surveillance

Laboratory testing confirms the syndromes of presumptive cases and helps in diagnosis of cases for case management.

9. Entomological Surveillance

Regular surveillance for vectors of diseaes under national vector-borne diseases control programme is being done to know vector density and sensitivity to *insecticide*.

NATIONAL SURVEILLANCE PROGRAMME FOR COMMUNICABLE DISEASES (NSPCD)

The Government of India launched NSPCD during 1997–98. The main objective was to strengthen the surveillance system of communicable diseases and developing capabilities at state level and district level so that disease outbreaks can be detected early in order to institute rapid response to avert morbidity and mortality. The programme was in operation in 101 districts in the country for monthy reporting of 20 CCDs. Now it has been integrated with IDSP.[3]

INTEGRATED DISEASE SURVEILLANCE PROGRAMME (IDSP)

In the year 2004, Government of India with World Bank assistance has launched a project called IDSP. The project intends to cover all states by phased manner.[4–6] IDSP is proposed to continue as integrated Disease Surveillance and Response Programme under NRHM with domestic budget in 12th plan.

Project Objectives

- To establish a decentralized district-based system of surveillance for communicable and non-communicable diseases so that timely and effective public health actions can be initiated in response to health challenges in the country in urban and rural areas.
- Integration of surveillance activities of various health programmes and share information across all disease control programmes and stake holders, so that valid data are available for decision making at district, state and national levels.

Specific Objectives

1 To integrate all existing surveillance activities of national disease control/eradication programmes at district level. The IDSP integrates both public and private sectors, integrates communicable and non-communicable diseases programmes, integrates both rural and urban health systems with medical colleges.

2 To establish system of data collection, collation, compilation, analysis and feedback by using information technology.

3 To improve laboratory support for disease surveillance.

4 To develop human resources for disease surveillance and action (rapid response teams).

5 To involve all stakeholders including private sector and communities in surveillance.

Project Activities

- Upgradation of laboratories.
- Upgradation of information technology and communication.
- Human resources and development (training—consultant/contract staff).
- Operational activities and response.
- Monitoring and evaluation.

Target Diseases for Surveillance under IDSP

a *Regular surveillance*

1 Malaria
2 Acute diarrhoeal disease (cholera)
3 Typhoid
4 Tuberculosis
5 Measles
6 Polio (acute flaccid paralysis)
7 Road traffic accidents (link up with police computers)
8 Plague
9 Meningoencephalitis/respiratory distress, haemorrhagic fevers, and other unusual clinical syndromes.

b *Sentinel surveillance*

1 HIV/HBV, HCV
2 Water quality monitoring
3 Outdoor air quality (large urban centres)

c *Regular periodic surveys:* For non-communicable diseases risk factors: Anthropometry, physical activity, blood pressure, tobacco, and diet.

Additional State Priorities

Each state may identify up to 5 additional conditions for surveillance, e.g. dengue, Japanese encephalitis, leptospirosis, filariasis, leprosy, diphtheria, leishmaniasis and tetanus neonatorum.

Scheme for Participation of Private Sector

It is estimated that 70% of first contact providers are in the private sector. The IDSP envisages partnership with health care institutions or selected sentinel private sites (SSPS) in the urban and rural areas to improve the *coverage* and sensitivity of surveillance.

Types of Surveillance in IDSP

(S) Syndromic: Syndromic surveillance is defined as the surveillance of diseases based on the presenting

symptom/s. Under IDSP, the health workers, village volunteers and non-formal practitioners are conducting syndromic surveillance. The cases identified through presenting symptoms are classified as 'suspect cases' of certain disease condition, e.g. a case of fever with rash, will be classified under the syndrome, fever with rash and not as measles. The lay case definition of disease should be widely circulated for this purpose. The clinical syndromes under surveillance are:

1 *Fever*
   i Less than 7 days without any localized sign.
   ii With rash
   iii With altered sensorium or convulsion.
   iv Bleeding from skin and mucus membrane.
   v More than 7 days with or without localized signs.
2 *Cough:* Cough for 2 weeks or more with/without fever.
3 *Acute flaccid paralysis* (AFP) in <15 years
4 *Diarrhoea:* Loose watery stools <2 weeks
5 *Jaundice:* Cases <4 weeks
6 *Unusual events* causing death or hospitalization. These syndromes are intended to pick up all priority diseases listed under IDSP for surveillance.[6–8]

(P) ***Probable:*** The medical diagnosis made on the basis of presenting symptoms and clinical signs by Medical Officer at a facility.

(L) ***Laboratory Confirmed:*** Clinical diagnosis confirmed by appropriate laboratory test.

Implementation—Reporting Units Participating in Regular Passive Surveillance under IDSP

The regular surveillance is passive in type and is being undertaken by Medical Officers.

For project implementation surveillance units with unique ID number have been set up at central, state and district levels.

Reporting units for disease surveillance

	Public health sector	Private health sector
Rural	Sub-centres, PHCs/CHCs, sub-district and district hospitals	Sentinel private practitioners and sentinel hospitals
Urban	Urban hospitals, ESI, railway and other hospitals, medical colleges	Sentinel private nursing homes, sentinel hospitals, medical colleges, NGOs and private laboratories

Data Management

Under IDSP report is collected on weekly basis—every Monday. The information is collected under "S" (Syndromic), "P" (Probable cases) and "L" Laboratory confirmed cases filled by health workers, clinicians and laboratory staff respectively. Weekly data gives time trends. Whenever there is rising trend of an illness in the area it is investigated by Medical Officers/Rapid Response Teams (RRT) to diagnose and control the outbreak. Data analysis and action are ensured by respective units. Emphasis is being laid on reporting of surveillance data form major hospitals both in public and in private sectors as also from infectious disease hospitals. To strengthen the transmission of data IDSP has established linkages with state and district headquarters and all Government Medical Colleges on a satellite Broadband Hybrid Network.

A 24 × 7 call centre has been established to receive disease alerts from anywhere in the country on a toll-free number, 1075 for verification and initiating appropriate action.[9]

Media Scanning and Verification Cell (MSVC)

This cell was established in July 2008 at NICD. Media scanning is one of the important systems of surveillance in detecting the early warning signals and giving feedback to surveillance units (SUs) for local action. Information published in leading national dailies on outbreak or unusual events is scanned by this cell for feedback to SUs by modern information technology. It supplements conventional disease surveillance system to detect outbreaks and appropriate action.

(A) METHODS OF DATA COLLECTION FOR DISEASE SURVEILLANCE

Data collection is the starting point of surveillance. The effectiveness of surveillance depends largely on quality of data, regularity of reporting diseases, timely reporting and ensuring adequate coverage. A surveillance system counts the same event consistently everyday. The criteria for diagnosing diseases under surveillance should be uniform and therefore "standard case definition of disease" has to be evolved and practiced by all reporting units of surveillance. For the purpose of surveillance "standard case definitions" of diseases like AFP, HIV/AIDS, measles, tetanus, diphtheria, pertussis have been evolved and it is expected that all participating units adhere to these definitions. Simple, standard forms for recording and reporting cases are in place to achieve uniformity.

(B) COMPILATION AND TRANSMISSION OF DATA

The cases that have been detected and recorded need to be compiled and transmitted to the next level on regular basis once a week or daily. This should be done on a fixed date from each type of unit. All reporting units/centres will provide zero reporting if no cases were detected. Zero reporting is mandatory to confirm that the conditions were looked for and not found. Use telephone, fax, e-mail, special messenger, police wireless—any method to report immediately. The designation of the person responsible for data compilation and transmission at each level has been identified (pharmacist, computer, statistical officer, lab technician and Medical Officer). The quality of data filled up by the health staff need to be *checked/looked* into by a senior before transmission. Data transmission is not a clerical job, it requires thinking, and examination to see whether signal is there. Computers cannot contact physicians and laboratory to obtain missing information and are no substitute for *looking, thinking, discussing* and taking action. The health workers, Medical Officers of PHCs and sentinel private practitioners will provide regular reports on prescribed formats on every Monday.

(C) ANALYSIS AND INTERPRETATION OF DATA

Data analysis: The process of analysis transforms raw data into *information for action.* Data are analysed by count, divide and compare (CDC) principle for time, place and person (TPP) description. CDC means count cases that meet case definition, divide cases by corresponding population denominator and compare incidence rates across time, places and persons (TPP).

Time analysis: Data by histogram (graph): Incidence by date of occurrence of cases over a short time period, or by weeks, months or by years. It gives seasonality and trends of the disease (rising, declining or stable trend) (Fig. 8.10).

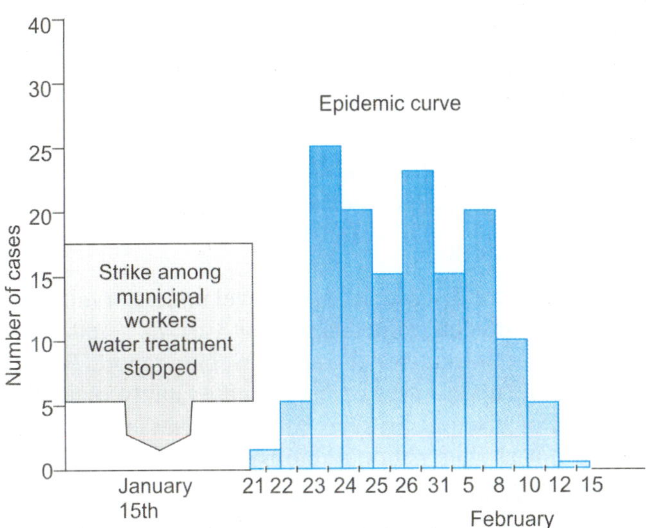

Fig. 8.10: Cases of acute hepatitis (E) by date of onset

Interpretation of graph (histogram) of acute hepatitis (E): Cases started occurring 3 weeks after he strike at the water treatment plant as the water treatment stopped and people consumed unsafe water and suffered jaundice. The source of infection persisted and continued to cause hepatitis E up to 12th February. Thereafter with interventions the cases declined.

- The epidemic curve shows the magnitude of epidemic over times as a simple, easily understood visual.
- The *shape* of the epidemic curve may provide clues about the pattern of spread in the population, e.g. *point* versus *intermittent* versus propagated.

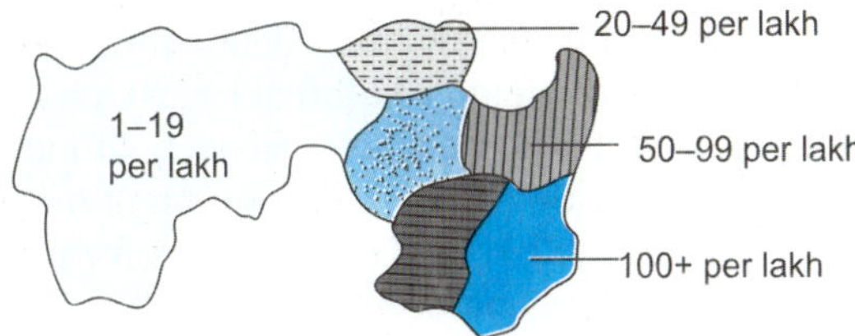

Fig. 8.11: Incidence map of acute hepatitis by blocks, attack rates per 1,00,000

- The curve shows where you are in the course of epidemic still on the upswing, on the down slope, or after the epidemic has ended.
- The curve can be used for evaluation of interventions.
- Outliers—cases that do not fit into the body of the curve—may provide important clues.
- The incubation period can be estimated from the curve and epicurve can be used to deduce a *probable time* of *exposure from* the *peak* and median of curve.

Place analysis: Data by incidence map.

Incidence maps take into account population size of affected block or locality (Fig. 8.11).

Table 8.14: Attack rate of hepatitis (E) by age and sex

Age groups	*Cases*	*Population*	*Attack rate per 1000*
0–4	1	1000	0.1
5–9	11	21000	0.5
10–14	40	70000	0.57
15–44	400	50000	8.0
45+	70	50000	1.4
Male	400	100000	4.0
Female	122	92000	1.3

Interpretation of incidence map: Cases were clustered in blocks supplied with river water (pumped from river bed).

Person analysis: Incidence table according to characteristics of a person, such as age, sex, vaccination status, etc.

Interpretation: Adult males were mostly affected in Table 8.1. The river water may have been supplied untreated in the area of the outbreak because of the strike at water treatment plant.

- Ensure completeness and timeliness of reports by all units to interpret performance of the reporting units.
- Weekly/monthly summary reports is presented as tables, graphs and maps which are easy to interpret and visualize. Incidence rates are required to compare reporting units.
- Compare with previous weeks/months/years to capture trend of diseases overtime. Weekly analysis compare the current week with data from the last three weeks to detect the epidemics at early stage and alert authorities for immediate action. Monthly and yearly analysis gives information on long-term trends, seasonal patterns and cyclical pattern of disease.

- Compare the weekly and monthly data with established thresholds levels to identify outbreaks early enough
- Comparison should also be drawn between various units for incidence and case fatality rate for current month.
- Compare between public and private units for trends in number of new cases and deaths.
- Compare reports between public health system and the laboratory.

Encourage data analysis at all the levels by medical officess, health supervisors and health workers, use different sources of information to cross validate (or triangulations). One can not combine cases reported on from 'S' and 'P' forms (syndromic and probable cases). The analysis is not complete until the most probable reason (hypotheses) for causation and spread of the disease is explained at each level and understood by those who collect these data. The data must be shared with people whose lives it affect most.

Ability to analyse and interpret data is an important skill in epidemiology for public health manager.

(D) ACTION

Surveillance without action is useless.

Outbreak of viral hepatitis needs superchlorination of water supply or boiling of water apart from personal hygienic measures at community level. Action must be built in the surveillance system. The purpose of investigation and analysis is thus not only to determine what happened but also to decide how to control current outbreak and how to prevent further outbreak in the future.

Action for the malaria surveillance is full therapeutic treatment, radical treatment and selective spray programme and to control breeding of vector as also to educate people. Similarly, action for outbreak of polio necessitates mass polio vaccination or outbreak response immunization.

(E) FEEDBACK

To ensure that reporting units at various levels remain motivated and involved in the surveillance process, there must be regular communication back from higher levels of programme management to lower levels. This can be done through communication: in-staff meetings, preparation of brief reports and publication of newsletters. The feedback should include comments on the performance and quality in recording and reporting of cases and suggestions in solving problems in collection of data.

A newsletter is one of the best way of communication of information back to the reporting units. The newsletter may contain the collection of morbidity and mortality reports. The reader will like to compare disease trends in their own areas with those of other districts or PHCs of the state/district.

Outbreak investigation, response and control—outbreak means unusual occurrence or unusual events. Surveillance detects the unusual by describing what is usual, everyday.

Detection of Outbreak (Unusual Events)

There are two ways to detect outbreaks

a *Event based surveillance:* Rumour register, community informants and media reports.

   Rumour register is a source of information from community. Medical officers should investigate all rumours of epidemic prone diseases recorded in rumour register. Key community informants should be identified and involved in reporting of *unusual events*. Media is important source of information.

b *Case based surveillance or routine surveillance data analysis:* One of the common way to early detection is review the data from the routine surveillance and check if it crosses threshold levels and triggers in IDSP, then public health *alert* is issued.

Warning Signs of an Impending Outbreak

- Clustering of cases or deaths in time and/or space.
- Unusual increase in cases or deaths.
- Even a single case of measles, AFP, cholera, plague, dengue or JE.
- Acute febrile illness of unknown aetiology.
- Occurrence of two or more epidemiologically linked cases of meningitis, measles.
- Unusual isolates
- Shifting in age distribution of cases.
- High vector density
- Natural disasters

Threshold for disease or cut off level under surveillance that triggers predetermined actions at various levels: This is based upon the number of cases in weekly report. Trigger levels depend upon—type of disease, case fatality, incidence and trend of disease: Triggers for each disease have been worked out at state/national/international level.

Malaria Triggers: Single case of smear-positive in an area where malaria was not present for a minimum of three months or slide positivity doubling over the last three months or single death from clinically/microscopically proven malaria.

Acute Watery Diarrhoea/Cholera Triggers: A single case of cholera or epidemiologically linked case of diarrhoea/a case of severe dehydration or death due to diarrhoea in a patient >5 years old. Clustering of cases particularly in village or ward where more than 10 houses having at least one case of loose stools irrespective of age.

Viral Hepatitis: More than 2 cases of jaundice in a village or 1000 population.

Measles: Two or more cases with fever and rash per village (1000 population).

Japanese Encephalitis: Even a single case of probable JE or two cases with fever with altered consciousness/ seizures in a village (1000 population).

Triggers lead to issue of an alert for actions at various levels.

Reporting of outbreak: Health workers report to Medical Officer. Medical officer report outbreak to the district level nodal officer. The first information report (FIR) is submitted to district surveillance officer.

Steps of an Outbreak Investigation

1 *Verification of the outbreak:* Much time may be wasted due to false alarm. Even if the outbreak is suspected from the routine surveillance data or through rumours/ media, it must be verified lest it may be a data entry error. The fastest way to verify is to contact the Medical Officer nearest to the location of outbreak and request him for confirmation of outbreak. First information report on form 'C' is filed by the reporting unit and submitted to district surveillance officer soon after the suspected outbreak in verified.

2 *Confirmation of outbreak (establish the existence of an outbreak)*: If there is an abnormal increase in number of cases as compared with past incidence or if the cases are epidemiologically linked or if some trigger events have occurred or if many deaths/hospitalization have occurred.

3 *Confirmation of etiology (verify the diagnosis):* Outbreak must be investigated to identify the specific cause by RRT (Rapid Response Team). Sample from first 10 cases are enough to confirm the etiology. Do not wait to confirm etiology, action must be prompt as soon as the outbreak is reported based on clinical diagnosis. Step 2 and step 3 are addressed at the same time.

4 *Find cases systematically and record information:* Search/identify cases at health facility—clinic, hospital, PHC, CHC or by *active* surveillance or survey of whole population. Line listing of all cases by onset date, age, sex, outcome, etc. is standard method adopted during epidemic investigation.

5 *Epidemiological investigation:* The basic aim of epidemiological investigations are to identify etiology, source of epidemic, route of transmission by using clinical diagnosis and laboratory support. Describe outbreak in terms of time, place and person (TPP) on the basis of count, divide and compare (CDC) principle.

6 *Generation of hypothesis:* The Rapid Response Team and local health teams, on the basis of TPP information gathered, will formulate a provisional hypothesis to explain the tentative cause of the outbreak. This will answers the following questions:

- What was the causal agent?
- What was the source of infection?
- What was the transmission pattern?
- Who were the people at risk?

7 *Verification of hypothesis:* This step involves case control studies. We study the chances of exposures in cases and controls in the population where epidemic has occurred. Odds ratio is calculated to establish weather association is causal or not.

8 *Response to an outbreak:* It has to be rapid response at local level; supported by rapid response teams of district or state. Action will differ with nature of epidemic (water-borne, vector-borne, food-borne, etc.).

9 *Report on outbreak (communicate findings):* The detail report is prepared as to controlling the present outbreak and prevention of outbreaks of similar nature in the future. The steps listed above may not follow the order or sequence, circumstances of the outbreak may dictate that a different order be followed. Control measures are implemented urgently.

SURVEILLANCE OF RISK FACTORS OF NON-COMMUNICABLE DISEASES[10,11]

(Tables 8.15 and 8.16)

The following major risk factors will be measured under IDSP: Tobacco use, alcohol consumption, raised blood

Table 8.15: Definitions for categories of relative weight

BMI	*Category of relative weight*
<18.5	Underweight
18.5–24.9	Normal weight
25.0–29.9	Grade 1 overweight
30.0–39.9	Grade 2 overweight
≥40.0	Grade 3 overweight

Source: WHO stepwise approach to NCD surveillance, 2005.

Table 8.16: Definitions and classification of BP levels

Category	*Systolic (mm Hg)*	*Diastolic (mm Hg)*
Optimal	<120	<80
Normal	<130	<85
High-normal	130–139	85–89
Grade 1 hypertension (mild) subgroup: Borderline	140–159, 140–149	90–99, 90–94
Grade 2 hypertension (moderate)	160–179	100–109
Grade 3 hypertension (severe)	≥180	≥110
Isolated systolic hypertension	≥140	<90

When an individual's systolic and diastolic BP falls into different categories, the higher category should apply.
Source: WHO stepwise approach in NCD surveillance, 2005.

pressure, obesity, diet, physical inactivity, diabetes mellitus and high serum cholesterol.

Definitions (American Diabetic Association): Diabetes mellitus: Fasting plasma glucose >126 mg/dl (fasting—at least 8 hours of overnight fasting).

- Impaired fasting glucose ≥111 to 125 mg/dl
- Normal fasting glucose <110 mg%
- Hypercholesterolemia: Serum cholesterol >200 mg%

THE WHO STEPWISE APPROACH FOR SURVEILLANCE OF RISK FACTORS IN NCD

Step is sequential process of gathering information on key risk factors from persons in age 15–64 years.

Step 1: Surveillance is based on self-reported information. The core module of Step 1 comprises markers of sociodemographic profile, data on tobacco and alcohol use, diet and age, sex, family history and physical activity.

Step 2: Adds simple physical measurements (e.g. blood pressure, height, weight and waist girth) to the Step 1 data. Step 1 and Step 2 are desirable and appropriate for most countries.

Step 3: Incorporates data collection at levels 1 and 2, but adds measurements obtained from biochemical analysis, (fasting blood glucose and serum cholesterol).

NCD Risk Factor Survey

The NCD risk factor survey Phase I was undertaken by ICMR in seven states (AP, TN, Kerala, Maharashtra, MP, Mizoram and Uttarakhand) in 2007–08. The risk factors included were—BMI, waist circumference, physical inactivity, diet, sociodemographic profile, fasting plasma glucose, cholesterol and consumption of alcohol and smoking/tobacco use.

Standard case definitions are given in respective chapters on CCDs and NCDs. A few case definitions are as follows.

ACUTE VIRAL HEPATITIS

Clinical Case Description

Acute illness typically including acute jaundice, dark urine, anorexia, malaise, extreme fatigue and right upper quadrant abdominal tenderness.

Biological signs include increased urine urobilinogen and >2.5 times the upper limit of serum alanine aminotransferase (ALT)[1].

Laboratory Criteria for Diagnosis

Hepatitis A: IgM anti-HAV positive.

Hepatitis B: Positive for HBsAg or IgM anti-HBc[2].

Hepatitis C: Positive for anti-HCV.

Hepatitis D: Positive for HBsAg or IgM anti-HBc plus anti-HDV

Hepatitis E: Positive for anti-HEV IgM.

Case Classification

Suspect case: As per clinical case definition.

Probable case: Not applicable

Confirmed case: A suspect case that is laboratory confirmed. For hepatitis A, a case compatible with the clinical description and with epidemiological link with a lab confirmed case of hepatitis A.

[1] Most infections occur in early childhood. A variable proportion of adult infections is asymptomatic.

[2] The anti-HBc IgM test, specific for acute infection, is not available in most countries. HbsAg, often available, cannot distinguish between acute new infections and exacerbations of chronic hepatitis B, although continued HBsAg seropositivity (>6 months) is an indicator of chronic infection.

MALARIA

Clinical Case Description

A case of fever which may be accompanied with, of the following:

- Headache, backache, chills, rigors, sweating, myalgia, nausea and vomiting.
- Splenomegaly and anaemia.
- Generalized convulsions, coma, shock, spontaneous bleeding, pulmonary oedema, renal failure and death (untreated falciparum infection).
- Generalized convulsions, coma, shock, spontaneous bleeding, pulmonary odema, renal failure and death (untreated falciparum infection) any case of fever in endemic area may be considered malaria.

Laboratory Definition of Malaria

Demonstration of malaria parasites in blood films or positive rapid diagnostic test for malaria.

Case Classification

Suspect case: Any case of fever (in an endemic area).

Probable case: A case that meets the clinical case definition.

Confirmed case: A suspect case with malaria parasites in blood film.

Measles	*Poliomyelitis*
Clinical case description Any person with: • Fever • Maculopapular (non-vesicular or without fluid) rash lasting for more than 3 days and	**Clinical case description** A case of AFP is defined as any child aged <15 years who has acute onset of flaccid paralysis for which no obvious cause (such as severe trauma or electrolyte imbal-

Contd...

Contd...

- Cough, coryza (i.e. runny nose) or conjunctivitis (i.e. red eyes)

Laboratory criteria for diagnosis

- Presence of measles specific IgM antibodies, or
- At least a fourfold increase in antibody titre in paired sample (acute and convalescent; collected at 14 days interval); or
- Isolation of measles virus

Case classification

Suspect case: A case that meets the clinical case definition.

Probable case: Not applicable.

Confirmed case:* A case that meets the clinical case definition and that is laboratory confirmed or linked epidemiologically to a laboratory-confirmed case

- For the purpose of epidemiological investigation, a clinically diagnosed measles case would be a case which has occurred within the last three months
- For operational purpose presence of measles outbreak should be verified if five or more than five clinically diagnosed cases of measles are identified in a block in a weak or in an area bordering several blocks or one or more than one death due to clinically diagnosed measles occur in a block in a weak

ance) is found, or paralytic illness in a person of any age in which polio is suspected

Cases of AFP without isolation of wild poliovirus may be classified as "polio compatible" if:

- Stool specimens were inadequate and
- Residual weakness was present 60 days after onset of paralysis or 60 days follow-up was not done (due to death or absence) and
- Expert review concludes that these cases could not be discarded as "non-polio" based on available data

Laboratory criteria for diagnosis

Wild poliovirus isolated from any stool specimen

Case classification

Suspect case: Syndromic case of AFP—fever with abrupt onset of paralysis of leg or arm

Probable case: Epidemiologically *linked case*

Confirmed case: A suspected case that is laboratory confirmed.

*Only for outbreak confirmation and during elimination phase.

TYPHOID

Clinical Case Description

Any person with fever for more than one week and with any of the following:

- Toxic look
- Coated tongue
- Relative bradycardia
- Splenomegaly
- Exposure to confirmed case
- Clinical presentation with complications.

Any person with an insidious onset of sustained fever, headache, malaise, anorexia, relative bradycardia, constipation or diarrhoea, and non-productive cough. Intestinal ulceration can produce intestinal haemorrhage or perforations. However, many mild and atypical infections occur.

Laboratory Criteria for Diagnosis

Isolation of *S. typhi* from blood, stool, or other clinical specimen. Serology—Typhi dot test +/Widal test.

Case Classification

Suspect case: A patient with fever of at least 38°C for 3 or more days.

Probable case: A clinically compatible case that is epidemiologically linked to a confirmed case in an outbreak.

Confirmed case: A suspect case with laboratory confirmed positive blood culture.

Carrier: *S. typhi* organisms persisting in stools or urine for >1 year after onset of disease.

OTHER DISEASES

Tetanus Neonatorum

Suspect case: History of normal suck and cry for first two days of life and history of onset of illness between 3 and 28 days of life and history of inability to suck followed by stiffness and/or jerking of muscles.

Probable case: History of normal suck and cry for the first 2 days of life and history of onset of illness between 3 and 28 days of age and history of inability to suck followed by stiffness and/or convulsions and often death.

Diphtheria

Suspect case: Sore throat, with grey patch or patches in the throat.

Probable case: Acute pharyngitis, acute nasopharyngitis or acute laryngitis with a pseudomembrane.

Confirmed case: Positive culture of *Corynebacterium diphtheriae*.

Pertussis

Suspect case: History or observation of repeated and violent coughing, with any one of the following: Cough persisting for two or more weeks, fits of coughing, cough followed by vomiting, typical whoop in older infants.

Probable case: History of severe cough and history of any one of the following: Cough persistent for two or more weeks, fits of coughing, cough followed by vomiting.

Confirmed case: Positive culture or immunofluorescence of nasopharyngeal secretions for *Bordetella pertussis* bacteria.

REFERENCES

1 Aga Khan Foundation. Surveillance of morbidity and mortality. PHC MAP Module 4. Geneva: Aga Khan Foundation Research Corporation. Centre for human services.

2 NICD. Manual on epidemiological surveillance procedure for selected diseases. New Delhi: NICD, GOI; 1984.

3 GOI. Annual Report 2003–04. New Delhi: MOH and FW, GOI; 2004.

4 GOI. Integrated disease surveillance project (IDSP) 2004–09. New Delhi: MOH and FW, GOI; 2004.

5 NICD. Surveillance of epidemic prone diseases. New Delhi: NICD; 1998.

6 GOI. National Child survival and safe motherhood programme—Conduct disease surveillance. New Delhi: MOH and FW, GOI; 1992.

7 NACO. Training module on the sentinel surveillance of HIV infection-based on WHO draft training module on surveillance of HIV infection. New Delhi: NACO, MOH and FW, GOI; 1993.

8 GOI. CD Alert. Monthly Newsletter of NICD, DGHS October 2005 Vol.9: (10). GOI.

9 GOI. NRHM Newsletter: Vol. 3, No. 3/4 Nov. Feb. 2008; GOI, New Delhi.

10 GOI. 2006 Integrated Disease Surveillance Project. Operational Mannual for District Surveillance Unit. DGHS, MOH and FW. Nirman Bhawan: New Delhi, GOI.

11 WHO. WHO STEPS surveillance manual, the WHO STEP-wise approach to chronic disease risk factors surveillance. Geneva, World Health Organization, 2005.

INVESTIGATION OF AN OUTBREAK OF JAUNDICE

Recognition of Cases and Reporting (Detection of Outbreak)

The present situation was urban resettlement and slum colonies. Initially, the people recognized their own signs and symptoms and reported to nearby health facility (Medical College, Rohtak and Civil Hospital, Rohtak). Subsequently, local press (newspapers) published the reports and drew the attention of civil and administrative authorities. Health workers of the urban slums like Revamping health posts and Anganwadi workers played marginal role in routine reporting as it is not built in the system of routine reports of urban areas. Similarly, private practitioners did not report the cases to district authorities. Press played major role in early reporting of this outbreak and district health authorities moved much later and appeared on the scene quite late. Outbreak requires recognition, reporting and rapid response; unfortunately the response of health authorities was late and people responded to their need themselves first of all. Over 400 cases of jaundice were recognized and reported from March 2000 to 30 Sept. 2000 (within a period of almost 6 months) to district health authorities from resettlement colonies (urban slums) of Rohtak town.

Verification of Outbreak

The Medical Officer of urban health post was contacted to verify the existence of outbreak. He confirmed the outbreak and identified the clustering of cases in five localities.

Establish the Existence of an Outbreak

People First

The existence of outbreak was established by ascertaining the facts from local people. People confirmed that it was an unusual occurrence, unprecedented as they recollected that such a large number of cases of jaundice has not been witnessed in the last 10 years or so. Health institutions and facilities did not provide basic epidemiological data on occurrence of jaundice of recent past (last year or preceding 2–3 years) because of nonexistence of system of surveillance in urban slums. Rapid Response Teams (RRT), which were pushed in, tracked the cases and gathered the essential data of affected persons and affected localities. Whole population of 5 localities which were affected worst, was surveyed through house to house visit in May 2000 by trained medical and paramedical personnel. Attack rates due to jaundice varied from 0.42 to 1.78% and worst affected locality was Naya Parav. Case fatality varied from 0 to 3.3% and overall case fatality was around 0.75% (Table 8.17).

Confirmation of Diagnosis

Since viral hepatitis is distinct clinical syndrome, it posed no difficulty in diagnosis. Standard case definition of acute febrile illness of short duration (fever) with malaise, anorexia, followed by jaundice, hepatomegaly and abdominal tenderness in right upper quadrant, increase in serum alanine aminotransferase (ALT) >2.5 times the upper limit and serum bilirubin >2 mg% was applied, limited number of blood samples were drawn and tested in laboratory of medical college, Rohtak, to confirm diagnosis.

Serological tests got done through national institute of communicable diseases indicated that outbreak was due to HEV. The samples were collected by postgraduates of community medicine and the outbreak was in fact investigated by them under the supervision of head of community medicine department of PGIMS, Rohtak. Jaundice was present in all the subjects, 74.4% of the subjects experienced fever before they noticed jaundice, 96.6% passed dark coloured urine, over 97% complained loss of appetite, vomiting was present in 69% and pain in right hypochondrium was experienced by 41% of individuals.

Table 8.17: Reported cases and deaths due to viral hepatitis in Rohtak town from 23.3.2000 to 30.9.2000

Locality	*Population at risk*	*Cases*	*Attack rates (%)*	*Deaths*	*CFR*
Janata Colony	14420	127	0.88	2	1.6
Shivaji Colony	7625	66	0.80	0	0
Naya Parav	1856	33	1.78	1	3.3
Kamla Nagar	3947	21	0.64	0	0
Vijay Nagar	4930	25	0.42	0	0
Other localities (56)	120000	128	0.10	0	0
Total	**152778**	**400**	**0.33**	**3**	**0.75**

Characteristics of Outbreak in Terms of Time, Place and Persons (TPP) Distribution

Cases were distributed in 61 localities of Rohtak town. Spot map indicated clustering of 272 cases in just 5 localities which were adjacent to each other and had piped water supply from water works "2". Most affected locality was Janata Colony slum from where 127 cases of jaundice were reported. Locality-wise attack rate and case fatality is reproduced in Table 8.17.

GEOGRAPHICAL DISTRIBUTION

The cases were plotted on spot map of Rohtak town (Fig. 8.12). This exercise indicated that the cases of jaundice were widely distributed. 61 localities were affected, however, clustering of cases was obvious in 5 localities which were contiguous to each other. Out of 400 cases, 272 (68%) cases were reported from these 5 colonies/ localities. This identified worst affected geographical area. This area was dependent for its water supply from water works "2" situated about 1 km away from these localities. The piped water supply was intermittent and it was a common practice to use online booster pumps, blocked sewer lines, poorly maintained water lines, leakages and contaminated with drain waste water in the affected localities.

New Ekta Colony which had no piped water supply and was dependant on shallow hand pumps escaped from the onslaught of outbreak of jaundice, no case was detected/reported from this locality. Similarly, localities such as Medical College Campus, University Campus were free from jaundice because of independent system of water supply.

Time Orientation (Epidemic Curve)

Datewise line listing of cases of occurrence of jaundice was recorded by the investigators. From these data, weekwise occurrence of jaundice was analyzed beginning from month of March 2000 till Sept. 2000. The data of weekly occurrence was plotted (Fig. 8.13). Frequency of occurrence was plotted against that week and a curve was drawn by joining the frequencies. Cases started occurring in the month of March and peak occurrence was observed in the third week of April and another peak was observed in the first week of May. The epidemic curve indicated that maximum occurrence was in the month of April and May (over 53% of cases). These are the hot summer months when acute water shortages are experienced in the area. The decline started in the second week of May probably due to interventions. Sporadic occurrence continued even in the month of September indicating that the hepatitis has established its roots in the form of an endemic disease. Serial interval indicated average incubation period of 15 days.

Age and Sex Distribution

Twenty-two percent of cases of jaundice were in children below the age of 14 years. Majority of cases (78%) were above the age of 15 years. Of these 78% around 77% were in the age bracket 15–59, and the remaining 1% were above the age of 60 years. Nearly two-thirds (66.5%) were males and 34.5% of sufferers were females. Most of the households reported a single case only.

Other Observations

Overall sanitary conditions in these localities were far from satisfactory. Piped water supply managed by public health engineering department was available to 92.5% of the households while 98% of households in New Ekta Colony were using shallow tube wells (hand pumps). Facility of sanitary latrines was accessible to 93.3% while open field defecation was practiced by 6.7% of households. 30.3% of the individuals did not wash their hands before eating, however, 93.3% of individuals washed hands with soap and water after defecation. Drinking water was stored in pitchers by 84% of households and was drawn by dipping hands and glass, ladle was used by 27.4% of the individuals. Boiling of water during the outbreak was accepted by 15% of the families.

Laboratory Investigations and Confirmation

During the outbreak period the water samples were collected for spot test of residual chlorine by orthotoluidine test and coliform count in the laboratory. Residual chlorine was absent in nearly one-third of the samples at household level, while 3 out of 5 samples of water were unfit for drinking because of unacceptable level of coliform organisms. District health authorities collected large number of water samples for orthotoluidine test and coliform count. Institutional investigation of admitted patients confirmed raised ALT to >2.5 times of upper limit and serum bilirubin to more than 2 mg% in many cases. Blood samples results from NICD and other laboratories indicated the outbreak of jaundice due to HEV. Out of three deaths, one death occurred in pregnant women.

INTERVENTIONS (RESPONSE TO AN OUTBREAK)

Superchlorination of water was done to ensure 0.5 ppm residual chlorine in the distribution system. Apart from this, home chlorination was resorted to whenever the orthotoluidine tests were found negative. Boiling of water at household level was accepted by literate and well to do people in these localities. People were educated to wash their hands with soap and water before eating and after defecation and also to store their water safe and draw the water by use of ladle. Anganwadi workers of ICDS, health workers, malaria workers played pivotal role in interpersonal communication. Public health department identified the leakage and corrected these, also chocked sewer were attended to urgently.

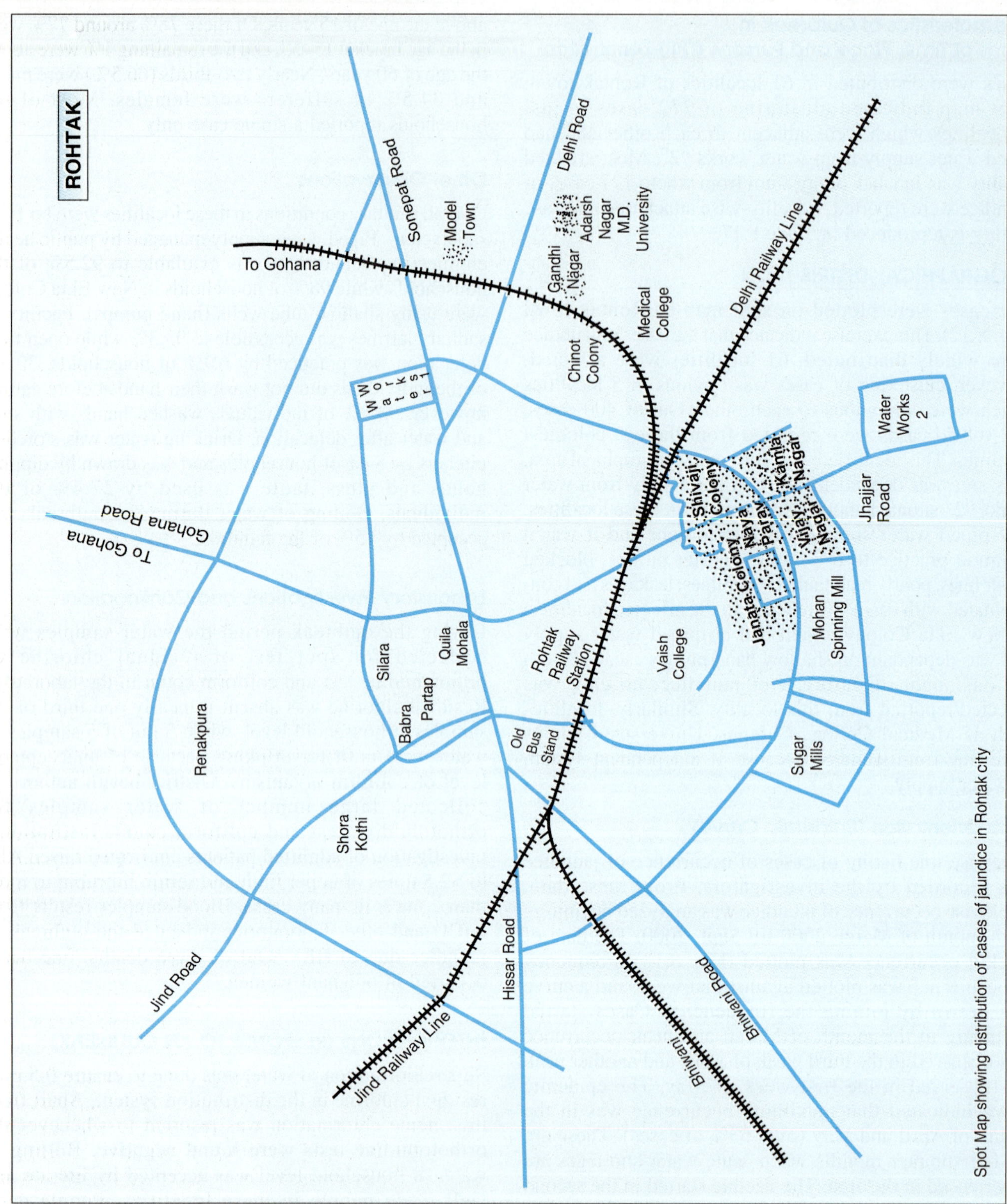

Fig. 8.12: Distribution of cases of viral hepatitis during outbreak (2000) in various localities of Rohtak city

Declaring the Outbreak to be Over

In theory it is laid down that the authority should declare the outbreak to be over only when there have been no new cases for the period of two incubation periods since the onset of last case. In the present situation outbreak was not declared as over. Active search was continued along with sanitary measures.

Even with all these measures sporadic cases due to hepatitis continued in the town. Maintenance of sanitation

8

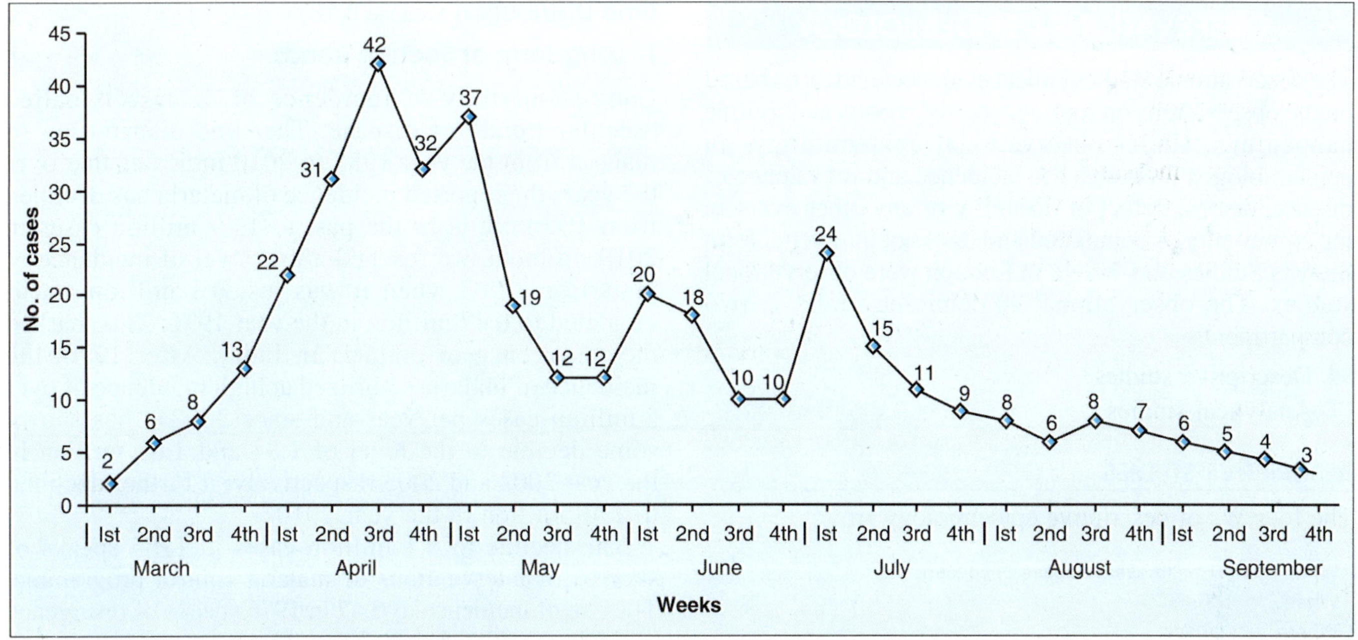

Fig. 8.13: Weekly incidence of jaundice from March to September 2000 in Rohtak town, Haryana (epidemic curve)

and sewerage system and ensuring safe water supply on sustainable basis is a real challenge. It requires regular monitoring of quality of water supply which is seldom ensured and these measures are undertaken only during outbreaks.

OUTBREAK REVISITED

In the year 2003, again 146 cases of viral hepatitis were reported in this town indicating breakdown of sanitation measures and failure of system of water supply and sanitation.

COORDINATION

The activities of investigation of outbreak of jaundice, its planning and implementation of interventions were undertaken jointly by the district health authorities, public health and engineering; ICDS sector, medical college and the people. The results of investigation were shared with all the participating sectors and with local people whose lives this outbreak affected most. The media was equal partner in dissemination of information to people. Each sector played its effective role during the outbreak and ensured utmost cooperation.

CONCLUSION

The present outbreak of jaundice (viral hepatitis) was most probably due to HEV; due to contamination of drinking water. Water works no. 2 was incriminated as those localities which drew water from water works no. 1 had very few cases in comparison to colonies which were dependent on water works no. 2. Of 272 cases of jaundice clustered in just 5 localities versus 128 cases spread over to 56 colonies, and some localities were free from jaundice while in other localities very few cases were detected. Case control study thus incriminated contamination of drinking water of water works no. 2. It was learnt that the water works no. 2 augmented the water supply of some areas and because of that the localities such as Model Town, Gandhi Nagar, Adarsh Nagar and Sector 14 were affected.

EPIDEMIOLOGICAL STUDIES, METHODS AND THEIR APPLICATION

There are various epidemiological methods used to study health problems or events in population. Some of the most commonly used epidemiological methods are:[1]

1 Observational epidemiology
   - Descriptive epidemiology
   - Analytical epidemiology
     – Ecological studies
     – Cross-sectional studies
     – Case control studies
     – Cohort studies

2 Experimental or intervention epidemiology
   - Randomized controlled trials
   - Field trials
   - Community trials

OBSERVATIONAL EPIDEMIOLOGY

The observational studies collect evidence/evidences based on the observations on routine records, reports and routine happenings. Under observational epidemiology, an epidemiologist measures the incidence and prevalence of disease, deaths, defect or disability or any other event in the community or population and does not intervene. John Snow's Studies on Cholera in London were observational studies. The observational epidemiology falls in two compartments:

1. Descriptive studies
2. Analytical studies

DESCRIPTIVE STUDIES

The four Ws of descriptive epidemiology are:

What	: Health event/disease of concern
When	: Time
Where	: Place
Who	: Person

The descriptive epidemiology follows the approach of count, divide and compare (CDC). CDC means identifying and counting cases, dividing number of cases by the size of population in which they occurred to arrive at rates and compare these rates over different time, place and different group of people. In essence descriptive epidemiology describes the health events in terms of time, place and person (TPP). This can be better understood in terms of 3 Ws, i.e. when (Time) did the disease occur—Date of onset of disease, where (Place) did it occur and who (Person) were affected most by the disease. Compiling, analyzing and interpreting data by time, place and person provides important clues to the causes or risk factors of disease, source of infection and mode of transmission, and these clues can be helpful in generating hypotheses.

The descriptive studies in epidemiology simply describe the occurrence of disease in the community and it measures the incidence, prevalence, trends and distribution of disease or diseases in population. Descriptive studies use data of routine reports or records or data of special surveys. Descriptive studies describe the health status of the community-based on parameters like under-five mortality, infant mortality, per capita income, life expectancy, total adult literacy, poverty rates, school enrolment, nutritional status, percentage of children immunized, percentage of population using improved drinking water sources and sanitation facilities, incidence of ARI and diarrhoea, prevalence of HIV/AIDS, etc. The descriptive studies are most commonly used to produce evidence-based data for appropriate action. Since time immemorial, the observations made on occurrence is the first step towards scientific investigations. In essence, the descriptive epidemiology describes the status of health, disease, nutrition and immunization in population.

Time Distribution (Table 8.18)

1. Long-term or Secular Trends

Long-term study of incidence of disease is called "secular trend" of disease. The time distribution of malaria from the year 1935 to 2010 indicates that over the years the reported incidence of malaria has declined from 100 million in the past to 1.49 million cases in 2010. In India, we reached a low level of incidence of malaria in 1965 when it was just 0.1 million and it escalated to 6.47 million in the year 1976. This marked the resurgence of malaria in India. After 1976, the incidence of malaria stabilized at high incidence of over 2 million cases per year and since 2002 it has shown some decline to the level of 1.84 and 1.65 million in the year 2002 and 2003 respectively; it further declined to 1.49 million in the year 2010.[2,3]

The decline to 0.1 million cases in 1965 speaks of success of interventions of malaria control programme. The rise of incidence to 6.47 in 1976 speaks of resurgence and failure of interventions/programme.

Impact of Observations

The epidemiological observations of high incidence of malaria in 1976 necessitated change in strategy of malaria

Table 8.18: Secular trend of malaria in India

Years	*Malaria cases in millions*	*P. falciparum cases*
1935	100	–
1947	75	–
1965	0.1	–
1976	6.47	0.75
1984	2.18	0.65
1986	1.79	0.64
1987	1.66	0.62
1988	1.85	0.68
1989	2.05	0.76
1990	2.02	0.75
1992	2.13	0.88
1993	2.21	0.85
1994	2.51	0.99
1995	2.93	1.14
1996	3.04	1.18
1997	2.66	1.01
1998	2.22	1.03
1999	2.28	1.14
2000	2.03	1.05
2001	2.09	1.01
2002	1.84	0.90
2003	1.87	0.86
2006	1.79	0.84
2007	1.51	0.74
2008	1.53	0.77
2009	1.56	0.84
2010	1.49	0.77

eradication programme and modified plan of operation was evolved (MPO of malaria) in 1977.

Further long-term trends of falciparum malaria (which is killer malaria) indicates rising trend that over the years and now over 50% of malaria is due to *Plasmodium falciparum* or *Pf* malaria. This observation is a cause of concern. Drug resistance in *Pf* malaria and insecticide resistance in mosquitoes has added more problems. Right now the epidemiological situation of *Pf* malaria is grim.

Application

By studying the disease like malaria over the years we can determine:

- The success or failure of national programme of malaria.
- It helps for re-planning and re-thinking about the strategies.
- It helps us to know the changing pattern of disease as falciparum malaria incidence has increased significantly in India.

2. Seasonal Distribution

The incidence of malaria is not uniform all over the year. The incidence rises in the months of July to October because of favourable conditions for transmission of malaria. After rains, the mosquito breeding and density of vector increases and transmission becomes favourable, hence the incidence rises. This is known as seasonal variations in malaria occurrence. Rise of malaria in these months is a caution to get ready with the system to fight disease: Mounting spray operation well before transmission period and adequate coverage with indoor residual insecticides, stepping up operations of surveillance in these months and raising the target of active case detection during transmission season. Thus, seasonal variations of malaria help us to gear up plans to fight against malaria.

3. Short-term Variations

Day of week and time of day: For occurrence of road traffic accidents, occupational diseases/exposures displaying data by day of the week or time of the day may be more informative. Pattern of these occurrences may suggest hypothesis and possible explanation.

Epidemic curve: Distribution of cases by date of onset or by hour of onset, the epidemiologist can draw an epidemic curve or histogram. In epidemic curve 'Y' axis shows number of cases and 'X' axis shows the date of onset. The shape and other features of an epidemic curve can suggest hypothesis about the time and source of exposure and the mode of transmission (*see* page 321).

The short-term fluctuation in the occurrence or incidence of malaria indicated that the disease has attained an epidemic proportion or outbreaks in certain years. Malaria is an endemic disease in the country. When it occurs beyond the expected level (usually compared with past year or past years occurrence) then we call this behaviour as an epidemic proportion of occurrence, i.e. "when the malaria occurrence is clearly in excess of normal occurrence or expected occurrence then it is termed as epidemic of malaria".

In the years 1994, 1995 and 1996 (Table 8.18), there were fluctuation in occurrence of malaria, as incidence of malaria in these years increased beyond two million, hence, these were the epidemic years for malaria in several places. The incidence of malaria suddenly increased as also the number of deaths reported (Tables 8.19 and 8.20).

Reported incidence of deaths due to malaria in the country from 1976 to 2010 (Table 8.19) indicates that during the years 1994, 1995 and 1996 the deaths were far excess than the previous years, hence, these deaths were clearly in excess of expected level. Therefore, these years (1994, 1995 and 1996) were epidemic years for malaria as many deaths were reported in these years from the states of Odisha, Rajasthan, Haryana, Madhya Pradesh, Maharashtra, Gujarat, Karnataka and Assam (Table 8.20). Unit of determining the outbreak of malaria should be district or community development block or CHC/PHC or subcentre (Section).

Table 8.19: Reported deaths due to malaria 1976–2010

Years	*Deaths*	*Years*	*Deaths*
1976	59	1993	354
1984	247	1994	1122
1985	213	1995	1151
1986	323	1996	1010
1987	188	1997	879
1988	209	1998	664
1989	268	2006	1707
1990	353	2008	935
1991	421	2009	1144
1992	422	2010	767

Table 8.20: Areas affected by malaria outbreaks 1994–2006

Years	*States*	*No. of districts affected*
1994	Rajasthan, Haryana, Manipur, Nagaland	13
1995	Maharashtra, WB and Assam	28
1996	Rajasthan, Haryana	8
1997	Gujarat, Goa and WB	4
1998	Goa, Maharashtra	2
1999	Andhra Pradesh, Assam, Bihar and WB	23
2000	Karnataka, UP and MP	5
2003	Rajasthan, Large epidemic—several districts	
2004	Assam, Goa, Haryana, Gujarat, Karnataka, Manipur and Maharashtra	44
2005	Assam, Goa, Haryana, Gujarat, Karnataka, Manipur, Maharashtra	48
2006	Karnataka and West Bengal	5

4. Cyclical Variations

Malaria has cyclic pattern. In unstable malarious areas outbreak/epidemic occur every 8–10 years under natural conditions. In effective and efficient control programme conditions cycle may appear after 15–20 years whereas under the partial implemented control programme situation the cycle may come after 5–7 years. Cyclical variations are observed as spikes or rise in incidence of disease at regular interval of one or two years in some diseases like measles as also in smallpox which has now been eradicated. This is probably due to accumulation of susceptible individuals, i.e. young children who received no vaccination/immunization, against measles. Measles outbreaks are generally due to accumulation of measles susceptibles children including both unvaccinated children and those who were vaccinated but failed to seroconvert, approximately 15% of children vaccinated at 9-month are not protected after measles vaccination. Similarly, meningococcal meningitis shows cyclic trends after every 8–12 years.

Place Distribution

Distribution of disease in a district, state or country, or a geographical area is significant determinant and provides clue for prevalence of special risk factors in that area.

Malaria as a disease is public health problem in India; its distribution is not uniform all over India. Some states show high incidence while some states have low incidence of malaria (Fig. 8.14).

During 2015, 1.12 million cases of malaria were reported from the country with 0.75 (67%) million being those of *P. falciparum*.

Two states, namely Odisha and Chhattisgarh, contributed 50% of total malaria cases, these were the high burden states for malara incidence (Fig. 8.14).

Four states—Odisa, Chhattisgarh, Jharkhand and Meghalaya contributed nearly 50% cases of *Pf* malaria in India in the year 2015.

These two states have high percentage of tribal people, health services are poorly developed, surveillance and treatment facilities not easily accessible because of lack of infrastructure facilities. Problem of drug resistance may be acute in tribal belts of these states.

Geographical mapping of malaria or geographical information system (GIS) of a disease provides useful information and helps classify the areas for different control strategies. Based on geographical distribution of malaria the problem areas were broadly classified as under.

Hard-core Areas (Tribal Areas)[5]

These are those areas where malaria control operations over the last four decades have failed to contain the disease, such areas have the following characteristics:

- These are mostly difficult terrain areas, large part of which becomes inaccessible during monsoon and subsequent flooding.
- The population is predominantly tribal.
- They have predominant *Pf* malaria.
- They have *stable malaria* with transmission period extending up to 9 months or more.
- These report bulk of deaths due to malaria in the country.

These areas comprise seven North and Eastern States, tribal areas of 87 districts of Andhra Pradesh, Bihar, Gujarat, MP, Maharashtra, Odisha and Rajasthan.

Epidemic Prone Areas

High-risk areas are considered to be those which are often prone to malaria outbreaks or epidemics. The periodic fulminating malaria epidemic contributes a large number of malaria deaths. North Western plains, semi-arid climatic zone with annual rainfall up to 100 mm and Indo-Gangetic plains are identified as major epidemic prone areas. During epidemic, the malaria deaths in these high-risk areas outnumber the malaria deaths reported from the rest of the affected states. These areas have *unstable malaria,* with seasonal variations.

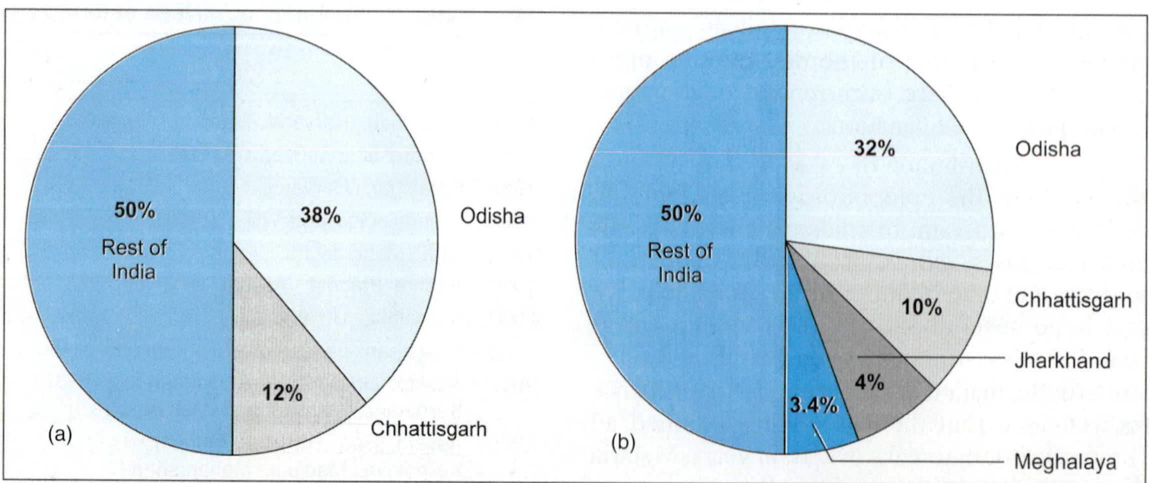

Fig. 8.14: (a) Distribution of malaria cases in India 2015, (b) distribution of falciparum malaria in India 2015

8

Project Areas

The development projects attract large number of migrant labour population from endemic areas bringing different strains of malaria parasites as well as non-immune population groups. The prolific increase in vector breeding places and increased man mosquito contact favours high transmission of malaria.

Example: Construction activities in metropolis, in and around Delhi, Gurgaon and Faridabad, migrant industrial labour and brick kiln labour are examples of project areas which become vulnerable population for many other problems apart from spreading malaria. Specific control strategies are required for such areas.

Urban Areas

Review of past data indicates that the following 15 cities are accountable for nearly 80% of cases of urban malaria scheme (UMS) of NMEP.

These cities are Delhi, Chennai, Kolkata, Mumbai, Hyderabad, Bengaluru, Bhopal, Ahmedabad, Jaipur, Lucknow, Chandigarh, Vadodara, Vishakhapatnam, Vijayawada and Kanpur. City of Chennai alone contributes half of malaria cases in Tamil Nadu.

These urban areas have unplanned and rapid growth, with prolific increase in slum population, large size of floating population, poor water management, civic by-laws for control of mosquito population are absent or not implemented and case finding mechanism is either absent or very poor and there is insufficient staff for antilarval activities. These urban areas require different strategies for control of malaria.

Triple Insecticide Resistant Areas

The ubiquitous rural vector, *Anopheles culicifacies* has become resistant to the conventional insecticides, namely DDT, BHC and Malathion in the Western belt of India specially Northern parts of Maharashtra and Karnataka and Southern parts of Gujarat. Alternate insecticides such as synthetic pyrethroids are considered for indoor residual spray in these areas.

Based on the observations and epidemiological situation the expert committee has used the epidemiological parameters to identify the worst affected areas in different malaria paradigms.

Rural Urban Distribution

The health indicators are usually low for rural areas as compared to urban areas. The distribution of diseases vary in urban and rural areas. Density of population is much more in urban areas, urban slums are worse than rural areas in many ways. The plan of action suggested for "high-risk" rural and urban areas for malaria is being implemented under National Programme of Control of Malaria. During the year 2007 in India, rural areas had very high share (92.6%) of malaria in comparison to urban areas (7.4%) (Fig. 8.15).

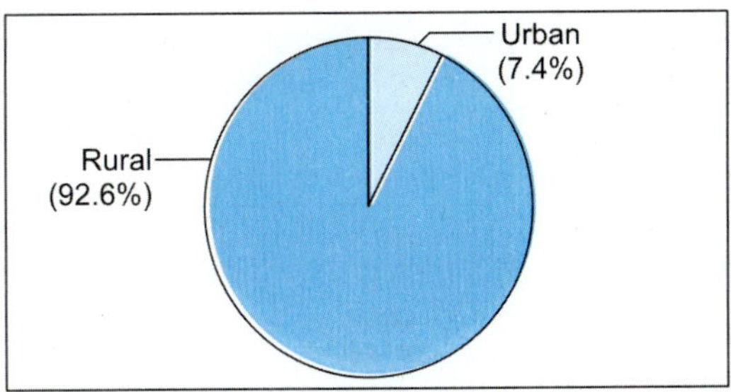

Fig. 8.15: Urban and rural malaria incidence recorded by malaria surveillance system under NMEP (2013)[4]

Person Distribution

The descriptive studies describe the distribution of disease according to characteristics of the person (host) like age, sex, race occupation, literacy, marital status, social class and health behaviour (lifestyle), resident or migrant, etc. The disease pattern varies with age of a person; diseases of infants, young children, adolescents, youths and adults and old age vary considerably. Common age classification for the purposes of epidemiology is as under: Under one year, 1–4 yrs, 5–14 yrs, 15–24 yrs, 25–34 yrs, 35–44 yrs, 45–54 yrs, 55–64 yrs, 65 yrs and over.

or

Age classification for special statistics of infant mortality: Under 7 days, 7–27 days. 28 days but under 1 year of age. For malaria control programme, age classification adopted is 0–1 year, 1–4 years, 5–8 years and 9–14 years and above 15 years for the purpose of distribution of drugs and study the incidence of fever and malaria in different age groups as also to calculate infant parasite rate which is an indicator of recent transmission of malaria in the community and it confirms local transmission of malaria during the current transmission period. Age incidence of a disease helps us to identify high *risk groups* or *vulnerables*, at which age to initiate immunization for measles, polio and other diseases.

$$\text{Infant parasite rate (IPR)} = \frac{\text{No. of infants found positive for malaria parasite}}{\text{Total no. of infants blood smears examined during survey}} \times 100$$

Age Distribution (Table 8.20)

Malaria affected all age groups in the rural community of this block. It means all age groups or whole of population is exposed to occurrence of malaria.

Sex Distribution

Similarly both sexes were affected, however, incidence of malaria in adult males was of high preponderance as compared to females, probably due to more outdoor exposure and outdoor sleeping habits (Table 8.21). This observation needs further studies and verification.

On the basis of observational or descriptive epidemiology, the evidence gathered *provides a ground for analytical*

8

Table 8.21: Age and sex distribution of malaria cases in a rural block[6]

Age groups (years)	Sex	Cases of malaria year 1996
0–1	M	4
	F	10
1–4	M	116
	F	97
5–8	M	239
	F	195
9–14	M	404
	F	209
15 and above	M	1432
	F	1183
Total		**3989**

Source: Health Centre PHC Chiri Population around 1,00,000.

epidemiology for testing of various hypotheses or speculations.

Hypothesis means a tentative theory or an assumption to prove or disapprove.

From the data of national malaria control programme following *hypotheses* can be developed why falciparum malaria is showing rising trends in India. What makes malaria to stay at high annual incidence of around two million cases?

Why there is variation of incidence and distribution of malaria in different states of the country?

To answer these questions or to prove/disapprove the *hypotheses* we use the knowledge of analytical epidemiology.

ANALYTICAL EPIDEMIOLOGY (WHY AND HOW?)

The analytical epidemiology analyses the relationship between the health status (incidence and prevalence of disease) with other variables or exposures or risk factors associated with occurrence and distribution. While descriptive epidemiology describes the health status and its distribution in population, the analytical epidemiology focuses on "determinants", *risk factors* and *reasons* for such situation or status in the population. Analytical epidemiology studies **cause to effect relationship** (*why* and *how* of health event). Analytical studies consist of the following.

a. Ecological Studies

Ecological studies are also known as *correlational studies*. The focus and unit of analysis in these studies is population or groups of people. These studies provide an indirect evidence or clue of some events.

1 National malaria eradication estimates on malaria morbidity (incidence) have been cross-checked, to the extent possible on the basis of consumption of antimalarials especially chloroquine phosphates and it has been suggested that a more realistic and safer assumption would be that 20–30 million episodes occur every year as against 2–3 million cases reported by NVBDCP. This provides an indirect evidence of incidence of probable malaria based on the sale of chloroquine tablets in the country.

2 The occurrence of deaths and injuries due to road accidents can be linked to increase in population of vehicles on road. For example, Table 8.22 provides clues to accidents in Delhi.

Table 8.22: Trends of fatal road accidents in Delhi

Year	Vehicles (lakh)	Road length (km)	Population (lakh)	People killed in accidents
1971	2.17	8380	43	NA
1981	5.61	15,490	62	1072
1991	19.23	22,487	94	1778
1996	27.93	25,948	114	2361
2001	35.89	25,948	137	1842
2004	44.00	25,948	160	1812
2011	72.28	Do	167	6937
2014	88.27	–	–	–

Source: Police Department, Delhi

As the population of vehicles increased on roads the number of fatal accidents went up in the national capital of Delhi. Many of the deaths in 2011 occurred at "black spots" at places, which have been notorious for years.

Ecological studies are quite attractive but the results are difficult to interpret. As in the above data as the number of vehicles increased the air pollution also went up and evidence of increased respiratory infections may provide some clue and correlations.

Ecological studies are rapid methods of getting clue for some evidences and based on the initial clues, the study can be enlarged.

b. Cross-sectional Studies

These studies are also called "prevalence studies". The hallmark of cross-sectional studies—these studies are done on part or sample of population representative of an area. In cross-sectional studies, the "exposure" and the "health effect" are measured simultaneously. In cross-sectional studies, it is not easy to measure the **cause** and **effect relationship.**

These studies are easier to conduct and results are available quickly with affordable cost.

Usefulness

- These studies provide quick estimate of burden of disease in the community.
- It also identifies individuals/population or groups at risk.
- Variation of disease or event in different geographical areas.

Examples of Cross-sectional Studies

There are innumerable examples. Most studies done (over 90%) are cross-sectional in nature. The major cross-sectional studies conducted in the country are:

1. National family health survey (NFHS I–IV) done once in five years. These provide data on key health and family welfare indicators such as fertility, use of contraception, mortality, coverage and quality of maternal and child health services by states.
2. National sample surveys (NSS).
3. District rapid household and facility surveys, under reproductive and child health programme, every alternate year, to know the utilization of services and coverage of services for mothers and children.
4. Sample registration survey (SRS) done every year provides state level estimates on birth, death and infant mortality rates.
5. Another example of cross-sectional survey is outbreak investigation and response. Since we have built the story of descriptive epidemiology on one disease, i.e. malaria it is worthwhile to discuss briefly utility of cross-sectional surveys in outbreak of malaria.

Outbreak Response

In the event of occurrence of outbreaks, the rapid response is essential. First response comes from local area and the district. The response or action consists of:

1. Stepping up of surveillance activities.
2. Additional laboratory support in the area of occurrence.
3. Ensuring adequate supplies of anti-malaria drugs.
4. Fogging and spray operations.
5. Mass fever treatment if indicated.
6. Deployment of additional manpower and material.
7. Involvement of community.

Warning System for Early Detection and Rapid Response to Outbreak

For prediction of outbreaks of malaria, we rely on surveillance system of active and passive case detection. Apart from this, regular monitoring of meteriological data like rainfall, temperature, humidity, etc. together with epidemiological situation of malaria are reviewed. Deviation from the normal trends in these variables may indicate increase in mosquitogenic potential, in that situation any lapse in control activities may lead to outbreaks of malaria. For accuracy and better prediction, these data need to be analysed locally at micro-level say a primary health centre or a section or a subcentre area. The exercise is not only data-based but also requires area specific information, both meteriological and epidemiological. Rainfall is single most important meteriological data along with epidemiological data for prediction of epidemic of malaria and averting impending outbreak. The exercise is useful for early warning signals.

Outbreak of malaria in district Betul, Madhya Pradesh in 2000: A team of National Institute of Communicable Diseases investigated "fever-related deaths" reported from 6 blocks of district Betul in October 2000.

General: Betul district is situated on Satpuda hills in Madhya Pradesh. The central part of district is plain, while the surrounding area is mostly hilly with thick forest. The annual rainfall is about 1043 mm and the temperature is favourable for survival of mosquitoes throughout the year.

Tribals constitute about two-thirds of the population. Of 65 deaths reported from 1st September to 5th October, 27(42%) occurred in persons having febrile illness. Bhimpur block reported 37% (24/65) of these deaths. Deaths occurred in all age groups with some preponderance in young adults (Table 8.23).

Table 8.23: Reported deaths in Betul district by various blocks, 1st September to 5th October 2000

Name of block	*Total deaths*	*Fever-related deaths*	*% Deaths with fever*
Chicholi	10	2	20
Bhimpur	24	11	45.8
Shakpur	10	5	50
Ghodadongri	12	3	25
Betul	5	3	60
Amla	4	3	75
Total	**65**	**27**	**41.5**

Source: NICD—outbreak investigation report.

The major presenting symptoms were moderate to high fever with chills and rigors, headache, bodyache, nausea and vomiting. In addition, severe cases had altered sensorium and were brought to health facilities in coma. No haemorrhagic manifestations were observed. The patients were treated with antibiotics and antimalarials. Only a few deaths occurred in admitted cases. The duration of illness was 2–3 days in most of cases.

A house-to-house survey was organized in a village on 11 October where a 9-year-old child had died on 6th October 2000. About 70% of population surveyed was found to have fever in the last two weeks. All age groups were affected and multiple cases were seen in many families. Of 33 blood smears collected from cases 24 (73%) were found positive for *Plasmodium falciparum* in the laboratories of NICD.

Eight blood samples tested for Hi antibody against JE and dengue viruses were found to be negative for these antibodies. These samples were also negative for antibodies against measles. Isolation of influenza group of viruses was attempted from throat swabs of 10 cases and one CSF sample without any positive results.

It is worthwhile mentioning that 34% of the blood smears collected from 88 cases in the affected areas during 6–9 September were positive for malarial parasites and 80% of them had vivax malaria. These and other epidemiological data indicated that vivax malaria continued to dominate up to September but gave way to falciparum malaria subsequently (Table 8.24).

Follow-up visits to the affected areas were made from 14–20 December 2000. Forty-two blood slides were collected from fever cases during the follow-up visits. Of the 42 slides collected, 36 (86%) were positive for malaria parasite. Thirty-four of positive slides showed *P. falciparum* (95%). By this time, at least 120 cases had died as shown in Table 8.25.

Conclusions

The district was endemic for malaria. The situation worsened in 2000 when falciparum malaria increased tremendously (Table 8.24) and caused many deaths because of:

- i Poor surveillance
- ii Inadequate insecticide spray coverage. These deaths could have been prevented had the surveillance mechanism been operative and guidelines of NAMP followed.
- iii The falciparum malaria was persisting which indicated the inadequate local capacity to deal with the situation.

This is an example of cross-sectional study during outbreak which has measured several exposures—like environmental conditions, surveillance operations, insecticidal spray, local practices, supervisory mechanism and spread of disease.

Table 8.24: Epidemiological situation of malaria in Betul district, 1999–2000

	1999	*2000*
Population (million)	1.44	1.47
Blood slides examined	3,12,440	3,96,019
No. of blood smears positive for malaria parasite	14,133	16,234
Slide positivity rate (%)	4.5	4.1
No. of blood slides positive for *P. falciparum*	3879	6668
Proportion of falciparum cases	24.4	41.07
No. of deaths due to malaria	0	30

Source: NMEP

Table 8.25: Distribution of total deaths in Betul by age due to fever

Age groups (years)	*No. of deaths*	*Percentage of deaths*
0–5	35	29.2
6–10	9	7.5
11–15	5	4.2
16–30	40	33.3
31–35	21	17.5
>45	10	8.3
Total	**120**	**100**

c. Case Control Studies

Purpose

The purpose of case control study is to investigate the **cause** or **probable exposure** or risk factors for that disease.

1. Case control studies focus on disease or sick persons. These studies are also simple and economical to carry out.
2. In addition to cases of disease, a suitable control group is also chosen/selected. Control group consists of people who are healthy and not affected by the disease, which is being studied.
3. The occurrence of **possible cause/exposure** is compared between cases and controls.
4. The case control studies collect data at more than one/ different points of time and are thus longitudinal in contrast to cross-sectional studies, which collect data at one point of time.

Steps in Case Control Study

The case control study follows the following steps:

- It begins with selection of cases of a disease. To select "case", we must adopt a standard case definition and include cases in the study as per standard case definition. *Example:* All adults 15–49 years who are HIV positive or adults who are positive for malaria parasite.
- The cases can be selected from a hospital or from the community.
- Selection of controls or healthy people: Again, controls can be close relatives of case or the controls can be selected from community or hospital/clinic (attendants coming with patients).

Controls should match with cases in respect of age, sex, social customs, culture and economic status and belong to the same background from where patient or case is selected. Preferably, controls should be chosen from the same population from where the cases are chosen.

Classical example of case control study is a marriage party of 150 men (Table 8.26).

Out of 150 persons who took part in marriage party, many suffered due to vomiting and diarrhoea and others escaped. Those who suffered were *cases* and those who did not suffer acted as *controls.*

Table 8.26: Association between ice cream consumption and development of diarrhoea and vomiting in the year 2004 in a marriage party

Disease		*Exposure (consumption of ice cream)*		
		Yes	*No*	*Total*
VOMITING AND DIARRHOEA	Yes	80	20	100
	No	20	30	50
	Total	**100**	**50**	**150**

The association of occurrence of vomiting and diarrhoea, with ice cream consumption can be measured by calculating the odds ratio (OR), which is the ratio of the odds (chances) of exposure amongst cases to the odds of exposure amongst *controls*. Odds ratio is sometimes called the *cross product ratio*.

From the data in Table 8.25, the odds ratio can be calculated by:

$$(80:20) \div (20:30)$$

$$\frac{80 \times 30}{20 \times 20} = 6$$

Measure of Association

It means that the cases were 6 times more likely than the controls to have consumed ice cream. Here in this example these were the natural controls who did not consume the ice cream. The association between consumption of ice cream and development of vomiting and diarrhoea is **causal** as the size of the risk ratio is more than 2. The odds ratio is very similar to risk ratio. Here there were natural controls, who did not consume ice cream.

In a rural community development block, 2700 births occurred in 100,000 population in the year 1996 of these 900 births weighed below 2.5 kg and the rest 1800 had birth weight of 2.5 kg and above (Fig. 8.16). We wish to test the following hypotheses:

- To ascertain the **causes** or **risk factors** of low birth weights in this block.
- Could it be due to moderate or severe anaemia in pregnant women, or could it be due to high parity (4 and above) or less birth interval. Are low birth weights common to primipara or to girls marrying in teen ages and having teen age pregnancy? To answer these questions or to test these hypotheses, we carry out **case control study.**

Definition of Case

- In this setting, the case is a live birth below 2.5 kg.
- Controls—live births in the same area above 2.5 kg.

We study the attributes or exposures like anaemia, parity, age of marriage, parity of women who gave birth to these children by interviewing or looking at the records and obtaining the history of these exposures. After ascertaining these exposures in *cases* and *controls* the data are compiled and analysis done (Table 8.27).

In this **contingency table** of 2 × 2, we depict the respective frequencies or numbers and calculate the odds ratio. The odds ratio of 5.44 indicate that mothers of low birth weight babies have over 5 times more chances of severe anaemia as compared to mothers of babies who have adequate birth weight. Thus, severe anaemia during pregnancy has **causal association** with low birth weights.

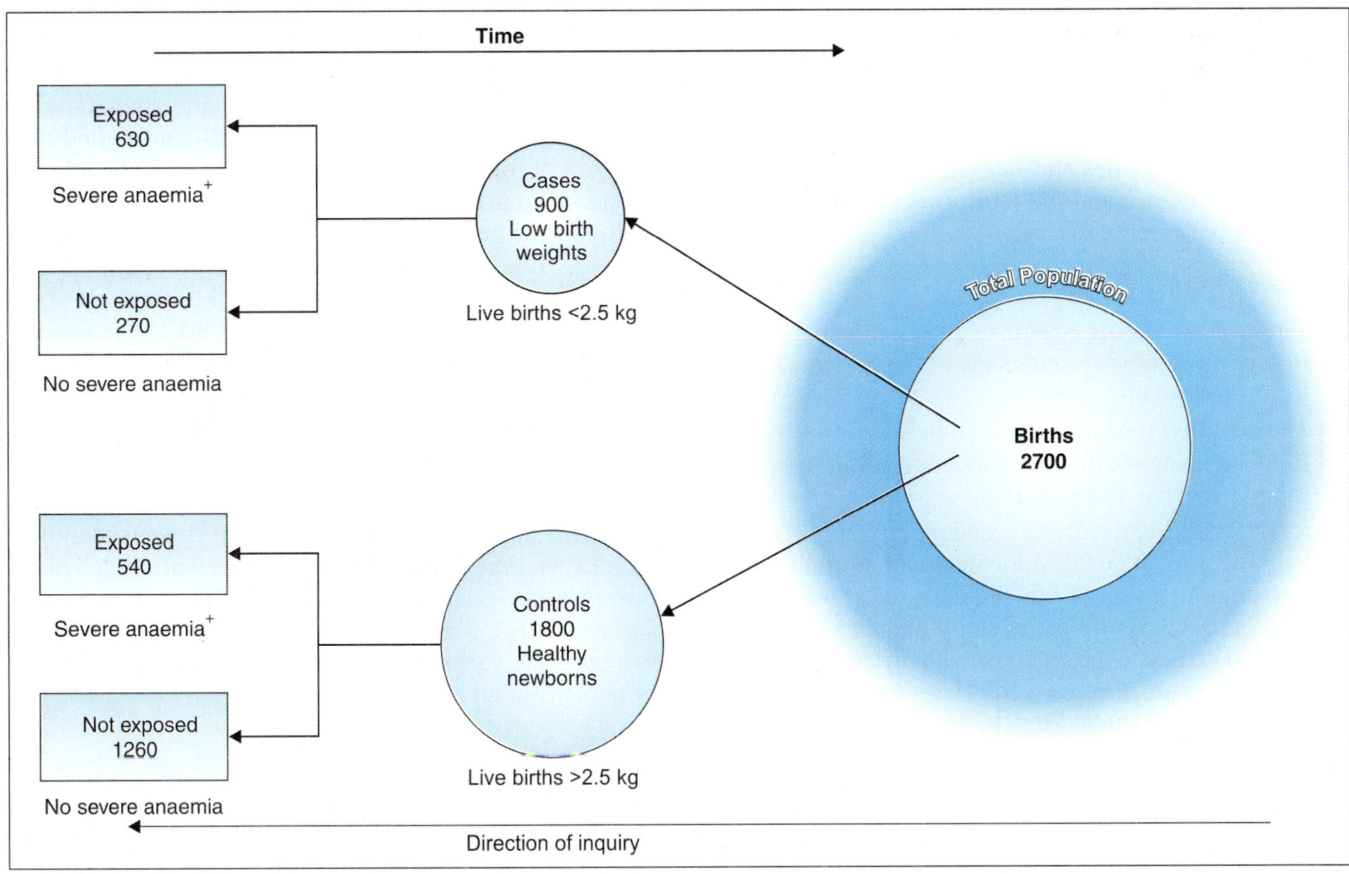

Fig. 8.16: Design of a case control study—severe anaemia of mother and birth weights

Table 8.27: Association between low birth weight and severe anaemia in pregnancy

Exposure			Birth weight		
			Yes <2.5 kg	No >2.5 kg	Total
ANAEMIA OF LESS THAN 7g	+	Yes	630	540	1170
	–	No	270	1260	1530
		Total	**900**	**1800**	**2700**

$$\text{Odds ratio} = \frac{630 \times 1260}{270 \times 540} = 5.44$$

d. Cohort Studies

The cohort study measures the incidence and for this reason cohort studies are also called as *incidence studies*. In cohort study, the focus is on *healthy population*. The healthy population is divided into two subgroups: One group is that which is exposed to the risk or risk factor is present in that subgroup and the second subgroup is free from risk or exposure. Both these groups, i.e. **exposed** and **non-exposed** should match each others in terms of age, sex, economic status and other attributes but for exposure.

Purpose

Cohort study has two purposes:

- To measure the incidence of disease.
- To find out the cause of disease.

Advantages

Cohort study provides the best information about the causation of disease and the most direct measurement of the risk of developing disease.

Disadvantages

- The cohort studies require long time period for follow-up of subjects and many of the subjects may be lost to follow-up.
- The cost involved may be too much.
- If the incidence of disease is low or it is rare very large sample size has to be studied.

Cohort studies are easier to conduct in young children, to study the growth and development and mortality in the first month or first year of life. Similarly, these are easier to conduct in pregnant women to study the outcome of pregnancy and associate the outcome with different variables.

Notable examples of global cohort studies are Framingham heart study, MONICA study on heart disease and Doll and Hill study on smoking and cancer.

Design of Cohort Study

8

During the year 1996 in a rural community development block in 1,00,000 population, 2700 births occurred. Of these 900 were low birth weights and 1800 weighed 2.5 kg or more. These two subgroups of births were followed for one-year period to study the effect of mortality/incidence of mortality in the first year of life. The hypothesis was that incidence of death is much more in babies who are born with low birth weights (Fig. 8.17 and Table 8.28).

The incidence of infant mortality (IMR) was 120 per thousand live births in low birth weight babies while IMR of 40 was observed in babies who had adequate birth weight. The incidence of IMR was three times higher in low birth weights as compared to normal birth weights after a follow-up period of one year. Thus, risk ratio of infant mortality ($I_E \div I_{NE}$) was measured as 120/40 = 3. Low birth weight was *cause* of high infant mortality.

The incidence of mortality can be obtained for different periods such as during the first 7 days of life, up to 28 days of life and 28 days to less than one year to capture early neonatal, neonatal and post-neonatal component of infant mortality.

Second Model (Table 8.29)

The cohort of young children was followed for one year period to study the incidence of morbidity. Once a week follow-up of young children was ensured at village level by Anganwadi workers and mothers themselves. The child weeks of follow-up were calculated as some children were entering and some were leaving and some were dying in the study group at different points of time, hence, person time in terms of weeks followed was used. For example, if a child could be followed up for 52 weeks that child contributed 52 weeks and a child who entered in the study group on the beginning of 51st week contributed only 2 weeks of follow-up. Follow-up period of each child was calculated and added up for all children. Total weeks of follow-up experience of all children were added up and this was used as denominator to calculate episodes of diarrhoea per child per 100-week of follow-up. Total weeks of follow-up for infants were 17,903, total episodes of diarrhoea were 2060, and episodes per year were 5.98 per infant in this study. Episodes of 2.63 per sick infant were arrived at in this study.[7] This is also known as **life table method of analysis.**

"Life expectancy of an individual is arrived at by cohort study. All births occurring at a point of time are followed up till such time that all die and the survival of each one at different age is calculated to arrive at life expectancy or if we apply the current age and sex specific mortality rates to a cohort at various ages we can arrive at life expectancy of persons in an area (*see* life table)."

Third Model (Table 8.30)

This cohort study measured the change of nutritional status of cohort of 570 under six children over a period of one year follow-up with intervention of supplementary and therapeutic nutrition under ICDS.

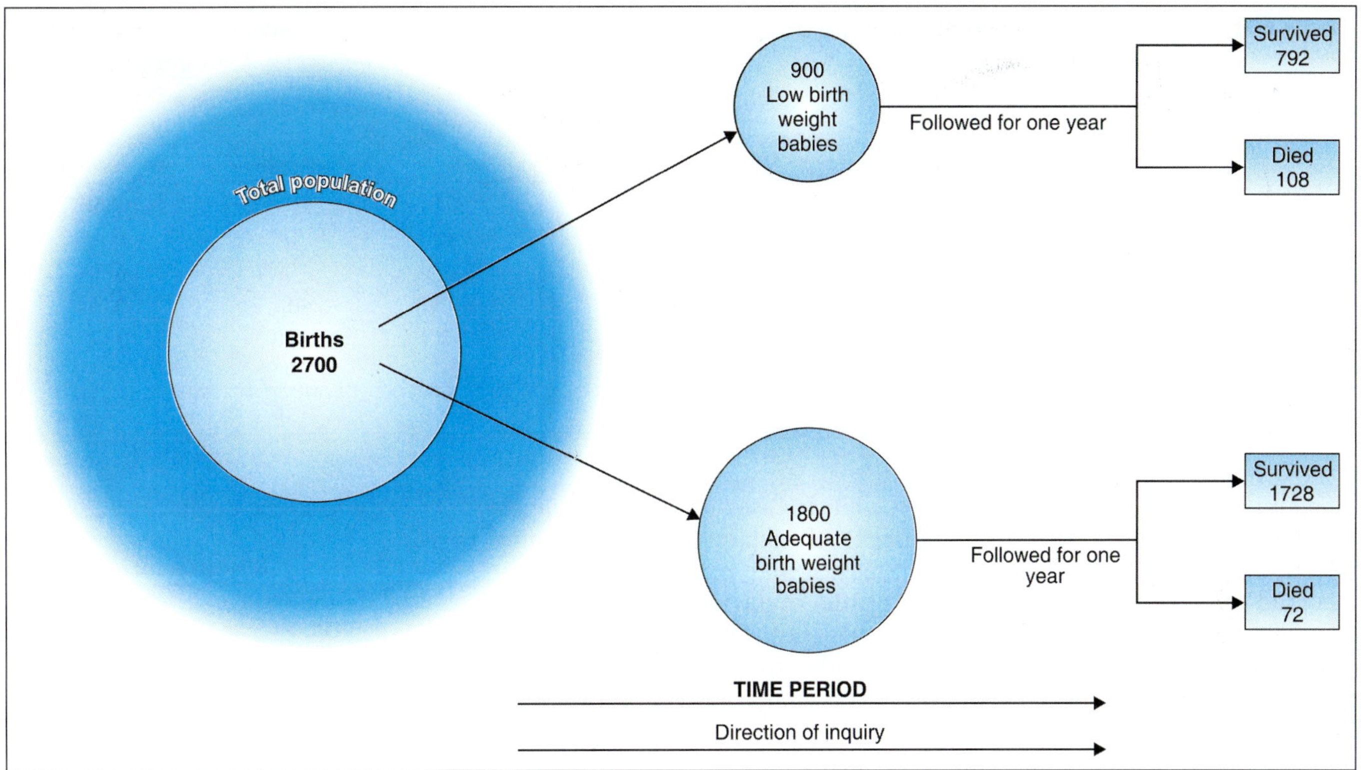

Fig. 8.17: Design of a cohort study

Table 8.28: One year follow-up of cohort of 2700 births in a rural block to study incidence of mortality in LBW

Birth weight (kg)	*Number*	*Survived*	*Died*	*Incidence of infant mortality*
<2.5	900	792	108	120
>2.5	1800	1728	72	40
Total	**2700**	**2520**	**180**	**67**

Out of 187 children who were normal in year 1979, 114(60.97) continued as normal while 39.07% deteriorated. Out of 202 grade I malnutrition 29.22% improved, 55.93% remained in the same grade while 14.36% deteriorated. Similarly, out of 118 grade II malnourished children 55.09% improved and 39.84% maintained the same grade while 5.07% deteriorated. Of 41 grade III children, 65.90% improved their nutritional status, 24.38% maintained and 9.72% deteriorated. Of 16 grade IV children all children, i.e. 100% improved their nutritional status (Table 8.30).

(a) Cohort Studies in Malaria

Infant parasite rate (IPR) is calculated as follows:

$$\text{IPR} = \frac{\text{No. of infants found positive for malaria parasite}}{\text{Total number of infants blood smears examined}} \times 100$$

This index gives great deal of information regarding malaria transmission in the area during the epidemiological year. Normally, infants do not have malaria infection at the time of birth, only in very rare cases in holoendemic areas, the transplacental infection may occur in infants.

Sometimes, a longitudinal survey of infant population is carried out. In this study, each infant is registered at the time of birth and followed for a period of one year. By this study, transmission period in an area can be arrived at.

During these longitudinal studies, the point of time when any of the infants in the cohort is found positive, the malaria transmission has deemed to have commenced 21–35 days prior to the date of positivity of the infant. In case, the

Table 8.29: Incidence of diarrhoeal episodes per year in a rural block April 1984 to March 1985[7]

Age groups (years)	*No. of children experiencing diarrhoea*	*Diarrhoeal episodes*	*Episode per sick child*	*Total weeks of follow-up*	*Episodes per year*
0–1	784	2060	2.63	17903	5.98
1–2	534	1370	2.56	12975	5.49
2–3	238	556	2.33	6892	4.19
0–3	1556	3986	2.56	37770	5.48

8

Table 8.30: Longitudinal follow-up of under six children to assess the outcome of nutritional status after one year of follow-up in a rural block

Year 1979 Baseline survey		*Repeat survey 1980*					
Gr.	*No.*	*Normal*	*Grade I*	*Grade II*	*Grade III*	*Grade IV*	*Not recorded*
Normal	187	114(60.97)	53(28.34)	16(8.56)	2(1.07)	1(0.53)	1(0.53)
Gr. I	202	59(29.22)	113(55.93)	24(11.88)	5(2.48)	0(0)	1(0.49)
Gr. II	118	20(16.95)	45(38.14)	47(39.84)	6(5.07)	0(0)	0(0)
Gr. III	41	2(4.86)	8(19.44)	17(41.60)	10(24.38)	4(9.72)	0(0)
Gr. IV	16	2(12.50)	1(6.25)	8(50.00)	5(31.25)	0(0)	0(0)
Not recorded	6	0(0)	0(0)	6(100)	0(0)	0(0)	0(0)
Total	**570**	**197**	**220**	**118**	**28**	**5**	**2**

infant is positive for *P. vivax*, it is 21 days, while in case of *P. falciparum,* it is 35 days. In the absence of malaria infection in the cohort of infants under study, it may be inferred that there was no or negligible malaria transmission during the epidemiological year. The epidemiologist can conclude that the area is either free of malaria or there was a very negligible malaria transmission. In case, the malaria control operations were being undertaken in the area, it could be concluded that they were able to interrupt the local transmission of malaria during the year of investigation.

(b) *Incidence of Malaria*

The active surveillance and passive surveillance under national malaria control programme generate epidemiological data on malaria incidence.

The surveillance data are continuous/longitudinal at fortnight interval and give the parasite distribution in the community for each fortnight. The annual parasite incidence rate during the year can be easily calculated from the surveillance data. Thus, the annual parasite incidence (API) is *incidence of malaria* in the community assessed on longitudinal basis.

$$\text{API} = \frac{\text{No. of blood smears found positive for malaria in one year}}{\text{Total population under surveillance}} \times 1000$$

The surveillance data under malaria is an example of incidence study or cohort study. Further the surveillance data gives accurate estimate of malaria incidence, endemicity, magnitude of malaria transmission and parasites distribution in different segments of the community including the parasite distribution by age, sex, etc. These parameters if utilized properly give a more reliable insight on malaria epidemiology of the area and help in formulation and evaluation of control measures.

Cohort Study in Leprosy (Tables 8.31 and 8.32)

This exercise was done in May 2004, for carrying out LEM (leprosy elimination monitoring). Cohort for the MB cases of leprosy registered during the period from 1st May 2001 to 30th April 2002 was analysed to determine total

Table 8.31: Case holding indicators for MB

Case = A person with clinical signs of leprosy (with or without bacteriological examination), who has yet to complete full course of treatment.
Cured = A patient who has completed a full course of MDT (12 doses for MB).
Defaulter = A patient who has not taken treatment consecutively for more than 12 months.
Left the control area = A patient who has left the area where he/she used to come for MDT treatment and has migrated somewhere else. This patient should be removed from the register (and therefore from the prevalence).

Number of MB cases from 1st May 2001 to 30th April 2002 Registered in area	**Number of MB cases cured**	**Number of MB cases defaulted**	**Number of MB still on treatment after completion of 12 doses of MDT**	**Left the control area**	**Died**
Total 18	**12**	**3**	**6**	**1**	**2**

Note: MB patients who had received more than 12 doses should be included in both columns (cured and still on treatment after completion of 12 doses).

Source of data: Leprosy treatment register and/or patient card for the period from 1st May 2001 to 30th April 2002.

Table 8.32: Case holding indicators for PB[8]

Case = A person with clinical signs of leprosy (with or without bacteriological examination), who has yet to complete full course of treatment.
Cured = A patient who has completed a full course of MDT (6 doses for PB).
Defaulter = A patient who has not taken treatment consecutively for more than 12 months.
Left the control area = A patient who has left the area where he/she used to come for MDT treatment and has migrated somewhere else. This patient should be removed from the register (and therefore from the prevalence).

Number of PB cases from 1st January 2002 to 31st Dec. 2002 Registered in area	**Number of PB cases cured**	**Number of PB cases defaulted**	**Number of PB still on treatment after completion of 6 doses of MDT***	**Left the control area**	**Died**
Total 40	**30**	**6**	**6**	**2**	**2**

*If a single skin lesion (SSL) case is treated with 6 MDT doses of PB as a PB case, he/she should be included in the cohort.
Note: PB patients who had received more than 6 doses should be included in both columns (cured and still on treatment after completion of 6 doses).

number of cases, total number cured and total number defaulted and total number still on treatment after completion of 12 doses.[8] Similarly, cohort for PB cases from 1st January 2002 to 31st December 2002 was chosen for outcome of treatment and case holding.

Similarly, cohort of new sputum smear positive cases of pulmonary TB can be followed up, to determine cure rate, sputum conversion rate, default and death rate.

EXPERIMENTAL EPIDEMIOLOGY

Experimental epidemiology is also known as intervention epidemiology. In this method, the interventions are undertaken which could be treatment, immunization, supplementary nutrition, therapeutic nutrition, specific nutrient like vitamin A, iron and folic acid, salt iodization, insecticidal spray, chlorination of water, etc. Similarly, new drug is tested for its effectiveness. Experimental epidemiology involves experimentation in the groups or community and usually the effects of an intervention are measured in two groups, namely **experimental group** and **control group.** The interventions are strictly determined by laid down protocol or plan. There are important ethical considerations in the conduct of these studies. If a drug is of proven value this is not denied to persons recruited in the experimental group.

There are three designs of experimental or intervention epidemiology:

1. Randomized controlled trials (RCTs)
2. Field trials
3. Community trials

RANDOMIZED CONTROLLED TRIALS (RCTs)

The randomized controlled trials are also known as randomized clinical trial.

Objective

Objective of RCT is to study the effectiveness of a new drug or a regimen in 'patients'.

Steps

1. First step in RCT is to prepare a plan of study or protocol what you wish to test or study.
2. Define study population.
3. Selection of participants by defined criteria as per plan.
4. Randomization of participants.
5. Treatment group and control group.
6. Follow-up of these groups.

Planning RCT

Define clear objectives of RCT, state the inclusion and exclusion criteria of case (case definition is essential to have valid conclusions). Determine the sample size, place, and period of study. The design of the trial must be written in advance whether it would be single blind, double blind or triple blind methods. In single blind method the investigator knows the treatment plan and it is not known to the patient to which group he belongs. In double blind trials, the investigator and the participants both do not know to which group the patient is allocated and the treatment plan. In triple blind trials, the investigator, participants and the person associated with analysis do not know the treatment plan and group allocation. The blinding is useful tool to avoid bias in the study. The plan of study must be approved by ethical committee of the institute.

Study Population

The study population varies according to nature of RCT. Most often the patients are chosen from hospital or from the community as per defined criteria as explained below. In choice of patients for domiciliary and home treatment; *open cases of tuberculosis* were chosen as **study population.**

Selection of Participants—Inclusion Criteria

Once we have defined study population out of open cases of tuberculosis those who fulfilled criteria for inclusion as participants were selected based on some of the criteria like age groups, severity of disease and treatment taken or not, etc. Thus, the participant patients must meet the criteria set by the investigator under the step planning of RCT. Further informed consent of the participant is essential for RCT.

Randomization

Subjects in a population are randomly allocated to groups. Once you have selected the study population the next step is to allocate the participants of study into:

1. Treatment groups
2. Control groups.

This should be done without any bias. You can adopt a lottery system, i.e. have predetermined chit or token specifying treatment or control word on it and as the case enters the study, draw a token and categorize the patient to either control or treatment group. Random table numbers can be used for randomization. Randomization is considered to be "sheet anchor" of RCT.

Treatment group and control group (intervention): The treatment group is put on a drug under trial and the control group is given no drug or given a placebo, which resembles with treatment drug in size and colour and looks identical with treatment drug.

If one wishes to determine the efficacy of two different drugs then subgroups can be made for allocation of these subgroups to drug A, B or C, etc. The treatment and intervention needs to be supervised very closely in the hospital.

Follow-up

The final outcome in two groups, i.e. treatment group and control group is observed with the passage of time or such time interval which has been predetermined. The outcome could be *cure* or *improvement* in the condition or *worsening* or no change in the condition or patient may die. Cure and all other outcomes are determined as per laid down criteria under the plan of study.

Analysis

The final outcomes are compared between the treatment group and control group or between various subgroups. It could be **meta analysis** of several RCTs done in different parts of the country.

Randomized Controlled Trials in Tuberculosis

Comparison of Home and Sanatorium Treatment

8

This study was undertaken by tuberculosis chemotherapy centre in Madras, as a controlled comparison of *Home* and *Sanatorium treatment* for one year and subsequently for another four years to study the emergence of relapse cases in these two groups.

Study Population

163 newly diagnosed and previously untreated sputum positive patients of pulmonary tuberculosis from poor section of the community in Madras city.

Randomization

These 163 cases were randomly allocated for treatment at *Sanatorium* or *Home* with the same chemotherapy, i.e. INH 200 mg and PAS 10 g in two divided doses per day. Patients in home series were given weekly supply of drugs to be administered by themselves at home with monthly supervision of their progress at the clinic and were visited at home by a health visitor every fortnight (supervised therapy).

Comparison

The patients in the sanatorium series had bedrest, good accommodation, balanced diet and nursing care. Thus, this was the comparison of treatment of patients in best *sanatorium conditions* with those in usual day-to-day *home conditions* of poor sections of the community.

Results

At the end of one year, 86% of patients treated at home converted to sputum negative and remained so (bacteriologically quiescent) as against 92% in sanatorium patients. Improvement in X-ray and closure of cavity were also of the same order in both the groups.

Follow-up

After one year, the sanatorium patients returned to their homes and the patients in both series were closely followed up for another 4 years to study the long-term results. Considering the overall relapse rate of disease in the two groups, it was found that 7% of patients in home series and 10% patients in sanatorium series had bacteriologically relapse over a 4-year period of follow-up.

Conclusion

It was conclusively proved that effect of treatment of patients at home was as good as treatment in an institution both in respect of immediate recovery and subsequent prevention of relapse and that good food, nursing care and isolation did not play any useful role in the treatment of tuberculosis. Domiciliary treatment has the added advantage of not causing any dislocation of the family during the period of patients treatment for tuberculosis. Supervised domiciliary treatment paved the way for present day DOTS under revised RNTCP and thus DOTS was born in India.

TB Attack Rates Among Close Family Contacts

This study was planned by the tuberculosis chemotherapy centre to determine the relative risks for contacts of patients treated at *home* and in the *sanatorium*.

256 close family contacts of patients treated in homes and 272 similar contacts of patients treated in sanatorium were intensively followed up by X-ray and bacteriological examination for five years. In each family, there was just one infectious case and the contacts in the two series were similar in all other aspects. Efforts of isolation of the index cases could be best studied by comparing attack rate in the two series in the first year when the index case of the sanatorium series was isolated in the hospital.

In the first year, 4.9% of the contacts in home series developed tuberculosis compared with 7.6% of contacts of sanatorium patients. Over the whole period of 5 years, 9.8% of contacts of patients treated at home developed tuberculosis as against 14.4% of *contacts* of patients treated in sanatorium. There was no difference of attack rates in the two groups even when the initially tuberculin negatives and initially tuberculin positives were analysed separately.

An interesting observation of the study was that the majority of cases in contacts occurred in children below 5 years of age and were detected within 3 months of diagnosis of the index case and there was suggestive evidence that in most of them the infection occurred before the index case was diagnosed.

Conclusion

There is no special risk to the contacts of patients treated at home with effective chemotherapy, the main risk to them being before the treatment has begun. Hence, *isolation* of patients in hospital/institution or at home is not required. What we require is effective chemotherapy treatment at the earliest.

Sociological Study of Awareness of Symptoms among Persons with Pulmonary Tuberculosis

About 2000 patients having evidence of inactive, probably active and active tuberculosis disease in their X-rays whose sputum results were also available (experimental groups) were age and sex matched with an equal number of persons with normal X-ray (control group) in 34 villages and 4 towns of Tumkur district in Karnataka. These persons were interviewed at random by social investigators for symptoms. Only such symptoms that were associated with pulmonary tuberculosis were taken into consideration. Of these cough for one month or more, fever for one month or more were analysed statistically. 79% of experimental group and 83% of the control group were satisfactorily interviewed.

Results

Cough was found to be the most important single symptom. 69% of sputum positives and 46% of X-ray positives had this symptom against 9% of the normal.

69% of the sputum positive, 52% of the X-ray positives, 29% of inactive and 15% of the controls had at least one of the above symptoms **(cough and fever more than a month).**

Analysis also showed that 95% of the bacteriologically positive cases were aware about their symptoms, 72% experienced cough and were worried about their symptoms and 52% of them actually took action at the existing health facilities under pressure of their symptoms.

Conclusion

Cough of more than a month was most important symptom in bacteriologically positive cases. It is now built in the programme that individuals or patients who have cough for 2 weeks or more with or without other symptoms should have 2 sputum samples examination done for AFB. Usually, at least 2% of adult outpatients in general OPD have cough for 3 weeks or more. Half or more than half of infectious cases in the community are already seeking services and knocking at the door of health services.

Clinical Trials in Malaria

Drug resistance in *P. falciparum* to chloroquine, as well as proguanil and pyrimethamine is attributable to selection under pressure of drug resistant mutants, which survive by utilizing alternative pathways.

Gradation of Response to Drugs

This has been explained in Chapter 12 under malaria.

Test Methodology in Drug Resistance Studies

The WHO recommended techniques of *in vivo* (7 to 28 days) are followed for observing the resistance status of *P. falciparum* parasites to chloroquine and other antimalarials, wherever the standard or extended tests are not operationally feasible simplified *in vivo* tests (day 0, day 2 and day 7) are also conducted.

Chloroquine is administered in the initial 3 days after collecting blood smear from day 0 to day 7 and then followed on day 14, day 21 and day 28. Urine test is repeated on day 1 or day 2 to confirm absorption of chloroquine.

Criteria for Selection of an Area

Area with intense malaria transmission showing predominantly *P. falciparum* infection, area with therapeutic failure to drug reported by physician, areas having malaria outbreaks, project areas with tropical aggregation of labour from endemic areas, area reporting high mortality due to malaria, etc. are chosen.

Inclusion Criteria

P. falciparum cases with minimum parasitaemia of 1000 asexual parasites per cu mm blood are selected for study through fever surveys and the fever cases attending the OPDs of PHCs/dispensaries. The screened cases without any evidence of history of consumption of chloroquine (confirmed by urine examination) prior to the test are selected for the study. Selected cases are then administered 25 mg of chloroquine per kg body weight in three divided oral doses of 10 mg, 10 mg, and 5 mg per kg body weight single dose over three consecutive days respectively.

Criteria for Declaration of Resistant Areas

A chloroquine resistant PHC will be characterized by detection of more than 25% of RII and RIII level cases in a minimal sample of 30 cases (*see* revised criteria).

It is observed that the percentage of sensitive cases markedly declined during the last 18 years from 89.8% in 1978 to 2.5% in 1997. The lowest sensitivity of 0.8% to chloroquine was observed in the year 1994.

Sensitivity Status of other Antimalarials

Large number of studies have been conducted with alternate drugs like amodiaquine, sulfa-pyremethamine, quinine, etc. Studies carried out from 1989 to 1997 in chloroquine as well as amodiaquine use in Northeast areas to determine the comparative efficacy of chloroquine and amodiaquine in treatment of *Pf* malaria indicate that amodiaquine has no advantage over chloroquine in resistant areas. Both the drugs have shown similar response and considering the toxicity associated with amodiaquine it has been withdrawn from the programme as per drug policy in 1995.

In vivo drug resistance studies with sulfapyrimethamine and quinine were conducted on 1127 and 209 cases respectively. Sulfapyrimethamine drug combinations were introduced as a second line of treatment in chloroquine resistant areas as per the NMEP drug policy. Study results have shown resistance to this drug combination in low proportion in the North Eastern states, West Bengal and Kolar district of Karnataka and in Bhopal city of Madhya Pradesh and Tripura.

Significance

The most important factor that determines the distribution of resistant strains is the prolonged drug pressure in the community with sub-therapeutic dosage of antimalarials. Efficacy of drug trials studies in malaria is *important to evolve national policy on drugs in malaria.*

Leprosy

A randomized controlled trial in leprosy has made revolution in treatment and has reduced the duration of treatment with multidrug therapy (MDT).

Outcome of multicentric study in India on efficacy of different treatment regimens have been accepted by WHO Leprosy Elimination Advisory Group (LEAG) in 1997 and 7th WHO expert committee on chemotherapy. The LEAG has endorsed the technical recommendations of the 7th expert committee on chemotherapy of leprosy and has urged all the national Governments to implement the same. Now the duration of treatment of MB has been reduced to 12 months and for PB cases for 6 months.

It is envisaged further to reduce the duration of MB treatment from 12 months to shorter duration.[9–11]

FIELD TRIALS

Field trials in contrast to clinical trials focus on healthy populations who are exposed to the risk of development of disease.

Example: Infants and young children who are at risk of developing measles in the community.

Trial of vaccine is conducted on healthy children or healthy population in the field. According to protocol, the study population is defined and participants are chosen and assigned to experimental group and control group and intervention is done. One group is immunized and other is non-immunized. These two groups are followed for a defined period (say one year or longer) and the outcome or incidence of disease occurrence in both groups is recorded and the results are compared in two groups. In field conditions such a situation already exists, some children are immunized and some do not accept the immunization and are left as unimmunized. This opportunity provides a chance to conduct field trials to determine the *efficacy of a vaccine*.

Example

The efficacy of measles vaccine is determined by field trials under ideal conditions, this vaccine has high proven efficacy (approx. 90%) and should not be denied to infants. Immunization services with a measles vaccine efficacy of 90% are protecting children as effectively as possible against measles. A vaccine efficacy of less than 80% means there is problem with the vaccine. This could be due to problem with the cold chain, the injection technique or the age at which the health worker is immunizing the children, and you should take action to correct it.

To calculate vaccine efficacy, we need to obtain following information from the health records.

- The size of study population—which are children 12–23 months of age since these children were under one year of age in the previous year.
- The coverage of measles vaccine in children.
- The number of cases of measles in immunized children, 12–23 months of age.
- The number of cases of measles in unimmunized children 12–23 months of age.

Size of Population

If a health centre has 30,000 population and the birth rate of the area is 30/1000, the size of study population (12–23 months children) can be calculated by 30,000 × .03 = 900.

8

1 Therefore, study population of 12–23 = 900
2 Measles immunization coverage in children 12–23 months of age = 40%
3 No. of measles cases in immunized children 12–23 months of age = 40
4 No. of measles cases in unimmunized children 12–23 months of age = 486
5 No. of immunized children in study population

$$= \frac{900 \times 40}{100} = 360$$

6 No. of unimmunized in study population = 540

Let us put these data in tabular form (Table 8.33).

Table 8.33: Efficacy of measles vaccine (field trials)[12]

Disease		No. of children (12–23)		
		Vaccinated	Non-vaccinated	Total
OCCURRENCE OF MEASLES DISEASE	Yes	40	486	526
	No	320	54	374
	Total	**360**	**540**	**900**

Attack rate of measles in immunized children $= \frac{40}{360} = \frac{1}{9}$

Attack rate of measles in unimmunized children $= \frac{486}{540} = \frac{9}{10}$

$$\text{Efficacy of measles vaccine} = \frac{\text{Attack rate in unimmunized } (-) \text{ Attack rate in immunized}}{\text{Attack rate in unimmunized}} \times 100$$

$$= \frac{\frac{9}{10} - \frac{1}{9}}{\frac{9}{10}} \times 100 = 88\%$$

Interpretation

The measles vaccine efficacy of 88% in field trials indicates that high efficacy is being achieved in field conditions. It means it confers protection to nearly 88% of immunized children and occurrence of disease—one in 9 children in immunized against 9 out of 10 in unimmunized further confirms its efficacy.

BCG Vaccine Trials

A field trial of BCG vaccine has reported the efficacy of BCG vaccine ranging from 50 to 60% all the world over. Thus, efficacy of BCG is variable. The reasons for this variation are not clear, but the conclusion is obvious—BCG vaccine will not control TB. It still has vital role in preventing serious disseminated disease in children and that is why it is incorporated in the universal programme of immunization in India and most developing countries.

COMMUNITY TRIALS

In these trials, the treatment groups are communities rather than individuals.

The best example of community trial is supply of iodized salt to community and reduction of prevalence of the problem of goitre in the community. The goitre prevalence rates were very high in Himachal Pradesh in 1953 as revealed through baseline survey of goitre in the community. A successful trial of providing iodized salt in phased manner indicated marked reduction of problem of prevalence of goitre in experimental population. The control groups in this study were communities in Himachal Pradesh not supplied with iodized salt or covered with iodized salt in phased manner subsequently (Table 8.34).[13]

Table 8.34: Community trials of iodized salt

Area	Prevalence of goitre 1956	Intervention 1962	Prevalence of goitre 1968	Prevalence of goitre 1994
Kangra	55%	Iodized salt	32.1%	7%
40 Districts of India	14–69% (1984–94)	Do	2–40% (2003)	

Some of the areas in Himachal Pradesh started receiving iodized salt as early as 1957 (Kangra Valley) after initial surveys in 1956, however, the national programme on control of goitre commenced in 1962. The prevalence of goitre was 55% in 1956 in Kangra Valley, which declined to low level of 32% in 1968 after the supply of iodized salt in Kangra Valley. Following this experiment, national programme on control of goitre was launched in 1962 and subsequently renamed as National Iodine Deficiency Disorders Control Programme (NIDDCP). The pilot study (1994) reported TGR of 7% in 4 selected blocks of district Kangra which further speaks of success of intervention.[13] A country wide study carried out by NIN and DGHS in 40 districts to assess the impact of iodization revealed that overall prevalence of total goiter rate declined from 14–69% during 1984–94 to 2–40% in 2003. TGR was >= 5% in 37 out of 40 districts.

COMMON ERRORS IN EPIDEMIOLOGICAL STUDIES

The focus of epidemiology is to measure diseases/events in the population. The measures must be accurate. The most epidemiological studies rely on part or sample of population, to arrive at true population value, sample value should reflect true value of population, which might not be so. Errors in epidemiological studies affect the sample value; hence, these errors should be minimized by observing the principles or rules of the study.

Common errors which can occur in the study are:

- Random errors (Non sampling errors)
- Sampling errors

Random Errors

These include individual biological variations, and measurement errors.

Biological Variations

The individual biological variations are well known since we study the part of population and that part of population may have different biological characteristics and may not be true representative of total population. The biological variations are related to age, sex, genetic make up and heredity, race and ethnicity.

Measurement Bias

The measurement of a disease may be inaccurate or may not be valid or in other words the measurement do not measure correctly what they intend to measure. Defective collection of information, it is called response error. There could be defective measurement or defective instrument (Proforma, Questionnaire) or defective diagnostic criteria. Laboratory results may differ from one lab to another. Therefore, standardization of technique of measurement or instrument is essential to avoid measurement bias. The instruments like blood pressure apparatus, weighing machine and laboratory test must be standardized.

Internal quality control by the testing laboratory itself is desirable and external quality control helps to establish reliability and validity of a test. HIV positive samples detected by one laboratory are cross checked at reference laboratory to enhance the quality control. Training of laboratory personnel helps avoid measurement errors apart from calibration of instruments.

Sampling Errors

These are due to wrong selection of participants from study population, which may not represent the characteristics of study population. The best way to reduce sampling errors is to increase the size of sample in the study and adopt ***Principle of randomization***. Determination of sample size for health studies has been published by WHO (Lwanga and Lemeshow 1991).

Selection Bias

The sample selected may be a biased sample and it may not be representative of true characteristics of population. Selection bias occurs when there are systematic differences between the characteristics of people selected for a study and characteristics of those who are not.

If the non-respondents are replaced by other individuals this results in selection bias. Selection biases are common in randomized controlled trials (RCTs). In a school health survey for prevalence of disease the sick children may be absent or stay at home on the day of survey or if one is studying the factory workers the sick might not have come at work place, unless follow-up visits are assured the results may be biased. In HIV sentinel surveillance, selection bias has been removed by including all consecutive new cases of STDs in the sample.

Participation Bias

If HIV testing is not unlinked/anonymous or if testing facility is located far way from clinic site then individual may not participate in study and this way participation bias results.

Confounding Bias

The confounder means a factor or character, which is equally important for causation of disease than the only one chosen factor to establish causal association. If one is studying the association of diet with occurrence of cardiovascular disease and the smoking is not being accounted for, the interpretation is biased one.

Common confounding factors are—age, social class and habit in epidemiological studies. Confounders can be removed by adopting the procedure of randomization, matching controls with experimental subjects and adhering to criteria of selection of cases and controls and by giving due weightage to confounding factors at the time of analysis.

Ethical Issues

The ethical issues in epidemiological studies are important and cardinal. The guidelines contained in the declaration of Helsinki and ethics and epidemiology, and international guidelines must be observed. The institutions where research is being pursued must have an ethical committee to regulate the ethical considerations. Before the studies are undertaken, the study plan must be approved by the ethical committee.

REFERENCES

1 Beaghehole R, Bonita R, Kjellstrom T. Basic epidemiology. Geneva: World Health Organization; 1993.

2 GOI. Annual Report 2003–04. New Delhi: MOH and FW, GOI; 2004.

3 Sharma RS, Sharma GK, Dhillon GPS. Epidemiology and control of malaria. First Edn. New Delhi: MOH and FW, GOI: National Malaria Eradication Programme; 1996.

4 GOI. Cases and deaths due to malaria in India National Health profile 2013.

5 GOI. Malaria Action Plan. New Delhi: MOH and FW, GOI; 1996.

6 Personal Communication. PHC Chiri Annual Report, 1997.

7 Lal S. Surveillance of acute diarrhoeal diseases at village level for effective home management of diarrhoea. Ind J Public Health 1994; 37(2).

8 NIHFW. Leprosy Elimination Monitoring (LEM) in India 2004. New Delhi: MOH and FW, GOI; 2004.

9 WHO. Leprosy Elimination Advisory Group (LEAG) Report. WHO Committee on chemotherapy; 1997 July 17; Geneva.

10 WHO. A guide to eliminating leprosy as a public health problem. First Edn., Geneva: Action Programme for the Elimination of Leprosy; 1995.

11 GOI/WHO. Validation of leprosy diagnosis in India. New Delhi: Leprosy Division. DGHS, MOH and FW, GOI; 2004.

12 GOI. National Child Survival and Safe Motherhood Programme Conduct Disease Surveillance. New Delhi: MOH and FW, GOI; 1992.

13 Sohal KS, Sharma TD, Kapil U. Assessment of Iodine Deficiency disorders using 30 cluster approach in district Kangra, Himachal Pradesh. Report by the technical group; 1999.

LEVELS OF PREVENTION

The word "Prevention" is derived from Latin "praevenire", "to come before". The prevention is anticipatory medicine. It comes before the disease occurs. Anticipatory actions or proactive measures are preventive in nature. Preventive actions can be taken at any stage of the spectrum of health and disease. Most of the preventive measures are focused on "healthy people", to ensure that they stay healthy and do not contract or develop disease or diseases. The goal of prevention is to "achieve health in for all" or "Health in all" to ensure adequate level of health which permits them to lead a productive and socially useful life (Fig. 8.18).

Clearly, the concern and focus of prevention is on "healthy people" to ensure that they stay healthy but the concept of prevention can be applied to unhealthy or sick also to restore their health at the earliest and to prevent deaths and disability in sick persons.

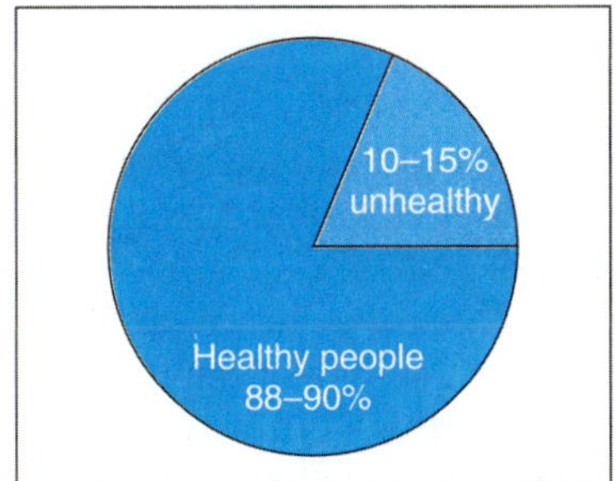

Fig. 8.18: Proportion of ailing persons

LEVELS OF PREVENTION IN EPIDEMIOLOGY

Following levels of prevention are applicable:

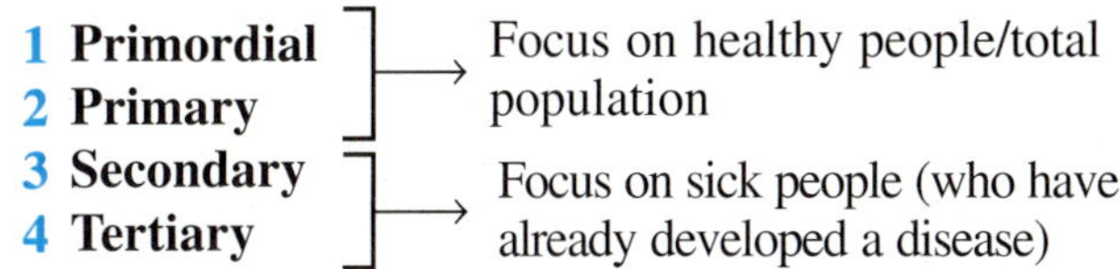

All these levels are important and complementary, although primordial prevention and primary prevention have the most to contribute to the health and well-being of the whole population.

Primordial Prevention

This is the real prevention, which does not allow the people to fall sick. The goal of primordial prevention is healthy nations, healthy population, healthy cities, towns and villages, healthy homes and healthy environments.

Aim

The aim of primordial prevention is to prevent the emergence of "unhealthy lifestyles" in population or to prevent the emergence of "risk factors" in the community.

Primordial prevention is a *strategy* to reduce risks and promote healthy lifestyles.

In developing countries with high mortality, 10 selected leading risk factors have been identified for appropriate actions, these are:

1 Underweight/malnutrition
2 Unsafe sex
3 Unsafe water, sanitation and hygiene
4 Indoor smoke from solid fuels
5 Zinc deficiency
6 Iron deficiency
7 Vitamin A deficiency
8 Blood pressure
9 Tobacco use
10 Cholesterol

The policy and legislation on tobacco and smoking have been adopted by many governments in the world including India. Tobacco epidemic can be prevented by effective legislation against tobacco. WHO global initiative has motivated many countries to adopt effective policy on tobacco.

People should not take onto smoking or adopt unhealthy lifestyles in relation to diets, exercise, and physical activity.

The world is living dangerously either because it has little choice or because it is making wrong choices. Today there are more than 7 billion people coexisting on this fragile planet. On the one side are many millions who dangerously face high and heavy concentrated burden from poverty, undernutrition, unsafe sex, unsafe water, poor sanitation and hygiene, iron deficiency and indoor smoke from solid fuels. On the other side lies unhealthy consumption, particularly tobacco and alcohol. The risks from blood pressure and cholesterol, strongly linked to heart attacks and strokes are also closely related to excessive consumption of *fatty, sugary* and *salty foods*. They become even more dangerous when combined with deadly forces of tobacco and excessive alcohol consumption. Obesity a result of unhealthy consumption coupled with lack of physical activity is itself a serious health risk.

India is facing a double burden of disease, i.e. infectious diseases due to lack of safe water, sanitation, and chronic non-communicable diseases due to *unhealthy lifestyles*.

Primordial Prevention Strategies

(a) At Government Level: Healthy Public Policies

The Government especially Health Ministry should play a stronger role in formulating risk prevention strategies which are population or community-based strategies.

- Provision of safe water and ensuring sanitation to rural, tribal and urban areas (The *Swachh Bharat Abhiyan*).
- Policy on nutrition to improve malnutrition by effective agriculture policy on "food for all and good nutrition for all" particularly improving the nutrition of most vulnerables: Infants, young children, adolescent girls, pregnant women and lactating mothers.
- National policy on promotion of healthy diets.
- Controlling food industry to prevent production and sale of junk foods, salt and transfats reduction in processed foods.
- **Tobacco, Alcohol and Substance Abuse:** Tobacco of course a major risk factor for cardiovascular diseases. In terms of intervention, the greatest tobacco-related improvements in population health would be a combination of tobacco taxation (sintax), comprehensive ban on advertising and restriction of smoking in public places and sale of cigarettes/bidis to children should be implemented. "legislations on tobacco" by all nations should be adopted in view of great health risks of tobacco.
- Policy on crop alternative to tobacco.
- Controlling/regulating behaviour of road users through Road safety Motor Vehicle Act—licensing for driving, use of safety belts and helmets.
- Prevention of air pollution (indoor and outdoor).
- Promoting non-health sectors involvement in developing policies for control of NCD and intersectoral coordination—Agriculture, Education, Food Industry, Women and Child Development and Ministry of Sports, etc.
- Protection of environments.
- Improved safety at workplace.

(b) At Community Level

- **Behaviour change communication** for healthy life styles.
- *Education:* Health education for adopting healthy behaviours through mass media focusing on predominant risk factors—undernutrition, unsafe sex, unsafe water and bad sanitation, high blood pressure, high cholesterol and overweight.

Thus, the primordial prevention can be achieved by combination of education and legislation on tobacco and food, promotion of physical activity, healthy and clean eating and observing personal hygienic practices. These measures should begin right during childhood period, continued during adolescence, and maintained in youth and adulthood period.

These measures will reduce emergence of risk behaviours in the population.

Primary Prevention

Once the risk factors have emerged in the community or unhealthy behaviours are practiced on large scale, the primary prevention has prime place.

Aim

The aim of primary prevention is to limit the *incidence* of disease by controlling underlying causes/risk factors.

or

To prevent the development of disease/diseases in population, by *modification* of *risk factors*.

Strategies of Primary Prevention

1. Health promotion.
2. Specific prevention/protection against disease, trauma and accidents.

1. Health Promotion

Health promotion means improving positive health in general by observing time honoured "best practices" like personal hygiene, brushing teeth, hand washing, avoiding smoking and alcohol, regular physical exercise, adopting healthy habits of eating, etc. *Best health practices (lifestyles)* are established and practiced in the family first of all and at school and work place and with peers in later life.

Measures for health promotion: Health promotion can be achieved through health education programmes, which could be formal and non-formal. Health education should be part and parcel of general education. Adequate nutrition, Universal exclusive breastfeeding improving environmental sanitation (safe water, safe disposal of human and animal excreta, reduction of air pollution), regular physical exercise and yoga promotes health and prevents diseases in population.

2. Specific Protection

- Immunization, against vaccine preventable diseases prevents many diseases. Most of the countries including India have national immunization programmes to prevent diseases. Immunization against polio was an important strategy for polio-eradication. Smallpox was eradicated by effective vaccination programmes. Hep B vaccine prevents liver cancer
- ***HPV:*** Vaccine prevents cervical cancer.
- Specific nutrients like mega doses of vitamin A and iron and folic acid tablets to young children, pregnant and lactating women and adolescent girls prevent blindness due to vitamin A deficiency and anaemia respectively. Iodine consumption by salt iodization prevents goitre/iodine defeciency disorders.
- ***Contraception:*** To prevent births contraceptives are used widely. This is the priority number one in India to limit the size of population by spacing and terminal methods of contraception.
- Prevention of HIV and AIDS as also STIs, hepatitis B by condom use are examples of specific protection.
- ***Accidents Prevention:*** Use of helmets and safety belts prevents head injuries and fatal accidents. Safety devices used in industries to prevent injuries and accidents are also example of specific protection against accidents and injuries.
- Avoidance of allergens, radiation by specific protection.

Approaches

We have two approaches in primary prevention, which are population-based and high-risk approach.

(a) Population-based Approach

In population-based approach, the intention is to cover the whole population for adopting healthy lifestyles through behaviour change communication. Universal immunization focuses on coverage of all infants. Similarly, in safe water for all the focus is whole population; universal elementary education is also population-based strategy. Other population-based approaches are legislation against smoking and tobacco and fixing legal age for marriage and risk reduction against HIV/AIDS, Universal Salt Iodization are the examples of population-based strategies to prevent diseases of national importance or epidemic prone diseases. Regulating salt content in manufactured foods, maintenance of healthy diets, reduction of salt intake and saturated fats, promoting physical activities and control of tobacco use are key population-based strategies.

Advantages

- Population-based approaches are useful and these make high impacts in reducing the incidence of diseases.
- The population approach does not require any screening programme to identify high-risk groups.
- Population based approaches are more rewarding in risk reduction in population and treating **underlying cause.**

(b) High-risk Approach

The focus of primary prevention in this approach is select individuals who have high-risk such as commercial sex workers or bridge population who practice high-risk sexual behaviour, and people with sexually transmitted infection (STD clinic attendees). This strategy is being followed in National AIDS Control Programme in the country.

Smokers are also high-risk individuals and similarly persons having family history of diabetes and hypertension are high-risk individuals.

Individual screening programmes for identification of high-risk individuals for coronary heart disease, hypertension and obesity have not met with much success. Screening is a costly affair and very few can afford it.

Focus on high-risk individuals will deal with only margin of the problem and will not have much impact on reduction of disease incidence or **underlying cause** in population. Individual measures to reduce risk-like screening for blood pressure, cholesterol, diabetes and weight and height measurement, may produce small effects as these involve lot of cost, and effect of individual approach pays least.

Advantages

High risk approach seems to be attractive as some argue that scarce resources should be used for high-risk people but this does not yield much results.

Conclusion

The distribution and determinants of risks in a population have major implications for strategies of prevention. Geoffrey Rose observed that in vast majority of diseases "natural history of disease presents us with continuum, not a dichotomy". Risk typically increases with across the spectrum of a risk factor. Use of dichotomous labels such as "hypertensive" and "normotensive" are therefore not a description of natural order, but rather an operational convenience. Following this line of thought, it becomes obvious that the "deviant minority" (e.g. hypertensive) who are considered to be high-risk are only part of risk continuum; rather than a distinct group. This leads to one of the most fundamental axiom in preventive medicine "a large number of people exposed to a small risk may generate many more cases than a small number of exposed to high-risk". Rose pointed out that wherever this axiom applies, a preventive strategy focusing on high-risk individuals will deal with only margin of the problem and will not have any impact on the large proportion of disease occurring in large proportion of people who are at moderate risk. For example, people with slightly raised blood pressure; suffer more cardiovascular events than the hypertensive minority. While the high-risk approach may appear more appropriate to individuals and their physicians, it can have only little effect at a population level. It does not alter the underlying cause of illness, relies on having adequate power to predict future disease, and requires continued and expensive screening for few high-risk individuals.

The relation between risk factors and disease events are continuous and most events occur in people in the middle range of risk factors distribution who are not normally judged as high-risk.

The effort expended on measuring risk factors in individuals is, therefore questionable (Robert Beaglehole). Screening for risk factors in individuals (checking blood pressure, overall check-up, check-up for diabetes and monitoring of cholesterol, etc.), cost time and lot of money and resources should be directed towards primary prevention based on population strategies of risk reductions.

In contrast, population-based strategies that seek to shift the whole distribution of risk factors have the potential to control population incidence. Such strategies aim to make healthy behaviours and reduced exposure into social norms and thus lower the risk in entire population. The potential gains are extensive, but the challenges are great as well, a preventive measure that brings large benefits to the community appears to offer little to each participating individual this may adversely affect motivation of population at large (known as **prevention paradox**). Population-based approach is most often applied to prevention of cardiovascular diseases.

Population-based strategies to reduce salt content of manufactured food, maintenance of healthy diets, promotion of physical activity and control of tobacco industry should be priority to control *epidemic* of cardiovascular diseases.

Secondary Prevention

This level of prevention is directed towards those individuals who have developed disease.

Aim

Aim of secondary prevention is to reduce *prevalence* of disease in the community by curing that disease.

The secondary prevention is valid in our country for early detection and prompt treatment of tuberculosis, leprosy, malaria, blindness and cancer in the country.

Strategies (Early Diagnosis and Prompt Treatment)

- The strategy of secondary prevention is to detect the disease at early stage and ensure prompt treatment to reduce its severity and duration. *Example:* Detection of malaria by active and passive fever surveillance offers prompt treatment in homes, similarly sputum examination of those persons having cough of 2 weeks or more helps early detection of tuberculosis and prompt treatment with DOTS strategy.
- By having screening programmes, we can detect the diseases at early stage. Screening of vision to detect refractive errors, to detect cataract, to detect precancerous lesions, blood pressure measurement for treatment of hypertension in middle-aged and elderly people. Similarly, growth monitoring of children and birth weighing can detect growth faltering at the earliest to treat it at that stage.
- Surveillance and screening programmes help early case detection and prompt treatment. Periodic medical examination of industrial workers and army personnel helps in early detection of disease and its prompt treatment. This aims at detect susceptible persons/workers and remove them from exposure before they suffer any permanent incapacitation.

Tertiary Prevention (Disability Limitation and Rehabilitation)

The tertiary prevention is the last level of prevention. It is applied when the individual has reached an advanced stage of disease. It indicates that the first two levels have failed.

Aim

- To limit the progress and development of complications of established disease.
- To reduce impairment and disability.
- To provide rehabilitation measures.
- To prolong life.
- To prevent deaths.

Disability Limitation

Once a disability (impairment, activity limitation, participation restriction) has occurred, measures can be taken to prevent its progression to handicap. Disability can be limited to minimum by advanced treatment at referral centres or established clinics by physiotherapy, and by training of disabled for self-care.

Rehabilitation

Once the disability has progressed to the stage of *handicap* then attempt is made to rehabilitate the individual. It is a restorative medicine using the remaining capacities of an individual and making him/her self-reliant and useful member in the community. The rehabilitation consists of physical, occupational and social rehabilitation measures. These are very costly. *Examples* of rehabilitation are—rehabilitation of paraplegics, amputees (those who have lost limbs), blinds, deaf, mentally retarded, leprosy cases and polio cases. These persons are being provided support for rehabilitation at established centres either by government or by voluntary organizations.

Example: Artificial limbs and foot, hearing aids, spectacles, wheel chair for mobility, speech therapy, crutches, etc.

Community-based rehabilitation (CBR) is the preferred approach wherein family and community takes responsibility and government provides support. CBR programmes are designed and run by local communities. CBR seeks to ensure that people with disabilities have equal access to rehabilitation and other services and opportunities—health, education, and livelihoods. Developed by WHO in 1980s CBR is practiced in more than 90 countries and represents move away from institutions towards community self reliance. Tertiary prevention is a costly and a challenging task.

HEALTH MANAGEMENT INFORMATION SYSTEM (HMIS)

Definition

HMIS is defined as a system that provides up-to-date, reliable complete and timely information to health managers, at various levels in order to make well-informed management decisions about programme performance and operations.[1]

HMIS is an important management as well as an epidemiological tool, which supports the management to make sound decisions. Most of the information reaches the programme managers in the form of routine statistical and management "reports". These reports, which are generally standardized in format and produced on a regular basis, constitute most visible part of health management information system.[1]

The data and information are not synonymous. What is information? The information is the outcome of data analysis and interpretation. Raw data becomes information when it is analysed processed and interpreted. The timely information thus generated is used for action and decision making at all the levels of management like home-based or client-based records and information → village-based → subcentre → PHC → CHC → District → State and national level. Information is needed at all these levels.

A formal system of reporting has been established in the health system. Every month a monthly progress report from the lowest level, i.e. "subcentre" and village level by ANM, 'ASHA', "Anganwadi centre" is processed and transmitted to higher level, i.e. PHC → CHC → District → State → Central Government.[2,3]

This forms the basis of the routine—regular information at all the levels for making decision and taking actions.

The health manager requires information on all aspects of the "system", i.e. information on inputs, processes and outcomes (outputs, effects and impacts) in order to make improvement in the delivery of services or programme. As inputs lead to development of services which lead to outcomes in the form of outputs, effects and impacts to achieve the set goal by the system.

Uses and User of HMIS

The main uses of the HMIS:

i To support decision making and taking actions.

ii To assess community health needs, e.g. community needs assessment approach (CNAA) under RCH can make use of HMIS for preparing subcentre action plans, e.g. who need immunization and how many need it.

iii To prioritize the health needs, e.g. under Community Needs Assessment Approach (CNAA) we prioritize or segment the eligible couples who need services for sterilization, spacing by contraception or priority is given to economical weaker sections.

iv To assess the performance of health workers or institutions like Subcentre → PHC → CHC → District or State.

v To monitor programme operations.

vi To evaluate the programme or to measure its success and failure.

vii For better planning of services and programmes at local level.

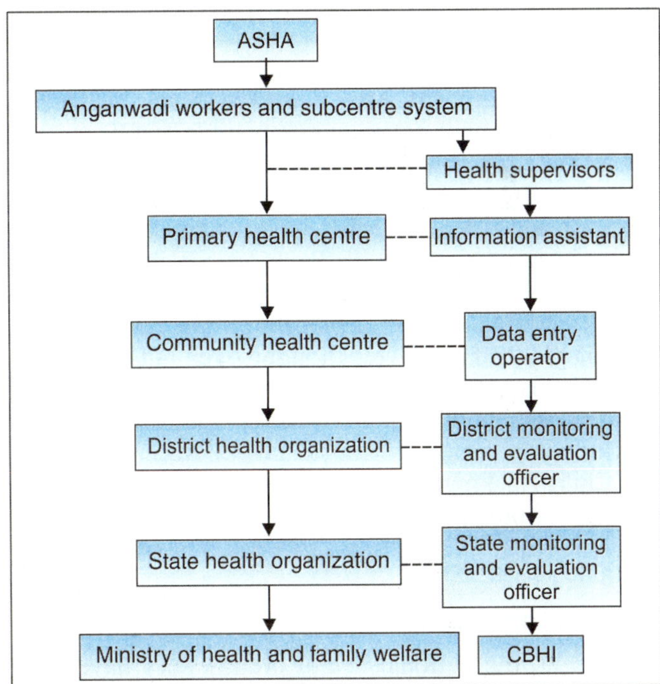

HMIS should be used at local level hence we have to build information use culture at the grass root level—subcentre and PHCs. Right now, health workers depend on formulae to prepare their action plans and they borrow the birth rate of the state and apply this to assumed population of subcentre to get a magic figure of antenatals, births, eligible couples, etc. If they have HMIS in operation, they can rely on it for planning the services at local level and sharing the information with local community.[4]

Health System Organization

The routine reports and information flows from village to national level as indicated in flow diagram. It is one-way traffic.

DEVELOPMENT OF HMIS IN INDIA

The deficiencies in information support to health for all (HFA) strategies in the country were identified as early as late 70s and it was decided to devise and implement effective management information and evaluation system (MIES) in the health sector.[3,4] It was also envisaged that the information system would reduce the unnecessary load of paper work by the peripheral health workers and streamline the system to avoid duplication of information or its unnecessary generation. The national health policy adopted by the Parliament in 1983 stated that "appropriate decision making and programme planning in the health and health-related fields is not possible without establishing an effective "health information system". A nationwide organizational set-up should be established to produce essential health information". It was also envisaged that this information system should be able to provide necessary support for local management of the health care so as to pave the way for effective decentralization of activities. Exercises in development of more effective HMIS continued and version 1.0 and 2.0 of HMIS were evolved in 1990. After a test run, it was decided in 1991 to implement computer compatible HMIS version 2.0 all over the country.[5] Then came the paradigm shift and target-free approach (TFA), which was adopted in 1996–97 and it led to further modification but retaining the basic structure of HMIS.[6,7] Under NRHM the HMIS formats have been revised and put into effect from Sept. 2008[8] (reporting format for subcentre). The HMIS system is well-planned and well thought over but its implementation is a problem because of problem of providing registers, stationary, training and lack of motivation besides lack of use of information at local level. Recently Mother and Child Tracking System (MCTS) has been launched to track every pregnant woman and Child by name.

HMIS IN INDIA

Records and Registers

At present, the national health programmes have their independent HMIS; however, at the level of village and subcentre, the reports are generated by subcentre health team. The key registers at subcentre level are:

- A Survey registers
  1. Subcentre village information
  2. Household information
  3. Eligible couple and children information
- B Continuous care registers
  1. Family welfare services
  2. Maternal care services
  3. Child care and immunization services
  4. Tuberculosis and leprosy control
  5. Malaria and blood smear and treatment
- C Other registers
  1. Home visit diary
  2. Clinic register (common ailments)
  3. Stock and issue register
  4. Birth and death register
  5. Accounts of untied funds and JSY *(Janani Suraksha Yojna)*

Attempts have been made by several states to reduce the number of registers and records. Similarly, Anganwadi workers have set of registers like household survey register, birth and death register, beneficiary register for mother and children, immunization, growth charts and weight book and stock registers.

Reports

The subcentre ANMs and Anganwadi workers are the responsibility centres for HMIS and they prepare monthly reports. The subcentre report provides information on inputs (health workers, material equipment, monthly stock position of drugs, vaccines received, functional status of equipment, etc.). It also provides information on processes and outputs or performance in terms of antenatal care, natal care, pregnancy outcome, postnatal care, newborn care, referral services, STI/RTI detection, immunization, disease surveillance, contraception services, malaria and tuberculosis output, and data on impact indicators like births and deaths. It also has information on interaction with the community, besides general information on population and eligible couples—parity-wise and age-wise. Similarly, Anganwadi worker provides useful information on health and nutrition services and impact measurement.

This information is generated every month and sent to PHC. The feedback on this information is provided at the sector level (circle) monthly meeting of health workers, Anganwadi workers (AWWs) and their supervisors.

Similarly, subcentre action plans are evolved at the level of subcentre once a year and submitted to higher levels. Monthly single reporting format for sub centre and equivalent institutions has been evolved to provide regular data/information to guide actions and decision making.

NATIONAL HEALTH MISSION (VERSION 1.1.6 UPDATED ON 16-2-15)

Monthly Single Reporting Format for Subcentre and Equivalent Institutions

State .... District .... Block/CHC

City .... Town/Village ....

Name of Subcentre/Facility ....

Facility type ....

Public/Private ....

Location Rural/Urban ....

Population .... Month/Year.

A. MATERNAL HEALTH

A1. Antenatal Care Services

- Total number of new pregnant women registered in the reporting month ....
- New pregnant women registered under *Janani Suraksha Yojna* ....
- Total number of pregnant women who received 3 ANC visits in the reporting month.
- Total number of pregnant women who have received 4th ANC visit in the reported month.
- Pregnant women given TT 1, 2 and TT booster dose.
- Pregnant women given full course of IFA tablets (100 tablets).
- Pregnant women initiated folic acid tablets within 12 weeks of pregnancy.
- Pregnant women given deworming tablet.
- Pregnant women initiated on calcium tablet.
- Pregnant women initiated on Vit. B_{12} tablet.
- Pregnant women initiated on Vit. C tablets.
- New cases of hypertension detected (BP >140/90) at facility.
- Pregnant women with anaemia Hb level 7–11 gm .... <7 gm (severe anaemia).
- High-risk/complicated pregnancies ....
- High-risk/complicated pregnancies referred.
- Pregnant women if preterm delivery between 24–34 weeks given at least one dose of inj. dexamethasone (antenatal corticosteroids) ....

A2. Deliveries

- Home deliveries ....
- Deliveries conducted at health facility ....
- Deliveries conducted at SC.
- Women discharged within 48 hours of delivery.
- Number counselled on infant and young child feeding practices (i.e. early initiation of breastfeeding, importance of colostrum, and exclusive breastfeeding for 6 months ....
- Number of complicated deliveries referred to higher facility ....
- **Janani Shishu Suraksha Karyakram** (JSSK).
- Number of pregnant women who delivered at health facility and received free drugs, consumables, free diet and diagnostics, referral transport services and C section.
- Delivery outcomes
  - Live births
  - Stillbirths
  - Abortions .... spontaneous/induced.
- Newborn children weighed at birth .... Birth weight <1200, 1200–1799, 1800–2499 and 2500 gm and above.
- Newborn care corner (NBCC) functional .... Yes/No.
- Number of newborn who required resuscitation
- Newborns administered **vitamin K** at the time of birth (within 24 hours).
- Number of newborn (birth weight 1800–2500) provided **Kangaroo Mother Care** (KMC).
- Postnatal care services (PNC) provided by ANM.
- On first, 3rd, 7th and 42nd day (four visits).
- Number of newborns who received 3 postnatal check-ups within 10 days of birth.
- Number of newborns referred ....
- Home-based newborn and postnatal care by ASHA/ANM-seven visits to neonate and visits to postnatal mother within 6 weeks of birth.
- Number of postnatals referred because of complications.

B. IMMUNIZATION AND CHILD HEALTH

B1. Immunization Services

- OPV zero dose (within 15 days).
- Hepatitis B (birth dose within 24 hours).
- BCG at birth or within one year
  - Pentavalent 1, 2, 3
  - DPT 1, 2, 3
  - OPV 1, 2, 3
  - Hepatitis B 1, 2, 3
  - Japanese encephalitis 1st dose (9–12 months)
  - Measles first dose (9–12 months).
- Fully immunized within 12 months of age (BCG, + Hep B 1, 2, 3 + OPV 1, 2, 3 + Measles Ist **or** BCG + OPV 1, 2, 3 + Pentavalent 1, 2, 3 + measles 1st dose).
- Fully immunized between 12 months to 23 months.
- BCG + DPT 1, 2, 3 and booster, OPV 1, 2, 3 and booster, Hep B 1, 2, 3 + measles 1 and 2 **or** BCG + OPV 1, 2, 3 and booster + pentavalent 1, 2, 3 + DPT booster 1 + measles 1, 2.
- Serious adverse events following immunization (AEFI).
- Number of sessions during the month

  1 Session per month for 1000 population in rural area.

  1 Session per month for 2000 population in urban slum area.

- Number of cases of childhood diseases (vaccine preventable and others) reported during the month (0–5 years).
- Vitamin A prophylaxis between 9 months and 5 years 9 doses.
- Children 1–5 years of age given albendazole tablet.

D1.

- IUCD insertions.
- Number of IUCD/PPIUCD removals.
- Number of oral pills (OP) cycles distributed.
- Number of emergency pills (EC pills) distributed.
- Number of condom pieces distributed.
- Number of pregnancy kits used.
- Quality of sterilization services complications/failures/deaths.
- Number of new eligible couples registered by ASHA for family planning.
- Ensuring spacing of 2 years after marriage.
- Ensuring spacing of 3 years after birth of first child.
- Number of beneficiaries receiving contraceptives at the doorstep.
- Number of ASHAs paid incentive for spacing/limitations.

J. OTHER SERVICES/HEALTH FACILITY SERVICES

J1. Patient Services

- No of Anganwadi centres reported VHNDs.
- **Outpatient services** OPD attendance (all).
- Laboratory testing .... Hb .... urine sugar .... urine albumin ....
- IMNCI (integrated management of newborn and childhood illness) .... 0–2 months .... and 2 months to 5 years ....
- **Infant and young child feeding practices** (IYCF practices)
- **Number of children assessed for malnutrition** on mother and child protection card (MCPC) .... or by mid upper arm circumference <11.5 cm SAM (severe acute malnutrition) MUAC ≥11.5 – 12.5 cm .... Number of SAM referred to NRC ....
- **Adolescent health weekly iron and folic acid tablets (WIFS)**
  - Number of adolescents (10–19 years) provided 4–5 tablets in schools ....
  - Number of adolescents (10–19 years) provided albendazole tablets in schools ....
  - Number of sanitary napkins pads sold to adolescent girls by ASHA ....
- **Preconception care package reporting.**
- Number of new beneficiaries registered at subcentre for preconception package services (those giving history of baby born with congenital abnormality, defect, stillbirth, low birth weight babies, intrauterine death.
- Those given folic acid tablets (30 tablets one month prior to conception).
  - Stock position of contraceptives, drugs, NBCC equipments and their functional status.
  - Mortality details—probable causes of death.
  - Monitoring and supervisory visits to facility by SMO/MOI/C-LHV/supervisor.

Deaths with probable causes in infants, maternal, adolescents and adults

S. No.	Name and village of deceased	Sex	Age	Cause	Code
1.					
2.					
3.					
4.					
5.					
6.					

LINE LISTING OF DEATHS

Mortality details: Each case is to be entered in a separate line. Only deaths occurring at the facility level to be reported giving the major probable cause of death.

Besides this, each PHC and CHC prepare their own report in terms of referral cases seen, outdoor and indoor patients report sent on annual morbidity and mortality format of ICD-10 in addition to report on 20 notifiable communicable disease and NCDs.

Reports or information of PHC and CHC which are sent to district every month, comprise:

1. Aggregated report of subcentre activities. Staff position—number of posts filled and vacancies category-wise, transport or vehicles, equipment and supply position.
2. Malaria report—monthly report of blood slides.
3. Tuberculosis report: Revised national tuberculosis control programme. Monthly report of logistics and microscopy.
4. School health report.
5. Epidemic and notifiable diseases under IDSP.
6. AFP—surveillance.
7. Family planning achievements.
8. Immunization report.

9. National child survival and safe motherhood programme report.
10. Input proforma for sterilization. Detailed report on sterilization cases (age, sex, caste, education and number of children).
11. Input proforma for IUD (age, caste, literacy and number of children).
12. Departmentwise achievement of family planning.
13. National programme on control of blindness monitoring.
14. Monthly report of PHC/CHC.
15. Medical termination of pregnancy.
16. Monthly expenditure statement.

In summary, the major sources of HMIS are

1. Routine service reports from subcentres → PHC → CHC → (primary health care services).
2. Routine reports of hospitals/dispensaries and railways, armed force services and others.
3. Integrated disease surveillance programme.
4. National health programmes data and information.
5. Sample registration system (SRS) once a year provides state and national estimates on fertility and mortality.
6. Civil registration system—continuous surveillance.
7. Model registration—survey of causes of death (rural) once a year up to 1994.
8. HIV sentinel survey (annual) once a year.
9. District level household survey report under RCH every alternate year.
10. National family health survey data (NFHS 1–4) once every five years.
11. Annual district health survey-2010 onwards.
12. Census—once every ten years.
13. Special surveys like survey to map out problem of tuberculosis (1958, 2003, 2013, etc.).
14. Administrative reports on accounts, personnel, etc.

Since the routine reporting and information system is inadequate, the policy makers and health administrators make use of other systems of information as indicated above (SRS, NFHS 1–4, census, sentinel data, hospital data and special data generated through surveys and studies). National Nutritional Monitoring Bureau, Hyderabad generates data on dietary consumption and nutritional status. Similarly, universities and medical colleges generated tremendous and robust data on maternal and child health under the banner of ICDS, which was fed back to the system to improve the content and quality of services for women and children.

Challenge is to make use of data locally and develop a mechanism that data which are collected, have lot of meaning to be used at local level for improving programmes performance and work schedules.

The most important source of HMIS is routine regular reports collected every month at local level which forms the basis for local decisions and actions. The most common problems with routine reporting system are:[9–11]

- These are incomplete and coverage of population may not be total.
- Quality of information is poor in respect of causes of death and weighing of children.
- The information is seldom used at local level by the health workers or by team leaders (Medical Officers).
- The information is not shared with the community. The subcentres should report on performance to panchayats, hospitals to *Rogi Kalyan Samitis* and District Health Mission to Zila Parishad. Annual district report card on people's health should be prepared and shared with people.
- The information is used as compliance and for transmission of reports to higher level only.
- The feedback to health workers who collect huge or voluminous data is not available and consequently there is no sustained motivation.
- The initial training and continuing education of health workers and Medical Officers is weak, not much emphasis laid on HMIS.
- There is a tendency to over—report the performance and figures are inflated quite often.
- Data gathered under RCH and other programmes are seldom analysed, poorly understood, and not acted upon locally for decision making or to improve the quality of services. The system remains data driven rather than **action driven.**
- The planning and management staff rely primarily on "gut feeling" to formulate ad hoc decisions rather than seek pertinent data base information support.
- The supply of registers and reporting formats are erratic and frequent stock outs is a common feature.
- CNAA and mother and child tracking system (MCTS) is the latest in its introduction. Thus, HMIS is an area with full of challenges. There is no easy solution insight. Some of the innovations have been done by many states and organizations which are:
  - Home-based or client-based records, e.g. immunization card or antenatal card, growth monitoring and Mother and Child Protection Card prepared by MOH and FW and Ministry of Women and Child Development records are available with mother.
  - Registers have been combined and one or two registers, which collect minimum information at the level of subcentre, have been produced to reduce the burden on health system and workers.
  - Computer systems have been introduced. The information is processed rapidly and disseminated quickly. Computer compatible reporting formats have been evolved by health and ICDS system and data are fed at Primary Health Centres and transmitted to CHC and District, State and Central Government.

ACTION

The system is data driven, reports are seldom read, least understood and data collected locally are seldom used for planning and evaluation purposes.[12–13]

There are frequent changes in the system as and when a new programme comes a new reporting format is introduced and sometimes workers are required to prepare separate reports for each programme, e.g. child survival and safe motherhood programme, universal immunization and EPI, reproductive and child health and much before this maternal and child health and family welfare programme had introduced special set of formats for reporting data and information.

The supervisors and team leaders have a tremendous role to make improvements in the HMIS. During their supervisory visits, monthly meetings or other periodical meetings, the sample check of household survey and verification of reports and records and spot correction can help to improve the quality of records. Community itself can monitor the quality of records maintained at the level of village or subcentre. Community based monitoring is a new beginning under NRHM. People have right to information and mothers or parents themselves can share the information of records and health and nutritional status of their children at the Anganwadi and subcentre. It is a wisdom if the information of an Anganwadi and subcentre is displayed at the village/community centre or at village headman's office for dissemination. This would generate a cycle—people may seek more information and that leads to improvement of system of information. The health workers, Anganwadi workers during each contact with the client/community (home visits—*Mahila Swasthya Sangh* meetings) should share the valuable information with each home and village community and stay connected with each home thus linking homes with health system for continuum of services.

Geographic information system (GIS): This envisages creation of an electronic database of health care facilities, educational institutions, training centres and other health care establishments in India. This data base will be used for mapping the health facilities using geographic information system for wider dissemination through CBHI website. National informatics centre will provide GIS mapping of government health facilities. The concept can be applied to endemic fluorosis and safe sources of water supply and many other areas of interest/diseases of national significance.

CIVIL REGISTRATION SYSTEM (CRS)

8

The details of the number of births and deaths occurring annually is very important not only for predicting the future course of population dynamics but also for a planned social and economic development of the country. Without the knowledge of such events any type of planning has to rely either on guess estimates of these events or on some indirect estimates provided by the demographers. In fact, CRS has a vital role to play in this respect and there may not be any viable alternative to it.[14] The sample registration system (SRS) of Registrar General of India (RGI) has become the best alternative to obtain satisfactory estimates of vital rates at the state and national level, but not at the level of smaller administrative units like districts, tehsils and blocks. By no means, however that this can replace or serve the purpose for which CRS is evolved.[15–17] CRS gives data not only at the national level, but also at the district and sub-divisional levels which are the basic units for the planning and implementation of health and family welfare services as well as several development programmes.

DEFICIENCY OF CRS

The vital events of births and deaths are grossly under registered. CRS does not provide complete information. We have to adjust CRS data by some indirect techniques for estimating the correct levels of fertility and mortality. Mention may be made that neither of these can help in providing the accurate information about the vital events at the district or lower levels of administration. In order to make it compulsory to register all births and deaths, an Act was made (Birth and Death Registration Act, 1969).

Birth and Death Registration Act, 1969

The registration of births and deaths has been made compulsory at the place of their occurrence with local registrar under whose jurisdiction it had occurred, throughout the country.

Responsibility of Reporting of Events

For domiciliary events the responsibility for reporting is assigned to head of the household or nearest relative or oldest adult male person. In case of institutional deliveries/deaths, the Medical Officer-in-charge of the institution and in respect of events in a jail, the jailors are responsible.

Responsibility of Registration

Local registrars have the responsibility to register these events. In rural areas, the registrars are Panchayat secretary, in-charge/revenue official/block development officer/primary health centre in-charge/health inspector/teacher of Government school. It varies from state to state. Village Panchayat holds the responsibility of registration of events and in its absence other agencies have been made responsible to register the events as indicated.

In urban areas, municipal committee/corporation holds the responsibility to register the events.

Structure

Local registrars—rural and urban areas as above. These agencies report the events to district registrar who happens to be District Health/Medical Officer or District Statistical

Officer or Deputy Commissioner/Collector or District Panchayat Officer. The district registrars report the events to chief registrar at the state headquarter. In most states, chief registrars are director health services besides economics and statistic chief at the state.

Birth and Death Certificates

Procedures for Registration

Events of birth and death should be registered within prescribed period of 21 days of occurrence, with the local registrar. After 21 days but with late fee, after 30 days and within one year with written permission of prescribed officer (usually district registrar) by producing an affidavit, after one year of occurrence by an order of executive magistrate with prescribed late fee.

Soon after the registration of birth or death, the registrar has to issue an extract (birth certificate) to the informant free of charge. Extra copies of the certificate can be obtained on payment of certain fee as prescribed in the state rules. Birth certificate now can be issued at PHC level.

Registration of Name of Child

Birth of a child can be registered even without the name of the child, if birth of a child was registered without name it can be entered into the register within 12 months of registration without any fee. After 12 months but within 15 years of registration with fee of ₹ 5.00. The registrar will issue a fresh certificate with name of the child.

Registration of birth and death of Indian citizens occurring outside India: The Indian Consulates register the births and deaths of Indian citizens occurring outside India as per provisions made in the Citizens (Registration of India Consulate) Rules 1956 under the Citizenship Act, 1955 and issue the birth and death certificate.

Maintenance of Records

Birth and death registers are permanent records and have to be retained forever. These registers along with the forms relating to the entries therein are retained by the registrar in his office for 12 months, after the end of calendar year to which they relate. Thereafter such registers and forms are transferred for safe custody to the designated officer. In rural areas, the registers are transferred to the district registrar and in urban areas; they are kept in municipalities/ corporation office.

Important

The events are to be registered at the *place of occurrence* and not at the *place of actual residence* of mother in case of birth and of person who died in case of death. Reliable data on actual level of birth and death (rates) are available from sample registration system (SRS), which collect this information for the usual *resident population*.

Live Birth Report

It gives information on date of birth, sex, name of child, place of birth, permanent residential address, father's and mother's name their literacy occupation and religion, age of mother in completed years at confinement, order of birth, number of live births including the birth registered, type of attention at delivery and the informant.

Death Report

It gives information on date and place of death, name of deceased, name of father/husband, age, sex, marital status, occupation, religion, nationality, permanent residential address, cause of death, whether medically certified (yes or no), kind of medical attention received if any and the informant.

Uses

Registration of births and deaths is a statutory activity. It has got both civil and statistical uses. It is useful for school admission, employment, foreign travel, mutation of property, death benefits, etc.

- It provides vital statistics (birth rates and death rates on continuous basis) at local level.
- Helps in formulating policies and programmes on health, fertility, family welfare, maternal and child health, safe motherhood, universal immunization. These records can be used effectively in the actual implementation of health care and family planning programmes at field level to accord priorities to eligible couples of high parity or non-acceptors, priority for spacing methods of contraception and for universal immunization.
- Causes of death help to formulate preventive programmes and interventions to reduce incidence of avoidable deaths of infants, young children maternal and other deaths.
- Besides these birth and death rates help to assess or measure the impact of health services or programme on reduction of fertility and mortality. It also helps to assess the health care needs of population especially of mothers and children, for delivery, postnatal care, etc.

Deficiencies in Registration Data

The common deficiencies are:

- Incomplete coverage of population and area.
- Under-registration of events.
- Quality of records in respect of causes of death is poor, besides incomplete information and not adhering to time schedule.

  Target is to register 100% of births and deaths.

Reasons

As 69% of population lives in rural areas, there is lack of appreciation and awareness. Access to registrar may not be easy. The cause of death is difficult to ascertain as deaths are not attended by qualified/trained person in rural set-up.

Measure to Improve the System

It is being improved by:

- Strengthening of organizational set-up at the state and district level and in the municipalities by setting-up of mechanical tabulation units (computer records).
- Effective coordination at various levels—health, ICDS, village Panchayats and Municipalities.
- Training of personnel, and compulsory production of birth certificates at the time of admission in school. A cautious approach is required as not to upset the programme of free and compulsory primary level education (universal elementary education). To begin with it can be introduced in urban areas.
- Introduction of medical certification on cause of death as per ICD-10: It is mainly possible in teaching and district hospitals and not in rural areas where we depend upon lay reporting system. Intensive training programme has been launched by RGI in the country on this aspect.

SAMPLE REGISTRATION SYSTEM (SRS)

Objective: The SRS is a large-scale demographic sample survey based on dual record system with the main objective of providing reliable official estimates of vital rates, at natural division level for rural and at state level for urban areas.

Coverage: It covers the entire country. The survey provides official estimates of birth rates, death rates, infant mortality rate and other fertility and mortality indicators and data on causes of death annually on continuous basis at the national and sub-national level.

Need: In the absence of dependable data from civil registration, the office of Registrar General India, initiated a scheme of sample registration of births and deaths in 1964–65.

The Main Components of SRS

1 **Baseline Survey:** The purpose is to obtain resident population of the sample unit. The base line survey is carried out prior to the start of continuous enumeration. This involves preparation of notional map of the area, house numbering, house listing and filling up of household schedule wherein the residential status of each individual and demographic particulars of each individual residing in the household, viz. name, sex, age, educational, marital status and relationship to head of household, etc. are collected. A list of pregnant women is also prepared at the time of base line survey.

2 **Continuous (Longitudinal) Enumeration of Vital Events:** The resident part-time enumerators—generally Anganwadi workers and teachers record all births and deaths occurring within the sample unit, in respect of all **residents** in the area as well as to those of *usual residents* occurring *outside* the sampling unit. The events in respect of visitors occurring within the sample unit are also listed but not taken into account while calculating rates. For ensuring complete netting, the enumerator uses different informants or sources—such as village priest, barber, village headman and midwife, to get information on the occurrence of vital events. Enumerator also maintains a list of pregnant women. Enumerator further ensures visiting all the households once in each quarter in rural area and once a month in urban area to complete the registration of events of births and deaths.

3 **Half-Yearly Survey (HYS):** HYS is carried out independently in each sampling unit by a full-time **supervisor.** He visits each household in the sample unit and records the particulars of births and deaths in respect of all the usual residents in half-yearly period (January to June or July to December) under reference. Simultaneously he updates the household list, household schedule and pregnancy status of women. While carrying out this survey the supervisor does not have access to the birth and death records of enumerator.

4 **Matching:** The events collected by half-yearly survey are matched with those of events collected by enumerator. The events thus are classified as fully matched, partially matched and unmatched.

5 **Field Verification of Matched and Partially Matched Events:** Every unmatched and partially matched event is verified by a visit to the concerned household either by a third person of jointly by the supervisor and the enumerator. Thereafter an unduplicated count of births and deaths is obtained.

6 **Sample Design:** The sample unit in a rural area is a village or a segment of it, if the village population is 2000 or more. In rural area of bigger states (population of 10 million or more) NSS natural division is the first geographical stratification or in rural area of smaller states the stratification is done on size of village having population less than 2000 forming stratum I and village with population 2000 or more forming stratum II. In urban areas, the sampling unit is census enumeration block (CEB) with population ranging from 750 to 1000. In urban areas, the categories of towns/cities have been divided into four strata based on the size classes, in constrast to the six strata in the earlier sampling frame. Towns with population less than one lakh contribute stratum I, towns/cities with population between 1 and 5 lakh fall under stratum II, towns and cities with population 5 lakh or more form stratum III and four metrocities of Delhi, Mumbai, Chennai and Kolkata as separate strata, viz. stratum IV.

At present SRS is operational in 7597 sample units (4433 rural and 3164 urban) spread across all states and union territories and covers about 1.5 million households and 7.52 million population.

The information collected in respect of births include place and date of birth, whether live or still, whether singly or multiple, sex, mother's residential status, i.e. whether usually resident or visitor, age and religion, type of medical attention at delivery, etc. Information collected in respect of deaths include date and place of death, residential status, age, sex, marital status, religion and medical attention before deaths as also cause of death.

The estimates on birth rate, death rates, infant mortality rate for urban and rural areas are published half-yearly in sample registration bulletins by RGI.

THE MODEL REGISTRATION SURVEY OF CAUSES OF DEATH

The Model Registration Scheme (MRS) was meant for ascertaining causes of death in the rural area of the country. The fieldwork is done by the paramedical personnel (called field agent), stationed at PHCs. The field agent is usually a sanitary inspector or health inspector. In each state, the number of primary health centres selected for this scheme was based on a norm of at least one centre per million population. All the districts in a state are represented. From 1999 'Survey of causes of death' has been merged with SRS and from 2001 onward it has become part of SRS Million Death Study (MDS) thus encompassing both rural and urban areas.

Objective: The objective of survey was to build up statistics on most probable causes of death for urban and rural India and its constituent states and union territories, using, "lay diagnosis reporting (post-death verbal-autopsy)" method through post-death enquiry based on symptoms, conditions, duration and anatomical site of disease as observed by family members of the deceased at the time of death.

Coverage: A well-designed verbal autopsy instrument has been developed and introduced in SRS.

Methodology: The survey is limited to the sample village population (2000–5000 persons) of the selected PHC. The Medical Officer in-charge of the PHC, recorder (statistical computer) field agent (paramedical staff—lady health visitor, ANM, sanitary inspector, etc.) and statistical officer are the main workers of the survey.

Local Informants

The field agent in the course of his duty contacts some locally resident informants regularly at short intervals. He obtains the addresses of the households where deaths occurred during the period that has elapsed since his last visit. He visits the concerned households and makes enquiries regarding the cause of death in accordance with a non-medical list (NML) prescribed for the purpose by WHO.

The list comprises a set of 10 major cause groups (including conspicuous symptoms) subdivided into numerous probable specific diseases.

The questions in the manual have been structured. The questions are designed in three stages of importance and sequence. In each cause group, stage I questions will isolate the cause of death relating to a specific major group of causes of mortality. There are ten such questions each relating to a major cause group. Questions in stage II bring the investigator closer to probable cause of death by aggregating similar symptoms of several specific causes under the major cause group. Questions in stage III are specific to a particular disease. These questions are framed such that they highlight to symptoms and conditions, duration or anatomical site of the disease, which would have been clearly observed (known from the deceased) at the time of a death by members of the family.

Structure of Questionnaire

The structural questionnaire has been divided into 10 major groups:

1. Accidents and injuries
2. Childbirth, pregnancy complications
3. Fevers
4. Digestive disorders
5. Cough (disorders of respiratory system)
6. Disorders of central nervous system
7. Diseases of circulatory system
8. Other clear symptoms
9. Causes peculiar to infancy
10. Senility

The non-medical list maintains comparability with major cause groups of WHO international classification of diseases (ICD).

To achieve the greater reliability, both qualitative and quantitative, the collected data are reviewed through a process of inspection and detection by an independent agency. All the events observed by field agent are reported back to PHC recorder for check-up. After the first check at recorder level, the Medical Officer in-charge of primary health centre further scrutinizes the cause of death of one out of every ten deaths in a month by personally visiting the household. This promotes the accuracy of data and motivates the field agent.

Limitation: There is very little direct supervision or check which can be instituted to verify the information collected and recorded by the field agent. The half-yearly survey and Medical Officer's check reports are only indirect means for achieving reliability of data.

The scheme should not be construed as substitute for proper medical certification of cause of death. In fact, wherever medical practitioner has attended to the deceased at the time of death, the cause of death has to be certified by the doctor and accepted by the field agent without any further interrogation. The scheme is meant only for rural area where deceased does not usually receive treatment from registered medical practitioners before death. The approach in the scheme is clearly that of "Lay reporting".

REFERENCES

1 GOI (1986). Manual on Integrated Management Information System for ICDS. Department of Women's Welfare, Ministry of Human Resource Development, Shastri Bhawan, New Delhi.

2 Management Training modules for Health Assistants (male and Female). "Module on Records and Reports". National Institute of Health and Family Welfare, New Delhi, 1987.

3 First report of the Expert Group on Health Information and Monitoring System. Directorate General of Health Services, October 1978.

4 Report of the National Seminar on Health Information System, Directorate General of Health Services, New Delhi, 5–7 Feb., 1979.

5 Health Management Information System (Version 2.0), Subcentre registers and reporting formats (Model). Government of India, Ministry of Health and Family Welfare, Nirman Bhawan, New Delhi, April 1992.

6 Manual on Community Needs Assessment Approach (Formerly Target Free Approach) in Family Welfare Programme, Department of Family Welfare, Ministry of Health and Family Welfare, Government of India, New Delhi, Jan. 1998.

7 Community Needs Assessment Approach (CNAA). Revised version of Forms and Formats. Proposed by the committee on CNAA to review formats and registers under CNAA constituted by the Ministry of Health and Family Welfare, Deptt. of Family Welfare, Government of India, Draft July, 2000.

8 GOI. NRHM. Health Management Information System Formats Version 1.0, MOH and FW, Government of India October 2008.

9 Evaluation of Quality of Maternal and Child Health Services at Primary Health Centre and suggested strategies for their Improvement. Feb. 1989. Indian Council of Medical Research; Ansari Nagar, New Delhi.

10 Improving the quality and coverage of Maternal and Child Health and Family Planning Services at Primary Health Centre level. An ICMR task force study. Indian Council of Medical Research, New Delhi; 1993.

11 Aga Khan Foundation (1993). PHC MAP Modules Assessing Information Need Module I Users Guide. AKF University Research corporation Center for Human services.

12 Design and Implementation of health information systems. World Health Organization, Geneva; 2000. Edited by Theo Lippeveld, Rainer Sauerborn, Claude Bodart.

13 Teaching Health Statistics. Lesson and Seminar Outline. Second Edition, Edited by Lwanga S.K., Cho-Yook Tye, O. Ayeni. World Health Organization, Geneva; 1999.

14 GOI (2000). Report of the working group on Registration of births, deaths and marriages. Primary and Secondary Education in relation to population stabilization. National Commission on Population. Government of India, Nov. 2000.

15 RGI Survey of causes of Death (Rural). Manual of Instructions (Part II Non-Medical List) vital statistics division, office of the Registrar General of India, Ministry of Home Affairs, New Delhi.

16 WHO (2002). World Mortality in 2000: Life Tables for 191 Countries. World Health Organization, Geneva.

17 RGI (2014). SRS Bulletin Sample Registration System. Volume, 49 No. 1, September 2014. Registrar General India.

EPIDEMIOLOGICAL BASIS OF NATIONAL HEALTH PROGRAMMES (NHP) IN INDIA AND LEARNING OF EPIDEMIOLOGY

Various national health programmes for specific communicable and non-communicable diseases and other problems have been launched in successive Five-Year Plan. The epidemiological basis/evidences for these programmes were as under:

i Wide spread geographical distribution of diseases.
ii High prevalence/incidence (high disease burden).
iii High mortality (premature deaths) and disabilities.
iv Occurence of epidemics and outbreaks.
v Rapid population growth and ageing.
vi Widespread undernutrition and emerging over-nutrition—obesity.
vii Changing lifestyles: Tobacco use, physical inactivity.
viii Deteriorating environments—leading to slums, vector breeding—poor waste management (garbage, human and animal excreta) indoor and outdoor air pollution.

Over the years these national programmes remained vertical and operated as single entity/stand alone programmes because of compelling needs. Now most of these programmes have been integrated under the umbrella of National Health Mission and are part of Public Health Care delivery system as also involving private sector and Non-Governmental Organizations and other sectors.

Common Objectives of NHP

- To reduce the incidence and prevalence of disease
- To prevent premature deaths and reduce mortality to acceptable low levels
- To prevent disabilities
- To eradicate/eliminate the disease is the ultimate objective
- To improve the nutritional status of vulnerables
- To promote healthy behaviours and lifestyles by BCC
- To improve the quality of life
- To stabalize population
- To improve environmental sanitation (promote hygiene, sanitary latrines, safe water and safe disposal of excreta)
- To strengthen the public health systems
- To establish surveillance system
- To promote research

- To achieve inter-sectoral coordination/convergence
- To involve private sector and NGOs
- To enhance community participation

Core Strategies/Interventions Adopted for NHP to Achieve the Objectives

1. **Education:** Behaviour Change Communication and Development of Healthy Lifestyles. Prevention of emergence of risk factors in population; and personal hygiene, periodic health check up and pre-placement examination.
2. **Improve nutrition:** Promote exclusive breast-feeding, complementary feeding, adequate feeding and supplementation of IFA and Vit A. Universal salt iodation and control infections, ensure food security—healthy eating and mass deworming.
3. Universal immunization
4. Early diagnosis and complete treatment as per standard treatment protocols.
5. Effective surveillance and screening programmes (Integrated Disease Surveillance Programme).
6. Integrated Management of Newborn and Childhood Illnesses (IMNCI).
7. **Treating and improving environments:** Safe water, safe excreta—disposal, source reduction for breeding (waste water and solid waste management). Integrated vector control and reduction of air pollution.
8. Maternal and Child Health Services (RMNCH) + A safe motherhood and child survival.
9. Population stabilization—contraceptive promotion
10. Curb use of illicit drugs—drug deaddication supply reduction and demand reduction strategies.
11. Health legislations and policies—to control tobacco, alcohol, drugs, food safety, regulate salt content of manufactured foods, enhance production and consumption of fruits and vegetables, promote physical activities.
12. Strengthening public health care delivery system (manpower, infrastructure and essential medicines/drugs). Engage private sector and NGOs.
13. Liquidation of reservoir of infection/disease (in zoonotic diseases), such as rats, pigs and birds or reduction of population of stray dogs by animal birth control.
14. Epidemic/disaster preparedness and managment.
15. **Prevention of injuries and accidents (intentional and unintentional):** Develop counselling services in school/college for life skill training, stress management and suicide prevention.
16. Observe universal precautions
17. Observe international health regulations.
18. Reduce illiteracy, ignorance and poverty
19. Research—health system, action and operational research.

These interventions focus on community and are population-based strategies, which treat underlying causes/determinants/risk reduction of disease or problem.

Message: Major aspects of epidemiology such as extent of health/disease problem, disease burden, incidence and prevalence, time trends, its geographical distribution, population affected most, case fatality, surveillance and case detection methods and evidence based interventions/strategies, programme management (planning, organization, implementation, monitoring and evaluation of programme) can be learned in a systematic manner by learning National Health Programmes. In a way all the national health programmes reinforce and enrich the learning of subject of applied epidemiology and their management aspects.

Knowledge of applied epidemiology helps to plan, organize, implement, monitoring and evaluation of all national health programmes besides applying evidence-based strategies/interventions (experimental epidemiology).

Various methods of epidemiology—descriptive, analytical and experimental epidemiology can be best learned through the National Health Programmes.

List of 20 communicable diseases reported every month by all health/medical institutions to CBHI: Acute diarrhoeal diseases including gastroenteritis, diphtheria, acute poliomyelitis—new cases, tetanus other than neonatal, neonatal tetanus, whooping cough, measles, pneumonia, enteric fever, hepatitis A, viral hepatitis B, viral hepatitis CDE, meningococcal meningitis, rabies, AIDS, syphilis, gonococcal infection, other STDs, and pulmonary tuberculosis.

List of National Health Programmes

A. National Health Programmes for Diseases

- NVBDCP: Malaria, dengue, chikungunya, Japanese encephalitis, filaria, kala-azar and KFD.
- Revised National Tubeculosis Control Programme (RNTCP).
- Leprosy: National Leprosy Eradication Programme.
- National Aids Control Programme and National Programme on prevention of Parent to Child Transmission.
- RTI/STI—National Guidelines.
- Polio eradication.
- Yaws eradication.
- National Programme for Prevention and Control of Deafness.
- National Programme for Prevention and Control of Rabies.
- National Programme for Prevention and Control of Antimicrobial Resistance.
- Programme for Prevention and Control of Leptospirosis.
- National Hepatitis Surveillance Programme.
- National Deworming Drives.

B. Water and Sanitation

- National Rural Drinking Water Supply and Sanitation Programme.
- National Programme for Prevention and Control of Fluorosis.
- National Guinea Worm Eradication Programme.
- National Diarrhoeal Disease Control Programme.

C. MCH and Family Planning

- National Family Planning Programme.
- Reproductive, Maternal, Newborn, Child and Adolescent Health (RMNCH + A).
- Integrated Management of Neonatal and Childhood Illness and Integrated Action Plan for Pneumonia and Diarrhoea in 4 states.
- India's Newborn Action Plan.
- *Navjat Shishu Suraksha Karyakram.*
- *Janani Shishu Suraksha Karyakram.*
- Universal Immunization Programme.
- Integrated Child Development Services Scheme (ICDS)—Mission.
- National Adolescent Health Programme (RKSK) and *Rashtriya Bal Swasthya Karyakram* (RBSK).

D. Nutrition

- School Health Programme.
- National IDD Control Programme.
- National Iron + Initiative.
- National Nutritional Anaemia Control Programme.
- National Programme for Control of Blindness (Vit A).
- Mid-day-meal Programme in Schools.
- Applied Nutrition Programme and Supplementary Nutrition Programmes.

E. Non-communicable Diseases (NCDs)

- National Programme for Prevention and Control of Cancer, Diabetes, Cardiovascular Diseases and Strokes.
- National Tobacco Control Programme.
- National Oral Health Programme.
- National Programme for Care of Elderly
- National Mental Health Programme.
- National Trauma Control Programme.
- National Programme for Prevention and Management of Burn Injuries.
- National Programme for Prevention and Control of Blindness.
- Drug Deaddiction Programme.
- National Organ Transplant Programme.

F. Others

- Integrated Disease Surveillance Programme.
- National Policy on ARI Control.
- National Health Mission—Universal Health Coverage.
- National Health Insurance Scheme (*Rashtriya Swasthya Bima Yojna*).
- National Disaster Management Authority and Disaster Management Act, 2005.
- National Guidelines on Hospital Waste Management.

NATIONAL HEALTH PROGRAMMES—CRITIQUE

The almost exclusive focus of policy implementation often masks the fact that all the disease conditions for which national programmes provide universal coverage account for less than 10% of all mortalities and only for about 15% of all morbidities. Over 75% of communicable diseases are not part of existing national programmes.

Overall communicable diseases contribute 24.4% of the entire disease burden, while maternal and neonatal ailments contribute 13.8%, non-communicable diseases 39.1% and injuries 11.8% now constitute the bulk of the country's disease burden.

Everyone of these national programmes require on one hand a robust public health system as their core delivery strategy, and on the other hand they can be considered as opportunities to strengthen health care systems and designed keeping this goal in mind. All services available under national programmes are free for all and universally accessed with fairly good rates of coverage.

CHAPTER

9

Applied Biostatistics

BIOSTATISTICS

Meaning of Statistics

Statistics means data or numerical observations.

What are data? Data mean set of related numbers or raw material for statistics. Data are the starting point in Epidemiology/Biostatistic studies/investigation. We collect data, analyze data into information and interpret the information for decision-making.

Biostatistics: The statistics related to living or human beings.

Vital statistics: Means data on vital events like births, deaths and marriages, etc.

Health statistics: Data related to health service system/ organizations and institutions. It includes all the data required for planning, implementation and evaluation of health services or health system.

The term data and information are often used synonymously. A distinction must be made between them. Data mean collection of facts. Information is the outcome of data analysis and interpretation. Information is used in programme management and in decision-making process. Thus data are abstract which when processed, provides information that is meaningful to the person receiving it. All reports which come with loaded data must be analyzed and processed to generate information for action, e.g. a subcentre reports 150 children were provided services it does not mean much unless it is processed into how many children were infants, preschool and school children and what was coverage level of infants for various services, what was the time period and were services adequate or inadequate? If data of 150 children is analyzed in that manner, it becomes useful information for action.

Types of Data

There are two types of data according to the strength of the scale of measurement:

1. Qualitative
2. Quantitative

1. Qualitative Data

a. These data have no magnitude or size.
b. These are not measurable on scale.
c. These are classified only by counting the units that have same attribute.

Example: Sex, colour and race.

Qualitative data/variables are measured either on nominal or an ordinal scale. Types of qualitative data:

(a) Qualitative Binary Data

The variable can only take two values, such as male or female, yes or no, cured or died, vaccinated or not vaccinated, exposed or not exposed, healthy or sick. These data can be presented by pie diagram or by simple table by frequency distribution.

(b) Qualitative Nominal Data

- The variable can take more than two values or any value.
- The information fits into one of the categories.
- The categories cannot be ranked.

Example: Nationality or State to which one belongs to, spoken language, blood groups.

Disease classification: Psychosis, neurosis, manic, and depressives, etc.

These data can be presented by frequency distribution in tabular form or by using a horizontal bar chart.

(c) Qualitative Ordinal Data

The variable can take a number of values that can be ranked through some gradient.

Example:

Birth order: First, second, third …
Severity of illness: Mild, moderate, severe …
Goitre grades: No goiter, grade I and grade II.

Nutritional status can be graded as normal, moderately underweight or severely underweight. Social status of a person/patient can be graded as upper, middle and lower class.

These data can be presented by frequency distribution table or by vertical bar diagrams.

2. Quantitative Data

These data have size or magnitudes. We can measure these data either on an interval or on a ratio scale.

Types of Quantitative Data

- Discrete
- Continuous

Quantitative Discrete Data

- Values are distinct and separated
- Normally, values have no decimal and are in whole numbers.

Examples: Number of sexual partners, parity, number of persons died of measles, number of households in community, number of beds in hospital and white cell count.

These data can be presented by frequency distribution table or by histogram. Date of onset of disease in epidemic can be displayed by histogram or epidemic curve and long-term trend by line diagram.

Quantitative Continuous Data

- These data can assume continuous, uninterrupted infinite number of possible values in any interval.
- Values may have decimals.

Examples: Weight, height, Hb level, temperature.

Quantitative Continuous Data can be measured by an interval scale, which is characterized by numerical unit of measurement, such that the difference between any two measurements is explicitly known in terms of an interval between the two measured points.

Examples: Body temperature is measured on an interval scale and unit of measurement is degrees Celsius (°C). Interval scale can have negative values as temperature can be –20°C.

The *ratio scale* has all the characteristics of the interval scale as well as true or absolute zero so that ratio between two values on the scale are meaningful or relative magnitude of the two measurements.

Examples: Height in meters and weight in kg.

No values exist below zero in this scale. The continuous quantitative variable/data can be presented by frequency distribution table or by diagram, such as histogram.

Data measuring procedure consist of instruments like weighting scales, thermometers, BP apparatus or clinical examination or combination of human and instruments.

Uses

The science of statistics along with epidemiology are used in health services system to assess the health needs of community, to plan services and to evaluate results of interventions or services and conduct research studies in the field of health as also for making decisions in health care delivery.

The hallmark of biostatistics is "variations" or uncertainties. Variation in characteristic occurs when its value changes from subject to subject, from time to time, or instrument to instrument, within same subject or from observer to observer. For example, no two individuals are similar. The blood pressure, weight, height, pulse rate, respiratory rate, biochemical levels like haemoglobin, blood sugar, blood counts and other values vary from one person to other. Blood pressure varies from person to person from morning to evening, before and during excitement or exercise, sitting and supine position, recording by different people and in measurement instrument. These variations are hallmarks in population. To fix a range of normal value for a community or individual, we take the help of science of statistics to compare two groups and populations.

SOURCES OF UNCERTAINTY OR VARIATION IN HEALTH

Uncertainty is caused by variations in:

- ***Biological factors,*** e.g. age, sex, birth order, and heredity determine the health and disease status in community.
- ***Environmental factors:*** Water supply, sanitation, socioeconomic status, stress, nutrition, addiction, smoking, availability, accessibility and use of services. The environments are major determinant of health and disease variations.
- ***Methodological factors:*** Observer variations, instruments, laboratory techniques, diagnostic tool, questionnaires.
- Chance or unknown factors.
- Incomplete information, imperfect tool, poor compliance of drug regimen and inadequate medical knowledge can lead to variations.

Any characteristic that can be measured or categorized is called variable.

Dependable variables are—weight, haemoglobin level, blood pressure and disease.

Indenpendent variables are—interventions like immunization, supplementary feeding/nutrients, and treatment.

SCALES OF MEASUREMENT

The four principal scales used to measure data are: the nominal, ordinal, interval and ratio scale.

1 ***Nominal:*** It is the scale in which names, labels or tags are given to distinguish one measurement from another on the basis of certain qualities or attributes.

Examples: Outcomes of a disease can be measured as survived or died, and outcome of treatment can be measured as cured, not cured. Psychiatric patient may be classified as psychotic, neurotics, manic, depressive or schizophrenics.

2 ***Ordinal:*** It is also called ranking scale. It has the characteristics of the nominal scales with implicit order relationship among measurements.

Examples: Social status of patients may be measured as upper, middle or lower class.

Goitre may be measured as no goitre, grade I and grade II. Nutritional status can be measured as normal, moderately underweight and severely underweight. The qualitative and attributive data is usually measured on nominal or an ordinal scale.

3 ***An Interval Scale:*** It is characterized by a numerical unit of measurement, such that the difference between any two measurements is explicitly known in terms of intervals between the two points.

Example: Body temperature is usually measured on an interval scale and unit of measurement is degree Celsius (°C). Body weight and height are measured on interval scale.

4 ***Ratio Scale:*** It has all the characteristics of the interval scale, so that the ratio between two values in the scale is a meaningful measure of relative magnitude of the two measurements.

Example: BMI-weight in kg over height in square metres, waist hip ratio, risk ratio. Quantitative data have numerical magnitude. They are measured on an interval or on a ratio scale.

SOURCES OF HEALTH DATA

From where to get facts and figures? In statistics or bio-statistics we must have data for analysis to generate information. From where to get data which is the basic requirement of statistics or biostatistics.

Data collection is the starting point for all kinds of statistics. It is not an easy task. Many sources of data are available and each source has its merits and demerits. Depending upon the need of data for health system, various sources are used. The health data can come from following sources:[1–5]

i People themselves—report outbreaks, diseases, births and deaths.

ii Routine records and reports of a health facility—subcentre, PHC, CHC and hospitals.

iii Routine reports and records of births and deaths at village level.

iv Health information of India—Published by CBHI Sample Registration System (SRS) of Registrar General of India—once a year provides information on fertility, i.e. birth rates, death rates at state and national level.

v Data of specific National Health Programme. Published in Annual reports by DGHS.

vi Survey data, of National Sample Survey Organization (NSSO).

- National Family Health Survey data (NFHS).
- General and special health survey (Singur, Calcutta, Tuberculosis-1958 and national survey on annual risk of tuberculous infection 2002 and 2009.

vii District level household surveys data under reproductive and child health—every alternate year—as also facility survey data besides annual district health survey data.

viii Surveillance data, e.g.

- HIV annual sentinel surveillance data.
- National polio surveillance project reports.
- Malaria surveillance and IDSP.

ix Census data (population count) after every 10 years.

x Media reports.

xi World Health Reports: Weekly epidemiological reports, annual statistical reports, etc.

We can categorize sources into two broad categories:

1 Primary sources or primary data which are collected by the individual or investigator himself by interview or by scientific study or by observations over a period of time or at a point in time.

2 Secondary data are those data 'which are not collected by the investigator himself but collected by some other source or institution, as mentioned above. The investigator makes use of secondary data which has already been published or reported or recorded.

People First

People themselves are great source of information and most of the time people report the events first, the official machinery comes to the scene much late. People's resources must be used. Rumour register kept at PHC level records rumours of disease/outbreaks which can be subsequently verified by health workers. This system was used in smallpox eradication programme.

Data Quality

High quality data mean that the data are accurate, reliable, complete, sufficiently precise, timely reported with integrity.

Accuracy: Valid data are data that have been accurately captured, that is, the data measures what they are intended to measure. Accurate data have minimum errors.

Reliable: It means data are consistent. If the process of data collection is repeated the data do not change.

Completeness: It means all indicators of all reporting units are being collected and reported.

Percision: This means the data have sufficient details (e.g. age group, sex and geographic area and exact unit of measurement).

Timeliness: Data are timely when the information is available on time (within prescribed timeline).

Integrity: It means no manipulation of data and ensuring confidentiality. Data error can happen while collecting data, during entry, during cleaning and validation of data.

Lot of data are collected or generated by health workers on routine basis. The health workers have with them data of each and every home/household, they have the information on water supply and sanitation, pregant woman, eligible couples and births and deaths, etc.

- The health workers do not make much use of the health data collected by them for local village or subcentre action plan; which is the requirement of RCH programme. These data are collected by the health system or health workers and used primarily for preparing reports for onward transmission to higher levels to satisfy the requirement of the system.
- Information is seldom shared with village community or people whose lives it affect most.
- There is no feedback to the workers or system who collect voluminous data on health and diseases.

VISIBILITY OF DATA

Most data collected lie dormant and lie as unprocessed and uncompiled. The data become visible if compiled and presented. The data collected can be made visible by tables and by simple diagrams (Graphs and Charts). A diagram is worth thousands words.

TABULATION OF DATA

Table means arranging data in rows and columns. If you measure the birth weight of 2700 newborns in a rural block it is raw data. These raw data must be compiled and summary data should be presented so that it can become visible summary (data reduction). Data in table is more precise.

Table 9.1 gives summary value of large number of observations. In table, the data becomes visible in summary form. One can draw inferences quickly.

Table 9.1 is a simple table providing summary of birth weights of 2700 newborn babies. We can quickly draw inferences that one-third of the babies had low birth weight in rural area and two-thirds of babies were born with adequate weight. This also provides a lead point for action as how to reduce the proportion of low birth weights in the community and with what interventions? Similarly, the data also may raise a question as to what factors or conditions are responsible for low birth weight babies in the community? If the health workers are able to interpret the data they are collecting, they will have a better understanding of the needs of their community, e.g. the health workers summarized the list of eligible couples in their area by tabular form for Community Needs Assessment Approach (CNAA) under reproductive and child health.

Table 9.1: Birth weights of newborns in a rural block 1997

Weight in kg	*No. of newborns*	*%age*
< 2.5 kg	900	33
> 2.5 kg	1800	67
Total	**2700**	**100**

The data on outdoor attendance of a primary health centre for the year 2004 was compiled and presented as simple counts in tabular form (Table 9.2).

This summary table presents the data on annual morbidity in OPD and one can interpret that the leading morbidity in this rural area was respiratory infections, followed by osteoarthritis, myalgia, fevers, accidents and injuries. According to morbidity, one has to arrange or plan for indent of medicines. One can also draw inference that acute communicable diseases were the major cause of morbidity in the area. One can draw year wise comparison to know the trends of morbidity in the area.

Contingency Table

Tables 9.1 and 9.2 are simple tables. Table 9.3 is contingency table. It is 2 × 2 table and it follows two way classification. Each cell has two attributes.

Example: Vaccinated and nonvaccinated children against measles and attack rate of measles disease in these two groups.

Each cell has two attributes—disease occurrence and vaccination status. This is also called cross-tabulation. For chi-square test of significance, we usually prepare 2 × 2 contingency table for qualitative characters; which is first step in χ^2 test.

Table 9.2: OPD morbidity at PHC—Chiri 2004

Disease	*Number*
Fevers	2495
Respiratory infections	4921
Diseases of bones and joints osteoarthritis, myalgia	3550
Accidents and injuries	1987
Conjunctivitis	857
Diseases of skin	239
Worm infestation	272
Diarrhoea	143
Cervical discharge and vaginal discharge	182
Tuberculosis	51
Others	2890
Total	**17587**

Table 9.3: Occurrence of measles in vaccinated and nonvaccinated children in a primary health centre area			
	Measles disease		
Vaccinated	Yes	No	Total
Yes	40	320	360
No	486	54	540
Total	**526**	**374**	**900**

Frequency Table

Frequency table is used to present quantitative data. Class intervals are presented in the first column and against that class interval the frequency is depicted in second column (*see* Table 9.4).

Life Table

This is a special kind of table to calculate life expectancy at birth and subsequent ages (Table 9.10) respectively.

Diagrams/Graphs: Displays Numeric Data in Visual Form

The frequency table or other tables can be presented by means of suitable diagrams such as histogram, bar charts, pie charts and line diagrams and scatter diagram.

Age and sex composition of an area can be presented by **population pyramid** (*see* under demography and population problem).

Histogram is diagrammatic presentation of the frequency distribution of quantitative variable with areas of rectangles proportionate to the class frequency. In histogram size of interval chosen can vary. Histogram is an area diagram (Fig. 9.1).

Interpretation of Bar Charts (Fig. 9.2)

The prevalence of malnutrition in India during 1998–99 was quite high as 47% of children below 3 years were

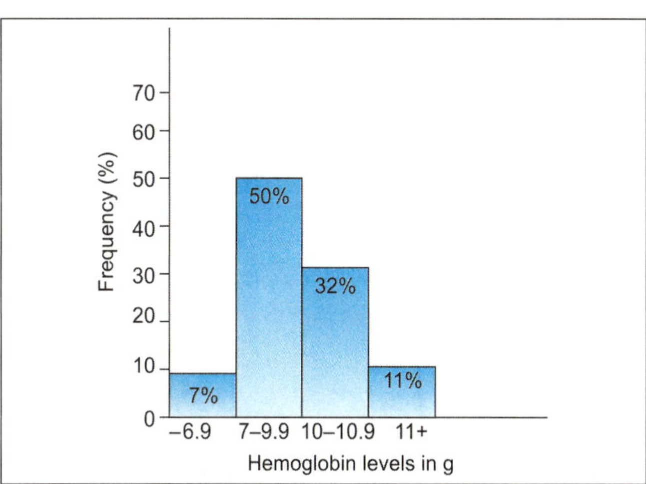

Fig. 9.1: Histogram showing levels of haemoglobin in adolescents in India

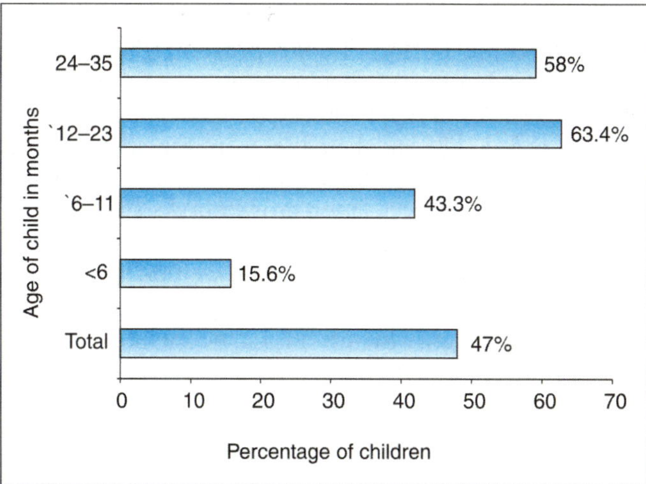

Fig. 9.2: Percentage of children under age three years who were underweight (NFHS-2) 1998–99

underweight. The malnutrition starts at 6 months of age and tends to increase as the child grows to age one and prevalence is maximum between 12 and 23 months of age, as 63.4% of children between 12 and 23 months were underweight.

PIE diagram provides visual impression of an event and is quite eye catching. Observer can immediately grasp the event or use of service by such diagrammatic presentation (Fig. 9.3).

Inference: 48% of eligible couples were using contraceptives. Female sterilization was the most popular and acceptable method. Men participation in contraceptive use tend to be low at 2% for sterilization and 3% for condom use. Overall the spacing methods are used by less number of women, only 2% used IUD and other 2% used pills. Spacing methods and men participation needs to be scaled up by IEC activities and increasing access to contraception (Fig. 9.3).

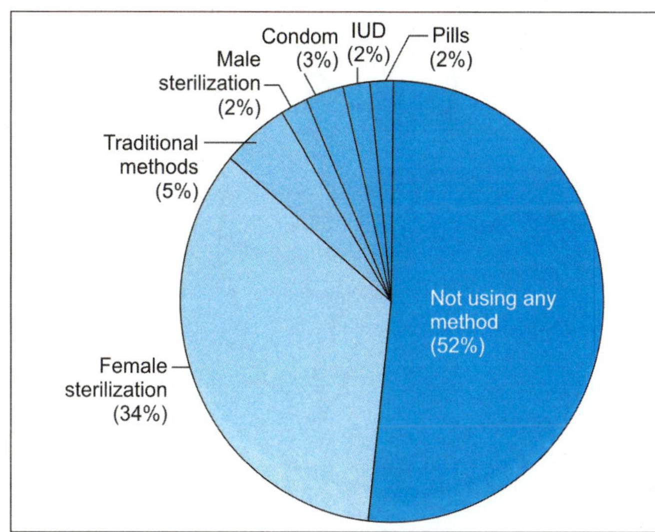

Fig. 9.3: Current use of contraceptives in India (NFHS-2)

Line diagrams are drawn to depict trends of an event over long time period. In the present line diagram (Fig. 4.5), it is evident that population growth rate in different decades in India witnessed marked increase from 1941–51 to 1971–81 and thereafter there was some respite, as for the first time in demography history the country observed decline in population growth in decade 1981–91 and the decline continued in next two decades as well (1991–2011). It means India's family welfare programme is making a slow but sure impact on population growth. Lowest decadal growth rate of 17.64 was observed in 2001–11.

Maps (Fig. 9.4)

Maps are used to depict the geographical distribution of disease or prevalence of disease in different geographical areas. Incidence maps help to compare events.

If there is clustering of cases of a disease it provides a useful clue for epidemiological investigation of an outbreak. Spread of outbreak can be shown on spot map of locality by marking dots for an event or disease.

Concentration or clustering of cases in an area draws an attention of affected locality and the epidemiological factors and conditions responsible for such a behaviour. Spot maps of an outbreak of hepatitis E is shown elsewhere (investigation of an outbreak of jaundice, *see* Fig. 8.10). Incidence maps make use of population.

Other Charts

Growth chart is a visual impression of growth of a young child. Direction of growth can be monitored and intervention can be undertaken at appropriate time. Growth charts are being used in ICDS to monitor the growth and prevent the occurrence of malnutrition in young children.

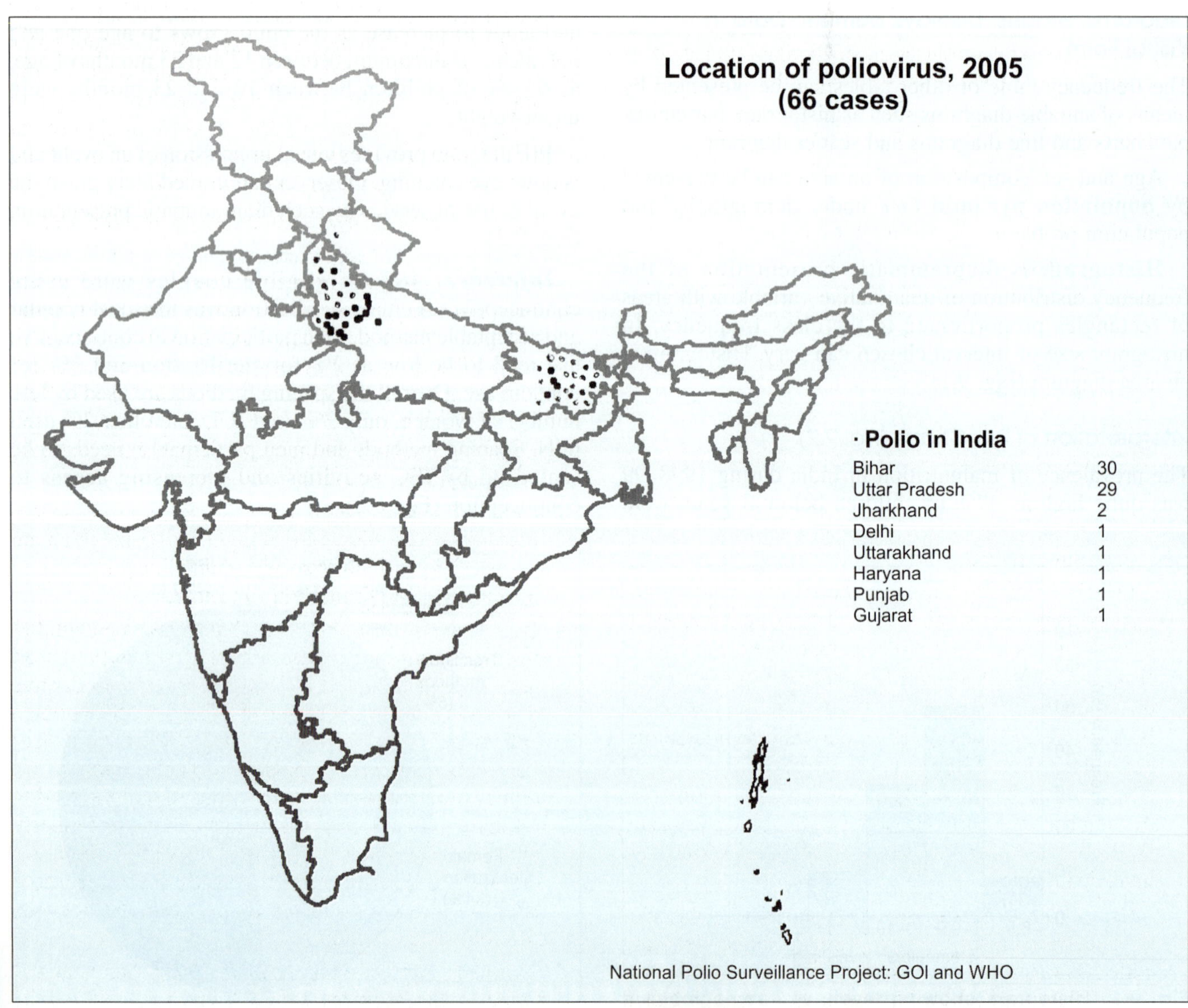

Fig. 9.4: Map of India showing distribution of confirmed cases of polio during the year 2005

Thus, growth charts are valuable tools to prevent malnutrition (*see* Figs 6.1a and b).

REFERENCES

1 CBHI. Health Information of India 2003. New Delhi: CBHI, GOI; 2004.

2 Registrar General India SRS. Sample Registration System Bulletin April 2004; 38(1).

3 International Institute of Population Sciences (IIPS)/ORC Macro. National Family Health Survey-2, 1998–99. Mumbai: IIPS; 2002.

4 GOI. Annual Report 2003–04. New Delhi; MOH and FW; 2004.

5 GOI. Census India 2001and 2011. New Delhi: GOI.

MEASURES OF CENTRAL TENDENCY

The most important information of the data collected, is to obtain one single value that describes the characteristic of the entire data. Such value is called '*central value*' or '*average*'.

Definition

"Average is an attempt to find out one single figure to describe whole of figures".......**Clark**

"The average is sometimes described as a number which is typical of whole group"...**Leabo**

Objectives of Averaging

1 To get single value representing entire data.
2 To facilitate comparison between different data.

Qualities of Average

1 Easy to understand.
2 Should be simple to compute so that it can be used widely.
3 Representativeness of all items and if one item is dropped or added in the data then the average must alter.
4 It should not be unduly affected by extreme observations.
5 It should be capable of further algebraic computations, e.g. subtraction, multiplication, addition, etc.
6 ***Uniqueness:*** Average should be properly defined so that it must have only one single value for a given data. It should not depend on personal variations and investigator bias.
7 ***Sampling stability:*** It means the stability of the averages calculated from different sets of data which are collected randomly should not differ significantly. As the difference will be less the average would be called more stable and vice versa.

SUMMARIZATION OF DATA, OR MEASURES OF CENTRAL TENDENCY

The data which an investigator or health workers or an organization collect has to be summed up. For example, if 1000 children have been weighed in the community, each child would have certain weight and we have 1000 observations. To give value for each and every child makes little sense. If we want to give only one value for all the 1000 observations on birth weight that would be 'summary value' of 1000 children. How can we do that? We calculate the average value of 1000 observations that would be one summary value of all these observations. Thus, we can say that "average" birth weight is 2.7 kg in this community that makes a lot of sense. This value speaks of entire data.

The "average" is most typical value of the observations as most of the values of the observations would be centering around it.

But the average has to be interpreted cautiously, e.g. average birth weight of 2.7 kg of 1000 observations does not mean that every child at birth would weigh 2.7 kg. Average though a valuable summary value of data hides many things underneath it; as many children in the community would have birth weight less than 2.7 kg and it is well known fact that in India 30–33% of children at birth have low birth weight and weigh less than 2.5 kg and many may be less than 2 kg and so on.

The most common *averages* available in India are:

1 ***Mean or average age of marriage for girls in India:*** It is 21.2 years. It is summary value of all marriages of girls occurring in India. It should be interpreted carefully. Marriage is early and almost universal in India. 30% of girls in age group 15–19 were married, 25% get married before the age of 15 and nearly 50% got married before the age of 18 (NFHS-2); the minimum legal age at marriage for girls set by Child Marriage Restraint Act of 1976.
2 ***Mean birth weight*** in India is 2.7 to 2.9 kg. But one-third of births are low birth weights in India which are below 2.5 kg, which is a major public health problem and cause of infant mortality in India.
3 ***Total fertility rate*** (TFR), which is an average number of children a woman would bear if she experienced current age-specific fertility rate during her reproductive years, was 2.9 births per women (NFHS-2). SRS quoted TFR of 3.3 in the year 1997. The TFR of 2.1 or less than that was observed in Kerala, Delhi, Puducherry, Tamil Nadu and Chandigarh while high TFR of 4.8, 4.4 and 4.2 were observed in states of Uttar Pradesh, Bihar and Rajasthan respectively. The TFR which is a summary value of fertility should be interpreted carefully in the light of variations observed between different states of India.
4 ***Similarly average income of ₹ 3000/-*** per year per capita at current prices is a ***summary value of income in India*** (2002–2003). This is to be interpreted very

carefully. Income of family of 5 would be ₹ 15,000/- per year. Based on this the families below poverty line (BPL) are identified for special programmes and economic uplift. The poverty line has been defined by World Bank as an income of $1/day per person or less. Planning Commission defines poverty line as a total household per capita expenditure sufficient to provide in addition, to basic non-food items—clothing-transport—a daily intake of 2400 calories per person in rural areas and 2100 in urban area. Family of 5 whose income is below ₹ 11,000/- per year are called, below poverty line families (in rural area) at 1991–92 prices. Recent estimates of poverty in India is 38%. Average size of household in India is 5.4 persons but average size of family is around 5 in India. However, in rural settings the average size of 7.0 person per household is not uncommon.

The common *averages* for summary values of data are:

- Mean (Arithmetic mean, geometric mean, weighted mean, harmonic mean)
- Median
- Mode
- Other measures of location are quartiles, percentile, and proportions.

Arithmetic Mean

It is most popular and most widely used measure of summation of data. It provides one summary value of the observations.

Definition: Arithmetic mean is the sum of all values of a set of observations divided by the number of observations.

The arithmetic mean (AM) is denoted by $\overline{X}$.

The haemoglobin level of 11 pregnant women was measured and the values of haemoglobin were as under:

7,8,9,10,11,11,11,12,13,14,15......................(i)

The sum of all the 11 values was = 121

The arithmetic mean was 121/11 = 11

Following are the haemoglobin levels of the 30 students in a class (in g%):

11,12,8,9,9,9,9,8,10,9,10,10,11,10,11,11,11,13,13,14, 13,13,13,12,12,11,8,8,9,8.............................(ii)

The simple arithmetic mean = Sum of all values/total no. of values

Sum of all values = 315

Arithmetic mean = 315/30 = 10.5 g%

Quantitative data: If the data is in the form of class intervals and frequency table, then the arithmetic mean can be calculated as follows:

Arithmetic mean of the sample = $\Sigma fm/\Sigma f$

If we tabulate the above data in the form of class intervals (Table 9.4) and prepare a frequency table then mean = 318/30 = 10.600 g%

Table 9.4: Showing distribution of Hb levels of students in a class (n = 30)

Class interval	Mid point of the class int. value (m)	Frequency (f)	fm
8–10 g%	9	15	135
11–13 g%	12	14	168
14–16 g%	15	1	15
		$\Sigma f = 30$	$\Sigma fm = 318$

As simple arithmetic mean discussed above gives equal importance to all the items, but, if the relative importance of the different items is different then we calculate—weighted mean. Weight—signifies the relative importance of an item.

Weighted Mean

The mean haemoglobin of all school children is found in two steps.

First step: Multiply the mean haemoglobin for each class by the corresponding number of children in each class (weights), and add-up the total thus obtained.

Second step: Divide the total cumulative haemoglobin of the school children by the total number of children in that school.

Class	No. of children	Mean Hb levels (in g%)
I	54	10.4
II	52	11.2
III	49	10.8
IV	48	12.1
V	48	10.7

then, the mean Hb levels of all the children = weighted mean =

$$= \frac{(10.4\times 54) + (11.2\times 52) + (10.8\times 49) + (12.1\times 48) + (10.7\times 48)}{54 + 52 + 49 + 48 + 48} = \frac{561.6 + 582.4 + 529.2 + 580.8 + 513.6}{251}$$

$$= \frac{2767.6}{251} = 11.02 \text{ g\%}$$

Thus, the weighted mean = 11.02 g%.

The non-weighted mean ignores the fact that the number of children in each class is not the same (i.e. unequal weights). In the above example, non-weighted mean would be (10.4 + 11.2 + 10.8 + 12.1 + 10.7)/5 = 11.04 g%.

Geometric Mean

It is defined as the *N*th root of the product of *N* observations.

Geometric mean = $N\sqrt{X_1 \times X_2 \times \ldots\ldots Xn}$

It is theoretically considered as the best average.

It gives us an idea about the average rate of changes occurring between observations.

For example population of India of last 5 decades:

$$\text{Arithmetic mean} = \frac{439 + 548 + 683 + 843 + 1027}{5} = \frac{3540}{5}$$

= 708 million

Geometric mean = $5\ \sqrt{439 \times 548 \times 683 \times 843 \times 1027}$

= $5\ \sqrt{142238}$ = 677 million

In this example, the geometric mean gives the better average because it considers the change in decadal growth rate as well.

Harmonic Mean

It is defined as the reciprocal of the arithmetic mean or the reciprocal of individual observations.

$$\text{Harmonic mean} = \frac{N}{1/X_1 + 1/X_2 .... + 1/X_n}$$

and for continuous series

$$\text{Harmonic mean} = \frac{N}{1/f(X_1) + 1/f_2X_2..1/f_nX_n}$$

Median

The median is that value which divides the observations or distribution into two equal halves or it is the central or middle value of a series of observations when the observed values are arranged in order of magnitude (ascending or descending order).

Haemoglobin level (g%) of 11 pregnant women was arranged in ascending order:

7,8,9,10,11,11,11,12,13,14,15.

In the above series of 11 values, the middle most value is 11 g hence, the median value of haemoglobin of eleven pregnant women is 11. Median is not affected by extremes of values. If the number of observations are even then the two central values are added up then average of these two values is calculated to derive the median value, e.g. haemoglobin levels of 30 students of a class are as follows:

11,12,8,9,9,9,9,8,10,9,10,10,11,10,11,11,11,13,
13,14,13,13,13,12,12,11,8,8,9,8.

Median = Central value of orderly arranged data.
First arrange the data in ascending/descending order.

8,8,8,8,8,9,9,9,9,9,9,10,10,10,10,11,11,
11,11,11,11,12,12,12,13,13,13,13,13,14.

Total no. of values = 30.

Central value (30/2).

Median = Value of central observation.

= ½ (value of 15th and 16th observations)

= 1/2 (10 + 11) = 21 / 2 = 10.5 g%

Merits and Limitations of Median

Merits

1 Extreme values do not affect median significantly.
2 Useful in markedly skewed distributions.
3 Most appropriate average in qualitative data.
4 Can be calculated graphically.

Limitations

1 It is necessary to arrange the data.
2 It is a positional average and value is not determined by each and every observation.
3 Not capable of algebraic treatment.
4 Value of median is affected more by sampling fluctuations.
5 It is erratic if the number of item is small.

Mode

Mode is the value of observation which occurs maximum number of times in the data, i.e. the observation with highest frequency. In the above example of haemoglobin distribution of 30 students, the mode is 11 g%.

- If the two observations are occurring with same frequency then the observations around which the values are more condensed is the mode value.
- If several observations are occurring equal no. of times and there is no clear cut mode and for such type of data and other data with moderately asymmetric distribution the mode can be calculated by using formula.

Mode = 3 median – 2 mean.

Merits and Limitations of Mode

Merits

1 By definition—mode is the most typical or representative value of a distribution.
2 Not unduly affected by extreme values.
3 Can be determined graphically.
4 Can be determined in open end distribution.

Limitations

1 The value of mode is not unique always. In some cases may have bimodal series.
2 Not capable of algebraic manipulations.
3 Not based on each and every item of series.
4 Not a rigidly defined measure. As there are several formulae for calculating mode.

Merits and Limitations of Average

Merits

Simplest to understand and easy to compute:

- Affected by the value of every item
- Defined by rigid mathematical formula

- It is relatively reliable
- It is calculated value and not related to position of variables in the series.

Limitations

1 Very small and very large values unduly affect the value of mean for a given sample and the effect is inversely proportional to the number of observations in the group.
2 Not always a good measure of central value. In case of 'U' shaped distribution, the mean is not likely to represent central value.

It is better to express all the "summary values" of the observation, i.e. mean, median and mode. If the distribution is symmetrical any of these (mean, median and mode) may be used. When the distribution is skewed it is better to use median.

The summary value of eleven pregnant women (haemoglobin) observations are—mean 11, median 11 and mode 11. Ideally the mean, mode and median should be at one point in symmetrical distribution. The above distribution can be called symmetrical distribution.

Advantages of Mean

The mean is most commonly used average out of all. It is most easiest to calculate and it takes into consideration all the values of observations.

Disadvantages of Mean

Mean is affected by extreme values of the variables, the value which differs too much from other values of observation affects the mean. In the above example of 11 observations if we add two more observations of lesser values say 6 and 4 the mean value is pulled down to 10 (131/13 = 10) as is evident:

4,6,7,8,9,10,11,11,11,12,13,14,15.

The median is not affected and it is still 11. The extremes of values are very rare or occur least.

Other related positional measures:

- Besides median, the other methods which guide us about the position of the observations are also there. These are deciles, percentiles, and quartiles.
- Based on particular method the data is divided into number of parts denoted by the method respectively.

For example, in deciles, the given data are divided into 10 parts.

In percentiles, the given data are divided into 100 parts.

In quartiles, the given data is divided into 4 parts.

And each unit of that method denotes the part of data.

For example, 1st decile denotes the 1st 1/10th part of the whole data, i.e. 1/10th of the observations lie before the 1st decile and 9/10th of the observations lie after the 1st decile.

Similarly, 50th percentile denotes that out of total 100 units in which the data are divided the 50 units are lying below and 50 units are lying above that value, i.e. the median value.

The deciles and percentiles are important positional measures in psychological and educational and health statistics. Percentile values are being used in drawing the growth chart—used for growth monitoring purpose.

On each growth chart there are three printed growth curves. The top curve on the growth chart is the median, the second curve is minus two standard deviations of the median and the third curve is minus three standard deviations of the median.

Quartiles

These are the observations in an array that divide the distribution into four equal parts.

25%	50%	75%	100%
1st quartile	2nd quartile	3rd quartile	4th quartile

25% of the observations will lie below 1st quartile and 75% lie above it and similarly 2nd quartile divides the observations in two halves and 3rd quartile have 75% of observations below it and 25% above it.

FREQUENCY DISTRIBUTION AND NORMAL CURVE

The frequency curve of a particular sample guides us about the distribution of variable in the sample and this curve may have infinite number of different shapes. Some important frequency distributions are as follows:

1 There can be distributions with trough in the middle instead of peak called bathtub distribution (Fig. 9.5).
2 Peak in the centre with tails symmetrical on both sides of peak called bell-shaped curve (Fig. 9.6).
3 'Skewed' distribution—skewing may be towards left or right and the direction of tail in the direction of skewing.

Characteristics of a Frequency Distribution

After drawing a frequency distribution, the next step is calculation of certain important values which may be used to describe the characteristics of that distribution and helps in making comparison with other distribution. These characters are:

1 Central tendencies, i.e. mean, median, mode.
2 Degree of spread or scattering of observations around the central value is called dispersion.
3 The pattern of scattering, i.e. dispersion around the central value, i.e. shape of the distribution asymmetry is called skewness.
4 The peaking or flatness of the distribution is called Kurtosis.

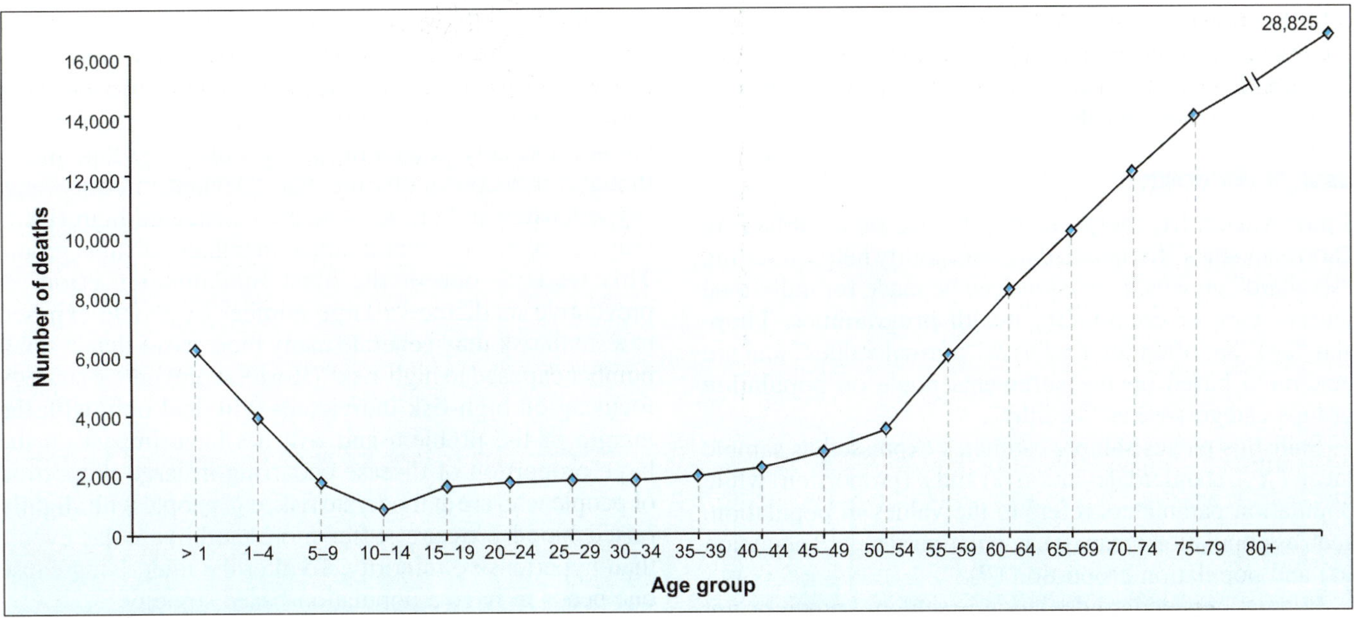

Fig. 9.5: Frequency distribution showing age wise distribution of 1,00,000 deaths in India in the year 2000. (Source: World mortality in 2000: life tables for 191 countries; WHO, 2002.)

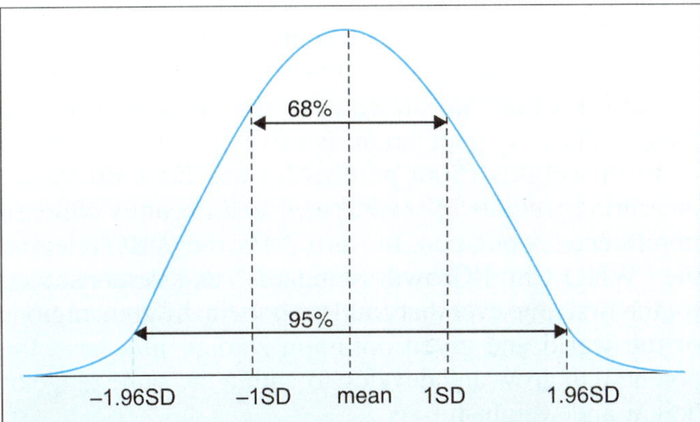

Fig. 9.6: The normal distribution curve

- Different types of frequency distributions will differ in the above mentioned four characteristics and each type of distribution will have its unique set of characteristics.

NORMAL DISTRIBUTION AND NORMAL CURVE

The variables or attributes which we study are generally distributed in the population/universe, in one way or the other. These are situations where study variables are of continuous nature, e.g. height, weight, blood pressure. To analyze a particular study, we need to apply some tests—tests of significance—to our study, which can be applied only if some assumption are fulfilled. One of the most important assumption is that the distribution of variable must follow normal or Gaussian distribution.

Normal or Gaussian Distribution

This is a special type of frequency distribution in a population which has following characteristics (Fig. 9.6):

1. The curve has a peak in the centre with two tails on either side.
2. The mean, median and mode of the distribution coincide and correspond to the peak of the distribution.
3. The curve is bell-shaped and bilaterally symmetrical around the mean of the distribution.
4. The proportion of frequencies lying on either side of the mean follows a specific pattern—which is proportion of frequencies lying within range of one standard deviation on either side of mean is 68.27% and within range of ±2 standard deviation is 95.45% and within sum of ±3 standard deviation is 99.73%.
5. Area under normal curve is unity (or one).
6. The standard deviation is one.

MEASURES OF VARIABILITY

Variability is a hallmark in statistics. The summary values of observations, such as average (mean, mode and median) are insufficient to describe the characteristics of population. Although measures of central tendency are very useful for summarizing a frequency distribution, they do not indicate the spread of values in population or group, e.g. average birth weight or one summary value of birth weight of 2.7 kg does not explain the spread of birth weights in population or around the summary value of 2.7 kg. Medical statistics have to decide whether to classify a newborn as low birth weight or of as normal or of adequate birth weight and to classify an individual as healthy or sick, suffering from particular disease or not, needing treatment or not. We need to have "cut-off" levels of different measurements. Measures of spread of values are essential for understanding, using and interpreting the concept of "normal" values, and for a complete description of a given health data set.

Uses of Variability

Thus, variability helps in describing or establishing "normal values" for health data. Variability helps in setting "standard" on which decisions can be made for individual patient care or community health programmes. These standards are often referred to as "normal values" and are generated based on measurements made on population groups categorized as "healthy".

Statistics means sample estimates expressed as sample mean ($\overline{X}$), standard deviation (*s*) and *p* (proportion) while population parameters refers to the values in population, such as population mean (μ), population standard deviation (σ) and population proportion (*P*).

Population standard deviation is seldom known or not known we usually derive the results from sample statistics to represent the value of population parameters.

In medical statistics, range of "normal values" is obtained by making use of mean value and standard deviation. Mean value of measures, such as serum cholesterol, blood glucose level, blood pressure, body mass index of sufficient large sample, representative of population are calculated and standard deviations are also calculated.

Normal Range

Most of the measurements in medical sciences are expressed in range within which most normal or healthy subjects will fall. No single or point value can be fixed. From sample mean value with the help of standard deviation, we derive the range of normal value. *Normal range* is expressed as mean ±2SD, it will cover 95% of values in the observation or 95% of healthy individuals in population will fall within this range of blood pressure, serum cholesterol and body mass index or any other measurement, provided it is Gaussian distribution or normal distribution curve where mean, median and mode are equal or near equal and standard deviation is one.

For mean ±2SD normal range there would be 2.5% of individuals on (either side) who will fall beyond the normal range. These would be labelled as abnormal values or abnormal individuals. It is quite possible that some of these individuals who have values or measurement beyond normal range may be absolutely healthy and similarly some unhealthy subjects may fall in normal range. Most of the normal range values expressed in medicine use mean ±2SD criterion.

Caution in Interpretation of Normal Range

9

The nature presents us with a process of continuum and not a dichotomy. Use of dichotomous labels, such as "Hypertensive and normotensive" therefore is not a description of natural order but rather a operational convenience. The relation between risk factors (blood pressure, serum cholesterol and body mass index) and disease events are continuous and most events occur in people in middle range of the risk factor distribution who are not normally judged high-risk. Following this line of thought, it becomes obvious that "deviant minority" e.g. (hypertensive and obese) who are considered high-risk is only part of the risk continuum, rather than a distinct group. This leads to one of the most fundamental axiom in preventive medicine "a large number of people exposed to a small risk may generate many more cases than a small number exposed to high-risk" (Rose). A preventive strategy focusing on high-risk individuals will deal only with the margin of the problem and will not have impact on the large proportion of disease occurring in large proportion of people who are at moderate risk, e.g. people with slightly raised blood pressure suffer more cardiovascular events than hypertensive minority. To alter the underlying cause one needs to have a population-based strategy.

Very often all measurements falling below/above a certain critical limit are classified as unacceptable and the critical limit is then known as "cut-off" point. The cut-off point is a selected boundary of acceptability and can be adjusted if necessary when resources for remedial action improve or diminish (Table 9.5).

Cut-off points are drawn after the measurements are made on healthy population. For example, median curve of birth weights (50th percentile) has been drawn by measuring weights of several well to do healthy children in reference population. In April 2006, the WHO released the "WHO Child Growth Standards" and demonstrated for the first time ever that children born in different regions of the world and given optimum start in life, have the potential to grow and develop to within the same range of height-and weight-for-age.

Two types of "normal" values are often used "point normal" values and "normal ranges". The point normal values are derived from summary values or averages (mean, median and mode). Normal ranges give the general level (in terms of an interval) of a measurement for healthy population group as described above. Some individuals in population will have exceptionally high or low value of particular measurement and still apparently healthy. These are called "outliers". Such measurements or values are not regarded as typical of population groups.

Table 9.5: Some examples of cut-off level

Measurement	*"Cut-off" point*
Birth weight	2500 g
Weight-for-age	–2SD to –3SD
Height-for-age	–2SD or 90% of reference median
Haemoglobin pregnant women	11 g
BMI	18.5
Blood pressure	140/90
Serum cholesterol safe level	200 mg/dl

Most biomedical normal ranges have been adopted to ensure that 95% of randomly selected healthy people would fall in within the limits. The normal distribution has extremely useful characteristics. Approximately two-thirds of values under a normal distribution curve fall within one standard deviation of mean and approximately 95% fall within two standard deviations of the mean. The normal values must refer to population to which it belongs to, because population of two places may differ biologically and environmentally.

Measures of Variation

The following are the common measures of variations or dispersion:

1. Range
2. Interquartile range
3. Standard deviation
4. Variance

1. Range

Difference between highest and lowest value in series of observations. It is calculated by $R = L - S$ where L is the highest value and S is the lowest value in the observations.

In 2700 births weighed, the highest value of observation was 3.8 kg and lowest was 1000 g. The values thus ranged from 1000 to 3800 g and range is 3800–1000 = 2800 g.

$$\text{Coefficient of range} = \frac{L - S}{L + S} = \frac{2800}{3900} = 0.72$$

Advantages

Range is simple to calculate, easy to understand, extreme values are dependent on sample size.

Disadvantages

It is not based on all observations as it takes no account of variability of observations between the two extreme values. It is not readily amenable to mathematical treatment. It should be used in combination with other measurements of variability.

2. Interquartile Range

Here the observations are divided into four quarters. The quartile 1 (Q1) indicates that 25% of the observations fall below it and 75% are above it and quartile 3 (Q3) indicates that 25% of values are above it and 75% are below it. The interval between Q1 and Q3 covers middle 50% of values of observations in the group. Unlike the range, the value given by interquartile range is unaffected by the occurrence of rare/extreme values and thus it makes a good measure of dispersion.

3. Standard Deviation (SD)

This is the best method and widely used measure of depicting variation or dispersion. It is *root mean square deviation*, where deviations have been taken from the mean. This equals the square root of variance, expressed in the units of original observations (Table 9.6).

4. Variance

Sum of squared deviations, taken from the mean, divided by the number of observations-n (or n-1 for an unbiased sample variance), expressed as square of unit of the original observations.

Table 9.6: Method of calculation of SD

Observations (X) Hb levels of 30 students	*Deviation from mean $(X-\overline{X}) = d$*	*$(X-\overline{X})^2$, i.e. d^2 square of deviation*
11	0.5	0.25
12	1.5	2.25
8	–2.5	6.25
9	–1.5	2.25
9	–1.5	2.25
9	–1.5	2.25
9	–1.5	2.25
8	–2.5	6.25
10	–0.5	0.25
9	–1.5	2.25
10	–0.5	0.25
10	–0.5	0.25
11	0.5	0.25
10	–0.5	0.25
11	0.5	0.25
11	0.5	0.25
11	0.5	0.25
13	2.5	6.26
13	2.5	6.25
14	3.5	12.25
13	2.5	6.25
13	2.5	6.25
13	2.5	6.25
12	1.5	2.25
12	1.5	2.25
11	0.5	0.25
8	–2.5	6.25
8	–2.5	6.25
9	–1.5	2.25
8	–2.5	6.25
$\Sigma x = 315$		$\Sigma d^2 = 97.75$

In above example: Mean = 10.5 g

$$\text{Variance} = \frac{\Sigma d^2}{X}$$

$$= \frac{97.75}{30} = 3.258$$

Standard deviation

$$SD = \sqrt{3.258} = 1.81$$

Standard deviation: Following are the haemoglobin levels of the 30 students in a class (in g %): 11, 12, 8, 9, 9, 9, 9, 8, 10, 9, 10, 10, 11, 10, 11, 11, 11, 13, 13, 14, 13, 13, 13, 12, 12, 11, 8, 8, 9, 8.

Steps in calculating SD

i Depict all the values or observations in column 1.

ii Calculate arithmetic mean

iii Find out deviation from mean for each value in column 2

iv Square the *deviations*

v Sum the *square* of deviation

vi Find out the *mean* of sum of square of deviation to arrive at 'variance'

vii Square *root* of variance is 'SD'.

Advantages

SD and variance are based on all observations. The deviations are taken from mean, i.e. the summary measure of central tendency. It is most widely used because of the properties of the theoretical normal distribution curve.

If repeated samples are taken from the same population the statistics or statistical measures, such as mean, median and standard deviation, vary between samples. The degree of variation depends upon both the amount of variation in the population and the size of the samples. One of the most important role of statistics is that, even if the underlying population is not normally distributed, the means of the samples themselves will be approximately normally distributed if the sample sizes are sufficiently large.

The standard deviation of the distribution of sample means is called *standard error of the mean*, it is calculated by dividing the standard deviation of a sample by the square root of the sample size.

$$SE = \frac{SD}{\sqrt{n}}$$

COEFFICIENT OF VARIATION

Definition

Standard deviation expressed as percentage of the mean (this is independent of the scale/unit of measurement).

This is used for comparison of relative variability of two distributions. It measures level of variability in the data relative to the average value. It is independent of any unit of measurement and thus useful for comparison of variability in two distributions having variables expressed in different units. It takes into account each value of the distribution.

$$\text{Coefficient of variation} = \frac{\text{SD}}{\text{Mean}} \times 100$$

In above example

SD = 1.81

Mean = 10.5 g%

$$\text{Coefficient of variation} = \frac{1.81}{10.5} \times 100 = 17.2$$

Relative or Standard Normal Deviate or Variate (Z)

It is measured in terms of SDs and indicates how much an observation is bigger or smaller than mean in units of SD? So *Z* will be a ratio calculated by subtracting mean from the measurement and divided by the SD the value thus obtained is *Z* score.

$$Z = \frac{\text{Observation} - \text{mean}}{\text{SD}} = \frac{X - \overline{X}}{\text{SD}}$$

for non-normal distribution

$$Z\ score = \frac{(\text{observed value} \div \text{M})^{\text{L}} - 1}{\text{L} \times \text{S}}$$

Where M is the reference median value which estimates the population mean. L is the power needed to transform the data in order to remove skewness (i.e. to normalize the data). S is the coefficient of variation (or equivalent).

The reference lines on the growth charts are called Z score lines because they are based on Z scores, also known as standard deviation (SD) scores. Z scores or SD scores are used to describe how far a measurement is from the median (average). These scores are calculated differently for measurements that are distributed normally and non-normally in the reference population.

The total area under normal distribution curve is taken as unity or *1* with mean = 0 and SD = 1. The mean of Z scores is always zero and SD is always one. Area of different values of *Z* under the curve is tabulated and available for interpretation. When *Z* test is applied to sampling variability the difference observed between a sample estimate and that of population is expressed in terms of SE instead of SD. The score of value of the ratio between observed difference and SE is called "*Z*". In case, the distance in terms of SE or *Z* score falls within ± 1.96 SE (95% confidence limit) it is zone of acceptance (Fig. 9.7).

SAMPLING

Statistics and epidemiology deal with "population" and we are interested in "population characteristics" and results must be applied to population, and all estimates should be related to population.

POPULATION

It means total population of a defined geographical area and it is called "Universe".

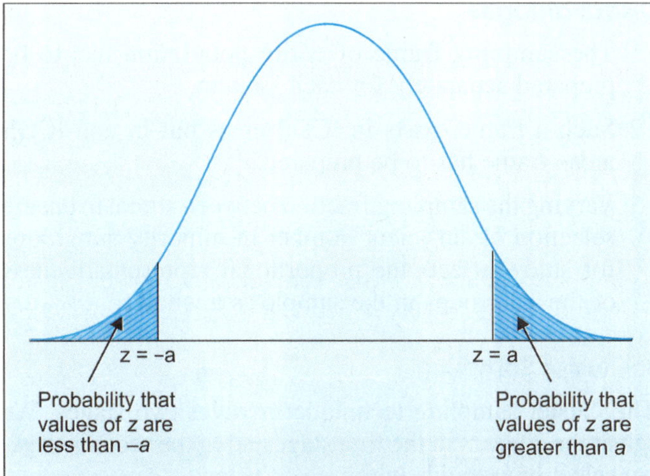

Fig. 9.7: Area under the normal curve

Sample

Sample is part of population or universe. Since it is not possible to study the entire population to arrive at an estimate, we therefore take "part" of the "whole" population.

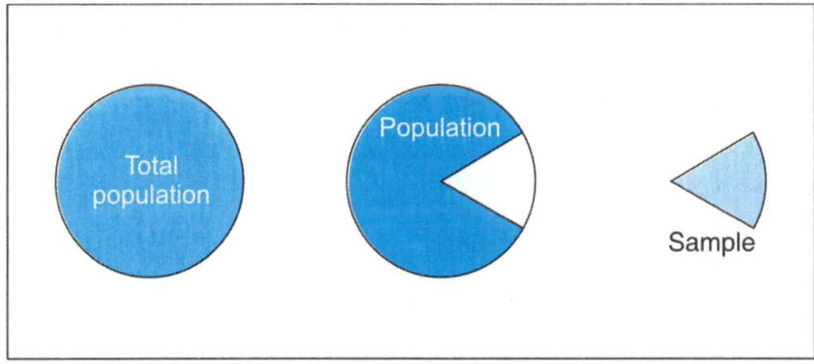

Sample is just one smaller segment of population as indicated in the above diagram.

Applications

All studies and surveys rely on "sample". It saves time; cost and results are quickly available for applications. The findings of sample will apply to population. Errors in the study may be due to small sample or biased sample (*see* errors in epidemiological studies—Chapter 8).

Sampling Unit

A household, a family, or an individual of specific characteristic are the natural units in the population. Family is the smallest unit in the population. All families in an area or a village set-up constitute units for study.

Sampling Frame

If all the natural units; say families or households are listed and they are assigned numbers this constitutes sampling frame. From this sampling frame, one can choose the desired number of sample units.

Ideally, every individual or family in the universe or population from which the sample is drawn should have a known chance of being included in the sample.

Sampling Fraction

It is the relation of the size of sample to the size of whole population from which it is drawn and can be expressed in terms of proportions or percentages.

Advantages

1. Sampling reduces demands on resources, such as finance, personnel and materials.
2. Results are obtained quickly with better accuracy.

Disadvantages

1. There is always a sampling error.
2. Sampling may create a feeling of discrimination.
3. It may be inadvisable where every unit in the population is legally required to have a record.

TYPE OF SAMPLING

1. Simple Random Sampling

Simple random sampling is the most acceptable and easy to understand method of sampling. You can consider this method to be the "gold standard" of sampling methods.

In simple random sample, every study unit has an equal chance of being included in the sample.

In this method, we list and number each unit, and mix up them thoroughly, and then select one unit at a time from the box until the required sample size is achieved. The given unit is selected only once without replacement.

Random selection from the sampling frame can be done by balloting or lottery system, by table of random numbers or employing a computer.

Advantages

1. Because every unit in the population has an equal chance of being included in the sample, the sample is assured of being representative and subject only to sampling error.
2. Estimates are easy to calculate.

Disadvantages

1. If the sampling frame is large, this method may be impracticable because of difficulty and expense of constructing or updating it in large scale surveys.
2. Minority subgroups of interest in the population may not be present in the sample in sufficient number for study.

2. Systematic Random Sampling

This is more simple and convenient method. In this, a systematic sample is formed by selecting one unit at random and additional units at evenly spaced intervals. (First requirement in this technique is to enlist the population completely may be on the basis of alphabetical, geographical or numerical order). The second requirement

is to calculate the interval called sampling interval or sampling ratio which is calculated by:

$$K = \frac{N}{n}$$

where N = total size of population
n = sample size.

In systematic random sampling method, all the sampling units in the population are numbered serially, e.g. if there are 1000 families in a village and we wish to select sample size of 100. Divide 1000 by 100 you get the answer (sampling interval) 10, it means you select every 10th family.

Next, you draw a random number less than 10 from a currency note or by lottery say if it comes 7. The first sampling unit will be 7th household or family and then you go on adding 10 to it to select rest of the families (7, 17, 27, 37, etc.). Thus in this technique, all the sampling units had known chance to be included in the sample. You have to just choose one number and the rest get selected automatically.

3. Consecutive Sampling—A Kind of Random Sampling

For annual HIV sentinel surveillance for antenatals clients consecutive sampling method is being used to remove selection bias. It is a kind of random sampling where sampling interval is zero. All individuals attending sentinel site facility who meet the defined selection criteria should be recruited in order they attend clinic. Starting with first individual, every successive eligible individual should be recruited in HIV sentinel surveillance till the desired sample size is achieved or the desired period is over.

4. Stratified Random Sampling

When the population is not homogeneous, we use this technique. The population is first divided into groups or strata according to characteristic of interest. *Example*: In a village, it is observed that there are two strata of population one stratum comprising over landowners and well to do people and second stratum is of landless or weaker sections of the community. If we wish to study the prevalence of malnutrition in this village, we will draw sample from two different strata.

Thus, first step is formation of strata in the village and second step is preparing the sampling frame for these strata. Then a simple random sample is selected from each stratum using the same sampling fraction.

Advantages

1. Every unit in a stratum has the same chance of being selected.
2. Using the same sampling fraction for all strata ensures proportionate representation in the sample of the characteristic being stratified.
3. Adequate representation of minority subgroup of interest can be ensured by stratification and by varying the sampling fraction between strata as required.

9

Disadvantages

1. The sampling frame of entire population has to be prepared separately for each stratum.
2. Such a frame exists in ICDS areas but in non-ICDS areas frame has to be prepared.
3. Varying the sampling fraction between strata, to ensure selection of sufficient number in minority subgroups for study, affects the proportional representativeness of the subgroups in the sample as a whole.

5. Cluster Sampling

The cluster sampling technique involves two stages. We select the clusters in the first stage and in the second stage, we select households within the cluster.

Sampling Frame

For cluster selection, we provide a list of clusters (villages for rural area and wards for the urban area) with the size of population. Once we know the number of clusters to be selected. It can be calculated randomly when the chance of every cluster being selected is equal. The chance of selecting one particular village will depend upon the population of each village.

Selection of Cluster

The tricky part of the cluster sampling is to make sure that everybody has the same chance to be selected as a sample. In cluster sample, this condition can be fulfilled by selecting different number of persons per cluster according to the population size of the clusters. However, selecting a different number of persons per cluster has other disadvantages; it becomes complicated for the field investigator and it becomes difficult to maintain quality control of the survey. The modification, which has been made to simplify cluster sample method without violating statistical assumption, is to weigh the cluster selection by their population size. With this modification, we can get a constant number of households per cluster without violating the equal chance of being selected of the person in our sampling frame. This method is also called selecting clusters with probability proportionate to size (PPS) method.[1,2]

1st Stage

- The villages or wards are listed in a column, each with its "size" of population in the next column.
- In the third column, the sizes are cumulated or cumulated population is worked out.
- Take the final entry in the third column (the total "cumulative size of population" and divide this by the number of clusters desired in the sample to give the sampling interval (SI). Usually we select 30 clusters but it could be any number (Table 9.7).

Table 9.7: Cluster sampling technique

Name of village	No. of households	Cumulative size	Cluster selection
001	200	200	
002	240	440	........X_1
003	160	600	
004	100	700	
005	260	960	
006	220	1180	
007	200	1380	
008	180	1560	
009	280	1840	
010	140	1980	
011	200	2180	
012	220	2400	
013	260	2660	
014	180	2840	
015	140	2680	
016	200	3180	.......X_2
017	240	3420	
018	220	3640	
019	200	3840	
020	160	4000	
021	450	4450	
022	230	4680	
023	500	5180	
024	400	5580	
.	600	6180	.........X_3
.	.	.	
.	.	.	
.	.	.	
.	.	.	
.	.	.	
.	.	.	
350	180	87,000	

$$\text{Sampling interval} = \frac{\text{Total cumulative population}}{30}$$

$$= 87000/30 = 2900$$

- Using table select a random number (*R*) between 1 and the sampling interval that has been calculated. The number you select must have the same number of digits as the sampling interval.

Find the first entry in the cumulative column which equals or exceeds *R*, this is the first selected cluster. Add the sampling interval to *R* to select the second cluster and continue to add the sampling interval until the selection is complete.

In the following example, the total "size" or total cumulative household population is 87,000, the number of clusters to be selected is 30.

Step 1: Calculate Sampling Interval (S1): Divide the total Cumulative Population 87,000 by 30 (Number of clusters) to be surveyed = 2900

Step 2: Choose a random number between 1 and sampling interval (in this example 2900) by using a currency note or random table number. Assume the random number selected was 0250.

Step 3: The first cluster in this example will be where the 0250 household is found based on the cumulative population column; in this example, village 002, because the 0250th household is within it.

Step 4: Continue to select clusters by adding the sampling interval cumulatively. In this example, to identify the second cluster, 0250 + 2900 = 3150, for the third cluster, 3150 + 2900 = 6050, the fourth 6050 + 2900 = 8950, and so on—till the 30th cluster is arrived. In cluster sampling, probability is proportion to size (PPS).

2nd Stage

Once the clusters have been selected, the next step is to select the households within these clusters. The households can be selected by using the simple random sampling method. It means that you should have a list of every household in the selected cluster and use the random number table to select the individual households.

In coverage evaluation survey of immunization, seven children between 12 and 23 months of age are selected by moving in one direction till the desired number of children are completed. Randomization at household level is not done because households are not numbered but we can use randomization by using register of Anganwadi worker, which is a perfect sample frame of all households or families in a village.

The two-stage cluster sampling method has been widely used in immunization coverage and diarrhoeal disease surveys as also in leprosy elimination monitoring surveys.

Advantages

1. Cuts down on the cost of preparing a sampling frame.
2. Cuts down on the cost of travelling between selected units.
3. Eliminates the problem of "packing" (in health surveys, especially those involving case finding and treatment, it is not unusual for neighbouring houses not included in the sample to transfer their households temporarily to a selected house).

Disadvantage

Sampling error is usually higher than for a simple random sample of the same size.

Pathfinder Surveys

"Pathfinder" method uses stratified cluster sampling technique, which aims to include the most important population subgroups likely to have differing disease levels. These surveys are used for assessment and planning of oral health.[3]

Index ages and age groups: The recommended age groups are 5 years for primary teeth, and 12, 15, 35–44 and 65–74 years for permanent teeth. The number of subjects in each index age group to be examined ranges from a minimum of 25 to 50 for each cluster or sampling site, depending upon the prevalence and severity of oral disease.

6. Multistage Sampling

The selection is done in stages. Cluster sampling is an example of multistage sampling. In the 1st stage, an area or village is chosen and in the second stage we choose households.

7. Lot Quality Assurance Sampling (LQAS)

This technique was traditionally used for quality assurance purposes in the industry but statisticians and epidemiologists found it suitable for assessing a variety of primary health care services, e.g. measuring immunization coverage.

In this technique, surveys would be carried in two or more sets with the same objective. All the different sets under study population will be different, i.e. belonging to different geographical areas and we will calculate the results from those sets of population with respect to defined objective and comparing the weighted results with the given assumptions which may be the same or different for different sets of population. Hence, we can find out that which set of population gives acceptable results and which set gives unfavourable results, requiring urgent interventions, e.g. LQAS was used to determine the low vaccination coverage areas in five cities in Bangladesh (Bulletin WHO, Vol. 79, 6, Geneva; 2001).

8. Non-random Sampling (Non-probability Sampling)

In this, the probability of selection of a particular item/individual is not fixed. The sampling unit is selected at its own with some units have very high chances of selection and other have zero chances.

9. Judgment Sampling

In this method of sampling, the choice of study units depends exclusively on the judgment of the investigator. This type of sampling is useful when:

- Number of sampling units in the universe are small.
- To study effect of some unknown factors on a population whose characteristics are known.
- In solving urgent public health/policy problems or everyday business problems where we cannot wait for probability sample designs.
- But this is not a scientifically proven appropriate method and does not follow basic laws of sampling.

10. Quota Sampling

It is a type of judgment sampling and is the most frequently used sampling technique among non-random sampling techniques. In this, the population/universe is divided into quotas according to some specific characteristics, e.g. age, socioeconomic status, religion, etc. and number of study units selected within each quota depend on personal judgment of the investigator.

- This is generally used in public opinion studies.
- But this does not follow laws of sampling.

11. Convenience Sampling/Purposive Sampling

The sample when obtained by selecting a part of population on which it is convenient to carry out a study. This method is also called the *chunk*.

- The population parts which are easily accessible and those population groups in which it is easy to conduct surveys or investigations are chosen irrespective of the representativeness of the population.
- Generally used for making pilot studies to have just a basic idea about the study variable.
- Biases are maximum in this sampling method and generally the results obtained are unsatisfactory in terms of drawing conclusions.

Sample Size Determination

Sampling for a Quantitative Characteristics

When sampling for a quantitative character (e.g. the mean level of hemoglobin in a population) one needs to state:

1 How precisely one wishes to estimate this mean level, that is the amount of sampling error that can be tolerated (d), in either absolute or relative term?
2 The standard deviation(s) of the distribution of hemoglobin in the population.
3 The chance the investigator is willing to take to get an unlucky sample giving a sampling error greater than d, a 5% chance or error (i.e. a 95% confidence interval) is conventional.
4 This means that $\overline{X} \pm d$ are the required 95% confidence limits, so that $d = 1.96$ SE, where SE of mean $= s/\sqrt{n}$. Hence, $d/1.96 = s/\sqrt{n}$, and therefore, the required (minimum) sample size for a large population given by: $n = (1.96)^2\, s^2/d^2$.

Example

An investigator wishes to estimate the mean hemoglobin level in a defined community. Preliminary information indicates that this mean is about 150 mg/L with a standard deviation of 32 mg/L. If a sampling error of up to 5 mg/L in the estimate is to be tolerated how many subjects should be included in the study?

Here $s = 32$ mg/L, and $d = 5$ mg/L

If the population is assumed to be very large, the required minimum sample size would be:

$$n = [(1.96)^2 \times (32)^2]/(5)^2 = 157.4.$$

If the community to be sampled has 1000 people the required minimum sample size would be:

$$n = (1.96)^2 \times (32)^2 / [(5)^2 + (1.96)^2 \times (32)^2/1000] = 136$$

Therefore, at least 136 people would have to be studied. For a larger community with, e.g. N = 3000 people, the required sample size would be:

$$n = (1.96)^2 \times (32)^2 / [(5)^2 + (1.96)^2 \times (32)^2 / 3000] = 149.5$$

At least approximately 150 people would have to be studied (WHO, 1999 Teaching Health Statistics).

Sampling for an Attribute or Qualitative Characteristics

When sampling for an attribute (to estimate the proportion of persons with a certain characteristic in a population) one needs to state.

- A rough approximation to the proportion (p) or prevalence rate.
- The sampling error that can be tolerated (d) in either absolute or relative term.
- The acceptable chance of an unlucky sample (conventionally 5%).

The minimum sample required for a very large population is then:

$$\text{SE of proportion} = \sqrt{\frac{Pq}{n}}$$

or

$$\text{Sample size } (n) = (1.96)^2\, p(1-p)/d^2$$

Example

If $p = 0.26$, and $d = 0.03$, then, for a very large population:

$$n = (1.96)^2 \times 0.26 \times 0.74 / (0.03)^2 = 821.2$$

Thus, the study should include at least 822 persons.

If the sample is to be drawn from a small population of, e.g. 3000 people, the required minimum sample could be obtained from the above estimate by adjustment as:

821.2 / (1 + 821.2/3000) = 644.7

Thus, the study should include at least 645 people.

REFERENCES

1 GOI. National Child Survival and Safe Motherhood Programme—Evaluate Service Coverage. New Delhi: MOH and FW, GOI; 1992.

2 WHO. Global Programme on AIDS. Evaluation of a National AIDS Programme—A methods Package. Geneva: WHO; 1994.

3 WHO. Oral Heath Surveys Basic Methods, 4th Edition. World Health Organization, Geneva; 1997.

CONFIDENCE INTERVAL[1,2]

Once the sample has been drawn, it can be used to estimate the characteristics of the underlying population. Because estimates vary from sample to sample, it is important to know how close the estimate derived from any one sample is likely to be to the underlying population value. One way to find this is to construct a confidence interval around the estimate, i.e. to construct a range of values surrounding the estimate, which have a specified probability of including the true population values. The specified probability is called the confidence level and the endpoints of confidence interval are the confidence limits.

Population means are always derived from sample means.

Population standard deviation (σ) is hardly ever known we use the standard deviation of sample means. From the normal standard distribution we know that normal range (mean ± 2SD) covers 95% of observation values.

Confidence Intervals of Means

Same concept can be applied to sample means.

$$\text{Mean} \pm 2\text{SE}$$

It is the range that would cover 95% samples to be more exact.

To calculate the confidence limits around the estimated population mean, it is necessary to have measures of: (1) Variation, such as the population standard deviation (σ), (2) the estimated mean ($\overline{X}$), (3) the sample size (n) and (4) the specified probability of including the true population value. If we assume that the underlying population is normally distributed with a known standard deviation σ, then the formula for calculating the limits of 95% confidence interval around the mean is as follows:

$$\text{Lower limit of CI} = \overline{X} - \frac{1.96\,\sigma}{\sqrt{n}}$$

$$\text{Upper limit of CI} = \overline{X} + \frac{1.96\,\sigma}{\sqrt{n}}$$

As an illustration, suppose in a random sample of 100 factory workers, the mean blood lead concentration ($\overline{X}$) was 90 µg/L. Suppose further that the level of concentration of lead in blood is normally distributed with a standard deviation of 10% (i.e. σ =10) then the limits of the 95% confidence interval around the estimate can be calculated as follows:

$$\text{Lower limit} = 90 - \frac{1.96 \times 10}{\sqrt{100}} = 88.04$$

$$\text{Upper limit} = 90 + \frac{1.96 \times 10}{\sqrt{100}} = 91.96$$

Thus, the confidence interval ranges from 88.04 to 91.96.

A sample estimate is usually presented along with confidence interval. It is important to realize that size of confidence interval is related to the sample size, the larger the sample the smaller is the confidence interval for a given confidence level. The size of confidence interval is also related to the confidence level specified.

Inference

Ninety-five percent chances are that the population parameter will lie within the confidence interval.

Major uses of Standard Error of Mean

1. To work out desired confidence interval or interval estimation within which the population mean (μ) would lie $\overline{X}$ ± 2SE.
2. Whether a sample has been drawn from a known population.
3. To determine statistical significance of difference of two means.
4. To determine sample size.

$$\text{Standard error of proportion SEP} = \sqrt{\frac{p \times q}{n}}$$

Where p is the estimated prevalence and q is 1–p and n is the size of sample.

Confidence Interval of Proportion

It is given by formula:

$$CI = p \pm \frac{Z\sqrt{p \times (1-p)}}{n}$$

Example

Calculation of 95% confidence interval around a prevalence estimate in STD clinic attenders who have syphilis serology, where a sample of 400 was used and 40 HIV positive sera were identified.

The prevalence is 40/400 or 10%, therefore, $p = 0.1$

The sample size is 400, therefore, $N = 400$.

For 95% confidence intervals, $Z = 1.96$

$CI = p \pm Z \times \sqrt{[p \times (1-p)/N]}$

95% $CI = 0.1 \pm 1.96 \times \sqrt{[0.1 \times (1-0.1)/400]}$

$= 0.1 \pm 1.96 \times \sqrt{(0.000225)}$

$= 0.1 \pm 1.96 \times 0.015$

$= 0.1 \pm 0.029$

$= (0.071 \text{ to } 0.129)$

Multiplying by 100 to convert to percent, the 95% confidence intervals are 7.1 to 12.9% for a prevalence estimate of 10% and a sample size of 400.

REFERENCES

1. Lwanga SK, Tye CY. Teaching Health Statistics Lessons and Seminar Outlines. Second Edn., Geneva: WHO; 1999.
2. Beaglehole R, Bonita R, Kjellstrom T. Basic Epidemiology. Geneva: WHO; 1993.

PROBABILITY

The literary meaning of probability is the chance and it is defined as "the average relative frequency with which an event is expected to occur in the given population/universe". Probability measures the degree of certainty and uncertainty.

SCALE OF PROBABILITY MEASUREMENT

Probability ranges from 0 to 1 (the minimum value is 0 and maximum is one). If an event which is sure to occur the probability is 1 and if an event is impossible to occur probability is 0. No probability is ever negative, e.g.

1. Probability of giving birth to a boy/girl in the given pregnancy is equal to 0.5.
2. Probability of getting head/tail on tossing of a coin = ½ = 0.5.
3. Probability of getting kings in a set of playing cards, etc. = 4/52 = 1/13

It is denoted by symbol **"P"**.

Probability of occurrence of a particular event can be calculated by the following formula:

$$P = n_p / N$$

Where n_p = no. of times the event happened/occurred.
N = Total no. of trials.

The 'Zero' represents—'absolute impossibility' of occurrence of an event and 'one' represents absolute certainty of occurrence, all the times.

It is also important to find out probabilities in complex situations where the same event is happening in more than one ways and events concerned are independent. For these conditions—two important rules of probability are helpful:

1. Addition rule.
2. Multiplication rule.

Addition Rule

If an event is occurring in mutually exclusive way in trial then the total probability of occurrence of that event in any of the trial is the sum of probabilities of the occurrence of that event in individual trials. Mutual exclusive events follow the addition rule of probability. Mutually exclusive events—events that cannot occur simultaneously or be present at the same time. Mutually exclusive events are birth of male or female child, blood groups A or B or O or AB; Rh positive or Rh negative, etc.

Addition rule: $P(A \text{ or } B) = P(A) + P(B)$ if A and B are mutually exclusive.

1. Probability of getting red or green coloured balls from a set of 20 balls—5 balls of each colour—red, green, blue and yellow, respectively.

The probability of getting red balls = 5/20 = ¼

Probability of getting green balls = 5/20 = ¼

As the event, is selection of either red or green balls and selection of red/green balls are mutually exclusive then the total probability of event = sum of individual probabilities = 1/4 + 1/4 = 2/4 = $^1/_2$

2. In a sample of 100 individuals consisting of 50 males and 50 females, out of which 10% of each are anaemics 5 males and 5 females are anaemics. To calculate the probability of selecting an anaemics either male or

9

female individual from that sample—following method is used:

Event—selection of anaemic individual (either male or female).

Probability of selecting male anaemic = 5 / 100 = $^1/_{20}$

Probability of selecting female anaemic = 5 / 100= $^1/_{20}$

Total probability = 1 / 20 + 1/20 = 2/20 = $^1/_{10}$

So, probability of getting anaemic individual either male or female from the given sample is $^1/_{10}$.

Multiplication Rule

Independent events follow the multiplication rule of probability.

Independent events: Two events are said to be independent, if the presence or absence of one does not alter the chances of other being present, or if the occurrence of one does not alter the chance of occurrence of the other, e.g. sex at birth and blood group and Rh blood group status.

Multiplication rule = $P(A \text{ and } B) = P(A) \times P(B)$ if A and B are independent events.

This rule is applied to two or more than two events occurring together, but not associated with each other, i.e. the events must be independent from each other, e.g. sex at birth and Rh factor are independent events and occur in any child.

Example

What will be the probability of child being male and Rh negative?

Probability of a child born being male = P_1 = ½

Probability of a child born being Rh negative = $P_2 = ^1/_{10}$ (10% of children at birth may be Rh negative)

Probability of child being male and Rh negative

$= P_1 \times P_2$

= 1 / 2 × 1/10

= 1 / 20 = 0.05

Example

What are the probabilities of getting male and female children when two children are borne one after the other, sequences could be:

Both males M and M = ½ × ½ = ¼

One male and one female = ½ × ½ = ¼

One female and one male = ½ × ½ = ¼

Both females F and F = ½ × ½ = ¼

Conditional probability: The chance of a particular event happening depends on the outcome of some other event. $P(B/A)$ = the probability that event B occurs, given that event A has already occurred.

If we want to determine the probability of occurrence of diabetes and hypertension both from a group of people then we have to calculate conditional probability. As, we know that a person can be diabetic and hypertensive both at a given time. So, the events are not mutually exclusive and in such conditions the probability of simultaneous occurrence of the events can be determined by calculating:

- Conditional probability.
- In these cases, the general use of multiplication rule is modified as:

Conditional probability of simultaneous occurrence of event A and B:

$$P(A \text{ and } B) = P(B) \times P(A/B) \text{ or } P(A) \times P(B/A).$$

Where $P(A)$ = Probability of occurrence of event A.

$P(B)$ = Probability of occurrence of event B.

$P(AB)$ = Simultaneous occurrence of events A and B.

$P(A/B)$ = Probability of occurrence of event A given that event B has already occurred is given by:

$$P(A/B) = P(AB)/P(B)$$

Bayes' rule: $P(A/B) = (P(B/A)\ P(A)/P(B)$

Baye's rule has been used frequently to evaluate the performance of diagnostic and screening tests, which are discussed under section of epidemiology (validity of screening test).

Binomial distribution: The binomial distribution is formed by the terms of the expansion of the binomial expression: $(p + q)^n$

When n = sample size, p = the probability of a "success", q = the probability of a "failure", and $p + q = 1$

Example

When $n = 2$ the terms of expansion of $(p + q)^2$ are $p^2 + 2pq$ and q^2

Similarly, we can calculate the probability of non-occurrence of a particular event and that will be called probability of non-occurrence, generally denoted by 'q' and is equal to 1–P.

Where 'P' is the probability of occurrence of the particular event.

Some Important Probabilities in use

- Probability of surviving at various ages are depicted in life table (Table 9.10).
- Probability of developing tuberculosis diseases in infected persons in lifetime is 10% (0.1).
- Probability of perinatal transmission of HIV is 30%.
- Probability of LBW is 30% in India.
  - a Concept and application of probability can be linked to validity of screening tests (sensitivity and specificity), i.e. probability of a positive test in people with the disease and probability of a negative test in people without disease. Probability of a person having the disease when the test is positive (positive predictive value) and probability of the person not having the disease when the test is negative (negative predictive value). These are also examples of conditional probability.

b Similarly, probability of person not falling within acceptable range or limits (sample mean ± 2SE). It is usually 5% (0.05).

c Probability of dying and survival at various ages in life table is most relevant to the concept and application of probability.

TESTING OF HYPOTHESIS

Testing of hypothesis refers to the process of selecting and using a sample statistic, i.e. mean, median, mode, standard deviation or standard error to draw conclusion about a population parameter, based on observations on a sample.

HYPOTHESIS

It is an assumption which we make about a population parameter, used as a basis for further investigation.

Assumptions

The most important assumptions to be followed by a particular sample after which we can apply tests of significance on those sample data are as follows:

i If the sample is large enough—then it must follow the principles of standard normal distribution.

ii If the sample size is small then the sample must follow the principles of some standard distribution which are not purely normal but are near normal distributions, e.g. student's 't' distribution, chi-square distribution, Fischer's "f" distribution, etc.

Different Steps in Hypothesis Testing

1 Making assumptions and setting up of a hypothesis.
2 Setting up suitable level of significance.
3 Setting up a test criterion (test of significance).
4 Computations and drawing conclusions.

1. Making Assumptions and Setting-up of a Hypothesis

First step in setting up of a hypothesis about a population parameter is that, we have to assume or estimate a certain value of population mean (μ) which is seldom available; then we collect sample data and calculate the information about that parameter, i.e. calculating sample mean. After this we have to formulate null hypothesis.

Null Hypothesis (H_0)

The hypothesis of "no difference" or more correctly, the hypothesis that the observed difference is entirely due to sampling error, i.e. it occurred purely by chance. In the test of significance, the "null hypothesis" is postulated to establish the basis for calculating the probability that the difference occurred purely by chance. When the difference is not significant, the null hypothesis is not rejected. When the difference is significant, the null hypothesis is rejected in favour of other hypothesis about the cause of the difference. The null hypothesis is never proved to be completely right or wrong, or true or false but is only rejected or not rejected at the probability level of significance concerned, e.g. 0.05 or 0.01. Thus a null hypothesis either rejected or not rejected. If the H_0 is rejected, the alternate hypothesis is not rejected.

- Null hypothesis (H_0) is hypothesis of "no difference". It is denoted by H_0. It means there is no difference between sample mean and population mean $H_0 = \mu$
- The alternate hypothesis is denoted by (H_a) and the sample mean is different or not equal to population mean $H_a \neq \mu$.

If null hypothesis (H_0) is rejected then the alternate hypothesis is not rejected and vice versa.

2. Level of Significance

It is the maximum tolerable probability of type 1 error. Since the type 1 error is quite serious particularly in the field of medicine when a therapeutic trial is done and a drug which is not effective is accepted on the basis of null hypothesis trial results. It is, therefore, necessary to fix a level of significance well in advance of the trial being conducted. We fix maximum tolerable probability for type 1 error (α) say 5% which is known as predetermined "level of significance" for α error (type 1 error).

The predetermined level of significance of α is the maximum tolerable chance of type 1 error.

What is p value: The *p* value is the actual probability of committing type 1 error.

- *p* value is based on statistical calculation, whereas level of α is fixed in advance or predetermined.
- If calculated *p* value is less than or equal to α result is inferred as statistically significant and we reject the null hypothesis (H_0).
- It p is greater than α, we do not reject hypothesis (H_0).

Type 1 error (α) is also called "rejection error".

3. Setting up of a Test Criterion

Next and the most important step is to select a proper test of significance which when applied to the given data give the results accurately. To select a particular test of significance, it is necessary to identify the probability distribution of the sample and appropriate test statistic is selected.

Example Student's 't', Fischer's 'f', 'chi-square', etc.

4. Computations and Drawing Conclusions

Final step in the testing of hypothesis is doing computations and drawing conclusion. In computation, the selected test statistic value is calculated, and is compared with the table value pertaining to that statistic at a given level of significance corresponding to the degree of freedom of the sample. Then we have to see whether the computed statistic values fall under zone of rejection or zone of acceptance.

- If the computed value lies in zone of acceptance then we say that hypothesis is accepted and if it lies in zone of rejection then we say that hypothesis is rejected (Fig. 9.8).

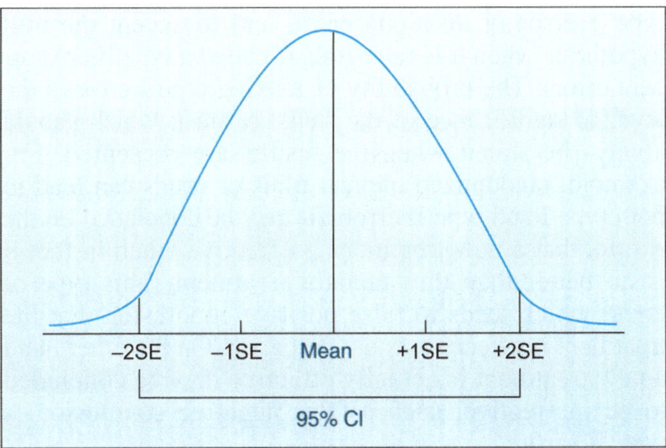

Fig. 9.8: Acceptance and rejection zone in a two failed test of significance at 95% level of significance

- If the value lies on the borderline zone then the best and wisest step is not to draw any conclusion but draw other sample and investigate again.

Errors in Hypothesis Testing

Error in hypothesis testing can mainly occur in 2 ways:
a Problems in sample selection.
b Limitation of a particular test of significance.

Errors Related to Sampling

If we want to compare the results between different samples, then we assume that all the samples drawn from the population are distributed randomly and bear same characters as the population/universe. But generally it is not true and minor variations in the 'statistic' calculated from different samples exist because the samples are not alike and we assume that distribution of the samples drawn from a population follows normal distribution called *sampling distribution* (just like normal probability distribution) and the standard deviation of sampling distribution is called standard error and is equal to standard deviation of the sample divided by square root of total no. of observations SE = $s/\sqrt{n}$

Errors Related to Limitations of Tests of Significance

There can be four possibilities in testing of a hypothesis.

- Hypothesis true—Accepted—correct decision.
- Hypothesis true—Rejected—Type I error (α error)
- Hypothesis false—Accepted—Type II error (β error)
- Hypothesis false—Rejected—correct decision.

Type I error is also called 'α' and is related to level of significance and type II error is called 'β' and type I error is much more serious than type II error.

Type I Error or 'α' Error (Alpha Error)

Type I (α) error is also called "rejection error". This error is committed when the null hypothesis is true and the study or trial rejects it on the basis of level of significance and *p* value. The name of type I error is an alpha (α) error and it has always a predetermined level of significance. Say at 5% (0.05). It means if we conduct repeated studies and trials there are 5% of chances that we may reject a true null hypothesis.

Type II Error or β Error (Beta Error)

When the null hypothesis is false and we have not rejected it, then type II error is committed unlike (α) error type II error has no predetermined level of significance.

STATISTICAL INFERENCE HYPOTHESIS TESTING

In hypothesis testing, the null hypothesis is either accepted or rejected, depending on whether the *p* value is above or below a predetermined cut-off point, known as the significance level of the test. If the *P* value is less than the cut-off point, the null hypothesis is rejected. If the *p* value is greater than or equal to the cut-off point, the null hypothesis is accepted. It is usual to choose either 0.05 (5%) or 0.01 (1%) as significance levels for testing the null hypothesis.

As an example, suppose it is known that in a particular country the weight at birth of male babies is normally distributed with a mean of 2.9 kg and a standard deviation of 0.5. Suppose further that a random sample of 100 male babies born to a particular ethnic subgroup was found to have a mean birth weight of 2.8 kg. We wish to determine whether the mean birth weight in the ethnic subgroup is different from the birth weight in the country as a whole. The null hypothesis would state that the mean birth weight of the ethnic subgroup is 2.9 kg.

In this example, the appropriate test statistic is z:

$$z = \frac{\bar{x} - \mu}{\sigma / \sqrt{n}}$$

where

$\bar{x}$ = Sample mean
μ = Known country mean
σ = Known standard deviation
n = Sample size.

For the above example: $z = \frac{2.8 - 2.9}{0.5/\sqrt{100}} = -2$

The statistic z has been constructed so that if the null hypothesis were true (i.e. birth weights in the population sampled were normally distributed with a mean μ and standard deviation σ), then the distribution of z over all possible samples of size n would be close to that of a normal distribution with mean 0 and standard deviation 1. An important characteristic of this distribution is that the area under the normal curve to the right of the line z = a (Fig. 9.7) can be interpreted as the probability with which values of z are grater than a. Similarly, the area under the curve to the left of the line z = – a gives the probability with which values of z are less than – a. Therefore, the *p* value associated with a particular value z = a, is equal to the area under the normal curve to the right of z = a, *plus* the area under the curve to the left of z = – a.

For the above example, consultation of the appropriate normal distribution tables found in many statistical textbooks (which give *p* values for areas under the normal curve associated with each value of z) indicates that the area under the curve to the left of z = – 2 is 0.023. Similarly, the area under the curve to the right of z = 2 is 0.023. Therefore, the *p* value associated with this value of z is 0.046. This can be interpreted as indicating that if the null hypothesis were true (i.e. birth weights in the ethnic subgroup are normally distributed with a mean of 2.9 and standard deviation 0.5), only 4.6% of all possible samples of 100 babies would have mean birth weights differing from 2.9 kg by 100 g or more.

If we had decided on a significance level of 5% for the statistical test, we would reject the null hypothesis and accept the alternative that the mean of the population is not equal to 2.9. However, had we decided on the 1% level of significance the null hypothesis would have been accepted. The phrase "statistically significant" is used to indicate that a result has led to rejection of the null hypothesis. It is important to keep in mind that the null hypothesis is never proven right or wrong but is only accepted or rejected at a given level of significance. The small *p* value may be consistent with a weak association, and a difference between two groups may fail to be statistically significant if the sample size is not large enough.

Many statistical tests involve the comparison of two quantities (in the example above, the sample mean was compared with the known country mean). Usually the statistical test allows for the possibility of differences in both directions (either quantity can be larger than the other; the country mean might have been greater than the sample mean or smaller than it). This is known as a two-side or two-tailed test. As in the example above, the *p* value is calculated on the basis of probabilities from both tails of the sampling distribution (thus, in the above example *p* was the sum of the probability of z > + 2 and z < – 2).

However, there are some situations in which there is interest in a difference in only one direction. For example, one may wish to test whether a specific treatment is better than a placebo (the case in which the treatment is worse than the placebo being of no interest). In this instance it would be appropriate to use a "one-sided" or "one-tailed" test. The calculation of the test statistic for a one-sided test is identical to that of the two-sided test. The difference between the two types of tests lies in the calculation of the *p* value. A one-sided test is based on probabilities from only one side or one tail of the sampling distribution, whereas a two-sided test sums the probabilities from both tails of the distribution. Therefore, the *p* value associated with the one-sided test is equal to half the *p* value associated with the two-sided test.

Two types of error are associated with the decision: to reject the null hypothesis when it is true (this is called type 1 error or an alpha error, and to accept the null hypothesis when it is false (this is called a type II error or beta error). The probability of making type I error is the level of significance of the statistical test; which should always be stated when the results are presented. For example, randomized clinical trials of drugs can lead to both type I and type II errors. It may be concluded on the results that a new treatment is effective when in fact it is no better than the standard treatment. This type of error, which leads to false positive conclusion that the treatment is effective, is a type I error. On the other hand a new treatment is actually effective may be concluded to be ineffective, such a false negative conclusion is type II error.

The probability of rejecting a null hypothesis when it is false is known as power of a statistical test. It is equal to one minus the probability of type two error (1 – β). The power of a test depends upon sample size—the larger the sample size, the higher the power, all else being equal.

The power of test is also dependent on the significance level chosen. For any given sample size, the higher the level of significance (i.e. the lower the probability level of a type I error), the lower is the power (the more likely a type II error will be made). It is common for studies to aim for a power of 0.8 at a significance level of 0.05. This means that the probability of a type II error (0.2) is four times the probability of a type I error (0.05), reflecting the fact that in most studies a type I error is considered much more serious than type II error. The power should be presented when a negative result is reported. The power of a test is an important consideration in the planning of an epidemiological study, since it indicates how likely the test is to have a statistically significant result under different circumstances (WHO, 1993).

Another set of useful statistical tests are known as t-tests, and are especially important for small samples. For instance, one can test the hypothesis that the mean of a population is equal to a predetermined value, μ, when the standard deviation of the underlying population is unknown, but the standard deviation of the sample is known. The appropriate formula is:

$$t = \frac{\overline{X} - \mu}{s/\sqrt{n}}$$

where 's' is the standard deviation of the sample and *t* has *n* – 1 drgrees of freedom.

This is similar to the z-test described above. However, the z-statistic is used when the standard deviation of the population is known, while the t-statistic is used when the standard deviation of the population is unknown and estimated by the standard deviation of the sample.

When the hypothesis is true and it is rejected we call it '(α)' or type I error. '(α)' error is related to level of significance. The actual probability of committing type I

9

error is called the p value. It is customary to attach special significance to 'p' values falling below 0.05 (5%), because it is generally agreed that less than 1 chance in 20 is a small risk of being wrong. Differences associated with p less than 0.05 are called "statistically significant" ($p < 0.05$) $p > 0.05$ means that it is "statistically non-significant" as the chances are more than 1 in 20 which is not a small risk but large risk of being wrong.

However, p value greater than 1 in 5 are usually reported as simply $p>0.20$, because nearly every one can agree that probability of an (α) error that is greater than one in five is unacceptably high.

Relationship between Testing of Hypothesis and Confidence Interval (CI)

The usual level of confidence interval is set up at 95%. The limits of confidence are fixed on either side of the mean, which we call as confidence limits, with predetermined probability. If the population mean has normal distribution then 95%, CI = mean ± 2SE, where SE refers to standard error of sample means ($SE_{\bar{x}}$). This covers almost 95% of the area of the curve (Fig. 9.8).

Choice of a Test

According to Sample Size

In small samples—with sample size 30 or less generally the normality assumptions do not hold good and certain other tests are required to analyse and test these data based on their probability distribution, assuming that to be near normal.

1. Small samples—sample size less than or equal to 30. Tests of significance of choice are:
   - Student's 't' test (paired and unpaired).
   - Analysis of variance (ANOVA)
   - Non-parametric tests
2. Large samples—all tests which can be applied on small samples plus along with
   - 'z' test.
   - Chi-square test, etc.

According to Type of Data

1. Quantitative data—'t' test, 'z' test, ANOVA.
2. Qualitative data—'chi-square' test, Kruskal—Wallis test, etc.

According to Probability Distribution

1. Normal distribution—'z' test.
2. Near normal distribution—'t' distribution—Student's 't' test.
   - Chi-square distribution—chi-square test.
   - Fisher's distribution—Fisher's 'f' test.

According to Number of Samples to be Compared

1. Comparison between two samples—'t' test, 'z' test, chi-square test.
2. Comparison between more than two samples 'chi-square test' (for qualitative data) 'ANOVA (analysis of variance) test' (for quantitative data).
3. The tests of significance most commonly used to analyze small samples are:

Student's 't' test: for comparing two quantitative data and is further of two types:

1. Paired student's 't' test.
2. Unpaired student's 't' test

Chi-square test—generally for qualitative data.

Others are:

- Non-parametric tests—Mann-Whitney, Wilcoxon's rank sum test, Kendall's 'S' test, McNemar's test, etc.
- ANOVA test, Fisher's 'f' test, etc.

Example: Hb levels of 72 boys and 54 girls students of MBBS 2004 were as depicted as below:

- Test whether the mean Hb levels of boys and girls differ or not.
- Mean Hb levels for girls (X) =

$$\frac{10 + 11 + \ldots\ldots + 9.5 - 11}{54} = \frac{561.50}{54} = 10.39 \text{ g\%}$$

- Mean Hb levels for boys (Y) =

$$\frac{10 + 17.5 + \ldots\ldots + 14 + 14}{72} = \frac{1043.20}{72} = 14.49 \text{ g\%}$$

Assumptions: The sample is adequate and we assume that Hb levels among boys and girls do not differ from one another.

Hypothesis

Null Hypothesis

There is no significant difference between the mean Hb levels of boys and girls.

Hb levels of 126 students of MBBS 2004 batch
Girls (X):
10,11,12.5,10.5,12,10,12.5,11.5,11,10.4,10,9.3,11,11,9.5,11,10.5, 11.5,10,9.5,11.2,11,9.2,9.2,10,10.8,11,10.5,10.1,9,10,9.5,12,10.5, 11,10,10,10,10,10.3,10,9,11,9.5,9.5,8.5,9,10.5,10.5,10.5,12,11,9.5, 11
Boys (Y):
10,17.5,14.2,15,14.1,14,14.5,14.7,14.5,13.5,14.5, 14.5,14,15,16, 14,14,15.2,14.2,14,14.2,14,14,14.8,14,14.5,13.3,15.5,14.5,15, 15.5,14.2,14.8,14,14,15.2,14,15,14,14,15,14.2,14.5,15.2,14,14.8, 15.2,14.6,14.7,14.2,14,13.9,14.9,14.5,14.5,14.5,14.5,14.1,15.3, 14.5,14.7,15,14.5,14.2,17,14.7,14.5,14.6,13.8,14.2,15,14

Alternative Hypothesis

Mean Hb levels of boys and girls differ significantly.

9

Level of significance for testing above mentioned hypothesis is fixed at 95%

Choosing a test criterion and a test of significance. Test criterion chosen for hypothesis testing is the mean and as the data are appropriate and quantitative, so test of significance chosen is:

Unpaired 't' test/'z' test.

$$\text{'t' statistic} = \frac{\overline{X}_1 - \overline{X}_2}{s_p\sqrt{(1/n_1) + (1/n_2)}}$$

$$\text{Standard deviation of Hb levels of girls} = \sqrt{\frac{\Sigma(X - \overline{X})^2}{N_{1-1}}}$$

$$\frac{\sqrt{(10-10.39)^2 + (11-10.39)^2 + \ldots\ldots + (11-10.39)^2}}{54 - 1} = 0.9117$$

$$\text{Similarly, SD of Hb levels of boys} = \sqrt{\frac{\Sigma(y - \overline{y})^2}{N_{2-1}}}$$

$$\frac{\sqrt{(10-14.4)^2 + (17.5-14.4)^2 + \ldots\ldots + (14-14.4)^2}}{72 - 1} = 0.8642$$

$n_1 + n_2 - 2 = 54 + 72 - 2 = 124$ df

In boys $\overline{Y} = 14.49$ and $s_1 = 0.8642$

In girls $\overline{X} = 10.39$ and $s_2 = 0.9117$

The pooled estimate: Sp = Pooled standard deviation

$$s_p = \sqrt{\frac{(n_1-1)s_1^2 + (n_2-1)s_2^2}{n_1 + n_2 - 2}} = \sqrt{\frac{(54-1)\times(0.86)^2 + (72-1)\times(0.91)^2}{52 + 74 - 2}}$$

$$= \sqrt{\frac{52.51 + 43.88}{124}} = \sqrt{\frac{96.39}{124}} = \sqrt{0.777} = 0.9$$

$$\text{'t' statistic} = \frac{10.39 - 14.49}{0.9\sqrt{(1/54 + 1/72)}} = \frac{-4.10}{0.9\sqrt{(0.0139 + 0.0185)}}$$

$$\frac{-4.10}{0.9\sqrt{(0.0324)}} = -25.37$$

Degree of freedom = 54 + 72 − 2 = 124

Table value of 't' statistic at 124 degree of freedom is 1.98.

't' calculated is >'t' critical

So, the difference is real and significant and hence, null hypothesis is rejected and alternative hypothesis is accepted.

Results: The Hb levels of boys and girls in MBBS 2004 batch differ significantly at $p < 0.05$.

Chi-square Test

- It is a type of non-parametric test.
- Not based on any assumption of any variable.
- Developed by Karl Pearson.
- Important applications of this tests of significance are as a test of:
  - Proportions
  - Association
  - Goodness of fit

Assumptions to be fulfilled:

1. Sample must be random.
2. Data should be qualitative.
3. Sample size should be > 30.
4. Data collected should be tabulated in the form of cross tabulation 2 × 2 contingency table.
5. If sample size is less than 30 then also chi-square test can be applied but only with Yates correction (in 2 × 2 tables) but can only be applied when the expected frequency in each cell is more than 5.
6. If the sample size is small and the expected frequency in any cell comes out to be less, then chi-square test (in 2 × 2 tables) can be applied but with a modification of Fisher's exact test.

Important Steps

1. Prepare 2 × 2 contingency table.
2. Calculation of expected value for each cell: Expected value for each cell can be calculated by the following formula.

$$E = \frac{\text{Corresponding row total} \times \text{Corresponding column total}}{\text{Grand total}}$$

3. 'Chi-square' statistic is calculated by the formula.

$$\text{Chi-square value } (\chi^2) = \frac{(O - E)^2}{E}$$

Where O = Observed value of the cell.

E = Expected value of the cell.

4. Fourth important step is to find out degrees of freedom so that comparison can be made with the table value corresponding to calculated degree of freedom.

Degree of freedom (df) = (R − 1) × (C − 1)

Where R = Number of rows.

C = Number of columns.

Example

The following data correspond to number of patients who were given treatment for tuberculosis under DOTS strategy and under non-DOTS strategy with corresponding number of cured patients.

Total patients = 310

Null hypothesis: Cure rate with DOTS and non-DOTS do not differ significantly in our study.

Alternative hypothesis: Cure rates for tuberculosis in patients receiving treatment under DOTS and non-DOTS strategy respectively differ significantly.

Levels of significance: Fixed at 95% level.

Selection of test criterion: Expected cure rate is the test criterion and test of significance chosen is 'chi-square' test because:

- Data is qualitative.
- Sample size > 30.
- Data tabulated in the form of cross tabulation.
- We want to test association between DOTS and non-DOTS strategy-cure rates.

Solutions/Computations

Table 9.8: Treatment outcome with DOTS and Non-DOTS

Treatment outcome	*DOTS*	*Non-DOTS*	*Total*
Cured	140	90	230
Not cured	20	60	80
Total	**160**	**150**	**310**

$$\text{Expected value of 1st cell} = \frac{\text{RT} \times \text{CT}}{\text{Grand total}} = \frac{230 \times 160}{310} = 118.7$$

say = 119

Similarly, expected values of other cells are calculated.

Treatment outcome	*DOTS*	*Non-DOTS*	*Total*
Cured	140 (119)	90 (111)	230
Not cured	20 (41)	60 (39)	80
Total	**160**	**150**	**310**

Note: Figures in parenthesis are expected values.

$$\text{Chi-square value for 1st cell} = \frac{(O - E)^2}{E} = \frac{(140 - 119)^2}{119}$$

$$= \frac{21^2}{119} = \frac{441}{119} = 3.7$$

and similarly chi-square value for other cells

$$= \frac{(90 - 111)^2}{111}, \frac{(20 - 41)^2}{41}, \frac{(60 - 39)^2}{39}$$

= 3.9, 10.7, 11.3 respectively.

Total chi-square value = 3.7 + 3.9 + 10.7 + 11.3 = 29.6

Degree of freedom = (R – 1) × (C – 1)

= (2 – 1) × (2 – 1) = 1 × 1 = 1

Making Comparisons

Table value of chi-square at degree of freedom '1' and 95% level of significance (i.e. $p = 0.05$) = 3.84.

Calculated chi-square value is 29.6 and is > 3.84.

Hence, the null hypothesis is rejected.

- Alternative hypothesis is not rejected.

Conclusions: There is a significant difference in the cure rates in patients of TB who were given treatment under DOTS and non-DOTS strategy.

DOTS regime achieves significant high cure rates in tuberculosis.

Non-parametric Tests

Most of the statistical tests of significance which we use require some important assumptions to be fulfilled, e.g.

- Distribution of random variable—either normal or near normal type of distribution.
- Estimations are based on meaningful sample statistic called a—parameter and testing of the hypothesis is generally based on these estimated parameters.
- But in several studies, these assumptions are not fulfilled, i.e. distribution of a random variable is markedly skewed and sample size of the study group is very small and estimation with respect to a particular parameter does not hold true and cannot be used as a basis of significance. So, for analyses of these types of study samples, different type of tests of significance are required, these are called distribution free or non-parametric tests.

Important non-parametric tests are as follows:

1. Chi-square test.
2. Sign test.
3. Rank sum test.
   - Mann-Whitney 'U' test.
   - Wilcoxon's rank sum test.
   - Kendall's 'S' test.
4. Rank correlation tests.

The most common of these tests is chi-square test (discussed earlier). The other important test is Spearman's rank correlation test.

Spearman's rank correlation coefficient: If we have a sample of individuals and we have two sets of values of observations of these n individuals then to see the correlation if it exists or not between these two sets of observations we calculate Spearman's rank correlation coefficient (r_s) and is calculated as:

$$r_s = 1 - \frac{6\sum_{i=1}^{n} d_i^2}{n(n^2 - 1)}$$

$$= 1 - \frac{6\sum d^2}{n^3 - n}$$

Where n = No. of individuals

d = Difference in paired ranks.

So, 1st ranks are allotted to observations according to their ranking in that particular lot.

Then pairing of ranks is done and difference 'd' is calculated, e.g. height and weight of 10 students of a class are as follows in Table 9.9.

Table 9.9: Height and weight ranks of 10 students

Students	A	B	C	D	E	F	G	H	I	J
Ht (in cm)	158	155	166	154	161	156	160	168	170	171
Wt (kg)	55	56	58	54	62	60	61	63	59	64
Ranking (Ht)	7	9	4	10	5	8	6	3	2	1
Ranking (Wt)	9	8	7	10	3	5	4	2	6	1
d^2	4	1	9	0	4	9	4	1	16	0

Spearman's rank correlation coefficient

$$(r_s) = 1 - \frac{6(4+1+9+0+4+9+4+1+16+0)}{10^3 - 10}$$

$$= 1 - \frac{6 \times 48}{990} = \frac{990 - 288}{990} = \frac{692}{990} = 0.698$$

Conclusion: Height and weight have positive linear correlation.

Regression

Regression analysis can be thought of as finding the best mathematical model for predicting one variable from another. One variable is considered to be dependent variable, its value varying according to one or more independent variables. The most common form of regression is linear regression in which the mathematical model is a straight line; the regression equation is the equation of the straight line that best fits the data.

Given data on a dependant variable *Y*, an independent variable *X*, regression analysis involves finding the "best" mathematical model to describe *Y* as a function of *X* or predict *Y* from *X*.

Uses

Regression analysis is a measure of the nature of association between two quantitative variables, e.g. age and blood pressure, gestational age and head circumference of newborn. Knowledge of this association helps predicting more accurately the value of the characteristic of an individual, when the value of other characteristic of that individual is known. Regression analysis helps in determining nature of association and prediction in conditions like:

Age of person and blood pressure, effect of temperature and heart rate, protein intake and growth rate of young children, intake of iron and folic acid in diet or as supplement and haemoglobin level, age and weight/height of young children.

Scatter Diagram

The weight-for-age of 12 preschool children is plotted on weight-for-age chart, we get 12 dots. These twelve dots follow a tendency on scatter diagram to cluster along a straight line, which we call as "regression line". This kind of relationship is linear relationship, i.e. as the age increases the weight also increases (Fig. 9.9). It depicts strong positive correlation. Thus, the scatter diagram indicates the nature and strength of the relationship.

The relationship could be strong negative correlation as depicted below (Fig. 9.10).

Regression equation : $Y = a + bx$

It is used to describe the dependence of one quantitative variable (*Y*) upon the other variable (*x*), while *a* and *b* are constants computed from data, *b* is the regression coefficient of *Y* on *x*.

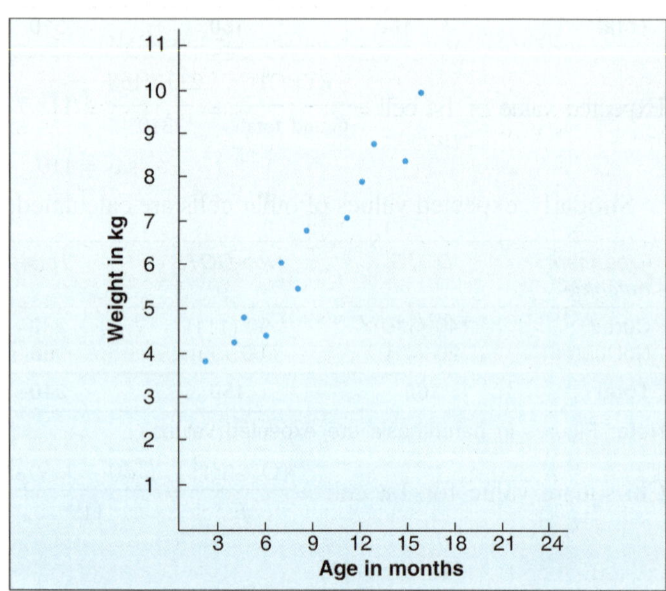

Fig. 9.9: Age and weight scatter of 12 healthy children

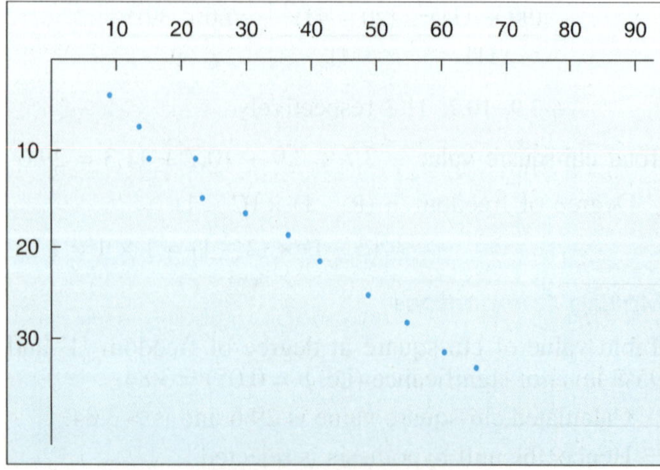

Fig. 9.10: Strong negative correlation

9

Pearson coefficient correlation (ϒ)

Pearson correlation coefficient is used as a measure of strength and direction of linear relationship. It has certain properties.

- Unit free (the coefficient r is an absolute number)
- Independent of change of origin and scale.
- Lies between – 1 and + 1.

It measures the strength of association between two quantitative variables. There are several limitations of Pearson coefficient correlation. It may conclude no relationship from zero correlation, while in fact strong nonlinear relationship may exist.

LIFE TABLE

Life table is a summary measure of age and sex specific deaths in a community (country). From life table, we can derive expectation of life at particular age (say at birth, at 1,2... and age 70, etc.). Expectation of life is defined as the estimated number of years a person is expected to live beyond certain age if he/she is exposed to current risk of mortality at different ages.

Uses

1. One important use is to determine expectation of life in a country. This is an important positive indicator of health status of a community. On the basis of life expectancy, we can compare the health status of one country with the other.
2. We can determine the number of survivors at different ages, which have several applications like old age pension, voters, number of women entering in reproductive health, children requiring schooling, basis of success of life insurance policies and number of adolescents requiring services.
3. Life table method of analysis is used for cohort studies in medicine/health. To know survival rates after cancer or other long-term diseases like diabetes, hypertension and stroke and coronary heart disease.
4. Life table can be used to calculate the Years of Potential Life Lost (YPLL) and to calculate disability adjusted life years, i.e. DALY. If the life expectancy of a person is 63 years at birth and he dies of heart attack at 50, then he has lost 13 years of potential life as a result of premature death.

CONSTRUCTION OF LIFE TABLE AND ITS PROPERTIES

***Principle*:** The life tables are constructed after each census (once in 10 years). We usually follow a cohort of 1,00,000 newborn babies and follow them through various ages (0, 1, 2, 3, 4, 5....15....25...75) till all die. During the course of follow-up, we also determine the number of persons surviving at exact age "x" and the total number of person years lived, to arrive at an average expectation of life.

For construction of life tables, the two basic things required are:

1. Actual population living in the specific age groups in the selected time.
2. Number of deaths occurring in these age groups in the given selected time.

Construction of life table rests on the assumption that the two distinct age patterns of mortality, i.e. observed and the standard patterns are related to each other.

The life table for the females for India is shown in Table 9.10 (WHO, 2002).

Column I (x to $x + n$)

Describes the age group intervals. The first one is 0–1 year, next is 1–4 years and then subsequent age group intervals are of 5 years each till 99 age and the last one is open ended interval with age group of 100 and above.

First two age intervals are divided so, because the mortality rate vary very significantly in first 5 years of age and we cannot assume the death rate to be equal for initial 5 years of life. Subsequently, grouping is done assuming the mortality remains equal for a particular age group interval.

Column 2 (l_x)

It is the cohort, who start their life at birth. It is hypothetical number. It is 1,00,000. This indicates the cohort who survives at exact age x, e.g. at birth this is 1,00,000 and at 1–4 years it is 93,623.

Column 3 (q_x)

It is the probability of dying at that age or it is the age specific death rate to which the cohort of life table is exposed to, e.g. in age group 0–1 year or during the first year of life the probability of death (infant mortality) is 63 / 1000 live births.

Column 4 (d_x)

The number of deaths, i.e. 6377 is arrived at by applying current infant mortality rate of 0.0638 to 1,00,000 which is approximately 6377 per 1,00,000. The survivors at the end of that age would be 93,623 (who live to see their first birth day).

Column 5 (L_x)

This column provides the information on number of person years survived/lived by individuals in different age intervals. For example, during age interval 0–1 year 93,623 individuals survived at the end of one year, since each of these 93,623 persons survives for one year period, contributes 93,623 × 1 year = 93,623 person years. Of 6377 infants who died, did not experience the mortality at one point in time and each one probably survived on an average of 3 months and hence contributed survival period of 1638 years. Therefore, if we add 1638 to 93,623 person years lived by individuals we get a total of 94,261 person years

Table 9.10: Life table for the females in India (2000) [Abridged Version]

1 Age (x to x + n)	2 l_x	3 $_nq_x$	4 $_nd_x$	5 $_nL_x$	6 T_x	7 e^0_x
0–1	1,00,000	0.0638	6,377	94,261	62,68,417	62.7
1–4	93,623	0.0376	3,524	3,66,035	61,74,156	65.9
5–9	90,099	0.0125	1,128	4,47,675	58,08,121	64.5
10–14	88,971	0.0066	588	4,43,384	53,60,446	60.2
15–19	88,383	0.0103	907	4,39,645	49,17,062	55.6
20–24	87,475	0.0139	1,213	4,34,345	44,77,417	51.2
25–29	86,263	0.0145	1,247	4,28,194	40,43,072	46.9
30–34	85,015	0.0151	1,281	4,21,874	36,14,878	42.5
35–39	83,735	0.0159	1,334	4,15,339	31,93,004	38.1
40–44	82,401	0.0222	1,883	4,07,421	27,77,665	33.7
45–49	80,568	0.0320	2,577	3,96,396	23,70,244	29.4
50–54	77,991	0.0440	3,432	3,81,374	19,73,848	25.3
55–59	74,559	0.0673	5,020	3,60,243	15,92,474	21.4
60–64	69,539	0.0998	6,937	3,30,350	12,32,231	17.7
65–69	62,601	0.1514	9,475	2,89,318	9,01,881	14.4
70–74	53,126	0.2173	11,545	2,36,767	6,12,563	11.5
75–79	41,581	0.3075	12,786	1,75,938	3,75,796	9.0
80–84	28,795	0.4262	12,273	1,13,290	1,99,858	6.9
85–89	16,522	0.5698	9,441	59,080	86,568	5.2
90–94	7,110	0.6824	4,852	20,996	27,488	3.9
95–99	2,258	0.8300	1,875	5,669	6,492	2.9
100+	384	1.000	384	823	823	2.1

Source: World mortality in 2000: life tables for 191 countries; WHO, 2002[1]

lived during 0–1 year age interval. Similarly, at age interval 60–64 there were 69,539 individuals alive at the beginning of this interval of these 69,539 persons 62,601 were still alive at the end of 64 years, since each of these 62,601 persons survives the entire period of 5 years. Contributes 62,601 × 5 = 3,13,005 person years, plus the person years contributed by those who died in 5 years in this age interval and adding these years to 3,13,005 person years we will get total of 3,30,350 person years lived in the age interval 60–64.

Column 6 (T_x)

It denotes total number of person years lived beyond their xth birthday by l_x persons alive on that birthday. It is obtained by summing column 5 from bottom upward.

Column 7 ($e^0{}_x$)

This gives the expectancy of life at the start of a particular age group, x.

Life expectancy at birth is expressed as:

$$e^0_o = \frac{\text{(Total number of person years lived after age x)}}{\text{Number of starters/survivors to age x}}$$

In the table under reference (life expectancy at birth) $= \frac{\text{Total number of person years lived } (T_0)}{\text{No. of starters } (l_0)}$

$$= \frac{6268417}{100,000} = 62.68 = 62.7 \text{ years}$$

$$\text{Life expectancy at age x} = \frac{T_x}{l_x}$$

$$= \frac{\text{Total number of person years lived beyond age x}}{\text{No. of persons entering the cohort at age x}}$$

$$\text{Life expectancy at age 1 year} = \frac{61,74,156}{93,623} = 65.9 \text{ yrs}$$

Similarly life expectancy at age 60 years

$$= \frac{\text{Total person years lived beyond age 60}}{\text{Persons entering the cohort at 60 years}}$$

$$= \frac{12,32,231}{69,539} = 17.7 \text{ years}$$

9

REFERENCE

1 WHO. World Mortality in 2002. Geneva: WHO; 2002.

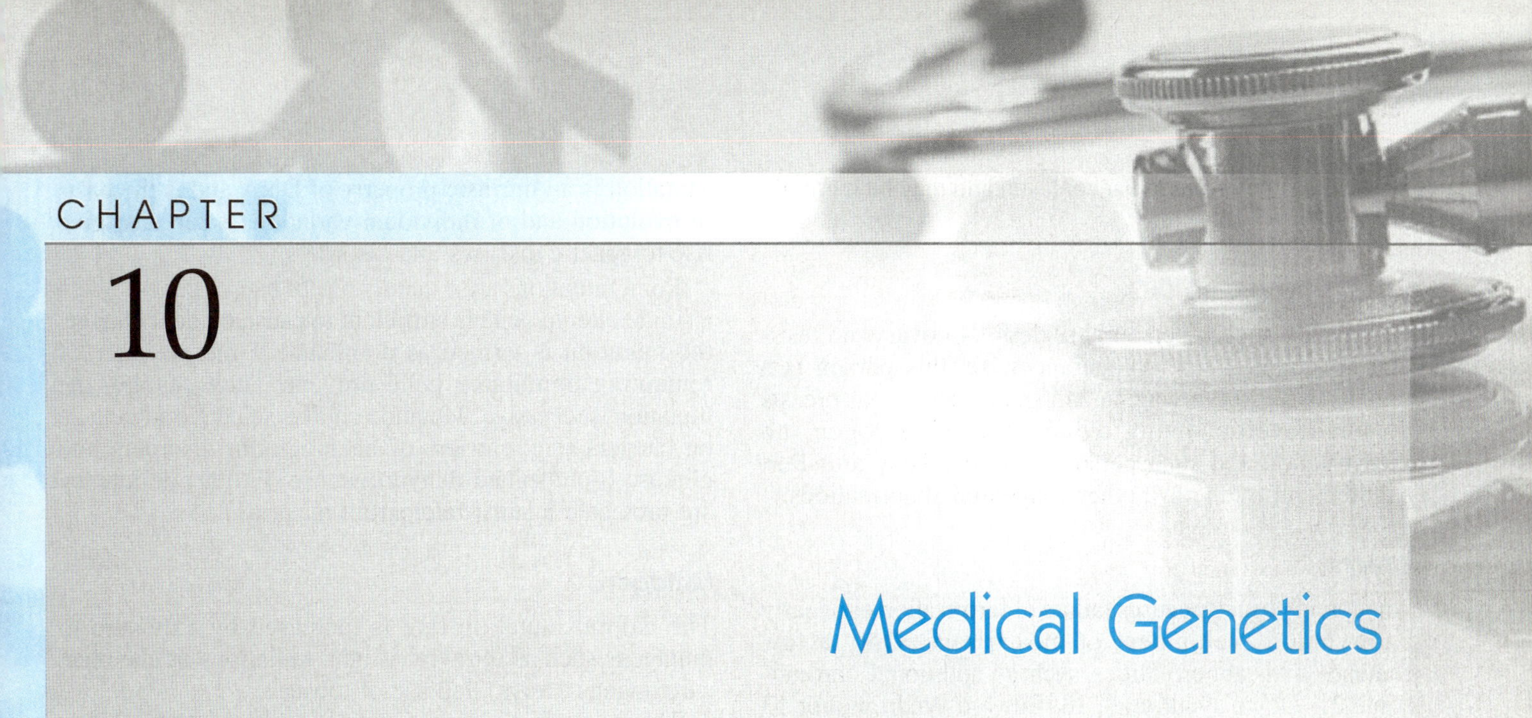

CHAPTER 10

Medical Genetics

INTRODUCTION

The major application of medical genetics is control of hereditary diseases. Research on human DNA is being coordinated internationally. The main medical application of DNA technology at present is in the diagnosis of genetic disorders, genetic counselling, screening and prevention of hereditary diseases.[1]

Nucleic acids are of two kinds; deoxyribonucleic acid (DNA) and ribonucleic acid (RNA). The DNA is the basis of life. DNA is found within the nucleus and mitochondria and RNA is found in cytoplasm. DNA is responsible for synthesis of RNA, duplication, and genetic copying and mutation. RNA synthesizes proteins.

Most human DNA is contained in 23 pairs of chromosomes in the cell nucleus. Each chromosome consists of a single DNA molecule associated with proteins. DNA is not confined to the nucleus, however, mitochondria also has an independent and characteristic DNA complement, inherited only through the mother.

Human beings have 46 (23 pairs) chromosomes of which 44 are autosomes and the rest two are sex chromosomes. In male, these sex chromosomes are XY and in female XX. The male and female chromosomal pattern can be depicted as 44 + XY = 46 and 44 + XX = 46

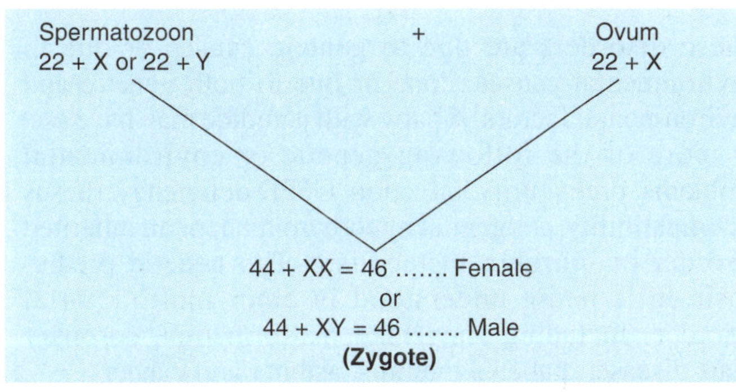

respectively. Due to reduction cell division (meiosis), in male and female gamete (spermatozoon and ovum) a gamete will contain 22 autosomes + 1 sex chromosome. In case of spermatozoon, it is 22 + X or 22 + Y and in case of ovum it is always 22 + X.

Thus, the spermatozoon (not the ovum) is the sex determinant factor.

Chromosomal Abnormalities

Two full chromosome sets are required for balanced gene expression leading to normal embryonic development and functioning. However, errors of cell division leading to aneuploidy (one or more chromosomes present in the many or too few copies) are common during gamete formation.

Normally, the unfertilized ovum should contain after reduction division 22 + X number of chromosomes, however, if the reduction of sex chromosome fails to occur, it will be 22 + XX. If such an ovum fertilizes spermatozoon of 22 + Y it can lead to:

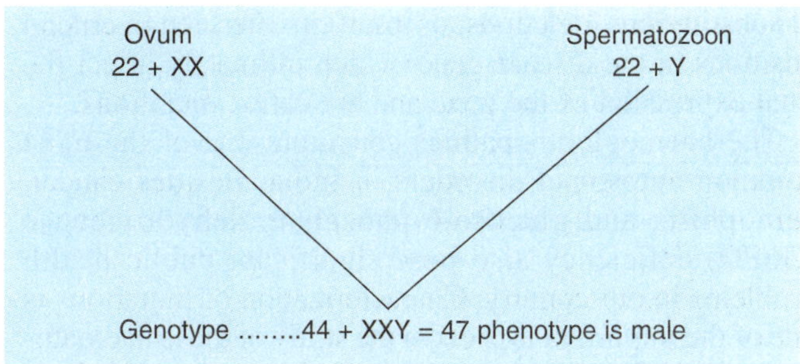

This is called Klinefelter's syndrome (XXY).

The person is genetically female because of presence of two X chromosomes. Phenotype of this individual is male (outward appearance) the penis, testis, vas, seminal vesicles are small with no spermatogenesis (sterility).

Sometimes they have gynaecomastia and may be mentally retarded.

Turner's Syndrome (XO)

Genetically such a person is sexless. No ovary, no testis and no gonadal sex. Appearancewise, this person is a female (have vulva, vagina and small uterus) but breasts do not develop owing to absence of estrogen, no menstruation and such person is sterile. They are short statured and often have other congenital abnormalities.

Effects

Aneuploidy usually causes failure of fertilization or of early embryonic development or miscarriage. Only a few foetuses with abnormalities such as additional chromosome 21 (Down syndrome), 18 (Edward syndrome) or 13 (Patau syndrome) or an additional, or missing sex chromosome, survive to birth.[2]

The frequency of chromosomal aneuploidy and hence of spontaneous abortions and of chromosomally abnormal infants, increases with maternal age.

Chromosomal rearrangements, in which two chromosomes exchange unequal proportion of their DNA, can also occur during gamete formation, and hence, is another important cause of genetic disease.

Demographic factors influence the incidence of chromosomal disorders because of their relationship with advanced maternal age. Where women continue having children up to the end of reproductive life, the birth incidence of chromosomal disorders may reach 6/1000 and of children with **Down syndrome** about 3/1000. Family planning and bearing children at appropriate age reduces the incidence of Down syndrome by 30–60%.

Mutation of Gene

In normal individual, several variations are seen in the genomic DNA sequence which are called polymorphisms. In individuals with genetic disorders, variations in the form of substitutions, deletions, or insertions are seen in crucial positions in the disease gene, which ultimately affect the final expression of the gene and are called mutations.

The haemoglobinopathies constitute one of the most common autosomal disorders in India. Besides cancer, hemophilia and glucose-6-phosphate dehydrogenase (G6PD) deficiency also pose significant public health problems in our country. Characterization of mutations is one of the important aspects in the study of these haematological disorders. Several powerful and sensitive molecular techniques are available to diagnose these disorders.

A mutation is a spontaneous change in the sequence or the complement of DNA. There are two broad groups of mutations, namely chromosomal abnormalities which are changes in chromosome number or arrangement and point mutation; which are changes in the sequence of DNA bases.

Mutation is an intrinsic property of DNA and is the basis of evolution and of individual variation, it can also give rise to genetic diseases and disorders.

Point mutations arise in only one of pair of genes. When a single altered gene is sufficient to cause evident change, the mutation is termed as dominant; if the presence of remaining unmutated gene prevents such change, the mutation is recessive. Mutation confers selective advantage on carriers (e.g. carriers of haemoglobin disorders and glucose-6-phosphate dehydrogenase (G6PD) deficiency are protected against falciparum malaria).

Mutagens

The natural mutation rate is increased by exposure to mutagens such as ultraviolet light, radiations or chemical carcinogens (drugs) and use of tobacco.

The frequency of mutation rises with parental age.

Genetic Diagnosis

- By taking family history in detail—as genetic disorders are inherited from parents to offsprings.
- By biochemical methods to detect marker or presence or absence of a particular protein.
- By molecular genetic and changes in DNA.

Single Gene Disorders

Single gene disorders are important causes of fatal or chronically disabling disease especially in childhood and have led to the development of the modern biochemical and DNA methods for investigating the genetic component in more common and complex disease categories.

Example: Huntington disease, haemophilia, phenylketonuria (PKU) follow clear-cut inheritance pattern that directly reflect the transmission of the abnormal gene.

The number of single gene disorders is very large more than 6000 are now known. When the gene involved is known, it may be possible to offer definitive carrier tests (biochemical or DNA) to determine which relatives are, and which are not carriers of mutated gene. Carrier then may choose different options to avoid passing of disorder to their offspring.

Multifactorial Disorders

These disorders are due to genetic causes or due to environmental causes alone or due to both genetic and environmental factors. A baby with jaundice may have one or more of the following genetic or environmental problems; prematurity, infection, G6PD deficiency, rhesus incompatibility, congenital hypothyroidism or an inherited disorder of bilirubin metabolism. The genetic predisposition is being understood in other multifactorial disorders including congenital malformation, coronary heart disease, diabetes mellitus, asthma and cancer.

Dominant Inheritance

Everyone inheriting a gene for dominant disorder is likely to be affected. Severe early onset dominant disorders (e.g. osteogenesis imperfecta or brittle bone disease) are caused by new mutations, arise without previous family history and are not passed onto descendants because they are fatal in early life. Parents of the affected child have a very low risk of the disorder recurring in subsequent pregnancies. Dominant conditions transmitted in families are usually of late onset, after reproductive age is reached (e.g. Huntington disease, adult polycystic disease of the kidney, family cancer syndromes, tuberous sclerosis, neurofibromatosis). Carriers of dominant genes have a very high reproductive risk, each of their children has 50% chance of inheriting the gene and suffering from the same disorder.

Recessive Inheritance

Recessive inherited disorders include haemoglobin disorder, cystic fibrosis, phenylketonuria and Werdnig-Hoffmann disease. Carriers are healthy themselves but have a reproductive risk. When partner carry the same mutated gene there is 1 in 4 chances in each pregnancy, that the child will suffer from the disorder. Most people carry one or two lethal recessive mutations, but these are usually transmitted through many generations without causing disease. Most children with a recessively inherited disease do not have a family history. About 50% of their first degree relatives will be carriers, but only a tiny fraction of the carriers present in the population can be identified by testing family members. Therefore, when a condition is common and carrier screening is feasible and useful, it is appropriate to offer it at the population level.

X-linked Inheritance

Most mutations on the X chromosome are transmitted through unaffected carrier females (with the X chromosomes) and affect mainly, but not exclusively males. Examples include hemophilia, Duchenne muscular dystrophy, fragile X mental retardation and glucose-6-phosphate dehydrogenase deficiency. In principle, about 60% of carriers of X-linked disorders might be detected by family studies, but a family history may be absent if the disorder has been transmitted in the female line for several generations or is the result of a new mutation. Female carriers are at high genetic risk, in each pregnancy there is a 25% risk of an affected son and 25% risk of a carrier daughter.

EPIDEMIOLOGY OF GENETIC DISORDERS AND SERVICES

Congenital Abnormalities and Genetic Disorders

Many environmental agents are known to cause congenital disorders "An agent which causes congenital abnormalities is called *teratogen*". Common teratogens include maternal infection with rubella, radiation during pregnancy, tobacco use and treatment with drugs during pregnancy.

The incidence and burden of congenital abnormalities is increasing. Out of every 100 babies born in India annually, 6 to 7 have a birth defect. In Indian context this would translate to 1.7 million birth defects annually out of 26 million births. This would account for 9.6% of all newborn deaths. Around 2 lakh babies are born with congenital rubella syndrome every year. Appropriate prevention and treatment strategies need to be developed (Table 10.1).

Haemoglobin disorders and G6PD deficiency are commonest single gene disorders. The carriers are protected against *Plasmodium falciparum* malaria. Both types of genetic disorders are endemic in tropics and subtropics and migration has distributed them widely. Haemoglobin disorders are often the first genetic condition to be recognized as public health problem in developing countries.

Consanguineous Marriages (Marriage between Cousins)

It is favoured by at least 20% of the world's population and probably more. This social *custom/practice* increases the risk of congenital malformation, stillbirth and childhood death. It increases the birth incidence of children with recessively inherited disorders.

Management of congenital disorders is by advanced surgical intervention, and it can treat about 40% of children and other diseases require social support and rehabilitation.

Prevention

It includes: Adopting contraception to limit the size of family (family planning), optimal maternal nutrition, prevention of rubella by immunization, genetic diagnosis and family counselling, early diagnosis and treatment when possible (e.g. for congenital malformations, phenylketonuria (PKU), congenital hypothyroidism, sickle cell disease) and prenatal diagnosis. It is estimated that use of all these approaches could prevent more than 75% of congenital abnormalities.

ROLE OF GENETIC PREDISPOSITION IN COMMON DISORDERS

Research related to human genome project will eventually lead to the identification of every gene that contributes to susceptibility or resistance to disease.

Recent progress in molecular genetics has shown that inherited predisposition is important in a number of common diseases which normally manifest in later life such as atherosclerosis, coronary heart disease, hypertension, diabetes mellitus and some rheumatic, oncological and mental illnesses, which appear at an early age and develop into severe disabilities in predisposed people.

Coronary Heart Disease

More recently risk factors identified include high levels of fibrinogen and possibly also homocystine (both of which

Table 10.1: Incidence of genetic disorders and congenital abnormalities up to the age of 30 years in a typical developed country[3]

Categories	*Estimates births per 1000*	*Commonest diagnosis*
Single gene disorders	**10.0**	
1. Dominant	7.0	• Familial hypercholesterolaemia • Adult polycystic disease of the kidney • Huntington disease • Neurofibromatosis • Chondrodystrophy
2. X-linked	1.33	• Muscular dystrophy • Haemophilia and Christmas disease • Colour vision disorders • X-linked mental retardation • Glutathione deficiency
3. Recessive	1.66	• Cystic fibrosis • Phenylketonuria • Amino acid disorders • Werdnig-Hoffmann disease • Thalassaemias
Chromosomal	**3.49**	
1. Autosomes	1.69	• >70% Down syndrome
2. Sex chromosomes	1.80	• Mostly Klinefelter and Turner syndrome
Congenital abnormalities	**52.80**	
1. Genetic component	26.60	• Congenital heart disease • Club foot • Congenital dislocation of hip • Pyloric stenosis • Cleft palate/lip
2. No genetic component	26.20	
Other multifactorial	**10.06**	• Strabismus • Inguinal hernia • Epilepsy • Diabetes • Mild mental retardation
Genetic unknown type	**1.20**	
Total genetic	51.34	
Total genetic + non-genetic congenital abnormalities	77.54	

Source: WHO Tech. Report Series 865.

are genetically influenced), high level of lipoprotein [Lp(a)] and apolipoprotein E4 (ApoE4) and polymorphism of apolipoprotein E. Non-apolipoprotein "candidate" genes (e.g. angiotensinogen converting enzyme-1) have also been identified. Similarly, genetic predisposition may be involved in as many as 10–25% of cases of cancer of colon and breast. At least one relatively common gene probably on chromosome 17, is known to predispose to breast cancer. A careful family history is a must in these cancers. Screening of relatives of breast and colon cancer for early detection and prompt treatment may be helpful.

Asthma

Asthma and allergy have a strong familial tendency and a specific gene that affects plasma level of IgE may contribute to susceptibility.

Diabetes Mellitus

Evidence for genetic element in IDDM comes from studies that show a higher concordance in identical twins (25–30%) than in non-identical twins (5–10%). Similarly, prevalence of IDDM is 3–6% among first degree relatives of people with disease, compared with 0.2–0.5% among the general population. Genes on the short arm of chromosomes, either within or close to the major histocompatibility (HLA) region are primarily responsible for genetic predisposition. Diabetes thus has strong familial tendency. Gene therapy and transplantation of pancreatic tissue may be future biological treatment.

Mental Disorders

Some mental disorders occur preferentially in people with inherited predisposition. Research continues for detection of responsible gene.

Alzheimer's Disease

A strong association has been found between the ApoE4 polymorphism on chromosome 19 and late onset Alzheimer's disease. The ApoE4 protein may participate in the disease process and homozygotes are at very high-risk of developing Alzheimer's disease by the age of 80.[1,3]

Approaches for Prevention

The various approaches for prevention of congenital and genetic disorders are given below.

Basic Public Health Measures

1. ***Rh group:*** Screening of women for rhesus blood groups (Rh group) allows appropriate management of at risk programmes by giving Rh negative women anti-D antibody after childbirth, miscarriage or termination of pregnancy. Perinatal mortality and chronic problems of rhesus hemolytic disease have significantly decreased in most developed countries by appropriate management (Table 10.2).
2. ***Congenital rubella:*** It can be prevented by immunizing children and non-pregnant women and routine testing of pregnant women for antibody; abortion is usually offered to women infected in early pregnancy. The incidence of congenital rubella has declined in Europe from 3.5 to 0.41% per 1,00,000 (Table 10.2).
3. ***Congenital toxoplasmosis:*** It can be prevented by advising pregnant women to eat only well-cooked meat and avoid contact with cat faeces. In some areas, vulnerable women are identified by antibody screening followed by surveillance (TORCH test explained elsewhere). Pregnant women and newborn infants with evidence of infection are treated with antibiotics to prevent damage to eye or brain from primary and later reactivated infection.
4. ***Risk of neural tube defects:*** Use of folic acid is promoted in planned pregnancies during the periconception phase (three months before and three months after conception) which can prevent neural tube defects and other congenital anamolies. National programme for prevention and control of anaemia in India helps to prevent these defects as all pregnant women are provided with iron and folic acid prophylaxis.
5. Pregnant woman with insulin dependent diabetes have an increased risk of bearing severely malformed child but this can be greatly reduced by meticulous control of blood sugar. A similar risk is associated with certain anti-epileptic drugs. Mothers with either risk are candidates for expert scanning for foetal abnormalities during second trimester.
6. ***G6PD deficiency:*** The incidence of newborn jaundice and exchange transfusion can be greatly reduced by screening of neonates, exposure of babies to light and education of population not to feed broad beans (which provokes a clinical reaction in G6PD deficiency) to children.

The stillbirths and neonatal deaths should be examined for an evidence of genetic problem to prevent further deaths. Measures like healthy diet and lifestyle may be rewarding.

Detection of Genetic Risks by Population Screening

Sporadic Disorders

It includes most congenital malformations and chromosomal disorders, the vast majority of affected children are born to parents with no known risk factor and the risk of recurrence is low.

It is essential to identify people at risk of developing disorder themselves and/or of passing a disorder onto their children. Population screening is helpful and reliable. There is usually a moderately increased risk for people with an affected relative, 1–6% in most multifactorial disorders, 1–2% for chromosomal disorders and women with IDDM.

Various screening programmes focus on preconception, antenatal, neonatal and for general population. Screening can be helpful in reducing the risk to foetus and identification of risk couples and affected foetus and for early detection and treatment.

Table 10.2: Established genetic population screening services[3]

Types of service	*Conditions*	*Preventive or screening action*
Primary prevention	• Rhesus haemolytic disease • Congenital rubella • Congenital malformation	• Postpartum use of anti-D globulin • Immunization of girls (MMR vaccine) • Addition of folic acid to the maternal diet (may prevent neural tube defect) • Control of maternal diabetes. Avoidance of mutagens and teratogens such as alcohol, certain drugs and possibly tobacco
Antenatal screening	• Congenital malformations	• Ultrasound fetal anomaly scan, maternal serum alpha-fetoprotein estimation (AFP) and amniocentesis
	• Chromosomal abnormalities • Inherited disease	• Noting maternal age and maternal serum factor levels • Checking family history, carrier screening for haemoglobinopathies, Tay-Sachs disease
Neonatal screening	• Congenital malformations	• Examination of the newborn for early treatment (e.g. of congenital dislocation of the hip) by ultrasonography
	• Phenylketonuria, congenital hypothyroidism, sickle cell disease	• Biochemical tests for early detection

Inherited disorders: These affect a limited number of families and are usually transmitted by healthy carriers who have a high-risk of passing the disorder to their children. Genetic counselling can be offered following diagnosis of either genetic disease or the carrier states in a family member.

Population-based screening enhances the significance at the public health level and can be high cost-effective as compared to family based approach (Table 10.2).

Genetic Family Studies

Genetic diagnosis has implications for whole family as well as for individual. While a correct diagnosis benefits individual patient, who can be given guidance on the management, natural history or prognosis, and put in touch with support group. It is also of value to other family members who can be offered genetic counselling.

Genetic Population Screening

A genetic population screening programme means to identify and counsel as many people at genetic risk as possible. A simple "primary screening test" is usually offered to the whole population to identify those groups at increased risk, who are then offered further tests for definite diagnosis. A screening programme is public health policy and it should meet epidemiological criteria: condition being serious, clear diagnosis available and sound knowledge of natural history of disease and effective method of treatment available with affordable cost.

Genetic Counselling

Genetic counselling is a coping mechanism. It recognizes the autonomy of the individual couple, each couple has the right to complete information and highest standard of confidentiality must be maintained. Genetic counselling takes time and most clinical geneticists work with number of trained associates. Genetic counselling involves serious decisions on the part of client. The decision such as to marry or not to marry, to produce a child or not to produce a child, what are the chances of child being abnormal with genetic defect, etc. are critical decisions. The main components of genetic counselling are:

- A correct diagnosis.
- Estimation of genetic risk; this often requires a pedigree and may call for investigations involving other family members.
- Provision of information on existence of risk and on any options for avoiding it. The options will depend upon:
  - The nature of disorder involved.
  - The prognosis and the availability of treatment or palliative care.
  - The chances that other family members may be at risk and in particular, of passing the risk onto children.
  - The possibility of avoiding risks to individuals own health.
  - Possibility of avoiding transmission of the risk to children.

Genetic counselling requires long-term contact and support. Every one who suspects a personal genetic risk or a risk of having offspring with a serious disease or malformation should have access to genetic counselling.

It is generally agreed that the genetic counselling should be "non-directive", this does not mean, however, simply giving information or facts and leaving them to make their own mind, rather, it implies that they should be actively helped to reach the decision that is right for them in their personal circumstances and according to their own moral code, not that of health worker (Table 10.3).

Molecular Genetics

DNA has many advantages for genetic diagnosis. It is easy to obtain since every cell of an individual or foetus contains

Table 10.3: Options open to carriers of an inherited disease

Time at which the risk is discovered	*Possible action*	*Frequency*
Before choosing partner (uncommon)	• Remain single • Avoid selecting another carrier as partner[a] • Select a partner in the usual way	• Uncommon • Very uncommon • Most uncommon
Before pregnancy (more common)	• Remain childless	• Common only for severe disease, when prenatal diagnosis is impossible
	• "Take a chance" • Use prenatal diagnosis • Use artificial insemination by donor or other form of assisted reproduction	• Common for less severe diseases • Very common • Very common
	• Separate and find another partner	• Very uncommon indeed
After birth of an affected child (most common)[b]	• Accept infant and treatment • Accept infant, but reject treatment • Reject infant	• Usual • Occasional • Occasional

[a] Relates only to recessively inherited disorders.
[b] The options that apply before first pregnancy also apply to pregnancies following the birth of an affected child.

10

the full DNA complement of that individual. Genes can be studied whether they are actively producing their product or not. A definitive diagnosis can usually be made, and essentially similar laboratory approaches can be used for the diagnosis of all genetic conditions. One important limitation of DNA diagnosis, however, is that many different mutations may underlie the same clinical disorder and it can be difficult to identify them all, particularly rare ones.

DNA Technology

DNA technology is advancing rapidly and it has been used in many ways for diagnosis, therapy and to identify carriers and the mechanism of evolution:

- The synthesis of DNA probes with specific sequences which allows genetic diagnosis.
- DNA sequencing methods for rapid analysis of unknown DNA and identification of mutations.
- New diagnostic techniques such as polymerase chain reaction (PCR) for amplifying known DNA sequencing. This allows a simple and rapid diagnosis using extremely small tissue samples.
- Techniques for synthesis of DNA that allows the production of known sequences of increasing length. Coding sequences produced in this way can be used for the production of therapeutic agents such as insulin, erythropoietin and factor VIII. They may also be used in the creation of transgenic animals and gene therapy.
- Positional cloning strategies using genetic markers, which are now defined along the entire human genome.
- *In vitro* methods for examining the proteins product of gene sequences with unknown functions.
- New cytogenetic techniques such as fluorescence in situ hybridization (FISH), which permits direct visualization of the relationship of the genes to one another in the nucleus of the living cell.
- Comparison between the DNA sequences of different genes and species. This helps elucidate the mechanisms of evolution.
- Insertion of coding DNA sequences into animal embryos to create transgenic animals: valuable for studying the roles of specific genes in multifactorial diseases.
- *Gene therapy:* Insertion of missing DNA sequences into individuals with genetically determined disorders.

The most recent revolution in biology has been the development of the recombinant DNA technology which has been used in synthesis of substances like insulin, growth hormone, interferon, factor VIII, factor IX, somatostatin and vaccines.

THE HUMAN GENOME PROJECT[1,3]

The sum total of genetic information of an individual which is encoded in structure of deoxyribonucleic acid (DNA), is called genome. The study of genome is called "genomics".

It is now believed that the information generated by genomics will, in the long-term, have major benefits for the prevention, diagnosis and management of many diseases which hitherto have been difficult or impossible to control. These include communicable and genetic diseases, together with other common killers or cause chronic ill-health, including cardiovascular diseases, cancer, diabetes, the major psychoses, dementia, rheumatic diseases and asthma.[3]

The human genome project is an attempt to systemize the research on mapping and isolating human genes that is already in progress in many countries, in order to create a single linear map of the human genome, with each coding gene defined and sequenced. Essentially, it is mapping and sequencing of gene in population.

Aim

The primary aim of human genome project is to advance knowledge and increase understanding of the way in which genes interact with each other and with the environment to generate normal structure and function; findings will also cover the individual variation that incidentally contribute to susceptibility to common diseases.

The DNA data obtained by mapping and sequencing will need to be correlated systemically with clinical and scientific data, which may be more difficult to obtain once relevant genes and their interactions, with each other and the environment have been defined. Scientific, clinical, epidemiological and psychological research will be required to determine gene function and to identify possibilities for prevention or treatment of particular disorders. "International collaboration is essential to ensure that clinically relevant information can be applied worldwide, and to permit international and inter-regional comparisons, quality control, technological simplifications and free exchange of reagents and clinical data. The burden of congenital and genetic disorders is frequently greatest in developing countries, where the emerging problems have a genetic component. It is important to encourage genetic studies in populations with specific problems such as thalassaemias and sickle cell anaemia and to ensure that technology and resources are generally available and to maintain international collaboration".

It is an important function of Human Genome Organization (HUGO) to ensure that data from the project are available to all, in an integrated and usable form.

THE HUMAN GENOME DIVERSITY PROJECT

As a part of the work of HUGO, the Human Genome Diversity Project (HGDP) is aimed at increasing understanding of human evolution. The major objective is to define the genetic relationships between human populations and interpret them in terms of natural selection, genetic drift, migration, etc. For example, the frequency and distribution of single gene disorders are related to history of human migration. The HGDP is not primarily concerned with health, but certain aspects of human genetic diversity related to health and disease are relevant to the project. For instance, difference between populations in the incidence of common disorders such as hypertension, atherosclerosis, diabetes and some forms of cancer and in the proportion of fit elderly people, suggest that the study of "genes for health" could be considered as part of HUGO strategy.

GENE THERAPY

Gene therapy means the introduction of gene sequence into cell with the aim of modifying the cell behaviour in a clinically relevant fashion. It can be used in many ways, e.g. to correct genetic mutation (as for cystic fibrosis), or to kill a cell (as for cancer) or to modify susceptibility (as for coronary artery disease). The gene may be introduced using a virus (usually a retrovirus or adenovirus) or by means of a lipid or receptor targeting. New system for gene delivery will be developed in due course of time.

EUGENICS

Galton propagated the idea of hereditary improvement of men and animals by such methods as selective breeding. Thus *eugenics* can be defined as improvement of human species or race by selective breeding. But we cannot advocate drastic eugenic policies as our knowledge in human genetics is still inadequate. It is not simple to propagate or transfer a particular character or desirable character (intelligence, height or colour or physique) to offsprings through genes as many environmental factors modify the behaviour of genes.

Positive Eugenics

It is being applied to animals in a prolific way. Improving cattle breeding by artificial insemination to have increase yield of milk and to have better quality of animals for other purposes. Improving yield of grains (wheat and rice) has been in practice for many years now, is another example of genetic manipulation for human welfare and survival. Positive eugenics in those persons who carry harmful hereditary factors of the risks of having affected children can be by limitation of family size or accepting other reproductive choices.

EUTHENICS

It means providing appropriate environments/suitable environments for genotype to express themselves fully. The environmental manipulations for development of genotypes is called euthenics.

GENETIC SERVICES

Genetic services are very rudimentary in our country. Greater attention needs to be paid to develop genetic services at the level of tertiary, secondary and primary health care. Community genetic services are relatively inexpensive and set against the great social and financial burden of chronic disease, highly cost-effective. One of the main problems in delivering genetic services appears to be difficulty of informing both the health professions and the community of the real significance of genetic problem.

PC-PNDT Act, 1974 and Medical Termination of Pregnancy Act, 1971 lays down the legislative framework of application of science of genetics in the country.[4]

Sex selective abortions need to be eliminated by implementation of PC-PNDT Act.[4] This is positive eugenics to have a balanced sex ratio and to avoid demographic catastrophy.

Antenatal clinics provide the opportunity to educate individual and family on genetics.

Screening of antenatal mothers for Rh grouping, avoidance of teratogenic drugs and radiation and promoting immunization against rubella before pregnancy is preventive genetics. Contraception for limiting the size of family and bearing children at right age is another example of positive and preventive genetics. Improving nutritional status and consumption of iron and folic acid tablets during pregnancy prevents anaemia as also neural tube defects. Use of ultrasonography to detect defective children is essentially a good screening activity. Early childhood development services in ICDS programme by providing environmental stimuli is an attempt to realize full potential of genetic endowment of young children. Malnourished children and children with mild mental retardation have progressively improved, and developed their IQ to desired level by early childhood education through environmental stimuli.[5]

THE PRECONCEPTION AND PRENATAL DIAGNOSTIC TECHNIQUES (PC-PNDT) (PROHIBITION OF SEX SELECTION) ACT, 1994 AND AMENDED RULES, 2003

Problem

The Prenatal Diagnostic Techniques (Regulation and Prevention of Misuse) Act, 1994 has since been amended to make it more comprehensive. The amended Act and Rules came into force with effect from Feb 2003 and the PC-PNDT Act has been renamed as "Preconception and Prenatal Diagnostic Technique (prohibition of sex selection) Act, 1994 to make it more comprehensive.

There is unfavourable female sex ratio and child sex ratio due to female foeticide and sex selective abortions. To achieve balanced sex ratio, the Government of India made PC-PNDT Act.

The Act provides for the prohibition of sex selection before and after conception and for the regulation of prenatal diagnostic techniques for the purpose of detecting genetic abnormalities, or metabolic disorders or chromosomal abnormalities or certain congenital malformations or sex-linked disorders and for prevention of their misuse for sex determination leading to female foeticide and for matters connected therewith.

Regulation of Prenatal Diagnostic Technique

No place including a registered genetic counselling centre or genetic laboratory or genetic clinic shall be used or caused to be used by any person for conducting prenatal diagnostic techniques except for the purpose specified below:

1. Chromosomal abnormalities
2. Genetic metabolic disorders
3. Haemoglobinopathies
4. Sex-linked genetic diseases
5. Congenital abnormalities
6. Other abnormalities as may be specified by the central supervisory board.

Following conditions must be fulfilled:

- i Age of the pregnant women is above 35 years.
- ii The pregnant women have undergone two or more spontaneous abortions or foetal loss.
- iii The pregnant women had been exposed to potentially teratogenic agents such as drugs, radiation, infection or chemicals.
- iv The pregnant women or her spouse has a family history of mental retardation or physical deformities such as spasticity or any other genetic disease.
- v Any other condition as may be specified by the board.
- vi Person conducting ultrasonography on pregnant women shall keep complete records as prescribed under the Act.
- vii No person including a relative or husband of the pregnant woman shall seek or encourage the conduct of any prenatal diagnostic techniques on her except for purposes specified above.

Prenatal diagnostic procedures cannot be conducted unless:

- All side and after effects of such procedures have been explained to the concerned pregnant women.
- Her written consent to undergo such procedures has been obtained in the language she understands.
- A copy of her written consent has been given to the concerned woman. Communication of sex of the foetus by words, signs or in any other manner to the concerned pregnant women or her relations or any other person is prohibited.

Determination of sex is prohibited in genetic counselling centre, genetic laboratory or genetic clinic and no person shall whatever means cause or allow to be caused selection of sex before or after conception.

Before conducting pre-implantation genetic diagnosis or any prenatal technique/test/procedure such as amniocentesis, chorionic villi biopsy, foetoscopy, foetal skin or organ biopsy or cordocentesis, a written consent in a language the person undergoing such procedure understands, shall be obtained.

Any person conducting ultrasonography/image scanning on a pregnant woman shall give declaration on each report on ultrasonography/image scanning that he/she has neither declared nor disclosed the sex of foetus of the pregnant women to anybody. The pregnant woman should before undergoing ultrasonography/image scanning declare that she does not want to know the sex of her foetus.

Who Can Do the Procedures?

Gynaecologist having experience of performing at least 20 procedures in chorionic villi aspiration per vagina, per abdomen, chorionic villi, biopsy, amniocentesis, cordocentesis, foetoscopy, foetal skin or organ biopsy or foetal blow sampling, etc. under supervision of an experienced gynaecologist or a sonologist, imaging specialist, radiologist, or registered medical practitioner having postgraduate degree or diploma or 6 months training or one year experience in sonography or image screening or a medical geneticist, may set up a genetic clinic/ultrasound clinic/imaging centre.

APPROPRIATE AUTHORITY

Under the Act, the appropriate authority has been decentralized at the district level. Civil surgeon/chief medical officer (CMO) has been designated authority under the Act to recognize and register an ultrasonography/genetic centre.

Registration of Genetic Counselling Centres, Genetic Laboratories or Genetic Clinics

Genetic counselling centre, laboratory or genetic clinic, including clinic, laboratory or centre having ultrasound or imaging machine or scanner or any other technology capable of undertaking determination of sex of foetus and sex selection can be opened unless it is duly registered under the Act. District civil surgeon/chief medical officer is appropriate authority to issue certificate of registration of place and machine.

Offence

Any medical geneticist, gynaecologist, registered medical practitioners or any other person who owns a genetic counselling centre, a genetic laboratory or a genetic clinic or is employed therein and renders his or her professional technical services there, whether on honorary basis or otherwise and who contravenes provisions of the Act or rules made under that and advertising relating to preconception and prenatal determination of sex or sex selection is punishable; with imprisonment up to 3 years and fine up to 10 thousand rupees and on any subsequent conviction, with imprisonment which may extend to 5 years and with fine which may extend to 50 thousand rupees. If any person who seeks the aid of any centre/ doctor or any person for sex selection or for conducting prenatal diagnostic techniques on any pregnant women, he shall be punishable with imprisonment up to 3 years and fine up to 50 thousand rupees for the first offence and for any subsequent offence with imprisonment up to 5 years and with fine up to 1,00,000 rupees.

THE MEDICAL TERMINATION OF PREGNANCY ACT, 1971 (AMENDED ACT, 2002 AND AMENDED RULES, 2003)

This Act is known as Medical Termination of Pregnancy Act, 1971

Pregnancies which can be terminated by a registered medical practitioners under the Act:[6]

a Where the length of pregnancy does not exceed 12 weeks.

b Where the length of pregnancy exceeds 12 weeks but does not exceed 20 weeks, if not less than two medical practitioners are of the opinion formed in good faith. That:

  i Continuation of pregnancy would involve a risk to the life of pregnant woman or of grave injury to her physical or mental health, or

  ii There is substantial risk that if the child was born, it would suffer from such physical or mental abnormalities to be seriously handicapped.

  iii If a pregnancy is alleged by the pregnant women to have been caused by rape the anguish caused by such pregnancy shall be presumed to constitute a grave injury to the mental health of pregnant women.

  iv When pregnancy occurs as a result of failure of a contraception used by married women or her husband.

No pregnancy of a woman, who has not attained the age of 18 years or who having attained the age of 18 years, is mentally ill person shall be terminated without the consent in writing of her guardian.

Most MTPs are done in private sector. Safe abortion services are denied to most of women in most of Government facilities hence women are compelled to seek services from unsafe providers and risk their lives.

REFERENCES

1 WHO. Genomics and World Health. Geneva: WHO; 2002.

2 Emery AEH, Mueller RF. Elements of Medical Genetics. Seventh Edition, Churchill Livingstone, London, Melbourne and New York (1988).

3 WHO. Control of Hereditary Diseases. Technical Report Series. Geneva: WHO; 1996. Series No.: 865.

4 GOI. Preconception and prenatal diagnostic techniques. (Prohibition of sex selection) Act, 1994 and amended Act, 2003. New Delhi: GOI; 2003.

5 GOI. ICDS Annual Report 2003–04. New Delhi: Deptt. of women and child development. Ministry of Human Resource Development, GOI; 2004.

6 GOI. The Medical Termination of Pregnancy Act, 1971 and amended Act, 2002. New Delhi: GOI; 2002.

CHAPTER

11

Medical Entomology and Control of Vectors of Diseases

Medical entomology deals with insects of medical importance. These insects are responsible for transmission of several diseases. Major vector-borne diseases have been discussed in Chapter 12. This chapter discusses the bionomics of insects or vectors of medical importance and diseases transmitted by these.

ANOPHELES MOSQUITOES

Life History

The mosquito passes through four distinct stages, i.e. egg, larva, pupa and adult, the first three being aquatic (Fig. 11.1).

Egg

Eggs are small dark bodies and are just visible to naked eye. Eggs are laid on water, leaves and stems of aquatic plants, mud and even on wet grounds. Anopheline eggs are always laid singly and separately; they float on the surface of water. Eggs are usually boat-shaped. Eggs are laid in clear water. Eggs can withstand considerable amount of desiccation, but large majority of eggs die when kept away from water for some time. The egg stage lasts for 2 days under the most favourable conditions.

Larva

The eggshell hatches and larva is released. The larva is very active and shows swift movements. *Anopheles larvae* are exclusively surface feeder and float just below the surface of water. Larva subsists on bacteria and organisms floating on the surface of water. The breathing apparatus consists of parallel air tubes in the body of larva at the tail end. Every species of Anopheles has preference for breeding places like collection of rain water, irrigation channels, and open cisterns. Usually, it prefers clear water. *An. sundaicus* prefers brackish water. Larval stage develops to pupa in 5 days. *Gambusia affinis* feeds on larvae and can be used as biological method to control larvae of mosquitoes. Similarly, Paris green and mosquito larvicidal oil (MLO) can be used as larvicidal material.

Pupa

Pupa is also active swimmer. It is a comma-shaped structure and sees with its eyes but cannot feed as the mouth parts are entirely suppressed. Pupal stage lasts for 24–48 hours and it all depends upon temperature and seasonal factors.

Adult

The period from oviposition to the emergence of first offspring is about 7–10 days in Anopheles. Adult starts mating on day one after emergence. Females usually mate only once but produce eggs at intervals throughout their life.

Biting Behaviour

Anophelines as a rule show a decided preference for either human (anthropophilic) or animal blood (zoophilic). Though both males and females can live on vegetable sap and carbohydrate food, a blood meal on the part of female anopheline is essential for maturation of the ovum. Anopheles is both *zoophilic and anthropophilic*. Keeping animals in and around dwellings affords protection wall to human beings.

Once the cattle sheds are sprayed with insecticide, the mosquitoes shift readily to dwellings and bite human beings. Under the insecticide spray policy, cattle sheds are now not taken up for spray activity.

Resting Habits

After feeding the blood meal, the female mosquitoes rest in some sheltered place for the purpose of digesting blood and development of ovum. Indoor resting habits are called endophilic. It is endophagic (feeding indoor).

Flight

Anophelines adult mosquitoes can cover long distances. An average flight range is 0.75–1.5 km. This is significant for effective control of mosquito vector breeding.

Lifespan

On an average, the lifespan of Anopheles in India is about a month. Hibernating mosquito may live longer (6 months or more).

Anopheles is an important vector in the epidemiology of malaria. The longer it lives the greater is the chance of its being infected and infective.

Species

1. *An. culicifacies* has a very wide distribution in India. It is most important vector in malaria transmission. It prefers clear water and breeds in open irrigation channels, river beds, pools, ponds, lakes, springs, and back water, burrow pits in fruit and vegetable gardens and even in wells. The larvae are also found in seepages and other collections of stagnant water.
2. It is more *zoophilic* than *anthropophilic*.
3. Adult culicifacies survive for about 4 weeks.

Infective Density of Anophelines

Infective density is the average number of infective anophelines per room per night. *Infective* mosquito is one, which shows sporozoites in their salivary glands, while *infected* mosquito is one, which shows any stage of malaria parasite (gametocytes, oocysts and sporozoites).

Bio-ecological Characteristics of Principal Malaria Vectors in India

An. culicifacies

It is vector of *rural* and peri-urban malaria in the North, South and Central India. Usually breeds in water not rich in organic matter, irrigation channels, river bed, pools, tanks, ponds, in rice fields, irrigation wells, and even brackish water, foot marks and cart tracks (wheel ruts), rain water collection in burrow pits along rail, canal and road, and rock pools.

Resting habits: Predominantly indoor rester—cattle sheds and human dwellings. Prefers pools with low disturbance places, some may rest outdoor after spray. Bites in dusk, peak time is 10.30 p.m. to 12.30 a.m. It is mainly zoophilic, indiscriminate feeder at high density. Flight range is normally 1 km and up to 3 km at high density.

An. stephensi

11

It is normally an *urban mosquito* and urban vector for transmission of malaria in urban and industrial areas. It prefers small collections of clean water for ovipositing such as overhead cisterns, wells, small water reservoirs, pools, springs, marsh and collection of rain water.[1–3]

Breeding: Urban areas—domestic and peridomestic water collection and underground tanks, wells, cisterns, fountain, ornamental tanks and artificial containers, water collection on roofs and withstands heavy pollution. It often breeds in large number in river beds.

It is also a vector of rural malaria in Rajasthan and breeds and rests in the water storage tanks called "tankar".

Resting habits: Differs widely but common places are—human dwellings and cattle sheds. Bites soon after dusk. Peak—4 to 6 a.m. It is indiscriminate feeder on human and cattle. Flight range is 1 km. However, it does not disperse to long distances from the breeding places.

An. minimus: In NE states, North West Bengal, breeds in streams.

An. fluviatilis: Foothills all along the Himalayan range seepage and in irrigation channels.

An. dirus: Deep forests in NE region breeds in streams.

An. sundaicus: Andaman and Nicobar island—breeds in brackish water. Rests often in human dwellings.

Control Measures

Integrated vector management under NVBDCP by insecticide indoor residual spray (IRS), larvicides, biological and environmental control measures (source reduction) are being adopted for control of mosquitoes.

CULEX MOSQUITOES

These mosquitoes are principal intermediate host of *Wuchereria bancrofti* (filaria) in India. This species is one of the commonest of Indian mosquitoes and is found everywhere in this country up to 6,000 feet or more. It alone is responsible for the winter and spring plague of mosquitoes experienced almost all over India. It is essentially a domestic and peridomestic species (Fig. 11.1).

Egg

Culex mosquitoes lay eggs in polluted water contaminated with sewage, e.g. in cesspools, septic tanks ground pools, cement pits, sewage farms and drains having high organic matter. The egg has micropollar process at one end. Eggs are laid in clusters which acquire the shape of raft consisting of as many as 200 eggs glued to each other. Egg stage lasts for 2 days when it hatches and larva emerges (Fig. 11.1).

Larva

The larva has long and narrow siphon tube. It has much slower and snake like movements. The respiratory openings

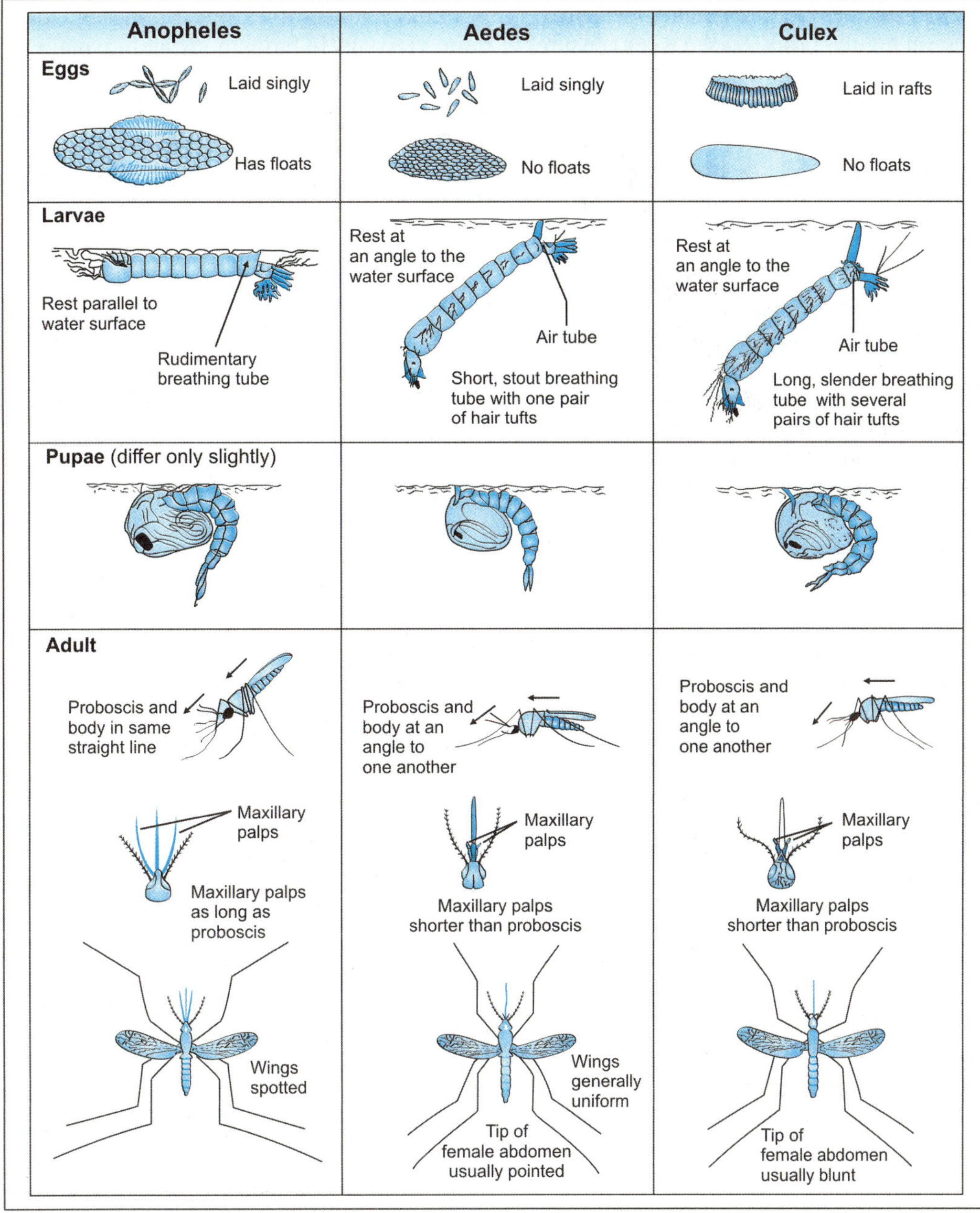

Fig. 11.1: Some of the main characteristics for differentiating Anopheles, Aedes and Culex (WHO)

lie at the end of siphon tube. Larva hangs from the surface, hence not a surface feeder. The larvae subsist on bacteria and other organic matter. Larval stage lasts for 5–6 days.

Pupa

It is a comma-shaped structure and this stage lasts for 2 days. The period from egg to adult stage takes 8–10 days. The egg, larva and pupa are aquatic stages.

Adult and Diseases Transmitted

Adult mosquito has head, thorax and abdomen.

In culex, the thorax makes an angle with the abdomen, i.e. it has a hunch backed appearance. The flight range is 1–3 km or even more from breeding area. The mosquito is very active during dusk and night. The female sucks blood and is anthropophilic (sucks human blood). *Culex quinquefasciatus* is prevalent universally and is most important vector of *W. bancrofti*. It is highly anthropophilic (prefers human blood). *Culex vishnui* group of mosquitoes are the most important in the transmission of *Japanese encephalitis* in India. The average lifespan of culex mosquito is about 21 days. The vector prefers mainly outdoor resting and outdoor feeding (exophilic and exophagic).

Control

Prevention of stagnation of sewage contaminated water, i.e. source reduction is best method. But this is difficult to achieve. Larvicidal measures are supplementary measures. Antilarval measures, on regular basis (once a week) ensure control of breeding but these are expensive. Paris green, kerosene oil or pyrethrum can be used as antilarval measures.

Control of adult mosquitoes is done by insecticidal spray, malathion fogging/ultralow volume spraying (ULV). Malathion fogging is restricted to urban and periurban areas. Integrated vector control measures are recommended.

AEDES AEGYPTI

It is the vector for dengue fever, chikungunya fever and yellow fever. It is known most commonly as tiger mosquito or container mosquito (because it breeds most commonly in containers). Once thought to be urban vector, it has now spread to vast rural areas of the country. *Aedes aegypti* index is being kept below 1 by effective control measures.

Breeding Habits

Aedes aegypti profusely breeds in desert coolers, storage tanks, earthen pots and other receptacles with rain water or stored clean water, in flower vases, neglected cups, tyres, broken glasses and discarded plastic containers.

Life Cycle

It completes its life cycle around human dwellings.

Female lays eggs in all types of man-made and natural containers. Egg is elongate, blackish in colour and the shell is highly chitinized. Eggs are glued to the surface in damp areas above water surface and generally 60–100 eggs are laid during each oviposition. Female distributes eggs in several containers. Within 24 hours the embryonic development takes place but eggs can withstand long periods of desiccation, up to 1 year. Eggs when flooded hatch rapidly leading to emergence of first instars larvae. There are three larval instars and larval development is completed within a week, but it all depends upon temperature. Pupal stage lasts for 24–30 hours leading to emergence of adult mosquito.

Adult Mosquito

Like all other mosquitoes adults have head-thorax and abdomen and six legs. The adult mosquito is ornamented with silvery white scales all over the body. The mosquito is of black or blackish brown colour with silvery spots and markings. Because it bites fearlessly, it is also called tiger mosquito (Fig. 11.1).

Bionomics

Adults seek dark and quiet places to rest on unsprayed objects such as clothes, curtains, bedrooms, bathrooms, kitchen, on walls, furniture, hanging articles, e.g. clothings, ropes and closets. Average survival for male is 20 days and that of female 30 days.

Female mosquitoes bite throughout the day and it is quite vigorous in biting and can bite many persons. Flight range is usually 400 meters, thermal death point is reached at 41–42°C. The vector density and other indices have been discussed in Chapter 12 under dengue fever. An infected mosquito is capable of transmitting virus to susceptible individuals for the rest of its life.

Diseases Transmitted

Infected mosquitoes transmit dengue and dengue haemorrhagic fever (DHF), chikungunya, yellow fever, as also Zika virus infection. Yellow fever is absent in India but dengue and DHF are common and occur in epidemic form from time to time.[4, 5]

Control

Source reduction measures involve: Do not allow breeding of mosquitoes in coolers, flower vases, discarded tins, broken bottles, tyres, plastic containers, etc. This requires people participation and not legislative measures. Thus, education of people is most essential.

During epidemic, vector control would require the use of space sprays to knock down the infective vector population. ULV and thermal malathion fogging may also be used under special situations for a limited period to fight the epidemic. Fogging should be done at least once weekly and fog should stay inside rooms for about 10–15 minutes for it to be effective. Most situations are not suitable for fogging hence main reliance should be on source reduction.

MANSONIOIDES (MANSONIA MOSQUITOES)

This mosquito is recognized by speckled wings and legs. These mosquitoes depend for their breeding on aquatic Plants (*Pistia stratiotes*) for the supply of oxygen. The eggs are laid in clusters on or under surface of the leaf of Pistia plant. The larvae and pupae do not come to the surface until shortly before the emergence of the mosquito.

Disease Transmission

Two species of this vector *Mansonioides uniformis* and *M. annulifera* transmit *Brugia malayi* infection of filariasis in India.[6]

Implications

For the control of this mosquito, the control of vegetation, i.e. removal of Pistia plant is significant to reduce the disease transmission. Clearance of pistial plants reduces the breeding (Fig. 11.2).

SANDFLIES

They belong to genus phlebotomus. The important species consist of *Phlebotomus argentipes*, *P. papatasi*, *P. sergenti*

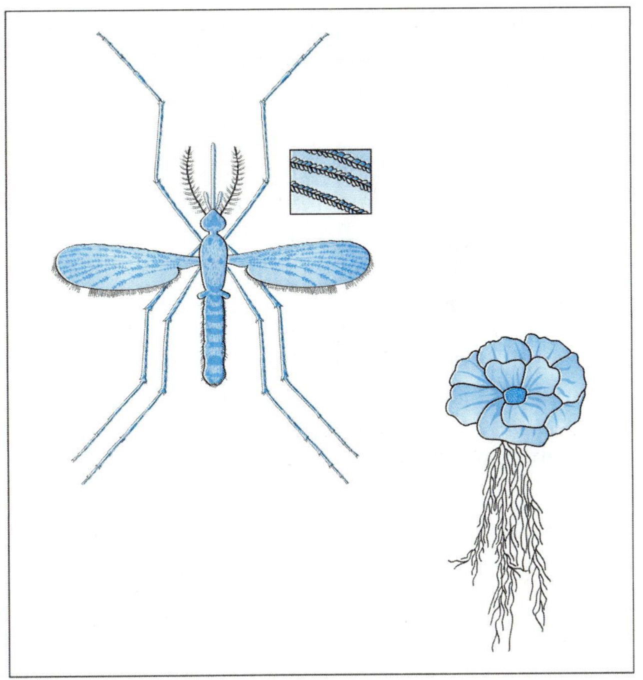

Fig. 11.2: *Mansonioides uniformis* female in flight and Pistia plant

and *P. braziliensis*. These are vectors for transmission of leishmaniasis (kala-azar or visceral leishmaniasis, oriental sore and Espundia). Sandflies also transmit the virus of sandfly fever.

These insects are small and of greyish yellow to brown colour, 1.5–3.5 mm long. Sandflies are not capable of flying any long distance but they move by hopping from one place to another. They have very short lifespan.

Head-thorax and abdomen is covered with hair. The antennae are long and filamentous and carry whorl of hair at the joints. The thorax is humped and bear a pair of wings which are hairy. The insect has 3 pairs of slender legs and are much longer in proportion to the size of the insect. Long legs are adapted for hopping. The abdomen has 10 segments and covered with hair and last two segments of abdomen are modified into sexual organs. Male and female insects can be distinguished on the basis of claspers which are present only in male insect (Fig. 11.3).

Life History and Bionomics

Eggs are laid on organic matter (animal's excreta and other decaying material). The eggs are torpedo-shaped and hatch

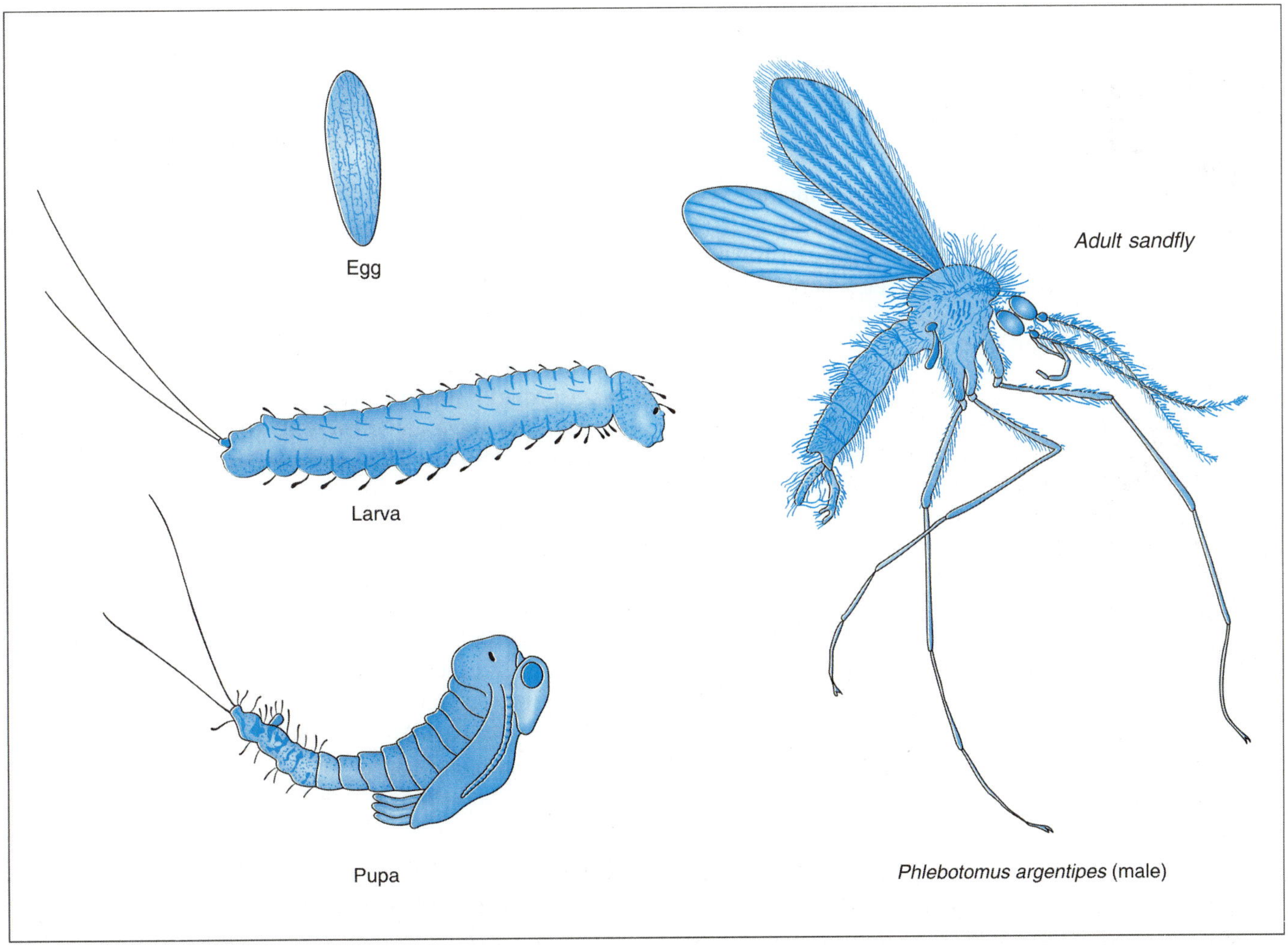

Fig. 11.3: Complete metamorphosis of a sandfly

out in 3–4 days in summer season and after one week in winter season. Larvae feed on organic matter and mature to pupa stage in 2 weeks time after undergoing three moultings. The larvae bear two anal spines. Cattle sheds are favourite breeding ground of sandflies, usually under the earthen ware feeding trough. Larvae can penetrate the soil to a depth of 3 or 4 inches in loose and sodden soil. Thus, most commonly larvae are found in cattle sheds and poultry houses. Blood meal is required by female for maturation of ova. Within 10–15 days, the pupa develops into adult insect. The whole life cycle takes about 30 days, the egg, larva and pupal stages requiring 4, 14 and 7 days respectively in most favourable conditions.

The female insect is blood sucker and male lives on plant juices. Female insect sucks blood of animals as well as man. Sandflies remain confined to their places of breeding and can cover only short distances. The man gets bitten accidentally when walking bare foot or coming in contact with soil infested with insect or contaminated with animal excreta (stables, poultry houses and cattle sheds).

Sandflies are active during night in the dark, usually attack the lower extremities and are capable of biting through thin clothes and can cross through meshwork of nets because of being very small. Lizards and spiders are the natural predators of sandflies.

Disease Transmission

Sandflies transmit *Leishmania donovani* from man to man as man is the only known reservoir of kala-azar. It is necessary that sandfly should survive at least for 8 days after the infected blood meal for development of infective form of *Leishmania donovani* (aflagellar forms). Sandflies feed on cattle, goats and man.

Control Measures

- ***Source control:*** Abolition of breeding grounds or short of it is frequent removal of animal dung from stable and cow sheds and improving sanitation. Cracks, crevices and holes must be closed by cementing techniques.
- ***Anti-adult measures:*** Residual insecticide like DDT spray is quite effective against adult insect. Widespread use of DDT under malaria control and eradication programme kept the population of sandflies under control. It was a collateral benefit of DDT spray under malaria programme. Sandflies have developed resistance to DDT and now synthetic pyrethroid are in use.
- ***Personal protection:*** Proper clothing—long trousers with socks, tops drawn over the trousers cuffs or ankles worn over them. Use of repellents is also helpful.

HOUSEFLY

Housefly belongs to order diptera. There are many species of which *Musca domestica* is distributed worldwide and known commonly as housefly. Housefly has retractile proboscis. In early summer and during monsoon, their population is enormous. Because of lack of sanitation in urban slums and rural areas they breed in a prolific manner. Apart from nuisance, the housefly act as a mechanical carrier for several diseases. Since open defecation is widespread and excreta around houses/homes is abundant, fly can carry on its body parts, part of faecal matter, garbage and disease producing germs and can shift these to food, and eatables which are left uncovered.

Diseases Transmitted

Flies are mechanical carriers and propagate disease germs which can be carried on hair, bristles, wings, foot pads, proboscis and it can regurgitate the germs in its saliva. The flies have been incriminated for spread of diarrhoeal diseases, cholera, typhoid fever, dysentery, intestinal worms, poliomyelitis, viral hepatitis A and E, enteroviruses, trachoma, conjunctivitis, anthrax, yaws and tuberculosis. Fly can deposit its eggs on wounds and causes myasis.

Life Cycle

Different stages in the life cycle of fly are—egg, larva, pupa and adult (Fig. 11.4).

Eggs

Eggs are laid by gravid female flies in garbage, human and animal excreta, which is rich in organic matter. Heaps of cow dung and garbage along with refuse dumped around houses and municipal dumping ground around peri-urban area provide most favourable breeding place for flies to breed. The eggs are glistening white and look like tiny grains of polished rice, oval in shape and measure about 1 mm in length. The fly generally deposit its eggs in dark places. A fly may lay 300–900 eggs in 3–6 batches and subsequent development depends upon temperature and moisture. The eggs hatch in summer after 8–16 hours and it may take longer time to hatch in winter. There are three larval stages. The larva moults twice. The larva is about half an inch in length and is quite active. Larva is without eyes or legs. The larvae burrow deep down to the garbage or loose soil up to variable depth before they pupate.

The larval stage lasts for 3–6 days when they migrate to dry soil and change to pupa.

Pupa

The pupa is barrel-shaped structure about 6 mm in length. The pupa is sluggish, it neither feeds nor grows. The pupal stage does not last more than 3–7 days and adult fly emerges

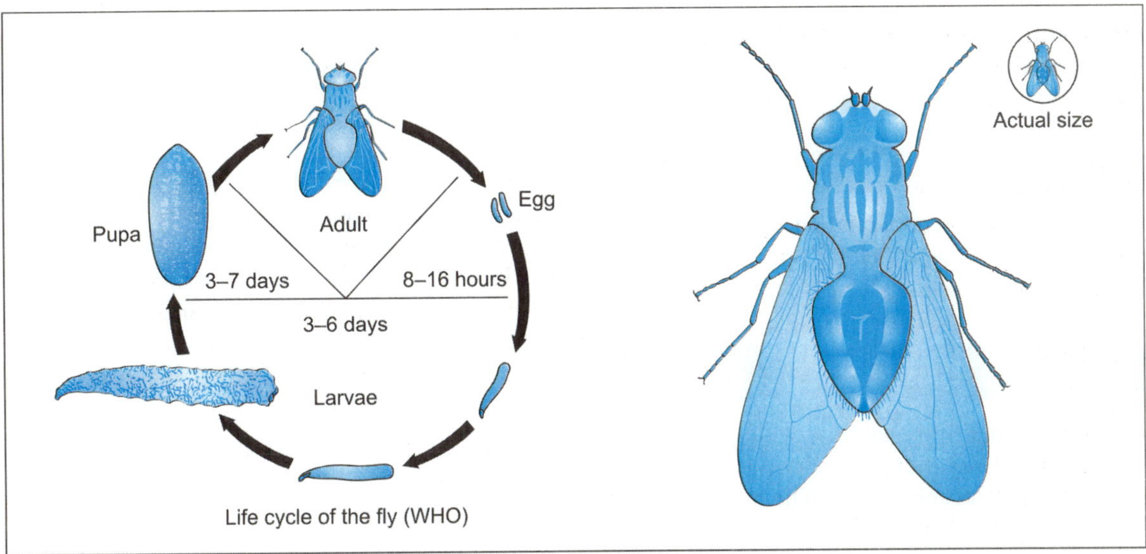

Fig. 11.4: Housefly—*Musca domestica*

out of it. Under favourable conditions, the whole life cycle of fly gets completed in 5 days time in summer and during winter it may take longer time, range is 6–42 days.

House dumps of garbage and refuse must be removed periodically and with such frequency which should not allow the fly to complete its life cycle. The garbage must be removed daily or at least once in 3 days to safer place to prevent breeding of flies.

Adult Fly

The adult fly measures about 6–9 mm in length and has labile proboscis which can be retracted and projected for feeding. The body of fly consists of head, thorax and abdomen and three pairs of legs. It has compound eyes and powerful wings to fly with speed and acrobatics. House flies are attracted to sweets—sugar and exposed food and it feeds intermittently and at times voraciously. After feeding, the fly cleans its head and proboscis with its armour, i.e. legs. It has habit of sitting on filthy material such as animal and human excreta, garbage, sputum and sores, etc. From time to time, it vomits and regurgitates its food on the substance, probably to soften the solid food and saliva helps such solids to be converted into liquid form.

The fly has restless nature, it is intermittent feeder, and it continuously defecates and vomits every now and then and it feeds indiscriminately on filth and articles of foods meant for human consumption. These habits of fly are highly conducive to the spread of pathogenic organisms. The total lifespan of adult fly is about 15 days in summer and 25 days in winter.

Fly Control and Prevention

Environmental Control (Control of Breeding)

1 It is difficult to eliminate flies altogether, however, their population can be reduced. Eliminate breeding places. Dumping of refuse, garbage and animal cow dung near dwelling should be avoided by developing scientific manure pits away from dwelling. Compost pits and manure pits of appropriate sizes can be developed near to the field. It means removal of garbage, refuse and animal excreta on daily basis to manure pit, which is not an easy task. It means more work for women. Men must participate.
2 Gobar gas plant installation is also effective measure to dispose off animal as well as human excreta, and we get excellent manure and user-friendly fuel for cooking.
3 Indiscriminate defecation promotes fly breeding. Promoting sanitary latrines will prevent fly breeding and prevent soil pollution and reduces the spread of hookworm and intestinal parasites apart from diarrhoeal diseases. Improving environmental sanitation is a long lasting measure to control flies.
4 Removal of garbage and refuse and safe composting by municipal authorities is the key function of civic authorities. This leaves much to be desired. The disposal grounds should have sanitary tipping and scientific approach (Bengaluru or Indore composting methods should be adopted). Municipal bodies have poor budget and this aspect is neglected. The system is well developed in some corporations.

Control of Adult Flies

Residual spray

1 The housefly has developed resistance to several organochlorine compounds. Residual spray with malathion and synthetic pyrethroids on resting sites such as manure dumps, and walls is helpful.
2 Pyrethrum 0.1% is useful for destruction of adult flies to suppress their population.

3 Poisonous solid baits containing 1–2% diazinon, DDVP and malathion have been successfully tried.
4 Sticky fly paper and swatting is useful.

Physical control: Use of light traps (electrocutors) are very useful in dining areas and public eating places.

Fly proofing: Using fly-proof containers and cupboards and covering the food with proper fly proof mesh. Doors and windows need fly proofing.[6]

FLEAS

Fleas belong to the order Siphonaptera; widely distributed all over the globe. They belong to two main groups 'Coombless flea' and 'Coombed flea'. The most important species are: *Xenopsylla cheopis*, *X. astia*, *X. braziliensis*.

Diseases Transmitted

X. cheopis transmits *bubonic plague* from rat to human beings and epizootic in rats.[7] Besides *X. cheopis*, *X. astia* and *X. braziliensis* can also be effective vectors. *Rickettsia typhi* is also transmitted from its rodent reservoir to man by the same rat fleas. Fleas can also transmit rat trypanosomiasis, cat and dog tapeworm, canine leishmaniasis and chiggerosis. Flea index of 1 or above is critical for potential outbreak.

Morphology

The adult flea is wingless, small insect and its body is laterally compressed, size varying from 1.5 to 6 mm, legs are long and powerful, these characters allow the insect to move freely in the hair of host. The cuticle is strongly chitinized. The flea lives on warm blooded animals (rats mostly) and mouth parts are adapted to suck blood of mammals; which is the only food for the insect. The body parts consist of head, thorax and abdomen and mouth parts are best suited for biting, piercing and sucking blood. Both male and female suck blood (Fig. 11.5).

Life History and Bionomics

The flea undergoes a process of complete metamorphosis through the successive stages of egg, larva, pupa and adult.

The eggs are often laid in rat holes, burrows, in rubbish, debris under carpets, and in granaries. The eggs are never laid on the body of the host. It continues to lay eggs throughout its lifetime. During the summer, it takes 4–5 days for eggs to hatch.

The larva is footless hairy caterpillar like maggot, extremely active and it thrives on animal's dropping or excreta. The larval body consists of head, thoracic and abdominal segments. The head carries a pair of antennae. The larva is devoid of eyes but very sensitive to light. Direct sunlight kills the larva. The flea larva moults twice and has three larval stages. The third stage larva spins a cocoon around it and becomes inactive. The normal larval stage lasts for 15 days then it transforms itself to pupal stage. The pupal stage in the cocoon lasts for 7–15 days and may be prolonged for a considerable time. The whole process of metamorphosis takes around 2–4 weeks but may be prolonged considerably if conditions are unfavourable.

The average flea is able to jump about 3 inches from the ground when gorged and 4 inches when starved. Fleas of both sexes thrive exclusively on blood meal which is necessary for their own nutrition and maturation of the ovum. Flea may leave the rat or when rat blood is not available it may attack man. Oviposition takes place within 24 hours of copulation. Fleas are very sensitive to light and air. They always hide under dark objects. The average lifespan of flea is 4 weeks approximately.

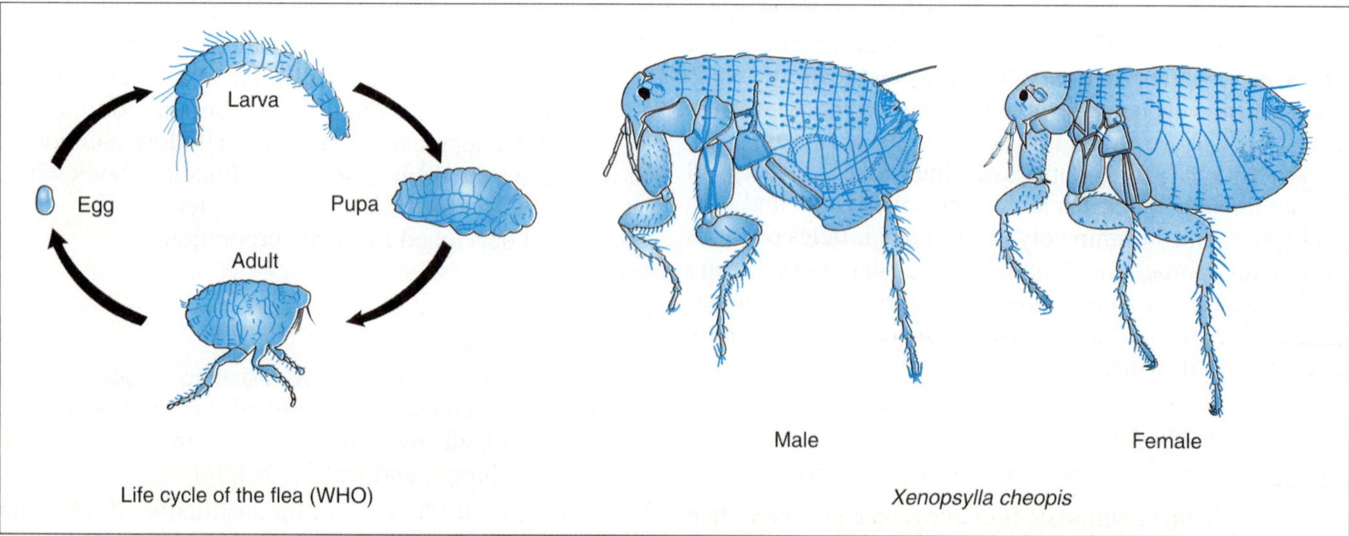

Fig. 11.5: Flea

Vector Control

Indoor residual insecticidal spray (IRS) at the lower one meter of the wall surface and adjacent floor area is effective. Choice of insecticide is diazinon or malathion. Dusting with diazinon 2%, malathion 5% or carbaryl 2% may be applied at a dosage of 2–3 g/sq. meter under grain bins or rat runs, and furniture. Dusting brings down flea density considerably.[8]

Dusting of pet dogs and cats also helps to get rid of fleas. Similarly, rodent control measures are helpful in reducing the population of rat flea. This is an indirect measure to control rat flea.

Murine Typhus (Endemic Typhus) or Flea-borne Typhus

It is an acute febrile illness caused by *Rickettsia typhi* and transmitted to human by the bite of infected *Xenopsylla cheopis*. The mode of transmission is by contamination of broken skin by rickettsia-laden faeces of flea and dried flea faeces gaining entry through conjunctiva or respiratory tract by aerosol. This is endemic in India as the animal reservoir, rats, are abundant in every town. It necessitates direct control measures against rodents and rat flea. In India, endemic typhus has been reported from Pune, Lucknow, Mysore, Kolkata, Golkunda, Karnal, Rewari and Kashmir.

CHIGGEROSIS

The flea *T. penetrans* has been reported from Western parts of India. This is originally South American species. It flourishes best in sandy soils. Domestic animals usually play the host to this flea and this flea has not been able to establish in India.

Disease Relationship

Tunga penetrans (flea) causes chiggerosis in man and domestic animals. It usually attacks sole of the foot and palm of the hand. The toes and fingers are affected. The female embeds itself into the skin of foot and it causes considerable inflammation and discomfort. Insect is treated and killed with 8% pyrethrum ointment over the affected part and dead fleas are removed.

LICE

The head and body lice belong to order Anoplura. These are parasites on mammals. They belong to genus *Pediculus*. The important species of human lice consist of *Pediculus humanus capitis* (head louse), *Pediculus humanus corporis* (body louse). The other louse is *Pthirus pubis* (crab or pubic louse).

Habitat

The head louse (*Pediculus humanus capitis*) infests the head-hair mostly around the occiput and behind the ears and neck region. Their population increases in winter months; but they persist throughout the year. Body louse infests the hair of chest, breast and axilla and is confined to the seams of clothes or fibres on which eggs are laid.

The crab louse infests the hair of pubic region, perineal region and even spread to abdomen, thighs and forearms and occasionally in eye lashes and eyebrows leading to blepharitis and conjunctivitis. Lice lead parasitic life and feed entirely on blood. In the absence of host, these will not survive. There are no constant differences between the head louse and body louse but for sizes. *P. capitis* is small as compared to *P. humanus corporis*. Body is pigmented in *P. humanus capitis* and pigmentation is absent in *P. humanus* corporis or body louse.[9]

Disease Transmission

Only body louse is a vector for the transmission of *Rickettsia prowazekii*, causing the epidemic typhus; *Rochalimaea quintana* causing trench fever, and *Borrelia recurrentis* causing relapsing fever. "Pediculosis" mean infestation of body parts with lice, it leads to irritation, scratching and intense scratching leads to secondary infection and it causes considerable inconvenience to man. They bite quite often at night which often interferes with sleep.

The bites are associated with local pigmentation of skin, and skin gets hardened and at one time it was known as vagabond's disease.

Morphology

The body of lice is flattened dorsoventrally, the integument is highly chitinized, wings are absent the mouth parts are well adapted for piercing of skin and sucking of blood and the metamorphosis is incomplete. Both male and female thrive on blood sucking, hence both can transmit the disease. The body of lice is elongate and divided into head, thorax and abdomen and they have 3 pairs of legs with strong claws. Female louse is much larger in size as compared to male louse (Figs 11.6 to 11.8).

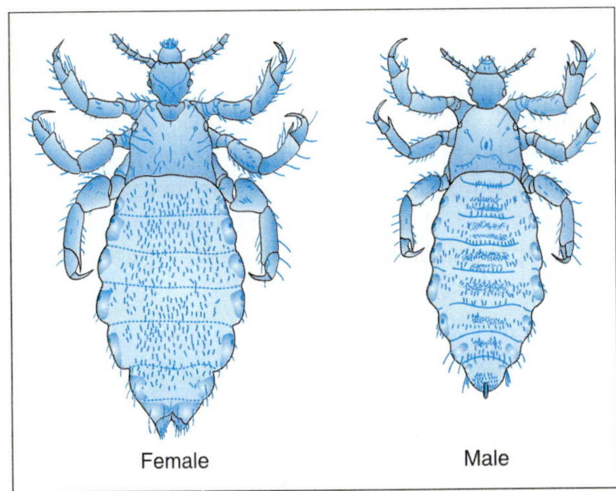

Fig. 11.6: *Pediculus humanus*

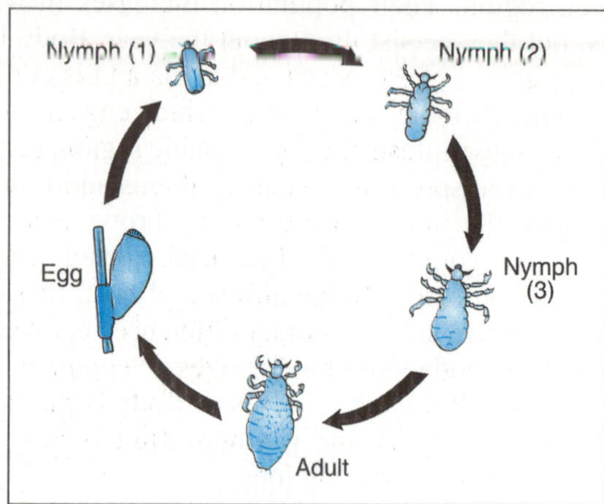

Fig. 11.7: Life cycle of the louse

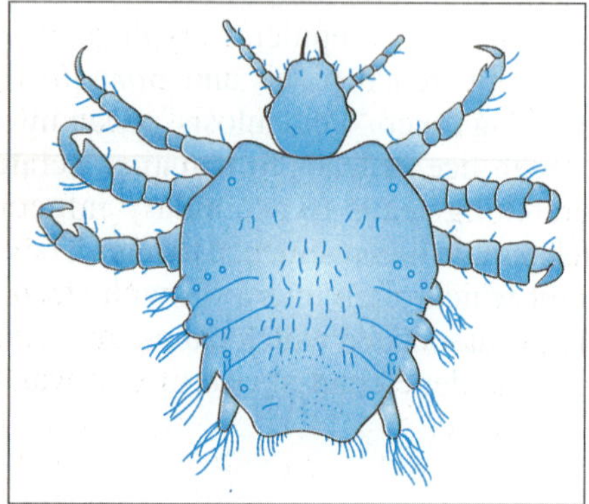

Fig. 11.8: *Pthirus pubis*, female

Life History and Bionomics

Oviposition usually begins 24–36 hours after the adult female emerges from the third larval skin. The egg is oval and pearly white and appropriately very large and these adhere to hair (called as nits) (Fig. 11.7). Body louse lays eggs in the seams of the vests or clothing. Only one egg is laid at a time. It takes 4 days time for egg to hatch under suitable temperature. When the larva or nymph emerges from egg shell the empty shell usually remains attached to hair for quite some time even more than 6 weeks. There are three larval or nymphal stages in the development cycle of pediculus and accordingly three successive moults occur before the insect acquires adult stage from immature nymph stage. On an average, a total period of 15–16 days is necessary between hatching of egg and appearance of the adult stage. Average lifespan of louse is 34 days.

Dissemination

The multiplication of louse depends upon the neglect of personal hygiene and wearing of underclothing days together. The dissemination occurs, because of close contacts and overcrowding and sharing of beds. The overcrowding in urban slums and metropolis is a common feature. Where many individuals stay in small shelter, the spread of louse is quite common. Conditions are favourable when the people congregate in refugee camps, and barracks. Spread is faster during famine and war conditions. By sharing beddings, clothes, blankets, towels, coombs and brushes the lice can be easily disseminated.

The *pubic louse* can be disseminated by *sexual contact* also.

Louse-borne Epidemic Typhus

Man is the sole reservoir of epidemic typhus. The causative organism is *R. prowazekii*. The disease is transmitted by human body louse *P. humanus corporis*. The organism *R. prowazekii* multiply intracellularly in the midgut of louse. Within a period of 10 days midgut cells rupture. A large number of rickettsiae appear in the body fluids and in the faeces of louse. The infection is transmitted by entry of infectious faeces, the gut contents and the body fluids of crushed louse through abrasion on the skin caused by scratching. The dried excreta can be inhaled and infection can also be transmitted through conjunctiva. The infected lice remain infective throughout their life. Infected lice die within 2–4 weeks.

Due to epidemic typhus, about 30 million cases and 3 million deaths occurred in Soviet Union between 1918 and 1922. This causes prolonged febrile illness lasting for days. The average incubation period is 6–15 days. The case is infectious to louse during the last 2–3 days of incubation period and throughout the febrile period which lasts for 12–14 days. In India, the endemic spot is Kashmir. In some who recover from the disease, the rickettsiae remain latent in the lymphoid tissues or organs for years. Such latent infection leads to recurrent typhus or Brill Zinseer disease.

TRENCH FEVER

It is transmitted from man to man by body louse (*Pediculus humanus corporis*). The causative organism is *Rochalimaea quintana* which grows in the gut of louse. When faecal matter of louse comes in contact with abraded skin the infection occurs.

Louse-borne Relapsing Fever

This disease is caused by *Borrelia recurrentis*, transmitted by body louse. The disease organisms can enter the body through abrasions, wounds or the mucous membrane when the infected body lice are crushed between finger nails or the teeth.

Weil-Felix test—commonly used test. The Weil-Felix test is helpful in establishing presumptive diagnosis in disease caused by members of typhus and spoted fever group of Rickettsiae. The sensitivity and specificity of Weil-Felix test is low as compared to specific serological tests for detection of IgM antibodies.

Prevention and Control

- Best way to prevent louse development is adequate personal hygiene, regular bathing and washing of clothes. Good personal hygienic practices keep away lice.
- When the louse infestation develops steam disinfection of clothing and sun drying of clothing along with shaving the hair helps to get rid of lice.
- 10% DDT powder dusting of garments of lousy individuals causes rapid reduction of infestation. If need be second application can be done after 10 days this will eliminate the infestation. 60 g of powder is needed for one application.
- Anti-lice shampoos are available which include Permethrin 1%, fenitrothion (0.2–0.4%), deltamethrin shampoo (0.03%). An emulsifiable concentrate known as NBIN containing 68% of benzyl benzoate, 6% DDT, 12% benzocaine and 14% tween 80 (an emulsifier) is also useful. After bath the emulsion is applied after diluting it five times. Treated person should not bathe for 24 hours. About 20 ml of this emulsion is required per person. Impregnation of garments can also be done with these emulsions.

ITCH MITES AND SCABIES

Itch mite (*Sarcoptes scabiei*) causes scabies in man. They are also called burrowing mites and are responsible for mammalian scabies. *Sarcoptes scabiei* is small globular in shape and of whitish colour. There is no definite segmentation of the body though it is clearly divided into two regions by a fold or the integument. The integument shows transverse striations and is provided with scales, hair and spines. The legs are short and stumpy and are arranged in two groups, each is provided with powerful claw. The mite is hardly visible to the naked eye but with hand lens it can be better appreciated (Fig. 11.9).

Life History

The female itch mite burrows into epidermis of skin. The parts of the body selected for burrowing and oviposition are well defined which include, interdigital spaces, the wrists particularly the ulnar margins, elbows, anterior folds of axilla, the penis, scrotum and buttocks, the back of the knee, ankles, toes and abdomen.

Oviposition commences almost with burrowing. Eggs are laid in burrows. The egg is ovoviviparous. The larvae emerge from eggshell after 3–4 days and on emerging from eggshell these quickly escape to the surface. It has a short life and it moults to form nymph in 2–3 days. The nymph digs into the hair follicle for the first time. A papule appears at the spot selected by the nymph for burrowing and it develops into vesicle. The appearance of vesicle synchronizes with the maturation of nymph to adult which takes 4–8 days. The whole life cycle gets completed in 9–15 days.

Scabies

The appearance of papule causes intense itching, irritation and this induces scratching and it enables the parasite to escape to the surface of the skin. The female after depositing the full complement of eggs dies at the blind end of the burrow. The itching is more intense at night than daytime. The transmission of scabies occurs by close contacts and prolonged contacts and sleeping on the same bed and sharing of linen is necessary for spread of disease. Most often all the family members are affected one after the other because they share same beds and clothing. Scabies run into family and invariably affects all family members. Its implication is that the treatment should be given to all family members; otherwise the infection tends to persist in the family. Infection does not provide any immunity.

Prevention and Control

Scabies is seasonal disease and affects those families and individuals who lack personal hygiene. Good personal

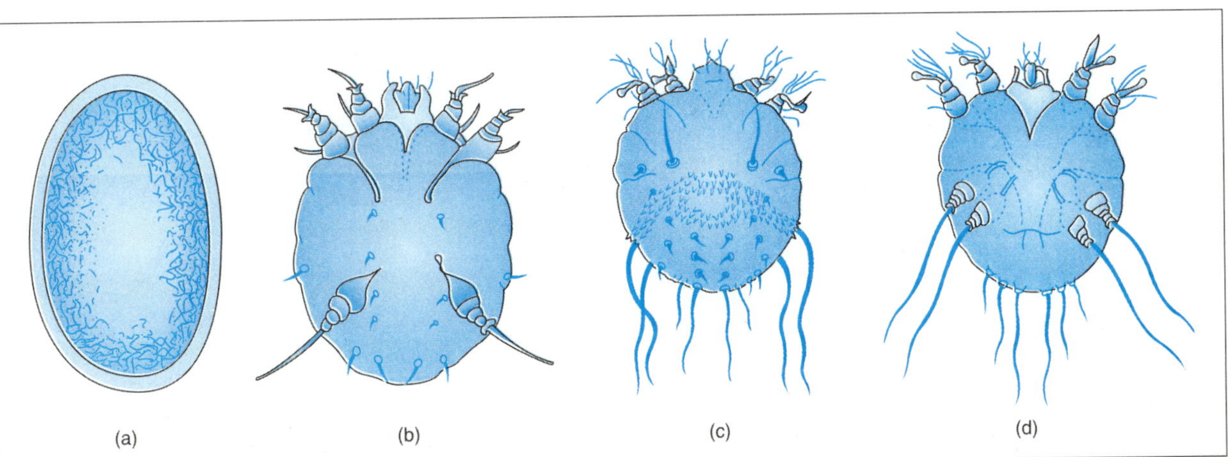

Fig. 11.9: Egg (a) and larva (b) of *Sarcoptes scabiei* (female) from man; dorsal and ventral aspects (c and d)

hygiene—regular bath and clean linen and clean undergarments and exposure of bed linen to sun, prevents scabies. Therefore, best prevention against scabies is personal hygiene.

Treatment

All the family members must be treated as scabies is household infection and affects all the family members. It is the household which needs to be treated. Beds and linen be washed and sun dried.

Treatment: After bath with soap and water the application of benzyl benzoate emulsion 25% all over the body; the body should be painted with this emulsion, below neck and avoiding application to eye. The application may be repeated after 12 hours and thereafter bath with soap and hot water be given. The clothes, bed linen should be washed and sun dried.

BITING MITES

Mites are known by several names such as chiggers, harvest mites, kedany or scrub mite and house dust mites. Numerous species of mite are parasitic on mammals and birds and occasionally attack humans. The trombiculid mites transmit typhus fever due to *Orientia tsutsugamushi* in Asia and Pacific.

Distribution

The most important species are:

1. *Leptotrombidium deliense* which is vastly distributed in Indian Subcontinent and South East Asia. In India, it is distributed in whole of the Shivalik ranges, Eastern and Western ghats and Vindhyachal ranges in central India. It transmits scrub typhus.
2. *Leptotrombiculum akamushi* is widespread in Japan.

Disease Relationship—Scrub Typhus

Biting mites can transmit a number of rickettsial diseases to humans, but the most important one is *scrub typhus*. It is caused by gram-negative bacterium of family Rickettsiaceae—*Orientia tsutsugamushi* and leads to high grade fever with chills, severe headache and lymphadenopathy. At the site of attachment of the infected larvae (Chiggers), a primary skin lesion consisting of a punched-out ulcer covered by eschar commonly develops before the onset of the fever attack. In severe cases with pneumonia and myocarditis, the mortality rate may reach 30 percent.[9]

Morphology

The adult trombiculid mite is 1–2 mm in size bright red or reddish-brown in colour, of velvety appearance and its body is densely covered with hair. The mouth parts are suited for bite and proboscis has cutting apparatus called chelicerae.

Life Cycle (Fig. 11.10)

The mite passes its life cycle through four stages: (a) Egg, (b) larva, (c) nymph, and (d) adult. Eggs are laid in the soil. After about a week, the egg hatches and larva emerges. Larva is very active. It moves actively in search of host such as rat, mouse, bandicoot and human host. Only larval stages are parasitic. The larva (Chigger) feed on lymph and tissue fluids of the animal host and remain attached to skin of the host for two days to a month. After feeding, the larva drops on the ground or loose soil it takes 7 days time to digest the food and to develop to next stage, i.e. nymph. The nymphal stage lasts for 14 days. After about 10 days adult mite with differentiated sex emerges. Overall it takes 6–12 weeks time for its development from egg. All stages except larva develop in soil. *Chigger index* of ≥0.69 per

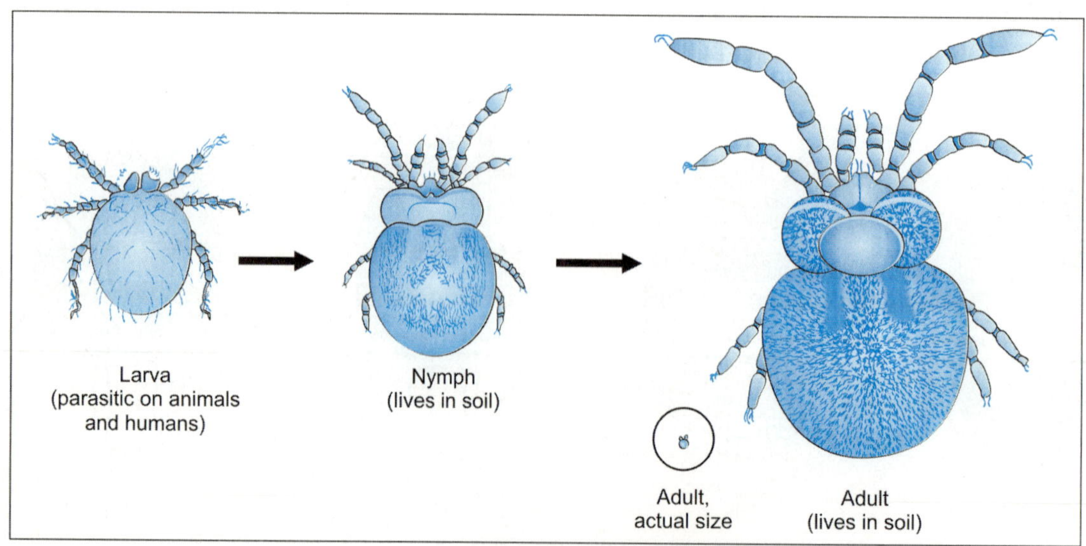

Fig. 11.10: Biting mite (Trombicula species)

host is critical indicator of implementation of vector control measures.

Animal Reservoirs

The animal reservoir for larval stage of mite are rats, mice, bandicoots, shrews and humans. These play host for larval mites. These animals also serve as reservoir of rickettsiae. Mite-borne scrub typhus is caused by rickettsial organism: *Orientia tsutsugamushi* which is transmitted to man by bite of infective larval mite. Man is accidentally involved when he comes in contact with infected larvae of mite in infested soil. Large number of cases occurred in army personnel during 1965 and 1971 conflict with Pakistan. In India, scrub typhus has been reported from Rajasthan, J & K, Vellore, Himachal Pradesh and Sikkim.

Control Measures

Infected persons can be treated with tetracycline or its derivatives. Prevention is possible by avoiding contact with mite and application of repellents to skin and clothing. Residual insecticide spray (malathion) in infested area is effective against mites.

TICKS

Ticks included in the order Acarina are divided into two families, Ixodidae and Argasidae. The family Ixodidae includes hard ticks and family Argasidae includes soft ticks. The hard tick is a jungle tick while the soft tick is domestic or household tick like a bedbug.

HARD TICKS

Hard ticks belong to superfamily Ixodidae. The common hard ticks in India which belong to genera ixodes; are *Dermacentor, Amblyomma, Haemaphysalis, Rhipicephalus, Hyalomma and Boophilus.*[6]

Diseases Transmitted

These ticks transmit Kyasanur forest disease (KFD), tick-borne relapsing fever, Q fever, lyme disease, Rocky Mountain spotted fever, tick typhus, Colorado tick fever and other viral haemorrhagic fevers and encephalitis. These ticks also transmit Tularaemia besides tick paralysis.

Morphology

The body is oval, segmentation into head-thorax and abdomen is obliterated. Hard ticks are readily recognized by their dorsal shield called scutum and also by the capitulum which lies anteriorly. The scutum may be ornate with grey or white pattern. The two sexes can be easily differentiated. The scutum or hard shield is derived from the integument and becomes highly chitinized. In male, it covers almost the whole back and this prevents the tick from increasing to any appreciable size, whereas in the female it covers only a small part of the back; thus allowing female tick to increase in size considerably. The females are thus much larger in size. At the anterior end, lies the false head or capitulum and posteriorly the abdomen. The capitulum has rectangular or hexagonal shape. From its anterior part project, the proboscis or beak which includes cutting instruments called chelicerae. Antennae are absent. Eyes may or may not be present. Metamorphosis is incomplete and sexes are separate. Both sexes thrive on blood alone and lead an intermittent parasite life during the major part of their cycle. The host range includes warm blooded and cold blooded animals. Majority of the ticks live on ground in forest. Adults have four pairs of walking legs. The larvae has three pairs of walking legs, while nymph has four pairs (Fig. 11.11).

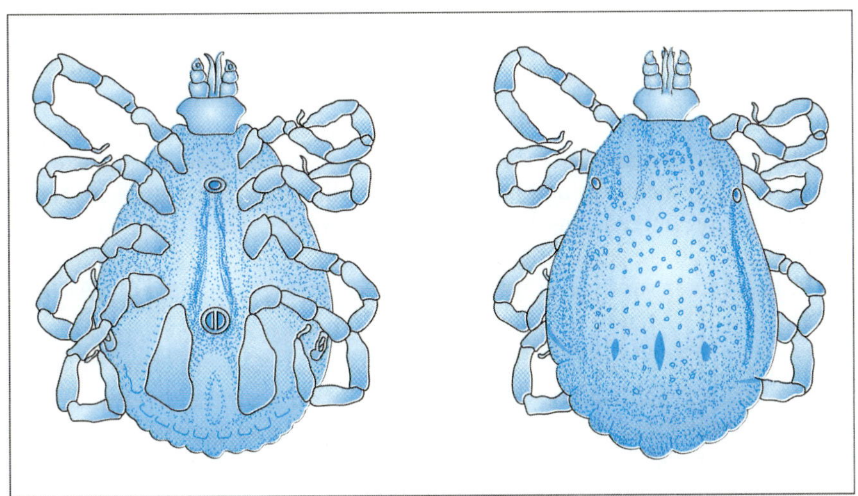

Fig. 11.11: Ventral and dorsal aspects of *Rhipicephalus sanguineus* (hard tick)

Life Cycle

The life cycle consists of four stages: Egg, larva, nymph and adult.

- After mating, the eggs are laid in cracks, crevices or on grass in vicinity where female tick has dropped off from the host. Large number of eggs are laid. The oviposition often occupies more than a week. The egg is proportionately large, round and brown in colour when ripe. Hard ticks deposit all their eggs in a single act of oviposition after which the female dies. The egg seldom hatches before three weeks. From the eggs emerges hexapod larva.
- Larva survives on ground and waits for appropriate host. It attaches itself to host to suck blood, and when its body is full of blood meal it drops on the ground and remains quiet till the blood gets digested. It moults and develops into next stage, i.e. nymph.
- In the same way as larva does, the nymph seeks a new host, feeds on blood and falls on the ground where it moults and get transformed into an adult. After fertilization and feeding has been completed the life history begins again. This is an instance of three host tick where adult, larvae and nymphal tick abandon their hosts after feeding. Thus, they require access to host on three occasions—in the adult, larval and nymphal stages.

Bionomics

Most members of genus *Rhipicephalus* and *Boophilus* spend whole of their life cycle on one host hence they are called "one host tick". It means adult, larva and nymphal stage thrive only on one host for their total development cycle.

- *R. evertsi* which is a two host-ticks undergoes metamorphosis from larva to nymph upon the host.
- Medically important hard ticks belonging to genera Ixodes, *Haemaphysalis* and *Dermacentor* are all "three host-ticks".
- In soft ticks genus Ornithodoros, each stage of the five moults is completed on different hosts and hence such ticks are called 'multiple host-ticks'. Adult may also feed intermittently on different hosts.

Vector Potential

Ticks are capable of producing disease in man by transmitting the viruses, rickettsia, spirochaetes and bacilli of infectious diseases. They also produce toxins in their saliva. Ticks feed entirely on blood and are persistent blood suckers. Wide range of host helps their survival in nature. Further transovarian transmission of infection sustains the infection for years. Ticks can survive the hardy environment.

Indian Tick Typhus

11

The disease is caused by *R. conorii* and is transmitted to man through bite of hard ticks such as *Rhipicephalus sanguineus* in Kashmir, *Ixodae ricinus* in Almora and *Haemaphysalis leachi* var *indica* in Manipur. The ticks are acquired by man from domestic animals like cattle, horses and dogs. The disease occurs in sporadic form in India and has been reported from many parts of the country namely Allahabad, Narsapatnam, Ratlam, Secunderabad, Bangalore, Jhansi, Pune and Lucknow.

SOFT TICKS

Soft ticks of genus Ornithodoros are important. In soft ticks the dorsal cover or scutum is entirely absent hence they are called soft ticks. The capitulum lies ventrally and mouth parts are not visible from above. Sexual diamorphism is absent (Fig. 11.12). They feed during night. Soft ticks are domestic and are able to live much longer without any food (even about a year). These are found in human dwellings and cattle sheds and attack man and animals during their sleep. They, however, live away from their hosts, like bed bugs, in cracks and crevices and only emerge at night to feed on the host.

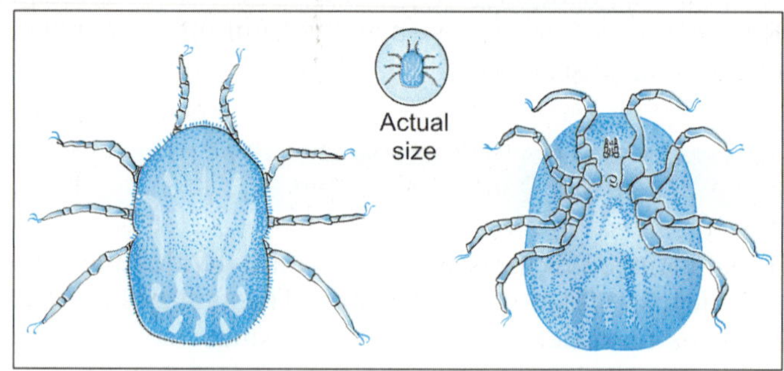

Fig. 11.12: Soft tick *Ornithodoros moubata*; dorsal and ventral aspects (WHO)

Disease Transmission

Soft ticks of genus *Ornithodoros transmit* various types of spirochaetes causing relapsing fever in certain parts of the world.

Relapsing fever is caused by *Borrelia duttoni* in Africa and it is transmitted by soft tick from man to man by the human tick called *O. moubata*. The tick serves as true intermediate host for this disease and the infection is transmitted through ovaries (transovarian) to their offsprings. *O. turicata* is prevalent vector in America. *O. lahorensis* is found in central Asia and North West India. In India, they are found in Kashmir and are known as *O. crossi*.

CONTROL OF TICKS AND MITES

Tick infested areas can be treated with appropriate insecticide. Since the hard ticks are in jungle it may not be possible. In human dwellings, the ticks can be controlled by regular spray operation or dusting with insecticide can be helpful. Suspension of 50% HCH water dispersible powder, one kg in 10 litres of water sprayed over 500 meters or Lindane 0.5 kg/hectare are also effective. It can be repeated after 8 weeks. This is useful if a camp is to be set-up for refugees or army or for persons who have to work in forests.

Premises or Dwellings

Application of HCH suspension on floors and wall surface on alternate days, malathion, fenitrothion or carbamate compounds can also be used as 0.5–1.0% spray or as 5–10% dust. Dogs and other pets can be treated by wash or spray containing 2.0% malathion.

Personal Protection

It includes wearing of shoes and proper clothing and application of repellent like dibutylphthalate (DBP), diethyltoluamide (DEET) and benzylbenzoate. These are applied to clothing and skin. Application to clothing is more effective.

RODENTS

Rodents in India are significant because of their nuisance and alarming population, besides losses of crops after harvesting. The rodents are reservoir of many diseases of public health significance. Rodent population (particularly rat population) is much more than human population. In view of this, it becomes necessary to control their population. Rats should be destroyed not only for the reason that they are principal reservoir of bubonic plague in man but also are responsible for economic loss.

COMMON RODENTS

- Common house mouse is known as Mus musculus.
- Roof rat is known as *Rattus rattus*.
- Sewer rat is known as *Rattus norvegicus*.
- Besides these, there are several wild rodents.

In *R. rattus,* the tail is often one and a quarter time long as the head and body combined, the eyes are large and prominent, the ears are large, muzzle narrow, tail uniformly dark, feet slender. The colour in the Indian species is usually brown. It is widely distributed in India. It is a domestic rat and is a good climber.

In *Rattus norvegicus,* the tail is almost 90% the length of head and body. It is a heavy bodied rat with large heavy tail, ears and eyes are small, the feet are large, heavy and flesh coloured, no long piles or bristles on the body. It is a drain rat and visits houses at night. It is also a burrowing rat and good swimmer (Fig. 11.13).

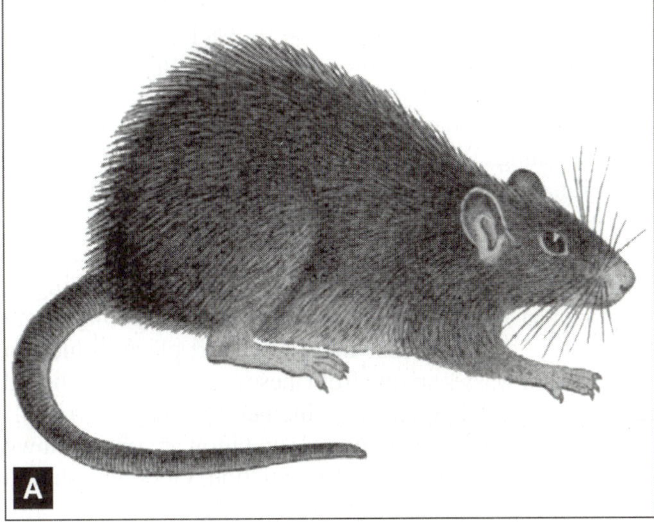

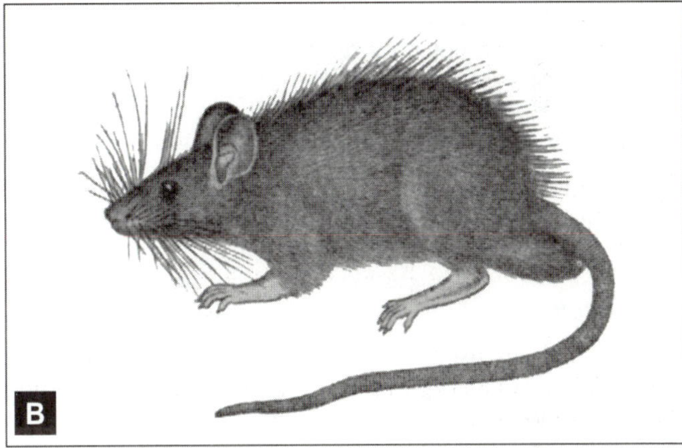

Fig. 11.13: (A) *Rattus norvegicus,* (B) *Rattus rattus*

Significance

Rodents are responsible for zoonotic diseases and they serve as reservoir of many zoonotic diseases the major zoonotic diseases related to rodents are:

i Rodents act as hosts to ecto- and endo-parasites causing human and animal diseases. Rat flea is most important ectoparasite of rats which transmits bubonic plague in man. Other bacterial infections transmitted through rodents are *P. tularensis* and salmonellosis.

ii Rat flea also transmits Murine typhus (endemic typhus). It is caused by *R. typhi.*

iii Wild rodents are reservoir of scrub typhus, when infective mite larva transmits infection to human beings accidentally.

iv *Allodermanyssus sanguineus* mite infest rats and transmits rickettsial pox.

v Tick typhus is also associated with rodents.

vi Transmission of three species of Spirochaetes namely *Leptospira icterohaemorrhagica*, *Spirillium minus* and *Borrelia recurrentis* and Dutoni, causing Weil's disease or leptospirosis, rat bite fever and relapsing fever respectively are related to rodents.

vii Virus of lymphocytic choreomeningitis, haemorrhagic fever, encephalitis and certain parasites like leishmaniasis, Chagas' disease are other infections associated with rodents.

ANTI-RODENT MEASURES

Environmental measures include town planning and slum clearance. Denying the rats to hide and access to food are the cardinal principles. Common places where rat population thrive in abundance include warehouses, provision houses, slaughter houses, hostels, restaurants and slum areas. In rural settings, rats thrive in granaries, cattle sheds, rooms, piggeries, horse stables which provide them abundance of food, breeding and places to hide. Each home in rural setting is a granary as grains are stored for months together till next harvesting. Thus, all homes are vulnerable and rats thrive on in abundance on these grains. Most engineering measures are required in these settings. Similarly, rat breeding is abundant at disposal grounds selected by the municipal corporation as it provides them food and place to hide in burrows. All wastes arising from these establishments should be disposed off hygienically, incineration is preferred. If high standards of environmental sanitation are observed we can reduce the menace of rat population. Godowns should be properly planned both regarding their sites and construction. These should be away from habitation. The godowns must be not only rat proof but also be equipped with arrangements for fumigation.

Temporary Methods

These include trapping of rats by baits. Traps are set along the rat runs or near the burrow. After trapping, the rats can be killed by various methods.

Rodenticides

Rodenticides are used after baiting exercises, subsequently the poison can be added to bait. Baits can be prepared by adding following poison:

- **Barium carbonate:** It is inexpensive, but toxic to man and cat. It can be mixed with wheat or rice flour or any pretested bait in the ratio 1:3 (one part powder of barium carbonate and 3 parts of flour). After mixing water, the mixture can be rolled into pills and used appropriately.
- **Zinc phosphide:** Widely used rodenticide. It can be used in the ratio of 1 part to 10 parts of flour (wheat or rice). It emanates garlic smell. Toxic to man. It is used in granaries, godowns and on docks.
- **Warfarin (a derivative of Dicumarol):** It is anticoagulant and causes slow death in rats. It is used in the ratio of 1 part of poison to 19 parts of dry-meal in flour or chapattis or bread crumbs. This is commonly used on board, the ships, and also in granaries. It is toxic to man.
- **Alpha-naphthylthiourea (ANTU) 1–3.5%:** It is specific for *Rattus norvegicus*. It is sprinkled in and around rat burrows, holes and runways.
- **Coumatetralyl:** The compound is available as Racumin tracking powder (0.75%) one part of poison in 19 parts of wheat flour can be used.
- **Fumigants:** Fumigants are widely applied in enclosed spaces such as ships, granaries, godowns and rodent burrows. Commonly used fumigants are sulphur dioxide, carbon disulphide, calcium cyanide (cynogas), carbon monoxide and methyl bromide. Cynogas has been widely used in India. Fumigation is done by mechanical devices.
- **Aluminium phosphide tablets (Al-phos):** 6 g tablet per rodent burrow is effective in field. The burrow should be sealed with wet soil after the bait is placed.

Note: All baits mentioned above are poisonous to human beings and domestic animals. These should be used with great precaution. Left out baits should be carefully counted and removed safely.

CYCLOPS OR WATER FLEA

These are minute creatures and popularly known as water fleas and they have the capability of swimming in water with jerky movements. They are visible to naked eye (Fig. 11.14).

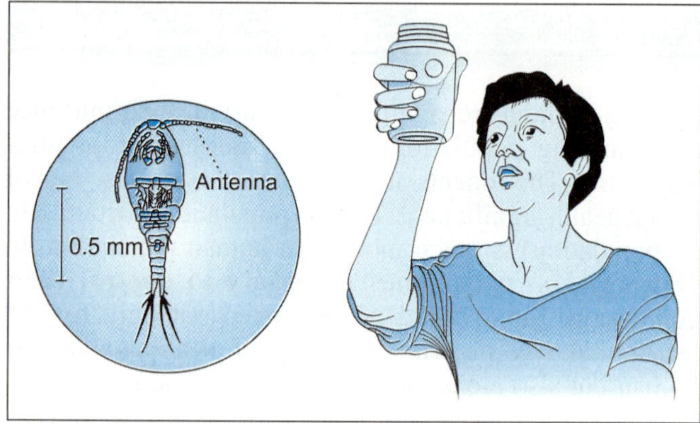

Fig. 11.14: Cyclops—intermediate host of guinea worm (WHO)

Disease Relationship

Cyclops are intermediate host of guinea worm (*Dracunculus medinensis*). The disease has been eradicated from India since 2000.

Cyclops exist almost over the globe and found in pools, tanks, ditches, step wells and ponds and thrive on spores of aquatic plants and algae and minute insects. These can be easily strained by piece of muslin cloth. Ordinary domestic strainer can be used to separate cyclops and to make drinking water safe. In fact, strainers were widely used as part of guinea worm eradication programme to make the water free from cyclops. Boiling of water also kills cyclops.

Characters

It is an insect which is demarcated into cephalothorax and abdomen. The head is fused with thoracic segment. It is pear-shaped. The head always carries two pairs of antennae. The other appendages of head consist of three pairs of jaw. The chiten is strongly calcified. The sexes are separate. The life cycle passes through the stages of egg, larva or naupilus and adult. The eggs can resist dry conditions and are blown by winds and contaminate water source at distant place.

Control

1. The cyclops can be easily filtered by a piece of muslin cloth or domestic nylon strainer. Strainer and muslin cloth can withhold cyclops.
2. Boiling of water can kill cyclops. Similarly, super-chlorination kills cyclops. Guinea worm has been eradicated now by provision of alternate sources of safe water supply and by education campaigns.

REDUVIID BUGS

It belongs to family Reduviidae and genus *Triatoma* and also called cone-nosed bug. It is much larger than bedbugs and found in all parts of the world. The body is elongate, the head is also elongate and eyes are placed well forward. It is a blood sucker. Size is about an inch or more in length and it attacks man. The bug thrives in old houses, crevices and holes.

Disease Relationship

It transmits *Trypanosoma cruzi* which produces Chagas' disease in South America. This parasite develops in the intestine of bug and man becomes infected due to faecal contamination of the wound.

Control measures: By observation of sanitation measures. The bugs are killed by insecticide like pyrethrum.

REFERENCES

1. GOI. Entomological activities under National antimalarial programme. Malaria and its control in India. Country Scenario. New Delhi: MOH and FW, GOI; 1999.
2. GOI/MOH and FW. Bio-ecological characteristics of principal malarial vectors in India. Epidemiology and control of malaria in India. New Delhi: MOH and FW, GOI; 1996.
3. Roy AP, Narasimham MVVL, Kalra NL. Indian society for malaria and other communicable diseases. Malaria—A brochure for Medical Officers. Misc. Publications 1991 June; 1(1).
4. ICMR. Summary report of the International Conference of Dengue Haemorrhagic fever and National Brain Storming session on Dengue. ICMR Bulletin 1994 May 5; 24(5).
5. Sharma VP. Ranbaxy Science foundation. Dengue haemorrhagic fever epidemic in Delhi. Some entomological aspects. Round table conference. 1996 December, Series I. New Delhi: India.
6. WHO. Vector Control. Methods for use by individuals and communities. Geneva: WHO; 1997.
7. NICD. Zoonotic diseases of public health importance. New Delhi: NICD; 2000.
8. WHO. Chemical methods for the control of vectors and pests of public health importance. Geneva: WHO; 1984.
9. GOI. NCDC, DGHS, Scrub Typhus and other Rickettsioses. Monthly News Letter of NCDC May–July 2009; 13:(1).

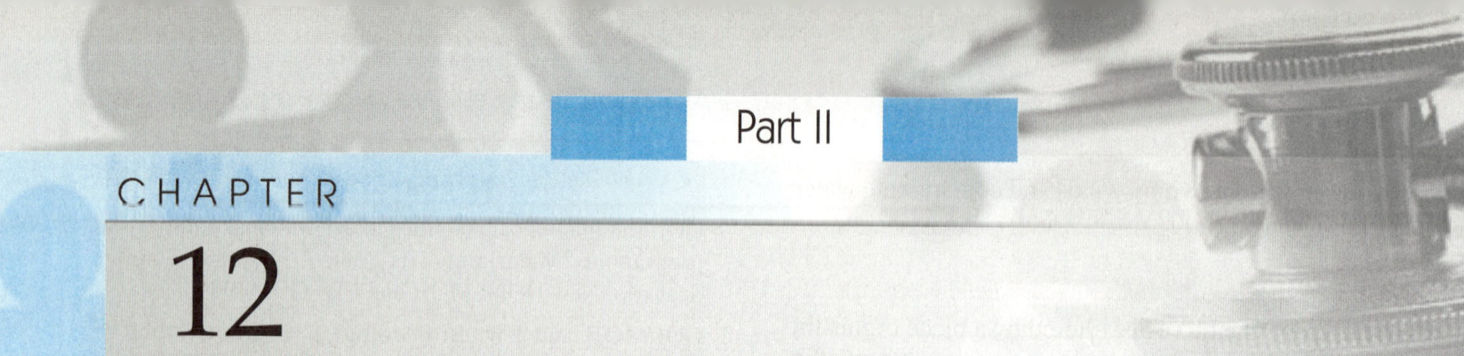

CHAPTER

12

Epidemiology of Communicable Diseases and Related National Health Programmes

HIV/AIDS

Acquired immunodeficiency syndrome (AIDS) is a leading cause of adult deaths in the world. Case fatality rate is 100%. HIV/AIDS has emerged as Pandemic and has become the leading cause of death in many parts of the world. Acquired immunodeficiency syndrome (AIDS) is caused by human immunodeficiency virus (HIV) and is a serious disorder of immune system. HIV destroys body defence mechanism or immune system against infection and threatens life. AIDS is a killer disease—no cure is known and no vaccine is available against it. HIV was first detected in India at Vellore in 1986.

Sustainable development goal for HIV and AIDS: Halt and begin to reverse by 2015, the spread of HIV and AIDS and **end** epidemic by 2030.

NATURAL HISTORY OF HIV/AIDS

The natural history of any disease refers to the stages through which a disease passes, in the absence of any intervention. Clear knowledge of natural history of a disease helps in identifying the stages vis-à-vis appropriate intervention to prevent or control the disease.

The natural history of HIV infection begins as soon as virus enters the body of a susceptible host through any of the routes of transmission as discussed subsequently (sexual, parenteral and perinatal).

Antibody test at this stage does not reveal the true status as it takes some time for formation of antibodies. Therefore, a person during this stage is not aware (even after testing) that he is infected and is capable of transmitting the virus to others. Even after the test becomes positive, the person still continues to look and feel healthy and remains asymptomatic for a number of years. Also, such a person continues to transmit infection to others, who may be unsuspecting, i.e. he/she is an HIV carrier. The *infectivity* of the virus is thus *lifelong*, though it may vary with time, being high:

- In the initial stages of infection
- In the late stages when clinical manifestations appear.

Progression to AIDS is variable. Evidence today suggests 20% of those infected will develop AIDS in 5 years, and 50% in 10 years and a decreasing proportion even after 10 years. The hallmark of HIV infection is progressive loss of a specific type of immune cell called T-helper or CD4 cells. When the CD4 count falls below 200, the person is said to develop AIDS.

Because of this long latent period in developing of clear-cut clinical manifestations, it is estimated that for every full-blown case of AIDS, there are 3–5 with ARC (AIDS-related conditions) and 50–100 infected with the virus but who are asymptomatic. AIDS is, therefore, often termed "The hidden epidemic" (Fig. 12.1).[1]

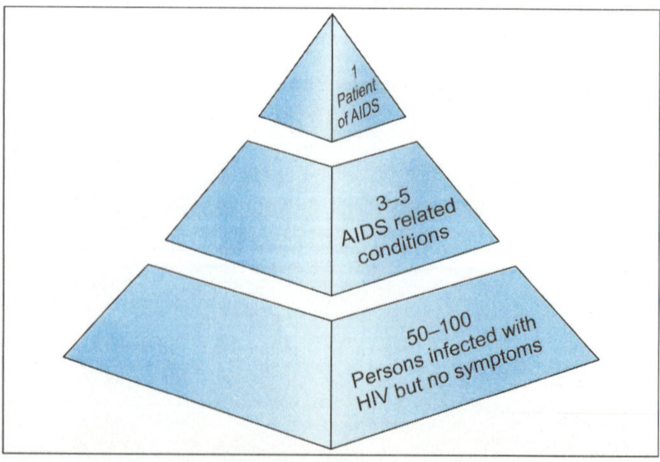

Fig. 12.1: Hidden epidemic (Iceberg phenomenon)

What is HIV Positive—Window Period?

The presence of antibodies against HIV in human body is termed as HIV positivity and the person is called HIV positive (seropositive). It takes 6–12 weeks after infection for antibodies to rise to detectable level. There is thus a *window period* during which infected person may transmit infection despite being seronegative.

EPIDEMIOLOGY OF HIV/AIDS

HIV and AIDS is a global problem: It is a modern epidemic and pandemic and it recognizes no boundaries. Since, it is a global problem, it requires global response.

Magnitude of Problem

At the end of 2014, people living with HIV were estimated around 36.92 million in the world more than ever before due to life prolonging effect of anti-retroviral therapy.[2]

New HIV infections in 2006.....2.9 million (2.7–3.1 million)[2], and 2.0 million new infections in 2014.

Deaths due to AIDS in 2014......1.2 million (WHO-UNAIDS Report, 2015).

HIV was leading cause of mortality and disease burden (DALYs) among adults (15–49 years of age) worldwide in the year 2003 leaving behind the ischemic heart disease, tuberculosis and road traffic accidents.

Global Distribution and Global Strategy 2016-21

Global burden of HIV in the year 2006 was around 32.4 million which increased to 36.92 million in 2014. While no country is free from HIV/AIDS, it is not uniformly distributed in the world. The worst affected region is Sub-Saharan Africa which is home to 25.80 million of HIV adults and children. Next comes Asia and pacific which accounts for 5.0 million HIV cases and India contributes over 2.11 million to this pool or India is the next big epicentre of HIV/AIDS after Africa (Table 12.1).

The joint United Nation's Programme on HIV/AIDS leads and inspires the world to achieve its shared vision of **zero** new HIV infections, **zero** discrimination and **zero** AIDS related deaths. Target by 2020: 90% people living with HIV know their status, 90% who know their status should be on ART and 90% on treatment have suppressed viral load.

Burden of HIV in India (Table 12.2)

India is facing multiple and diverse epidemics. India is large diverse country with regions that are primarily

Table 12.1: Global distribution of HIV/AIDS

	Adults and children living with HIV, 2014		
Region	*HIV case load (million)*	*Country*	*HIV prevalence levels in adults 15–49 years (%) in 2014*
Sub-Saharan Africa	25.80	Botswana	25.2
		Zimbabwe	15.0
Middle East and North Africa	0.24	Malavi	10.0
Asia and the Pacific	5.00	Zambia	12.4
Latin America	1.70	South Africa	18.9
		Kenya	5.3
Caribbean	0.28	**India**	**0.3**
Eastern Europe and Central Asia	1.50	Nepal	0.2
Western and Central Europe and North America	2.40	USA (2011)	0.6*
		Canada (2011)	0.3*
Global burden	**36.92**	Thailand	1.1

Source: UNAIDS global and regional statistics, 2014 and UNICEF – 2016*.

Table 12.2: Trends of HIV in India in different population groups

Population groups	*2003*	*2004*	*2005*	*2006*	*2007*	*2008–09*	*2010–11*	*2014–15*
STD	5.68	5.54	5.66	3.73	3.59	2.21	–	Discontinued
Antenatals	0.80	0.95	0.90	0.60	0.49	0.49	0.42	0.35
FSW	10.33	9.43	8.44	4.90	5.06	4.94	2.67	2.2
IDU	13.15	11.16	10.16	6.92	7.23	9.19	7.17	9.9
MSM	8.47	7.47	8.74	6.41	7.41	7.30	4.43	4.3
Trukers	–	–	–	2.37	2.87	1.57	2.59	–
Migrants	–	–	–	1.60	3.61	2.17	0.99	–

Prevalence figures in Percentages source, NACO—India.

experiencing low level and concentrated epidemics. High prevalence rates of > 5% have been observed in high-risk core groups and bridge population (concentrated epidemics).

There is no generalized epidemic in India (i.e. prevalence rate > 5% in antenatals).

There are 'HOT SPOTS' (high prevalence pockets) in each state which needs to be targeted for interventions on priority basis.

Until 2005, the rising trend of HIV in India was obvious. Though the epidemic was introduced late in India it has spread very fast and no state is free from HIV.

During the year 2006 reported HIV prevalence rate of 0.36% was down from last year's (2005) 0.9% in adults. Accordingly the disease burden due to HIV/AIDS in India was 2.47 million adults, down from 5.21 million in the year 2005. This was due to application of improved method of estimation of HIV by using the internationally comparable workbook method and using multiple data sources namely expanded sentinel surveillance system, NFHS III, integrated biological and behavioural survey (IBBS).

Until year 2005, HIV estimates in India were produced mainly using sentinel surveillance data which was the only large dataset available. During the year 2006 by use of additional data sources in addition to the improved methodologies have resulted in a lower and a more robust estimate of HIV in India. The new methods developed for revised estimates have also been used to "back calculate" the prevalence for years since 2002 based on new set of assumptions and measures. These figures allow a fair comparison of year on year trends in HIV prevalence. The calculation of figures for several years using the new model helps us understand that new **lower estimates** do not mean a sharp decline in the epidemic. The estimated adult prevalence in the country was 0.26% at the end of 2015, with HIV load of 2.11 million. The prevalence rate of HIV in the country has stabilized over the last few years (Table 12.3).[3]

Epidemiological Situation of HIV/AIDS in India[4-5]

One of the important application of HIV sentinel surveillance data is estimation of adult HIV prevalence, number of people living with HIV, new HIV infections (incidence), AIDS related deaths and treatment needs.

National Adult HIV Prevalence

- The adult (15–49 years) HIV prevalence level at national level has continued steady decline from estimated level of 0.38% in 2001 to 0.26% in 2015 with approximately 2.11 million people living with HIV (Table 12.3).
- **Among the states:** Manipur has shown the highest adult HIV prevalence of 1.15%, followed by Mizoram 0.80%, Nagaland 0.78%, Andhra and Telengana 0.66%, Karnataka 0.45%, Gujarat 0.42% and Goa 0.42%.
- The estimated number of new annual HIV infections has declined by 66% over the past decade from 2.51 lakh in 2000 to 86000 in 2015—a sign of reversal of epidemic in India (Fig. 12.2), around 1.48 lakh people died of AIDS related causes in 2007 in India which have declined to 67600 in 2015 (54% decline).
- Sex disaggregated data for number of people living with HIV is estimated at approximately 61% male and 39% female. The HIV infection by age is estimated at 6.54% among children below the age of 15 years, 86% among adults aged 15–49 years and the remaining 7% among people over 50 years of age.
- While declining trends have been noted at national level among general population, female sex workers and men who have sex with men, stable trends are recorded among Injecting Drug Users (IDUs) warranting increased attention to emerging pockets of IDU in different states (Punjab, Delhi, Maharashtra, Manipur, Mizoram, Chandigarh and Odisha)—Table 12.2.
- Around 57% new infections are occurring in low prevalence states of North India, Haryana, Uttarakhand, Chhattisgarh, Gujarat, Jharkhand and Odisha. Higher prevalence in rural than urban population, higher

Table 12.3: Trends of adult HIV prevalence in India (2001 to 2015)

Year	Prevalence rate(%)	HIV burden in million
2001–03	0.38	2.51
2007	0.34	2.22
2008	0.32	2.19
2009	0.31	2.17
2010	0.30	2.15
2011	0.29	2.14
2012	0.28	2.12
2013 and 14	0.27	2.11
2015	0.26	2.11

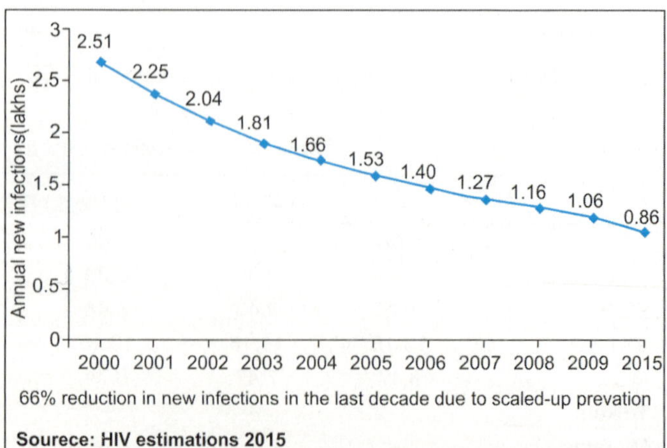

Fig. 12.2: Evidence of programme impact

12

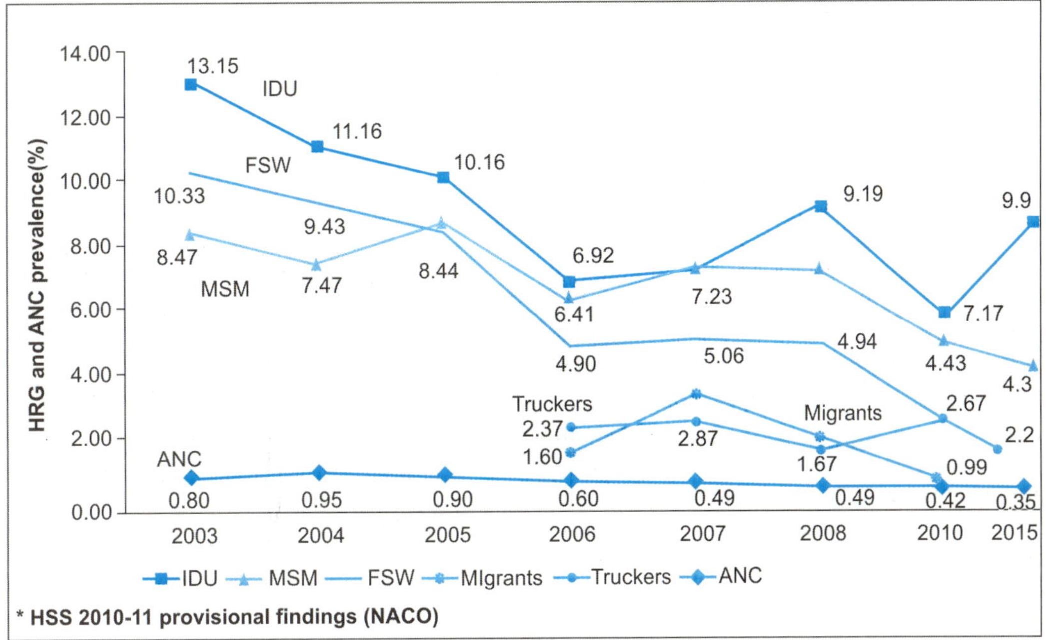

Fig. 12.3: HIV: Declining trends in general population and high-risk groups

prevalence among pregnant women with migrant spouses and very low levels of HIV prevalence among HRG, coupled with evidence generated beyond HSS, towards possible role of Single Men Migration in the spread of epidemic in some of these states.

HIV Prevalence in Core High Risk Groups (IBBS—2014–15)

India is known to have concentrated HIV epidemic in FSW, MSM and IDU. The IBBS provides critical information for the first time on representative HIV prevalence data among FSW, MSM and IDU from many more states and regions across the country. This critical evidence based information is helpful to National Programme to prevent further transmission and control of HIV (Fig. 12.3).

HIV Prevalence: Among FSWs at the national level was recorded as 2.2%. In Maharashtra it was 7.4%, and 6.3% in Andhra Pradesh. Other high prevalence states with higher than 5% prevalence rate were the group of states of Manipur, Mizoram, and Nagaland where prevalence was recorded as 5.9%, followed by FSWs in Karnataka with similar prevalence of 5.8%. All other groups of states recorded HIV prevalence less than 2%

HIV Prevalence among MSMs recorded at national level was 4.3%, MSMs in Andhra Pradesh recorded HIV prevalence of 10.1%, in Gujarat and Goa 6.8% and other group of states of West Bengal, Odisha and Jharkhand it was 6.7%, in Maharashtra 4.9% and in Karnataka 4.1%. In all other states and group of states the HIV prevalence was 3% or less.

HIV Prevalence among IDUs at the national level was 9.9%. In the group of states of Bihar, UP, and Uttarakhand it was 27.2%, closely followed was the state group of Delhi and Rajasthan (21.8%). Other states/group of states where HIV prevalence was more than 10% were: the state group of Chhatisgarh and MP (13.6%) and state of Manipur recorded 12.1% prevalence, Mizoram recorded 10% and state group of Odisha, Jharkhand, and West Bengal and State group of Punjab and Chandigarh recorded 9.7% of prevalence and other group of states with more than 5% of prevalence were Haryana, Himachal and J & K (7.3%). Among all other states prevalence was less than 5%.

HIV Prevalence among Youth

The prevalence of HIV in young people indicates high prevalence in Sub-Saharan Africa—1.3% of male against 3.1% female were infected in the year 2011, while in South and South East Asia prevalence in male and female was 0.1%. The prevalence has come down almost 50% when compared with baseline year of 2001.

Parent to Child Transmission

Of 17 sub-Saharan countries reporting on prevention of mother to child transmission (PMTCT), 12 have almost no ARV prophylaxis programme with HIV prevalence among newborn babies of infected mothers reaching 25%.

Incidence[6–8]

Globally, 7000 new HIV infections occur per day most among youth and women. About 900 of these were in children below 15 years of age. In 2014 around 2.0 million were newly infected with HIV, a reduction of 36% since 2000. Young people aged 15–24 years accounted for 40% of all new adult (15+) HIV infections. In India incidence

12

(new infections) were estimated to be 86000 million in the year 2014. Prevalence of 0.11% of HIV in young persons in India is proxy for incidence in young persons.

In India, HIV prevalence among young people (15–24 years) at national level is estimated at 0.11% unlike adult HIV prevalence where HIV prevalence among male is around 1.5 times that among female, in young population HIV prevalence is equal among men and women at 0.11%. HIV prevalence in young people has declined from 0.30% 2000 to 0.11% in 2011.

The age of first infection in 15–19 years, and the prevalence of HIV in this age group provides indirect evidence of new infections. It was however stable to increasing among 15–19 years of age in certain high prevalence states. Among the Southeren states Andhra Pradesh and Karnataka had a higher prevalence in 2008–09 than 2007 (Table 12.4). In the North Eastern states there was an increase in prevalence only in Nagaland other than Arunachal Pradesh. Other states in which prevalence of HIV increased in 2008 were Himachal Pradesh, Punjab, Odisha and Jharkhand.

India is young and 50% of its population is young between 15 and 24 years old who are "sexually active" if the incidence of HIV is to be reduced, this age bracket must be targeted for information, education and communication on HIV/AIDS.[9–10] They should have access to HIV information for adopting healthy lifestyles and behaviour. This group requires special targeting.

Sex Distribution

In sub-Saharan Africa, men and women are affected in equal proportion. In India, 60% of HIV infections are among men, 40% are in women and 6.54% among children. Men are more mobile and indulge in high-risk sexual behaviour (unsafe sex) and transmit infection to their faithful wives.

Urban-rural Ratio of Estimated HIV Infections

During 2005, the proportion of rural infections was 58.7% against 41.3% urban. It signifies the spread of infection in rural population.

Pattern of Transmission

Thailand's thorough monitoring of epidemic indicated "waves" of HIV transmission:

- The first wave of epidemic transmission in mid-1980s emerged among homosexual men through sexual transmission (men having sex with men or MSM).
- The second wave of transmission was seen among injecting drug users.
- The third wave was observed among commercial sex workers (CSW) as 30% of CSWs were positive by 1993.
- The fourth wave was observed in male STI patients, largely clients of CSWs.
- The fifth wave was evident from increasing HIV infection among the wives and girl friends of CSW clients. As high as 8% of pregnant women in Chiang Mai, Thailand were HIV positive in 1994.
- The sixth wave of transmission is now emerging as mother to child transmission (MTCT), i.e. mothers infected with HIV giving birth to HIV positive children. A similar pattern is emerging in India.

In Manipur (Eastern India), the epidemic unfolded among injecting drug users and 73% of them were positive for HIV in 1995.

Table 12.4: HIV prevalence in antenatal clinic attendees age 15–19 years (%)

Year	India	Nagaland	AP	Karnataka	Mizoram	Manipur
2006	0.49	–	–	–	–	–
2007	0.7	1.1	1.0	0.8	0.9	0.9
2008–2009	0.6	1.4	1.1	0.9	0.6	0.4

Bridge Population in HIV Transmission

Individuals who have sexual partners in the core high-risk group (HRG) and other partners are called "bridge population" because they form a transmission bridge from HRG to general population. HIV infection is transmitted from HRGs to general population through bridge population (Fig. 12.4).

In the context HIV pandemic, the concept of "bridging" refers to the group of people who connect high-risk and low-risk population. Single male migrants (SMM) and long distance truckers (LDT) and men who have sex with commercial sex workers and also with monogamous wives are an example of bridging population. Estimated number of SMM and LDT is 9.2 million in India. The larger the bridging group, the greater is the risk of transmission to general population. Population-based approach to change the behaviour of men who are sexually active and have unsafe sex with multiple sex partners is

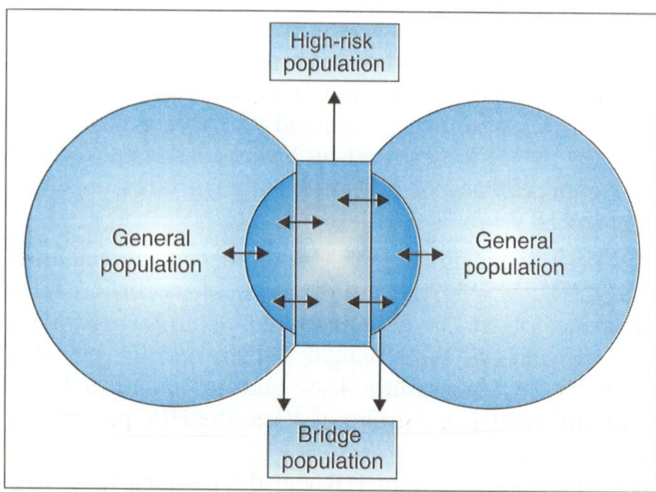

Fig. 12.4: Dynamics of HIV transmission

sound epidemiological approach. As the unprotected sexual intercourse whether men with men or women with men is the most common way of transmitting HIV, between *85 and 90% of new infections are transmitted through unprotected sexual intercourse*. Understanding the sexual behaviour of different sections of the population is the key to designing an effective response to the epidemic. Commercial sex workers are high-risk groups to contract and transmit HIV through sex, the clients of sex workers are the link or "*bridge*" for HIV transmission between the sex workers and the general population. Behavioural sentinel surveillance has been done in India to know the sexual behaviour of "*bridge*" population (Table 12.6).[9]

Modes of Transmission of HIV in India (Fig. 12.5)

The primary driver of HIV epidemic transmission in India is *through unprotected sexual intercourse* (88.2%). Sexual intercourse whether heterosexual or homosexual is the major route of transmission. HIV can be transmitted through any individual act of unprotected sexual intercourse, i.e. any penetrative sexual act in which condom is not used and where one partner is infected with HIV. The risk of becoming infected through an act of unprotected sexual intercourse depends upon:[11]

- The likelihood that the sex partner is infected, the probability that a person has become infected with HIV is in general proportionate to the number of unprotected sex acts, and the number of high-risk partners with whom the person has had sexual contact in recent years. Multiple sex partners is a risk. Sex with stranger and commercial sex workers is an invitation to HIV.
- ***Type of sex act:*** All unprotected acts of sexual penetration (anal, vaginal, oral) carry a risk of HIV transmission because they bring sexual secretions directly into contact with exposed mucus membrane. Injury to the mucus membrane of the rectum, the vagina or the mouth may help the virus to enter into the bloodstream. "Receptive" partners are thus at a greater risk than "insertive" partners in acts of intercourse. However, HIV can also be transmitted through unbroken mucus membrane.

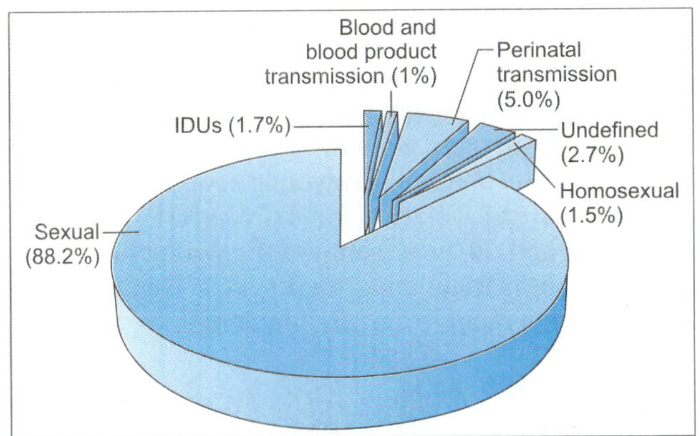

Fig. 12.5: Modes of transmission of HIV in India (2012–13)

- The amount of virus present in the blood or sexual secretion (semen, vaginal or cervical secretions) of the infected partner. Individuals with HIV infection become more infectious as they progress to HIV related diseases and AIDS. There is also an early period of high infectiousness around the time of seroconversion.
- Presence of other sexually transmitted diseases and/or genital lesion in either partner: HIV can be transmitted sexually even when neither partner has any of the other sexually transmitted disease. However, there is strong evidence that men and women with genital ulcer disease or urethral discharge are at increased risk of acquiring and transmitting HIV.

Injecting drug use (IDU) transmission is 1.7%, blood and blood product transmission is *1% and perinatal transmission* is 5%, homosexual transmission is 1.5% and the rest of 2.7% is undefined. Mode of transmission is important information for various interventions or programmes against HIV. Where to put our money and which is the sure bet to contain HIV/AIDS; these informations are the basis of the national programme.

Blood-borne Infection

HIV-infected blood, blood products (unsafe blood), transplanted organs or tissues and the use of improper sterilized needles and syringes that have been in contact with infected blood can transmit HIV. This is the most efficient way of transmission of HIV. Even a small transfusion of infected blood results in virtually 100% seroconversion. Screening or HIV testing of blood in all blood banks is thus mandatory.

Mother to Child Transmission (MTCT) or Vertical Transmission

HIV-infected women can transmit HIV to her foetus or infant before, during or after birth. A pregnant women with HIV infection has approximately 20–45% chance of passing the virus to her foetus or newborn baby. There is an evidence that infection can occur as early as the first 12–15 weeks of gestation. 60% of perinatal infections are *in utero* or during the birth process. It is estimated that 40% of perinatal infections occur through breastfeeding. The HIV prevalence in pregnant women is more than 1% in many districts of India which are categorized as high prevalence districts, children born to such mothers will increase the prevalence of HIV in childhood period. HIV will increase childhood mortality and gains achieved through other intervention will be demolished by HIV.

Agent Factors

Agent: HIV, the virus which causes AIDS is lentivirus, one of the subfamily of retroviruses. They have a unique enzyme, reverse transcriptase, which copies the viral ribonucleic acid (RNA) into deoxyribonucleic acid (DNA); which is integrated into host cell chromosome. Hence, HIV persists within cells for years and cannot be eradicated from host cells with any of the currently available anti-retroviral drugs. There are two types of HIV, HIV-1 and HIV-2. Both have many strains. The virus is fragile and gets killed by sunlight, hypochlorite solution and boiling.

Reservoir of Infection

People harbouring HIV in their body are the reservoirs of infection. They may be asymptomatic healthy carriers or full blown AIDS cases. Around 50% of people with HIV infections are likely to develop AIDS within 10 years after first becoming infected. In developing countries, the interval between infection and disease is probably shorter. Person infected with HIV looks normal and healthy for many years.

Sources of Infection

Body fluids like blood, semen, vaginal fluids which contain HIV are the major sources of infection. Contaminated milk may be source of infection from mother to child transmission. Saliva and tears are not considered to be epidemiologically important sources of transmission.

Host Factors

Age, sex (adolescents and youths indulging into unsafe sex), drug abuse, presence of STD in sexual partners and sex with CSWs, are risk behaviours which play an important role for HIV transmission in population. In addition, the literacy level and access to information on HIV and AIDS is an important determinant.

Sociocultural Factors

Urbanization, migration of young people in search of job and leaving their families in rural area and indulging into unprotected sex with CSWs and strangers expose the migrants to risk of HIV and STDs. Similarly, persons who are away from family for days together such as single men migrants, drivers, truckers, army personnel and others are exposed to the risk of unsafe sex.

Commercial Sex Workers (CSWs) and HIV

Prostitution is illegal in India; however, commercial sex work occurs in all parts of the country. In metropolitan cities, sex work tends to be well-organized and operate in well-defined "red light" areas, however, commercial sex work is widespread even in smaller towns, it occurs on major trunk roads, in residential areas, streets, hotels, beaches, massage parlours and call girls operate in posh areas. Thus, commercial sex work is a big industry and generate a lot of money. Because of poverty, many girls from rural areas migrate to bigger cities, such as Mumbai, Kolkata, Chennai and Delhi to work as CSWs and exchange sex for money. CSWs have little power of negotiating and cannot compel their clients to use condoms. Depending upon the area, the CSWs attract lot many clients and contract varied kinds of STI/STDs. Around 60–80% of CSWs have one or the other STDs. Although many CSWs use contraception for prevention of pregnancy, condom is not a popular method of contraception. HIV positive rates are higher in CSWs, because of unsafe sex and prevalence of STDs including hepatitis B surface antigen positivity which is more dangerous than HIV. Treatment seeking behaviour of CSWs for STD is variable and many of them do not seek early treatment.[12]

In Sonagachi, the oldest and largest red light area of Kolkata, the CSWs themselves organized a successful project of condom distribution and ensuring its use and sought early treatment for STDs. This approach had positive impact after 6 years, condom use increased to 90%, the VDRL positivity rate declined from 25 to 12% and HIV showed insignificant/minimum increase. This peer-based approach model demonstrated the worth of self-esteems and self-reliance to control STDs and HIV.[9]

Migration

Many young men migrate from rural areas to urban industrial and big cities as unskilled labourers in search of livelihood, leaving their families behind. Away from home they often have unprotected sex with CSWs. These men get infected and take HIV back to their home and infect their monogamous faithful wives.

Sexually Transmitted Diseases and HIV

STDs have nexus with HIV transmission. Sexually transmitted infections are quite common in India. Prevalence rates of syphilis among pregnant women range from 1 to 5% and it is estimated that approximately 40 million new cases may occur in the country every year. Overall prevalence of STDs varies in men and women, 5.6% of men and 4% of women may have STDs. High prevalence of STD indicates high prevalence of unprotected sexual intercourse; premarital and extramarital sex with commercial sex workers. Factors that determine sexual behaviour are the most important determinants of the spread of STDs. Integrating HIV control with STDs control makes a lot of sense to achieve better results. Thus, controlling STDs is one of the key strategy of HIV control programme.

Vulnerability of Adolescents and Young Adults

About 40% of all new infections of HIV arise in young people (15–24 years), already the prevalence of HIV in age group 15–19 years is showing unfavourable trends.[6] Adolescent health and health of young people should focus on "access to information on HIV/AIDS, modes of transmission and do away some of the wrong beliefs and misconceptions". Regulating their sexual behaviour will have tremendous impact on HIV epidemic.

Economics of HIV/AIDS

Economic losses due to HIV/AIDS are tremendous to individual, family, community and nation. At national and international level, it affects trade and at family level it depletes the budget of the family, due to heavy cost of treatment of AIDS and opportunistic infections. The nation has to spend its budget on this avoidable disease.

Discrimination and Stigma

HIV and AIDS discrimination and stigma prevails and many of them hide their HIV status and go underground. Human Rights Organizations and NGOs are working to eliminate discrimination and stigma but the impact is minimum. HIV positive persons are thrown out of the jobs, family and friends desert them and the person is left to his/her own fate, hospitals and doctors avoid them; by and large and their social life comes to halt.

Health Impact (Tuberculosis and HIV/AIDS)

Globally, 9.6 million people get sick with tuberculosis every year and nearly 1.1 million die of the disease. Most of these cases are reported from 5 countries—Bangladesh, India, Indonesia, Myanmar and Thailand. Between 56 and 80% of AIDS patients in the region have TB, making TB the **most common opportunistic infection** associated with HIV.

In India, 30% of population is infected with TB, although the majority of people who become infected with tuberculosis never develop TB disease, as the body has the ability to fight with TB bacteria which remains dormant. HIV infection is the most important risk factor for TB infection to become active disease. The rate of progression from TB infection to TB disease is 10–30 times higher among individuals with HIV and TB infection than among individuals with only TB infection.

Although not all HIV infected person get TB, it is most common and most important **life-threatening opportunistic infection.** TB can accelerate the progression of HIV to AIDS by accelerating the decline of CD4 counts and creating six- to seven-fold increase in HIV viral load as compared to those without TB. HIV produces multidrug resistant TB. In India, dual burden and epidemic of TB and HIV is a fatal combination, hence aggressive and integrated control of HIV and TB is imperative.

Expectation of Life

HIV/AIDS is a major global health emergency. It is a number one killer of adults the world over. It has reduced life expectancy. Untreated disease caused by HIV has a case fatality rate of 100%. It has made many children orphans.

Coverage of Adults with Antiretroviral Therapy (ART)

Nearly 41% of eligible adults have been covered in all WHO regions. WHO took a lead by initiating narrowing the AIDS treatment gap by providing 3 million people in developing countries with combination of ARV therapy by the end of 2005 (known as the "3 by 5" target).[2] In India 9.19 lakh PLHIV (40%) were on ART by 2015.

Revised guidelines by WHO in 2010: ART should be started in all adolescents and adults including pregnant women with HIV infection and CD4 counts of $\leq$ 350 cells/m^3.

The new strategy by WHO calls for early treatment of all HIV infected persons to stop HIV transmission to partner. This means treating people whose immune system is not depleted to the level that usually requires therapy. The increase in access to antiretroviral therapy is poised to drive the number of people newly infected further downwards, as people living with HIV become less infectious.

United Nations General Assembly Special Session on HIV/AIDS[13]

It was organized in June, 2001 at New York to address the problem of HIV/AIDS in all its aspects to secure a global commitment to combat it in a comprehensive manner and follow-up action and progress has been reported in 2003. Targets adopted by the countries included:

1. Reduction of HIV infection among young people (15–24 years) by 25% in most affected countries by 2005 and 25% reduction globally by 2010 (core indicator for countries with generalized epidemic).
2. Prevalence of HIV-infected infants born to HIV-infected mothers; target was 20% reduction by 2005 and 50% reduction by 2010.

National Surveillance System in HIV

There are two kinds of surveillance systems in HIV/AIDS:

a. Biological surveillance—Biological specimen (Blood) collection for HIV sentinel surveillance (HSS), Syphilis Survey (Prevalence of STD)
b. Behavioural Surveillance Surveys (BSS)—This includes information/knowledge and risk perception on HIV/AIDS, sexual behaviours and exposure to HIV/AIDS services.

Uptil now the biological surveillance and behavioural surveillance were being done separately or independently with different periodicity, different geographical units of study and population covered did not match. Thus there was no scope for linking behaviours with HIV outcomes for better understanding of vulnerabilities and risk profiles.

Hence combining Biological and Behavioural surveillance or Integrated Biological and Behavioural Surveillance (IBBS) is useful for better tracking of behaviours leading to HIV.

HIV SENTINEL SURVEILLANCE (HSS) IN INDIA

The HIV sentinel surveillance is collection of epidemiological information of sufficient accuracy and completeness regarding the distribution and spread of HIV infection for planning, implementation, monitoring, prevention and control of HIV and AIDS programme.[14] This is called biological surveillance.

There are five steps in surveillance, i.e. collection of data, compilation, analysis, action and feedback. In essence, the surveillance is information for action.

Objective: During first phase of surveillance, objective was to know or validate the presence of HIV epidemic in India. Presence of HIV infection was confirmed in 1986 when three commercial sex workers (CSWs) were found positive at Vellore.

Serosurveillance (1987–97): Commenced in 1987 through 62 surveillance sites and 9 reference centres in different parts of the country. Serosurveillance centres were established in medical colleges under ICMR. High-risk groups were targeted for surveillance activities.

Objective: During this phase of surveillance, the objective was to know the geographical spread of HIV infection and to determine major modes of HIV transmission. The serosentinel activities though commenced in 1994 through 55 sentinel sites which were confined mostly to high-risk groups in urban areas, however, these sites were inadequate for sentinel surveillance to get adequate picture of overall HIV situation.

Results: This activity indicated that HIV infection was widespread in India and reached almost all parts of the country by 1997 and heterosexual transmission was the major mode of HIV transmission.

Sentinel Surveillance 1998 Onwards[15]

The *objectives* of surveillance were redefined. From 1998 onwards, *objective* of sentinel surveillance was to monitor trends of HIV infection in different populations and geographical areas.

HIV sentinel surveillance objectives:

- To monitor the trends of HIV epidemic/infection in the country (tracking of epidemic) overtime.
- To monitor the distribution and spread of HIV prevalence in different population sub-groups (ANC, FSW, MSM, IDU) and different geographical areas.
- To estimate the burden of HIV infection.
- To assess the impact of interventions.
- To identify emerging pockets of HIV epidemic in the country.

Organised sentinel surveillance commenced in 1998 through 180 sentinel sites and subsequently increased to over 1359 sites in the year 2010 covering most districts in India.

POPULATIONS FOR SENTINEL SURVEILLANCE/ TRACKING OF EPIDEMIC

12

The HIV sentinel surveillance (HSS) system in India involves carrying out cross sectional surveys at regular intervals among selected population groups. These populations are also referred to as "sentinel groups".

In order to meet the objectives of sentinel surveillance the focus is on critical populations that are selected on the basis of epidemiological considerations and the current understanding of local HIV transmission dynamics. From the programme point of view, sentinel site should be selected to include the populations of greatest importance to local epidemic from both sexual and parenteral transmission perspective.

Population for Sentinel Surveillance

1. *Low-risk groups:* Antenatals.

   Pregnant women represent the sexually active segment of general population, and hence taken as proxy for monitoring HIV among general population. Facilities for antenatal care are available across the country at different levels of health care system and hence are feasible for implementation. At ANC clinics routine blood specimen collection is done for syphilis and haemoglobin testing, a part of which can be used for HIV testing.

   Objective: The main objective of ANC surveillance is to know the extent of spread of HIV among general adult population. Prevalence of HIV in pregnant women who attend ANC is most often used as a proxy for general population. In low level and concentrated epidemic in India, ANC attendees represent women who do not typically engage in risk behaviour themselves.

ANC Attendees

Eligibility Criteria for Inclusion of ANC Attendees in HSS

Inclusion criteria:

- Age 15–49 years
- Pregnant woman attending the antenatal clinic for the first time during the current round of surveillance.
- A pregnant woman should be recruited only once during a round of surveillance. To ensure this verify the date of her previous visit to ANC clinic. If the date of her previous visit to ANC clinic falls during the current round of surveillance, she should be excluded from the sample.
- Women, who are already registered with the antenatal clinic but are visiting the clinic for the first time during the current round of surveillance are eligible for inclusion.

2. *High-risk groups:* Female sex workers, men having sex with men, injecting drug users, single male migrants, and long distance truckers.

Objective: The main purpose of HIV surveillance in populations with high-risk behaviours is to detect emerging epidemics, monitor HIV trends and to evaluate programme impact. India being large and diverse country and facing multiple and diverse HIV epidemics in various states/ districts. The epidemic in India is at low level and concentrated in high-risk groups. In these diverse epidemics HIV infections are more likely to emerge first of all among high-risk groups, such as FSW, MSM and IDU, who constitute core high-risk groups and are most critical populations to target for the surveillance and prevention activities.

Eligibility Criteria

The following criteria should be evaluated while assessing the eligibility of high-risk individuals for inclusion in surveillance.

Eligibility Criteria for Inclusion in HSS at HRG Sites

Inclusion Criteria

1 Fulfil the case definition (as detailed below)
2 Age between 15 and 49 years

Exclusion Criterion

Already approached and administered informed consent once in the current round of surveillance.

Case Definitions for HIV Sentinel Surveillance

1 ***Female sex worker (FSW):*** Women who are engaged in consensual sex for money or payment in kind, as a means of livelihood in the last 6 months.
2 ***Men who have sex with men (MSM):*** Men who had anal or oral sex with a male partner in the last one month.
3 ***Injecting drug user (IDU):*** Men and women who use addictive substances or drugs for recreational or non-medical reasons, through injections, at least once in the last three months.
4 ***Transgender/eunuch (TG):*** Person whose identity does not conform unambiguously to conventional notions of male or female gender roles, but combines or moves between these.
5 ***Single male migrant (SMM):*** Single male, living at place other than "place of usual residence" without his spouse or family, for the purposes of work and visiting his home town at least once a year.
6 ***Long distance trucker (LDT):*** Truckers who travel more than 800 km one way between source and destination.

Sentinel site is defined as "a designated service point/ facility where blood specimens and relevant information are collected from a fixed number of eligible individuals from a specified population group over a fixed period of time, periodically, for the purpose of monitoring the HIV epidemic". Examples of sentinel site are, antenatal clinic, drop in centre or STD clinic or NGO clinic, etc.

It is essential to follow uniform eligibility criteria for recruiting individuals in every round of surveillance to facilitate comparison of HSS results overtime for determining trends.

Testing Strategy

The unlinked anonymous testing (UAT) strategy is being used, as it minimizes participation bias. In this type of testing, a part of the blood sample originally collected for other purposes is used for testing of HIV. For example, at ANC clinic when blood sample is collected for VDRL or Hb a part of it can be separated out and sent to the laboratory after removing all the personal identifiers, such as name, OPD number and address, etc. so that the HIV test result cannot be linked with the individual.

In unlinked anonymous testing (UAT) results cannot be communicated to participants, which denies them an opportunity to know their HIV status and receive HIV services, such as PPTCT, ART and care and support services. Thus, it is ethically difficult to justify UAT unless all UAT sites are also providing ICTC, and PPTCT services.

Predetermined Sample Size

For antenatal clinic sites, a sample of 400 consecutive women (15–49 years) attending the antenatal clinic for the first time during the sampling period (fixed period from July to September or any time duration fixed) will be tested. Sample size for high-risk groups, i.e. for FSW, MSM and IDU is 250 each consecutive or by random sampling method. If the quota is met before 12 weeks elapse, the sampling should stop. If the sample is not met during the 12 weeks period, that is no problem and the sampling should again stop.

Sampling method: Consecutive sampling method is followed in HIV Sentinel Surveillance (HSS). From the start of surveillance, all individuals attending the sentinel site facility who are eligible for inclusion in surveillance as per defined criteria, should be recruited in order they attend the clinic or sentinel site.

- Every successive individual should be recruited in HSS till designated sample size is achieved or designated period of three months is over, whichever is earlier. In consecutive sampling the sampling interval is zero.
- This sampling method removes all chances of *selection bias* or *exclusion bias* based on individual preferences and other reasons. It is convenient and easy to follow
- In high-risk groups consecutive sampling or random sampling method is used. In high-risk group informed consent/assent is also obtained.

Blood sample: 5 ml of blood sample is collected from antenatal and in high-risk groups dried blood spot (DBS) method is used where drops of capillary blood are collected through finger prick using a sterile lancet, on a special protein saver card and dried subsequently to prepare the dried blood spot specimens. The DBS specimens are sent to testing laboratories where serum is eluted from DBS and used for testing.

Test Protocol

The test protocol adopted in HIV sentinel surveillance: First test of high sensitivity and second test of high specificity if first test is positive. 5 ml of blood sample is (clinic based sentinel groups) drawn under aseptic conditions. HIV testing is done in designated laboratory and external quality control is ensured by sending all HIV positive samples and 5% of negative samples for cross checking to reference laboratory.

After each round of surveillance data was *collected*, *compiled* and *analysed* to find out the trend of HIV infection in these groups. Data are analysed for prevalence and estimates, distribution of HIV age-and sex-wise, rural-urban distribution as also by literacy and marital status, etc. Based on the prevalence of HIV infection, the states have been classified into high, moderate and low prevalence states. Based on the analysis of 1999 sentinel surveillance data collected from 180 sites, HIV prevalence in adult population have been broadly classified into following groups.

Group I

High prevalence states included Maharashtra, Tamil Nadu, Andhra Pradesh, Karnataka, Manipur and Nagaland where the infection has crossed 1% or more in antenatal women.

Group II

Moderately prevalence states include Gujarat, Goa and Puducherry where HIV infection has crossed 5% or more among high-risk groups but the infection is below 1% in antenatal women.

Rest of the states are low prevalence states which fall into category of highly vulnerable and vulnerable states.

Group III

Highly vulnerable states include states where the HIV infection in any of the high-risk group is still less than 5% and is less than 1% among antenatal women. These states are Bihar, HP, Kerala, MP, Punjab, Rajasthan, UP, West Bengal, Chhattisgarh, Jharkhand, Odisha, Uttarakhand and Delhi. In these states, number of migrant labourers are maximum and health infrastructure is weak.

Group IV

Vulnerable states are J & K, Haryana, Mizoram, Sikkim, Meghalaya, Tripura, Andaman and Nicobar, Chandigarh, Dadra and Nagar Haveli, Daman and Lakshadweep and Arunachal Pradesh. These states have poor HIV data.

12

The basic unit of implementation HIV will now be the district. Accordingly based on the epidemiological and vulnerability criteria, 609 districts in the country have been categorized into four categories based on the sentinel surveillance data for the last 3 years (2004–2006).

The categorization of districts based on vulnerability is useful in planning differential package of services for each category of district. Institutional arrangements and capacities will be strengthened of the SACS as well as the district AIDS prevention and control units (DAPCUs) set up in A and B category of districts (Table 12.5).

Table 12.5: Categories of districts

- Category A (156 districts): *High prevalence* (more than 1% ANC/PPTCT prevalence in district at any time in any of the sites in the last three years)
- Category B (39 districts): *Moderate prevalence* or Concentrated epidemic (less than 1% ANC/PPTCT prevalence in all the sites during last 3 years associated with more than 5% prevalence in any HRG group—STD/CSW/MSM/IDU)
- Category C (296 districts): *Highly vulnerable* (less than 1% in ANC prevalence in all sites during last 3 years with less than 5% in all STD clinic attendees or any HRG with known hot spots. Increased presence of vulnerable population—migrants, truckers, large aggregation of factory workers, tourists, etc.)
- Category D (118 districts): Low/*unknown vulnerability* (less than 1% in ANC prevalence in all sites during last 3 years with less than 5% in all STD clinic attendees or any HRG or no or poor HIV data with no known hot spots/unknown)

Epidemiological profiling of HIV/AIDS situation at district/sub-district level using data triangulation: Under NACP-III, the resources for HIV prevention, care and support are allocated largely based on district classification into A, B, C and D categories. Now many more data sets at district and subdistrict level prevalence among pregnant women and non-pregnant individual are available through VCTC and PPTCT centres besides annual sentinel surveillance. Use of more than one method or source of information and then check if the information obtained from different methods agrees—this is called 'Triangulation'. Triangulation excercises have been undertaken to generate district level prevalence in general population for district action plan at local level (epidemic scenario and programme response) to produce a report card on HIV for each district in the country.

Results of Surveillance—HIV Burden

HIV sentinel surveillance estimates of 2015 in India indicate HIV prevalence of 0.26% in adult population, down from last year's 0.27%. The estimated burden due to HIV in India for the year 2015 was 2.11 million people living with HIV/AIDS.

The infection has spread from urban to rural and from the high-risk groups to the general population. The epidemic continues to shift towards women and younger age group, since about 40.5% of all HIV infections occur in women. This also increases the HIV transmission from parent (mother) to child and augment the incidence of paediatric HIV. The NACP recognizes the feminine face of HIV and accords it the highest priority.

National Family Heath Survey-3 on HIV Prevalence

Community based survey in 2006 revealed that 0.28% of adults were infected with HIV, including 0.35% in urban area and 0.25% in rural areas. Prevalence in men being 0.35% and in women 0.22%. prevalence rate in Manipur and Andhra Pradesh were 1.13% and 0.97% respectively.

AIDS Case Surveillance

Objectives of AIDS case surveillance were:

- To ensure reporting of AIDS cases as per standard AIDS case definition.
- To improve skills of physicians for diagnosis of AIDS.
- To monitor the clinical profile of AIDS cases in terms of opportunistic infections.
- The overall objective is to capture disease burden due to AIDS and to evolve strategy to assess the requirements of ART and other resources; manage such cases in hospitals/*community care centres with ART*. Community care centres are managed by NGOs.

Physicians responsible for AIDS reporting and management (PRAM) have been trained.

Definition of AIDS

Case definition for AIDS in India was revised in Oct. 1999. The new case definition is as follows:

Case definition of AIDS in children (up to 12 years of age):

Two positive tests for HIV infection by ERS (ELISA/RAPID/SIMPLE) in children above 18 months or confirmed maternal HIV infection for children less than 18 months. And presence of at least two major and two minor signs in the absence of known causes of immunosuppression.

Major Signs

- Loss of weight or failure to thrive which is not known to be due to medical causes other than HIV infection.
- Chronic diarrhoea (intermittent or continuous) >1 month duration.
- Prolonged fever (intermittent or continuous) >1 month duration.

Minor Signs

- Repeated common infections (e.g. pneumonitis, otitis, pharyngitis).
- Generalized lymphadenopathy.
- Oropharyngeal candidiasis.
- Persistent cough for more than 1 month.
- Disseminated maculopapular dermatosis.

Case Definition of AIDS in Adults (for Persons Above 12 Years of Age)

1. Two positive tests for HIV infection by ERS test (ELISA/RAPID/SIMPLE).
2. Any one of the following clinical criteria:
   - Significant weight loss (>10% of body weight) within last one month/cachexia (not known to be due to a condition other than HIV infection). And chronic diarrhoea (intermittent or continuous) >1 month duration or prolonged fever (intermittent or continuous) >1 month duration.
   - **Tuberculosis:** Extensive pulmonary, disseminated, miliary or extrapulmonary tuberculosis.
   - Neurological impairment preventing independent daily activities, not known to be due to the conditions unrelated to HIV infection (e.g. trauma).
   - Candidiasis of the oesophagus (diagnosable by oral candidiasis with odynophagia).
   - Clinically, diagnosed life-threatening or recurrent episodes of pneumonia, with or without etiological confirmation
   - Kaposi's sarcoma
   - Other conditions:
     - Cryptococcal meningitis.
     - Neurotoxoplasmosis.
     - CMV retinitis.
     - *Penicillium marneffei*
     - Recurrent herpes zoster or multidermatomal herpes infection.
     - Disseminated molluscum contagiosum.

Age and Sex Distribution of AIDS Cases in India

The first HIV and first AIDS case in India was reported in the year 1986 and it reached almost in every state and UTs by 1997.

The number of AIDS cases reported in India represent only a small fraction of actual AIDS cases. The reported cases do not tell anything about the magnitude of the problem. This is due to under-reporting by states and lack of diagnostic skills are given below.

Cumulative number of AIDS cases in India (NACO)

Year	1986	1995	1999	2000	2001	2003	2005	2007	2009
Cases	01	2108	7012	13304	31000	61201	117716	197812	268180

The disease is affecting mainly the people in sexually active and economically productive age groups (15–49 years) as nearly 86% of cases are in this age bracket. The disease is more common in men than women. Large number of cases have been reported from Maharashtra and Tamil Nadu. The **major opportunistic infection** (OI) in the AIDS patient is tuberculosis indicating dual epidemic of AIDS and tuberculosis in India. The other OI are—candidiasis, cryptococcus and toxoplasmosis.

AIDS case surveillance data can supplement the HIV surveillance data in monitoring the epidemic and could contribute to the planning of hospital and home/community-based care for AIDS patient under the programme. HIV infection reporting is much better suited than AIDS case reporting to current programme requirements (WHO, 2008). AIDS cases reporting does not meet current programme needs hence has been discontinued.

SURVEILLANCE FOR SEXUALLY TRANSMITTED INFECTIONS (STIs)

STIs are markers of HIV risk behaviours (unsafe sex) and therefore surveillance for STIs serves as an early warning signal of emergence of HIV epidemic. Present practice of HSS through STD/STI clinics collect biased data, which is incomplete and irregular as most patient seek treatment through private practitioners and very few utilize the government STD clinics.[16] Around 1131 STI clinics have been established in the country under National AIDS Control Programme at district and sub-district level. These clinics need to be upgraded for service quality and reporting system must be improved. If that is done the data and information generated from these clinics can fill a gap and we can generate information on trends of STIs for appropriate interventions and actions. The present day HSS surveillance through STI clinics is questionable. Syphilis screening test for antenatals can generate a lot of information and it should be encouraged.

Behavioural Surveillance Survey (BSS)

Behavioural surveillance surveys initiated in 1995 (preventive indicators surveys) and repeated in year 2001 and 2006 highlight important facets of the country's bid to curtail the epidemic.[17–19] BSS collects information on awareness, knowledge, beliefs and practices in respect of HIV/AIDS.

Behavioural surveillance survey has been replaced with integrated bio-behavioural survey (IBBS) model.

National IBBS Programme[18]

Launched in 2014 to generate evidence on risk behaviours among: High risk Groups (FSW, IDU, MSM and Migrants) to support programme planning and prioritization of programme effects at district, state and national levels as also programme evaluation.

What is IBBS

Collection of Biological and Behavioural information from Core High-Risk Groups for **actions**.

Table 12.6: National integrated biological and behavioural surveillance (IBBS) in high-risk groups (HRGs) 2014–15

Indicators/HRGs sample size	*20707 FSWs (%)*	*23081 MSMs(%)*	*19902 IDUs(%)*
• Heard of HIV/AIDS	95	95	96
• *Comprehensive knowledge of HIV transmission and prevention	42.5	45.5	42.6
• Had misconception about route of transmission	26.8	20.9	26.1
• Tested for HIV in last 12 months	99	99	92
• HIV prevalence level	2.2	4.3	9.9
• Medium age of first sexual act.	18 years	16 years	19 years
• Median age of initiation of sex work	22 years	17 years	20 years initiation of drugs
• Sexual partners and condom use patterns			
A. Regular sex partners/clients	82	54	70
– Condom use in last sex act	91	82	41
– Consistent condom use in last one month	68	50	16
B. Casual/occasional partners /clients	79	48	28
– Condom used in last sex act	94	83	55
– Consistent condom use in last one month	74	54	29
– Have heard of STI (Genital ulcer/discharge/warts)	84	78	76
– Self reported STIs symptom in last one year	50	21	16
– Treatment sought for STIs	49	51	66
– Stigma, discrimination by friends/family	27	17	50
– Exposure to programme services in last one year	90	78	81
– Interpersonal contacts with peer educators/ORWs	71	61	80
– Shared needles and syringes	–	–	15–20
– Injected in groups	–	–	83

*Comprehensive knowledge—knows any two methods of prevention of sexual transmission, rejecting two most common local misconceptions and being aware that a healthy looking person can be infected with HIV.

Specific Objectives

- To analyse and understand HIV related behaviours and HIV prevalence among key risk groups in different ragions by linking behaviours with biological findings.
- To measure and estimate change in HIV related behaviours and HIV prevalence among key risk groups, between baseline and endline for NACP-IV.
- Generate district level behavioural estimates for HRG, which was major information gap under NACP-III for effective targeting and planning.

Key Findings

HRG's were quite young in their prime productive age of 30 years, had high level of HIV/AIDS awareness as over 95% of them have heard about HIV/AIDS. Comprehensive knowledge on route of transmission and prevention practices was low at 43% and 20–26% had misconception on HIV. Over 92% had been tested for HIV in the past one year. HIV prevalence levels were 2.2% in FSWs, 4.3% in MSMs and high of 9.9% in IDUs. 54–82% of HRGs had regular sexual partners/clients and consistent condom use rate in such sexual partnership varied from low of 16% in IDUs to 68% in FSWs. Casual/occasional sex partners/ clients varied from 28–79% and consistent condom use rate in this kind of partnership was low in IDUs—29%, 54% in MSM and high of 74% in FSWs.

Awareness level of STI was high at 76–84%, and self reported STIs (Genital ulcer/sore, discharge/warts) in the last one year was high in FSWs 50%, in MSMs it was 21% and 16% of IDUS reported one or the other STIs. Treatment for STIs was sought by 49–66% of HRGs and stigma and discrimination was reported by 17–50%. Exposure to programme interventions was high varying from 78–90%. Over 15–20% of IDUs shared needles and syringes and majority—83% injected in groups and one third of them injected Heroin. Prevention of parent to child transmission was known to over 63% of FSWs.

Mapping

Mapping of HRGs and migrants population has been done twice in India in 2006 and 2009. Last mapping completed in India in 2009 in 21 states. The estimated size of core high risk group was 1.47 million (female sex workers, men having sex with men and injecting drug users) besides 9.2 million bridge population (truckers and migrants). Strategy for migrants has been revised, linking it with source districts for prevention, care, support and treatment.

Female Sex Work Patterns and Implications

Commercial sex work is being propagated from generation to generation in the state of Rajasthan and Karnataka in close communities—Nats and Kanzer (in Rajasthan). These communities live in close knit families at the outskirt of a village or nearby high way. Nats and kanzers were landless and marginal community with poor socio-economic status. Traditionally, these communities earned their livelihood by way of entertaining people through special skills—singing, dancing, performing stunts: balancing on rope way and rope way walking and performing acrobatics and aerobatics as also indulging in sex work. The birth of a girl child is most welcome in Nats Community. The girl children are brought up very well and graduated to sex work by their parents. Most girls in these communities do not get married, but trained to pursue sex work, which is most often home based. Income generated from sex work sustains the life of family and whole family thrives on income generated through sex work. Most Nats families have now become rich as they own a good house with all modern amenities—television, car, mobile telephones and refrigerators. These young female sex workers have established a strong network in Mumbai and far flung places like Dubai to fetch more money by sex work tourism. Daughter marriage in Nats Community means—selling the girls for lump sum money.

Whole of Jaisinghpura village in Tonk district in Rajasthan is inhabited by 55 Nats families 2 km away from main village SODA. It is their stronghold and a kingdom for female sex work. Village Jaisinghpura is located close to religious place Diggi where lot many people keep on visiting Diggi temple throughout the year. Most tourists, truckers and young people from cities frequent young female sex workers at this village. Similarly, Bandersundri village on Jaipur, Ajmer highway—a hub of female sex workers of Nats Community is a long distance trucker's paradise and transit station for sexual activity. Similarly, Village Malpura in district Alwar close to national highway is a hub of female sex workers.

Sex work in the state of Karnataka can be linked or associated with Devadasi tradition. In several areas of Northern Karnataka families dedicate one of their daughter, to temple, to appease gods. The daughters so dedicated are called Devadasis and once dedicated they are not allowed to get marry for the rest of their lives. They serve the sexual needs of priests and wealthy married men. Many of these Devadasis have become commercial sex workers. Peer educators involved in the programme are sex workers, as were their mothers and grandmothers before them (ICHAP, 2004).

PREVENTION OF HIV

The only cure for HIV is prevention. Since, HIV/AIDS is incurable and it is fatal in the long run, population-based preventive strategies are imperative to reduce the spread of HIV epidemic. Preventive strategies include:

- Information, education and communication to establish healthy lifestyles in adolescents and young people. No sex before marriage, no extra-martial sex and having one faithful uninfected sexual partner. Say no to drugs and have safe injection if it is must.

- Safe blood saves life and prevents HIV. Voluntary donors are safe donors. Professional donors are risky donors. HIV testing of blood and organs for transplantation is mandatory.
- Promote voluntary testing and counselling.
- Change behaviour of high-risk groups (who are most vulnerable to contract and transmit HIV) by targeted intervention of controlling STDs and promoting use of condoms and safe sex with unknown or strangers.
- Control of STDs/STI effectively. Most STDs are curable.
- Safe sex by correct and consistent use of condoms.
- Prevention of drug abuse.
- Aggressive control of TB.
- Safe injection (safe needle, safe syringes).
- Adopt universal prevention practices.
- Safe disposal of hospital and dangerous waste.
- Prevention of vertical transmission (PPTCT).

Prevention of Parent to Child Transmission (PPTCT)

The PPTCT services now provide 'universal access' to all pregnant women for HIV screening, diagnostic, prevention and treatment services. As such the key goal is to ensure the integrated PPTCT service delivery with existing reproductive and child health (RCH) programme to achieve zero new HIV infections among children and mothers alive well. Currently only 40% Antenatals are covered.

When the mother is pregnant and HIV positive; prevention can still be applied. The objectives of PPTCT are:[20]

i Providing access to voluntary counselling and testing services, including pretest and post-test counselling.

ii **Anti-retroviral prophylaxis:** The national strategic plan for PPTCT services using multidrug ARV in India was developed in May 2013 for nationwide implementation in phase manner based on new WHO guidelines. Multidrug regimen has the potential to dramatically reduce HIV transmission from mother to child to less than 5% as compared to 10–12% using single dose Nevirapine. Henceforth all HIV positive pregnant women will be started on more efficacious multi-drugs – Tenofovir (TDF) 300 mg + Efaviranez (EFV) 600 mg + Lamivudine (3 TC) 300 mg life long, and all HIV exposed infants will be provided one dose of syrup Nevirapine daily for minimum of 6 weeks.

iii Modify midwifery practices to minimize the risk of PPTCT, e.g. avoidance of rupture of membranes, episiotomy and oral suction of newborn infant.

iv Ensure safer infant feeding practices.

Other strategies of PMTCT:

- Primary prevention of HIV among future parents.
- Improved access to family planning services and information for HIV positive parents.

NATIONAL PROGRAMME ON PREVENTION OF PARENT TO CHILD TRANSMISSION (PPTCT)

Transmission of HIV from parent to child can occur during pregnancy, at the time of delivery or after delivery through breastfeeding. Around 5–10% of PPTCT is estimated to occur during pregnancy. An estimated 10–20% of PPTCT occur intrapartum when fetus comes in contact with maternal blood or cervical secretions. Around 10–20% of PPTCT occur at some point during breastfeeding. There is 20–45% chance that the child of an HIV positive mother will also be infected with HIV. In India, *parent to child transmission of HIV (perinatal transmission) accounts for 5.4% of country's HIV/AIDS cases.*

Linkages between VCTC (ICTC) and PPTCT

- Spouses of HIV positive men and pregnant women who visit the VCTC must be informed about the availability of PPTCT services.
- A strong referral system to PPTCT sites need to be established.
- Maintain record of clients referred from VCTC for PPTCT.

PPTCT centres function with Obstetrics and Gynaecology department; with the facility of female *counsellor* and back up of laboratory support for HIV testing and other support services and care.

INDIA'S RESPONSE TO HIV/AIDS EPIDEMIC

NATIONAL AIDS CONTROL PROGRAMME (NACP) PHASE I (1992–99)[21]

The National AIDS control project was the first project in India to develop national public health programme on HIV/AIDS prevention and control, and was implemented between 1992 and 99.

The ultimate objective of the project was to slow down the spread of HIV, to reduce future morbidity and mortality and the impact of AIDS by initiating major effort in prevention of HIV transmission.

National AIDS Control Programe

Key timelines are indicated (Fig. 12.6).

NACP Phase III (2007–12)[22]

Goal

Primary goal of NACP III was to halt and reverse the spread of HIV epidemic in India over the next 5 years by integrating programmes for prevention, care, support and treatment. This will be achieved through four *strategic objectives* are given as follows.

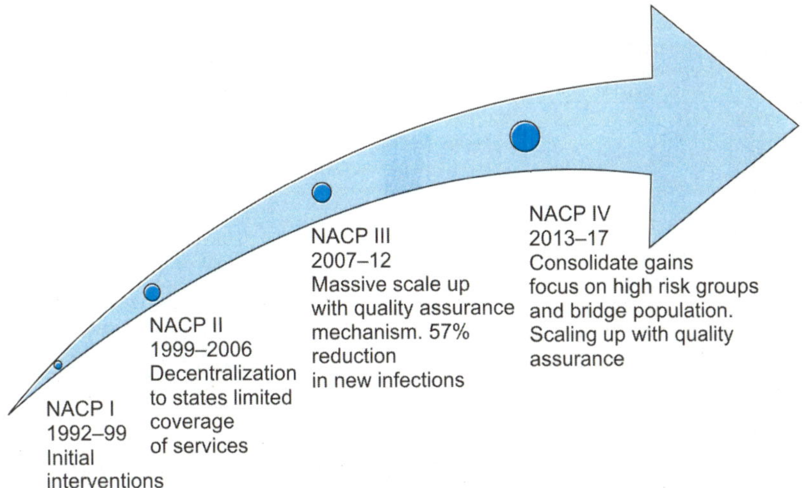

Fig. 12.6: National AIDS Control Programme timelines

Strategic Objectives

1. Prevention of new infection in high-risk groups and general population by:
   - Saturating coverage of high-risk groups with targeted interventions (TIs).
   - Scaling up interventions in the general population.
2. Increasing the coverage of people living with HIV/AIDS for care, support and treatment.
3. Strengthening the infrastructure, systems and human resources in prevention, care, support and treatment programmes at the district, state and national levels.
4. Strengthening a nationwide strategic information management system (SIMS).

Specific Objectives[23-26]

The specific objective is to reduce new infections as estimated in year 1 of the programme by:

- 60% in high prevalence states so as to obtain reversal of the epidemic.
- 40% in the vulnerable states so as to stabilize the epidemic.

Implementation Structure

The NACP is implemented through 35 State AIDS Control Societies (SACS) in the states and UTs. In addition, there are three Municipal AIDS Control Societies in Mumbai, Chennai and Ahmedabad. A major structural reform has been initiated under NACP III by constituting District AIDS Prevention and Control Units (DAPCUs) with a team of field functionaries in A and B category districts for decentralized programme implementation across 189 districts.

NATIONAL AIDS CONTROL PROGRAMME (NACP) PHASE IV (2013–17)

Based on the lessons learned and achievements made in phases I, II and III, India has now developed the IVth national AIDS control programme implementation plan (2012–17). India is committed to achieve sustainable development goal of 'ending the epidemic of HIV/AID by 2030' and reversing the spread of HIV/AIDS.

The programme strategy would be two pronged: Intensification of prevention interventions for HRGs and bridge population and integration of prevention, (including mother to child transmission) testing, counselling and treatment services among the *general population*, including pregnant women, *with routine RCH programme*. The State AIDS Control Societies and District AIDS Prevention and Control Units (DAPCU) will be integrated into the National Health Mission (NHM).

Primary goal: To accelerate the process of reversal of epidemic in India.

Key Priorities of NAPC IV

- Preventing new infections by sustained interventions and effectively addressing emerging epidemics.
- Preventing parent to child transmission (PPTCT).
- Focusing on IEC strategies for behaviour change and demand generation for HIV services.
- Providing comprehensive care, support and treatment to people with infection (affected people).
- Reducing stigma and discrimination
- Ensuring effective use of strategic information system at all levels.
- building capacities of NGO and civil society partners especially in states of emerging epidemics.
- Integrating HIV services with the health system in a phased manner.
- Mainstreaming HIV/AIDS activities with all key central and state ministries and departments.

Goal by 2017 (12th Plan)

Reduce **new infections** to **zero** and provide comprehensive care and support to all persons living with HIV/AIDS and treatment services to all those who require it.

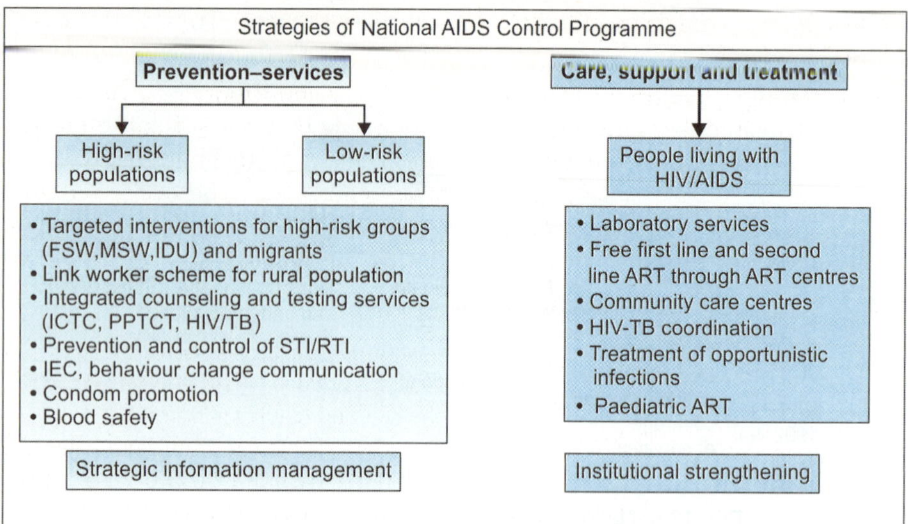

Strategies/Programme Components

Intensifying and consolidation of prevention services:

1. Targeted interventions
2. Link worker scheme
3. Prevention and control of STI/RTI
4. Care, support and treatment and lab services
5. Basic services
6. Information education and communication
7. Condom promotion
8. Blood safely
9. Mainstreaming
10. Strategic information management including integrated biological and behavioural surveillance (IBBS).

1. Targeted Interventions

a. Targeted interventions (TI) for high-risk groups or most at risk population: This is the highest priority in NACP IV. It is planned to cover 90% of HRGs.

Aim: Targeted intervention (TI) projects aim at to interrupt HIV transmission form core high-risk groups to bridge population and to general population (prevention of new infections).

The core high-risk groups and their sex partners are at greater risk of acquiring and transmission of HIV infection because of risky behaviour and insufficient capacity or power to decide to protect themselves.

Focus of TIs and Coverage

Primary focus is *saturating the coverage* of estimated 1.47 million *core high-risk groups* (female sex workers, Men who have sex with men, Transgenders/Hijras Injecting drug users) and an estimated 9.2 million vulnerable *bridge population* namely migrants and long distance truckers, with targeted interventions. Accordingly 1705 TIs sites have been set-up to cover 90% of estimated core high-risk groups and bridge population with primary prevention services.

Evidence for TIs

HIV epidemic in India is concentrated among high-risk groups (HRGs). High prevalence levels of HIV have been observed in female sex workers (2.2%), men having sex with men (4.3%), injecting drug users (9.9%) and transgender (8.82%). **Bridge population** like migrants and long distance truckers who constitute major proportion of clients of sex workers also show high HIV prevalence of 0.99% and 2.59% respectively. Therefore, these groups are being targeted for targeted interventions (TIs). TIs are NGO based, peer led preventive interventions to provide preventive services including:

- Detection and treatment for sexually transmitted infections (STIs) by regular medical check-ups for STIs once in three months and syphilis and HIV testing twice a year.
- Condom distribution and promotion
- Behaviour change communication to increase demand for services and products.
- Creating an enabling environment free of stigma and discrimination and break silence surrounding issues related to sexuality.
- Linkage to Integrated Counseling and Testing Centres (ICTCs).
- Linkage with care and support services for HIV positive HRGs.
- Specific interventions for IDUs
  - i Distribution of clean needles and syringes
  - ii Abscess prevention and management
  - iii Opioid substitutes therapy (OST)
  - iv Linkage with detoxification/rehabilitation services
- Specific interventions for MSM/TGs—provision of lubricant materials and condoms.

- Specific interventions for FSWs—provision of female condoms (on pilot basis).

Female sex workers who are brothel based, street based, home based, lodge based, dhaba based, bar girls, etc. are being covered with specific intervention strategies as mentioned above.

Objective is to reduce new infections in HRGs and keep prevalence level as low as possible.

Implementation of TIs: TIs are peer led interventions implemented through community based organizations in partnership with NGOs. TIs would be in the form of clinics at drop in centres, drug de-addiction or harm reduction centre or any other facility where high-risk groups can seek services and information.

b. TIs for clients of sex workers–bridge population in NACP III and IV

Migrant intervention: NACO has revised migrant intervention strategy with specific reference to linking migrants with services and information on HIV prevention, care and support *at source* (at their village), at *transit* (places like rail or bus stations where large number of migrants board train or bus to their places of work) and the *destination* (the places of work). NACO has identified 122 districts with high out-migration across 11 states for *source interventions*. At source interventions are to be managed by two block level supervisors (male and female) with support from ASHAs, ANMs, SHGs and PRIs. They will reach out to families of migrants with information and services. At 75 transit locations the part-time outreach workers have been placed. They conduct group sessions on HIV prevention and distribute migration kits containing information booklet on services available at major destinations, condoms, notebook, ball pen, comb, etc.

Long Distance Truckers Interventions: 2.1 million truckers covered for providing STI care services, condoms and risk reduction counseling.

2. Link Workers Scheme for HRGs in Rural Areas

Based on the annual surveillance data of 2007 it was estimated that 57% of HIV infected were in rural areas of India. 163 highly vulnerable A and B category of districts have been identified across 20 states to "Reach out to HRGs" and their partners, pregnant women and vulnerable groups in rural areas by providing information on HIV, condom promotion and distribution and referrals to counselling, testing and STI services. Male and female link workers and red ribbon club members reach out to cover rural HRGs and vulnerable with the help of ASHA, ANMs, Anganwadi workers and their supervisors. Convergence and linkage with NRHM would enhance the coverage of rural HRGs on long-term basis. NACP which is being pursued as a vertical programme has to be integrated into general health care delivery system to reach out to rural population of HRGs and general population.

3. Prevention and Control of Sexually Transmitted Infections (STIs)

This is the third most important priority in NACP. The base line survey carried out in the year 2003 by NACO indicated that at any given time 6% of the adult population in the country suffers from STI, but small number of clients report in STI clinics in government set-up. The NACO and Reproductive and Child Health Programme Phase II have prepared national guidelines on prevention, management and control of sexually transmitted infections. Based on enhanced syndromic case management (ESCM) 1131 designated STI/RTI clinics at PHC, CHC Sub-district, District and teaching hospitals, and 3565 preferred private providers (PPP) for community based STI services to the high risk population have been set-up. NACO has branded the STI/RTI clinics/services as "Suraksha Clinics" and has developed a communication strategy for demand generation for these services. Pre-packed STI/RTI/colour-coded drug kits have been provided. Early diagnosis, appropriate and complete treatment of STI/RTI reduces transmission rate of HIV infection by more than 40%.

4. Comprehensive Care Support and Treatment (CST) for People Living with HIV (PLHIV) and AIDS

The care support and treatment programme under NACP includes—comprehensive management of PLHIV with respect to treatment and prevention of opportunistic infections, **anti-retroviral therapy** and psychological support, home based care, positive prevention and impact mitigation. Interventions for PLHIV include:

i Free laboratory services for CD4 testing and other investigations.

ii Free first and second line anti-retroviral treatment (ART) through 520 ART centres, 1074 link ART centres and ART plus centres. Given the low level of coverage of ART, focus will be on assuring *universal access* to first line and second line ART drugs in phase IV.

iii Paediatric ART for children.

iv Early infant diagnosis for HIV exposed infants and children below 18 months.

v Nutrition and psychological support through 350 care support centres (CSCs).
   - Treatment of opportunistic infections—tuberculosis candidiasis, cryptococcus and toxoplasmosis.
   - Drop in centres for PLHIV networks.

5. Basic Services

a. Integrated Counseling and Testing Centers (ICTCs)

Only an estimated 25–30% of people who are infected know their HIV status; thus there is need to extend access to counselling and testing facilities to increase demand generation to cover the rest of 70%. Scaling up of voluntary testing to reach at least 21 million tests per year by 2011 in public sector and another 21 million tests by private sector has been planned. Aim is to have ICTC for each CHC.

Uptil now 15606 ICTCs have been set up in the country, (4818 stand alone and 10788 facility integrated ICTCs).

b. Prevention of Parent to Child Transmission (PPTCT)

Universal HIV testing for all pregnant women covering 90% is promoted as part of basic Ante-natal care package. HIV positive pregnant women are provided Anti-retroviral drug prophylaxis, life long.

c. Prevention Interventions for General Population

Prevention remains the mainstay of NACP. Despite the high number of HIV positive persons in the country, over 99% of the population is uninfected. NACP will place the highest priority on preventive efforts and integrate prevention with care, support and treatment. The programme aims to reduce *new infections* in all categories and prevent spread of HIV from high risk groups (HRGs) to the general population. A **behaviour change strategy based** on an effective information education and communication (IEC) campaign supported by appropriate service is being implemented.

d. HIV-TB Co-ordination (Cross Referral, between NACP and RNTCP Early Detection of HIV/TB Cases and Treatment with ART and ATT

e. National Paediatric AIDS Initiative

Around 7% of HIV infections are in children below 15 years of age. In order to provide comprehensive care and support (including ART to children infected and affected by HIV), the NACO has launched National Paediatric AIDs initiative on 30th November, 2006. For this initiative NACO along with Indian Academy of Paediatrics, UNICEF, WHO and Clinton Foundation, has developed guidelines for paediatric ART including diagnosis in children. Currently, paediatric drugs are provided at all ART centres. Care and support, for children living with HIV/AIDs, orphans and vulnerable children, forms an integral part of NACP.

6. Information, Education and Communication

The focus of IEC strategy has shifted from awareness generation to behaviour change communication. The key priorities of NACP communication strategy are:

Motivate behaviour change in populations at risk, including the high-risk groups and the bridge populations.

- Raise awareness level about risk and need for behaviour change among vulnerable and general population specially youth and women in >90%.
- Generate demand for increase utilization of HIV/AIDS related health services.
- Create an enabling environment that encourages HIV related prevention, care and support activities and reduces stigma and discrimination at individual, community and institutional level.
- Out of total budget nearly 67% has been spent on prevention programmes.

Activities

The **Adolescence Education Programme** (AEP) is a key intervention to build 'life skills' of young people and help them cope with negative peer pressure, develop positive behaviour, improve sexual health and prevent HIV infection. The focus of AEP is high school classes IX and XI to cover 1,12,000 schools. University Talk AIDS Programme focused on college students to raise the level of awareness and behaviour change.

- Red Ribbon Express (RRE) train was a unique experience. Red Ribbon Express Project exhibition has been launched to build awareness on HIV/AIDS in school and college youths and general population.
- 95% of young women and men who constitute 40% of country's population, will be accessed by collaborating the activities with Ministries of Youth Affairs, Human Resource Development (HRD), Women and Child Development and Ministry of Social Justice and Empowerment (MSJE), among others, volunteer networks and youth friendly information centres. Women in reproductive age, youth and adolescents will be the prime focus for multi-media (TV and Newspaper).

7. Condom Promotion

Since 88% of HIV infections are transmitted through unsafe sex, consistent and correct use of condom promotion programme is central to HIV/AIDS prevention at the intervention level. The use of condom is promoted as a protection against STIs and HIV/AIDS in addition to family planning. Despite high awareness and increase in condom availability during NACP I to III, its use remain at less satisfactory level. Routine condom use, ensuring adequate and convenient supply and promotion of negotiating skills for condom use amongst high-risk groups and others are important aspects of NACP. NACO has launched a massive targeted **condom social marketing programme** in 361 districts mapped on the basis of HIV prevalence and family planning needs. About 11,025 condom vending machines have been installed and another 11,000 are in the process of being installed. 3.5 billion condoms are targeted to be distributed through 3 million outlets under NACP. NACO has scaled up female condom programme in the state of Delhi, Haryana, Punjab, UP, MP, Assam, Karnataka, Gujarat, and Chhattisgarh.

8. Blood Safety

It aims to provide adequate and safe blood. For ensuring blood safety which is one of the efficient modes of transmission, over 1137 blood banks have been modernized till date to ensure blood safety through promotion of voluntary blood donation and a system of mandatory screening of every unit blood for HIV, hepatitis B and C, malaria and syphilis. Its objectives are to reduce blood-borne transmission to less than 0.5% from the current level of 1% and to increase voluntary blood donation from present level of 84 to 90%.

9. Mainstreaming HIV for Multi-sectoral Response

HIV needs a multisectoral response and strategy. Mainstreaming means "integrated, inclusive and multisectoral approach [that] transfers the ownership of HIV/AIDS issues—including its direct and indirect causes, impacts and responses to various stakeholders, including the government, the corporate sector and civil society organizations". Department of AIDS control is collaborating with various key ministries/departments (Higher Education, Coal, Petroleum and Natural Gas, Department of Youth Affairs, Sports, housing and Urban poverty alleviation and department of Defence). The whole purpose of mainstreaming is to reduce vulnerabilities, risks, discrimination, stigma and use of services and information, social protection besides integrating HIV/AIDS related programmes with existing health services.

10. Strategic Information Management System (SIMS)

One of the key strategy of NACP IV—is SIMS. The SIMS generates and manages critical information on the entire spectrum of HIV epidemic and its control, vulnerabilities and risk behaviours predisposing HIV transmission, Pattern of spread of the epidemic and factors contributing to it, disease progression, treatment requirements and regimens, planning and implementation interventions, monitoring service delivery and tracking beneficiaries, programme gaps and ways to overcome them, and effectiveness and impact of the programme. Another key function of SIMS is to promote data use for policy making, programme planning, implementation and review at National, distrist and Reporting unit levels.

HIV Testing in National HIV/AIDS Control Policy

- There is an active debate in the country on the issue as to whether there should be mandatory testing of people suspected of carrying HIV infection. Considerable thought has been given to this issue. Government of India has earlier issued a comprehensive HIV testing policy and the following issues are reiterated here:
  - No individual should be made to undergo mandatory testing for HIV.
  - No mandatory HIV testing should be imposed as a precondition for employment or for providing health care facilities during employment.
  - Adequate voluntary testing facilities with pretest and post-test counselling should be made available throughout the country in a phased manner. There should be at least one HIV testing centre in each district in the country which can be done in a phased manner.
  - In case a person likes to get his HIV status verified through testing, all necessary facilities should be given to that person and results should be kept strictly confidential and should be given to the person and with his consent to the members of his family. Disclosure of the HIV status to the spouse of the person will entirely depend on the person's willingness to share the information. However, the person should be encouraged to share this information with the spouse and family as it helps the person in getting proper home-based care when he is afflicted with AIDS.
  - In case of marriage, if one of the partners insists on a test to check the HIV status of the other partner, such tests should be carried out by the contracting party to the satisfaction of the person concerned.
- The HIV testing policy adopted in the NACO is found to be appropriate for the different types of testing that have to be done. At present, people are tested for:
  - Screening in blood banks
  - Epidemiological surveys
  - Confirmatory testing for clinical management and voluntary testing.
- In the case of screening for blood donation, a single test by rapid/ELISA is done to eliminate the possibility of HIV positive blood. In the case of epidemiological surveys also the same procedure is adopted, i.e. with one or two tests either with ELISA or rapid or simple with high sensitivity.

REFERENCES

1 NACO. Training module on HIV Infection and AIDS for Medical Officers. New Delhi: National AIDS Control Organization, MOH and FW, GOI; 2000.

2 UNAIDS, 2014 and 2015 Global and regional statistics. UNAIDS Fact sheet on HIV/AIDS, 2011 and 2014 and 2015.

3 NACO, ICMR (NIMS). Technical Report India HIV Estimates 2012.

4 GOI. Behind the numbers. A newsletter of the National AIDS Control Organization, MOH and FW. Vol III, issue 3. July-Sep 2007, New Delhi.

5 NACO. HIV Sentinel Surveillance 2010–11, A Technical Brief, India's voice against AIDS, Department of AIDS Control, MOH and FW, Government of India; September 2012.

6 NIHFW and NACO. Annual HIV sentinel surveillance country report 2006, MOH and FW; New Delhi.

7 GOI, NACO Annual Report 2009–10. Department of AIDS Control Ministry of Health and Family Welfare, Government of India, New Delhi.

8 UNAIDS. Follow-up of the 2001. United Nations General Assembly Special Session on HIV/AIDS. Progress Report

on the Global Response to the HIV/AIDS Epidemic. New York: UNAIDS; 2003 and 2010–2011.
9 WHO. Beyond 2000 Responding to HIV/AIDS in the New Millennium. New Delhi: WHO Regional Office for South East Asia; 2001.
10 Youth and HIV/AIDS: Can We Avoid Catastrophe? Population Reports Feb 2002; 50(12).
11 NACO. Specialist Training and Reference Modules. New Delhi: NACO; 2000.
12 Narain JP, Jha A, Lal S, Salunke S. Risk Factors for HIV Transmission in India. AIDS 1994; 8 Suppl. 2: 577–82.
13 UNAIDS. Summary of the Declaration of Commitment of HIV/AIDS. United Nations General Assembly Special Session on HIV/AIDS. New York: UNAIDS; 2001.
14 NACO. Training Module on the Sentinel surveillance of HIV Infection. New Delhi: NACO, GOI; 1993.
15 NACO. HIV Annual Sentinel Surveillance Estimates Conducted by NACO and Nodal Agency NIHFW. New Delhi: NACO, GOI; 1998–2015.
16 GOI. National guidelines on prevention, management and control of reproductive tract infections including sexually transmitted infections, MOH and FW; August 2007.
17 NACO, Nationwide Behavioural Surveillance of General and High-risk Groups Conducted by ORG-MARG. New Delhi: NACO; 2001–2 and 2006.
18 GOI: NACO (2015) National Integrated Biological and Behavioural Surveillance (IBBS) India—High Risk Groups 2014–15.
19 WHO. Global Programme on AIDS. Evaluation of a National AIDS Programme. A Methods Package Prevention of HIV Infection. Geneva: WHO; 1994.
20 UNAIDS. HIV Voluntary Counselling and Testing: A Gateway to Prevention and Care. UNAIDS Case Study. New York: UNAIDS; June 2002.
21 NACO. National AIDS Control Programme Phase I. New Delhi: NACO, GOI; 1992–9.
22 NACO. National AIDS Control Programme Phase II. New Delhi: NACO, GOI; 1999–2004.
23 GOI HIV/AIDS epidemiological surveillance and estimation report for the year 2005, NACO, MOH and FW. GOI, April 2006.
24 GOI: NACO. National AIDS Control Programme in India, Phase IV (2012–17), NACO, MOH and FW. GOI; 2013.
25 GOI Annual Report 2007–08. MOH and FW, GOI; New Delhi.
26 GOI: NACP III. To halt and reverse the HIV epidemic in India, 2007. NACO, MOH and FW; New Delhi.

REPRODUCTIVE TRACT INFECTIONS INCLUDING SEXUALLY TRANSMITTED INFECTIONS

12

Sexually transmitted diseases (STDs) remain a major public health problem in many parts of the world.

The term "sexually transmitted disease" (STD) is used for all infections that are mainly transmitted through sexual contact, during unprotected vaginal, anal or oral intercourse. Some are also transmitted from mother to child, before, during and after birth and through unsafe blood, blood products, donated organs or tissues and contaminated needles.

Recently, the term sexually transmitted diseases (STDs) has been replaced by the term sexually transmitted infections (STIs). Since 1999, the term sexually transmitted infection has been adopted by WHO as it covers *asymptomatic infections as well.*

Spectrum of Sexually Transmitted Infections (STIs)

STIs are group of communicable diseases which are predominantly transmitted by sexual contact. Traditionally, the following diseases were considered as STI: *Gonorrhoea, syphilis, chancroid, lymphogranuloma venereum and granuloma inguinale.*

The spectrum however has been enlarged to include several additional diseases such as genital herpes, venereal warts (due to Human Papillomavirus), cytomegalovirus, hepatitis B virus, chlamydia, candidiasis, trichomoniasis, bacterial vaginosis, non-gonococcal urethritis, nonspecific genital infection and most dreaded of them all HIV/AIDS, besides pelvic inflammatory disease (PID), epididymitis/orchitis, pediculosis pubis and scabies.

Clinical Spectrum of RTIs/STIs (Syndromes)

Clients having RTIs/STIs usually present with:

i Vaginal or urethral discharge
ii Vesicular and/or non-vesicular genital ulcers.
iii Inguinal bubo
iv Lower abdominal pain/scrotal pain
v Genital skin conditions.

Epidemiology of STIs

Global Disease Burden

According to current WHO estimates, there occur more than 333 million cases of curable STDs every year throughout the world. About one million new infections occur everyday. Most STIs are curable and preventable.

Problem of STD/STIs in India

Reproductive tract infections (RTIs) including sexually transmitted infections (STIs) present a huge burden of disease and adversely impact the reproductive health of people. They cause suffering for both men and women around the world, but their consequences are far more devastating and widespread among women than men. The exact data on STI prevalence in India especially in general population is lacking.

India has high incidence of STDs with an estimated incidence rate of 5% or 40 million new cases per year. Results of STI community-based prevalence study (NACO

2003) indicate prevalence rate of STI to be 6% in adult population in India. Based on these estimates, 30 million adults are infected with STI and half of them are likely to be symptomatic. The estimates also indicate that about 33–40% of women have symptom of RTI/STI at any given point of time but only 1% complete the treatment of both partners.[1–3]

Prevalence of self-reported and clinically diagnosed gynaecological morbidity among women:

There were marked variations in prevalence of self-reported RTI which ranged from 55 to 84%, while clinically diagnosed conditions ranged from 4 to 62% for vaginitis, 8–48% for cervicitis, 2–46% for cervical erosion and 1–24% for pelvic inflammatory disease. Community-based studies in India (Tables 12.7 and 12.8) are limited.[4]

STDs in High-risk Groups

The prevalence of STIs and RTIs among high-risk groups is very high. Up to 60–80% of CSWs in major cities such as Mumbai, Pune, Delhi and Chennai have STIs suggesting that frequent unprotected sexual intercourse is widespread. Similarly, prevalence of STIs is much higher in injecting drug users, prisoners and migrant workers (industrial workers)[4] and in men having sex with men.

Risk Behaviours and Practices Associated with STIs

1 **Urbanization, industrialization and migration:** Many young persons migrate to urban areas in search of livelihood leaving their families in rural areas. Similarly, long distance truckers and cleaners are away from their families for days together and many other persons whose occupation is such that they have to be away from home and families. Such persons often have unprotected sex with FSWs and consequently acquire STIs. Behaviour of such persons determines the occurrence of STIs.

2 **Multiple sexual partners and extramarital and premarital sexual intercourse** with strangers without use of condom or irregular use of condoms make them more vulnerable to STIs. Around 9% of men had non-regular sexual partners and practice high-risk behaviour.

3 **Poverty:** Driven by extreme poverty, many of the young girls migrate to cities and adopt the profession of CSWs and exchange sex for money. These girls have little negotiating power and cannot force their clients to use condoms. Legally, prostitution is banned but female sex workers (FSW) have established in major cities and on highways. FSW contract and transmit STIs to their clients. FSW seldom seek early treatment for STIs. "Call girls" in cities is a prolific business for exchange of sex for money.

4 **Behaviour of adolescents and youth:** Sexual activity gets initiated during the period of adolescence, uncontrolled and unprotected sex makes them most vulnerable to STIs. Their knowledge and access to information will determine the spread of STIs. Many of the adolescents and young people have poor knowledge of STIs and their transmission.

5 **Illiteracy:** Knowledge is power but it is missing with many, and illiteracy is widespread in India. Illiterates have poor access to information, including information on STIs occurrence and transmission and consequences of STIs.

6 **Occupation:** Industrial workers, migrant labourers and adolescent unemployed youths are most vulnerable groups for STIs.

Table 12.7: Self-reported symptoms of RTI

	Study 1	*Study 2*	*Study 3*	*Study 4*	*Study 5*	*Study 6*	*Study 7*
Sample size	654	500	756	840	440	1103	788
Menstrual problems	60	33	41	58	65	59	NA
Excessive discharge	13	50	31	22	22	57	26.8
Lower abdominal pain	13	17	21	9	16	NA	27.0
Lower backache	30	5	39	24	NA	30	50.4
Dysparunia	7	2	NA	NA	1	NA	NA
One or more conditions	55	65	74	65	NA	84	64.7

Table 12.8: Clinically diagnosed morbidity of RTI

	Study 1	*Study 2*	*Study 3*	*Study 4*	*Study 5*	*Study 6*	*Study 7*
Sample size	650	500	756	548	385	324	414
Vaginitis	62	4	15	11	13	10	13.5
Cervicitis	48	14	40	13	24	8	NA
Cervical erosion	46	2	21	5	10	20	16.1
PID	24	1	16	8	11	8	5.9
Prolapse	0.5	17	18	5	3	NA	8.8
One or more infections	NA	43	74	26	70	43	40.4

7 **Stigma and treatment seeking behaviour:** Since STIs carry a stigma and discrimination, people tend to hide such infection and do not seek treatment or seek treatment from quacks. Partner notification is rare. Only women came forward to seek treatment during intensive campaign of family health awareness.

8 **Partner notification** and failure to get sexual partners treated simultaneously leads to **recurrence** of infection and maintenance of infections and continuation of transmission.

9 Many of STIs remain asymptomatic and awareness of signs and symptoms and importance of STI treatment is poor as revealed by behavioural surveys.

Consequences

The STI could lead to infertility, ectopic pregnancy, pelvic inflammatory disease (PID); HIV infection is potentially fatal, congenital syphilis, congenital malformation, cervical cancer, fetal wastage, low birth weight, ophthalmia neonatorum, blindness and systemic infections and economic burden is also very high. Presence of STIs also compromises with contraceptive acceptance and continuation.

STIs produce considerable wastage of manpower, besides untold misery, both directly and indirectly through the complications they produce. The new entrant in the spectrum of STI named as acquired immunodeficiency syndrome (AIDS) has increased the significance of prevention and control of STIs.

Reproductive tract infections (RTIs) include three types of infections:

1 **Endogenous infections**, which are caused by overgrowth of organisms normally present in the genital tract of women and men; such as bacterial vaginosis (BV), candidiasis, vulvovaginitis prostatitis and epididymitis.

   As endogenous infections are not primarily sexually transmitted, clinical and public health actions as applied to STI may not apply to them. Treatment of partners is not recommended for non-sexually transmitted infections. Patient education and reassurance are important.

2 **Sexually transmitted infections (STIs):** Such as gonorrhoea, syphilis, trichomoniasis, genital herpes, genital warts (due to Human Papillomavirus) and those due to chlamydia and human immunodeficiency virus (HIV) infection. Here treatment of sexual partner is important as public health measure.

3 **Iatrogenic infections** that are associated with medical procedures such as transfusion of unsafe blood or blood products and unsafe injections.

Syndromic Approach in Management of STI

1 The traditional approach to diagnosis of a presumed STI was through etiological diagnosis established by microscopy and laboratory cultures and serological tests. This approach was expensive and slow in obtaining the results and leads to delay in initiation of treatment. It requires sophisticated laboratory equipment and trained manpower. Many of the clients of STI are lost as they may not come again to the facility or clinic.

2 Moreover most clients of STI are seen and attended by private sector (private practitioners and clinics) who have limited diagnostic facilities. Clinical diagnosis without any test would be cheaper but it is inaccurate and incomplete in majority of instances.

3 The limitation of this approach has led to the development and advocacy of a third strategy, which is known as "syndromic approach".[5]

The "syndromic approach" is a simple practical tool to improve diagnosis and treatment. The simplified syndromic-based approach, developed and promoted by WHO and is currently being used in large number of countries in the developed world.

Under the syndromic approach, the diagnosis of STI is based on identification of consistent group of symptoms and easily recognized signs (syndromes) and provision of effective treatment that will deal with majority of organisms responsible for producing each syndrome. Majority of STIs fall under the categories of, genital ulcer, vaginal discharge and urethral discharge, inguinal swelling and lower abdominal pain. Most STIs patients consult a doctor or health care providers with complaints related to above mentioned syndromes.

Advantages

The major advantages of syndromic approach are:

1 Diagnosis and treatment is done in one visit.

2 It can be implemented on large scale even at the primary health care level, being simple, rapid and inexpensive.

3 It requires minimum training and can be applied by health workers.

4 Patients are treated for possible mixed infections by addressing all the important causes of a syndrome.

Essentials of Syndromic Case Management (SCM)

It necessitates history taking, clinical examination, correct diagnosis, early and effective treatment, With *single oral dosages wherever possible*, counselling on sexual behaviour, voluntary testing for HIV, provision and promotion of condoms, partner notification and treatment, case reporting and follow-up; hence it is much more than mere treatment therefore, we call it Enhanced Syndromic Case Management (ESCM).

Criticism of Syndromic Approach

The syndromic approach is too simple for a physician, unscientific procedure, it does not use a provider's clinical skill and experience.

- It wastes a lot of drug.
- It promotes development of antibiotic resistance.
- Simple laboratory tests should be included.

Relationship between HIV and STI

STI and HIV have nexus:

- The predominant mode of transmission of both HIV and STI is through unprotected sexual intercourse.
- The same risk behaviour, which predisposes for STI also predisposes for HIV infection. Thus, many of the measures for prevention of STI and HIV are the same.
- Target groups for intervention are the same.
- STI clinic services provide an important access point for person at high-risk for both STI and HIV infection, not only for diagnosis and treatment but also for education and prevention.
- STI also facilitates the acquisition and transmission of HIV infection. In the presence of a genital ulcer, the risk of acquiring and transmission of HIV increases up to ten times while it is fivefolds in the presence of genital discharge. Most of the STIs causing ulcer or discharge are easily curable. Treatment and control of STI/RTI reduces the transmission rate of HIV infection by over 40%. Control of STI/RTI is the most cost effective means of preventing *new HIV infections*.
- Surveillance of trends in STI incidence and prevalence can be useful indicators of changes in sexual behaviour, and are easier to monitor than trends in HIV seroprevalence and are therefore valuable for determining the impact of HIV/AIDS control programme.
- The severity of STI and their manifestations and infectivity, in the presence of HIV infection, goes very high and the response to therapy decreased.

Prevention of STDs/STIs

The following guidelines can be helpful to prevent STIs/STDs.[6–8] Most STIs are *curable* and *preventable*.

- *Use of condoms:* Educate about correct and consistent use.
- Have one faithful uninfected sex partner.
- Avoid sex with partners who have genital rashes, redness, sores or discharge.
- Stay away from casual sex/reduce sex partners.
- Most STIs are curable. Early treatment is always desirable to prevent complications and further spread of infection. Sexual abstinence during the course of treatment is helpful.
- Good quality, non-stigmatizing services for diagnosis and treatment of STI should be provided in the existing health system in an integrated manner. Collaboration with private, industrial corporation and NGO sectors and re-orientation of specialized STD clinics can help to reduce the incidence of STI.
- Partner notification and treatment helps.
- Promote voluntary counselling and testing for HIV, syphilis and hepatitis B.
- Immunization against hepatitis B.
- Safe injections and safe blood.

STI Control Component of National AIDS Control Programme in India

Objectives

- To reduce STI cases (incidence and prevalence) and thereby control HIV transmission by minimizing the risk factors.
- Prevent the development of short- and long-term morbidity and mortality due to STIs.
- The other objectives are—to offer counselling and testing services for HIV/AIDS, besides behaviour change communication and screening asymptomatic women (contraceptive users and antenatal clients).

Policy on Control of STIs

The Ministry of Health and Family Welfare, Govt. of India, has adopted a policy to integrate STIs control into existing health care and reproductive and child health (RCH) services, both in the public and in the private sector. Special emphasis is being placed on the integration of comprehensive STI case management at primary health care level to provide non-stigmatized services. The policy also emphasizes on the cooperation and collaboration with private sector as well as non-governmental organizations for control of STI.

Strategies

- Convergence with National AIDS Control Programme (NACP) is envisaged in provision of these services.
- National AIDS Control Programme Phase III and IV includes services for management of STIs as a major programme strategy for prevention of HIV. The strategy for implementation plan (2012–17) includes expanding access to package of STI management services both in general population groups and for high-risk behaviour group by engaging private sector.
- Under RCH II there is commitment for implementing the RTI/STI services at sub-district level, i.e. in at least 50% of the PHCs and all FRUs, including drugs, training, disposable equipment and provision of laboratory technicians.

NATIONAL GUIDELINES ON PREVENTION MANAGEMENT AND CONTROL OF RTIs/STIs-2007[2]

The enhanced syndromic case management (ESCM) is comprehensive approach for STI management endorsed by WHO for resource limited setting. This is being practiced in major part of the world. The approach classifies the STIs into syndromes, which are easily identifiable group of symptoms and signs and provides treatment at first visit, with no or minimal laboratory tests. It also provides the other important components of STI case management, namely—treatment compliance and follow-up, counselling, partner treatment and condom promotion, apart from voluntary testing for HIV at Integrated Counselling and Testing Centre.

Management of STI/RTI is one of the major strategy for HIV control in India under National AIDS Control Programme. Under NACP II, the STI services were provided through designated STI clinics at the district level and medical colleges. Under NACP III, this has been expanded to primary health centres (PHCs) and community health centres (CHCs) in convergence with RCH II under National Rural Health Mission. Large number of general population is reached by involvement of private practitioners and overall service utilization being enhanced through demand generation for STI service.

Services of contracted preferred private practioners are made available to high risk groups at community level.

Pre-packed STI/RTI kits: Pre-packed colour-coded kits (kit 1–7) have been provided for free supply at all Govt. STI/RTI clinics, CHCs, PHCs and TI NGOs for enhanced syndromic case management (through standard treatment protocols). Treatment with single oral doses is a preferred strategy.

NACO is supporting 1131 designated STI/RTI clinics which are providing STI/RTI services based on enhanced syndromic case management. NACO has branded the STI/RTI clinics as "Suraksha clinics" and has developed a National communication strategy on STI/RTI service delivery for demand generation; one counselor is provided to each of these designated clinic besides one laboratory technician.

Flowcharts 12.1 to 12.4 describe the clinical syndrome, specific RTIs/STIs under the syndrome and the causative organisms of RTI/STI syndrome. Differential diagnosis of the condition is also mentioned wherever possible. Special emphasis is laid on syndrome specific partner management and management issues specific to pregnancy.

These can be used easily to make rapid decision by different health workers, supervisors, nurses and doctors.[6-8]

RTI/STI *among special populations*. STIs including HIV are most common among young people aged 15–24 (including adolescents) and more so in young women. Adolescents are being covered in the RCH II, though adolescent reproductive and sexual health (ARSH) strategy.

Core high-risk groups like female sex workers (FSWs) and men having sex with men (MSM) and injecting drug users (IDUs) show higher prevalence of STIs than general population. Nearly 50% of FSWs suffer from any one symptom of STIs which increases HIV transmission. Targeted interventions (TIs) for high-risk groups under NACP III and IV provide services for RTIs and STIs. (Medical check ups for STIs once in 3 months and syphilis and HIV testing twice a year) through drop in centres/clinics managed by Non-Governmental Organizations and 3565 prefered private providers (PPP).

Surveillance of STI

Syndromic surveillance of STI is being encouraged through regular reporting of STIs every month by "Suraksha clinics". Laboratory support and counseling services have been made available at STI clinics.

Integrated Counselling and Testing Centres (ICTCs) and their Role in STI Prevention and Management

Clients with STI have shown high-risk sexual behaviour. Based on this high-risk behaviour, the health care workers should inform the client about the links between STIs and HIV and should encourage all clients to undergo an HIV test as the risk of HIV among STD is up to 10 times higher. At ICTC, the STI client will receive comprehensive and accurate information on HIV/AIDS and HIV counselling to facilitate an informed choice regarding an HIV test.

REFERENCES

1 NACO. Training module on HIV infection and AIDS for Medical Officers. New Delhi: MOH and FW, GOI.

2 GOI. National guidelines on Prevention, Management and Control of Reproductive Tract Infections Including Sexually Transmitted Infections, coordinated by NIRRH–ICMR: MOH and FW, GOI; August 2007.

3 NACO—Operational guidelines for Programme Managers and service providers for strengthening of STI services, NACO, May 2007, New Delhi.

4 UNFPA. Reproductive tract infections in India. The HIV/AIDS connection. New Delhi; UNFPA; Nov 1999.

5 WHO. Management of sexually transmitted diseases at District and PHC level. Regional Publication, SEARO, 1997; 25.

6 WHO. Guidelines for the management of sexually transmitted infections. Geneva: World Health Organization, 2003.

7 NACO. National AIDS Control Programme in India. Simplified STI and RTI treatment guidelines (Flow charts). New Delhi: MOH and FW, Govt. of India.

8 NACO. Specialists training and reference module NACO II (1999–2004). New Delhi: MOH and FW, GOI.

Flowcharts for Management of RTI/STI Syndromes

Flowchart 12.1: Management of urethral discharge/burning micturition in males

SYNDROME: URETHRAL DISCHARGE IN MALES

RTIs/STIs: GONORRHEA, CHLAMYDIAL INFECTION, TRICHOMONIASIS

Causative organisms
- *Neisseria gonorrhoeae*
- *Chlamydia trachomatis*
- *Trichomonas vaginalis*

History of
- Urethral discharge
- Pain or burning while passing urine, increased frequency of urination
- Sexual exposure of either partner to high-risk practices including orogenital sex

Examination
Look for
- The urethral meatus for redness and swelling
- If urethral discharge is not seen, then gently massage the urethra from the ventral part of the penis towards the meatus and look for thick, creamy greenish-yellow or mucoid discharge

Laboratory investigations (if available)
- Gram stain examination of the urethral smear will show gram-negative intracellular diplococci in case of gonorrhea
- In non-gonococcal urethritis more than 5 neutrophils per oil immersion field (1000X) in the urethral smear or more than 10 neutrophils per high power field in the sediment of the first void urine are observed

Treatment
As dual infection is common, the treatment for urethral discharge should adequately cover therapy for both gonorrhoea and chlamydial infections
Recommended regimen for uncomplicated gonorrhoea + chlamydia
Uncomplicated infections indicate that the disease is limited to the anogenital region (anterior urethritis and proctitis)
- Tab. cefixime 400 mg orally, single dose plus
  Tab. azithromycin 1 g orally single dose under supervision
- Advise the client to return after 7 days of start of therapy

When symptoms persist or recur after adequate treatment for gonorrhoea and chlamydia in the index client and partner(s), they should be treated for *Trichomonas vaginalis*
If discharge or only dysuria persists after 7 days
- Tab. Secnidazole 2 g orally, single dose (to treat for *T. vaginalis*)

If the symptoms still persists
- Refer to higher centre as early as possible

If individuals are allergic to azithromycin, give Erythromycin 500 mg four times a day for 7 days

Syndrome specific guidelines for partner management
Treat all recent partners
- Treat female partners (for gonorrhoea and chlamydia) on same lines after ruling out pregnancy and history of allergies
- Advise sexual abstinence during the course of treatment
- Provide condoms, educate about correct and consistent use
- Refer for voluntary counselling and testing for HIV, syphilis and hepatitis B
- Schedule return visit after 7 days

Management of pregnant partner
Pregnant partners of male clients with urethral discharge should be examined by doing a per speculum as well as a per vaginal examination and should be treated for gonococcal as well as chlamydial infections
- Cephalosporins to cover gonococcal infection are safe and effective in pregnancy
- Tab. cefixime 400 mg orally, single dose
  or
  ceftriaxone 125 mg by intramuscular injection
  +
  Tab. erythromycin 500 mg orally four times a day for 7 days
  or
  Cap. amoxycillin 500 mg orally, three times a day for 7 days to cover chlamydial infection
- Quinolones (like ofloxacin, ciprofloxacin), doxycycline are contraindicated in pregnant women

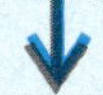

Follow-up
After seven days
- To see reports of tests done for HIV, syphilis and hepatitis B
- If symptoms persist, to assess whether it is due to treatment failure or re-infection
  For prompt referral if required

Colour-coded kit 1—Grey

Flowchart 12.2: Management of genital ulcers

SYNDROME: GENITAL ULCERS

RTIs/STIs **SYPHILIS** **CHANCROID** **GENITAL HERPES**

Causative organisms
- *Treponema pallidum* (syphilis)
- *Haemophilus ducreyi* (chancroid)
- *Klebsiella granulomatis* (granuloma inguinale)
- *Chlamydia trachomatis* (lymphogranuloma venereum)
- *Herpes simplex* (genital herpes)

Examination
- Presence of vesicles
- Presence of genital ulcer—single or multiple
- Associated inguinal lymph node swelling and if present refer to respective flow chart

History
- Genital ulcer/vesicles
- Burning sensation in the genital region
- Sexual exposure of either partner to high-risk practices including orogenital sex

Ulcer characteristics
- Painful vesicles/ulcers, single or multiple – Herpes simplex
- Painless ulcer with shotty lymph node – Syphilis
- Painless ulcer with inguinal lymph nodes – Granuloma inguinale and LGV
- Painful ulcer usually single sometimes associated with painful bubo – Chancroid

Laboratory investigations
- RPR test for syphilis
- For further investigations refer to higher centre

Treatment
- If vesicles or multiple painful ulcers are present treat for herpes with Tab. acyclovir 400 mg orally, three times a day for 7 days
- If vesicles are not seen and only ulcer is seen, treat for syphilis and chancroid and counsel on herpes genitalis

To cover syphilis give

Inj: Benzathine penicillin 2.4 million IU IM after test dose in two divided doses (with emergency tray ready)
(in individuals allergic or intolerant to penicillin, doxycycline 100 mg orally, twice daily for 14 days)
+
Tab. azithromycin 1 g orally single dose or
Tab. ciprofloxacin 500 mg orally, twice a day for 3 days to cover chancroid
Treatment should be extended beyond 7 days if ulcers have not epithelialized, i.e. formed a new layer of skin over the sore

Refer to higher centre
- If not responding to treatment
- Genital ulcers co-existent with HIV
- Recurrent lesion

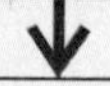

Syndrome specific guidelines for partner management
- Treat all partners who are in contact with client in last 3 months
- Partners should be treated for syphilis and chancroid
- Advise sexual abstinence during the course of treatment
- Provide condoms, educate about correct and consistent use
- Refer for voluntary counselling and testing for HIV, syphilis and hepatitis B
- Schedule return visit after 7 days

Kit 3: White: Genital ulcer, non-herpetic ulcers

Kit 4: Blue: Patient allergic to penicillin, non-herpetic ulcer

Kit 5: Red: Herpetic ulcers

Management of pregnant women
- Quinolones (like ofloxacin, ciprofloxacin), doxycycline, sulfonamides are contraindicated in pregnant women
- Pregnant women who test positive for RPR should be considered infected unless adequate treatment is documented in the medical records and sequential serologic antibody titers have declined
- Inj Benzathine penicillin 2.4 million IU IM after test dose (with emergency tray ready)
- A second dose of benzathine penicillin 2.4 million units IM should be administered 1 week after the initial dose for women who have primary, secondary, or early latent syphilis
- Pregnant women who are allergic to penicillin should be treated with erythromycin and the neonate should be treated for syphilis after delivery
- Tab. erythromycin 500 mg orally four times a day for 15 days
- (Note: Erythromycin estolate is contraindicated in pregnancy because of drug related hepatotoxicity. Only erythromycin base or erythromycin ethyl succinate should be used in pregnancy)
- All pregnant women should be asked history of genital herpes and examined carefully for herpetic lesions
- Women without symptoms or signs of genital herpes or its prodrome can deliver vaginally
- Women with genital herpetic lesions at the onset of labour should be delivered by caesarean section to prevent neonatal herpes
- Acyclovir may be administered orally to pregnant women with first episode genital herpes or severe recurrent herpes

Flowchart 12.3: Management of vaginal discharge in females

SYNDROME: VAGINAL DISCHARGE

VAGINITIS | **TRICHOMONIASIS** | **CERVICAL HERPES** | **CERVICITIS**

Causative organisms
Vaginitis
- *Trichomonas vaginalis* (TV)
- *Candida albicans*
- *Gardnerella vaginalis, Mycoplasma* causing bacterial vaginosis (BV)

Causative organisms
Cervicitis
- *Neisseria gonorrhoeae*
- *Chlamydia trachomatis*
- *Trichomonas vaginalis*
- *Herpes simplex virus*

History
- Menstrual history to rule out pregnancy
- Nature and type of discharge (amount, smell, color, consistency)
- Genital itching
- Burning while passing urine, increased frequency
- Presence of any ulcer, swelling on the vulval or inguinal region
- Genital complaints in sexual partners
- Low backache

Kit 2: Green

→

Examination
- Per speculum examination to differentiate between vaginitis and cervicitis
  (a) *Vaginitis*
  Trichomoniasis—greenish frothy discharge
  Candidiasis—curdy white discharge
  Bacterial vaginosis—adherent discharge
  Mixed infections may present with atypical discharge

  (b) *Cervicitis*
  Cervical erosion/cervical ulcer/ mucopurulent cervical discharge
  - Bimanual pelvic examination to rule out pelvic inflammatory disease
  - If speculum examination is not possible or client is hesitant treat both for vaginitis and cervicitis

→

Laboratory investigations
(if available)
- Wet mount microscopy of the discharge for *Trichomonas vaginalis* and clue cells
- 10% KOH preparation for *Candida albicans*
- Gram stain of vaginal smear clue cells seen in bacterial vaginosis
- Gram stain of endocervical smear to detect gonococci

↓

Treatment

Vaginitis (TV + BV + Candida)
- Tab. secnidazole 2 g orally, single dose or
  Tab. tinidazole 500 mg orally, twice daily for 5 days
- Tab. metaclopramide taken 30 minutes before Tab. secnidazole, to prevent gastric intolerance
- Treat for candidiasis with Tab. fluconazole 150 mg orally single dose or local clotrimazole 500 mg vaginal pessaries once

Treatment for cervical infection (chlamydia and gonorrhoea)
- Tab. cefixime 400 mg orally, single dose Plus
  Azithromycin 1 gram, 1 hour before lunch. If vomiting within 1 hour, give anti-emetic and repeat
  - ➢ If vaginitis and cervicitis are present treat for both
  - ➢ Instruct client to avoid douching
  - ➢ Pregnancy, diabetes, HIV may also be influencing factors and should be considered in recurrent infections
  - ➢ Follow-up after one week

Management in pregnant women
Per speculum examination should be done to rule out pregnancy complications like abortion, premature rupture of membranes

Treatment for vaginitis (TV + BV + Candida)

In first trimester of pregnancy
- Local treatment with clotrimazole vaginal pessary/cream only for candidiasis. Oral fluconazole is contraindicated in pregnancy
- Metronidazole pessaries or cream intravaginally if trichomoniasis or BV is suspected

In second and third trimester oral metronidazole can be given
- Tab. secnidazole 2 g orally, single dose or
  Tab. tinidazole 500 mg orally, twice daily for 5 days
- Tab. metoclopramide taken 30 minutes before Tab. metronidazole, to prevent gastric intolerance

↓

Specific guidelines for partner management
- Treat current partner only if no improvement after initial treatment
- If partner is symptomatic, treat client and partner using above protocols
- Advise sexual abstinence during the course of treatment
- Provide condoms, educate about correct and consistent use
- Schedule return visit after 7 days

Flowchart 12.4: Management of lower abdominal pain in females

SYNDROME: LOWER ABDOMINAL PAIN

Pelvic inflammatory disease (PID)

→

Causative organisms
- *Neisseria gonorrhoeae*
- *Chlamydia trachomatis*
- *Mycoplasma, Gardnerella,* Anaerobic bacteria (Bacteroides SP, gram-positive cocci)

History
- Lower abdominal pain
- Fever
- Vaginal discharge
- Menstrual irregularities like heavy, irregular vaginal bleeding
- Dysmenorrhoea
- Dyspareunia
- Dysuria, tenesmus
- Low backache
- Contraceptive use like IUD

→

Examination
- General examination: Temperature, pulse, blood pressure
- Per speculum examination: Vaginal/cervical discharge, congestion or ulcers
- Per abdominal examination: Lower abdominal tenderness or guarding
- Pelvic examination: Uterine/adnexal tenderness, cervical movement tenderness

Note: *A urine pregnancy test should be done in all women suspected of having PID to rule out ectopic pregnancy*

→

Laboratory investigations if available
- Wet smear examination
- Gram stain for gonorrhoea
- Complete blood count and ESR
- Urine microscopy for pus

Differential diagnosis
- Ectopic pregnancy
- Twisted ovarian cyst
- Ovarian tumor
- Appendicitis
- Abdominal tuberculosis

↓

Treatment (outclient treatment)

In mild or moderate PID (in the absence of tubo-ovarian abscess), outclient treatment can be given

Therapy is required to cover *Neisseria gonorrhoeae, Chlamydia trachomatis* and anaerobes
- Tab. cefixime 400 mg orally BD for 7 days + metronidazole 400 mg orally, twice daily for 14 days +
- Doxycycline, 100 mg orally, twice a day for 2 weeks (to treat chlamydial infection)
- Tab. ibuprofen 400 mg orally, three times a day for 3–5 days
- Tab. ranitidine 150 mg orally, twice daily to prevent gastritis
- Remove intrauterine device, if present, under antibiotic cover of 24–48 hours
- Advise abstinence during the course of treatment and educate on correct and consistent use of condoms
- Observe for 3 days. If no improvement (i.e. absence of fever, reduction in abdominal tenderness, reduction in cervical movement, adnexal and uterine tenderness) or if symptoms worsen, refer for inclient treatment

  Caution: *PID can be a serious condition. Refer the client to the hospital if she does not respond to treatment within 3 days and even earlier if her condition worsens*

→

Syndrome specific guidelines for partner management
- Treat all partners in past 2 months
- Treat male partners for urethral discharge (gonorrhoea and chlamydia)
- Advise sexual abstinence during the course of treatment
- Provide condoms, educate on correct and consistent use
- Refer for voluntary counselling and testing for HIV, syphilis and hepatitis B
- Inform about the complications if left untreated and sequelae
- Schedule return visit after 3 days, 7 days and 14 days to ensure compliance

Management of pregnant women

Though PID is rare in pregnancy
- ➢ Any pregnant woman suspected to have PID should be referred to district hospital for hospitalization and treated with a parenteral regimen which would be safe in pregnancy
- ➢ Doxycycline is contraindicated in pregnancy

  Note: Metronidazole is generally not recommended during the first three months of pregnancy. However, it should not be withheld for a severely acute PID, which represents an emergency

↓

Hospitalization of clients with acute PID should be seriously considered when:
- The diagnosis is uncertain
- Surgical emergencies, e.g. appendicitis or ectopic pregnancy cannot be excluded
- A pelvic abscess is suspected
- Severe illness precludes management on an outclient basis
- The woman is pregnant
- The client is unable to follow or tolerate an outclient regimen
- The client has failed to respond to outclient therapy

Note: All clients requiring hospitalization should be referred to the district hospital

Kit 6: Yellow

TUBERCULOSIS (TB)

Tuberculosis is an infectious disease in human beings caused by *Mycobacterium tuberculosis* (MTB). Other *mycobacteria*, namely *M. bovis* and *M. africanum* are rarely implicated in human beings. TB is curable.

Tuberculosis has existed in India since the earliest days. In 1500 BC, the *Rigveda* described the illness as *Rajayaksma*, "King of diseases". Today India accounts for 23.3% of all new cases of tuberculosis in the world, a figure that is likely to increase as India's population grows and the HIV epidemic progresses (Fig. 12.7).[1–4]

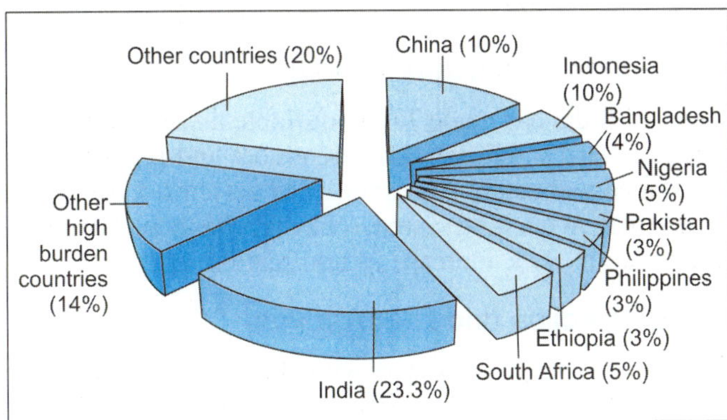

Fig. 12.7: India accounts for nearly one-quarters of the global TB burden (WHO Geneva; WHO Report 2015—global tuberculosis control; surveillance planning and financing)

EPIDEMIOLOGICAL FEATURES

Global Burden of Disease

In 2014, there were an estimated 9.6 million incident cases of TB (range 9.1 to 10 million) globally equivalent to 133 cases per 100000 population, of these 80% occurred in developing countries. Higher global totals for new TB case in 2014 were due to improved notification. There were an estimated 13 million prevalent cases (range 11–14 million) of TB in 2014. This is equivalent to 174 cases per 100000 population. In 2014 an estimated 1.1 million deaths occurred among HIV negative cases of TB. This is equivalent to 16 deaths per 1,00,000 population.[1]

'To stop TB partnership' target of halving TB prevalence rates by 2015 compared with 1990 has been achieved in 3 WHO regions and 9 high burden countries.

Indian Scenario—Disease Incidence

Though India is the second most populous country in the world, India has more new TB cases than any other country. In 2014, out of the estimated global **annual incidence** of 9.6 million TB cases, 2.2 (2.0–2.3) million were estimated to occur in India, of whom one million were infectious cases. Thus, India contributed to 1/4th of global incidence. Point **prevalence** of tuberculosis in India is 2.5 million cases.

Tuberculosis is one of India's most important **public health problem.** National tuberculosis sample survey by ICMR conducted in 1955–58 revealed:[5]

- That 1.6% of people were having active and probably active tuberculosis disease based on the radiological evidence or X-ray positive.
- 0.4% were having active pulmonary tuberculosis disease and were sputum positive (infectious cases).
- Rural population suffered equally as urban.
- Elderly population suffered more than younger ones.
- Distressingly high prevalence of tuberculosis, 1.4% continued even in year 2000. Sputum positive TB prevalence was estimated in the range of 4–5/1000 during 10th five-year plan (2002–2007).[6]

Estimation of Burden of Tuberculosis in India for Years 2000 and 2009

Annual Risk of Tuberculous Infection (ARTI)

The annual risk of tuberculous infection (ARTI) is one of the most sensitive epidemiological indicator of TB burden in the community as it expresses the overall impact of various factors affecting the transmission of tubercle bacilli, i.e. the load of infectious cases in the community, duration of infectiousness and efficacy of case finding and treatment programme.

ARTI represents the proportion of population that gets newly infected or reinfected with tubercle bacilli over the course of one year. Prior to year 2000 the ARTI was 1.7%. Currently, the average ARTI in the country as a whole is estimated to be 1.5%. It has been estimated that for every 1% annual risk of tuberculosis infection, there are about 50 new pulmonary sputum smear-positive (NSP) cases per 100,000 population per year. Out of all new TB cases 85–90% are pulmonary and 10–15% are extrapulmonary. Of the new pulmonary TB cases 50% are expected to be sputum positive. This means that, with ARTI of 1.5% there will be 75 new smear-positive cases, 75 new smear-negative cases, 38 retreatment cases and 15 extrapulmonary cases totalling to 203 cases per lakh population per year. Total patients registered for treatment include new sputum smear-positive cases, new smear-negative cases, new extrapulmonary cases, smear-positive retreatment cases and others.

India accounts for nearly one-fourth of the global incidence of tuberculosis, thus prevalence of tuberculosis disease in India is very high. Every year in India nearly 15–18 lakh (1.5–1.8 million) people develop tuberculosis and approximately 8 lakh is the incidence of sputum smear-positive cases every year.

National, annual risk of TB infection (ARTI) survey conducted between (2000 and 2003) by National Institute of Tuberculosis, Bengaluru and Tuberculosis Research Centre, Chennai derived a National ARTI of 1.5% from zonal estimates in children age group 1–9 years. ARTI in different zones varied from 1.0–1.9%. This study has provided robust data on the epidemiology of TB in India and will serve as the baseline data for calculating case detection rates in the future and the assessment of the long-term epidemiological impact of RNTCP.[7]

Based on nationwide sample survey of annual risk of tuberculosis infection (ARTI) by NTI and TRC and recent prevalence of disease in adults (>15 years) and children (0–14 years) during 2000–2003, the burden of disease was estimated by: Prevalence of disease corresponding to 1% of ARTI multiplied by the corresponding ARTI estimates from the nationwide ARTI survey for rural and urban areas of four survey zones. These estimates of prevalence then multiplied by adult population in the respective areas. The prevalence amongst children was estimated in the same way.[6] Based on the latest ARTI Survey in 2007–09. ARTI has been reduced to 1.1%. Accordingly, the incidence rate of TB will be revised in the country to the level of 149 cases per lakh population per year (55 new-smear-positive cases, 55 new smear-negative cases, 28 retreatment cases and 11 extrapulmonary cases).

Burden of TB in 2000 as Per ARTI-2000

The estimated number of bacillary cases was 3.75 million, of which 1.7 million were smear-positive cases and 2.05 million smear-negative, culture positive cases. X-ray abnormals were estimated to be 12.9 million. The number of abacillary cases was estimated to be 3.9 million (30% of 12.9 million X-ray abnormals) and for extrapulmonary cases burden was 0.8 million (20% of 3.8 million bacillary cases). A total of 8.5 million burden of TB cases was estimated (Gopi et al., Sept 2005, Table 12.9). Based on ARTI data, estimated new smear-positive cases per 1,00,000 population for North Zone was 95, East Zone and South Zone was 75, West Zone is 80 and for Odisha it was 85.

Deaths: Tuberculosis is captain of deaths in India (Table 12.10)

Table 12.9: Estimated burden of tuberculosis in India for the year 2000 (in million)

Type of cases Year 2000	*Number*	*(95% CI)*
Bacillary cases	3.8	(2.8–4.7)
Abacillary cases	3.9	(2.9–4.8)
Extrapulmonary cases	0.8	(0.6–0.9)
Total cases	*8.5*	*(6.3–10.4)*

Table 12.10: TB burden in India and world (2014)[8]

Indicators	*World*	*India*
Population	7.23 billion	1295 million
Incidence (all cases including HIV)/100000	133	167
Incidence (new SS+)/100000	–	49
Prevalence (including HIV)/100000	174	195
Mortality excluding HIV/100000	16	17
Incidence HIV positive (%)	12	5.0
New cases multidrug resistance (%)	3.3	2.2
Case detection rate (%)	63	66

Source: WHO Report 2015.

Nearly 2.2 lakh die of tuberculosis every year or 740 everyday. TB kills more people in India than HIV, STD, malaria, leprosy and tropical diseases combined. It is most important killer of adults in India than any other infectious disease. Thus, tuberculosis has acquired the status of epidemic in India, because of the widespread and high burden (high prevalence) and high mortality rates of tuberculosis.[1] Incidence and prevalence of TB in the year 2014 is presented in Table 12.10 (WHO).

WHO in 1993, declared TB as a global emergency and advocated that all countries adopt and implement the WHO recommended Directly Observed Treatment, Short course (DOTS), considered by the World Bank as one of the most cost-effective strategies to control tuberculosis (World Bank report 1994).

Notification of TB Cases in India

Govt. of India has made TB a notifiable disease from May 2012 onward to ensure early treatment and prevent drug resistance and establish surveillance systems. Case based online patient tracking system (Nikshay) has been launched, which led to 29% increase in notification in 2015.

Risk of Infection and Infection Rate

Number of people infected with the tubercle bacilii are estimated to be 1.7 billion in the world; of which 1.3 billion live in developing countries. Global prevalence of tuberculosis infection was 32% (year 1999). In India, 30% *of people are infected with TB*. Pool of infected people determines the disease occurrence. TB is most important opportunistic infection in HIV positives.

Prevalence of tuberculosis infection in India is 30%, i.e. 30% of Indian population has been infected with tubercle bacilli but these persons are healthy and non-infectious. Annual risk of becoming infected with TB is 1.1%.

Tuberculosis infection means entry, multiplication and establishment of TB bacilli in the macrophages of lung alveoli, which get destroyed in the process of interaction between host and the organism. Within 2–4 weeks after infection, the host immune system mounts a specific cell-mediated immunity that arrests infection in more than 90% of individuals. Thus, TB infection means that tubercle bacilli are viable within the body but are not multiplying. People who have TB infection but not TB disease are not infectious and hence cannot spread the disease to others.

Risk of Development of Disease

In majority of individuals, i.e. 90%, the body's defence mechanisms arrest the infection and only 10% of infected people develop the disease during their lifetime. The chances of developing disease are maximum during first 2 years following infection.

India has large pool of TB cases (pulmonary tuberculosis) who continue to spit the organisms and thereby contaminate the air around. Most people in India are thus exposed to the risk of developing tuberculous infection and disease. Risk of developing disease in infected person is increased many folds in the presence of HIV infection.

The prevalence of infection varies by age and sex in the community, increasing rapidly in males than females after childhood. Infection rate below 4 years of age varies from 1 to 5% and above the age of 55 over 62%. The objective of reducing infection rate below 1% in children below 14 years appears to be a distant dream in India.

Repeated exposure of individuals to cases of tuberculosis increases the chances of infection. The density of population and size of family and crowded localities like urban slums have higher rate of infection than planned developed areas. Poor ventilation and crowded living conditions favour more infection and more disease. Individual habits and practices also influence the spread of disease. Indiscriminate coughing and spitting by infectious individuals contaminate the nearby air and environment and poses threat to individuals in the family and close contacts. You can have history of suffering of grandfather, father, son, wife and daughter. Infection and disease persist in the family if the sufferer is not treated or partially treated as he/she acts as source of infection.

Covering mouth and nose with piece of cloth during coughing is very effective method of reducing the probability of spread and transmission of disease. Similarly, improved ventilation reduces the risk of transmission of disease.

Reservoir and Source of Infection

The pulmonary tuberculosis case with sputum smear-positive acts as reservoir and source of infection. India harbours a large reservoir of tuberculosis as indicated that every year we detect 1 million sputum positive cases, disease burden of bacillary cases in India is very high. Large pool of sputum positive cases in India is a risk factor to other healthy population in urban and rural areas; more so in urban slums.

Mode of Transmission

It is lung-to-lung transmission. When a sputum smear-positive case coughs, sneezes and laughs, talks or sings, the bacilli are sprayed into air as infectious droplets. These droplets dry up rapidly and remain suspended in air for several hours. People in the vicinity or nearby contacts may inhale these droplets containing virulent TB bacilli. These bacilli may reach alveoli of lung and begin to multiply in damaged macrophages and carried to different parts of lung by other macrophages and phagocytes or lymphatics and through circulation may reach to other parts of body like brain, kidney, spine, and other parts. People living with sputum smear-positive cases and having longer and continuous contact have more chances of developing infection. A single untreated patient can infect 10 or more people in a year.

Acquiring tuberculosis by ingestion of milk has become rare because of boiling and pasteurization of milk.

Treatment Success Rate (Fig. 12.8)

RNTCP has more than trippled the treatment success rates from 25 to 88% and it has reduced the relapse rates just 3% as compared to 45% in patient put on unobserved treatment.

One smear-positive case if left untreated can infect 10–15 other persons each year creating a self-perpetuated pool of infection hence the imperative need of prompt treatment of all known cases with DOTS.

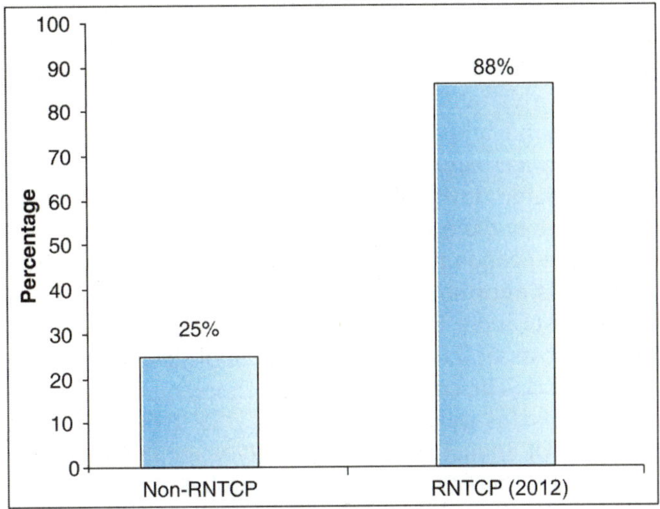

Fig. 12.8: Treatment success rate

Mortality from Tuberculosis in India (Fig. 12.9)

The mortality rate of TB which was 38 per lakh in 1990 has declined to the level of 17 per lakh in 2014 a decline of 55% after successful DOTS strategy however in sputum positive cases mortality has decreased from 29% to 4%

High mortality is reflection on failure to diagnose, inadequate treatment or delayed treatment. Mortality can be reduced by effective DOTS strategy and its implementation all over the country. Tuberculous patient with HIV infection have more chances of deaths (14% against less than 4% in HIV negative TB cases) and development of multidrug resistant TB. Case fatality is more in tuberculous meningitis and miliary tuberculosis. Smear-positive cases are more likely to die in comparison to smear-negative cases and those who take inadequate treatment are likely to die more often. Without treatment about 50% of people with active TB will die within two years. Tuberculosis is nearly 100% curable now with DOTS and this has reduced TB deaths 7-fold in India from 29% to around 4% in comparison to pre-RNTCP era (Fig. 12.9)[2].

TB and Poverty (Economic Impact of TB)

TB and poverty are closely related. Malnutrition, overcrowding, poor ventilation and sanitation factors associated with poverty increase both the risk of infection and

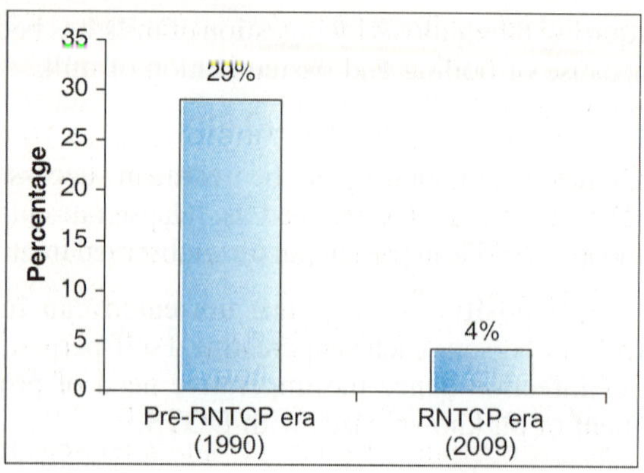

Fig. 12.9: Mortality from sputum + tuberculosis in India

probability of developing clinical disease. Poverty and TB form a vicious circle; TB decreases a person's work capacity and adds burden of treatment expenses and thereby exacerbating their poverty. TB is serious obstacle to sustainable development. Because more than 80% of patients are in the economically productive age group (15–44 years), the economic and social cost to them and to their families is enormous.

TB costs India Rs. 12,000 crore annually. Other non-disease costs of TB are 3,00,000 school dropouts due to parents' TB. The cost to patient for shopping of diagnosis and successful treatment averages US$ 100–150, more than half of annual income of a daily wage labourer.[8] On an average 3 months of work time are lost if an adult has TB; resulting in loss of 20–30% of annual household income, and an average of 15 years of income is lost if the patient dies from disease.

Indirect cost to society: US$ 3 billion per year, direct cost US$ 300 million.

Loss of 100 million productive workdays per year due to illness alone. Each year India loses more than 13 billion productive workdays due to TB deaths.

More than 1,00,000 women are rejected by their families on account of TB (TRC, IJTLD, 1999; 3: 869–77).

HIV and TB: The Deadly Combination

HIV and TB form a lethal combination, each speeding-up the other's progress. In India, 30% of people are infected with tuberculous infection, who are healthy and if such infected person acquires HIV, the chances of developing active TB increase to 60%, whereas an HIV negative person infected with TB bacillus has only a 10% life time risk of developing TB. Thus, HIV infection accelerates development of tuberculosis disease in infected person and thus HIV gives a push to TB epidemic and increases disease burden substantially. The number of HIV positive persons in India in the age group (15–49 adults) was estimated to be *2.11 million* (2015 sentinel surveillance report). The HIV epidemic readily increases the incidence of TB in India. HIV positive TB patients have mortality rates that are 2 to 4 times higher than those of HIV negative patients.

Active TB disease is the commonest life-threatening opportunistic infection occurring among HIV positive persons. TB shortens the survival of patient with HIV infection. HIV infected persons become full-fledged cases of AIDS with the superimposition of TB. TB is a leading cause of death among AIDS patients. In a developing country like India, the potential burden of new cases attributable to HIV could overwhelm budget and support services as has already happened in those countries heavily affected by the HIV epidemic.

Incidence of HIV + TB in India is 5%. India is facing dual epidemic of HIV and tuberculosis, which are deadly combination.

The alarming evidence is that the HIV epidemic can facilitate the emergence of multi-drug resistant strain of *Mycobacterium tuberculosis* and this has serious implications for TB control as DOTS strategy may be hit and may become ineffective to cure the TB and alternate drugs have to be found which may be costlier and beyond reach.

Risk Factors for Developing TB[9]

The following conditions appear to increase the risk that TB infections will progress to disease:

- Infection with HIV is most powerful risk factor.
- Contacts of sputum positive patient
- Alcohol abuse and IV drug use
- Recent TB infection (within the past 2 years)
- Chest X-ray suggestive of previous TB
- Diabetes mellitus
- Silicosis
- Prolonged therapy with corticosteroids
- Immunosuppressive therapy
- Certain types of cancer (e.g. leukaemia, Hodgkin's disease)
- Tobacco use
- Malnutrition.
- Indoor air pollution, urbanization and migration.

Mantoux Test (Tuberculin Test)

Tuberculosis infection rate in the community can be determined by tuberculin test. Tuberculin test is the only available tool to determine TB infection. The international unit of tuberculin recommended by WHO was standardized in 1951 and is called tuberculin PPD RT 23. A dose of two tuberculin units (TU) of PPD RT23 is recommended for surveys, 0.1 ml of PPD is injected intradermally to raise a wheel of 8 mm on the forearm by tuberculin syringe. The results are read after 48–72 hours. The diameter of induration is measured, if it is more than 10 mm the test is considered to be positive. The test is very sensitive but not specific. Determining the prevalence of tuberculosis infection is seriously hampered by the presence of cross-reactions due to environmental bacteria and BCG vaccination. Global prevalence of infection is around 32% and in India prevalence of TB infection is 30%.

NATIONAL TUBERCULOSIS CONTROL PROGRAMME (NTCP)

The epidemiological findings of National sample survey (1955–58) by ICMR formed the basis of National policy for control of tuberculosis in the country. It served as base for working out resources and manpower.

National Tuberculosis Institute (NTI) was established at Bangalore to formulate National Tuberculosis Control Programme of India. NTI used the findings of Tuberculosis Chemotherapy Centre now Tuberculosis Research Centre (ICMR), Madras. Home treatment and sanatorium treatment were equally effective as at the end of one year 86% of patient treated at home converted to sputum negative and remained so (bacteriologically quiescent) as against 92% in sanatorium patients.[5] Improvement in X-ray and closure of cavity were also of the same order in both the groups. Treatment modality of INH 200 mg and PAS 10 g per day was followed. Relapse rate at the end of 4 years of follow-up in home series and sanatorium series were 7% and 10% respectively. It was thus conclusively proved that effect of treatment of patients at home is as good as of treatment in an institution. This gave revolution to *domiciliary treatment* of tuberculosis. Further it was established that there was no special risk to the contacts of patients treated at home and treated at sanitorium over the follow up period of 5 years, with effective chemotherapy, hence *isolation of patients* in hospital or at home is not required.

Further most patient of active tuberculosis, 69% of sputum positive cases had symptoms and sought treatment from nearby facility.[10–13]

These evidence-based findings, formed the basis of National TB control programme in the country.

NTI, Bangalore formulated *district tuberculosis programme* in 1961 and it was implemented by Government of India in 1962 as a centrally sponsored scheme.

The programme was aimed at early case detection in symptomatic patients seeking health care through sputum microscopy, X-ray and effective domiciliary treatment with standard chemotherapy. BCG vaccination was used on mass scale to cover population below 25 years of age and subsequently the focus shifted to infants and BCG vaccination was integrated with expanded programme for Immunization (EPI).

The major components of control programme were:

- District TB centres as support to peripheral units and function as referral centre for entire district.
- Case detection by microscopy centre set-up at each PHC by TB multipurpose worker.
- Training of district teams or key personnel.
- Supply of drugs and reagents for laboratory besides microscopes.
- BCG vaccination by BCG team located at district.
- Monitoring of programme through routine reports.

Target worked out for the district was treatment of 1500 sputum positive cases per year.

At the beginning of programme, it was estimated that infection rate due to tuberculosis was around 50% in population. At the prevalence rate of 1.6%, it was estimated that about 9 million persons were having radiologically active tuberculosis disease and about quarter of them, i.e. about 2 million were infectious; excreting tubercle bacilli in their sputum and most of them had symptoms.

Case holding and cure rates: In SEARO region only 30–50% of those diagnosed with TB were cured and the remainder continued to transmit the infection. Each untreated/uncured patient infects approximately 10 persons per year, thus increasing the pool or source of infection. Incomplete treatment may result into resistance to anti-TB drugs.

India's National Tuberculosis Control Programme (NTCP) was established in 1962 and provided a system of 446 Distt. TB centres, 330 TB clinics and more than 47,000 hospital beds for TB control throughout the country. After more than 3 decades of operation, it established the infrastructure for TB treatment in India.[14]

Outcomes

- The emphasis of NTCP remained on case detection.
- Case detection rate and case holding rate was low.
- Treatment completion rate was only 30%.
- The programme did not make a significant impact.
- There was no dent/decline in morbidity and mortality due to TB after three decades of implementation.

Incorporation of short-term chemotherapy, which shortened the duration of treatment to 9 months was started in selected districts in 1983.

REVISED NATIONAL TUBERCULOSIS CONTROL PROGRAMME (RNTCP) PHASE - 1

NTCP was reviewed in India in 1992 and revised national tuberculosis control programme (RNTCP) was drawn and formally launched in March 1997 with phased coverage in various states throughout India.

The Objectives of RNTCP

1. To achieve and maintain a high cure rate of at least 85% among new sputum smear-positive patients already detected thereby interrupting the chain of transmission.
2. To achieve and maintain at least 70% detection of new sputum smear-positive cases.

   However, the target for case detection should only be attempted once the cure rate of 85% is achieved among new smear-positive cases already detected.
3. Reduce annual incidence and mortality due to tuberculosis by 50% by 2015.

National Strategic Plan for RNTCP in 12th Five-Year Plan 2012–17

Vision: "TB free India" "Reaching the unreached"

AIM: "Universal access" to quality diagnosis and treatment for all TB patients.

One of the major policy decision taken by RNTCP in the year 2010 is to change the focus of the New Smear-positive (NSP) detection of at least 70% to the concept of 'Universal Access' to good quality diagnosis and treatment for all TB patients. There is now a global consensus that the twin objectives of 70/85 alone is not enough to achieve adequate reduction of TB burden at the pace with which epidemiological impact is expected. Today's missed smear-negative case may be tomorrows smear-positive case. Hence it is extremely important for TB control programme to focus on early and complete detection of *all TB cases including smear-positive* and *smear-negative* TB cases. Strategies must ensure that all TB patients have access to early case detection and effective treatment.

Targets/Objectives

i Early detection and treatment of at least 90% of estimated TB cases in the community including HIV associated TB.

ii Successful treatment of at least 90% of all new TB patients, and at least 85% of all previously treated TB patients.

iii Reduction of default rate of new TB cases to less than 5% and in retreatment cases to less than 10%.

iv Initial screening of all re-treatment smear-positive TB patients for drug resistant cases and provision of treatment services for MDR-TB patients.

v Offer HIV counseling and testing for all TB patients and linking HIV infected TB patients to HIV "care and support". Treat all HIV infected TB patients with ART irrespective of CD4 count.

vi Extend, RNTCP services to patients diagnosed and treated in private sector.

***Sustaintable development goals*:** There is shift from 'STOP TB strategy' to 'End TB strategy' by 2030, i.e. reduce TB deaths by 90%, new cases by 80% and eliminate catastrophic expenditure".

The principles of DOTS were first formulated in India. During 1950s and 1960s, pioneering studies conducted at the Tuberculosis Research Centre (TRC), Chennai demonstrated the safety and efficacy of domiciliary treatment of TB, the efficacy of intermittent treatment with Anti-TB drugs, and necessity and feasibility of direct observation of treatment. In 1960s, studies at National tuberculosis institute (NTI) Bangalore, documented the efficacy, feasibility and importance of case detection by sputum microscopy in primary health care institutions. These findings laid the foundation of the DOTS strategy, which has been adopted by 180 countries worldwide. In India, DOTS is implemented as the revised national tuberculosis control programme (RNTCP).[14–16]

DOTS is a strategy for ensuring high cure rate in patients with tuberculosis. In the RNTCP, more than 8 out of 10 patients have been treated successfully. Thus, cure rate of over 85% has been achieved and results of treatment have been quite encouraging. Once infectious cases have been detected, the health workers or any other person other than family member who is acceptable and accessible to the patient and accountable to the health system can be **treatment observer.**

Principles of DOTS (Components of RNTCP)

Political and administrative commitment: TB is leading cause of death among adults. It kills more women than all causes associated with childbirths combined and leaves more orphans than any other infectious disease. Tuberculosis can be cured and epidemic reversed, it should have topmost priority. Govt. of India is committed to it. The priority must continue and expanded at state, district and local level.

Good quality diagnosis: Sputum smear microscopy is the best test for diagnosis of pulmonary tuberculosis.

Ensuring accessibility to designated microscopy centre at CHC level. Designated microscopy centres have been established at CHC level in India.

Good quality drugs: Regular uninterrupted supply of anti-TB drugs. In RNTCP, a Patient-Wise Boxes (PWB) of medicines for the entire course of treatment is earmarked for every patient registered, ensuring the availability of the full course of treatment to the patient. Hence in RNTCP the treatment never fails on account of non-availability of drugs.

Short course of chemotherapy given in a programme of directly observed treatment short-course (DOTS) chemotherapy. The heart of DOTS programme is "directly observed treatment" in which a health worker or other trained person who is not a family member watches as the patient swallows the anti-TB medicines in their presence. This strategy achieves high cure rates and prevents drug resistance. However, directly observed treatment (DOT) is not just supervised swallowing but a service to the patient. It helps to develop human bond between the patients and the treatment observer, which increases the probability of the patient completing treatment. With short course chemotherapy it is easier to prevent drug resistance by using directly observed treatment, and achieve high cure rate. Currently, DOTS is being practised in over 180 countries.

Systematic monitoring and accountability: To monitor initiation of DOTS within one week of diagnosis, sputum conversion rate, cure rate and case detection rate. There are two means of monitoring the success of treatment. First, sputum is examined during the course of treatment to monitor the progress and cure of patients. Second, a revised recording and reporting system rigorously monitors and evaluates the outcome of every patient treated at different levels of the health system, and if any area is not achieving 90% sputum conversion rate at the end of 3 months and 85% cure rate, supervision is intensified.

Major Organization Change for DOTS Programme

State TB cell
↓
Distt. TB Centre—Distt. population—1.9 million
↓
TB Unit (TU) 1 per 5 Lakh population
(*Staff:* Medical officer, senior treatment supervisor, and senior TB laboratory supervisor)
↓
Microscopy centre 1 per 1,00,000 population
↓
DOT centre-DOT Providers-MPW, NGO, PP

The major organizational change is the creation of *sub-district level*—the Tuberculosis unit (TU) for the systematic monitoring and supervision of diagnosis and treatment aspects of the programme. One TB unit has been established for 5 lakh population. State TB control societies and district TB control societies have been formed to give more ownership to the states and districts. Ideally a microscopy centre (MC) be established at each PHC as against one designated MC for one lakh population at CHC.

Strategy of Case Detection under RNTCP

New guidelines effective from April 2009: Every patient who has **cough for 2 weeks** or **more** with or without other symptoms should have 2 sputum samples examined (spot, and early morning) microscopically for AFB at Designated Microscopy Centre (DMC).[17] Ideally all the 2 specimens should be collected within 2 days.

- As against the previous guidelines which considered a person to be a pulmonary TB suspect with cough for 3 weeks, or more, now a person with **cough for 2 weeks or more** would be considered as a *pulmonary TB suspect*.
- Screening of all patients with TB risk factors, change of TB suspect definition in high-risk groups to cough of any duration or fever with night sweats.
- The number of specimen required for diagnosis of smear-positive pulmonary TB is two, compared to three in the previous guidelines, with one of the two, being a morning sputum specimen.
- **One specimen out of the two** is enough to declare a patient as smear-positive TB, as against two out of the three samples as per the previous guidelines.
- Smear-positive TB is further classified as a new or retreatment case based on their previous treatment history, and appropriate therapy is prescribed.
- Patients in whom both specimens are smear-negative should be prescribed symptomatic treatment and broad spectrum antibiotics for 10–14 days. In such cases, antibiotics such as fluoroquinolones (ciprofloxacin, ofloxacin, etc.), which are active against TB should not be used. If the symptoms persist after a course of broad spectrum antibiotics, repeat sputum examination (2 samples) must be done for such patients.
- If one or more repeat sputum specimen is positive, the patient is diagnosed as having smear-positive pulmonary TB. If none of them is positive, a chest X-ray is taken, and if findings of the X-ray are consistent with pulmonary TB, the patient is diagnosed by the physician as a case of sputum negative pulmonary TB.
- Patients suspected of extrapulmonary TB, and patients who are contacts of sputum smear-positive patients, should have their sputum examined for AFB if they have *cough of any duration*.
- Extrapulmonary TB cases will be diagnosed by the physicians and referred to DTC/chest clinic or MO TB control. Procedure undertaken to arrive at the diagnosis must be mentioned on the treatment card. X-ray-based evaluation causes over diagnosis of TB. NTI, Bangalore found that nearly 40% of cases diagnosed and put on treatment on the basis of X-ray did not actually have tuberculosis. At present, sputum smear microscopy is the best test for diagnosis of pulmonary tuberculosis.

One sputum collected on spot when a patient is suspected of having TB. Second specimen is early morning specimen.

Usually, at least 2–3% of new adult out-patients in general OPD have cough for 2 weeks or more. Medical officer should ensure sputum examination of all such suspected TB cases. On an average 10% of TB suspects are expected to have sputum smear-positive pulmonary TB.

If good diagnostic practices are followed as indicated above it is expected that among the new pulmonary TB cases at least 50% will be sputum smear-positive cases.

Treatment Outcome and Type of Patients

- ***Cured:*** Initially sputum smear-positive patient who has completed treatment and had negative sputum smears, on at least two occasions, one of which was at completion of treatment.
- ***New:*** A patient who has never had treatment for TB or has taken anti-TB drugs for less than one month.
- ***Relapse:*** A patient cured for TB by a physician or completed treatment but who reports back to the health service and is found to be bacteriologically positive.
- ***Transfer out:*** A patient who has been transfered to another tuberculosis unit/district and whose treatment outcome is still not known.
- ***Failure:*** A smear-positive patient who remains smear-positive at 5 months or more after starting treatment.

Failure also includes a patient who was initially smear-negative but who becomes smear-positive during treatment.

- *Treatment after default:* A patient who received anti-TB treatment for one month or more from any source and returns for treatment after having defaulted, i.e. not taken anti-TB drugs consecutively for two months or more and found to be smear-positive.
- *Others:* Patients who do not fit into above mentioned type. Reasons for defining a patient as "other must be specified".
- *Treatment completed:* Initially sputum smear-positive patient who has completed treatment, with negative smear at the end of intensive phase/two months in the continuation phase but none at the end of treatment is declared as treatment completed or sputum smear-negative TB patient who has received full course of treatment and has not become smear-positive during or at the end of treatment or extrapulmonary TB patient who has received full course of treatment and has not become smear-positive during or at the end treatment.
- *Defaulted:* A patient after treatment initiation has interrupted treatment consecutively for >2 months.
- *Died:* Patient who died during the course of treatment.

Initially Category I regimen was provided to new smear-positive PTB, 'seriously ill' new smear-negative PTB and extrapulmonary TB cases. However, the eligibility to Category I treatment widened as RNTCP included:

- All new cases who were HIV infected irrespective of type of TB, site or severity.
- All new cases of TB in pediatric cases except primary complex and minor forms of EPTB.

This resulted in a marked decline in the number of patients being placed in Category III treatment. WHO treatment guidelines, 4th edition, 2009 recommended against the omission of ethambutol in intensive phase for new patients in view of the elevated levels of INH resistance among new patients and lack of testing for INH resistance among them.

In the light of these facts, and the recommendations of JMM 2009, meeting of National Experts (NTI, September 2009) and National Task Force for Medical Colleges (October 2009), it has been decided to have only 2 first line TB treatment regimens in future and discontinue the 3-drug Category III regimen from the guidelines.

Treatment Regimen and Discontinuation of Category III

For the purpose of treatment TB patients are classified into two groups namely, "New" or "Previously Treated", based on the history of previous treatment.

Determine the Category of Treatment (Table 12.11)

New (Category I): All new sputum smear-positive, new sputum smear-negative, new extrapulmonary and new others.

Treatment: Treatment is given in *two phases*. The *intensive phase* (IP) consists of isoniazid, rifampicin, pyrazinamide and ethambutol given under direct observation thrice a week on alternate days and lasts for

Table 12.11: Category of treatment (national guidelines)

Treatment groups	*Type of patient*	*Regimen**	
		Intensive phase (IP)	*Continuation phase (CP)***
New (Category I) (Red)	New sputum smear-positive New sputum smear-negative New extrapulmonary New others	$2(HRZE)_3$	$4(HR)_3$
Previously treated (Category II) (Blue)	Smear-positive relapse Smear-positive failure Smear-positive treatment after default, and others**	$2(HRZES)_3$ $1(HRZE)_3$	$5(HRE)_3$
Category IV MDR–TB cases Category V XDR–TB cases		6–9 (Km Lvx Eto Cs ZE)*** 6–12 (Cm PAS, Mfx, High dose–H Cfz, Lzd, Amx/CLv)***	18 (Lvx Eto CsE) 18 (PAS Mfx, High dose–H, Cfz, Lzd, Amx/CLv)

* The number before the letters refers to the number of months of treatment. The subscript after the letters refers to the number of doses per week. H: Isoniazid (600 mg), R: Rifampicin (450 mg); Z: Pyrazinamide (1500 mg), E: Ethambutol (1200 mg), S: Streptomycin (750 mg). Patients who weigh more than 60 kg receive additional Rifampicin 150 mg. Patients more than 50 years old receive streptomycin 500 mg. Patients in categories I and II, who have a positive sputum smear at the end of the initial intensive phase receive an additional month of intensive phase treatment. Adult patients who weigh less than 30 kg receive drugs in patient-wise boxes from the weight band suggested for paediatric patients.

** For patients with TB meningitis, disseminated disease and spinal TB with neurological complications, continuation phase may be up to 7 months.

*** Km: Kanamycin, Lvx: Levofloxacin, Eto: Ethionamide, Cs: Cycloserine, Cm: Capreomycin, Mfx: Moxifloxacin, Cfz: Clofazimine, Lzd: Linezolid, Amx/CLv: Amoxyclav.

2 months (24 doses). This is immediately followed by the *continuation phase* (CP), which consists of 4 months (18 weeks; 54 doses) of isoniazid and rifampicin given thrice a week on alternate days—the first dose every week being directly observed. If the sputum smear is positive after 2 months of treatment, the four intensive phase drugs are continued for another one month (12 doses) before starting the 4 months (18 weeks) of *continuation phase*. If the sputum smear is positive after 5 or more months of treatment, the patient is declared as a *Failure* and is placed on CAT II treatment afresh. Failure rate should be less than 5%.

Previously treated (Category II): These include smear-positive relapse, smear-positive failure, smear-positive treatment after default, and others.

Treatment: Treatment is given in two phases. *The intensive phase* consists of 2 months (24 doses) of isoniazid, rifampicin, pyrazinamide, ethambutol and streptomycin all given under direct observation thrice a week on alternate days, followed by one month (12 doses) of isoniazid, rifampicin, pyrazinamide and ethambutol, all given under direct observation thrice a week on alternate days. This is immediately followed by the *continuation phase*, which consists of 5 months (22 weeks; 66 doses) of isoniazid, rifampicin and ethambutol given thrice a week on alternate days, with at least the first dose of every week being directly observed. If the sputum smear is positive after 3 months of treatment, the four oral intensive phase drugs are continued for another one month (12 doses) before starting the 5 months *continuation phase*.

Drugs are supplied in patient-wise boxes (PWB) containing the full course of treatment, and packed in blister packs. The PWB have a colour code indicating the category—Red for Cat I, Blue for Cat II. In each PWB, there are two pouches—one for *intensive phase* (A) and one for *continuation phase* (B). For the *intensive phase*, each blister pack contains one day's medication. For the *continuation phase*, each blister pack contains one week's supply of medication. The combipack drugs for extension of the intensive phase are supplied separately. Information on dosage is provided in Table 12.12.

Table 12.12: Dosages for adults

Medication	Dose (thrice a week)***	Number of pills in combipack
Isoniazid	600 mg	2
Rifampicin	450 mg*	1
Pyrazinamide	1500 mg	2
Ethambutol	1200 mg	2
Streptomycin	0.75 g**	–

*Patients who weigh 60 kg or more are given an extra 150 mg dose of rifampicin.

**Patients over 50 years of age are given 0.5 g of streptomycin.

***Adult patients who weigh less than 30 kg receive drugs in patient wise boxes from the weight brand suggested for paediatric patients.

Dosages for children are given below. Treatment regimen for children with active TB are similar to those of adults. Children are rarely sputum smear-positive. Ethambutol in young children is safe and to be used as per RNTCP regimen (WHO).

Dosages for children

Drugs	Therapy per dose (thrice a week)
Isoniazid	10–15 mg/kg
Rifampicin	10 mg/kg
Pyrazinamide	35 mg/kg
Streptomycin	15 mg/kg
Ethambutol	30 mg/kg

Regimen for Non-DOTS Treatment in RNTCP Areas

Up to 1% of patients may get non-DOTS treatment in RNTCP areas, because of migration and adverse effects of drugs.

However, it is an admission of failure of the programme. Since patients who receive non-DOTS treatment are more likely to default and die, all efforts should be made to phase out non-DOTS treatment, as has already been done in many areas. This is important to ensure the success of RNTCP. For this to occur, convenient, patient centred treatment observation is essential.

The prescribed regimen and dosages are given below:

Treatment	Type of patient	Regimen
Non-DOTS Regimen 1	New sputum smear-positive cases Smear-negative pulmonary, seriously ill Extrapulmonary, seriously ill	2 SHE⁺ 10 HE
Non-DOTS Regimen 2	Smear-negative cases not seriously ill Extrapulmonary not seriously ill	12 HE

S–Streptomycin H–Isoniazid E–Ethambutol

Non-DOTS Regimen 1 (R_1): Twelve months conventional chemotherapy regimen, with streptomycin given in the first 2 months. This is given to patients who are:

- New cases of smear-positive pulmonary TB.
- Seriously ill cases of smear-negative and extrapulmonary TB (meningitis, disseminated TB, tuberculous pericarditis, peritonitis, bilateral or extensive pleurisy, spinal TB with neurological complications, intestinal and genitourinary TB).

The treatment consists of 12 months conventional chemotherapy. The initial intensive phase lasts for 2 months and the continuation phase for 10 months. Isoniazid and ethambutol are self-administered by the patient daily for 12 months. Streptomycin is administered daily in the initial intensive phase.

Dosage for adults is one tablet of isoniazid (300 mg) and one tablet of ethambutol (800 mg) everyday. The dosage for streptomycin injection is 0.75 g per day (0.5 g for those over 50 years of age and those who weigh less than 30 kg) receive dosages calculated as per body weight.

Non-DOTS Regimen 2 (R_2): Twelve months conventional chemotherapy regimen, without streptomycin for:

- All patients with smear-negative pulmonary TB who are not seriously ill.
- All patients with extrapulmonary TB who are not seriously ill.

The treatment consists of 12 months conventional chemotherapy. Isoniazid and ethambutol are self-administered by the patient daily for 12 months. The dosage for adults is isoniazid (300 mg) along with ethambutol (800 mg) per day.

Implementation Status of DOTS in India

Universal Coverage Achieved

India has been world leader in designing the tuberculosis control programme and advocating DOTS and domiciliary treatment. We have world class standard institutions like NTI and Tuberculosis Research Centre at Bangalore and Chennai, respectively. But 30 years of operation of NTCP could achieve treatment completion rate of only 30%. With the revised strategy, the coverage of the programme of RNTCP which incorporates DOTS have reached to 1114 million population of 632 districts by March 2006. Entire population of the country in 36 States and Union Territories has thus been covered.[16] DOTS in India is the largest programme in the world. Results of the DOTS treatment have been quite encouraging as 88% of patients have been successfully treated. Hopefully it is sustained and positive impact is made to reduce the disease burden (Table 12.13 and Fig. 12.10).

Private Health Sector in RNTCP

Many patients at least half of the total tuberculosis patients may seek services from private practitioners of various systems. Public sector reach is limited to cover the entire load of tuberculosis in the country. Of necessity it becomes imperative to involve private practitioners and non-governmental organization (NGO) by imparting training or orientation of professional associations and NGOs on recent advances in RNTCP and strategy of DOTS, national policy of drug regimen in tuberculosis and diagnostic criteria adopted as also free availability of anti-tubercular drugs. They can be accredited as peripheral health institutions (PHI) providing care and where they fulfill the criteria of designated microscopy centres also. Special public–privatee mix (PPM) scheme for *urban slums* has been recently introduced to enhance coverage and case detection. Involvement of private practitioners has strengthened the RNTCP and established uniform practice on diagnosis and regimen of drug. Govt. of India and RNTCP is striving hard to establish public–private partnership (PPP) but this requires tremendous efforts, apart from regular contacts and monitoring of progress and mid-course correction.

Under RNTCP, 291 medical colleges have been involved. RNTCP centres have been set-up in various

Table 12.13: Treatment categories and sputum examination schedule (national guidelines)

	Treatment regimen		Sputum examination for pulmonary TB			
Category of treatment	Type of patient	Regimen*	Pre-treatment sputum	Test at month	IF result is	THEN
New (Category I)	New sputum smear-positive New sputum smear-negative New extrapulmonary** New others	2(HRZE)3 4(HR)3	+	2	–	Start continuation phase, test sputum again at 4 and 6 months
					+	Continue intensive phase for one more month, test sputum again at 3, 5 and 7 months
			–	2	–	Start continuation phase, test sputum again at 6 months
					+	Continue intensive phase for one more month, test sputum again at 3, 5 and 7 months
Previously treated (Category II)	Smear-positive relapse Smear-positive failure Smear-positive Treatment after default and others***	2(HRZES)3 1(HRZE)3 5(HRE)3	+	3	–	Start continuation phase, test sputum again at 5 and 8 months
					+	Continue intensive phase for one more month, test sputum again at 4, 6 and 9 months

*The number before the letters refers to the number of months of treatment. The subscript after the letters refers to the number of doses per week. H: Isoniazid (600 mg), R: Rifampicin (450 mg), Z: Pyrazinamide (1500 mg), E: Ethambutol (1200 mg), S: Streptomycin (750 mg). Patients who weigh more than 60 kg receive additional Rifampicin 150 mg. Patients more than 50 years old receive streptomycin 500 mg. Patients in categories I and II who have a positive sputum smear at the end of the initial intensive phase receive an additional month of intensive phase treatment. Those who weigh less than 30 kg receive dosages as per body weight.

** Examples of seriously ill extrapulmonary TB cases are meningitis, disseminated TB, tuberculous pericarditis, peritonitis, bilateral or extensive pleurisy, spinal TB with neurological complications and intestinal and genitourinary TB.

*** In rare and exceptional cases, patients who are sputum smear-negative or who have extrapulmonary disease can have relapse or failure. This diagnosis in all such cases should always be made by an MO and should be supported by culture or histological evidence of current active tuberculosis. In these cases, the patient should be categorized as 'Others' and given category II treatment.

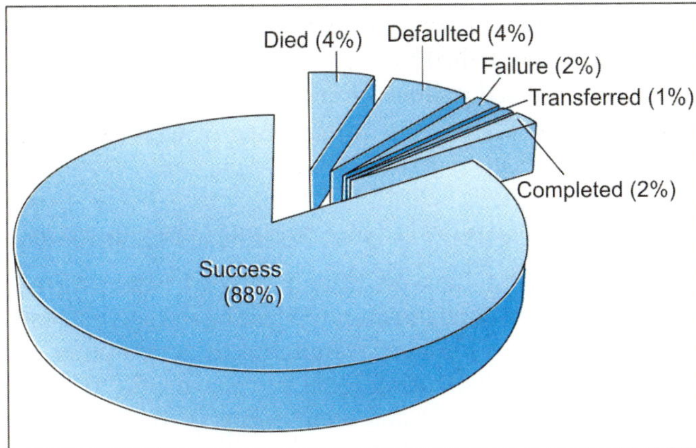

Fig. 12.10: Treatment outcome under RNTCP (2014)

medical colleges and in phased manner all the medical colleges will be covered on priority basis. Their potential will be used in training and continuing education, conducting operational research, monitoring and supervision, information education and communication activities, private sector participation, quality assurance of drugs and sputum microscopy. Additionally, colleges are providing services for the management of complicated cases and developing model DOTS centres.

CHEMOPROPHYLAXIS

Recent infection with TB bacilli is one of the risk factors for disease development. The younger the child, the higher is the risk of breakdown of infection to disease. Therefore, child contacts of smear-positive TB cases especially those below 6 years of age, must be screened for symptoms of tuberculosis. If the symptoms are present the child should be given a full course of anti-TB treatment if diagnosed as TB case. For asymptomatic children below 6 years of age who stay with smear-positive case, TB chemoprophylaxis with isoniazid (10 mg per kg body weight) should be administered daily for a period of six months. This is regardless of BCG vaccination.

RNTCP PHASE II (2006–2011)

RNTCP Phase I lasted till september 2006 and it achieved the target of full coverage of population by March 2006. The second phase of the RNTCP commenced on 1st October 2006 for a further period of 5 years and is being assisted by the World Bank and the Department of International Development (DFID). Phase II of the RNTCP is a step towards achieving the TB-related millennium development goal (MDG)/targets. The goal of TB control programme is to decrease mortality and morbidity due to TB and cut transmission of TB. DOTS remain the core startegy. The second phase of RNTCP will consolidate, maintain and further improve the achievements of the first phase.

It aims to further universal access to good quality care for TB patient to achieve early and complete case detection to cover marginalized groups in hard to reach areas through continuation of all activities of Phase I. The following new activities have been envisaged in the Phase II of RNTCP:

- Implementation of DOTS Plus for MDR TB cases.
- TB/HIV collaborative activities.
- Setting up of state level intermediate referral laboratories (IRL).

The RNTCP has adopted the recently published "International Standards for TB Care (ISTC)" for better management of TB in India.[18–20]

Multidrug Resistant Tuberculosis (MDR-TB)–Cat IV

Multidrug resistant tuberculosis (MDR-TB) refers to strains of tubercle bacilli that have developed resistance to two most effective anti-tubercular drugs available—Isoniazid and Rifampicin. MDR-TB can be diagnosed only in specialized laboratory. The treatment of MDR-TB requires at least 24–27 months of supervised chemotherapy, which is 200 times more expensive and often highly toxic with a high failure rate. In a country like India, MDR-TB is almost equivalent to a death sentence, as very few patients have financial capacity or the resourccs to complete the required long-term regimen.

MDR-TB is a symptom of underlying poor programme implementation. The priority of TB control programme should be to prevent MDR-TB by effective primary treatment with DOTS. Effective implementation of DOTS can prevent MDR-TB in India that is the only way out.

In India, preliminary results show the prevalence of MDR-TB to range from 0.5 to 3% (Average 2.2%) among previously untreated patients. Among previously treated patients the MDR-TB was around 14–17%. These findings indicate the need for DOTS and need to achieve high cure rates among new patients.[1,3]

WHO Global TB Report 2013 estimates that 73000 cases of MDR-TB emerge annually in India.

Extensively Drug Resistant TB (XDR-TB) Category V

It is defined as resistance to at least Isoniazid and Rifampicin (i.e. MDR-TB), plus resistance to any of the fluoroquinolone and at least one of the second line injectable drugs (Amikacin, Kanamycin or Capreomycin).

DOTS PLUS

DOTS Plus, conceived by the WHO and several of its partners, is a strategy for management of multidrug resistant TB (MDR-TB). The RNTCP views the treatment of MDR-TB patients as a 'standard of care' issue. Under RNTCP phase II, it is planned to have a network of DOTS plus sites; as per international guidelines, capable of enrolling and providing care and management up to 5000 'new' multidrug resistant tuberculosis cases a year. To provide treatment service for MDR-TB patients, the RNTCP is establishing a network of state level quality assured culture and drug susceptibility testing (DST). Intermediate reference laboratory (IRL) in each state by 2009–10. DOTS plus is thus a comprehensive management strategy that includes the five components of DOTS strategy. It takes into account of specific issues such as use of second line TB drugs to tackle areas having significant high prevalence of MDR-TB. DOTS plus works as a supplement to standard DOTS strategy, to address both drug susceptible and MDR-TB in areas with significant levels of MDR-TB. Having a successful DOTS based TB control programme in place with a default rate of <5% and availability of an accredited mycobacteriology laboratory in the state, is a prerequisite for considering DOTS plus in an area. DOTS plus services for management of MDR-TB have been rolled out in 31 states and 43 accredited laboratories have been established.

Key features of RNTCP for programmatic management of drug resistant TB (PMDT) in India:

Diagnosis of MDR/XDR-TB—National Guidelines

- *Decentralized diagnosis and treatment services:* 43 RNTCP certified culture—DST laboratories are functioning with rapid molecular test (Line Probe Assay—LPA) available in 31 of these labs.
- *Diagnosis:* Clinical indication to offer drug susceptibility testing (DST).
  - i Initially all failure of first line regimen, and contacts of known MDR TB case (Criteria A).
  - ii *Subsequently:* + All smear-positive re-treatment cases at diagnosis, any smear-positive follow-up case (Criteria B).
  - iii *For XDR-TB:* If culture is positive at 6 months and culture reverted cases (Criteria C).

Major Initiatives

TB/HIV Coordination

Globally, the HIV epidemic is worsening the TB situation by increasing the number of TB cases and accelerating the spread of the disease. HIV increases the person's susceptibility to TB infection and tuberculosis increases morbidity and mortality in HIV infected persons. HIV is the most potent risk factor for progression of TB infection to disease.

National Framework for joint TB/HIV collaborative activities at national, state and district level has developed "Intensified HIV-TB package" in 2008, which has been rolled out in 28 states. Linkages of RNTCP and NACP activities at ICTCs, ART centres and TB clinics/TB centres have been established to improve service delivery for TB and HIV infected patients. Early initiation of ART for all HIV infected TB patients irrespective of CD4 count will help enhance survival.

Information-Education and Communication (IEC)

RNTCP emphasizes on decentralized planning and implementation of health communication initiatives. States and districts develop need based annual action plans and implement activities using local popular media to spread information about TB and availability of free diagnosis and DOTS treatment. Communication facilitators have been engaged for IEC. 24th March of every year is cellebrated as "World TB Day".

Other Initiatives

Other initiatives like Public–private Mix in RNTCP, involvement of NGOs, Medical colleges/TB hospitals and other sectors (ESI, Railways, CGHS hospitals and corporate hospitals), greater level of access of TB to urban slum areas has been introduced under Public–private Mix.

Impact of the Programme

- TB mortality in the country has come down from over 38/lakh population in 1990 to 17 lakh population in 2014 a decline of 55%.
- The prevalence of all forms of TB in the country has declined by 58% from 465/lakh population in 1990 to 195/lakh population by the year 2014.
- Incidence has declined from 216 to 167 per lac per year (23% decline).
- Repeat population survey conducted by National Institute of Tuberculosis Research indicate annual decline of prevalence of disease by 12%. Thus India could achieve MDGs by 2015 by halving prevalence and mortality.

FROM STOP TB STRATEGY TO END TB STRATEGY BY 2030

From 2016 the goal is to 'end global TB epidemic' by implementing "the end TB strategy". Adopted by the World Health Assembly in May 2014 and with targets linked to the newly, adopted "sustainable Development Goals", the strategy serves as a blue print for countries to:

- Reduce deaths by 90% by 2030 (compared with 2015 levels).
- Reduce incidence by 80%.
- Ensure elimination of catastrophic cost.

Tuberculosis is no longer a dreaded disease. It is nearly 100% curable by early and prompt treatment by DOTS. Disease burden in India has been reduced by effective coverage of total population with RNTCP and DOTS. India has been leader in developing DOTS strategy and now it has come back to India, better than ever. Effective implementation of DOTS has saved millions of lives in India.

REFERENCES

1 WHO Report 2015—Global Tuberculosis Control.
2 GOI. TB India 2002. RNTCP Status Report. New Delhi: Central TB Division, DGHS, MOH and FW; 2002.
3 GOI. RNTCP Status Report. Every Breath Counts-Stop TB Now. New Delhi: GOI; 2004.
4 Narain JP. Tuberculosis epidemiology and control. 1st edition. New Delhi: WHO Regional Office of SE Asia, 2002.
5 Barua BNM. Tuberculosis in India. New Delhi: Central Health Education Bureau, DGHS; 1977.
6 Planning Commission. Tenth Five-Year Plan 2002–07, Vol I; Sectoral Policies and Programmes. New Delhi: GOI; 2002.
7 PG Gopi, R Subramani, T Santha, V Chandrasekaran, C Colapan N Selvakumar and PR Narayanan. Tuberculosis Research Centre, Chennai, IJMR 122, September 2005; pp 243–8.
8 WHO. Global Tuberculosis Control Surveillance, Planning and Financing. Geneva: WHO; 2009 and 2013.
9 WHO. Research for action—understanding and controlling TB in India. New Delhi: WHO Regional Office for SE Asia; 2000.
10 Harris HW. The natural history of tuberculosis, New Delhi: WHO Regional Office of SE Asia; 2001.
11 Pamra SP. Lectures on Tuberculosis, New Delhi: The TB Association of India.
12 Proceedings of Silver Jubilee Celebration; 1985: NTI, Bangalore.
13 NTI. Sociological aspects of TB—Summaries of published literature (1939–2000). Mumbai; Foundation for Research in Community Health.
14 The TB Association of India. Blue print for tuberculosis control in India, New Delhi: The TB Association of India; 1979.
15 GOI. Managing the Revised National TB Control Programme in your area—A training course-modules 1–4, New Delhi: DGHS, GOI; 2002 and 2005.
16 GOI. TB India 2001 RNTCP Status Report. New Delhi: Central TB Division, DGHS; MOH and FW; 2001.
17 Government of NCT of Delhi. Diagnosis of smear-positive pulmonary TB. New guidelines from Ist April 2009.
18 GOI. RNTCP performance report India. First Quarter 2006. Central TB Division, DGHS, MOH and FW; Nirman Bhawan, New Delhi.
19 GOI. TB India 2006. RNTCP Status Report. DOTS for all. All for DOTS. Central TB Division, DGHS, MOH and FW; Nirman Bhawan, New Delhi, 2006.
20 GOI. Towards Universal access to TB Diagnosis and treatment 2010, MOH and FW: GOI, New Delhi.

LEPROSY

It is one of the oldest disease known to mankind. Leprosy is a chronic infectious disease caused by bacteria: *Mycobacterium leprae*; an acid-fast, rod-shaped bacillus. When *M. leprae* was discovered by GA Hansen in 1873, it was the first bacterium to be identified as causing disease in man; however, treatment became available only in 1940s with the introduction of dapsone. Leprosy is *least infectious* out of the communicable diseases. It mainly affects the skin, peripheral nerves and occasionally the mucosa of respiratory tract. It is a *curable disease*.

Global Distribution

It once affected every continent and it has left behind a terrifying image in history and human memory of mutilation, rejection and exclusion from society. Now the global prevalence has been reduced by 90%. By the end of year 2000, leprosy has been eliminated as a public health problem at the global level by reducing the prevalence level to 0.88/10000. Now, early in 2003, 110 countries have reached the elimination target at the national level and leprosy remains a public health problem in only 12 countries. Leprosy burden is now concentrated in the five most endemic countries (Brazil, India, Madagascar, Mozambique and Nepal) which account for 83% of prevalence and 88% of detection worldwide. The combined prevalence in these countries is about 4/10,000 population.[1]

Magnitude of Problem in India and Present Status

The national prevalence of leprosy during March 1981 was 57.6/10000 population and it declined to 0.84/10,000 population as on December 2005 and 0.68/10,000 in March 2014. Leprosy is endemic in India and India's contribution of leprosy caseload in the world was about 58%. In the year 2004, 13 states were identified as endemic states in India (Andhra Pradesh, Bihar, Chhattisgarh, Delhi, Jharkhand, Karnataka, Madhya Pradesh, Maharashtra, Odisha, Tamil Nadu, Uttaranchal, Uttar Pradesh and West Bengal) (Table 12.14).[2,3]

Overall prevalence of 0.68/10,000 has been reported by the end of March 2014, thus India has achieved elimination goal of leprosy but it remains problem in 2 states/UTs (Chhattisgarh and Dadra and Nagar Haveli). 34 states/UTs have achieved the status of leprosy elimination.

From 2005–2015 the National Leprosy Eradication Programme recorded 1.25 to 1.35 lakh new cases per year giving Annual New Case detection rate of 0.998 per 10000 population. We have 150 high endemic districts.

Reservoir

Man is the only known source of infection for *M. leprae*.

Transmission

Leprosy is transmitted from one untreated multibacillary patient to another healthy person via droplet infection or skin lesion. The major sites from which bacilli escape from body of an infectious patient are the nose and mouth.

Nose appears to be major site of entry of bacilli. It is acquired through prolonged exposure and only a small proportion of population is affected. Leprosy is not highly infectious disease. Leprosy affects all ages and both sexes.

Incubation Period

The disease has very long period of incubation or latency running into several years varying from 6 months to 30 years. On an average, incubation period is between 3 and 5 years.

Types of Leprosy

- Proportion of multibacillary (MB) and paucibacillary (PB) is variable but in the community 20–30% cases are of MB leprosy and rest are PB cases.
- Around 15–20% of leprosy cases are in children (below 15 years). Childhood leprosy is significant because the proportion of new child cases detected in a year is an important indicator of recency of transmission of disease in the community.
- Leprosy is not hereditary disease and it is acquired and caused by germ.

Leprosy is serious public health problem in Chhattisgarh, and Dadra and Nagar Haveli where prevalence rate is more than 1/10,000. In Delhi, the high prevalence rate was due to migration from these high endemic areas and high proportion of re-registered MB cases continuing MDT beyond fixed duration of 12 months in tertiary care hospitals (Table 12.14).[4]

Annual new case detections (ANCDs) significantly declined after effective MDT application, however, in India which contributes 58% of global annual new case detection, the Annual new case detection (ANCD) is stable at very high level which may be due to re-registration of cases or several operational and administrative shortcomings.

Social Stigma and Disabilities

The leprosy has been notorious amongst the infectious disease to inflict social stigma and out-casting and desertion. Physical disabilities of claw hand, claw foot and autodissolution of fingers and toes as also disfigurement of nose and face are well-known consequences of untreated leprosy cases and delay in treatment. Now with early treatment with modern drugs—MDT the disabilities have almost disappeared or considerably reduced. Social impact of leprosy is much more than medical impact. Attitude of people and community, family and relatives towards leprosy cases are still unfavourable. Discrimination and stigma prevails widely in rural and urban areas.[3] United Nations General Assembly in 2010 resolved to eliminate discrimination against persons affected by leprosy.

Grading Disabilities in Hands and Feet

Grade 0: No anaesthesia, no visible deformity or damage.

Grade 1: Anaesthesia present but no visible deformity or damage.

Grade 2: Visible deformity or damage present in hand or foot or damage in leprosy includes ulceration, shortening disorganization, stiffness or loss of part or all of hand and foot.

Eyes

Grade 0: No eye problem. No evidence of visual loss.

Grade 1: Eye problem due to leprosy present but vision not severely affected.

Grade 2: Severe visual impairment (vision worse than 6/60, inability to count fingers at 6 meters).[4]

Eye problems due to leprosy include corneal anaesthesia, lagophthalmos and iridocyclitis. Rehabilitation of disabled is a challenge. Early detection and prompt treatment with MDT prevents disabilities. Government and NGOs are undertaking many rehabilitation programmes for leprosy cases.

Diagnosis of Leprosy

A case of leprosy is diagnosed by eliciting cardinal signs of leprosy through systematic clinical (and wherever possible bacteriological) examination.

Cardinal signs: At least one of the following cardinal signs must be present to diagnose leprosy.

1. Hypopigmented or reddish skin lesion(s) with definite loss of sensation.
2. Involvement of peripheral nerves as demonstrated by definite thickening with loss of sensation and weakness of the muscles of the hands, feet or face.
3. Demonstration of *M. leprae* in the lesions. The first two cardinal signs can be identified by clinical examination alone, while the third can be identified by examination of the slit skin smear.

Leprosy patches can be pale or reddish or copper coloured, can be flat or raised, do not itch, usually do not hurt, lack sensation to heat, touch or pain and can appear anywhere.

Table 12.14: Prevalence rate and new case detection rate in various states as per LEM-2004

Indicator	*Bihar*	*Odisha*	*Chhattisgarh*	*Jharkhand*	*Delhi*	*UP*	*Maharashtra*	*WB*	*AP*	*TN*	*Uttarakhand*	*MP*	*Karnataka*	*Total*
Prevalence rate	5.2	3.0	4.6	4.6	4.0	3.5	3.0	2.9	1.7	1.4	2.0	2.0	1.3	3.1
New case detection rate	7.9	5.1	5.9	7.1	3.2	4.7	4.3	2.4	4.0	2.4	3.3	2.6	2.1	4.5

A case of leprosy: A leprosy patient is one who has a skin patch or patches with a definite loss of sensation and has not completed a full course of treatment with multidrug therapy (MDT).

New leprosy case: A leprosy patient who has never taken MDT drugs anywhere in the past.

Re-registered case: A case of leprosy, partially or fully treated with MDT in the past at any health facility and who is re-registered again as a new case for treatment.

Leprosy defaulter: A patient who has not collected treatment for 12 consecutive months is a defaulter and should be removed from prevalence.

Cured patient: A patient who has completed a full course of fixed duration of MDT (6 months for PB and 12 months for MB) is cured.

Released from treatment (RFT): A cured person is released from treatment (RFT)

Lepromin test is of academic interest. This detects cell-mediated immunity. The test is positive in tuberculoid leprosy and negative in lepromatous leprosy. Lepromin antigen by intradermal injection of 0.1 ml is deployed for this test and test is read after 48 hours and 21 days after injection. If the area of redness is more than 10 mm it is considered as positive. The widespread BCG vaccination has produced cell-mediated immunity in Indian population and interpretation of lepromin test in children may be difficult.

Classification of Leprosy

Leprosy has been a subject of several classifications but WHO recommends only two classifications for the purpose of treatment. Diagnosis of leprosy is mainly based on clinical signs and symptoms. In pre-MDT era, skin smears were routinely used for classifying a case of leprosy as PB or MB. WHO has made clear that skin smears are not a prerequisite for managing leprosy elimination programme and there is no need to maintain or establish skin smear services exclusively for leprosy. The clinical system of classification for the purpose of treatment includes the use of number of skin lesions as the basis for grouping the leprosy patients into MB and PB. If in doubt, the patient should be treated with MB regimen. Use of skin smears should be limited to referral centres only for special investigations (suspicion of resistance, complex and relapse cases) and research purposes.

1 *Multibacillary case (MB):* 6 or more skin lesions with loss of sensation.
2 *Paucibacillary case (PB):* Up to 5 lesions with loss of sensation.

Some programmes classify leprosy using other systems of classification. For the purpose of treatment, this is not necessary. However, if used, multibacillary (MB) leprosy includes both lepromatous (L) and borderline (B) leprosy in the Madrid classification and LL, BL, BB and some BT leprosy in the Ridley and Jopling classification. Paucibacillary (PB) leprosy includes indeterminate (I) and tuberculoid (T) leprosy in the Madrid classification and I, TT and BT leprosy in the Ridley and Jopling classification.[5]

Multidrug Therapy (MDT) in Leprosy[5–7]

Leprosy is *curable* by MDT which is available free of cost at health facilities. Since its introduction in 1982, MDT has remained highly effective in varying field conditions for the following reasons:

- It cures leprosy and stops transmission.
- Relapse rates are low (less than 1%).
- There is no reported resistance to combined drugs.
- Side effects are negligible.
- Disabilities are prevented through early treatment.
- Health workers can be easily trained to administer the drugs.
- It is easy to administer as it is taken orally.
- It is conveniently available in blister packs containing 4 weeks treatment.
- The drugs can be stored under ordinary storage conditions.

MDT was important technical advance to prevent primary and secondary drug resistance to dapsone. MDT treatment is provided in blister packs, each containing 4 weeks treatment. Specific blister calendar packs (BCP) are available for multibacillary (MB) and paucibacillary (PB) leprosy for adult and children.

- Standard adult treatment regimen for MB leprosy is:
  - Rifampicin 600 mg once a month
  - Clofazimine 300 mg once a month and 50 mg daily
  - Dapsone 100 mg daily

  Duration 12 months
- The standard adult treatment for PB leprosy is:
  - Rifampicin 600 mg once a month
  - Dapsone 100 mg daily

  Duration 6 months
- Standard child (10–14 years) treatment regimen for MB leprosy is:
  - Rifampicin 450 mg once a month
  - Clofazimine 150 mg once a month and 50 mg every other day
  - Dapsone 50 mg daily

  Duration 12 months
- The standard child treatment regimen for PB leprosy is:
  - Rifampicin 450 mg once a month
  - Dapsone 50 mg daily

  Duration 6 months

Children under the age of 10 should receive appro-priately reduced doses of the above drugs as per body weight.

The efficacy of MDT has been clearly demonstrated by extremely low relapse rate (average 0.1% per year for PB and 0.06% per year for MB) following successful completion of treatment; these figures are based on reports from a number of countries and information available at

WHO. In addition, the MDT is highly acceptable because of low frequency of side effects. The available evidence shows that there is significant reduction in the frequency and severity of reversal reactions (Type 1) and erythema nodosum leprosum (ENL) reactions (Type 2) in leprosy patients on MDT.

Rifampicin is an exceptionally potent bactericidal agent against *M. leprae*. A single dose of 600 mg is capable of killing more than 99.9% of viable organisms. The rate of killing is not proportionately enhanced by subsequent doses. Rifampicin also exerts a delayed antibiotic effect for several days, during which the organism is incapable of multiplying. The high bactericidal activity of rifampicin makes a single monthly dose of the drug feasible and cost-effective for leprosy control programme.

Persisting *M. leprae*, by definition, are those viable organisms that are fully susceptible to antileprosy drugs but survive despite adequate treatment with these drugs. The phenomenon probably occurs because these organisms are in low or dormant metabolic state. The evidence to date indicates that persisters do not play an important role in the occurrence of relapse among leprosy patients treated with MDT.

Clofazimine is a repository drug, i.e. it is stored in the body after administration and is then slowly excreted. A loading dose of 300 mg is given once a month to ensure that the optimal amount of Clofazimine is maintained in the body tissues, even if the patient misses his/her daily dose.

Accompanied MDT: Accompanied MDT has been designed to help patients who have to interrupt their treatment because of their inability to attend the health facility regularly or due to geographical distance. These patients are provided more doses of MDT in case patient is not likely to come for next collection.

Recent advances are continuing to further shorten the duration of treatment of leprosy. Universal MDT of MB six blister calendar packs for all kinds of leprosy (PB and MB) has been successfully tried in India and abroad.

Red coloured urine after MDT is due to the colour of rifampicin, which is taken once every month. This lasts for only a few hours after taking drug. Darkening of skin is due to clofazimine used daily for treating MB patients. This is harmless and will disappear within a few months after completing the treatment. Patient must be assured that these are harmless. In case of allergic reactions, patient should be treated at nearby health facility with prednisolone.

NATIONAL LEPROSY ERADICATION PROGRAMME (NLEP)

The Govt. of India launched the leprosy control programme in the year 1955. Eradication means complete absence of the disease and the organism that causes it throughout the world. At present, we lack the tools both to protect people from developing leprosy and to diagnose and treat the disease in its subclinical form, hence eradication is difficult proposition. On the contrary, elimination is feasible and practical proposition. In 1983, a new strategy based on MDT was introduced and the programme was renamed as National Leprosy Eradication Programme (NLEP). In 1991, the world health assembly passed a resolution to eliminate leprosy as a public health problem by the year 2000.

Elimination was defined as a prevalence rate of less than 1 case per 10000 population although this has been achieved at global level by the end of 2000, extra efforts are still needed to achieve the goal at national level in some countries. India eliminated leprosy in December 2005

Special Efforts for Leprosy Case Detection and Prompt MDT

Modified leprosy elimination campaign (MLEC) was an attempt to intensify case detection and prompt MDT in the entire country during the year 1997–1998, 2000 and 2002–2003. Paramedical workers were involved to identify suspect cases, which were subsequently confirmed by medical officers of health facility. During these operations, (campaigns) 4.63 lakh, 2.13 lakh and 1.65 lakh patients were detected and treated with MDT respectively. This was active search of cases from house to house and voluntary reporting of cases (VRC). Active search was resorted in areas with prevalence rate >5/10,000 and VRC were adopted in areas with PR less than 5.

The elimination strategy is based on detecting and treating all cases with MDT and thereby reducing the disease burden to a very low level. At this level, the transmission of *Mycobacterium leprae* is likely to be reduced to such an extent that the occurrence of new cases in the community would gradually decrease. The key will be to ensure that all new cases continue to have access to MDT services. Leprosy is one of the few infectious diseases to meet the strict criteria for elimination:

- There is only one source of infection, untreated, infected human being.
- Practical and simple diagnostic tools are available: leprosy can be diagnosed on clinical signs alone.
- The availability of an effective intervention to interrupt its transmission: multidrug therapy (MDT).
- Under natural conditions, "incident cases" (new cases in which the disease has recently developed) make up only a small fraction of the prevalence pool. Below a certain level of prevalence, any resurgence of disease is very unlikely.

Goal: Reduce prevalence less than 1 per 10,000 population and incidence to zero in all districts.

Component of National Leprosy Elimination Programme

a Case Detection and Management by Universal access to MDT through primary health care delivery system—as also through secondary and tertiary care facilities.
b Integrating leprosy services (diagnosis, treatment and recording and reporting of cases) with general health services. Leprosy elimination should no longer be vertical health programme. This would enhance the access and coverage of population.
c Renewed emphasis on prevention of disability and medical rehabilitation.
d Monitoring leprosy programme through acceptable indicators (prevalence rate, annual new case detection rate, case holding, treatment completion rate, child cases, female cases, MB and PB cases and deformity rate) through simplified information system (SIS).
e Behaviour Change Communication (BCC) activities at all the levels of health care delivery system to disseminate messages that leprosy is curable and MDT treatment is available free of cost at all health facilities.
f Training and retraining of health workers and medical officers and specialists to make them responsible for elimination of leprosy.

Epidemiological Achievements

The goal of leprosy elimination at national level (i.e. prevalence rate of <1 case per 10,000 population) as set by National Health Policy 2002 had been achieved in December 2005. In year, 1981 the country had prevalence rate of 57.6 cases per 10,000 population which has come down to 0.68 per 10,000 population in 2014–15 March. 34 states/UTs have achieved the status of leprosy elimination. Remaining two states/UTs (Chhattisgarh, Dadra and Nagar Haveli) are having prevalence rate of 2–4 per 10,000 and contribute to 27.8% of country's caseload. Out of 1.26 lakh new cases of leprosy detected in 2013–14 March, the proportion of MB cases was 49%, female (37%), children (9.7%) and grade II disability (3.0%). Global Goal is reduction of grade 2 disability to less than 1 per million by 2020.

National Sample Survey 2011: In 2006, India boastfully declared it had eliminated leprosy achieving the WHO target of <1 case per 10,000 population, but a National Sample Survey has shown an alarming trend—annually 1.4 new cases have been detected per 10,000 population in the year 2010. After the government's eliminations declaration active search for patient was stopped and leprosy programme was integrated with general health services.

Involvement of NGOs in Leprosy Elimination

Non-governmental organizations (NGOs) have been involved in leprosy elimination since time immemorial. Their contribution in reducing the disease burden and disabilities has been remarkable. More than 290 NGOs are working in the field of leprosy throughout the country; of which 54 are getting grant in Aid from Govt. of India. Another 35 NGOs have been given recognition for conducting reconstructive surgery (RCS) and are given reimbursement for undertaking major RCS operations on disabled leprosy patients at the rate of Rs. 2500 per surgery.

International Organizations

The NLEP is being supported by WHO, DANIDA for anti-leprosy (MDT) drugs to the country with assistance from NOVARTIS besides support to leprosy cell in the state and centre. Danish International Development Agency (DANIDA) as a bilateral agency is supporting the leprosy programme in India since 1986.

World Bank supported NLEP project has been in operation since 1993–94. The project has been completed to achieve elimination of leprosy at national level through integration of leprosy services and provision of MDT.

Global Alliance for Elimination of Leprosy and "The Final Push" Strategy[6,7]

At the initiative of WHO, the Global Alliance for Elimination of leprosy (GAEL) was established in November 1999. After eliminating leprosy at global level, the next challenge was to eliminate disease at the national level from every country in the world by the year 2005. It was expected that about 2.5–2.8 million cases will be detected and cured during the period 2000–2005. The key elements of the final push strategy were:

- Integration of leprosy services into general health services to improve access to treatment
- Capacity building to enable general health care staff to diagnose and treat leprosy
- Improve logistics to ensure adequate stocks of MDT at health services
- Change society's perception of leprosy and motivate people to seek timely treatment
- Ensure high cure rates through flexible and patient friendly drug delivery systems
- Simplify monitoring to keep track of progress towards elimination.

Leprosy Elimination Monitoring (LEM)

The objectives of LEM is to assist the decision makers and programme managers to assess the progress towards leprosy elimination by providing additional information on elimination indicators such as prevalence rate, annual new case detection rate, case holding, accessibility of MDT services, integration of leprosy with general health services, quality of MDT blister packs, adequacy of MDT, and information and education level of community on leprosy, etc. Three rounds of LEM have taken place from 2002–2004. According to LEM, the overall prevalence rate has declined to 3.1 and new case detection rate was 4.5 during the year 2004.

Validation of Leprosy Diagnosis by Specialists

During the year 2003, the total number of cases over reported by the health staff were 27.9% (9.4% wrongly diagnosed, 13.5% re-registered and 5% non-existent). These figures of over-reporting are a real concern. When applied to the entire country it represents a large number of cases, as well as MDT supply. During the year 2004, the figure of over-reporting was 33.3% (due to re-registration 18.7%, wrong diagnosis 9.4% and non-existent cases 5.2% respectively).

Focus: Since 2004–05, focus of attention under NLEP has shifted from endemic states to high priority districts and blocks based on prevalence rate (PR). Focused Leprosy Elimination Plan (FLEP-2005–07) and focused Block Leprosy Elimination Awareness Campaign (BLAC) was launched in these areas.[8]

- Out of 657 districts 497 districts have achieved elimination by march 2015.
- A total of 150 districts have been identified as high endemic districts for special action at block level and in 2 urban areas.

Urban leprosy control programme has been implemented since 2005 under which assistance is being provided by Government of India to 524 urban areas having population size of more than one lakh.

Disability prevention and rehabilitation: For prevention of disability of hands and feet patients are given dressing material, supportive medicines and microcellular rubber (MCR) footwear. There are 31 physical and medical rehabilitation institutes, besides 11 district rehabilitation centres in 10 major states. Community based rehabilitation (CBR) is the preferred strategy.

Future Strategy

Although the prevalence has come down at national level yet the number of new cases are being detected every year. The new cases would continue to occur. Now the thrust is to provide quality leprosy services and use *treatment completion rate* as monitoring indicator under NLEP. Besides quality leprosy services through existing health care system enhance disability prevention, and rehabilitation services, reduce stigma, discrimination against persons affected with leprosy apart from capacity building and strengthening monitoring and supervision.

REFERENCES

1 Govt. of NCT of Delhi. Leprosy status in National Territory of Delhi 2003. Leprosy Control Cell, Directorate of Health services. Govt. of NCT of Delhi—F-17, Karkardooma Delhi.

2 GOI. Annual Reports 2011 to 2014, MOH and FW: Govt of India; New Delhi.

3 GOI (2004). Leprosy Elimination Monitoring in India. Survey Report, GOI, WHO and NIHFW, New Delhi.

4 GOI (2004). Leprosy Elimination Monitoring in Delhi. GOI, World Health Organization and NIHFW, New Delhi.

5 GOI (1999). Learning Material on Leprosy for capacity building of Medical Officers, Working in Hospital/ PHC/CHC and Dispensaries. DGHS, MOH and FW (Leprosy Division), Govt. of India and International Federation of Anti-Leprosy Association (ILEP), New Delhi.

6 WHO (2003). The Final Push Strategy to Eliminate Leprosy as a Public Health Problem—Questions and Answers. Second Edition, World Health Organization (WHO), Geneva.

7 WHO. Guide to eliminate leprosy as a public health problem. Leprosy elimination group of World Health Organization (WHO), Geneva.

8 GOI (2013). National leprosy Eradication Programme. Triuning manual for medical officer. Central lapray Division, DGHS, MOH and FW. Nirman Bhawan New Delhi.

12

VECTOR-BORNE DISEASES

World health day 2014 "small bite big threat": Major vector-borne diseases are being discussed here, other vector-borne diseases have been discussed in Chapter 11.

NATIONAL VECTOR-BORNE DISEASE CONTROL PROGRAMME (NVBDCP)-2003

The National Vector-Borne Disease Control Programme is comprehensive umbrella programme for prevention and control of vector-borne diseases namely—malaria, filaria, kala-azar, Japanese encephalitis, dengue fever and chikungunya which is now covered under the overall umbrella of NRHM. The NVBDCP was launched in 2003–04. The programme is being implemented by the states through existing health care infrastructure. The general strategy for prevention and control of vector-borne diseases under NVBDCP is described below:

1 **Disease management:** Including early case detection with active, passive and sentinel surveillance and complete effective treatment, and strengthening of referral services.

2 **Epidemic preparedness** and rapid response.

3 **Integrated vector management** (for transmission and risk reduction) by: Indoor residual spray (IRS) in selected high-risk areas, use of insecticide treated bednets (ITN), and Long lasting Insecticidal Nets (LLINs) use of larvivorous fish, anti-larval measures in urban areas including bio-larvicides, and source reduction by minor environmental engineering methods.

4 **Surveillance:** Surveillance of NVBDCP is an important epidemiological tool to control the spread of NVBD and predict epidemic, to investigate epidemic and to ensure rapid response.

5 **Entomological surveillance:** Under NVBDCP entomological surveillance in the programme is being carried out by entomological zones and entomological set up at regional offices. The parameters being collected are—vector density, and susceptibility status (adults test and larval test).

6 **Supportive interventions** including behaviour change communication, (BCC), public–private partnership and Intersectoral convergence, human resource development through capacity building, operational research including studies on drug resistance and insecticide susceptibility, monitoring and evaluation through periodic review/field visits and improving management information system (MIS) besides involvement of Panchayati Raj Institutions. Using standard treatment Protocols for treating vector-borne diseases at various levels is another important component.

7 **Vaccination only against JE**

8 **Annual Mass drugs administration (only against Lymphatic Filariasis).**

MALARIA

Malaria has been recognized as significant public health problem in India. League of Nations in 1930 estimated that one-third of global population suffered due to malaria and in 2015—over 50% of global population was exposed to the risk of malaria. Recent estimates indicate that 214 million cases and 0.438 million deaths occur per annum due to malaria worldwide, 88% of which occur per annum in tropical Africa (World Malaria Report, 2015). Malaria parasite was discovered in 1880 by Laveran a French army surgeon. Later in 1898, working in India Sir Ronald Ross reported that disease was transmitted through mosquitoes.

Malaria is an acute infectious disease caused in humans by 4 species of Protozoa, genus *Plasmodium* and transmitted by various species of mosquito genus *Anopheles*. The disease is characterized by a cyclical course with periods of acute febrile attacks and paroxysm free intervals.

Species of Human Malaria

There are 4 species of human malaria namely—*Plasmodium vivax*, *P. falciparum*, *P. malariae* and *P. ovale*, which is rare. The fourth species namely *P. ovale* has been recently recorded in some tribal areas of Odisha.

- The *Plasmodium vivax* is the most common and considered to be widespread. Relapses are common in *P. vivax* (due to persistence of exo-erythrocytic phase in liver) and hence relapsing malaria is feature of *P. vivax* usually. Relapse rate in vivax malaria in India is around 30%. As a rule, *P. vivax* infection and *P. ovale* have similarities and cause relapses.
- Of late, *P. falciparum* has taken over *P. vivax,* almost 50% of malaria in India is now *P. falciparum*. There are no relapses with *P. falciparum*, but it is killer malaria. Deaths in malaria are due to *P. falciparum*. *P. falciparum* in showing resistance to chloroquine, which is widespread in North Eastern States of India, Odisha, Karnataka and Gujarat.

Magnitude of Problem

Recent estimates indicate that all over the world there are between 350 and 500 million cases of malaria per year and over 1.5–2.7 million deaths due to malaria worldwide. The vast majority of this disease burden, over 90% falls on Sub-Saharan Africa where there are one million deaths per year. Children under-five are the worst affected.[1]

Past *Scenario of Malaria in India*

Malaria was a major scourge in India contributing 75 million cases and about 0.8 million deaths annually, prior to the launching of national malaria control programme (NMCP) in 1953. The objective of NMCP was to reduce the incidence of malaria to such a level that it ceased to be a public health problem. The major strategy adopted for NMCP was indoor residual spraying (IRS) with DDT. Encouraged by the results and achievements of NMCP the Government of India launched national malaria eradication programme (NMEP) in 1958. The objective was to root out malaria parasite from India. The major strategy was surveillance along with indoor residual spray (IRS). The NMEP was initially a great success with malaria incidence dropping to 0.1 million cases and no deaths due to malaria reported in 1965. The resurgence of malaria in the country resulted in escalation of incidence to 6.4 million cases in 1976. The resurgence was mainly due to various operational, administrative and technical reasons, including emergence of **drug resistance** in the parasite and **insecticide resistance** in the **vector.** In 1977, the *Modified Plan of Operation* (MPO) was implemented with immediate objective of preventing deaths due to malaria and reducing morbidity due to malaria. The national programme was integrated with primary health care delivery system. Under the MPO selective use of IRS was recommended. IRS was used in areas with annual parasite incidence (API) >2 in addition to early diagnosis and prompt treatment. The malaria incidence declined to 1.66 million in 1987. Due to paucity of resources in many states, however, allowed spray operations in areas with API >5 only. By 1996 there was another upsurge with 3.03 million cases and 2803 deaths and in many areas outbreaks/epidemics of malaria were reported.[2,3]

Since the focus shifted from eradication to control, the programme was renamed as National anti-malaria programme (NAMP) during the year 1999. In view of wide-spread outbreaks/epidemics of other vector-borne diseases like dengue, chikungunya, Japanese encephalitis and kala-azar in India, it become necessary to launch an integrated programme of vector-borne diseases to tackle these emerging problems (outbreaks and epidemics). Accordingly, NAMP was repositioned and modified and renamed as National vector-borne disease control programme (NVBDCP) in 2003. The NVBDCP became an integral part of the National Rural Health Mission in 2005 for prevention and control of malaria, filariasis, kala-azar, Japanese encephalitis, dengue and chikungunya.

Malaria Epidemics

Malaria outbreaks occur in various parts of the country. Malaria in India is mostly unstable and outbreaks are caused mostly by infection due to *P. falciparum*. The reasons for these outbreaks have been identified as inadequate surveillance and inadequate antilarval measures in urban areas. Epidemics in various parts of the country have been reported from 1994 to 2006 with large number of cases and many deaths in the state of Rajasthan, Gujarat, Goa, West Bengal, Andhra Pradesh, Assam, Bihar, Uttar Pradesh, Madhya Pradesh, Karnataka, Haryana and Manipur. To meet the challenge of malaria epidemics in the country one of the key strategy for prevention and control of malaria under the strategic action plan is "Epidemic preparedness and early response" by Rapid Response Teams (RRTs).

Malaria Paradigms/Ecotypes

There is considerable heterogeneity in malaria transmission characteristics between and within the states of the country and therefore many ecotypes and paradigms of malaria have been recognized during 1994. The expert committee classified the problem areas under the following paradigms.[4]

1. Hard Core Areas (Tribal Areas)

These areas comprise seven North Eastern states, Odisha, Jharkhand, Chhattisgarh and foci in other states:

- These areas have predominantly tribal population and difficult terrains and are inaccessible during rains and floods.
- They have predominant falciparum malaria.
- These areas have *stable malaria* with *high endemicity* and transmission period extending up to 9 months or more.
- These areas report bulk of deaths due to malaria in the country.
- The main recommended measures in these areas are IRS/ITNs/LLINs.

12

2. Epidemic Prone Areas

These are prone to malaria epidemics, North Western plains, semi-arid climatic zone with annual rainfall of 100 mm and Indo-Gangetic plains are identified as major epidemic prone areas (Punjab, Haryana, Western UP and Rajasthan). These areas have *unstable malaria*.

The main measures against malaria are anti-larval measures in some areas, one round of IRS in selected villages, space spray and IRS in case of outbreaks.

3. Project Malaria

The development projects attract a large number of labour population from endemic areas bringing different strains of malaria parasite as well as non immune population groups. These pockets contribute large proportion of malaria cases.

4. Urban Malaria

It is a distinct paradigm which contributes 10% of total malaria. Larvicides are provided by Central Government under urban malaria scheme, salary of staff is borne by the State Government. The main measures against malaria in this paradigm are Chemical and biological larviciding, environmental measures, ITNs/LLINs, house screening, other personal protection measures and focal spray of IRS in areas where this is possible (mainly single storey buildings).

5. Malaria in Organized Sector

In organized sector/army/road construction/tea gardens. They require IRS, ITNs/LLINs, in some situations personal protection and chemoprophylaxis.

6. Border Malaria

Border malaria has been recognized as a distinct epidemiological paradigm because of several reasons such as transmigration, illegal movements across the borders, inadequate infrastructure difficult terrain and inadequate communication and antimalarial activities. As a result, border malaria is being now monitored separately. Collaborative meetings with neighbouring countries are held periodically to review border malaria continuously. Similarly, interstate border malaria problem is reviewed regularly.

- **Stable malaria:** Areas showing consistently high incidence of malaria. Transmission occurs throughout the year, falciparum malaria dominates, peak is in November and December, areas are tribals, endemicity is high and predominant vectors are *A. culicifacies* and *An. fluviatilis*.
- **Unstable malaria:** Endemicity is low; transmission is seasonal, *P. vivax* malaria dominates, fluctuation in incidence are marked, these areas are epidemic prone areas and main vector is *A. culicifacies*.

Present Epidemiological Situation of Malaria

Malaria is one of the major public health problem in India. Annual parasite rate (API), which was 11.2 in 1976 has come down to 0.90 in 2015 but some states continue to have API of 5–10 and even more than 10. Around 1.5 to 2 million laboratory confirmed cases are being reported in the country per annum. Out of total malaria cases over 50% are *P. falciparum* malaria. Officials reporting of cases and deaths due to malaria is poor and actual numbers are estimated at 10–20 times of the reported cases and deaths, due to weakness of surveillance system and limitation in laboratory facilities. The WHO has estimated that malaria was responsible for 10.6 million cases and 15,000 deaths in India in 2006. Geographical distribution of malaria in the country is quite uneven (Fig. 12.11). Over 66% of total malaria case load was contributed by Odisha, Jharkhand, Chhattisgarh, MP, and rest of the states contributed 34% of cases during 2014.

The epidemiological situation of malaria from 1976 to 2015: Reported malaria incidence declined from 6.47 million cases to about one million cases per year (Tables 12.15 and 12.16).[5]

Increase in Falciparum Malaria

- From 1995 onwards, the incidence of killer malaria—falciparum malaria has risen and over 53% of malaria in the country is falciparum malaria (Table 12.16).
- The worst affected states due to falciparum malaria are Odisha, Chhattisgarh, Jharkhand, Assam, MP, Meghalaya, West Bengal and Tripura.
- Growing incidence of insecticide resistance in the vectors.
- Problem of *drug resistance in parasites* particularly falciparum malaria *resistance to chloroquine*. Problem of drug resistant malaria poses significant challenge and it is widespread.
- High incidence of malaria in tribal population—overall 30% malaria cases and over 50% *P. falciparum* cases are in tribal areas.
- In seven North Eastern states, we have higher proportion of *P. falciparum* cases and drug resistant malaria.
- In some areas, anaemia due to malaria is rampant.

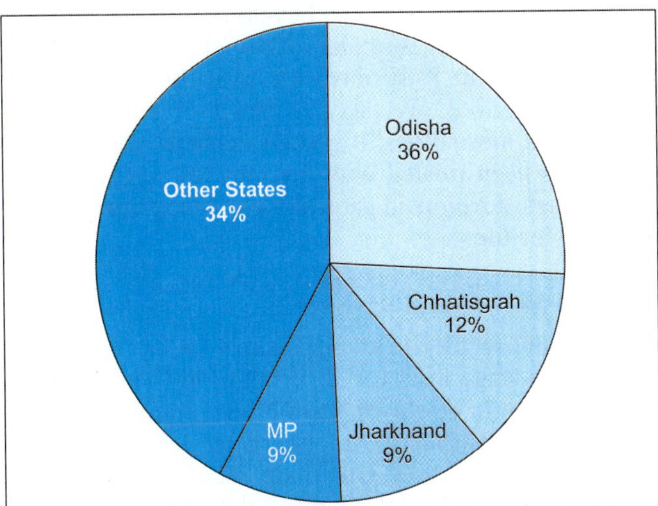

Fig. 12.11: Distribution of reported malaria in India–2014

Table 12.15: Epidemiological situation of malaria in India

Year	Total malaria cases (in million)	API	P. falciparum cases (in million)	Reported deaths due to malaria
1976	6.47	11.24	0.75	59
1984	2.18	3.08	0.66	247
1985	1.86	2.57	0.55	213
1986	1.79	2.43	0.64	323
1987	1.66	2.21	0.62	188
1988	1.85	2.42	0.69	209
1989	2.05	2.66	0.76	268
1990	2.02	2.57	0.75	353
1992	2.13	2.58	0.88	422
1993	2.21	2.65	0.85	354
1994	2.51	2.19	0.99	1122
1995	2.93	3.29	1.14	1151
1996	3.04	3.48	1.18	1010
1997	2.66	3.01	1.04	879
1998	2.22	2.44	1.03	664
1999	2.28	2.41	1.14	1048
2000	2.03	2.09	1.05	932
2001	2.09	2.12	1.01	1005
2002	1.84	1.82	0.90	973
2003	1.87	1.82	0.86	1006
2004	1.92	1.84	0.89	949
2005	1.82	1.68	0.81	963
2006	1.79	1.66	0.84	1707
2007	1.50	1.39	0.74	1311
2008	1.53	1.36	0.78	1055
2009	1.56	1.36	0.84	1144
2010	1.60	1.37	0.83	1018
2011	1.31	1.10	0.67	754
2012	1.01	0.88	0.53	519
2013	0.88	0.72	0.46	359
2014	1.10	0.89	0.72	562
2015 (P)	1.13	0.9	0.75	287

Transmission

From man to man, the malaria is transmitted by mosquitoes. *Anopheles* are most important vectors for malaria transmission in India. Out of 9 species of Anopheles 6 are primary vectors of malaria in India.[6]

An. culicifacies: Primary rural vector all over the country except North East. It is monsoon associated vector. This vector is responsible for 60–70% of transmission of malaria.

An. stephensi: Primary urban vector in large parts of the country including industrial areas.

An. fluviatilis: Primary rural vector in hilly and forest areas of the country and is responsible for 15% new cases of malaria.

An. minimus: Primary vector in North Eastern region and West Bengal.

Table 12.16: Proportion of *P. falciparum* cases in India, 1980–2015

Year	Proportion (%) of Pf cases
1980	20.3
1985	29.2
1990	37.3
1995	38.84
1998	46.35
1999	49.96
2000	51.54
2001	48.20
2002	48.74
2003	45.85
2004	46.47
2005	44.32
2006	47.08
2007	49.11
2008	50.81
2009	53.72
2010	52.12
2011	51.0
2012	50.0
2013	53.0
2014	65.5
2015	67.1

Source: NVBDCP

An. dirus: Primary vector in regions of evergreen forests in North East.

An. sundaicus (A. epiroticus): Primary vector in Andaman and Nicobar islands and coastal areas, breeds in brackish and salty water.

An. philippinensis: Secondary vector in rice field ecosystem of North East Region.

An. annularis: Secondary vector in rice field ecosystem in Uttar Pradesh and coastal areas of Odisha.

An. varuna: Secondary vector in Eastern Ghats (Andhra Pradesh) Bihar and Kerala.

Transmission Dynamics in Malaria

Transmission depends on agent, host, vector and environmental factors, apart from availability of health services.

Host factors include—innate resistance to malaria, duffy antigen, blood groups, haemoglobinopathies, nutritional status, and asymptomatic malaria cases. Habits of host like clothing, sleeping habits, use of bed nets, occupation, animal keeping, migration of population for construction or project work, and for search of job in industrial areas.

Factors related to vectors are vector density, flight range, feeding habits, resting habits, biting time and sensitivity to insecticides, besides entomological inocculation rate (EIR), i.e. the average number of infectious bites by malaria infested mosquitoes delivered to an individual human resident in that area in a period of one year.

Due to difficulties in measuring EIR parasite rate in young children is used as proxy for transmission intensity.

Environmental factors in malaria include humidity, rainfall, altitude, and geographic contours.

Agent factors include parasite load, and sensitivity to drugs.

Factors of services—availability and surveillance operation also determine the transmission dynamics.

After feeding of human blood, the mosquitoes tend to rest on surface of wall and if the walls and ceilings are sprayed with residual insecticides, the mosquitoes will die within few hours to few days depending upon the duration of contact with the insecticide. This will only happen if mosquito is endophilic and endophagic (i.e. indoor biting and indoor resting habits). If mosquito vectors of malaria are exophilic and/or exophagic (outdoor biting and outdoor resting) the vector will survive. Aquatic stages of mosquito (eggs, larvae and pupae) are most vulnerable to chemicals like Paris green, insecticides and oils which are frequently used as antilarval measures in urban setting to control the mosquitoes population. Breeding places should be minimized or eliminated (source elimination). The source elimination is real prevention but it is most difficult to achieve.

Incubation Period

It is the time between the infective bite and the appearance of clinical symptoms. In *P. falciparum*, it is 12 days range being 9–14 days. In *P. vivax* it is 15 days range being 12–17 days and in *P. malariae*, it is 28 days range being 18–40 days.

Cycle in Mosquito

The development of parasite involves two hosts. The cycle in mosquito (invertebrate) and cycle in man (vertebrate). Cycle in mosquitoes is sexual cycle and it gets completed on an average in 8–10 days (we call this as extrinsic incubation period). We take advantage of this period as the infected mosquitoes, if come in contact with surface which has been treated with insecticides, will be killed Sporozoites develop in mosquitoes. Mosquito remains infective for life.

Cycle in Man (Asexual Cycle)

Asexual phase of life cycle occurs in humans. Pre-erythrocytic stage lasts for 10–15 days in liver followed by erythrocytic cycle of 48–72 hours and man gets malaria after 12–15 days or longer after getting infective bite from mosquitoes (intrinsic incubation period). Gametocytes develop in red blood cells. Malaria parasite destroys Red Blood Cells.

Incubation Interval

Incubation interval is defined as the period between infectivity of one person (case) to the infectivity of another person to whom the former case has transmitted the infection.

Extrinsic plus intrinsic incubation period is called incubation interval. Incubation interval in case of *P. vivax* is 21 days while for *P. falciparum* it is 35 days. Thus, surveillance cycle of fortnightly with less than one incubation interval is justified to capture the secondary cases before the commencement of next cycle.[7]

Proportion of falciparum malaria cases out of total reported cases has gradually increased from about 20% in 1980 to over 67% in 2015 (Table 12.16). This increase over the years is due to several factors: changing ecosystems; creating foci of enhanced malaria transmission, shifting of falciparum foci, and introduction of developmental projects, and resistance to chloroquin.

NATIONAL MALARIA CONTROL PROGRAMME

Govt. of India launched NMCP in the year 1953. The objectives of the programme were:

- To reduce the incidence of malaria to a level at which it would cease to be a major public health problem.
- To hold down malaria transmission at low level indefinitely by each state.

Principal Activities

Residual insecticidal spray of human dwellings and cattle sheds with DDT, plus limited treatment of malaria.

Malaria control teams of the state malaria organization were to carry out surveys and monitor the malaria incidence in control area through 193 malaria control units.

No organized chemotherapeutic measures were taken up under NMCP but wherever the patient reported to a medical facility, drug was made available for treatment of malaria.

Encouraged by success of the programme (reduction of API by 62% and child parasite rate by 73%), the nation evolved *National Malaria Eradication Programme* (NMEP) in 1958.

Goal of Eradication

"The ending of transmission of malaria and elimination of reservoir of infective cases in a campaign limited in time and carried to such a degree of perfection that when it comes to an end there is no resumption of transmission."

Phases of NMEP

NMEP had four phases:

1. Preparatory
2. Attack
3. Consolidation as part of vertical programme of malaria eradication
4. Maintenance phase was to be taken by general health services of the state.

Preparatory Phase

Activities comprised of mapping up of problem by survey, working out requirement of men, money and material, recruitment of staff, training and preparation of manuals.

Attack Phase

During this phase, it was envisaged total coverage both geographically in terms of the population with residual insecticides or antilarval operations where technically indicated for cessation of malaria transmission.

Under the eradication campaign, the spraying operation was based on total coverage basis to include every roofed structure for a period varying from 3 to 5 years in most parts, however in India, because of epidemiological necessity it went on till 1967.

Focal Spray

- Focal spray activities were limited around a "positive case" of malaria spraying 50 houses around the "positive case" during transmission season "with a view to interrupt the transmission and spread of malaria".
- Case detection through passive surveillance, presumptive and radical treatment for liquidation of malaria reservoir were introduced in this phase.
- Introduction of surveillance mechanism

Consolidation Phase

Case detection through surveillance (active and passive) system as also presumptive and radical treatment was established and continued in this phase. The number of slides collected at least equivalent to 1% of the population per month during the months of malaria transmission be ensured. The other activity in consolidation phase was field epidemiological investigation of malaria cases carried out to discover and deal with source of infection.

Criteria for entry of units to consolidation phase: "The incidence of malaria of 0.5 per 1000 population per year where active and passive cases detection were effective.

Under Indian programme conditions, this was laid down as "0.1 case per 1000 population per annum—API (annual parasite incidence)".

Maintenance Phase

Maintenance phase would last as long as malaria exists in the world. State health services would maintain vigilance activities to prevent entry of malaria case and to carry out epidemiological investigations.

Results

NMEP showed spectacular results and by 1965 annual malaria incidence came down from 75 million cases to an all time low of 0.1 million cases and no death reported.

Collateral Benefits

As a result of widespread insecticides spray, plague disappeared and kala-azar was controlled. However, the success lasted for short period. From1968 onwards, there were setbacks and resurgence of malaria. By 1976, highest ever incidence of 6.47 million cases was recorded in India.

In 1977, attempts at malaria eradication were given up and phasing was done away. A modified plan of operation (MPO) was adopted under revised policy in view of the epidemiological situation of malaria (1976).

MODIFIED PLAN OF OPERATION (MPO)-1977

Objectives

- Prevention of deaths due to malaria
- Reduction of morbidity due to malaria
- Maintenance of industrial and green revolution due to freedom from malaria as well as retention of achievements gained so far.
- Establishment of drug distribution centres (DDCs) and fever treatment depots (FTDs) and initiation of operational research and training.

Activities

The programme covered all states and union territories. The predominant activities were:

1. Selective insecticidal spray with appropriate insecticide during transmission period in rural areas having API of two or above.
2. Surveillance by fortnightly blood smear collection by home visits from fever cases, their examination and treatment of fever/malaria cases with antimalarial drugs.
3. In urban areas: Recurrent antilarval operations.
4. Attempts were made to intensify these activities in rural areas in identified districts through Swedish International Development Authority (SIDA) by providing additional inputs under *P. falciparum* control programme.
5. Decentralization of laboratory services to the PHC level.
6. Establishment of DDCs/FTDs.

Fever Treatment Depots (FTDs)

Fever treatment depots were established under (MPO) Modified plan of operation (1977) to enhance the surveillance programme since multipurpose health workers had to cover large population. Since coverage of large population was beyond their reach and the fortnightly home visits were missed, an alternate strategy was evolved. Now ASHAs have been given the responsibility of FTDs in difficult, remote/inaccessible and tribal areas.

STRATEGIC ACTION PLAN FOR MALARIA CONTROL IN INDIA (2007-12)

The Focus in this Phase was to Effectively Control Malaria by Different Strategies

The national strategy on prevention and control of malaria has lately undergone a *paradigm shift* with the introduction of rapid diagnostic tests (RDTs) which has enabled early diagnosis of falciparum malaria cases and complete treatment by trained health workers and volunteers in the most remote areas of the country. This has resulted in availability of effective treatment in all parts of the country, thereby facilitating prevention of severe malaria and also breaking the transmission. **Emergence** of **chloroquine resistance** in falciparum malaria has led to rolling out of Artemisinin based combination therapy (ACT) as the first line of treatment of *P. falciparum* cases. Drug policy on malaria has been revised in 2013. Indoor residual spray (IRS) has been the mainstay of vector control in the programme, along with introduction of use of long-lasting insecticidal nets (LLINs) into the programmes. Modern concept of monitoring and evaluation have now been incorporated into the programme which takes into account of newer interventions like RDT, ACT and LLINs.

Overall Objectives of Programme

- Prevention of deaths due to malaria.
- Prevention of morbidity due to malaria.
- Maintenance of ongoing socioeconomic development.

Specific Objectives

- To achieve API of less than 1 in the 12th five-year plan.
- At least 50% reduction in mortality due to malaria.
- To halt and begin to reverse the incidence of malaria by 2015 as per millennium development goals.

STRATEGIC PLAN FOR MALARIA CONTROL IN INDIA 2012–17

It means scaling up malaria control interventions with a focus on high burden areas and categorized strategic interventions for achieving **pre-elimination status.**

National Goals

- Screening all fever cases suspected for malaria (60% through quality microscopy and 40% by RDT).
- Treating all P. falciparum cases with full course of effective ACT and primaquine and all P. vivax cases with 3 days chloroquine and 14 days primaquine.
- Equipping all health instituations (down to PHC level) microscopy facility and RDT for emergency use and

injectable artemisinin derivatives, especially in high-risk areas.

- Strengthening all district and sub-district hospitals as per IPHS with facilities for management of severe malaria cases in malaria endemic areas.
- At least 80% of those suffering from malaria get correct, affordable and appropriate treatment within 24 hours of reporting to the health system, by the year 2017.
- At least 80%of those at high-risk of malaria get protected by effective preventive measures such as ITNs/LLINs or IRS by 2017.
- At least 10% of the population in high-risk areas is examined under surveillance system annually (ABER >10%).

Impact Indicators

- To bring down annual incidence of malaria to less than 1 case per 1000 population at national level by 2017.
- At least 50% reduction in mortality due to malaria by the year 2017, taking 2010 as baseline

Target: To achieve by the end of 2017

- API < 1 per 1000 population

Strategic Plan (Fig. 12.12)

From control of malaria to 'pre-elimination stage'. Considering the feasibility of malaria eliminatin defined as **no indigenous transmission**, it is proposed to change to focus of strategies based on endemicity level. This will facilitate in achieving the long-term goal of elimination. This necessitates the stratification of states based on incidence as to decide and execute area specific interventions which would lead to reduction of incidence in high endemic areas and sustain reduction in low endemic areas to pave the way for the country to enter into the "pre-elimination stage". To reach "pre-elimination stage" entire country would require adequate inputs in terms of technical logistic and financial support. Accordingly, the states have been stratified as under in Table 12.17.

Table 12.17: Definition of 3 categories of states

No	Category	Definition
1	Category 1	States with API less than one, and all the districts in the state are with API less than one
2	Category 2	State with API less than one and one or more districts reporting API more than one
3	Category 3	States with API more than one

Following broad strategies of different categories have been approved by the technical advisory committee (TAC) for the programme as shown in Table 12.18.

Table 12.18: Malaria control strategies in the three categories of states

Category	Strategies
1	• Case based quality surveillance with foci for active, passive and sentinel surveillance • Screening of migrants in these areas • Integrated vector management (IVM) by involvement of village health and sanitation committees, other PRIs and MNREGA schemes • Supportive interventions including IEC and BCC activities
2	• Epidemiological surveillance and disease management (3Ts—Test, Treat and Track) • Screening of migrants in these areas • Integrated vector management (IVM) by source reduction through minor engineering, environmental management and focal spray • Supportive interventions including IEC and BCC activities with the involvement of private health care providers, community involvement and NGOs
3	• Epidemiological surveillance and disease management: by EDCT • Management of severe malaria cases by strengthening of district and sub-district hospitals and quality referral services • Integrated vector management (IVM) by IRS and LLIN distribution so as to saturate the entire high risk population • Supportive interventions.

For Areas Having Perennial Transmission (More than 5 Months in a Year)

- Two rounds of IRS with DDT/SP or 3 rounds with Malathion, depending on vector susceptibility and priority distribution of LLINs as per the guidelines.

For Areas Having Seasonal Transmission (Less than 5 Months in a Year)

- One round of IRS with DDT before start of transmission
- Focal spray whenever and wherever needed
- Priority distribution of LLINs as per guidelines.

NATIONAL FRAMEWORK FOR MALARIA ELIMINATION IN INDIA 2016–2030

The national framework for malaria elimination in India 2016–30 was launched in February 2016.

Vision

Eliminate malaria nationally and contribute to improved health, quality of life and alleviation of poverty.

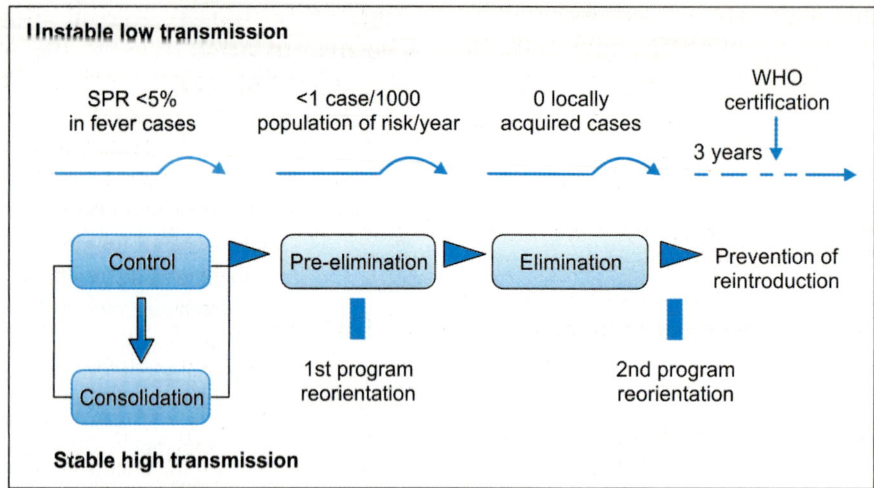

Fig. 12.12: Progress towards malaria elimination

Goals

In line with the WHO global technical strategy for malaria 2016–2030 (GTS) and the Asia Pacific leaders Malaria Alliance Malaria Elimination Roadmap, (APLMA) the goals of the national Framework for malaria Elimination in India 2016–2030 are:

- Eliminate malaria (zero indigenous cases) throughout the entire country by 2030; and
- Maintain malaria—free status in areas where malaria transmission has been interrupted and prevent re-introduction of malaria.

Objectives

The framework has four objectives:

- Eliminate malaria from all 26 low (Category 1) and moderate (Category 2) transmission states/union territories (UTs) by 2022.
- Reduce the incidence of malaria to less than 1 case per 1000 population per year in all states and UTs and their districts by 2024.
- Interrupt indigenous transmission of malaria throughout the entire country, including all high transmission states and union territories (UTs) Category 3) by 2027; and
- Prevent the re-establishment of local transmission of malaria in areas where it has been eliminated and maintain national malaria-free status by 2030 and beyond.

STRATEGIC APPROACHES

1. Programme Phasing

Programme phasing is necessary, because certain parts of the country belong to different phases and malaria transmission must be lowered before it is possible and rational to investigate each case. This prioritization does not mean that efforts to eliminate malaria in low endemic areas (Category 1) will be put on hold, only that such efforts will go on simultaneously with efforts to reduce malaria transmission in high endemic areas (Category 3).

As detailed in Table 12.19 below states/UTs will be subdivided into four categories with annual parasite incidence (API) as primary criteria and other malaria indicators, such as the annual blood examination rate (ABER) and slide positivity rate (SPR) as secondary criteria. Subsequently, category specific milestones and targets will be set and specific strategies will be implemented.

The intensified control phase will aim to bring malaria incidence down in all high-transmission districts (Category 3) to an API of less than 1 case per 1000 population at risk, when elimination can be considered.

In areas that are in the per-elimination phase (Category 2), particular attention will be paid to **revision of the surveillance system** and development of an elimination programme that must be completed before entering into the elimination phase.

Setting up a case—and foci-based surveillance with population-based reporting from all public health facilities

Table 12.19: Classification of states/UTs based on API as primary criteria

S. No	*Categories of states/UTS*	*Definition*
1.	**Category 0:** Prevention of re-establishment phase	States/UTs with zero indigenous case of malaria (currently, no State/UT)
2.	**Category 1:** Elimination phase	States/UTs (15) including their districts reporting an API of less than 1 case per 1000 population at risk.
3.	**Category 2:** Pre-elimination phase	States/UTs (11) with an API of less than 1 case per 1000 population at risk, but some of their districts are reporting an API of 1/1000 or above
4.	**Category 3:** Intensified control phase	States/UTs (10) with an API of 1 case per 1000 population at risk or above

and full participation of the private sector assuming well developed health **service, mandatory reporting of/ notifying each case** of malaria, and strong conviction that nothing is being missed is crucial and a core function in the elimination phase (Category 1) states and UTs with an API of less than 1 case per 1000 population at risk in all districts.

Finally, all states/UTs which have achieved elimination through interruption of indigenous transmission of malaria will qualify of the prevention of re-establishment phase (Category 0), with the main focus on sustaining malaria elimination status and preventing onward transmission.

2. District as the Unit of Planning and Implementation

Apart from the category to which they belong, each state/ UT will be advised to further classify their districts so that even if a given state/UT is not yet in the elimination phase, but has some districts with an API of less than 1 case per 1000 population at risk, those district(s) may be considered eligible for initiating elimination phase activities provided they meet the secondary criteria. In addition, states/ UTs may also sub-classify districts into community health centres into sub-centres, and sub-centres in to villages for localized planning and implementation based on API.

3. Focus on High Transmission Areas

In the year 2014, five out of 36 states/UTs contributed to more than 70% of the total malaria cases in the country. These were Odisha (36%), Chhattisgarh (12%), Jharkhand (9%), Madhya Pradesh (9%) and Maharashtra (5%). Historically, the above mentioned states and north-eastern states such as Meghalaya, Mizoram, Nagaland, which have wide coverage of forest, hilly, tribal and **conflict-affected areas**, contributed the majority of malaria in the country.

4. Special Strategy for *P. vivax* Elimination

As per the World Malaria Report 2015, more than 80% of the global *P. vivax* burden is contributed by 3 countries including India. *P. vivax* malaria is a serious challenge to malaria elimination efforts within the country due to a multitude of reasons. The parasite can survive in cooler climates, is less responsive to conventional methods of vector control, is more difficult to detect using conventional diagnostic tools, treatment of liver stage parasites requires a 14 day course of primaquine which can produce some serious side effects. Moreover, as significant proportion of *P. vivax* cases are being reported from urban areas. Special measures such as good quality microscopy to detect all *P. vivax* infections, operational research to estimate prevalence of G6PD deficiency in the population, appropriate vector control measures and ensuring good compliance to 14-day radical treatment with primaquine in affected individuals will be undertaken to address this challenge.

Strategies

The overall objectives of the malaria elimination programme are rapid reduction of transmission in areas with high malaria incidence; interruption of malaria transmission in low transmission areas; and prevention of re-establishment of malaria in areas where transmission has been interrupted.

The broad strategies of the malaria elimination framework are:

A Early diagnosis by surveillance and radical treatment
- Case-based surveillance and rapid response

B Integrated vector management (IVM)
- Indoor residual spary (IRS)
- Long-lasting insecticidal nets (LLINs)/insecticide treated bed nets (ITNs)
- Larval source management (LSM)

C Epidemic preparedness and early response

D Advocacy, coordination and partnerships

E Behaviour change communication and community mobilization

F Monitoring and evaluation

G Programme planning and management.

A. Epidemiological Surveillance and Case Management in Malaria

Surveillance is an important epidemiological tool in malaria. It means early case detection of malaria and complete treatment (EDCT). Surveillance precisely means "information for action" for effective control and prevention. Steps in malaria surveillance includes collection of data on fever and malaria, analysis, interpretation and dissemination of relevant information for action at various levels.

Malaria surveillance in India in the past was traditionally a system based mainly on slide results, which has been refined over many years. It relied on surveillance of fever cases in community by means of active fortnightly case detection conducted by the MPHW (M). Active case detection implies that the MPHW (M) makes house to house visits and covers all households in a fortnight in subcentre area or 5000 population. He looks for occurrence of fever cases between the current and previous visit. Blood smears of all fever cases were collected and sent to laboratory for examination along with administration of presumptive treatment with chloroquine. A target of Annual Blood Examination Rate (ABER) of 10% of population was fixed based on annual fever incidence in the population/ community. Active case detection by MPHW (M) formed the backbone of surveillance. With over a half century of programme implementation it has been realized that shortages of MPHW (M) (over 50–60% vacancies) resulted in poor surveillance in terms of coverage and quality. Poor surveillance resulted in inability of the system to generate "timely information on fever alerts for action" and consequently outbreaks/epidemics of malaria were reported.[6]

Malaria surveillance is based on active case detection (ACD) and passive case detection (PCD)

Active Case Detection

- **(ACD)** is carried out by trained health workers (multi-purpose health workers male) through fortnightly house to house visits and testing people with current or recent fever and chills in the past 14 days with bivalent RDTs. If the RDT result is positive, appropriate treatment is initiated and the blood slide/smears are discarded, and if RDT is negative, the blood slide is forwarded to laboratory for examination. Results of microscopy must be made available and communicated within 24 hours.
- **Passive case detection (PCD)** is carried out among fever cases who report themselves to a health facility or health volunteers for treatment of fever at PHC, subcentre and ASHA/AWW or health volunteer, with bivalent RDTs. Thick and thin blood smears are also prepared.

Surveillance in Category 3 (Intensified Control Phase)

- **ACD** is carried out by trained health workers (MPHWs) with bivalent antigen detecting RDTs through fortnightly house to house visits
- **PCD** is carried out by trained health care volunteer by ASHA/USHA/CHV or at subcentre/PHC/CHC with bivalent antigen detecting RDTs.
- **PCD** at PHCs CHCs/hospitals/medical colleges is done by microscopy, however bivalent antigen detection RDTs are used in emergent situations, odd hours, non availability of lab technician or until microscopy centre is made functional
- **PCD** in health providers in private and other sectors is done through microscopy (where results can be made available within 24 hours) or by bivalent antigen detecting RDTs.
- If a fever case is found to be positive for malaria treatment is initiated within 24 hours of detection and complete treatment is ensured.
- Sentinel surveillance and referral system should be strengtheried to find out reasons for development of severe malaria, improve case management and prevent deaths due to malaria.

Surveillance should sustain monthly blood examination rate (MBER) of minimum 1.5% during transmission months.

Surveillance in Category 2 (Pre-elimination Phase)

- Same as for category 3 given above. In addition, more focused attention in project areas and construction sites and among migrant populations and slum populations.
- The monthly blood examination rate (MBER) should be sustained at minimum of 1% during transmission months.

Surveillance in Category 1 (Elimination Phase)

Malaria should be made notifiable

- ACD is carried out by trained health care workers (MPHWs) by house to house fortnightly visits and collecting smears for microscopy. However in areas where microscopy results can not be available, bivalent antigen based RDTs are used and RDT negative patient strongly suspected of malaria are cross checked by microscopy.
- PCD is carried out by trained health care volunteers like ASHAs/AWWs or at subcentre, PHCs and CHCs, including private and other sectors by blood smear collection for microcopy. However in areas where microscopy results are not made available within 24 hours, or in emergency situation RDT will be used. RDT negative patients strongly suspected of malaria will be cross checked by microscopy.
- If fever case is found to be positive for malaria it should be notified to District/State/Regional officer for following actions:
  - Initiate treatment within 24 hours of detection and ensure complete treatment.
  - Detailed case investigations are carried out and case is classified as imported or indigenous. Case investigations should be completed within 3 days of detection.
  - Contact survey should be carried out by blood smear collection for microscopy in the surrounding 50 households by ASHA/MPHW/Technical supervisor.
  - If additional cases are found on contact survey the area. Should be expanded and appropriate action initiated within 7 days.

The ABER should be sustained at minimum of 7% in perennial transmission areas and minimum 5% in seasonal transmission areas.

Surveillance in Category 0 (Prevention of Re-establishment Phase)

Malaria should be made notifiable

All fever cases meeting the definition of suspected malaria should be investigated using microscopy. All positive malaria cases should be notified to District/State/Regional and directorate of NVBDCP and actions taken as enumerated above under elimination phase as also foci based adult vector control interventions—in and around 50 houses of positive case—space spray followed by IRS.

Screening at points of entry at international and interstate borders should be established for the purpose of cross reporting, enumeration of cases and public health action.

Case-based Surveillance

Each confirmed case of malaria in category 0 and 1 state requires both detailed epidemiological case and Focus based investigation by rapid response team. Each case and focus is investigated and classified.

Case Investigation

Case investigation must be completed within 3 days of notification. The case investigation is done to decide whether case is **indigenous** or **imported**. The correct epidemiological classification of malaria cases is crucial in malaria elimination.

Focus Investigation

Focus investigation means describe the characteristics of the geographical area (Geographical reconnaissance) where the case has occurred to determine population at risk and factors contributing to malaria transmission. The focus is classified into active focus, (current or history of transmission during the past two calendar years) cleared up focus (No cases present) and pseudo focus (conditions not suitable for transmission.

Sentinel Surveillance

Sentinel surveillance is necessary for events which are not being captured by the regular system of surveillance or reporting, viz. severe cases of malaria, their management and on malaria deaths and effectiveness of antimalarial drugs being used. Further, to track these events in the light of introduction to RDTs and ACT for falciparum malaria, it is expected that changes in API would occur and these improvements lead to decrease in incidence of severe malaria and malaria deaths. Thus, monitoring of these latter events may indicate the availability and efficiency of primary level services. The hospitals with large OPDs and in-patient case load have been chosen as sentinel sites. A minimum of two sentinel sites will be selected in each high endemic district to provide reliable data on *trends of severe malaria* and *deaths*. Sentinel Site Medical Officer (SSMO) will be incharge of all activities regarding malaria in the sentinel sites. Trained laboratory technicians will be placed at sentinel sites.

Entomological surveillance: It supplements and supports case based surveillance and focus investigation. It collects information on vector species, vector density and sensitivity to insecticide and potencial breeding places.

Lot Quality Assurance Sampling (LQAS) Surveys

LQAS survey is a tool to monitor the quality and coverage with interventions. The malaria programme has introduced LQAS Surveys for generating information on important process and outcome indicators at the block level with the aim of mid-course correction. At present LQAS are being carried out in seven North Eastern States. LQAS are ideally done on quarterly basis for category 2 and 3 states.

Early Diagnosis and Complete Treatment (EDCT)

The primary purpose of case management is to shorten the duration of illness, prevent the development of severe disease and death. EDCT reduces parasite load in the community, and thereby interruption of transmission. It also minimizes the risk of selection and spread of drug resistant parasites.

Therefore, case management for malaria must be based on early diagnosis, which is followed immediately by complete effective treatment.

Recognition of Malaria

People living in malaria-endemic areas will be informed that any febrile disease might be malaria and that malaria can rapidly become a very dangerous disease. They also need to be informed about where they can obtain quality care for malaria. This is particularly important for migrants to endemic areas (for example, temporary labour) who may be ignorant both of what malaria is and where treatment is available.

Diagnosis of Malaria

A patient with fever and no other obvious cause of fever is considered as a case of "Suspected Malaria". Any volunteer, health worker or health professional observing a case of "Suspected Malaria" must immediately initiate a diagnostic test by:

1. Microscopy of blood for malaria parasite
2. Rapid diagnostic test (RDT).

Objective: To ensure that by 2012, at least 80% of fever cases suspected to be malaria are diagnosed either by RDT or by microscopy within 24 hours of the first contact to health services.

1. Microscopy

It is highly sensitive and specific, detects parasites at low densities, quantifies parasite load, and also useful to distinguish the various species of malaria parasite and their different stages of life cycle. Microscopy of stained thick and thin smears remains the gold standard for confirmation of diagnosis of malaria. The microscopy tests involve staining and direct visualization of the parasite under the microscope whether from peripheral smear study or Quantitative Buffy Coat (QBC) test.

Microscopy will be required for diagnosis of *P. vivax*. cases occurring even in remote and hard to reach areas, till the time RDTs to detect *P. vivax* cases are introduced in the programme.

- Ensure functional microscopy in all facilities in high malaria burden areas.

- Introduce use of RDTs by the health volunteers, i.e. ASHAs in villages where the microscopic results cannot be made available within 24 hours, i.e. in remote and hard to reach and in health facilities without microscopy.

2. Rapid Diagnostic Test (RDT)

Apart from clinical and microscopic examination, the rapid diagnostic tests (RDTs) have been developed. These tests are based on detection of antigens derived from malarial parasite in lysed blood, using immunochromatographic methods. Most frequently, they deploy a dipstick or test strip bearing monoclonal antibodies directed against the target parasite antigens. The test can be performed in about 15 minutes. Several commercial test kits are currently available.[8] Some RDTs detect *P. falciparum* only, while others detect *P. falciparum* and the other malaria parasites on two separate bands, no RDT has been reported to differentiate between *P. vivax, P. ovale* and *P. malariae*.

Wherever a microscopy result can be made available within 24 hours, microscopy will be maintained as the only routine method, as its sensitivity and specificity is very high. If a microscopy results cannot be made available within 24 hours in *P. falciparum* predominant areas, RDKs have been supplied and used for early diagnosis. The criteria for selection of these villages or subcentre areas for RDTs are:

- *P. falciparum* % ≥30 and TFR (test falciparum positivity rate) is ≥1%.
- Consistently high API of more than 5 and deaths are reported.
- Inaccessible areas—cut off during transmission season, areas with limited road and public transportation facility.
- Antimalarial treatment is given only on the basis of a positive diagnosis. The RDT is done in front of the patient and a slide is taken. If the RDT is negative the slide is sent for microscopy. If it is positive, the patient is treated for falciparum or vivax malaria, and the slide is discarded in order to reduce the load on the microscopy services.

Mixed infection cannot be ruled out in such cases, but the risk is low. The large scale introduction of *P. falciparum* RDT is likely to lead to exaggerated estimates of *P. falciparum*.

The tests have sensitivity level of about 95%. RDT have short shelf-life of 12 months these may deteriorate at high ambient temperatures. HRP_2 antigen can persist for up to 4 weeks after clearance of asexual parasitaemia through treatment. False positive tests are therefore common, especially in patients with recent history of treatment. RDTs should therefore *not be* used for following up patients after treatment. If a patient, who has been treated, is febrile within one month after the treatment and the RDT is positive, the patient may have malaria. If possible, the diagnosis should then be confirmed by microscopy. NVBDCP has introduced use of RDTs by health volunteers, i.e. ASHAs in villages to solve the problem of early diagnosis of *P. falciparum* ASHAs have been given ACT. The programme also plants to supply RDT kits to private providers in return for data. RDTs will be used in PHC and other facilities only in emergency for treatment of severe malaria cases requiring immediate medical attention in the absence of the laboratory technician (LT). Bivalent RDTs (which detect and differentiate *P. falciparum* and *P. vivax*) have been introduced from 2013 onwards.

If RDT for only *P. falciparum* is used, negative cases showing signs and symptoms of malaria without any other obvious cause should be considered a "clinical malaria" and treated with chloroquine in full therapeutic dose of 25 mg/kg body weight over three days. If a slide result is obtained later, the treatment should be adjusted according to species. In circumstances neither RDT nor microscopy is available "clinical malaria" cases should be treated with chloroquine in full therapeutic doses.

Limitation of RDTs

These tests are more expensive, detection of all 4 species is limited to some RDTs, quantification of parasite not possible, differentiation between *P. vivax*, *P. ovale* and *P. malariae* not possible and differentiation between sexual and asexual stages not possible. It should be noted that *P. falciparum* HRP_2 based kits may show positive result up to three weeks of successful treatment. Presently, NVBDCP supplies RDT kits for detection of *P. falciparum* as microscopy results are not obtainable within 24 hours of sample collection in remote areas.

NATIONAL DRUG POLICY ON MALARIA (2013)[9]

Effective treatment of malaria under the national drug policy aims at:

- Providing complete cure (clinical and parasitological) of malaria cases
- Prevention of progression of uncomplicated malaria into severe malaria and thereby reduce malaria mortality
- Prevention of relapses by administration of radical treatment
- Interruption of transmission of malaria by use of gametocytocidal drugs
- Preventing development of drug resistance by rational treatment of malaria cases.

Treatment of Uncomplicated Malaria

1 It is stressed that all fever cases should be suspected of malaria after ruling out other common causes and should be investigated for confirmation of malaria by

Microscopy or Rapid Diagnostic Kit (RDK) so as to ensure treatment with full therapeutic dose with appropriate drug to all confirmed cases.

2 The malaria case management is very important for prevention of serious cases and deaths due to malaria. So, the private healthcare providers should also follow the National Guidelines for teratment of malaria as per the Drug Policy 2013

3 P. vivax cases should be treated with chloroquine for three days and Primaquine for 14 days. Primaquine is used to prevent relapse but is contraindicated in pregnant women, infants and individuals with G6PD deficiency.

Note: Patients should be instructed to report back in case of haematuria or high colored urine/cyanosis or blue coloration of lips and Primaquine should be stopped in such cases. Care should be taken in patients with anaemia.

4 P. falciparum cases should be treated with ACT (Artesunate 3 days + Sulphadoxine-Pyrimethamine 1 day). This is to be accompanied by single dose primaquine preferably on day 2.

5 However, considering the reports of resistance to partner drug SP in North Eastern States, the Technical Advisory Committee has recommended to use the Co-formulated tablet of Artemether (20 mg)-Lumefantrine (120 mg ACT-AL) as per the age-specific dose schedule for the treatment of Pf cases in North Eastern States. (Not recommended during the first trimester of pregnancy and for children weighing <5 kg)

6 Production and sale of Artemisinin monotherapy has been banned in India

7 Pregnant women with uncomplicated P. falciparum should be treated as follows:

- 1st Trimester: Quinine
- 2nd and 3rd Trimester: ACT

Note: Primaquine is contraindicated in pregnant woman

8 In cases where parasitological diagnosis is not possible due to non-availability of either timely microscopy or RDT, suspected malaria cases will be treated with full course of chloroquine, till the results of microscopy are received. Once the parasitological diagnosis is available, appropriate treatment as per the species, is to be administered.

9 Presumptive treatment with chloroquine is no more recommended.

10 Resistance should be suspected if in spite of full treatment with no history of vomiting, diarrhoea, patient does not respond within 72 hours, clinically and parasitoogically. Such cases not responding to ACT, should be treated with oral quinine, with Tetracycline/Doxycycline. These instances should be reported to concerned District Malaria/State Malaria Officer/ROHFW for initiation of therapeutic efficacy studies.

Treatment of Vivax Malaria

Diagnosis of vivax malaria may be made by the use of RDT (Bivalent) or microscopic examination of the blood smear. On confirmation following treatment is to be given:

Drug Schedule for Treatment of P. vivax Malaria

1 **Chloroquine:** 25 mg/kg body weight divided over three days i.e.

10 mg/kg on day 1,

10 mg/kg on day 2 and

5 mg/kg on day 3.

2 **Primaquine*:** 0.25 mg/kg body weight daily for 14 days.

* Primaquine is contraindicated in infants, pregnant women and individuals with G6PD deficiency.

14 days regimen of Primaquine should be given under supervision.

Dosage (in mg) chart for treatment of Vivax malaria

Age	*Day 1 CQ (150 mg base)*	*Day 2 CQ (150 mg base)*	*Day 3 CQ (150 mg base)*	*Day 1 to 14 PQ (2.5 mg)*
Less than 1 year	75	75	37.5	0
1–4 years	150	150	75	2.5
5–8 years	300	300	150	5
9–14 years	450	450	225	10
15 yrs or more	600	600	300	15
Pregnancy	600	600	300	Nil

***Note*:** CQ 250 mg tablet is having 150 mg base

Treatment of Falciparum Malaria

Diagnosis of falciparum malaria may be made by the use of RDT (Monovalent or Bivalent) or microscopic examination of the blood smear. It is imperative to start the treatment for falciparum malaria immediately on diagnosis. The treatment for falciparum malaria is as follow:

In other States (other than North-Eastern States)

1 **Artemisinin based combination therapy (ACT-SP)*:** Artesunate (AS), available as 50 mg tablets are given for three days, and Sulfadoxine-Pyrimethamine (S-P) tablets, containing 500 mg Sulfadoxine and 25 mg pyrimethamine are given for one day, as shown in the dosage chart (Table 12.20).

All tablets for a day should be taken together, swallowed with water. In addition, Primaquine (PQ Large) tablets should be given on the second day.

Dose Schedule for Treatment of Uncomplicated P. falciparum Cases

1 **Artemisinin based combination therapy (ACT-SP)*:** Artesunate 4 mg/kg body weight daily for 3 days Plus Sulfadoxine (25 mg/kg body weight)–Pyrimethamine (1.25 mg/kg body weight) on first day.

* ACT is not to be given in 1st trimester of pregnancy.

2 **Primaquine*:** 0.75 mg/kg body weight on day 2.

With the introduction of different coloured Blister Packs for different age groups, treatment by the field level staff has been made easy. The colour code for different age groups for Packing of Tablet ACT + SP has been given in Table 12.20.

Table 12.20: Dosage chart (in mg) for treatment of falciparum malaria with ACT-SP

Age group (years)	1st day		2nd day		3rd day
	AS	SP	AS	PQ	AS
0–1 Pink Blister	25	250 + 12.5	25	Nil	25
1–4 Yellow Blister	50	500 + 25	50	7.5	50
5–8 Green Blister	100	750 + 37.5	100	15	100
9–14 Red Blister	150	1000 + 50	150	30	150
15 and above White Blister	200	1500 + 75	200	45	200

Note: SP is not to be prescribed for children <5 months of age and should be treated with alternate ACT

In North-Eastern States (NE States)

1 ACT-AL Co-formulated tablet of Artemether (20 mg)-Lumefantrine (120 mg)* (Table 12.21).

*ACT-AL is not to be prescribed for children weighing less than 5 kg and first trimester of pregnancy.

Treatment of uncomplicated P. falciparum cases in pregnancy

1st Trimester: Quinine salt 10 mg/kg 3 times daily for 7 days.

Quinine may induce hypoglycemia; pregnant women should not start taking quinine on an empty stomach and should eat regularly, while on quinine treatment.

2nd and 3rd Trimester: Area-specific ACT as per dosage schedule given above, i.e. ACT-AL in North Eastern States, ACT-SP in Other States.

Primaquine (PQ) prevents transmission of falciparum malaria to others by its ability to kill gametocytes. PQ tablets should be taken after a meal; not on an empty stomach. Children less than the age of one year and pregnant women should not be given Primaquine. As pregnant women having falciparum malaria require different medicines, they should be directed to go to the nearest PHC or hospital immediately, without delay.

Treatment of mixed infections (P. vivax + P. falciparum) cases

All mixed infections should be treated with full course of ACT and Primaquine 0.25 mg per kg body weight daily for 14 days.

- **In North-Eastern States:** Treat with: Age-specific ACT-AL for 3 days + Primaquine 0.25 mg per kg body weight daily for 14 days.
- **In other States:** SP-ACT 3 days + Primaquine 0.25 mg per kg body wt. daily for 14 days (Table 12.22).

Treatment of *P. ovale* and *P. malariae*

In India these species are very rarely found in a few places. *P. ovale* should be treated as *P. vivax* and *P. malariae* should be treated as *P. falciparum*.

Treatment of Mixed Infections

All cases of mixed infection are to be treated as Pf as per the drug policy applicable in the area plus primaquine for 14 days.

Treatment of Severe Malaria

Full doses parentral artesunate is the treatment of choice for all severe malaria followed by a full dose of ACT orally. Treatment of asymptomatic cases detected by microscopy. Treat according to species

Chemoprophylaxis

Chemoprophylaxis should be administered only in selective groups in high *P. falciparum* endemic areas. Use of personal protection measures including insecticide treated bed nets (ITN)/long-lasting insecticidal nets (LLIN) should be encouraged for pregnant women and other vulnerable population including travelers for longer stay. However, for longer stay of military and paramilitary forces

Table 12.21: ACT-AL recommended regimen by weight and age group in NE states

Co-formulated tablet ACT-AL	*5–14 kg (>5 months to <3 years)*	*15–24 kg (≥3–8 years)*	*25–34 kg (≥9–14 years)*	*>34 kg (>14 years)*
Total dose of ACT	20 mg	40 mg	60 mg	80 mg
Total dose of AL	120 mg	240 mg	360 mg	480 mg
Pack size				
No. of tablets in the packing	6	12	18	24
Give	One tablet twice daily for 3 days	Two tablets twice daily for 3 days	Three tablets twice daily for 3 days	Four tablets twice daily for 3 days
Colour of the pack	Yellow	Green	Red	White

Table 12.22: Dosage chart for treatment of mixed (vivax and falciparum) malaria with ACT-SP. (Doses in mg)

Age	Day 1		Day 2	Day 3	Day 1–14
	AS tablet	SP tablet	AS tablet	AS tablet	Primaquine tablet
0–1	25	250 + 12.5	25	25	0
1–4	50	500 + 25	50	50	2.5
5–8	100	750 + 37.5	100	100	5
9–14	150	1000 + 50	150	150	10
15 years or more	200	1500 + 75	200	200	15

Tablet SP (Sulfadoxine 500 mg and Pyrimethamine 25 mg)

in high *P. falciparum endemic* areas, the practice of chemoprophylaxis should be followed wherever appropriate, e.g. troops on night patrol duty and decisions of their Medical Administrative Authority should be followed.

Short-term Chemoprophylaxis (up to 6 Weeks)

Doxycycline: 100 mg once daily for adults and 1.5 mg/kg once daily for children (contraindicated in children below 8 years). The drug should be started 2 days before travel and continued for 4 weeks after leaving the malarious area.

Note: It is not recommended for pregnant women and children less than 8 years.

Chemoprophylaxis for Longer Stay (more than 6 weeks)

Mefloquine: 250 mg weekly for adults and should be administered two weeks before, during and four weeks after exposure.

Note: Mefloquine is contraindicated in individuals with history of convulsions, neuropsychiatric problems and cardiac conditions. Therefore, necessary precautions should be taken and all should undergo screening before prescription of the drug.

New-Drug: India has developed indigenously first anti-malarial drug "Synriam" which beats all current available options of affordability, compliance and relief. The drug provides quick relief for uncomplicated *Plasmodium falciparum* malaria in adults.

In April 2012, Ranbaxy launched India's first new drug Synriam™. The synthetic antimalarial is the next generation non-artemesinin. Synriam contains arterolane maleate 150 mg and piperaquine phosphate 750 mg. One tablet daily for 3 days is the dose.

B. Integrated Vector Management (IVM)[10,11]

IVM is a process for managing vector population in a way to reduce or interrupt transmission of disease. The aim of IVM is to reduce number of bites by infected vector of malaria. The NVBDCP aims to achieve effective control by biological, chemical and environmental interventions of proven efficacy. Integration of IVM is done by using identical vector control methods to control malaria and leishmaniasis in rural areas and malaria and dengue in urban areas to achieve cost-effectiveness and synergy. The measures of vector control includes:

- **Measures to control adult mosquitoes:** By indoor residual spray (IRS).
- **Anti-larval measures**
- **Personal protection:** Use of bed nets including insecticide treated nets (ITNs).

The national malaria control programme is currently using IRS as the primary method of vector control in rural settings, and anti-larval measures in urban areas. Insecticide treated bed nets have been introduced in the programme, and the programme envisages to scale up their use as vector control option for full population coverage which replace IRS in areas, where operational factors indicated that this method alone will give sufficient impact.

Indoor Residual Spray (IRS)[10,11]

Residual spraying is used for indoors, meticulously sprayed on walls and other surfaces of the interiors. The endophilic malaria vectors that rest inside the houses after taking a blood meal are killed when they come in contact with the insecticide and thus transmission is prevented.

IRS is at present carried out in high-risk areas with coverage of 80 million population. DDT is the insecticide of choice; in areas where **vector** has shown **resistance** to DDT, the alternatives are malathion and synthetic pyrethroids. Two rounds of spraying are done for DDT and synthetic pyrethroids to provide protection during the entire transmission season and in the case of malathion, three rounds of spraying is required.

Dose of DDT: 1 g/m^2 DDT (75% WP): $\frac{2}{3}$: 10 : 500, i.e. 2/3 kg of 75% DDT in 10 liters of water sprayed over 500 square meters (approximately equivalent to three houses).

Dose of DDT (50% WP): 1g/m^2: 1:10 : 500, i.e. 1 kg of 50% DDT in 10 liters of water sprayed over 500 square meters. Residual effect is 10–12 weeks.

Dosage of malathion 25% WP 2 g/m^2, i.e. 2 kg in 10 liters of water for 500 square meters (Three houses). Residual effect is 6–8 weeks.

Dosage of Deltamethrin (Synthetic Pyrethroids) 2.5% WP: 20 mg/m^2, i.e. 400 gm in 10 liters of water for 500 square meters. Residual effect lasts for 10–12 weeks.

Category-wise vector control measures

Category of subcentre	*Vector control measures*
Category 0 (no case)	• Mapping of potential vector breeding sites • Vector prevalence and density monitoring • Environmental modification/manipulation for source reduction by VHSC. And UVBD scheme • Biological control by larvivorus fish • Foci based adult vector control in and around 50 houses of positive case–space spray followed by IRS
	Category 1, 2, and 3 States
Subcentres with API <1	Same as in category 0 above
Subcentres with API ≥ 1	• Universal coverage with LLINs of all subcentres with API > 1 • In subcentres with API > 1 if not covered with LLIN, two regular rounds of supervised IRS • In LLIN covered subcentre, if there is an upsurge of cases, efforts to be made to increase compliance rate of LLIN usage • In outbreak situations—one additional round of IRS • Antilarval measures in urban areas in outbreak situation slum clusters can also be covered with IRS • Larval control through source reduction, biological and Environmental measures
Low endemic subcentre, i.e. with 0 or < 1 API should be treated as category 1	

Planning of IRS: The first round of spray in an area is usually done to coincide with the time of build-up of vector populations which precedes the malaria transmission season.

Objectives: To achieve at least 80% coverage of households in targeted high-risk areas with spray of effective insecticides.

Operational design: During the strategic plan period IRS coverage will be targeted primarily at achieving a minimum of 80% coverage of IRS eligible population living in high endemic areas. These are the areas not targeted for community wide coverage with LLINs or conventional ITNs. It is possible that as LLINs are scaled up, the eligible population will become smaller, but the rate at which this will happen cannot be determined in advance.

Surveillance on **insecticide resistance will** form a critical component for taking decision on the insecticide to be used. Therefore, surveillance by National Institute of Malaria Research and Zonal entomologist will be used. DDT is one of the persistent organic pollutant and its widespread use in agriculture leads to environmental pollution and it enters to food chain. In accordance with the Stockholm Convention on *Persistent Organic Pollutants* reliance on DDT will be reduced by adopting other effective methods. But efforts will be made to progressively scale down its use.

Problem: Coverage rates for IRS tends to be low and refusal rates are very high and the impact with low coverage is minimal besides **insecticides resistance.**

Other Methods for Malaria Vector Control

The breeding of Anopheles mosquitoes can be reduced by a variety of physical, chemical and biological methods of larval control. In most situations these anti-larval measures have lesser impact than IRS and ITNs/LLINs which reduce the longevity of adult mosquitoes. However, in some areas, larval control can play an important role; either or as an adjunct to IRS and ITNs.

Mosquito Larviciding

Petroleum oils and Paris green are effective and are still used in some countries. Biocides (*Bacillus thuringiensis* serotype H-14 and *Bacillus sphaericus*, Larvivorus fish, monomolecular films) and insect growth regulators are finding increasing application in mosquito control programme. However, the main reliance is still on the chemical larvicides like organophosphates and pyrethroid insecticides. Recurrent use of Temephos (Abate) once a weak as larvicide in towns is quite popular.

Biological Control

a. Fish as Mosquito Control Agent

One of the most widely used biological control agents against mosquito larvae is the fish *Gambusia affinis*, the top water minnow or mosquito fish. The fish other than Gambusia, which has received the most attention as mosquito control agent is *Poecilla reticulata*; the common guppy. There is much evidence that *P. reticulata* is not as effective at controlling mosquito larvae as *G. affinis*. The guppy though reproduces more rapidly than mosquito fish, but is not as effective in controlling mosquito larvae.

b. Role of Bacteria in Mosquito Control

Bacillus sphaericus and *Bacillus thuringiensis israelensis* (Bti) have been used against mosquito larvae. These are in pilot use under the programme.

Environmental Control Methods

Source reduction: These are measures which prevent the breeding of mosquitoes or eliminate their breeding sites. If such measures are long-lasting or permanent like physical transformation of land, water and vegetation, they are often referred to as *environmental modification* (filling of sites, and improving drainage). When such measures have a temporary effect, and need to be repeated, they are known as *environmental manipulation* (observing dry days, removal of water plants, shading, cleaning and draining of pots, and stream flushing, etc.).

Use of Insecticide Treated Nets (ITNs)

Highly endemic areas of eleven states where API is above 1 and have achieved high coverage of bednets, have been chosen on pilot basis to promote use of ITNs.

Synthetic pyrethroids are used for impregnating bed nets. This compound is technically effective to repel or kill the vector. It is biodegradable and does not recycle in nature. This method has been found to be cost-effective.

Dosage of 25 mg/sq metre of deltamethrin/lambdacyhalothrin or 50 mg/sq metre of cyfluthrin is recommended. Thus, 1 g of deltamethrin (2.5%) or 0.5 g of cyfluthrin (10%) or 0.25 g of lambdacyhalothrin will be required per sq metre. The water absorbing capacity of the net is determined by trial and error method.

Residual effect: When not washed, the impregnated nets have the efficacy for 6 months. These can be provided to people on subsidized rates. There is need for strong partnership between Govt., NGO, industry and community for up-scaling of specific malaria control activities including use of ITN*s*.

ITNs Including LLINs (Long-lasting Insecticidal Bednets)

ITNs have emerged as an important tool in malaria control. Long-Lasting Insecticidal Nets (LLINs) are mosquito nets which have the insecticide incorporated in their fibre, so that it is not removed by as many as 20 washes. Because these nets have an even and quality controlled insecticide application, they are generally more effective than conventional ITNs.

Furthermore the LLIN is more cost-effective (as it can be used for 3–5 years) than conventional bed nets which need to be treated with insecticide once or twice a year. It is reiterated that ITNs are now becoming one of the main methods for control of malaria transmission. In population targeted for bednets, coverage must be as close to 100% as possible and the delivery should be a free public service.

ITNs and IRS are the two key methods of vector control promoted on large scale in the country. It is planned to scale up use of LLINs over the coming years and simultaneously reduce the reliance on use of conventional bednets treated with insecticides.

Objective: To ensure that at least 80% of people sleep under effective ITNs/LLINs in target areas by 2017.

Strategies

- Rapid scale up of ITN/LLIN coverage through a mass distribution campaign. Every eligible household will be supplied with family size LLINs @ 1 nets per 2 persons or use overall ratio of 1 LLIN for every 1.8 persons.
- Retreatment of plain nets with synthetic pyrethroids done free of cost to the community.
- BCC to ensure regular use of ITN/LLINs.
- Social marketing of LLINs.
- Vulnerable community plan (VCP).

The NVBDCP has taken a conscious decision to use either IRS or bed nets in a given area which means area chosen for one method will usually not to be covered by the second method of vector control.

Efficacy and Effectiveness of ITNs

Bednets whether impregnated or not act as physical barrier reducing the risk of the user getting any night-biting mosquito. ITNs like IRS, also reduce the longevity of vectors. A number of studies have shown that ITNs have a community effect, when the coverage is 60% or higher. While studies in Africa have focused on children under 5 years and found that their all cause mortality is reduced by 18% by ITNs, studies in Asia have focused on malaria morbidity in all age groups and found that is typically reduced by 50% by ITNs.

C. Epidemic Preparedness and Early Response

The aim of the NVBDCP including malaria is to prevent or identify epidemics/outbreaks in incipient stages and to prevent them from progressing into full blown epidemics. Prevention requires high level of preparedness and is closely linked with the integrated disease surveillance project (IDSP). The major causes of occurrence of outbreaks/epidemics are—climatic/environmental changes conducive to vector breeding, unplanned urbanization, population migration to and fro endemic areas, lack of manpower and facilities for malaria surveillance and resistance to anti-malarials and insecticides; lack of drugs and other commodities.[12]

Definition of outbreak/epidemic: Occurence of malaria cases in excess of the number expected in a given place and time. (Two standard deviations above the mean number of cases in preceding 3 years).

Detection of Malaria Epidemics

The MO-PHC should keep a constant watch on parasite load by continuous monitoring of the number of fever cases and distribution of *P. vivax* and *P. falciparum*. Epidemiological factors which may assist in early prediction of an outbreak are given below:

- Increase in fever cases (fever proportion of one-third or more of new OPD cases) and severe malaria cases.
- Increase in fever incidence in the population (as informed by health workers and CHVs) or through weekly fever trends available through IDSP.
- Increase in malaria incidence (as compared to that of same month of previous years).
- Increase in test positive rate, *P. falciparum* %, proportion of gametocytes to other stages, increase in resistance, non-response to antimalarial, increase mortality, and increase in consumption of anti-malarials.

Fever alert surveillance for malaria has been integrated with the IDSP. Fever cases are being reported in the "Weekly Fever Report" from PHC to District nodal officer of IDSP and DMO/DVBDCO. If an increase in fever incidence is observed, nodal officer of IDSP will send an alert to the DMO and MOPHC. Similarly, the DMO/ DVBDCO will inform the nodal officer of IDSP if any increase in fever incidence is observed. Once a strong degree of suspicion is aroused, the following steps need to be taken:

- Conduct a rapid fever survey and collect blood slides/ conduct RDT to find the test positivity rate (TPR) to assess the magnitude of disease occurrence.
- Compare the trend of malaria incidence in the area during the year under investigation, i.e. month wise malaria incidence, to preceding 5 years.
- The weekly/monthly data should always be compared with established threshold levels. Monthly/weekly mean should be calculated for the previous 5 years (excluding the month/week in which there was on epidemic).
- Compare the test positivity rate (TPR) obtained in the rapid fever survey and TPR of the current month to the TPR of the same month of the previous year.
- Increasing trends of malaria/fever over a short duration, i.e. weekly analysis should compare the current week data with data of previous three weeks.
- Collect information on supportive factors like climatic conditions, vulnerability, vector density and entomological factors, etc. If the following findings result from the analysis of above data, an epidemic/ outbreak is confirmed if there is:
    - i Increase in TPR (doubling) in the current period as compared to the same period of previous year and or >5% increase in TPR in period under investigation.
    - ii Increasing trend of malaria incidence in the months of the current year as well as compared to corresponding months of the previous years.
    - iii Increase vector density and positive findings of other supportive factors.

12

Criteria for Detection of Epidemic by use of Threshold Levels

There are four methods for calculating the weekly/monthly epidemic threshold level.

- Weekly/monthly mean for the past 5 years plus 2 standard deviations.
- **Upper third quartile:** This method involves placing the values of particular month/weak for the past 5 years in a series–minimum value, second lowest, median value, second highest and highest value. If the current month/week's cases exceed second highest value for the past 5 years it indicates that the epidemic threshold has been crossed.
- Cumulative sum (C-SUM) method, which is the mean of previous, current and following month/weak's data for the past 5 years.
- C-SUM refined by adding a 95% confidence interval (1.96 SD).

Prevention and Control of Malaria Epidemics[12]

The district should be prepared to respond rapidly to an outbreak/epidemic the requirements are:

- **Constitution of rapid response teams (RRTs):** RRTs should be constituted in collaboration with IDSP at district level and at local level such as PHC/CHC. The main function of RRT is to undertake urgent epidemiological and entomological investigations and provide emergency supplies and material, mobility as also additional manpower besides on the spot training.

Actions/Response

- **Rapid fever survey:** In every affected village/area all fever cases are identified and their blood smears are examined promptly by setting up field laboratory at the site of occurrence of outbreak. In areas where microscopy is not possible RDT should be performed.
- **Mass survey:** In case the affected population is relatively small, a mass survey of the entire population may be carried out in every village irrespective of fever status. Children must be included in such surveys. Mass survey of entire population should be completed within 7–14 days (within one extrinsic incubation period) to prevent secondary cases. All groups should be covered—children, pregnant women and migrants. Mass survey are difficult to conduct.
    - i Blood smears collected should be examined within 24 hours or alternatively RDT should be conducted.
    - ii All positive cases should be given radical treatment at the recommended doses according to the slide or RDT result.
    - iii If the initial results indicate a positivity rate above 30% among fever cases (either blood smear or RDT it may be considered to treat all fever cases as soon as blood samples has been collected).

iv In areas where ACT has been rolled out and initial investigation reveal that the current outbreak is predominantly due to *P. falciparum*, treatment of cases may be started with ACT, even before the result arrive.

Space Spray

- Every house in the affected area/village should be covered.
- Indoor space spray with pyrethrum should be carried out for 7–10 consecutive days or till IRS is completed in all houses of the locality. The equipment to be used for space spray is the hand operated micro-discharge fogging machine or hand operated atomizers (Flit pump).

IRS

- IRS should be started simultaneously with indoor space spray.
- The insecticide of choice will be the insecticide to which the local vector is susceptible according to best available information. All rooms of all houses and mixed dwellings will be sprayed to achieve full coverage (minimum of 80% of houses).

Entomological Investigation and other Vector Control Measures

The zonal entomological team should carry out vector density studies by entomological surveillance. They should point out prolific breeding places requiring immediate action such as antilarval measures along with IRS. Status of vector susceptibility to insecticide can be done on later date. The zonal team report their findings to RRT.

Follow-up Action

- Continue close surveillance for one month (twice the incubation period) after the outbreak has been contained (as demonstrated by epidemiological indices).
- Strengthen case detection and treatment services at all levels in the vicinity by ensuring that laboratories are fully functional, surveillance workers are deployed and supplies are ensured.
- Investigation to find out whether the epidemic was due to influx of migrants, break down of regular malaria control operations or natural calamities like floods, or heavy rain.

The final epidemic containment report should be submitted to higher levels.

D. Supportive Interventions Advocacy, Coordination

Capacity building: Recruit training, induction training, on the job training and off the job training for skill development apart from motivation is built into the programme.

Intersectoral coordination between various sectors happen through various coordination committees constituted at various levels by regular and periodical meetings at policy, planning and implementation level.

Reproductive and child health: Antenatal care services are utilized in distribution of LLINs to pregnant women in some areas of the country. Malaria is also included in integrated management of neonatal and childhood illness (IMNCI).

Community participation and behaviour change communication activities are organized for various components of the programme—early diagnosis and complete treatment, IRS, bednet distribution, referral services, bednet impregnation with insecticide, larval control and source reduction. All these areas need active community participation as also behaviour change to promote healthy practices for prevention and control of malaria and other vector-borne diseases.

Advocacy, Coordination and Public-Private Partnership

Most patients turn to private practitioners once they have fever. Training of private practitioners on standard treatment protocols and guideline on malaria, national drug policy on malaria and sharing information education material with them can go a long way in prevention and control of malaria. Involvement of NGOs, Faith based organizations and community based organization as well as PRIs is imperative need for the success of the programme.

E. IEC Strategy for Malaria Action Programme (MAP)

Behaviour change communication and community mobilization.

Objective is to create awareness among the members of the community about causes, prevention, treatment and management of malaria cases leading to the reduction of morbidity and mortality (mortality nil and morbidity 0.5 cases per 1000 per annum).

Specific Objectives

1. To create awareness on the reduction in the frequency of contact between man and mosquito.
2. To create awareness among masses, about the measures which bring about reduction in parasite load in the community.
3. To create awareness on the methods, which can bring about reduction in mosquitogenic conditions leading to reduction in mosquito density.

The education to individual family and community has to be part of primary health care. Interpersonal communication and mass-media communication can play effective role. Observing antimalaria month every year in June is intensification of education measures before transmission season.

Since June 2005 it has been envisaged that antimalaria month (AMM) campaign would not be confined to that specific month of June alone like earlier, but would be implemented in phases throughout the year.

In-depth—Review report 2007 and Joint monitoring mission report-2007 have reflected inadequate knowledge, awareness, and inappropriate practices in high-risk areas particularly those that are rural and tribal having deficient health system. The BCC strategic plan is aimed at to cover at least 80% of population by 2012 for improving knowledge, awareness and practices in relation to malaria.

Study, undertaken nationwide, provides an evidence that much needs to be done to build awareness against malaria and improve practices at household and community level.[13]

During the NMEP spray operation people perceived, that NMEP goal is "mosquito eradication" rather than parasite elimination. Govt. of India gave a slogan "*Macchar Rahega Par Malaria Nahin*" (there will be no malaria despite mosquito being there). People are ignorant about breeding of mosquitoes.

F. Monitoring and Evaluation in Malaria[14,15]

Regular reports generated by the programme forms the basis of regular monitoring and evaluation of the programme. Weekly reports of IDSP, fortnightly and monthly report at various levels covering different aspects of the programme are used locally for early response and planning activities. Monitoring indicators for disease surveillance, integrated vector management, IRS and programme management have been developed.

Monitoring Indicators used in Disease Surveillance and Case Detection

1. Disease burden and impact: Indicators are total fever cases, malaria cases, *P. falciparum* cases and deaths due to malaria every month and cumulative for the year can be obtained/accessed from M-1, M-4 and SC, PHC M-4 data.
2. Monthly blood examination rate (MBER)

$$(\text{MBER}) = \frac{\text{Number of blood smears examined + RDTs positive in a month}}{\text{Total population under surveillance}} \times 100$$

MBER should be more than 1% of population in the transmission season.

3. Annual blood examination rate (ABER)

$$(\text{ABER}) = \frac{\text{Number of blood smears examined + RDTs positive in a year}}{\text{Total population under surveillance}} \times 100$$

ABER would include fever cases screened through slides as well as RDTs. Minimum target of ABER is 10% of population. Both MBER and ABER measure the *incidence of fever* in the community. Based on fever incidence health worker male should collect 1% of slides (50 slides) per month in allocated population of 5000 or 500 slides per annum. This indicator measures the performance of the health worker male, further ABER is an indicator of operational efficiency of the programme. **Increase in fever proportion** (fever proportion of **one-third or more of new** OPD cases) is the indicator in early prediction of an outbreak of malaria in the community. The MO i/c of a PHC can monitor the fever incidence at PHC as well as in the community from the regular fortnight/ monthly report or community report/complaints.

4. Annual parasite incidence (API)

$$(\text{API}) = \frac{\text{Total number of blood smears positive for malaria parasite + RDTs positive for malaria parasite in a year}}{\text{Total population under surveillance}} \times 1000$$

The API measures the incidence of malaria in the community. Areas with API more than 2 are classified as *high-risk* areas and qualify for selective spray of IRS. Technical advisory committee on malaria in 2002 further rationalized the criteria for undertaking IRS on priority basis—all areas with more than 5 API should be covered with IRS (suitable insecticide) where ABER is 10% or more, taking sub-centre area as a unit. Thus, API helps to identify *high-risk* areas to decide priority for spray activities. API is dependent upon effective surveillance and it is valid if ABER of 10% is achieved in the area. Over the years, the API which was more than 11 in 1977 has declined to the level of 0.72 in the year 2013 which speaks the impact of the intervention.

5. Annual falciparum incidence (AfI) rate

$$(\text{AfI}) = \frac{\text{Total number of blood smears positive for } p.falciparum \text{ malaria parasite + RDTs positive for } p.falciparum \text{ malaria parasite in a year}}{\text{Total population under surveillance}} \times 1000$$

AfI like API measures incidence of *P. falciparum* malaria (killer malaria) in the community. This index measures disease burden due to *P. falciparum* malaria.

6. Test positive rate (TPR)

$$(\text{TPR}) = \frac{\text{Total number of blood smears positive for malaria parasite + RDTs positive for malaria parasite}}{\text{Total number of blood smears examined + positive RDTs}} \times 100$$

This is independent of surveillance activity, therefore a better indicator for measurement of disease burden and impact. TPR of 5% or more in routine surveillance should always raise alarm. TPR indicates disease burden in the community, month-wise or year-wise. It is also good indicator for endemicity. Whenever the case detection mechanism is inadequate this is dependable parameter to determine progress of containment measures. It is more reliable than API even for those years when ABER fluctuates from year to year. TPR and API tend to be close to each other. Increase in TPR (doubled) in the current period as compared to the same period of previous year and/or TPR in routine surveillance is 5% or more is indicative of outbreak/epidemic of malaria. If the TPR is low but the fever rate is high it indicates a disease problem, which is not malaria. In this case, the possibility of inadequate laboratory microscopic services should also be considered and improved accordingly (if required). High TPR in areas with high and stable transmission of malaria is not considered an outbreak.

7 Test falciparum rate (TfR)

$$(\text{TfR}) = \frac{\begin{array}{c}\text{Total number of blood smears positive for}\\ \textit{P. falciparum}\text{ malaria parasite + RDTs}\\ \text{found positive for }\textit{P. falciparum}\end{array}}{\begin{array}{c}\text{Total number of blood smears}\\ \text{examined + positive RDTs}\end{array}} \times 100$$

It is independent of surveillance and indicates *P. falciparum* preponderance. It measures disease burden due to *P. falciparum.* Declining trend will indicate impact of intervention. Area with TfR of more than 1% qualifies for RDT.

8 *P. falciparum* percentage (*P. falciparum*%)

$$(\textit{Pf.}\%) = \frac{\begin{array}{c}\text{Total number of blood smears positive for}\\ \textit{P. falciparum}\text{ malaria parasite + RDTs}\\ \text{positive for }\textit{P. falciparum}\end{array}}{\begin{array}{c}\text{Total number of positive blood}\\ \text{smears + positive RDTs for malaria parasite}\end{array}} \times 100$$

It measures disease burden due to *P. falciparum* malaria in the area. Over the years the disease burden due to *P. falciparum* malaria in India has increased and reached to over 65% in the year 2014. In some tribal districts in Jharkhand and Odisha the proportion of *P. falciparum* may be 70–80%. Rising trend of *P. falciparum* is indicative of drug resistance, inadequate surveillance programme and weak or non-functional health facilities and difficult access to services. Priority for IRS and ITNs is for those areas which have high burden due to *P. falciparum.* Different control strategies are required for those areas showing high burden due to *P. falciparum* malaria. RDT kits have been supplied in those villages or subcentres which show *P. falciparum*% >30. Passive surveillance has been stepped up in these areas.

9 *Infant parasite rate:* Discussed elsewhere.

10 Percentage of community level facilities equipped with RDT in the last reporting period. This indicator can be obtained by:

$$\frac{\text{ASHAs/other community volunteers equipped with RDT}}{\text{Total ASHAs/other community volunteers}} \times 100$$

This is a process indicator for RDT. Frequency of this indicator is once in a quarter or once a year.

11 *Utilization of ACT:* Number of *P. falciparum* cases treated with ACT. Now under Drug Policy 2010 and 2013, all *P. falciparum* cases should be treated with ACT.

Monitoring Indicators for IVM (Integrated Vector Management)

i Percentage of spray equipment in working condition.
ii Percentage of spray squads engaged against the requirement
iii Bed nets distributed
iv Bed nets treated
v Insecticide use—average insecticide per bed net
vi Percentage of eligible population covered by ITN. It should be 80% or more.
vii IRS coverage of eligible population: It should be 80% or more.
viii IRS coverage: Targeted rooms% (should be 80% or more)

Monitoring Indicators used for Programme Management

- Number of RDTs and ACTs planned versus received and used.
- Percentage of staff in place
- Percentage of staff trained for use of RDT/ACT.
- Percentage of diagnostic facilities functional for microscopy and RDT in the last reporting period.
- Percentage of fever cases with access to complete diagnosis and treatment.

The Major Externally Supported Projects[16]

Additional support for combating malaria is provided through external assistance in high-risk areas of malaria under following projects:

1 World Bank aided Roll Back malaria and enhanced malaria control project (EMCP)—1997–2005 in tribal areas of 8 states.

2 Global fund for Aids, TB, Malaria (GFATM) supported intensified malaria control project (IMCP) July 2005 to June 2010 in 106 districts of 10 states namely 7 North-Eastern states and selected high-risk areas in Odisha, Jharkhand and West Bengal. The cardinal features of GFATM projects were strengthening of surveillance, manpower, rapid diagnostic test (RDT) for early diagnosis of malaria and complete treatment with Artesunate combination Therapy (ACT) along with ITN and LLINs as personal measures. These measures helped to achieve decline in malaria incidence by 34.7%.

3 World bank supported project on malaria control and kala-azar elimination (March 2009 to December 2013).

The project is being implemented in 93 malarious districts of 8 states and 46 kala-azar districts in these states. Additional support provided in this project are rolling out of ACT for treatment of *P. falciparum* Cases, LLINs affected villages, RDT kits besides strengthening of monitoring and supervision, public–private partnership is one of the important strategies to be implemented in project districts.

Urban Vector Borne Disease (UVBD) Scheme

The UVBD under NVBDCP is being implemented in 131 towns with population more than 40,000 in 19 states and union territories. Since 1971, protecting 130 million population. The UMS aims at:

a To prevent deaths due to malaria
b Reduction in transmission and morbidity.

Epidemiological Situation

About 10% of total cases of malaria and deaths were reported from urban areas during 2008 to 2013 in the country.

The control of urban malaria lies primarily in the implementation of urban by-laws to prevent mosquito breeding in domestic and peridomestic areas, and government buildings. Larvicides are applied on weekly basis in water bodies that are unsuitable for fish use. The Government of India supplies larvicides to municipalities under Urban Malaria Scheme. The UMS is implemented by the state authorities, including salary of staff employed for spraying the larvicides.

Urban malaria continues to pose problems because of unplanned rapid urbanization, migration of labour for construction or jobs in the industrial set-up of urban location. The urban malaria vector is *A. stephensi*, breeds in stored water and domestic containers. Construction activities and aggregation of labour provide ideal opportunities for transmission of urban malaria. Fifteen large cities in India account for nearly 80% of cases of urban malaria scheme.

The norms for establishment of UMS are as follows:

- The town should have minimum population of 40,000.
- API should be 2 or above.
- Town would promulgate and strictly implement the civic by-laws to prevent/eliminate domestic and peridomestic breeding places.

Staffing pattern: A biologist is an overall in charge, is provided to supervise and monitor the scheme. Regular antilarval staff for each of 2.56 sq. km sector consists of superior field worker one, field workers two and a field worker for desilting, deweeding and minor levelling. Each ward has one malaria inspector and one insect collector.

Under UMS, the following strategies are followed:

Parasite Control

- To provide treatment to patients through passive surveillance by institutions such as hospitals, dispensaries and malaria clinics. One malaria clinic for 50,000 population is proposed in high-risk urban areas for early diagnosis and prompt treatment with the support of laboratory technician.

12

Vector Control

- ***Source reduction:*** Minor engineering methods like deweeding, desilting and levelling, etc. (environmental manipulation).
- Recurrent antilarval measures by larvicide like temephos (Abate) in towns once a week or mosquito larvicidal oil—MLO (Malariol), or kerosene oil.
- Biological control measures using larvivorus fish like gambusia and guppy fish.
- Awareness campaigns such as observance of anti-malaria month in June every year.
- ***Aerosol-space spray:*** 50 houses in and around every positive case are sprayed with 0.1% pyrethrum.

It is worth pointing that urban health services are weak and not well organized in slum population and accessibility and availability of primary health care is inadequate. Local bodies do not have enough funds and do not control slums development. Hence, urban slum population is high-risk population for malaria because of high density of population, overcrowding, and favourable breeding grounds for mosquito. Hence, urban malaria clinic must be located in urban slum area and urban health posts and RCH projects in slum areas can enhance malaria detection and ensure prompt treatment to reduce morbidity and deaths.

Drug Resistance/Sensitivity in Falciparum Malaria

Drug sensitivity status in the country was being assessed by conventional WHO *in vivo* protocol till 2002.

Interpretation of Conventional WHO Standard in vivo Field Test (7 Days Test)—Old Protocol

S/R I—If no asexual parasites are found by day 6 and none are present on day 7, the infection may be either sensitive (S) or resistance at R I level.

R I—If asexual parasites disappear for at least 2 consecutive days but return and are present on day 7 they are resistant at R I level.

R II—If asexual parasitaemia does not clear but is reduced to 25% or less of the original pretest level during the first 48 hours of treatment, the parasites are resistant at R II level.

R III—If asexual parasitaemia is reduced by less than 75% during the first 48 hours or if it continues to rise, the parasites are resistant at R III level.

New Criteria for Drug Sensitivity/Resistance[17]

From 2002 to 03 WHO protocol on "therapeutic efficacy of antimalarial drugs in uncomplicated *P. falciparum* malaria" is being followed for assessment of drug sensitivity status. In the new protocol, both clinical and parasitological responses are being assessed. The classification of response to treatment has been modified and is interpreted into 3 categories, i.e. adequate clinical and parasitological response (ACPR), early treatment failure (ETF) and late treatment failure (LTF). Till date drug policy was changed for primary health centres reporting 25% or more total treatment failure (ETF + LTF) to chloroquine (first line of treatment) in a sample of minimum 30 *P. falciparum* test cases. NVBDCP has lowered the cut off point (presently from 25 to 10% of total treatment failure) for initiating the process for switching over to ACT combination (AS + SP) therapy in areas of chloroquine resistance. The reasons attributed for implications using drug with low efficacy is that once the drug resistance has emerged in a locality, the continued use of the failing drug will result in the rapid spread of drug resistance in the area.

Classification of treatment outcomes:

Intense-transmission area

Early treatment failure (ETF)
• Development of danger signs or severe malaria on day 1, day 2 or day 3 in the presence of parasitemia • Parasitemia on day 2 higher than day 0 count irrespective of axillary temperature • Parasitemia on day 3 with axillary temperature ≥37.5°C. • Parasitemia on day 3 ≥25% of count on day 0

(a) Late treatment failure (LCF)
• Development of danger signs or severe malaria after day 3 in the presence of parasitemia, without previously meeting any of the criteria of *early treatment failure* • Presence of parasitemia and axillary temperature ≥37.5°C on any day from day 4 to day 14 without previously meeting any of the criteria of *early treatment failure*

(b) Late parasitological failure (LPF)
Presence of parasitemia on day 14 and axillary temperature <37.5°C, without previously meeting any of the criteria of *early treatment failure* or *late clinical failure*

Adequate clinical and parasitological response (ACPR)
Absence of parasitemia on day 14 irrespective of axillary temperature without previously meeting any of the criteria of *early treatment failure or late treatment failure or late parasitological failure*

Source: WHO 2003 assessment and monitoring of antimalarial drug efficiency for the treatment of uncomplicated falciparum malaria. WHO, Geneva.

Note

***Late clinical failure*:** There is a single definition of late clinical failure—regardless of transmission intensity. However, minor variations exist—because of differences in recommended duration of follow-up (14 days for intense transmission areas, 28 days for low to moderate transmission areas).

From 1978 to 2002, 16,833 *P. falciparum* cases have been subjected to conventional *in vivo* test (as per old protocol). Of these, 13,053 (77.5%) were sensitive to chloroquine, 2361 (14.0%) showing resistance at R I level, 813 (4.8%) at R II and 612 (3.7%) at R III level.

Therapeutic efficacy studies have been initiated from 2002 onwards so far 2527 *P. falciparum* cases have been tested against chloroquine. Of these, 1522 (60.2%) have shown adequate clinical and parasitological response (ACPR) and 1005 (39.8%) have shown treatment failure (both ETF + LTF). Out of 168 cases studied with sulpha-pyrimethamine, 151cases (90%) have shown adequate clinical and parasitological response.

G. Programme Planning and Management

The Programme planning and management has been decentralized to the village level and subcentre level. Annual district action plans for malaria elimination are prepared by aggregation of villages, subcentres, PHCs and CHCs plans. Ideally it should be part of district health action plan developed under National Health Mission. Every annual plan is based on the experience of previous year. Village health and Sanitation and Nutrition Committees should be involved in planning process district annual plan on malaria elaborates population to be covered, status of health facilities, human resources, epidemiological situation of malaria, high-risk areas and population, information on outbreaks in the previous year, estimation of RDT, ACT and LLIN requirement, microplanning for IRS, training activities, BCC activities, commodity requirement, cash assistance and budget. District plans converge into State Plans and National Plans is evolved by directorate of NVBDCP at the national level. Management and accountability at each level is critical to achieve the elimination goals and targets to defeat malaria.[18]

REFERENCES

1 GOI. Malaria and its control in India. Country Scenario. New Delhi: NAMP, MOH and FW; 1999.

2 Directorate of National Malaria Eradication Programme (India). Operational manual for malaria action programme, New Delhi, 1995.

3 GOI. Annual Report 2007–2009. New Delhi: GOI Ministry of Health and Family Welfare.

4 GOI. NMEP Malaria Action Programme; Based on Expert Committee Report, New Delhi. GOI: NMEP, DGHS, MOH and FW; 1995.

5 NICD. NVBDCP—Status of malaria in India up to 2009.

6 Ray AP, Narasimhan MVVL, Kalra NL. Malaria—A Brochure for Medical Officers. Indian Society for Malaria and Other Communicable Diseases 1991; 1(1).

7 Sharma RS, Sharma GK, Dhillon GPS. Epidemiology and control of malaria in India. First edition. New Delhi: Government of India, MOH and FW: NMEP, DGHS, 1996.

8 WHO. Malaria Diagnosis, New Perspectives WHO. Report of a Joint WHO/USAID Informal Consultation. Geneva: WHO; 1999.

9 GOI. National Drug Policy on Malaria (2010 and 2013). Directorate of NVBDCP, DGHS, MOH and FW, 22 Shamnath Marg, Delhi.

10 ICMR Bulletin. Chemical insecticides in malaria vector control in India New Delhi, ICMR 2002; 32(10).

11 Haq S, Yadav RS, Kohli VK. ICMR Bulletin. Developing larvivorus fish network for mosquito control in urban areas. New Delhi: ICMR 2003; 33(7).

12 Govt. of India (GOI). Some Important Outbreaks of Malaria of India during 2000. New Delhi, CD Alert 2001; 5(1).

13 Aggarwal OP, Bhasin SK, Chaturvedi S, Sharma AK. A study of Knowledge Attitude and Practices regarding malaria in Indian Population. National Anti-malaria Programme. New Delhi: MOH and FW, GOI; 2001.

14 GOI. Operational manual for Implementation of malaria programme 2009. Directorate of NVBDCP, DGHS, MOH and FW. GOI; New Delhi.

15 GOI. Strategic Action Plan for malaria control in India 2007–2012 "Scaling up malaria control interventions with a focus on high burden areas". Directorate of NVBDCP, DGHS, MOH and FW. GOI: 22 Shamnath Marg, Delhi.

16 WHO. Roll Back Malaria (RBM) Advocacy Guide WHO/CDS/RBM. WHO 2000; 26.

17 WHO. Assessment and Monitoring of Antimalarial Drug Efficacy for the treatment of uncomplicated Falciparum Malaria. WHO; Geneva, 2003.

18 GOI, MOH and FW, National Framework for malaria Elimination in India 2016–30. Directorate of NVBDCP, DGHS New Delhi.

FILARIA

Filaria is a vector-borne disease; it covers wide range of manifestations. Of all, lymphatic filariasis deserves utmost attention because of its wider implications in terms of disease burden, deformity and disability, social stigma and economic loss. Lymphatic filariasis is a vector-borne parasitic disease caused by lymphatic dwelling nematode parasites namely *Wuchereria bancrofti*, *Brugia malayi* and *Brugia timori known as filariae*. The filariasis manifests as progressive lymphoedema leading to disfiguring elephantiasis, hydrocele and loss of respiratory function due to tropical pulmonary eosinophilia.

Global Disease Burden

12

Globally, there are nearly 1400 million people in 73 countries living in areas endemic for lymphatic filariasis and are exposed to the risk of infection. There are 120 million clinical cases of filariasis either having latent microfilaraemia or chronic filarial disease. *W. bancrofti* accounts for 90% of all filarial cases in the world followed by *B. malayi* and *B. timori*.[1] India contributes 40% of global burden of lymphatic filariasis.

Problem of Filariasis in India

The disease is widespread and endemic in many states. Nearly 650 million people are living in endemic states and are at risk of infection.

The line listing of lymphoedema and hydrocele cases were initiated since 2004 by door-to-door survey of filaria in 250 filaria endemic districts. The updated figures till October 2014 revealed 8 lakh lymphoedema and 4 lakh hydrocele cases (Total of 12 Lakh cases with clinical manifestations).[1,2]

Distribution

Rural-urban

Initially, filariasis was thought to affect urban and peri-urban areas only, but rural areas are equally affected with the disease, hence the control measures, which are predominantly restricted to urban areas, have to cover the rural areas as well. The filaria infection and disease affects children and adults. Children show high prevalence of filaria antigenaemia making them important target for intervention.

Social and Economic Effect of Filariasis

Lymphatic filariasis mostly affects economically weaker sections of people living in urban slums and rural areas and makes them poorer. The disease produces progressive physical deformities in limbs (lower legs and upper limbs) and reduces the work capacity of affected individuals. Lymphatic filariasis is the second leading cause of permanent physical disability in human beings next only to mood disorders. As over 1.2 million people are suffering from disease and various grades of lymphoedema the economic losses are colossal. Economic loss due to filariasis has been estimated to be Rs. 5000 crore per annum. Apart from economic loss, the affected person carries a social stigma and is looked down upon by the society.

Reservoir of Infection

Individuals who have circulating microfilaria in their blood are known as carriers of microfilaria. We had in India around 29.7 million microfilaria carriers who were potent source of infection to other healthy individuals in the area. India has large reservoir of infection, being maintained in the endemic areas. The goal of filaria elimination is to reduce this reservoir to a minimal acceptable level. These individuals should be targeted for intervention programme. National programme of filaria control and elimination is focusing on mass drug administration (MDA) for interruption of transmission.

Transmission

Filariasis is a vector-borne disease. *Culex quinquefasciatus* is the vector of bancroftian filariasis. In India 99.4% of infections are caused by *W. bancrofti*. In endemic areas, the vector breeds in polluted water, high humidity is favorable for breeding. This vector is endophilic (rests inside the house after blood meal) and anthropophilic (bites human being). The transmission is seasonal. The density of this vector is low in summer season and is on peak in monsoon and post-monsoon period. Vector for *Brugia malayi* is Mansonioides group of mosquitoes. This form of filariasis is confined to a limited geographical area of Kerala. *Mansonioides annulifera* and *M. uniformis* are the major vectors for *B. malayi,* these breed in polluted water ponds with vegetation of *pistia stratiotes* (a kind of plant or hyacinth). The larvae of the vector have special affinity with *Pistia plant*.

The parasite cycle in the mosquito begins when the microfilariae are picked up by the vector mosquitoes during their feeding on the infected person (microfilaria carrier).

The microfilaria in mosquito develops into three stages and under optimum conditions of temperature and humidity; the duration of the cycle in mosquito (extrinsic incubation period) is about 10–14 days. When the infective mosquito feeds on other human host, the infective larvae are deposited at the site of mosquito bite from where the infective larvae get into lymphatic system. In the human host, the infective larvae develop into adult male and female worms. The adult worm survives for about 5–8 years or sometime as long as 15 years or more.

Incubation interval: Variable usually long incubation period of several years. The time interval between the introduction of infective larvae and first appearance of detectable microfilaria is known as "Pre-patent" period. It usually varies from 1 to 1½ years. The peak prevalence of infection occurs in age bracket 20–30 years, which can be considered as target age for case detection.

Epidemiological Indices for Filaria to Estimate Filaria Endemicity

1 ***Microfilaria (Mf.) rate:*** Percentage of persons whose blood smears are positive for Mf. If it is 1 or more than 1% the area is chosen for mass drug administration.
2 ***Disease rate:*** Percentage of persons having visible lymphoedema, hydrocele (clinical signs of filaria). 12.0 lacs have clinical disease in India.
3 ***Average endemicity rate:*** Percentage of persons showing Mf. in the blood or disease manifestation (Mf. % plus disease %) or both.
4 ***Average Mf. density:*** Mean number of Mf. per 20 cmm of blood.
5 ***Average infestation rate:*** Average number of Mf. per positive slide.
6 Vector density per man hour.
7 ***Infected vector rate:*** Percentage of mosquitoes showing any stage of Mf. (L1/L2/L3 stages).
8 ***Infective vector rate:*** Percentage of mosquitoes showing *Mf. larvae* stage three only (infective larvae).
9 ***High endemic districts:*** Mf. rate 1% and above.
10 ***Low endemic districts:*** Mf. rate below 1%.
11 Coverage levels achieved with MDA. It should be above 80% for 5–6 years.

NATIONAL FILARIA CONTROL PROGRAMME (NFCP)

India mounted its NFCP in 1955. Currently, the programme covers 52.93 million population of 20 endemic states/UTs. Though the total at risk population is around 600 million, of this 120 million is the urban population. Currently (April 2005) there were 206 filaria control units, 199 filaria clinics and 27 filaria survey units to cover 52.93 million population in endemic areas. Only high endemic areas (Mf rate >5%) have been chosen for large scale control mearsures because of limited resources, for following activities:

Activities

- Recurrent weekly antilarval operations and biological control of vector through larvivorus fish.
- Source reduction through environmental and water management.
- Diagnosis and treatment of microfilaria carriers and management of cases in filaria clinics.
- IEC for community awareness.

Detection of Carriers

This is being done through night blood survey before MDT as Mf. appears in peripheral circulation during night. Surveillance operations during night (8.30 pm to midnight) are difficult and unpopular.

Because of these problems, a need was felt for development of rapid, specific, sensitive and reproducible diagnostic methods for field application for the detection of infection (microfilaraemia or adult parasites) both in humans and in vector mosquitoes. A rapid day blood immunochromatographic card test (ICT) has been found highly specific and more sensitive in India in comparison with the night blood smear examination. Although it is costlier, it has the advantage of on the spot, day blood detection of parasite carriers in large number (compared to night blood smear examinations).

Surveys: Microfilaria survey in all the implementation units (districts) is being done through night blood survey before MDA. The survey is done in 4 sentinel and 4 random sites collecting total 4000 slides (500 from each site) to know the prevalence of microfilaria in an area and to decide MDT.

NATIONAL FILARIA ELIMINATION PROGRAMME (NFEP)[3–7]

Filariasis has been identified as one of the 6 diseases (among over hundred considered); which could be targeted for elimination/eradication based on the epidemiological considerations.

- Human beings are the only reservoir of infection.
- Diethylcarbamazine (DEC) is the effective drug acting on the parasite is available without report of resistance over 5 decades. Mass annual single dose with selective vector control could eliminate infection by interruption of transmission.

Goal: To achieve less than one percent microfilaria prevalence in all the districts.

ELIMINATION OF LYMPHATIC FILARIASIS (ELF) BY 2015

The elimination has been defined as "Lymphatic filariasis ceases to be a public health problem, when the number of microfilaria carriers is less than 1% and the children born after antigenaemia."

India aimed to achieve the goal of LF elimination by 2015. The programme was initiated on pilot basis in 13 out of the 250 endemic districts during 1996–97 with DEC alone and thereafter with DEC and Albendazole. The Programme has been gradually scaled up to cover all the 250 endemic districts spread over in 20 states and UTs targeting 600 million population at risk.

World Health Assembly (WHA) passed a resolution in 1997 for global elimination of lymphatic filariasis by 2020. India's National Health Policy—2002 has targeted elimination of lymphatic filariasis by following strategies:

Anti-Parasitic Measures

Mass Drug Administration (MDA) (for Interruption of Transmission)

- Supervised annual mass drug admmistration (MDA) of single dose of DEC + Albendazole for a minimum five rounds or more to the eligible population (except pregnant women children below 2 years of age and seriously ill persons) to interrupt transmission of filarial.
- Home based management of Lymphoedema cases and upscaling of hydrocoele operations in identified CHCs/ district hospitals/medical colleges.

Antivector measures to continue in all NFCP towns as complementary to antiparasitic measures and microfilaria carries detected in filarial clinics and elsewhere to receive standard dose of DEC @ 6 mg/kg per day for 12 days.

- Information, education and communication for protective and preventive measures for filaria control.

Drug Dosage Schedule—Streamlined (Table 12.23)

Annual supervised single dose mass chemotherapy with DEC, agewise dose schedule: The single day mass DEC treatment will be as per the existing dose, i.e. 6 mg/kg body weight. Since, it is not feasible to weigh every individual in the field to calculate the exact dose to be administered, it is convenient to adjust the dose schedule as per different age groups adopted in the programme.

Note

i The advantage of streamlined DEC dosage is that the number of tablets are less and the three doses can easily be remembered by the peripheral drug administrator (Table 12.23).

ii In 7 districts (6 in Tamil Nadu and one in Kerala) under co-administration, 400 mg albendazole is administered along with DEC to all the eligible population (2 years and above age groups except pregnant women and critically ill persons).

Individual Treatment

The Mf. carriers detected in filaria clinics and elsewhere will receive standard dose 6 mg/kg body wt/day for 12 days.

Adult and children above 10 years of age are given full dose 6 mg/kg body weight and children below 10 years are given half of the adult dose.

Use of DEC fortified salt is another intervention recommended for filaria control.

Approach: "Supervised drug administration by door to door visit supplemented with drug administration at booth" on a single day with three days mopping operation in all 250 endemic districts since 2004.

Inclusion Criterion for MDA

The MDA was launched in 2004. The selected district or PHC should meet the criteria of 1% or more microfilaria rate for inclusion under MDA.

DEC is as effective as ivermectin in drastically reducing the levels of transmission. Mass drug administration

Table 12.23: Streamlined DEC drug dosage schedule

Age in years	*Dose of DEC 100 mg each*	*No. of tablets*
<2	Nil	Nil
2–5	100 mg	1
6–14	200 mg	2
15 and above	300 mg	3

12

(MDA) or fortified salt requires effective methods of delivery system, through primary health care, integrated child development services (ICDS) and involvement of non-governmental organizations apart from massive education of people.

National Filaria Day (NFD)

Convincing healthy persons and carriers of Mf. to consume DEC on National Filaria Day (NFD) once every year for 5–7 years or more can eliminate lymphatic filariasis, in community. Integrated control of vector and mass chemotherapy can achieve better results.

Coverage level: Actual consumption of DEC tablets by more than 85% of population is the most critical aspect in this programme to achieve success. Persistent coverage of above 80% for 5–7 years can reduce the microfilaria rate and thereby interrupt the transmission in community.

Selective Mass Therapy

Only persons who are Mf. positive are given single dose of DEC 6 mg/kg body wt. per annum in known endemic areas of lymphatic filariasis.

Advantages of MDA

Advantages of single dose mass therapy:

i It avoids the cost of mass blood examination.

ii All members of community receive treatment and compliance rate is enhanced.

iii It is as effective as 12 days therapy for public health measure.

iv It has lesser side effects.

v It involves decreased delivery cost.

vi It does not require complex management infrastructure.

vii It can be integrated into existing primary health care system for delivery.

viii Single dose mass treatment annually has either eliminated or markedly reduced the transmission of lymphatic filariasis in some countries.

Side Effects of DEC

a Those due to drug itself: Headache, anorexia, nausea, abdominal pain, vomiting, dizziness, weakness and lethargy. These symptoms begin within 1–2 hours of taking drug and persist for few hours.

b Those due to allergic reactions due to destruction of microfilariae and adult worms: Fever, local inflammation around dead worms.

Disability Prevention and Control (for Relief of Sufferings)

This intervention aims at:

- Home-based management of lymphoedema by assisting lymph flow through elevation, exercises, bandages and personal hygiene.
- Prevention of acute inflammatory episodes by preventing secondary bacterial infection by use of soap and water, hygiene, skin care and treatment of "entry lesion".
- Hydrocele management by surgical repairs.
- Disability prevention and control clinics have started functioning at Varanasi, Calicut and Rajahmundry in endemic states.

Achievements

- MDA with DEC and albendazole has been scaled up 53 districts have stopped MDT after sucessfully passing TAS.
- 203 districts out of 250 endemic districts have achieved microfilaria prevalence less than 1%

Coverage of MDA and Microfilaria Rates-Trends

Years	2004	2005	2006	2007	2014
• Population coverage (%)	72	76	82	83	46.42–85.60
• Microfilaria rate (%)	1.24	1.02	0.98	0.64	0.52 to 0.44

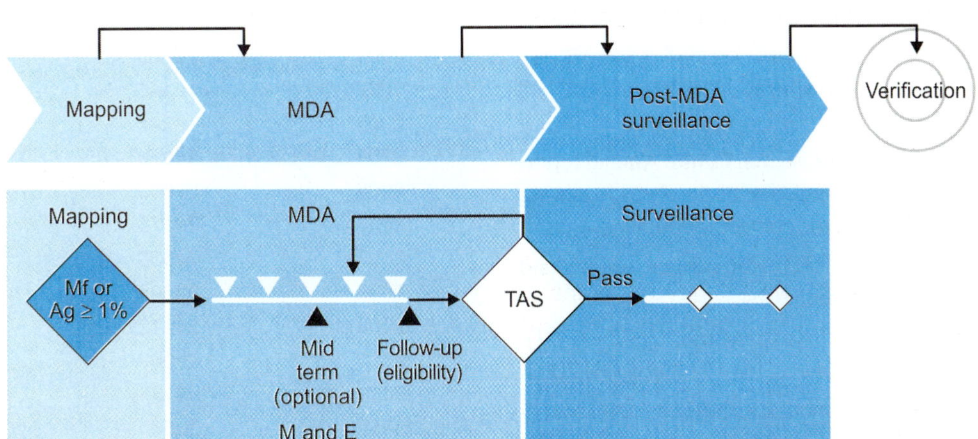

Fig. 12.13: Steps for interrupting transmission of lymphatic filariasis by mass drug administration (MDA) as described by WHO in 2011

12

- The coverage levels have increased over 80% and microfilaria rates have steadily declined to 0.44% over the years.[8, 9]

Transmission Assessment Survey (TAS)[10]

Effective monitoring and evaluation are necessary to achieve the goals of LF elimination. After mass administration of medicines, programme must be able to assess whether the interventions have succeeded in lowering the prevalence of infection to a level at which transmission is no longer likely to be sustainable. Transmission Assessment Survey (TAS) is a decision making tool which is designed to provide a simple, robust survey design for documenting that the prevalence of lymphatic filariasis among 6–7 year old children is below a predetermined threshold. It provides the evidence base that MDA can be stopped and to assure that program has achieved elimination goal. Area passes TAS if it has successfully implemented MDA for minimum of five years with at leastor more than 65% of population coverage in each round and have achieved microfilaraemia rate of less than 1% or that of antigenaemia of 2% at all sentinel sites (Fig. 12.00). All such districts which have successfully completed TAS are put under post MDA surveillance.

Morbidity survey: Door to door morbidity survey in non endemic districts by ASHA to detect LF foci.

The problems faced: Inadequate coverage of population and poor compliance of drug therapy is a big problem. Carriers of Mf. are healthy individuals and other healthy people in high endemic areas refuse to take drug.

Actual consumption (compliance) should be considered as major criterion rather than drug distribution.

REFERENCES

1 ICMR. Mathematical modelling for optimizing and predicting outcome of intervention measures for the control of lymphatic filariasis. ICMR Bulletin 2002 Jan; 32(1).

2 ICMR. Clinical features, pathogenesis and management of lymphatic filariasis. ICMR Bulletin 1998 May; 28(5).

3 ICMR. Prospects of Elimination of Lymphatic Filariasis in India. ICMR Bulletin 2002 May–June; 32 (5 and 6).

4 ICMR/WHO. Vector Control Research Centre Annual report 2000. WHO collaborating centre for research and training in integrated methods of vector control, 2000.

5 GOI. Annual Report 2002–2003. Ministry of Health and Family Welfare, Govt. of India, 2004.

6 Planning Commission. 10th Five-Year Plan 2002–07 (II). Sectoral Policies and Programmes, New Delhi: GOI; 2002.

7 NICD Lymphatic Filariasis Elimination. Disability Prevention and Control—An important intervention CD Alert. Monthly Newsletter of NICD, DGHS, Govt. of India, 2001 July; 5(7).

8 GOI. Operational guidelines on elimination of lymphatic filariasis, Directorate of NVBDCP, DGHS, MOH and FW, GOI, 2005.

9 GOI. MOH and FW; GOI Annual Reports 2004–12.

10 GOI, MOH and FW, DGHS, NVBDCP, National Roadmap for Elimination of Lymphatic Filariasis 2015.

KALA-AZAR (VL)

Kala-azar (*Visceral leishmaniasis*) is caused by *Leishmania donovani* is confined to man only with no animal reservoir.

It is a vector-borne disease transmitted by sandfly belonging to genus *Phlebotomus*.

Distribution

It is worldwide distributed affecting 88 countries. About 350 million people are exposed to the risk of VL. India Bangladesh, Nepal, Sudan and Brazil contribute 90% cases of visceral leishmaniasis (VL). According to WHO estimates, more than 10 million are affected globally and 50% VL cases are from Indian subcontinent.

Indian Scenario

Presently kala-azar is endemic in 54 districts, 33 districts of Bihar, 11 in West Bengal, 6 in UP, 4 in Jharkhand are endemic and reporting cases of VL or kala-azar. Total cases and deaths reported from 1992 to 2014 are depicted in Table 12.24. Cutaneous leishmaniasis has been reported from Himachal Pradesh and Uttarakhand as well. Over 130 million population is exposed to the risk of kala-azar

Table 12.24: Trends of kala-azar in India[1]

Year	Cases	Deaths
1992	77102	1419
1996	27049	687
1997	17419	255
1998	13627	226
1999	12886	297
2001	12239	213
2002	12140	168
2003	18214	210
2004	24479	155
2005	32803	157
2006	39178	187
2007	44533	203
2008	33598	151
2009	24212	93
2010	29000	105
2011	33187	80
2012	20600	29
2013	10140	15
2014	9241	11

in the endemic areas. KA has been declared a notifiable disease in Bihar and west Bengal.

The causative agent for VL and PKDL in India is the Leishmania donovani. There are two distinct stages in the life cycle of parasite.

i Amastigote (aflagellar) or Leishmania stagewhich occurs in man. Man is the only host of Leishmania donovani in India

ii Promastigote (flagellar) or Leptomonad stage occurs in gut of sandfly and artificial culture.

The parasite (Leishmnia donovani primarily affects reticuloendothelial system and found in abundance in bone marrow, spleen and liver.

Vector

Visceral leishmaniasis or kala-azar is transmitted by the bite of infected female sandflies. **Phlebotoms argentipes** is the only known vector of kala-azar in India.

Incubation Period

Generally it varies form 1–4 months but in realty the range is from 10 days to 2 years (in India range is 4 months to one year). Extrinsic incubation period in vector is 4–25 days which is the time required for the vector to become infective after an infective blood meal.

Outbreaks and Resurgence

Resurgence of kala-azar has been a perpetual problem in Bihar and UP.

Indian Scenario

In India, two types of leishmaniasis are prevalent: visceral leishmaniasis (VL) and cutaneous leishmaniasis (CL). VL is usually fatal when untreated. CL is disabling disease when lesions are multiple. Post kala-azar dermal Leishmaniasis (PKDL) is a condition in which *L. Donovani* invades cells of skin.

NATIONAL KALA-AZAR (KA) ELIMINATION PROGRAMME

Kal-azar elimination is on top priority under WHO neglected Tropical diseases.

Centrally sponsored kala-azar control programme has been operative since 1991 for control of disease in endemic areas. The programme has been successful in reducing the morbidity and mortiality due to kala-azar as is evident through decline in annual incidence and 99%of reduction of deaths in 2014 as compared to 1992 (Table 12.24). Based on the recommendations of the expert committee in 2003 the government of India approved 100% central assistance for kala-azar elimination by 2015. Out of 514 KA endemic blocks 320 have achieved the target of elimination.[2–4]

Elimination: Elimination is defined as reducing the annual incidence of kala-azar to less than 1 case per 10,000 population at the sub-district level (block PHC)

Goal: The national goal is elimination of KA by 2015.

Objective

- Reducing the incidence of KA in the endemic communities.
- Reducing case fatality due to KA
- Treatment of Post kala-azar dermal leishmaniasis (PKLD) to reduce the parasite reservoir.
- Prevention and treatment of KA-HIV, TB Co-infection.

Strategies

- Early diagnosis and complete treatment (EDCT)
- Integrated vector management and vector surveillance
- Advocacy, communication for behavior impact and intersectoral convergence
- Capacity building
- Programme management (supervision, monitoring and evaluation).

Early Diagnosis and Complete Treatment (EDCT)

EDCT includes diagnosing a case early along with complete treatment to interrupt transmission. This strategy will reduce case fatality. The starting point for early diagnosis is to follow uniform suspect case definition.

- **A suspect case:** History of fever of more than 2 weeks and enlarged spleen and liver not responding to anti-malaria treatment in an endemic area.
- All patients with above symptoms should be screened with rapid diagnostic test (rk 39) and if found positive should be treated with effective drug.
- Or a patient with above symptoms clinically examined by doctor and found positive on screening with rapid diagnostic test (rk 39).
- Or in case with past history of Kala-azar or in those with high suspicion of Kala-azar but with negative RDT test result-confirmation of Kala-azar can be done by examination of bone marrow/spleen aspirate for LD bodies at district hospital.

Treatment

Injection liposomal amphotericin B (LAMB) in single day singal dose of 10 mg/kg as the first choice of treatment regimen. Other treatment regimen are:

i Combination of miltefosine and paromomycin injection

ii Amphotericin B emulsion

iii Capsule miltefosine for 28 days.

iv Injection amphotericin B (15 injections on alternate day).

- Post kala-azar dermal leishmaniasis are to be treated with:
  - i Liposomal amphotericin B 5 mg/kg by infusion two times per week for 3 weeks for a total dose of 30 mg/kg or
  - ii Miltefosine: 100 mg orally per day for 12 weeks or
  - iii Amphotericin B deoxycholate: 1 mg/kg over 4 months 60–80 doses.

Surveillance for EDCT[5-6]

KA disease surveillance is useful in planning IRS through mapping of areas to be sprayed and monitoring trends of kala-azar incidence.

Passive surveillance is the mainstay of the programme. This means regular, timely and accurate reporting (collection of information for action) on kala-azar cases who seek diagnosis and treatment form health facility in the Government, Private or NGO sector (PHC, CHC, District Hospitals).

Active Surveillance (Active Case Search)

Active surveillance implies active search of Kala-azar and PKDL case. Active surveillance in India at present is being done on **Quarterly active search basis.** Health workers and volunteers visit households to find out individuals with fever of more than 2 weeks duration. Suspected cases are referred to PHC for clinical examination and rapid diagnostic test for confirmation of diagnosis and treatment initiation.

Surveillance of Post Kala-azar Dermal Leishmaniasis (PKDL)

Surveillance of PKDL cases in important as PKDL cases serve as reservoir of disease transmission during the inter-epidemic period. Reporting of PKDL cases is an integral part of the programme for diagnosis and complete treatment.

Vector Surveillance (Entomological Surveillance)

Vector surveillance (sand fly) means identification of breeding places, critical density of vector and control measures.

Integrated Vector Management (IVM)

The main objective of IVM is to reduce longevity of the adult vectors, eliminate breeding sites, decrease contact of vectors with humans and reduce the density of vector, sand fly. IRS is the mainstay of vector control for breaking human-vector-human cycle of transmission. Vector control is carried out by undertaking two rounds of spray annually with 50% DDT at a dose of 1 g/m^2 of wall surface inside walls of rooms up to height of 6 feet and full coverage of cattle sheds. In view of tolerance/resistance to 50% DDT it has been decided to use synthetic Pyrethroids (SP) in seven districts reporting DDT tolerance as also high endemicity of kala-azar during 2015. More areas will be covered with SP in phased manner.

12

Programme Management (Supervision, Monitoring and Evaluation)

This involves coordination between centre and state and different sectors including private health sector and NGOs. Programme management is vital for success of elimination of KA. There is need to strengthen surveillance system for KA and PKDL including line listing of cases at village level to identify hot spot areas (villages reporting five or more cases in previous or current year), and update areas for microplanning for spray operations. Involvement private sector to capture complete burden of diseases. Since the emergence of VL–HIV and TB Co-infection is posing threat on achievements, surveillance of VL-HIV cases is important apart from early and long-term follow-up of KA and PKDL, Cases (6 and 12 months respectively) as well as informationon on relapses. Evaluation or validation of elimination will pave the way towards further reducing KA burden in the community.

Advocacy, Communication and Social Mobilization for behavioural Impact and Intersectoral Convergence

Information on KA must be communicated to people in endemic areas to promote community participation for effective utilization of services provided under the programme. Interpersonal communication by health workers and available media/channels of communication including local channels should be used effectively and maximally

Capacity Building

Continuing education/training of health volunteers (ASHAs) health workers, medical officers, and health managers and other stakeholders on newer strategies of KA elimination is essential to achieve the targets and goals of elimination apart from continuum of services.

REFERENCES

1 GOI. Annual Reports 2008–09 to 2012–13. New Delhi. MOH and FW, GOI.

2 WHO. Formulary based on 13th model list of essential medicines 2003: Geneva: WHO; 2004.

3 Planning Commission. Tenth Five-Year Plan 2002–07. New Delhi: GOI; 2002.

4 GOI. CD Alert. Monthly Newsletter of NICD, DGHS, January 2006; (10) 1.

5 NHM, NVBDCP, Operational Guidelines on Kala-azar (Visceral Leishmaniasis) elimination in India 2015.

6 MOH and FW and DGHS, DNVBDCP; National Road Map for Kala-azar Elimination 2014

DENGUE/DENGUE HAEMORRHAGIC FEVER

Problem

Dengue fever is an outbreak prone viral disease in many parts of the world and is *re-emerging* global health problem.

Dengue infection causes a spectrum of illness that ranges from mild, nonspecific viral syndrome to severe and fatal disease. Dengue fever is an acute febrile illness caused by a flavivirus, which has four serotypes: DEN 1, DEN 2, DEN 3 and DEN 4 respectively.

Distribution

Dengue is *re-emerging* a major national and international public health problem. The geographical distribution is worldwide and it has expanded with speed and number of cases have dramatically increased in the recent past. Dengue is now endemic in more than 141 countries of the world and threatens the health of about 50% of the world's population (4 billion).[1] Unprecedented outbreak of dengue haemorrhagic fever (DHF) swept the National Capital of Delhi in 1996 and thereafter upsurge of cases in many other parts of India during 2003, 2005, 2006 to 2014 have occured.

Extent

Over 1.2 million cases were reported to WHO in 1998, the greatest number ever for a single year. There are an estimated 60–100 (58.40 million cases in 2013) million infections annually, including 0.25–0.5 million cases of dengue haemorrhagic fever (DHF). Dengue costs world about $8.9 billion annually.

Dengue in India: Dengue is endemic in 31 states/UTs with population of over 1100 million at risk. Recurring outbreaks of DF/DHF have been reported from various states/UTs.

Although dengue fever (DF) is known to be endemic in India for over two centuries as a benign and self-limiting disease detected first in vellore in 1956. Etiology of disease was discovered only in 1945 by Sabin who isolated the first dengue virus from soldiers who became ill in Kolkata. The first major outbreak of dengue fever/DHF, which was investigated systematically occurred in Calcutta in 1963 and 1964, DEN 2 virus was isolated in first peak and chikungunya virus was isolated in second peak.

Since 1960, more than 50 outbreaks have been reported to or investigated by the National Institute of Communicable Diseases in different parts of the country.[2]

1996 epidemic of dengue and dengue with haemorrhagic fever (DHF) and dengue shock syndrome (DSS) was worst of its kind, which affected 16517 persons and 545 deaths were reported. Similarly, outbreaks in the year 2003 claimed 215 lives (Reported data),[3–6] 157 deaths in 2005, 184 deaths in 2006, 89 deaths in the year 2009, 110 deaths in year 2010 and 242 deaths in 2012 and 137 deaths in 2014 (Table 12.25). The disease is spreading to newer geographical areas every year.

Epidemiology

DF/DHF is caused by group B arbovirus (flavivirus) and it includes four serotypes (DEN 1, 2, 3 and 4). Epidemics are mostly due to DEN 2. Infection with one type provides lifelong homologous immunity but does not provide protection against the other serotypes. Each person can have as many as four dengue infections in their lifetime, one with each type of virus. The second infection with different type of virus usually results in a severe form of illness, possibly due to sensitization effect of the first one. All four serotypes were seen co-circulating.

Reservoir: Only human reservoir, i.e. case of dengue fever/DHF. No extra-human reservoir of any consequence is known in India. Incubation period is 4–7 days.

Transmission: Dengue fever is transmitted by the bite of an infected female mosquito—*Aedes aegypti*. The mosquito has characteristic white stripes on the back and legs. It usually bites during daytime, early morning and late afternoon. The mosquito becomes infected by biting a patient with dengue infection. The mosquito becomes infective after 8–10 days of taking infective blood meal. Once the mosquito becomes infected, it remains so for lifelong. There is evidence that vertical transmission of

Table 12.25: Reported cases and deaths due to dengue/DHF in India[2] from 1996 to 2014

Year	*Cases*	*Deaths*
1996	16,517	545
1997	1215	37
1999	944	17
2000	650	7
2001	3306	53
2002	1926	33
2003	12,754	215
2004	4153	45
2005	11,985	157
2006	12,317	184
2007	5534	69
2008	12,561	80
2009	15,535	89
2010	28,292	110
2011	18,860	169
2012	50,222	242
2013	75,808	193
2014	40571	137

Source: Annual Report 2003–04 and 2009 MOH and FW GOI and National Health Profile 2005 and 2008 to 2015

dengue from infected female mosquitoes to the next generation occurs through eggs which is known as tranovarian transmission.

Vector: Predominant vector for DF/DHF is female *Aedes aegypti* and less often *Aedes albopictus*. This is also called tiger mosquito.

Risk Factors for Transmission/Resurgence

- Unplanned and uncontrolled urbanization, migration, and population growth.
- Lack of mosquito control measures such as source reduction.
- Poor solid waste management and widespread use of plastic cups, containers, etc.
- Increased population movements.
- Poor public health infrastructure.

Urban–rural distribution: The DF/DHF, which was primarily confined to urban areas or cities is no longer true. It is spreading fast to rural areas as well because of favourable conditions in rural areas and changing lifestyles.

Seasonality: Mostly dengue and DHF are seasonal and peak incidence is observed from mid-August to November.

Re-emerging threat: Dengue had been known to be endemic in India for over two centuries as a benign and self-limiting disease. But in the recent years, the disease has changed its course and manifesting in a severe form as DHF/DSS with increasing frequencies, outbreaks of DHF/DSS have become a perpetual affair.[7–9]

Mortality

DF is benign and self-limiting disease but it has acquired a killing instinct. During 1996, epidemic of Delhi, 4% case fatality was reported even with best of care in best of hospitals. The mortality has been reduced to 0.3% after the national guidelines issued in 2008 and 2015. The goal during 12th plan is to sustain case fatality rate of less than one percent.

Risk of Dengue/DHF and DSS

Dengue infection causes spectrum of illness ranging from subclinical to severe and fatal disease, typical DF is self-limiting with symptomatic treatment. DHF and DSS cases are to be monitored till their recovery. The risk of DHF is approximately 0.2% during the first dengue infection but increases 10 folds during infection with second serotype of dengue virus. However, the circulation of multiple dengue serotypes does not always produce DHF. It has been estimated that during outbreaks between 150 and 200 mild or silent dengue infection occur for each case of DHF/DSS seen in the hospital.

NATIONAL MIDTERM PLAN FOR PREVENTION AND CONTROL OF DENGUE AND CHIKUNGUNYA (2011-13)

Objectives:

- To reduce the incidence of dengue and chikungunya to bring down disease burden.
- To reduce case fatality rate due to dengue

Key eight elements (Octalogue) of midterm plan:

1. Surveillance—disease and entomological
2. Case management
3. Vector management
4. Outbreak response
5. Capacity building
6. Behavior change communication
7. Intersectoral coordination
8. Monitoring and evaluation

1. Surveillance

The objective of surveillance for dengue and chikungunya are to:

- Monitor trends, distribution and spread of disease over time
- Detect cases early for timely intervention
- Measure the disease burden
- To assess the social and economic impact
- Evaluate effectiveness of prevention and control measures.

Dengue and Chikungunya surveillance has two components—Epidemiological and Entomological surveillance.

Epidemiological Surveillance of Dengue Fever (DF)

It is an integral part of Integrated Disease Surveillance Programme (IDSP). For effective epidemiological surveillance of DF uniform data collection as per standard case definition would be carried out on prescribed formats. All suspected, probable and lab. Confirmed cases should be recorded and reported. The disease surveillance includes clinical diagnosis, monitoring of fever trends and sero-surveillance. The medical OPDs of hospitals as principal site for monitoring the clinical cases of DF as per standard case definition and fever cases for an increase/clustering and send samples of suspected/probable cases for sero-surveillance. Data collection, compilation, analysis, interpretation and feedback as also follow-up action are carried out in a systematic and organized manner. Reporting units (facilities such as Subcentres, PHCs, CHCs and Sentinel Hospitals) report once every week on Monday in non or low transmission period and on daily basis during transmission period/outbreaks.

Proactive Surveillance

The most important component of proactive surveillance is serological surveillance designed to monitor dengue virus transmission during inter-epidemic periods and to provide continuously on where transmission is occurring and what virus serotypes are involved. This information helps to detect the introduction of virus into new areas.

For carrying out proactive surveillance and enhancing diagnostic facilities, 347 sentinel surveillance hospitals (SSH) with laboratory support have been set-up in endemic areas and further for advanced diagnosis and back up support 14 Apex Referral laboratories have been identified and linked with SSH. To make them functional test kits are provided free of cost. Further rapid response by concerned health authorities is ensured on report of any suspected case from SSH, to prevent further spread of dengue and chikungunya.[10,11]

Lab Surveillance

Government of India recommends use of ELISA based **antigen detection** test—NS 1 for diagnosing cases from first day onwards to 5th day of onset of fever and **antibody detection** test—IgM capture ELISA (MAC ELISA) for diagnosis of cases after 5th day of onset of disease for confirmation of dengue infection. Due to lack of validation use of rapid diagnostic tests is not recommended under the programme.

Entomological Surveillance and Larval Indices

Vector surveillance should be regular, this helps in identifying areas for initiating control measures and assess impact. The larval indices used to determine the intensity of dengue vector are:[12–14]

- ***House index:*** Percentage of houses positive for larvae or pupae of *Aedes aegypti*. House index provides information on extent of breeding.
- ***Breteau index (BI):*** Number of positive containers for *Aedes aegypti larvae* per 100 houses inspected. BI is used as yardstick for evaluation of control strategy.
- ***Container index:*** Percentage of water holding containers positive for *Aedes* breeding. It is mostly utilized for drawing vector control strategies. However, a single water container found positive for *Aedes* breeding warrants for immediate action for source reduction.
- ***Adult landing/biting rate:*** *Aedes* mosquito can be collected on a human bait and landing rate/bait/hour is calculated. Adult collection in endemic areas is not envisaged as the adult may be infected with virus.

Epidemiological interpretation of various entomological indices[12]

Entomological index	*High-risk of transmission*	*Low-risk of transmission*
I Breteau index	> 50	< 5
II Larval house index	> 10%	< 1%
III Landing/biting rate	> 2 per man hour	< 2 per man hour

Breeding

The life cycle of *Aedes aegypti* is closely associated with the lifestyle of man, more so related to water storage practices.

It is a container mosquito. *Aedes aegypti* breeds profusely around houses in artificial water collection. It can breed efficiently in small collection of water in desert coolers, over head tanks, discarded buckets, tyres, plastic cans, flower vases, broken bottles, earthen pots and other receptacles with rain water or stored clean water stagnating for more than a week.

Eggs are laid above water surface and within 24 hours embryonic development takes place. Eggs can withstand dry conditions without water even up to one year. Mature eggs hatch within a few hours leading to emergence of first instar larva and there are three larval instar and larval development is completed within a weak; they then change into round pupal stage. Pupal stage lasts for 24–30 hours after which the adult mosquito emerges ready to bite. Life cycle is completed in 7–9 days.

Bionomics

It is a daytime biter. Adult female mosquito feeds on human blood (*Aedes aegypti* is highly anthropophilic) Commonly adult seek dark, cool and shady places to rest in bedrooms, bathrooms, kitchen, on unsprayed objects such as clothes, curtains and other hanging fabrics, and furniture. Flight range is 400 meters. At low temperature below 16°C, and above 41–42°C, the mosquito cannot survive.

Vector density of 10–30 per man hour was observed in Delhi epidemic of 1996.

2. Case Management[15]

There is no therapeutic drug for management of dengue and chikungunya. However, symptoms are treated with paracetamol. Aspirin should not be used. Currently no vaccine is available. Supportive therapy is extremely important in dengue particularly preceding or during shock when the blood volume and serum electrolytes are so labile (DHF/DSS). A hematocrit run every one or two hours will indicate whether whole blood, plasma, glucose in saline or other electrolytes are needed parenterally.

3. Vector Management

Aedes aegypti is the main vector for dengue and chikungunya in India. It can be managed by following measures:

Environmental Management for Source Reduction

a. Environmental modifications: Physical transformation of land (land filling) water and vegetation to reduce vector habitats without causing any adverse effect to human environment. Changes to environmental modification are normally long lasting such as improved water supply of sufficient quantity and quality and mosquito proofing of overhead tanks apart from improving drainage system as also solid waste management.

b. Environmental manipulations: Those requires repeated activities in time bound manner such as covering domestic water storage containers, weekly draining and cleaning of flower pots/ vases, coolers, ant-traps, drums, used tyres, birds baths, pets watering dishes and observing dry days. Individual, family and community participation is essential for these activities.

Personal Protection by

a. Clothing: Full sleeves shirts and full trousers with stocking may protect the arms and legs which are preferred sites for mosquitoes bites.

b. Mats, coils and aerosols: Household insecticidal products namely mosquito coils and aerosols are used extensively for personal protection against mosquitoes. Electric vaporizer mats and liquids vaporizers are more recent additions.

c. Repellents: Such as chemical repellent—DEET (N, N Diethyl—*m*-tolumide) can provide protection for few to several hours.

d. Insecticide treated mosquito nets (ITNs and LLIN) have limited utility since vector species bite during day. However, nets can be used to protect infants and in hospital set-up.

e. Legislation: Such as International Health Regulations and municipal by-laws including mandatory notification of dengue fever are helpful control measures.

4. Outbreak Response

Ensure epidemic preparedness: Dengue fever and chikungunya outbreaks evolve quickly, requiring emergency actions to control infected mosquitoes in order to interrupt or reduce transmission and to reduce or eliminate breeding sites of *Aedes aegypti*. In order to meet such emergencies it is essential that persons at all levels—household level, at school, at community level and public health personnel actively contribute to prevent the spread of epidemic. Two major components of outbreak response are:

a Early diagnosis and case management to decrease dengue deaths.

b Emergency vector control measures to curtail transmission of dengue/chikungunya by:

i Constitution of rapid response teams (RRT)

ii Investigation of outbreak by RRT:

To establish the existence of an outbreak from routine reports of sentinel surveillance hospitals/ facility, i.e. line listing of cases and comparison with past occurrence, verification of diagnosis by laboratory, find cases systematically by adopting standard case definition and analyze data by count, divide and compare as also by time, place and person to substantiate the outbreak, develop hypothesis, confirm hypothesis and initiate control and preventive measures, communicate findings with authorities along with recommendations of control measures besides managing media.

Vector Control during Outbreak/Epidemic

For control of epidemics, vector control is considered to be one of the important strategies to interrupt or reduce transmission. Adult mosquitoes can be controlled by the use of chemical insecticides. *It should be emphasized, however, that rapid and effective source reduction or elimination of breeding sites of vector mosquitoes will achieve the same results.* Moreover, larval control is more economical and provides sustainable control by eliminating the source of newly—emergent adult mosquitoes. Chemical space sprays are not effective in most of the conditions and it is rare that an epidemic will be controlled by using these methods. Because of their visibility however, people think the government is doing something. This often creates a false sense of security and prevents implementation of the community as well as individual efforts outlined above.

Indoor residual spray (IRS) is generally not very effective against *Aedes aegypti* because of their habit of resting on unsprayed objects such as clothes, curtains and other hanging fabrics rather than on walls and ceiling.

There are two main types of space spraying for adult mosquito control:

a. Indoor Space Spraying

Insecticidal aerosols are used for killing of adult mosquitoes during outbreaks. For indoor space spraying 2% pyrethrum extract after dilution with Kerosene (1:19) is sprayed with flit pump or hand operated fogging machine fitted with micro discharge nozzle. Advantage of Pyrethrum space spray are—it is non-toxic to humans, spray equipment is simple, and vectors have not developed resistance to this natural product so far. Insecticidal action does not last long, hence the spray need to be repeated frequently (once a weak).

b. Outdoor Space Spraying

i. Ultra low volume (ULV): Spray (cold fog) with technical malathion. The insecticide is broken down into fine droplets of a volume median diameter (VMD) 40–80 microns, producing a cloud of insecticide droplets that remain suspended in air. The ground equipment mostly used for ULV spray includes portable motorized knapsack blowers and cold aerosols generators.

ii. **Thermal fogging:** Here insecticide is vaporized, which condenses to form a thick cloud of droplets on contact with cooler air when it comes out of the machine. It generates highly visible fog. Thermal fogging is quite expensive because it requires large volume of kerosene oil as solvent. Insecticide of choice for fogging is malathion/ pyrethrum.

Larval control measures include: Removal, disposal or burrying of all unused tins, cans, jars, bottles, tyres, coconut shells and emptying desert coolers once a week. In case water containers cannot be emptied, Temephos (1 ppm) should be applied on a weekly basis. Ensure mosquito proofing of overhead tanks and underground reservoirs.

5. Capacity Building-training

Training in laboratory techniques: MAC-ELISA and NS 1, diagnosis and case management by using standard guidelines, vector surveillance and surveillance of dengue and chikungunya disease as a part of IDSP should be actively persued; besides epidemic/outbreak response.

6. Behaviour Change Communication

IEC activities are crucial for community sensitization and participation. People need to be educated about the disease, mode of transmission, availability of treatment and adoption of control measures. The activities have to be intensified particularly to effect changes in practice of storage of water and personal protection measures (use of insecticide treated nets and repellants) and source reduction. Special campaigns may be carried out with the involvement of mass media—TV, Radio and outdoor publicity besides involving NGOs, etc.

7. Intersectoral Coordination

The prevention and control measures requires close collaboration and partnership between the health sector and private sector, Municipal bodies, PRI, Non-governmental organization, Media, Education and Administrative authorities to enforce civil by-laws for vector control measures, such as source reduction, antiadult measures as also solid waste disposal.

8. Monitoring and Evaluation

Monitoring of disease surveillance indicators, trends, distribution and spread through routine surveillance programme reports and special studies as also measuring vector indices besides inputs, processes and outcomes are essential to improve the programme.

Standard Case Definition for Surveillance

Dengue virus causes two forms of clinical syndromes namely—classical dengue fever (DF) and DHF/DSS. Dengue fever is self-limiting disease and represents the majority of cases of dengue infection. In some situations, it manifests in severe forms as dengue haemorrhagic fever (DHF) and dengue shock syndrome (DSS). Case fatality can be high in DHF and DSS. Primary or first infection in non-immune persons usually causes dengue fever. Subsequent dengue infection by different serotype causes more severe illness like DHF/DSS. Standard case definition is essential for epidemiological surveillance of dengue fever and essential for outbreak investigation purposes.

Case Definition of Dengue Fever (DF)

Suspect case (Clinical features of DF)

An acute febrile illness of 2–7 days duration, with two or more of the following manifestations: headache, retro-orbital pain, myalgia, arthralgia, rash, haemorrhagic manifestations.

Probable DF/DHF

A case compatible with clinical description (clinical criteria) of dengue fever during outbreak:

or

Non-ELISA based NS1 antigen/IgM positive (A positive test by RDT will be considered as probable due to poor sensitivity and specificity of currently available RDTs).

Confirmed Dengue Fever

A case compatible with the clinical description of dengue fever with at least one of the following:

- Isolation of dengue virus (virus culture +) from serum, plasma leucocyte.
- Demonstration of IgM antibody titre by ELISA positive in single serum sample.
- Demonstration of dengue virus antigen in serum sample by NS1–ELISA.
- 1gG seroconversion in paired sera after 2 weeks with four fold increase of IgG titre.
- Detection of virus nucleic acid by polymerse chain reaction (PCR).

For early diagnosis ELISA based NS1 kits have been introduced under the programme which can detect the cases from first day of infection. IgM capture ELISA tests (MAC-ELISA) can detect the cases after 5th day of infection.

Case Definition of Dengue Haemorrhagic Fever

a A case with clinical criteria of DF

b Haemorrhagic tendencies evidenced by one or more of the following—positive tourniquet test, petechiae,

12

ecchymoses or purpura, bleeding from mucosa, gastrointestinal tract, injection sites or other sites and haematemesis or melaena, *plus*

c Thrombocytopenia (less than 1,00,000 cells per mm^3 *plus*

d Evidence of plasma leakage due to increased vascular permeability, manifested by one or more of the following—a rise in average haematocrit for age and sex ≥20%, a ≥20% drop in haematocrit following volume replacement treatment compared to baseline, signs of plasma leakage (pleural effusion, ascites, hypoproteinaemia).

Case Definition of Dengue Shock Syndrome

- All the above criteria for DHF, *plus*
- Evidence of circulatory failure manifested by rapid and weak pulse and narrow pulse pressure (≤20 mm Hg) or hypotension for age and cold clammy skin and restlessness.

DENGUE CASE CLASSIFICATION AND MANGEMENT LEVELS 2015 (Fig. 12.14)[16]

Platelet transfusion is not the mainstay of treatment with DF. In general there is no need to give prophylactic platelets

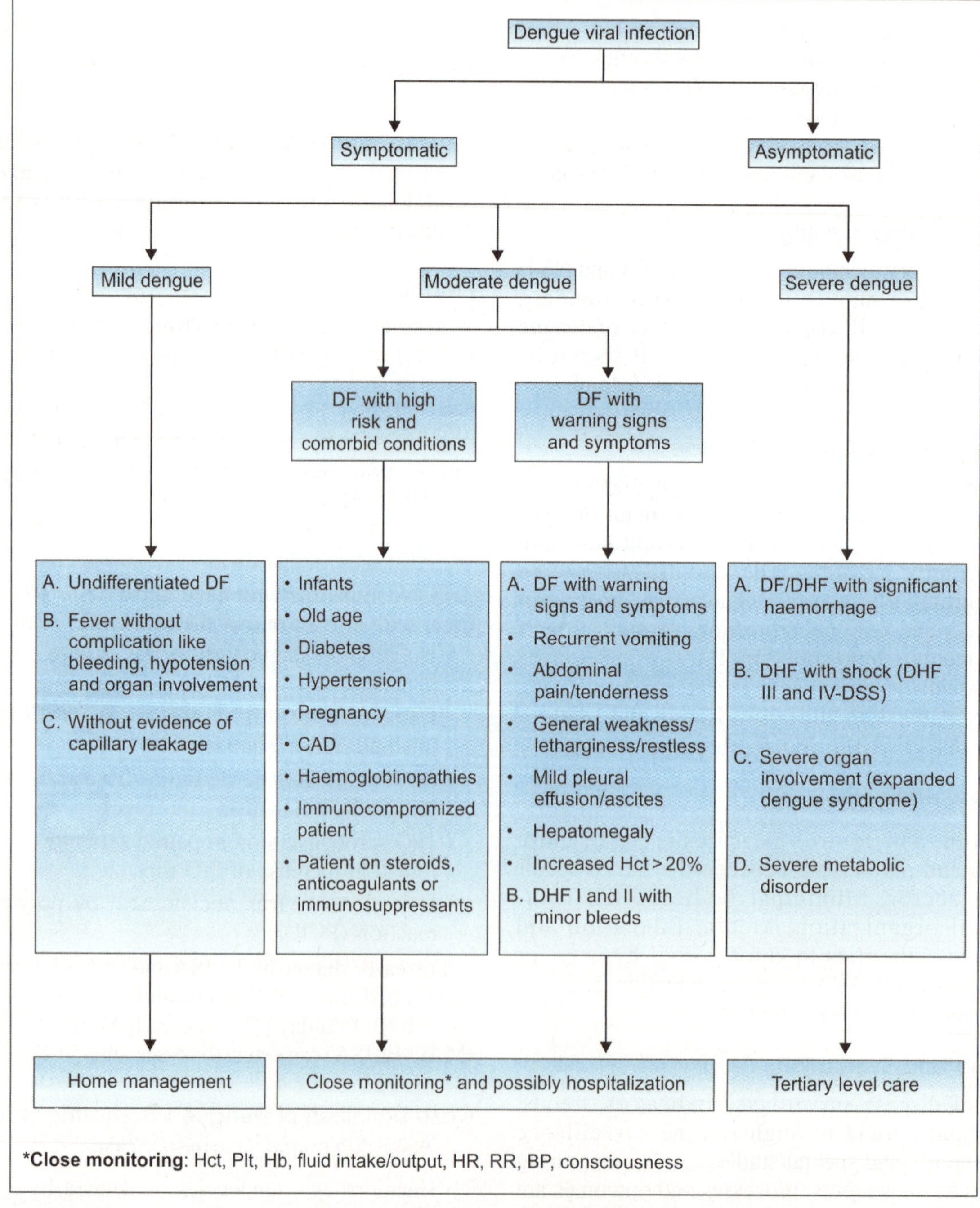

Fig. 12.14: Dengue case classification and mangement levels

even if platelet count is <10000/mm^3. Management guidelines are indicated in flow diagram.

Grading of DF/DHF

***DF:** Fever of 2–7 days with two or more of following—headache, retro orbital pain, myalgia arthralgia with or without leucopenia, thrombocytopenia and no evidence of plasma leakage.

DHFI: Above criteria plus positive tourniquet test and evidence of plasma leakage. Thrombocytopenia with platelet count less than 100000/cu.mm and Hct rise more than 20% over baseline.

DHFII: Above criteria plus some evidence of spontaneous bleeding in skin or other organs (black tarry stool, epistaxis, gum bleeds) and abdominal pain. Thrombocytopenia with platelet count less than 100000/cu.mm and Hct rise more than 20% over baseline.

DHFIII (DSS): Above plus circulatory failure (weak rapid pulse, narrow pulse pressure < 20 mm Hg, hypotension, cold clammy skin, restlessness). Thrombocytopenia with platelet count less than 100000/cu.mm and Hct rise more than 20% over baseline.

DHFIV (DSS): Profound shock with undetectable blood pressure or pulse. Thrombocytopenia with platelet count less than 100000/cu.mm and Hct rise more than 20% over baseline.

Prevention and Control (Summary)

Dengue fever is preventable disease: There is no vaccine or anti-viral drug available against dengue infection. Mortality can be minimized by early diagnosis and prompt symptomatic management of cases. Control of the mosquito vector is currently the only option available for reducing dengue and DHF.

Since *Aedes aegypti* is a container habitat species, breeds in artificial containers and receptacles. People should be encouraged to:

- Emptying water containers once a week.
- Keeping the permanent water containers covered with tight lid or cover.
- Removing waste material suitable for breeding.

Thus, source reduction of breeding places by people can go a long way. In the event of outbreak, source reduction and antilarval measures may be supplemented by anti-adult measures to interrupt the transmission of dengue.

Lessons Learned from Dengue Epidemic in Delhi

We must accept and face the reality that dengue has come to stay in India, and would surface again and again and that to prevent future outbreaks in the absence of any specific antiviral treatment or vaccine, preventive community-based measures are the key to success.

- Delhi study indicates that usefulness of platelet infusion did not seem to affect the outcome.
- Bleeding tendencies: Gastrointestinal bleeding do not necessarily correlate linearly with platelet counts.
- Due to unfamiliarity of the health professionals with DHF/DSS extensive continuing education programmes are essential.

REFERENCES

1 GOI. Dengue/DHF: Calls for an immediate public health action. CD Alert. Monthly Newsletter on Communicable Diseases. NICD, DGHS, GOI, April 2000; 4(4).

2 GOI. Annual Report 2003–04. Ministry of Health and Family Welfare. GOI, DGHS, New Delhi, 2004 and 2006–07.

3 University College of Medical Sciences and GTB Hospital, Department of Medicine, Delhi. Update on Dengue Fever. Delhi, May 3, 1997.

4 GOI. Dengue Haemorrhagic Fever. CD Alert. Monthly Newsletter on Communicable diseases. NICD, DGHS, GOI, New Delhi, 1997: 1(3).

5 Ranbaxy Science Foundation. Dengue Outbreak in Delhi, 1996. Round Table Conference Series No. 1, December 1996. Ranbaxy Science Foundation. New Delhi, India, March 1997.

6 UNICEF. Indian Medical Tribute. Special Release Jointly with UNICEF in Public Interest Medical Communication Network, November 1996.

7 GOI. Standard Case Definitions for Epidemic Prone Communicable Diseases. CD Alert. Monthly Newsletter of NICD, DGHS, GOI. New Delhi, March 2001: 5(3).

8 GOI. Epidemic preparedness—Dengue Fever, Dengue Haemorrhagic Fever and Dengue Shock Syndrome, CD Alert. Monthly Newsletter of NICD, DGHS, GOI: New Delhi, June 2001; 5(6).

9 GOI. Viral Haemorrhagic Fever Potential Threat to Public Health. CD Alert. Monthly Newsletter of NICD, DGHS, GOI, New Delhi, August 2000; 4(8).

10 GOI. Annual Report 2012–13, MOH and FW, Government of India, New Delhi.

11 GOI Mid-term Plan 2011 for Prevention and Control of Dengue and Chikungunya. Directorate of NVBDCP, 22 Shamnath Marg, Delhi.

12 GOI. Meet on Disease Surveillance and Infections Disease Outbreaks, Prevention and Control. CD Alert. Monthly Newsletter in Communicable Diseases. NICD, DGHS, GOI: New Delhi, August 1999; 3(2).

13 GOI. Emerging, Re-emerging New Infections. CD Alert. Monthly Newsletter on Communicable Diseases NICD, DGHS, GOI: New Delhi, 1997; 1(1).

14 NICD-WHO, Guidelines for Prevention and Control of Dengue 2006. Zoonosis Division, NICD (DGHS), Delhi.

15 DGHS, MOH and FW 2008. Guidelines for clinical Management of Dengue HF and DSS. Directorate of NVBDCP, Shamnath Marg, Delhi.

16 GOI, WHO, DGHS, DNVBDCP, NHM, National Guidelines for clincial management of dengue fever, 2011 and 2014.

CHIKUNGUNYA FEVER

Chikungunya is a debilitant non-fatal acute viral disease presenting with acute fever associated with severe arthralgia/arthritis (painful and stiff joints), followed by other constitutional symptoms and rash, lasting for a period of 1–7 days. The usual incubation period is 2–3 days. Fever rises suddenly and often reaches 39–40°C.

Causative Organism

Chikungunya fever is caused by *chikungunya virus* which is a group IV (+) (RNA) virus belonging to family Togaviridae with genus *Alphavirus* and species *Chikungunya*.

Transmission

Chikungunya virus is transmitted to humans through the bite of an infected *Aedes aegypti* mosquito.

In **Africa** CHIK virus is transmitted by *Aedes* mosquito (*Aedes africanus*, *Aedes luteocephalus*; *Aedes opok* and *Aedes furcifer, Aedes taylori*, *Aedes cordillieri*). In Africa, the non-human primates (vertebrates) such as cercopithecus, monkeys or baboons amplify and maintain virus circulation in natural cycle and ensure survival of virus and local spill-over into human population by mosquito.

Asia: Transmission in Asia follows different pattern: It is primarily transmitted from human to human by infected *Aedes aegypti* and monkeys have little role in amplification of the virus.

CHIK activity has been reported in Thailand since 1958, with outbreaks in 1962 and 1980.

Epidemiology

Global

The outbreak of CHIK was reported in Port Klang in Malaysia in 1999, in 2005–06 in La Reunion, 2,04,000 people may have been infected by chikungunya virus since March 2005. Since Jan. 2006, other countries in South West Indian Ocean (Mayotee, Mauritius and Seychelles) have reported chikungunya cases.

India

Chikungunya outbreaks in India have been reported since 1963 (Table 12.26). Outbreaks typically result in large number of cases but deaths are rarely encountered. After a silent period of about three decades, outbreaks of chikungunya started in Andhra Pradesh in 2005 as also in Maharashtra and Karnataka. During the year 2006, over 1.39 million suspected fever cases of chikungunya and 2001 confirmed cases were reported and similarly 59535 suspected fever cases of chikungunya and 1876 confirmed cases were reported in 16 states and UTs (AP, Karnataka, Maharashtra, Tamil Nadu, MP, Gujarat, A and N Islands, Delhi, Rajasthan, Puducherry, Goa, Odisha, West Bengal, Lakshadweep, Uttar Pradesh and Haryana) in 2007.

During the year 2008 about 95,091 suspected cases and 2425 confirmed cases were reported. During the year 2009 around 73,288 suspected cases were reported. Similarly, 48,176 suspected cases in year 2010 and 20,402 cases in 2011 were reported. Incidence declined in the year 2012, 2013 and 2014

Chikungunya fever is usually self-limiting disease resolving with time and requires supportive treatment. There is no specific treatment or vaccine.

Diagnosis

Confirmatory diagnosis comes through laboratory tests. Chikungunya fever should be suspected when epidemic disease occurs with characteristic *triad* of *fever*, rash and *rheumatic manifestations*.

Table 12.26: Chikungunya outbreaks in India 1963–2014

Year	*Locality*	*Important characteristics*
1963	Calcutta	• Cases in lakhs, 37% haemorrhagic manifestation and 200 deaths
1964	Madras	• Cases in lakhs, 5.8% haemorrhagic manifestation
1973	Maharashtra	• Small outbreak, no haemorrhagic manifestation
2005*	Andhra Pradesh	6421 cases, no haemorrhagic manifestation and deaths
Dec 2005*	Maharashtra	34,725 cases, no haemorrhagic manifestation and deaths
Dec 2005	Karnataka	18,529 cases, no haemorrhagic manifestation and deaths
2006	16 states and UTs	1.39 million suspected cases and 2001 confirmed cases
2007	16 states and UTs	59535 suspected cases and confirmed cases 1876
2008	17 states and UTs	95091 suspected and 2425 confirmed cases
2009	12 states and UTs	73288 suspected cases
2010	17 states	48176 suspected cases and 4890 confirmed cases
2011	20 states	20402 suspected cases
2012		15977
2013		18639
2014 (P)		15445

* Source: Reference no. 1–3

Attack rates in affected states

States	*Attack rate in different villages*
Andhra Pradesh	2.3–39.1%
Karnataka	4–45%

Case Definition

Suspect Case

An acute illness characterized by sudden onset of fever with joint pain, headache, backache, photophobia, arthralgia and rash.

Probable Case

As above and positive serology.

Confirmed Case

A probable case with any of the following:

- Fourfold HI antibody difference in paired serum samples.
- Detection of IgM antibodies.
- Virus isolation from serum.
- Detection of chikungunya virus in sera by RT–PCR.

Under NVBDCP IgM capture ELISA is being used for diagnosis.

For serology: Acute sample—collected up to 5 days after the onset of illness. Convalescent or paired sample should be collected 10–14 days after the first sample. For isolation of the virus and RT–PCR, samples should be collected within first 5 days of illness. These should immediately be transported (within 48 hours) to the referral laboratory in cold (preferably frozen) chain system.

Prevention and Control

1 Vector control by elimination of breeding sites or source reduction is the best control method. *Aedes aegypti* is container mosquito and breeds in receptacles and containers having water.
   - All water tanks, cisterns, barrels, trash containers, etc. need to be covered tightly with a lid.
   - Remove or empty water in old tyres, tin cans, buckets, drums, coolers bottles or from other places where mosquitoes breed.

2 Use of insecticide treated mosquito curtains/nets be advocated to avoid mosquito bites.

3 Insecticide spray should be done to kill mosquitoes. Fogging operation is recommended with 2% pyrethrum diluted with kerosene in the ratio of 1:19, space spray during outbreaks/epidemics or in high-risk villages/wards.

4 Epidemiological and entomological surveillance is helpful in early recognition and response as elaborated under dengue surveillance.

5 Education of people by media and by interpersonal communication.

REFERENCES

1 GOI. MOH and FW. Annual Report 2008–09 pp. 91–92, New Delhi.

2 GOI. Chikungunya fever. CD Alert. Monthly Newsletter of Communicable diseases. NICD, DGHS, GOI: New Delhi, Feb 2006; 10(2).

3 GOI. CBHI, National Health Profile 2008, Nirman Bhawan New Delhi.

JAPANESE ENCEPHALITIS—ACUTE ENCEPHALITIS SYNDROME (AES)

Japanese encephalitis (JE) is a disease of public health importance because of its epidemic potential and high case fatality rate. In patients who survive, complications may lead to lifelong sequelae.

Japanese encephalitis (JE) is an Acute viral infection of the central nervous system. JE is caused by flavivirus transmitted by *Culex vishnui* group of mosquitoes. JE is a zoonotic disease. It affects central nervous system.

Global Distribution

It was first recognized in Japan in 1924 when it was named as Japanese B encephalitis, but now it is universally known as Japanese encephalitis. JE has been reported from Nepal, Bangladesh, Bhutan, Burma, China, Republic of Korea, Pakistan, Sri Lanka and Thailand in the form of outbreaks, sporadic cases and endemic occurrence.

Distribution in India

The JE virus activity was first noted in India way back in the year 1952 and JE disease first in 1955 in Vellore and Puducherry. JE virus was first time recovered from human beings in 1958. Till 1970, the disease was confined to Southern states of India. Thereafter the disease outbreaks/epidemics were reported from other states and by 1978; cases were reported from as many as 26 states and union territories (Table 12.27). The disease is endemic in in 171 ditricts in 19 states of which Assam, Bihar, West Bengal, Tamil Nadu and UP have been reporting outbreaks. In India, the disease is endemic in Southern India and cases occur sporadically throughout the year, while in North India disease occurs in the form of epidemics during summer and monsoon months.

Worst affected states are Uttar Pradesh, Karnataka, Andhra Pradesh, Tamil Nadu, West Bengal, Assam, Bihar, Goa, and Manipur. 98 districts are reporting JE regularly every year in these states and it is estimated that 375 million population in these states is exposed to the risk of JE. Reported cases may be an under-estimate of the total problem of JE as many cases go unreported, because of lack of surveillance activities.[1]

Outbreaks of JE in India[2–6]

JE is killer disease with high case fatality rate. Occurrence of JE outbreaks regularly in India in 11 states, which are worst affected, indicate that JE is active and is being maintained in these geographical areas. It also reflects that JE control measures have not been effective or were inadequate to contain JE. The worst JE outbreak was reported from Uttar Pradesh in 1986 when 7500 cases and

Table 12.27: Year-wise AES/JE cases, deaths and CFR, India, 1978–2014

Year	Cases	Deaths	CFR (%)
1978	7463	2755	36.9
1979	2845	926	32.5
1980	3478	1436	38.3
1981	3894	1167	29.9
1982	3516	1261	35.9
1983	1716	581	33.4
1984	3370	1405	41.7
1985	2490	916	36.8
1986	7500	2627	35.0
1987	3515	1346	38.3
1988	6867	2404	35.0
1990	2916	1291	44.3
1991	4071	1530	37.6
1992	2432	888	36.5
1993	2291	923	40.3
1994	1243	640	51.5
1995	2974	942	31.7
1996	2244	593	26.4
1997	2516	632	25.1
1998	2120	507	23.9
1999	3427	680	19.8
2000	2591	556	21.0
2001	2061	479	23.2
2002	1765	466	26.5
2003	2568	707	27.4
2004	1714	367	21.41
2005	6727	1682	25.0
2006	2872	663	23.15
2007	4110	995	24.0
2008	3855	684	18.0
2009	4975	779	17.2
2010	5167	679	13.9
2011	8249	1169	14.0
2012	8344	1256	15.0
2013	7825	1273	17.0
2014	10867	1719	15.8

2627 deaths (CFR 35%) were recorded from only 8 districts. Maximum number of outbreaks have been reported from Gorakhpur and Deoria districts of UP. Outbreaks of JE in Gorakhpur have been reported since 2005 in which many deaths were reported. Over 500 deaths per outbreak due to JE were reported from UP mostly in Gorakhpur in 2011, 2012, 2013 and 2014.

The most disturbing character of JE is frequent outbreaks with *high case fatality* and prolonged morbidity. Outbreak investigations necessitates age and sex-wise line listing of cases adhering to standard case definition besides collection of information on vector density and laboratory confirmation of cases. Since integrated surveillance system is weak the outbreak prediction is difficult. Early recognition of outbreaks and rapid response at local level is the only mechanism to contain the outbreaks of JE.

Case Definition of Acute Encephalitis Syndrome (AES)

Clinically a case of AES is defined as a person of any age, at any time of the year with the acute onset of fever and a change in mental status (including symptoms such as confusion, disorientation, coma or inability to talk).

and/or

New onset of seizures (excluding simple febrile seizures). Other early clinical findings may include an increase irritability, somnolence or abnormal behaviuor greater than that seen with usual febrile illness.

Case Classification

- ***Suspect:*** A case that is compatible with the clinical description.
- ***Probable:*** A suspected case with presumptive laboratory results.
- ***Confirmed:*** A suspected case with confirmatory laboratory results.

Laboratory Criteria for Diagnosis

Presumptive: Detection of an acute phase antiviral antibody response through one of the following:

Elevated and stable serum antibody titre to JE virus through ELISA, haemagglutination—inhibition or virus neutralization assays or IgM antibody to the virus in serum.

Confirmatory: Detection of JE virus, antigen, genome in tissues, blood or other body fluids by immunochemistry or immunofluorescence or PCR or JE virus specific IgM in the CSF

or

Fourfold or greater rise in JE virus—specific antibody in paired sera (acute and convalescent phases) through IgM/IgG, ELISA, haemagglutination inhibition test or virus neutralization test.

Rural Urban Distribution

In India, most of the cases and outbreaks have been reported from rural areas (over 90%) but outbreaks have also been reported from peri-urban areas. These outbreaks have been associated with monsoon, paddy fields in paddy cultivation, and presence of animal reservoir hosts.

The disease shows a scattered distribution with 1–2 cases reported per village. Presence of one clinical case in the community suggests that 250 to 1000 people have inapparent infections. Thus cases of JE represent tip of the iceberg.

Age and Sex Distribution

It is predominantly a disease of children living in rural areas/periurban and semiurban areas. Available data of various outbreaks in India reveal that vast majority of cases occurred in children less than 15 years of age. If the infection of JE occurs for the first time in an area, all the age groups are affected.

Males are affected more as compared to females because of more exposure.

Reservoir and Transmission

Primarily JE virus circulates and multiplies among pigs and birds. In nature, the cycle of JE is maintained in pigs and birds. Man is incidentally involved in this cycle.[2]

Pig-to-pig cycle: Pig-to-pig cycle is maintained by *Culex vishnui*. Pigs are major vertebrate hosts. Pigs develop viraemia but do not manifest any symptoms. The pigs act as amplifying hosts.

Bird's Cycle

Ardeola grayii (pond heron) and *Bubulcus ibis* (cattle, egret) play definite role in maintenance of virus in nature.

Man

Man is involved in the cycle incidentally. When the mosquitogenic potential increases after monsoon and flood resulting into high density of vector. The virus is transmitted from pigs to man through mosquitoes. Man-to-man transmission is unknown. Man is the dead end of transmission of JE.

Vector

Many types of mosquitoes transmit this disease but *Culex vishnui* group of mosquitoes (*Culex tritaeniorhynchus*) are the most important in the transmission of JE in India. The mosquitoes are zoophilic and once infected remain infected for life.

Virus

The JE virus belongs to genus *Flavivirus* and family Togaviridae within the same genus are also present the viruses of dengue fever, Kyasanur forest disease and yellow-fever and West Nile.

Incubation Period

It ranges from 5 to 15 days. The extrinsic incubation period in vector mosquitoes is 9–12 days.

Case Fatality Rate (CFR)

Case fatality rate varies from 20 to 40%. Over the years the CFR has declined but it is still very high at about 25% in affected children.

Sequelae

About 30–40% patients who survive/recover from acute episode may have neurological sequelae like mental impairment, severe emotional instability, personality changes and paralysis.

Seasonal Variation

The JE outbreaks are most commonly observed during rainy and post-rainy seasons. Peak period is August to October. If the environments are suitable, the infection is maintained at low level throughout the year (Southern states).

NATIONAL PROGRAMME FOR PREVENTION AND CONTROL OF JAPANESE ENCEPHALITIS/ACUTE ENCEPHALITIS SYNDROME (2014)

On the recommendations of Group of ministers the GOI approved National Programme for prevention and control of JE.

Goals and Objectives

i To strengthen and expand JE vaccination in affected districts.

ii To strengthen surveillance, vector control and timely referral of serious and complicated cases.

iii To increase access to safe drinking water and proper sanitation facilities to the target population in affected rural and urban areas.

iv To estimate disability burden due to JE/AES, and to provide adequate facilities for physical, medical, neurological and social rehabilitation.

v To improve nutritional status of children at risk of JE.

vi To carry out intensified IEC/BCC activities.

Strategies[7-11]

Coverage: During phase one out of 171 JE endemic districts in 19 states 60 districts in 5 statss (Assam, Bihar, Tamil Nadu, UP and West Bengal) will be covered.

Multipronged strategy has been adopted

Convergence of ministries—like Ministry of Health and Family Welfare with other ministries. Considering the risk of transmission of AES through contaminated drinking water (Entero-viral infection), Ministry of Drinking Water and Sanitation for provision of safe drinking water and proper sanitation are critical for prevention and control of AES, Women and Child Development for providing high quality nutrition to children, Ministry of Social Justice and Empowerment for establishement of District Disability Rehabilitation Centres, Minsitry of Housing and Urban Poverty Alleviation for safe water and sanitation, Ministry of Human Resources Development for Providing Eduction and skills to disabled children.

Ministry of health and family welfare is the nodal agency for JE. Following Programe Components have been recommended by group of ministers (GOM).

a Strengthening and expansion of JE vaccine.
b Strengthening of Public Health activities.
c Better clinical management of JE/AES cases.
d Physical medicine and rehabilitation.
e Establishing of district counselling centres.
f Monitoring supervision and coordination.
g Research-cum intervention project.

Component of Strengthening of JE Vaccine

One dose of live attenuated JE vaccine 0.5 ml to all children between 1–15 years in campaign mode was given in all high risk district in 2006. Following the campaign the vaccine has been integrated into UIP. 132 districts have already been brought under JE vaccination as part of universal immunization programme. Further new districts will be covered in phased manner. Since 2013 two doses of live attenuated JE vaccine (AS–14–14–2) at the age of 9 months and at the age of 16–24 months are included under universal immunization programme.

Adult JE vaccine: Govt of India has decided to extend age for JE vaccine to adults in high burden districts.[7–11]

Component - 2 Strengthening of Public Health Activities

District level model action plan has been developed for 60 priority districts. This plan focuses on, vector control, disease surveillance, advocacy meeting, behavior change communication and IEC; monitoring and supervision, setting up of department of physical medicine and rehabilitation at medical colleges (neurorehabilitation component), district disability and rehabilitation centres and paediatric intensive care unit (PICU).

Vector Control

JE vectors are exophilic (outdoor resting habits) and endophagic in nature. The risk of transmission increases when the human dwellings and animal sheds particularly piggeries are situated close to each other. Vector control using indoor residual spray is technically not feasible because of outdoor resting habits of vector, due to vast and enormous breeding habitats like perennial ponds, paddy fields and other water bodies, anti larval measures are also not feasible. Therefore vector control using ULV (ultra low volume) fogging with malathion is the only method for vector control and can be used during JE epidemics also.

Epidemiological Surveillance

Syndromic Surveillance for JE is recommended.

Case definition of suspect case:

- Acute onset of fever, not more than 5–7 days duration
- Change in mental status with/without
  - New onset of seizures (excluding febrile seizures)
  - (Other clinical findings–may include irritability, somnolence or abnormal behavior greater than that seen with usual febrile illness)

In an epidemic situation fever with altered sensorium persisting for more than 2 hours with a focal seizure or paralysis of any part of the body is encephalitis.

Purpose

The purpose of JE surveillance is to:

- Assess disease burden area wise—incidence of JE and deaths.
- To detect epidemic/outbreak at the earliest.
- To determine trend of JE.
- To determine geographical distribution and vulnerable population.

Sentinel Surveillance

The key component of AES surveillance system is the referral hospital with laboratory facility to diagnose JE with at least one site per district with laboratory facility in endemic areas. This unit will regularly generate information on JE by line listing of all confirmed cases.

Sentinel sites without laboratory facility and other informer units will be linked with IDSP and district laboratory. Weekly or daily report during epidemic are generated. All notified cases are verified and investigated by specially trained district rapid response Team/district surveillance officer. Early warning signals are generated form surveillance data and advance warning is given to the area.

Outbreak Investigation and Response

JE is a disease of epidemic potential and has high case fatality rate. JE patients who survive may have life long sequelae. The rapid response teams are mobilized for containment measures. Clinical management of suspected JE cases at referral centre is essential to reduce case fatality. For early response involve local community. Ensure vector control measures by fogging with malathion technical in all affected villages and Urban areas; besides use of bed nets and personal protective measures to prevent mosquito bites.

Isolation or destruction of amplifying host (pigs) is not advised. Main axe falls on destruction of pigs during outbreaks such a measure is not practicable, and is counter productive as the vector which is primarily zoophilic shifts to human beings and bites human beings and transmits more infections.

REFERENCES

1 GOI. Annual Reports 2009–13. New Delhi: MOH and FW, GOI; 2009–2013.
2 Sehgal S, Bhatia R. Japanese Encephalitis. New Delhi: NICD; 1988.
3 NICD. Japanese Encephalitis—Control Mechanism requires strengthening. CD Alert March 2000; 4(3).
4 NICD. Epidemic preparedness—Japanese Encephalitis. CD Alert April 2001; 5(3).
5 Planning Commission. Tenth Five-Year Plan 2002–07 (II)— Sectoral Policies and Programmes. New Delhi: GOI; 2002.
6 GOI. National Health Profile-2005: CBHI, DGHS, MOH and FW; GOI.
7 GOI. NRHM. Newsletter, Feb-March 2006; 1, MOH and FW; Govt of India.
8 GOI. MOH and FW; GOI Annual Report 2006–07, pp. 74–75.
9 GOI. MOH and FW, Annual Report 2007–12.
10 NICD and WHO 2006 Guidelines Prevention and Control of Japanese Encephalities. Zoonotic Division, NICD (DGHS), 22 Shamnath Marg, New Delhi, 2006.
11 GOI, MOH and FW, DGHS, NVBDCP, National programme for prevention and control of JE/AES Operational Guidelines 2014.

KYASANUR FOREST DISEASE (KFD)

Prevalence/Incidence and Geographical Distribution of KFD

The KFD is geographically confined to a few districts of Karnataka state in India. The affected districts are Chickmaglur, Dakshin Kannada, Shimoga, Uttar Kanada and Udupi Distt. Shimoga and Chickmaglur are worst affected. The worst year was 1983 when 2167 cases and 148 deaths were reported and since then the KFD is endemic in the state of Karnataka forest area (Table 12.28).

KFD is a tick-borne infection and is localized to Karnataka only. Monkeys are recognized as amplifying hosts for KFD but monkeys die of KFD infection and cannot maintain virus in nature. Man is affected incidentally by tick bites in the forest area. Man is the dead end host of KFD. Severe infections may cause violent headache, high fever, nausea, coma and death.

Prevention: No specific treatment is available. Prevention requires, avoidance fields and forests infested with ticks, use of repellents, use of impregnated clothing and removal of attached ticks.[1]

Table 12.28: Reported cases and deaths due to KFD in India (Karnataka state)

Year	Cases	Deaths
1983	2167	148
1984	884	150
1985	366	12
1986	780	14
1987	228	10
1988	322	6
1989	1550	22
1995	174	1
1996	140	3
1997	75	4
1998	47	1
1999	10	0
2000	30	3
2001	59	2
2002	98	6
2003	306	11

YELLOW FEVER

Yellow fever is an acute, viral infectious disease of short duration and varying severity, transmitted between humans by infected mosquitoes.

Distribution

The disease affects people of all ages and occurs in tropical areas, mainly in sub-Saharan Africa and Central and South America. No case has been reported in Asia including India, although the mosquito vector is found in India.

Problem

An estimated 2,00,000 yellow fever cases with 30,000 deaths occur each year, almost all in sub-Saharan Africa and America. Over 508 million people in 33 countries are at risk of infection in this area.

Transmission

Yellow fever is primarily disease of monkeys and it maintains three cycles in nature.

1 ***Sylvatic or jungle cycle:*** The yellow fever virus mainly occurs in population of monkeys in dense forests and gallery forests in Africa and South and Central America. It is transmitted from monkey-to-monkey by forest dwelling mosquitoes (*Aedes* species in Africa, Haemagogus and *Sabethes* in South and Central Africa). Jungle or Sylvan yellow fever is enzootic in Africa.
2 ***Rural cycle:*** These mosquitoes occasionally bite humans when they enter forests and may thus transmit the virus from monkey reservoir to the human population. In Africa monkeys sometimes in jungle leave the forest in search of banana plantations and may then infect the local species which in turn infect humans living or working on plantations.
3 ***Urban cycle:*** People infected in or near forests can carry the virus to rural or urban areas where *Aedes aegypti* or related mosquitoes can pick it up and transmit it among the human population. Such situation

can result in serious epidemics and many deaths. Man-to-man cycle in urban and rural areas is maintained by *Aedes aegypti* mosquitoes.

In America, urban outbreaks used to be very severe but have not occurred since 1954. However, the risk remains and cases are reported each year among people working in forests. In Africa, urban and rural outbreaks are occasionally reported from areas near forests and may cause thousands of deaths. People working in forests also become infected regularly. Urban yellow fever outbreaks are still reported from Africa.

Occurrence

It is endemic disease in Africa, South and Central America and it can occur in epidemic proportion in these areas.

Endemic zone in Africa: Angola, Zambia, Tanzania, Zaire, Rwanda, Burundi, Kenya, Somalia, Ethiopia, Sudan (part) Central African Republic, Congo, Cameroon, Equatorial Guinea, Nigeria, Sao Tome and Principe. Togo Benin, Ghana, Burkina Faso, Liberia, Sierra Lone, Guinea Bissau, Senegal, Gambia, Côtd'ivoire, Mali (part) Niger (part), Liberia, Chad (part), and SaoTome and Principe.

Endemic zone in South and Central America: Brazil, Bolivia, Peru, Equador, Colombia, Panama, Venezuella, Guyana, Suriname, and French Guana.

Case Fatality

The case fatality rate in endemic region is under 5% but, may reach 50% among non-indigenous groups. *Aedes aegypti* mosquitoes transmit yellow fever in urban and certain rural areas and other *Aedes* mosquitoes transmit the infection from monkey to man in Africa. In the forest of South America, transmission is by *Haemagogus* mosquitoes. The blood of patient is infective for mosquitoes before the onset of fever and for the first 3–5 days of illness. It is highly communicable where many susceptible persons and abundant vector mosquitoes coexist.

There is evidence in some areas of endemicity that the virus is maintained in mosquitoes population through transovarial transmission in the absence of vertebrate reservoir.

Incubation period: It is 3–6 days.

Clinical Features

Many infections are mild. Typical attacks have a sudden onset with fever, headache, backache, prostration, nausea and vomiting. As the disease progresses, the pulse weakens and albuminuria and anuria may occur. Haemorrhage and jaundice follow the period of fever and vomiting.

In 15% of patients it can lead to shock (bleeding from mouth, nose, eyes and/or stomach), and kidneys and liver failure. Persons recovering from yellow fever have lifelong immunity against reinfection.

12

There is no specific drug treatment effective against the yellow fever virus, but with supportive care most patients can survive.

Epidemic can be controlled by vaccinating all persons living in affected areas, by space spraying with insecticides against adult mosquitoes and by appropriate larval control measures. Non-immunized person can reduce the risk of infection by protecting themselves from mosquito bite with protective clothing, repellents and screens to prevent day time biting.

Prevention and Control

Surveillance: Yellow fever is international notifiable disease by WHO hence, regular surveillance helps to keep a track and control this disease by controlling environments.

Vector surveillance: Vector surveillance is being done to keep the vector density low (*Aedes aegypti* index being kept below 1). Ships and aircrafts coming from endemic areas are made free of mosquitoes by appropriate measures.

Valid vaccine certificate: As per international health regulations, yellow fever vaccine certificate is mandatory for persons coming from endemic areas to India or other areas where disease is absent. Similarly, persons going from India or areas free of yellow fever to endemic areas should have valid yellow fever vaccination certificate.[2–4]

Prevention

Yellow fever is best prevented by immunization which is recommended for all persons working in or visiting forests where yellow fever occurs. Immunization is also indicated for people in urban or rural areas at risk.

Vaccination

Yellow fever vaccine is a live attenuated virus vaccine which contains the viable attenuated yellow fever 17D strain virus. Adults and children 6 months of age and older can be vaccinated against yellow fever in endemic areas. A single dose by subcutaneous route confers immunity for 10 long years. The validity of vaccination starts after 10 days of primary vaccination and on the day of booster. It is valid for 10 years.

Dose: A single dose of 0.5 ml, for all ages confers immunity after 7 days of administration. Yellow fever vaccine has very high efficacy, the antibodies may persist for 30–35 years but revaccination within 10 years is still required by the international health regulations for travel to and fro endemic areas.

Storage: 0°+8°C. Long-term storage should preferably be at –15° to –25°C.

Contraindication: It is contraindicated in infants below 4 months and pregnant women. If pregnant women must travel to areas where the risk of yellow fever is high, vaccination should be given after 6 months of pregnancy.

Quarantine: If a person entering the receptive area without valid vaccine certificate or before the vaccine certificate becomes valid that person is a 'suspect' and is quarantined for 6 days under mosquito free conditions and his movements are restricted.

REFERENCES

1 WHO. Vector control methods for use by individuals and communities, Prepared by Jan A. Rozendall. World Health Organization, Geneva, 1997.

2 WHO. International Health Regulations (1969). Third Annotated Edition. World Health Organization, Geneva.

3 WHO. Teaching Health Statistics Lessons and Seminar Outline. Second Edition. World Health Organization (1999). Edited by S.K. Lwanga, Cho-Yook Tye and O. Ayeni.

4 WHO. International Health Regulations (2005), Second Edition. World Health Organization, Geneva.

WATER-BORNE DISEASES (WBDs)

WBDs are dirty water disease; those caused by water that has been contaminated by human, animals and chemical wastes.

DIARRHOEAL DISEASES

Diarrhoea is a killer disease in young children. One in six deaths in children under the age of 5 are estimated to be due to diarrhoea.

Definition

Diarrhoea is the passage of loose, liquid or watery stool. In many regions, acute watery diarrhoea is defined as passage of three or more loose or watery stools in 24 hours period with or without dehydration. However, it is the recent change in consistency and character of stools rather than the number of stools that is more important. Passage of even one watery stool in a young child constitutes diarrhoea. In most cases, mother knows what is abnormal stool for her child. Frequent passage of normal stool is not diarrhoea. Similarly, passage of frequent formed stool, passage of pasty stool in breastfed infants and passage of stool during or immediately after feeding due to initiation of gastrocolic reflex are not to be considered as diarrhoea.[1]

WHAT CAUSES DIARRHOEA?

Acute watery diarrhoea is caused by a variety of infectious agents whose action alter intestinal function by different mechanisms. Enterotoxigenic strains of *Escherichia coli* and *Vibrio cholerae* colonize the mucosal surface and produce enterotoxins, which causes increased mucosal secretion, without any apparent damage to mucosal cell. Enterotoxins stimulate enzyme adenyl cyclase in the enterocytes. The latter promotes active losses of electrolytes and water from the intestinal cells.

The viruses, multiply within the mucosal cells of the intestine and produce patchy and transient mucosal damage. The following common organisms produce acute watery diarrhoea:

1 ***Escherichia coli:*** It produces heat labile (LT) and heat stable (ST) enterotoxins. The *Escherichia coli* could be:
   a Enterotoxigenic *E. coli* is major cause of acute watery diarrhoea.
   b Localized-adherent *E. coli* (LAEC).
   c Diffuse-adherent *E. coli* (DAEC).
   d Enteroinvasive *E. coli* causes dysentery type of diarrhoea.
   e Enterohaemorrhagic *E. coli* (EHEC).

Vibrio cholerae produces enterotoxins.
- Shigella .... invasive produce
- *Campylobacter jejuni* .... invasive
- Salmonellae, other than *S. typhi* .... invasive.
- *Cryptosporidium* .... invasive.

2 ***Viruses:*** Rotavirus .... invasive.
3 ***Parasites:*** *E. histolytica* .... invasive, produces dysentery; *Giardia duodenalis* .... non-invasive.

One-third to half of acute watery diarrhoeas are due to bacteria, one-third are due to viruses and in the remaining one-third the causative organisms cannot be pin pointed. In India, Rotavirus and enterotoxigenic *E. coli* account for nearly half of total episodes among children. Only a small proportion of all acute watery diarrhoeas (5–10%) are due to cholera. In 5–10% of all cases of diarrhoea, the shigellae invade the mucosal cells and cause necrosis resulting into passage of blood and mucus in the stool (dysentery). *Campylobacter jejuni* also is an invasive organism. Infestations with *Entamoeba histolytica* and *Giardia duodenalis* result in subacute and chronic illness.

Electrolytes: Normally the small intestine secretes, rather than absorbs water. In acute diarrhoeal infection (diarrhoeal diseases), the volume secreted is large and cannot be fully absorbed by the colon, so the watery diarrhoea continues even if the oral intake stops. Whatever may be the etiology the hallmark of acute watery diarrhoea is loss of electrolytes and water from the body.

Epidemiolgy of Diarrhoeal Diseases

Age group affected: Infants and young children are commonly affected by acute watery diarrhoea. Children between 6 months to 2 years of age are most vulnerable to diarrhoeal diseases. Diarrhoea is *a major disease* in young children. Economically weaker sections are affected most.

Risk Factors (Determinants) in Diarrhoea

Low birth weight babies, severely underweight children and Bottle-fed babies have more chances to develop diarrhoea because of unclean bottles or teats. Similarly, unclean or soiled hands or unwashed hands can contaminate food or water with germs. Flies can also bring dirt and germs to uncovered food. Drinking contaminated water results in diarrhoea. Thus unclean food, milk, unsafe water, unclean hands and unclean utensils are the predominant risk factors for acute watery diarrhoea in the community. All these risk factors are unhealthy behaviours or unhealthy practices at household level.

Magnitude of the Problem

In 1980 in developing countries, an estimated 5 million children under 5 years of age—about 10 every minute—died as a consequence of diarrhoeal disease. These deaths were an outcome of the some 1000 million episodes that occurred among the 338 million children in this age group and were undoubtedly more frequent in poorer families (WHO).[2] In 2002 Globally 15.2% of under 5 died due to diarrhoea

Diarrhoel diseases accounted for 17.9% of deaths in children age group 1–4 in the year 2010–13 (Table 12.29).

Problem in India: NFHS-2 data highlights morbidity profile of under 3 years, which includes; fever (27%), acute respiratory infections (17%), diarrhoea (13%) and underweight (43%) and often due to combination of these conditions.[4]

Diarrhoeal diseases are major public health problem among children under the age of 5. Around 8–11 million cases are being reported annually in India (Table 12.30). About 6–10% of under—five children experienced diarrhoea in the two weeks preceding the survey (NFHS 3–4).

Distribution: It is widespread mostly in urban slum areas with poor sanitation.

Acute diarrhoeal disease is one of the major causes of morbidity and mortality in India especially among infants and children under 5 years of age. In a prospective study undertaken in rural setting of ICDS block in Rohtak district, it was observed that young children below the age of 3 years, on an average, experienced 4–6 episodes of diarrhoea per year.[5–7]

Table 12.29: Top 10 causes of death in age 1–4 year during (2010–13)

Rank	Cause of death	Deaths (%)		
		Male	Female	Person
1	Pneumonia	17.6	18.9	18.2
2	Diarrhoeal diseases	16.3	19.4	17.9
3	Injuries	18.5	15.3	16.6
4	Other noncommunicable disease	11.8	9.4	10.6
5	Malaria	7.4	6.5	7.0
6	Fever of unknown origin	6.5	6.2	6.3
7	Other infectious and parasitic d	3.9	4.2	4.0
8	Congenital anomalies	3.9	3.2	3.5
9	Meningitis/encephalitis	3.5	3.5	3.5
10	Ill defined or cause unknown	3.3	3.1	3.2
	All other remaining causes	3.7	10.4	8.9
	Total	**100.0**	**100.0**	**100.0**

Source: SRS—2010–13

Table 12.30: Reported incidence of acute diarrhoeal diseases in India, 2000 to 2011

Year	No. of cases reported
2000	88,70,507
2001	92,87,758
2002	94,41,456
2003	1,05,10,476
2004	1,04,87,238
2005	1,04,78,459
2006	1,02,13,917
2007	1,09,93,639
2008	1,12,31,039
2009	1,19,84,490
2010	1,07,42,327
2011	1,02,31,049
2013	1,14,13,610
2014	1,16,73,018

Source: National Health Profile 2008 to 2015. CBHI, DGHS, MOH and FW, GOI, 2015.

Many studies have also indicated that most of diarrhoea cases in the community, 90% show no signs of dehydration, 10% of them may have some dehydration and only one in hundred patients may have severe dehydration and require treatment at health centre or hospital. Therefore, it was estimated that about 50–100 million diarrhoea patients may be requiring rehydration therapy at health facility.[8]

Severity (consequences): Young children between 6 and 12 months of age are affected severely with diarrhoea and account for high mortality as compared to older children and adults. Diarrhoea kills 1.5 lakhs children every year in India due to dehydration. Dehydration leads to loss of water and electrolytes (sodium chloride, potassium and carbonates) from the body. Dehydration occurs where water and salt are not replaced adequately. This can lead to shock and death. Diarrhoea also produces undernutrition and growth failure in young children. Diarrhoeal disease constitute one of the important "nutritional leak" in young children. Even a brief episode of diarrhoea leads to the loss of 1–2% of body weight. Undernutrition in diarrhoea occurs due to loss of nutrients and because of withholding of food during episode of diarrhoea by family/parents. Frequency and quantities of supplementary foods are seldom increased during convalescent period.

Common Beliefs and Practices in Diarrhoea[9–12]

Working mothers commonly hold the belief that their "body heat" gets into child's body through breast milk. After long hours of hard work in the field and farm, if mothers immediately offered breast milk to their babies, on return, they develop loose motions. There is thus a general tendency to refrain from breastfeeding within half an hour to one hour after return from the fields.

- Doctors and health workers consider loose motions as an illness which leads to serious consequences. However, most mothers generally describe diarrhoea as normal occurrence or at the most a minor illness and rarely more serious.
- Diarrhoea is believed to be a consequence of teething or considered as normal occurrence during "teething". There is a common saying that a child during teething should have bouts of loose motions, fever and red eyes (conjunctivitis). Accordingly diarrhoea is considered to be normal body response to impacted tooth and hard gums. Quite often mothers give weak tea with butter or ghee or milk and ghee to young children (which is good practice). Lot of butter or ghee (oil) is rubbed on the head with a belief that it helps facilitate eruption of teeth.

Diets: During diarrhoea in infants, dietary restrictions are imposed on lactating women. They are not allowed to eat pulses, vegetables, groundnuts, halwa (sweet wheat porridge), jaggery as these are thought to be heavy and heat producing foods and liable to cause diarrhoea in breastfed infants, through mother's milk. Quite often mother in law and elderly ladies consider that these food items cause tense-abdomen, excessive crying and diarrhoea.

Good foods/best practice: Rice and green gram porridge (*khichri*), curd (dahi) are encouraged as these foods are considered to be light and easily digestible but quantities and frequency of feeding is reduced.

Feeding: Most mothers restrict feeding/stop feeding during diarrhoea. Mother avoid giving milk, butter milk, staple cereals, vegetables, sugar, jaggery and fried foods during diarrhoea. All supplementary foods are stopped or drastically cut down during diarrhoea. Generally less eating is preferred during diarrhoea. Frequency of feeding and quantity of food is reduced by as many as 80% of mothers.

Use of antibiotics: NFHS-2 indicates that nearly 68% of children continue to be pushed in antibiotics during diarrhoea; though the providers (practitioners) were trained on ORT, their practices have not much changed. The use of anti-diarrhoeal drugs is widespread across most socioeconomic groups. Though over 80% of practitioners knew that antibiotics are harmful in acute watery diarrhoea yet 80% of them prescribed antibiotics.

Rather than directly combating the beliefs held locally an effort should be made to incorporate these local beliefs into positive messages about diarrhoea.

Messages

1. Oral rehydration salt (ORS) cools the body and removes heat from body.
2. Diarrhoea can kill children by draining too much liquid from the body, so it is essential to give plenty of liquid to drink. ORS is best drink.
3. A child with diarrhoea needs more food and frequent breastfeeding.
4. A child who is recovering from diarrhoea needs an extra meal everyday for at least two weeks.
5. Medicine other than ORS should not be used except on medical advice.
6. Diarrhoea can be prevented by breastfeeding, by immunization against measles by using sanitary latrines, by keeping food and water clean and by washing hands before eating.

Classification of Diarrhoea[13–15]

It is done on the basis of clinical syndromes:[9]

ASK: Does the child has diarrhoea? If yes ask: The age of the child. What is the frequency and duration of diarrhoea? Is there blood in the stool? Diarrhoea is classified as:

- Acute watery diarrhoea.
- Dysentery (blood in the stools)/bloody diarrhoea
- Persistent diarrhoea.
- ***Acute watery diarrhoea:*** Acute watery diarrhoea starts suddenly and is characterized by passage of loose watery stools. Most episodes of acute diarrhoea recover or are self-limiting, within 3–7 days. More than 75% of all diarrhoeal episodes in the community are acute watery episodes.
- ***Dysentery:*** This is diarrhoea with visible blood and mucus in the faeces. The presence of blood may also be accompanied with abdominal cramps, fever, anorexia and rapid weight loss. Shigellae group of organisms produce dysentery.
- ***Persistent diarrhoea:*** An acute episode of watery diarrhoea or dysentery which lasts for **more than 14 days** is classified as persistent diarrhoea. It is because of persistent colonization of microbes in small intestine due to recurrent intestinal infection or due to protein energy malnutrition, reduced immunity or defence mechanism and/or dietary allergies and carbohydrate intolerance. Incidence of persistent diarrhoea is around 5%, i.e. 5% of acute diarrhoeas may persist beyond 2 weeks. Protozoal infections with *Giardia lamblia* and *Entamoeba histolytica* and inadequate treatment of diarrhoea are other important causes of persistent diarrhoea.[1]

Classification of Dehydration

Look and feel: Does the child have signs of dehydration?

Assessing dehydration: Degree of dehydration is usually classified as, *no dehydration, some dehydration and severe dehydration on the basis of history, observation (looking) and clinical assessment (Table 12.31).*

Laboratory Investigations

Clinical assessment is sufficient to initiate appropriate therapy. Routine determination of etiology of diarrhoea in

Table 12.31: Assessing severity of dehydration

Signs	*Classification of dehydration*	*Treatment plan*
Not enough signs to classify as some or severe dehydration	*No dehydration*	**Plan A**
Two of the following signs: • Restless, irritable • Drinks eagerly-thirsty • Sunken eye • Skin pinch goes back slowly	*Some dehydration*	**Plan B**
• Lethargic or unconscious • Unable to drink or drinking poorly • Sunken eye • Skin pinch goes back very slowly	*Severe dehydration*	**Plan C**

a laboratory is neither necessary nor practical. Stool culture is of little value in routine management of diarrhoea. The management of case of diarrhoea is based on the clinical assessment of the disease.

Principles of Management of Acute Diarrhoea

Irrespective of the etiology, acute watery diarrhoea requires fluid and electrolytes replacement to correct dehydration. In the early stages of diarrhoea when ORS packets are not immediately available, home available fluids (HAF) and water can be used. The first response to diarrhoea should be *drinking lot of fluids* and continue *breastfeeding* and *feeding* whatever is liked by the child or parents consider best for the child.

Feeding

Feeding must be continued during all types of diarrhoea and quantities and frequency should be increased during recovery (convalescent period) to avoid any adverse effect on nutritional status.

Rational use of Drugs

ORS is the drug of choice for all cases of diarrhoea. It is lifesaving when used timely, in adequate quantities. ORS has saved million of lives. Only a small proportion of cases of diarrhoea (dysentery, cholera and associated illnesses) need specific antimicrobials. Amoebiasis and giardiasis are rare in children and drug therapy should be started only when trophozoites of *E. histolytica* or *Giardia* are seen in the faeces. Irrationale use of antimicrobials or antibiotics can worsen the diarrhoea and may lead to loss of life of young child.

Anti-diarrhoeals (anti-motility drugs, binding agents, stimulants, steroids and other drugs) have no place in the treatment of diarrhoea and must not be used. Since anti-diarrhoeals have no clinical benefits and are potentially dangerous, their marketing has been banned in India.

Fluid Therapy (Best Solution is ORS)

Fluid and electrolytes replacement is necessary for all types of acute watery diarrhoea and is the mainstay of treatment of case with diarrhoea. ORS is the best available solution for fluid and electrolytes replacement. ORS has been the most important technological advance of the 20th century as this modality has saved millions of lives of young children. The first response of mother in diarrhoea should be drinking home available fluids (HAF). Drinking HAF should become the habit and it must be institutionalized in all families and all homes where the diarrhoea strikes. Best drink (ORS) can be started as soon as it is available.

Home Available Fluids (HAFs)

HAFs are best means to prevent dehydration. HAF should be given frequently; and also after each loose stool to prevent dehydration. A good HAF is one which is safe when used in large quantities. Some of these fluids which are commonly used in the homes are time tested and have sound physiological basis. Examples are:

- *Food-based solutions* like rice water or rice conjee with salt, dal or dal water with salt, butter milk or curd with salt. and certain soups with salt.
- *Home available fluids* which can be used are lemon water, soup, coconut water and plain water.
- Water is a good home available fluid if taken with food. These fluids are more effective when given along with food (i.e. feeding should be continued), thus providing for starch (ultimately glucose) and protein (ultimately amino acids); to promote sodium and water absorption from gut. *These fluids together with food provide oral rehydration therapy* (ORT).
- In younger infants, *breast milk* is an ideal fluid and should be frequently given.

Soft drinks, plain glucose water, sweetened fruit juices and sweetened tea should not be used. These have high osmolarity and can lead to worsening of dehydration.

Oral Rehydration Salt (ORS)

ORS prevents and treats dehydration from diarrhoea irrespective of cause or age group affected. It is a balanced and the best mixture of glucose and electrolytes for use in treating and preventing dehydration, potassium depletion and base deficit due to diarrhoea. Glucose in ORS helps in transporting sodium and water across the intestinal membrane during diarrhoea. Glucose thus promotes/increases the absorption of sodium and water from the intestine.[10–15]

Basis of ORS and Mechanism of Action

In most diarrhoeas, the absorptive capacity of gut is retained and nutrients such as glucose, amino acids and dipeptides tend to be absorbed in majority of cases. As glucose is absorbed in the gut, sodium is carried along and also gets absorbed, even though it is being actively lost in secretory diarrhoea due to the effect of enterotoxins. ORS helps absorption of glucose and sodium. Sodium also promotes absorption of water. This is the physiological basis of oral rehydration therapy.

The ORS packet supplied under the national programme has a light blue colour and has the national LOGO. If ORS from other sources are used, the packet should be checked to confirm that it has the right composition. Packets with a high glucose content (more than 20 g per litre), should not be used as these can lead to osmotic diarrhoea and worsen the condition of child. Packets containing colouring and sweetening agents like saccharine should also not be used.

Reduced osmolarity ORS with sodium 75, chloride 65, glucose anhydrous 75, potassium 20, citrate 10 mmol/litre with total osmolarity of 245 mmol/litre has been recommended by **WHO, UNICEF,** IAP and MOH and FW as universal ORS solution. This solution has improved efficacy for treatment of children with acute non-cholera diarrhoea (Table 12.32).[16]

Table 12.32: Composition of reduced osmolarity ORS*

Ingredient	*Weight (g)*
Sodium chloride	2.6
Glucose-anhydrous	13.5
Potassium chloride	1.5
Trisodium citrate, dihydrate	2.9

*To be used in one litre of potable water

Because of improved effectiveness of reduced osmolarity ORS solution, especially for children, with acute, non-cholera diarrhoea, WHO and UNICEF, now recommend that countries to use and manufacture the above formulation in place of previously recommended ORS solution with a total osmolarity of 311 mOsm/litre. From now on reduced osmolarity ORS of 245 mmol/litre is being used in the programme. India is the first country in the world to introduce reduced osmolarity ORS.

National Guidelines/Policy on Management of Diarrhoea

In early stages, when fluid loss is less than 5% of the body weight, children may not show any clinical signs of dehydration, but may still have subclinical or incipient dehydration. The purpose of fluid therapy in such cases is to prevent dehydration by giving HAF and ORS.

Policy guidelines: ORS should, however, be advised to all such cases when they are brought to the health facility and mothers must be advised on how to prepare ORS solution and how much ORS should be given. The quantities of fluids to be given are shown in **Plan A**.

Treatment Plan A—Prevention of Dehydration

i. *Replacement of Ongoing Losses to Prevent Dehydration* (Table 12.33)

Mother or caretakers of children without physical signs of dehydration **(no dehydration)** visiting health care providers should be educated to give ORS for replacement of ongoing losses to prevent dehydration and use increased amount of culturally appropriate home available fluids (HAF) and food based solutions.

Show the mother how much ORS to give after each stool in addition to usual fluid intake. Give her enough ORS packets for 2 days.

Give a teaspoonful every 1–2 minutes for a child under 2 years. Give frequent sips from a cup for an older child.

If the child vomits wait for 10 minutes. Then give the solution slowly (a spoonful every 2–3 minutes). If diarrhoea continues after the ORS packets are used up, tell mother give home available fluids or return for more ORS. Mother should continue feeding during diarrhoea.

ii. *Provision of Normal Daily Fluid Requirement*

The normal daily fluid requirement should be continued, i.e. breast milk and for those not taking breast milk, the milk they were providing (full strength animal milk or infant formula). Other fluids consumed by the child and plain water should be continued. Semisolid foods should be offered at frequent interval.

Treat Diarrhoea at Home

Mother or caregivers hold the key for prevention of dehydration at home. Response of mothers in acute diarrhoea is critical to prevent dehydration and deaths. Hence, counselling of mothers, by health workers, AWWs, ASHAs on their home visits or contact with mother, to practice 4 rules of Home Treatment: Give extrafluid, continue feeding including breastfeeding, give zinc and when to return to facility.

Table 12.33: Plan A—for prevention of dehydration*

Age	*Amount of ORS to be given after each liquid stool*	*Amount of ORS to provide for use at home*
• <6 months	50 ml	Give one packet for no dehydration and two packets for children with dehydration
• 7 months to less than 2 years	50–100 ml	
• 2 years up to 10 years	100–200 ml	
• 10 years or more	As much as wanted	

*ORS is appropriate for both prevention and treatment of dehydration

12

1 Give extrafluids (as much as the child will take)
   a Breastfeed frequently and for longer at each feed if passing frequent watery stools:
      - For less than 6 months age give ORS and clean water in addition to breast milk.
      - If six months or older give one or more of the home fluids in addition to breast milk.
   b If the child is not exclusively breastfed
      In addition to ORS give one or more of the acceptable and available food based or home available fluids. It is especially important to give ORS at home when:
      - The child has been treated with plan B and plan C or
      - The child cannot return to the clinic if the diarrhoea gets worse.

2 Continue feeding—counsel the mother
   - Up to 6 months of age exclusive breastfeeding at least 8 times in 24 hours. Do not give any other food or fluids except ORS/ORT. Continue breastfeeding during diarrhoea.
   - *6 to 12 months:* Breast feed as often as the child wants. Give at least one *katori* serving at a time (3–5 times per day) of mashed roti/rice/bread mixed in sweetened undiluted milk/or mashed roti/rice/bread mixed in thick dal with added ghee/oil or Khichri with added oil/ghee. Add cooked vegetables also in serving.
   - *12 months up to 2 years:* Breastfeed as often as child wants. Give at least $1\frac{1}{2}$ *katori* serving 5 times per day of above mentioned recipes.
   - *2 years older:* Give family food at least 3 meals each day and nutritious food between meals such as banana/biscuits and seasonal fruits. Teach your child hand washing before feeding.

3 Give zinc supplements—Government of India Policy, 2006.
   While ORS remains mainstay of therapy during acute diarrhoea, zinc as an adjunct to ORS has an additional benefit in reducing duration and severity of diarrhoea. All cases of diarrhoea should receive zinc in addition to ORS. A uniform dose of 20 mg of elemental zinc should be given to all children 6 months and older and should be started as soon as diarrhoea starts and continued for a total period of 14 days. Children aged 2 months up to 6 months should be advised 10 mg per day of elemental zinc for a total period of 14 days. Dispersible tablets or syrup can be used. These tablets can be dissolved in breast milk or water. Iron interferes with zinc absorption.

4 *When to return:* The mother should be advised to take the child to the health worker/doctor if the child does not get better in 5 days or immediately if the child develops any of **danger signs**—Many watery stools, repeated vomiting, marked thirst, eating or drinking poorly, fever and blood in stool. If this level of prevention of dehydration succeeds some dehydration will not occur and plan B would not be needed and child recovers soon.

Treatment Plan B—Patients with Physical Signs of Dehydration: Rehydration Therapy

Some dehydration indicates failure of level one—to prevent dehydration in diarrhoea. All cases with obvious signs of dehydration need to be treated by trained health workers (AWW/ASHA/ANM trained in IMNCI) or in a health centre or hospital. Oral fluid therapy must be commenced promptly and continued during transport. The fluid therapy for dehydration has three components: At ORS corner.

1 Correction of existing water and electrolyte deficit (dehydration) by rehydration therapy.
2 Replacement of ongoing losses due to continuing diarrhoea.
3 Provision of normal daily fluid requirement.

1 **Guidelines for correcting dehydration by rehydration therapy.**
   - 75 ml/kg of ORS in first 4 hours (patient's age to be used only when the weight is not known) should be started immediately as shown below:

More ORS sould be offered if the child wants it. 100–200 ml clean water should be given during this period to infants up to 6 months who are not breastfed.

Plan B—for treating some dehydration with ORS. Approximate amount of ORS solution to be given in first 4 hours

Age *Weight in kg*	*Up to 4 months* *<6 kg*	*4 months up to 12 months* *6–<10kg*	*12 months up to 2 years* *10–<12 kg*	*2 years up to 5 years* *12–19 kg*
• ORS in ml	200–400	400–700	700–900	900–1400
• Approximate local measure (glass)	1–2	2–3	3–4	4–6

Breastfeeding should be encourged and continued during rehydration and start semisolid foods soon after deficit replacement.

Show the mother how to give ORS solution.

Give frequent small sips from a cup. If the child vomits wait for 10 minutes, then continue but more slowly. Continue breastfeeding.

After 4 Hours

In most children dehydration gets corrected with ORS. Reassess the child and again classify the child for dehydration and select the appropriate plan to continue treatment. Begin feeding the child in the clinic.

If the mother must leave before completing treatment: show her how to prepare ORS solution at home. Show her how much ORS to give to finish 4 hours treatment at home. Give her enough ORS packets to complete rehydration. Also give her 2 packets of ORS as recommended in plan A.

Explain the 4 Rules of Home Treatment:
Give extrafluids
Continue feeding
Give zinc
When to return

2 **Guidelines for maintenance fluid therapy** (replacement of ongoing losses)

This begins when signs of dehydration disappear, usually within 4 hours. Follow plan 'A' for replacement of ongoing losses to prevent dehydration. ORS in volumes equal to diarrhoea losses should be offered. Approximately 10–20 ml per kilogram body weight for each liquid stool. ORS should be continued in this manner till diarrhoea stops. Plain water should be offered in between.

3 **Continue feeding and when to return** (provisions of normal daily fluid requirement)

Counsel mother for continued feeding as given under plan 'A' and when to return as given under plan A.

How Effective is ORT?

In infants and children with clinical evidence of some dehydration, oral rehydration therapy is effective in 95–97% of cases.

Plan C:* *Treatment of severe dehydration with rapid IV rehydration

Severe dehydration results because of failure of level 1, i.e. prevention of dehydration and level 2, i.e. timely correction of some dehydration. Severe dehydration is an emergency hence to be treated quickly by intravenous therapy.

Plan C: Intravenous fluid therapy in severe dehydration 100 ml/kg of Ringer's lactate solution/normal saline divided as follows:

While the drip is being set up, ORS solution should be given if the child can drink.

The best IV fluid solution is Ringer's lactate (Hartmann's solution). An ideal preparation would be Ringer's lactate with 5% dextrose. However, if not available, normal saline solution (0.9% NaCl) can be used. Dextrose/plain glucose on its own is not effective.

Plan C

Age	*First give 30 ml/kg in*	*Then give 70 ml/kg in*	*Total 100 ml/kg*
<12 months	1 hour*	5 hours	6 hours
Older children	30 minutes*	$2\frac{1}{2}$ hours	3 hours

* Repeat once if radial pulse is still very weak or not detectable.

Reassess the child every 1–2 hours. If hydration status is not improving give the IV drip more rapidly. Also give ORS (about 5 ml/kg/hour) as soon as the child can drink usually after 3–4 hours (infants) or 1–2 hours (children).

Reassess an infant after 6 hours and a child after 3 hours, classify dehydration. Then choose the appropriate plan (A, B or C) to continue treatment.

If the treatment facility is far away rehydration can be started with nasogastric tube or by mouth with ORS solution: Give 20 ml/kg/hour for 6 hours (total of 120 ml/kg). Reassess the child after 1–2 hours.

Nutritional Management of Acute Diarrhoea

Diarrhoea worsens nutritional status. Diarrhoea is an important 'nutritional leak' in young children because of (a) decreased food intake and maternal food withholding and (b) intestinal malabsorption of macronutrients and some micronutrients. Anorexia is restricted to acute febrile phase only and up to 80% of recommended daily intake is accepted by infants even during very acute phase of diarrhoea. Anorexia does not affect intake of breast milk. Full caloric intake during diarrhoea is safe and advantageous. There is no physiological basis for resting the bowel during or following acute diarrhoea. Fasting further reduces the digestibility of food in the intestine and is dangerous in already malnourished children. Recovery from diarrhoea is not simply cessation of liquid stools but achievement of catch up growth. A higher than recommended intake of food during convalescence is consumed by affected children and it facilitates catch up growth.

- Children should continue to be fed during acute diarrhoea, because feeding is physiologically sound and forms the component of ORT, helps prevents dehydration, early recovery and minimizes the deterioration of nutritional status.
- In acute diarrhoea breastfeeding should be continued uninterrupted even during rehydration with ORS.
- Staple foods should be enriched with fats/oils or sugar to provide more energy. *Khichri* with oil, rice with milk or curd, mashed potatoes with oil and lentil are good foods.
- Animal milk does not need to be diluted during any phase of diarrhoea. Milk cereal mixtures, e.g. dalia, and milk rice mixture is good food.
- During recovery an intake of at least 125% of normal should be with nutrient dense food.

Persistent Diarrhoea (PD)

Diarrhoea that starts as an acute episode and lasts at least 14 days is said to be persistant diarrhoea. This excludes celiac disease and tropical sprue. The predominant causes of persistant diarrhoea are:

- Persistent *infection* with one or more enteric pathogens.
- Malabsorption particularly of carbohydrates and fat and due to combination of malnutrition and enteric infection.
- Infrequently dietary protein intolerance.

The major consequences of PD are growth faltering, worsening of malnutrition and death during subsequent illness or diarrhoea.

Management

- Prevent dehydration and treat dehydration if present
- Treat undernutrition
- Treat infection with specific antibiotics
- Give single dose of vit A as per age
- Give zinc sulphate 20 mg per day for 14 days.

Nearly two-thirds of persistent diarrhoea patients can be treated at home. In the presence of dehydration and severe malnutrition and presence of systemic infection hospital treatment is indicated.

Milk cereal mixtures, milk or curd cereal mixtures are tolerated well in persistent diarrhoea.

Drug Therapy in Acute Diarrhoea

Antimicrobial drugs are not required for treatment of cases of acute diarrhoea because these are caused by viral agents or by *Escherichia coli* that act by liberating enterotoxins (ETEC). Clinical studies have shown that antibiotic therapy does not offer any significant clinical benefit in ETEC associated diarrhoea.

The only specific clinical indications for use of antimicrobial agents are:

- Cholera and Bloody diarrhoea

Cholera

Cholera should be suspected when a child older than 5 years develops severe dehydration from acute watery diarrhoea, or any patient older than 2 years has acute watery diarrhoea where cholera is endemic.

Treatment: Treatment of dehydration is the mainstay.

Initial treatment of dehydration from cholera should follow the guidelines given above for patients with some or severe dehydration. For patients with severe dehydration and shock, the initial intravenous infusion should be given very rapidly to restore adequate blood volume.

Antimicrobial for treatment: Antibiotic of choice is Doxycycline single dose 50 mg for children 2–4 years and 100 mg for children 4–5 years. Alternate antibiotic is Tetracycline. After rehydration zinc should be given for 14 days.

Bloody Diarrhoea

The episode of diarrhoea is termed bloody diarrhoea or dysentery when visible blood is present in the stool. Terms like bloody diarrhoea, dysentery, bacillary dysentery and invasive diarrhoea are often used interchangeably. Bacillary dysentery is used for dysentery caused by shigella and distinguishes shigellosis from amoebic dysentery.

Antimicrobial Therapy in Bloody Diarrhoea

Antimicrobial therapy is the mainstay of treatment of bloody diarrhoea and is targeted towards shigella as it is the commonest cause of bloody diarrhoea. WHO recommends ciprofloxacin as the drug of choice, 15 mg/kg twice a day for 3 days. Second line of drug is ceftriaxone 50–100 mg/kg once a day, intramuscular for 2–5 days. Azithromycin 6–20 mg/kg once a day orally for 1–5 days. Treat dehydration and give zinc.

Acute Diarrhoea in Severely Malnourished Child

Severe malnutrition is defined as presence of severe wasting (less than 70% weight-for-height or < –3SD) and/or edema and mid upper arm circumference <11.5 cm.

Basic format for assessing dehydration remains the same for SMN however there are some signs that are not reliable. In SMN child usually has dry mouth and absent tears because of atrophied salivary and lacrimal glands. Skin turgor is not useful sign in SMN. Signs that are useful for assessing dehydration are: Eagerness to drink (sign of some dehydration), weak or absent radial pulse and decreased or absent urine flow (sign of severe dehydration).

Fluid Therapy in SMN with Dehydration

Give the low osmolarity ORS orally or by nasogastric tube, much more slowly than you would when rehydrating a well-nourished child.

Other Oral Rehydration Therapy (ORT)

Sugar Salt Solution (SSS): 40 g sugar (Sucrose) and 4 g of salt (Sodium Chloride) in one litre of water makes an excellent rehydration solution and is effective replacement when ORS is not available.

Food-based Solutions

Food-based solutions are those that are commonly used in homes and have a sound physiological basis (i.e. contain acceptable concentrations of starch and sodium). Examples are rice water with salt, dal or dal water with salt, butter milk (Lassi) with salt and certain soups with salt.

Home Available Fluids (HAF)

Plain clean water (preferably given with food), lemon water, soup, coconut water are classified as home available fluids. A second catergory may include fluids like rice kanji, dal without salt. Many of these fluids lack glucose precursors or salt or both. Therefore, these fluids are likely to be effective only in the presence of continued feeding which provides starch (ultimately glucose) and protein (ultimately amino acids) to promote absorption of luminal sodium. These fluids together with food provide ORT (oral rehydration therapy).

Components of ORT: ORS Plus Home fluids (Food based solutions and Home available fluids) plus sugar salt solution plus continued feeding. ORT is used for prevention as well as treatment of dehydration.

Prevention of Diarrhoea

Exclusive breastfeeding: Encourage exclusive breastfeeding up to 6 months of age. Breastfeeding prevents diarrhoea and ensures adequate growth of child. Avoid bottle feeding.

Hand washing: A systematic review estimated that safe disposal of excreta alone can reduce diarrhoeal diseases by 36%, and a separate review of the effects of *hand* washing with soap on diarrhoea found a 45% reduction.[17] Taken together this suggests that the safe disposal of excreta combined with associated hygiene could reduce the incidence of diarrhoeal deaths by 65%.[18,19]

Clean food: Eating clean food and freshly cooked food prevents diarrhoea.

Clean water and sanitation: Drinking safe water after chlorination and safe storage of water at home is necessary to prevent diarrhoea and this measure reduces diarrhoeal morbidity by 26% (WHO 1992). Improved water supply and safe disposal of excreta of children and adults is long-term goal in prevention of diarrhoea.

Immunization: Measles immunization prevents measles and thereby measles induced diarrhoea in young children.

Vit. A: Prophylactic doses of vitamin A in young children builds protection of epithelium and it has a role in prevention of diarrhoea.

Nutrition: Improved nutrition of young children prevents malnutrition and thereby reduces the development of persistent diarrhoea. Improved nutrition increases the fighting power against infections in general.

Rotavirus Vaccine in Diarrhoea Prevention

Rotaviruses are leading cause of severe, dehydrating diarrhoea in children aged <5 years globally, and causes approximately 40% of childhood diarrhoea hospitalization worldwide and around 39% in India in children less than 5 years of age. Rotavirus diarrhoea kills 122000 to 153000 children every year in India mostly under 2 years.

Live, oral monovalent rotavirus vaccine (Rotarix®) has been licensed in India and other countries. Government of India has introduced rotavirus vaccine under UIP as a 3 dose oral vaccine along with OPV 1st, 2nd and 3rd dose, in a phased manner in a few states and districts as per vaccine availability by 2016. It prevents only rotavirus diarrhoea and not other diarrhoeas in young children hence prevention remains the mainstay.[20]

NATIONAL DIARRHOEAL DISEASES CONTROL PROGRAMME (NDDCP) AND POLICY ON MANAGEMENT OF DIARRHOEAL DISEASES[21-23]

Recognizing the problem of acute watery diarrhoea in children the 31st World Health Assembly in May 1978, called for a concerted attack on diarrhoeal diseases as part of global commitment to primary health care and health for all by the year 2000 AD. The WHO diarrhoeal diseases control programme was launched soon thereafter.

During the 6th five-year plan, it was realized that cholera constituted only 5–10% of morbidity and mortality due to diarrhoeal diseases. The need to seriously consider other diarrhoeal diseases was felt. National Cholera Control Programme (NCCP) was renamed as National Diarrhoeal Disease Control Programme (NDDCP).

In view of the recommendations of World Health Assembly Diarrhoeal Disease Control Programme was launched in India in 1981 with main emphasis on short-term objective of reduction of mortality through effective introduction of oral rehydration therapy (ORT). Now it is integral part of Integrated Management of Childhood Illness (IMCI) strategy and integrated action plan for pneumonia and diarrhoea.

Goal

- Reduce diarrhoeal associated mortality in children under the age of 5 by 30% by 1995 and by 50% by 2010 (NHP 2002).
- Reducing case fatality rate to less than 1%.

Long-term goal was to decrease morbidity due to diarrhoeal diseases through improvement in environmental health by providing potable water and sanitation facilities. Since 1985–86 with the inception of National ORT programme the focus of activities has been on strengthening of case management of diarrhoea for children under the age of 5 and improving *maternal knowledge* and practices related to use of home available fluids, use of ORS and continuing feeding.

Strategies

i Ensure standard case management of diarrhoea (including dysentery and persistent diarrhoea) by training of medical and other health personnel.
ii Promote standard case management practices among private practitioners through Indian Medical Association and Indian Academy of Paediatrics.
iii Improve maternal knowledge on home management of diarrhoea and recognition of danger signs for seeking immediate medical care. Intensified diarrhoea control fortnights were leunched in July 2014 and 15

ORT use Rate (Coverage Evaluation Survey-2009)

Free supply of standard ORS packets at village level through subcentres, contained in subcentres drug kit "A" have been provided. Though ORS is most important advance of 20th century only 43% of children who suffered from diarrhoea were treated with ORS packets. While 56.3% used any ORT or increased fluids and gruel. Around 47% of prescriptions of diarrhoea included ORS, while tonics, antidiarrhoeal drugs and injections continued to be prescribed in same proportion (UNICEF Survey-2009).

Revised Guidelines for Management of Diarrhoea

The revised guidelines for management of diarrhoea issued by Government of India and the Indian academy of pediatrics recommend low osmolarity ORS, plus zinc (10 mg elemental zinc for infants 2–6 months and 20 mg per day for children ≥6 months for 14 days) and continued feeding of energy dense feeds in addition to breastfeeding. The guidelines emphasize the importance of home available fluids, hand washing and other hygiene practices. Antimicrobials are recommended only for gross blood in stools or *Shigella* positive culture, cholera, associated systemic infection, or severe malnutrition.[24–25] Apart from reducing duration and severity of the treated episode of acute diarrhoea, zinc has the potential to decrease hospital admission rates by 15–20%, decrease child mortality by 3–5%. Water dispersible zinc tablets are available for use.

REFERENCES

1 Ghai OP. Understanding and Managing Acute Diarrhoea in Infants and Young Children. In: Ghai OP. Essential Paediatrics; New Delhi.

2 WHO/UNICEF. The management of diarrhoea and use of oral rehydration therapy—A joint WHO/UNICEF statement. Geneva: WHO; 1983.

3 WHO. World Health Report. Geneva: WHO; 2003.

4 IIPS and ORC Macro. National Family Health Survey, NFHS-2 and 3. Mumbai: IIPS; 2000 and 2006.

5 Lal S. Assessment of health and disease situation—Surveillance of acute diarrhoeal diseases at the village level. Regional Scientific meeting, International Epidemiological Association; 1986 Feb. 25–28: Jhansi (UP).

6 Lal S. Surveillance of acute diarrhoeal diseases at village level for effective home management of diarrhoea. Ind. J. Pub Health Apr-June 1994; 38 (2): 65–8.

7 Central Technical Committee. Survey—Evaluation and Research, 1975–1995. New Delhi: ICDS/CTC.

8 GOI. Diarrhoeal diseases status in urban and rural areas of India, 1985. New Delhi.

9 WHO. Guidelines for cholera control programme for control of diarrhoeal diseases. Geneva: WHO; 1985.

10 Ayres D. Diarrhoea knowledge can save lives. Health for all 2000 AD. The count down has begun. Geneva: WHO; 1985.

11 Shiva M. A taste of tears. New Delhi: Voluntary Health Association of India; 1984.

12 GOI. Training of doctor on treatment of diarrhoeal diseases and programme management—National diarrhoeal disease control and ORT programme. Calcutta: NIC and ED, ICMR.

13 GOI. National child survival and safe motherhood programme. Programme intervention. New Delhi: MCH division MOH and FW; 1994.

14 Pierce NF, Hirschhorn. Oral fluids—a simple weapon against dehydration in diarrhoea. WHO chronicle 1977; 31: 87–93.

15 ICMR. Treatment of diarrhoeal diseases—A guide for basic health workers. Calcutta: Cholera Research Centre.

16 WHO. Reduced osmolarity oral rehydration salt (ORS) formulation. Report of meeting of experts organized by WHO/UNICEF. UNICEF House, New York; WHO; 2001.

17 Esrey SA, potash JB, Roberts L, shift C. "Effects of improved water supply and sanitation on ascariasis, diarrhoea, dracunculosis, hookworm infection, schistosomiasis and trachoma". Bulletin of WHO, 1991; 69 (5): 609–621.

18 Government of India, Monthly Newsletter of NICD, DGHS water-borne diseases July and August 2006, 10: 7–8.

19 Curtis V and Cairncross S. 'Effect of washing hands with soap on diarrhoea risk in community: a systemic review'. The lancet infectious diseases 2003; 3:275–81.

20 GOI. Operational Guidelines, Introduction of Rotavirus vaccine in UIP in India. Immunization Division MOHFW Dec. 2015.

21 ICMR. National diarrhoeal disease, control programme India. Management of acute diarrhoea. Calcutta: NIC and ED ICMR; 1982.

22 WHO. World Health Report, 2002—Reducing risk and promoting healthy life. Geneva: WHO; 2002.

23 WHO. People first, water and sanitation later—community partnership in the international decade. Geneva: WHO; 1987.

24 GOI. Policy on management of diarrhoeal diseases amongst children under-five through promotion of ORT. New Delhi: MOH and FW; GOI.

25 Govt. of India, use of zinc in NPDDCP, MOH and FW, Dept. of Family Welfare Child Health Division. Nirman Bhawan, New Delhi, 2nd Nov 2006.

26 GOI. Revised guidelines for management of diarrhoea in Children for Medical officers and Health Workers—India, August 2007.

CHOLERA

Cholera has re-emerged as a major infectious disease in the recent past with a global increase in its incidence. Cholera is one of the acute diarrhoeal diseases and accounts for 5% of total diarrhoeal diseases in India. Hence, clinical management should be essentially the same as for acute diarrhoea from other causative organisms. *Vibrio cholerae* is the causative organism of cholera. *Vibrio cholerae* is a facultative anaerobic, Gram-negative, non-spore forming curved rod-shaped organism actively motile and widely distributed. Toxigenic *V. cholerae* produces cholera enterotoxin (CT) which disrupts the ion transport by intestinal epithelial cells.

Vibrio cholerae of 01 biotype *El Tor* has replaced the age old *V. cholerae* 01 biotype classical. With the exception of classical cholera outbreak in Madhya Pradesh in 1970, no large scale outbreak of cholera due to biotype classical has been reported after 1965. In fact hardly any classical *V. cholerae* has been isolated in India after 1980. The epidemiology of cholera took a dramatic turn when *V. cholerae* 0139 Bengal emerged as new strain of cholera in Madras in 1992.

EPIDEMIOLOGY OF CHOLERA—SALIENT FEATURES

Occurrence

Cholera occurs in endemic, epidemic and pandemic forms.

Between 1817 and 1923, six pandemics of cholera originated in Indian subcontinent. The classical biotype was responsible for 5th and 6th pandemics and is believed to have been associated with the earlier pandemics as well, although there is no hard evidence.

The seventh pandemic which started from Indonesia in 1961 which invaded India in 1964 was due to *V. cholerae* 01 biotype *El Tor*. Similarly, the current eighth pandemic is attributable to 0139 serogroup. A new cholera epidemic erupted in Madras, Southern India, in October, 1992 and rapidly spread eastward. The causative organism for this outbreak was *V. cholerae* non-01, which produces cholera toxin and is now known as the 0139 serogroup. *V. cholerae* strains were isolated from Calcutta and Bangladesh and this may be the beginning of eighth pandemic (Bhattacharya et al. 1993; Nair et al. 1994). The classical *V. cholerae* has been displaced by biotype *El Tor* all the world over. The epidemiology of cholera took a dramatic turn when *V. cholerae* 0139 Bengal emerged as a new strain of cholera in Madras in December, 1992; it spread rapidly far and wide and became a major cause of epidemics in India and Bangladesh. After 1992, both the strains biotype *El Tor* and 0139 continue to exist. The new strain remained confined to South Asia. Since imported cases due to *V. cholerae* 0139 have been reported from many countries including USA, Germany and Japan, and therefore, the new strain still poses a global threat.[1]

Epidemics

Current Global Scenario (Table 12.34)

Cholera has *re-emerged* as a major infectious disease in the recent past; with a global increase in its incidence. In 1994, cholera cases were notified from 94 countries—the highest ever number of countries in one year (WHO 1995). Two disturbing aspects of global cholera picture in 1990s have been dramatic and unexpected reappearance of epidemic cholera caused by *V. cholerae* 01 *El Tor* in Latin America after 100 years absence from the region and unprecedented appearance in 1992 in Southern India of an epidemic strain of *Vibrio cholerae* non-01, classified as *V. cholerae* 0139 Bengal. It indicated that cases have increased in all the continents in the last few years; due to changes in environments which have created conditions favourable for cholera outbreaks worldwide. Cholera is International notifiable disease and its occurrence is regularly reported to WHO. Trade embargo or restrictions are imposed on countries that report cholera, which are unfounded and discouraging for correct and adequate reporting. WHO has never documented any outbreak of cholera resulting from commodities imported from cholera endemic areas. Cholera outbreak in Haiti reported 60,240 cases and 1415 deaths up to 20th November, 2010 with case fatality rate of 2.3%.

Table 12.34: Global cholera situation, 1991–2013

Year	No. of countries reporting cholera	No. of cases	No. of deaths	CFR (%)
1991	59	5,94,694	19,295	3.2
1992	68	4,61,783	8072	1.7
1993	78	3,76,845	6781	1.8
1994	94	3,84,403	10,692	2.8
1995	78	2,08,755	5034	2.4
1996	71	1,43,349	6689	4.7
1997	65	1,47,425	6274	4.3
1998	74	2,93,121	10,586	3.6
1999	NA	2,22,475	8423	3.8
2006	52	2,36,896	6311	2.6
2008	–	1,90,130	5413	2.7
2009	45	2,21,226	4946	2.24
2010	33	3,17,534	7543	2.37
2011	58	5,89,854	7816	1.3
2013	47	1,29,064	2102	1.63

Current Situation in India (Table 12.35)

Many outbreaks of cholera (epidemics) have been reported in various states in India from 1975 to 2014 which have been investigated by NICD.[2] These epidemics were associated with contamination of water supplies. Contamination of water sources occur regularly due to discharge of raw sewage from cities in rivers, during natural calamities—floods, earthquakes or during mass gatherings (Kumbh-mela, ritual baths, refugee camps and religious festivals). People may drink contaminated river water and carry holy river water in bottles/cans to their homes.

Available data indicate that cholera is endemic (persisting) in India. Reported cases and deaths due to cholera in India from 1950 onwards are presented in Table 12.35. This is in fact gross underestimate of real incidence because of under reporting of cases and deaths and poor surveillance system. The mortality has been considerably reduced because of better case management with ORS. Case fatality which was around 44% in 1955 has been reduced to less than 1% because of improved management.[3]

Endemicity

Cholera is endemic in West Bengal, Odisha and Chennai (Madras) and in many other countries in the world. The endemicity is linked with the warm and humid conditions and salinity of water. Epidemics are typically abrupt but self-limited. Asymptomatic carriers of cholera are common.

Reservoir of Infection

Man is the only known reservoir of infection. Patient remains infectious usually for a few days after recovery

Table 12.35: Notified cases and deaths of cholera in India from 1950 to 2014

Year	Cholera		Year	Cholera	
	Cases	Deaths		Cases	Deaths
1950	1,76,307	86,993	1985	5813	154
1956	39,759	17,121	1986	4211	71
1957	56,007	22,996	1987	11,423	224
1958	66,076	28,180	1988	8957	215
1959	1,14,937	5418	1989	5044	72
1960	14,167	5250	1990	3704	87
1961	47,637	16,334	1991	7088	150
1962	27,165	9403	1992	6911	55
1963	56,988	20,209	1993	9437	53
1965	42,385	12,947	1994	4973	32
1967	13,658	3122	1995	3432	9
1968	22,587	4472	1996	4425	34
1969	19,280	3757	1997	3173	18
1970	17,268	3801	1998	7151	10
1972	21,344	2908	2000	3879	18
1973	40,855	5308	2001	4178	6
1974	30,997	2189	2002	3455	10
1975	21,955	2320	2003	2893	2
1976	17,492	861	2005	3155	6
1977	9091	538	2006	1939	3
1978	10,708	263	2007	2635	3
1979	5638	312	2008	2680	1
1980	8717	309	2010	5155	9
1981	6073	200	2011	2341	10
1982	4693	217	2012	1688	2
1983	9202	432	2013	1127	5
1984	2642	68	2014 (P)	969	5

from clinical symptoms. Occasionally, the carrier stage may persist for several months.

Transmission

Even before the cholera organism was discovered; the transmission of cholera through contaminated water was described in 1853 in London by John Snow's pioneering epidemiological investigations. Cholera is transmitted or spread through contaminated water and food with faecal matter. Water supply system or source when contaminated due to sewage or by dirty hands at household level is a risk factor for occurrence of cholera. A high dose of more than 10^4 organisms is usually required to produce clinical disease.

Incubation Period

It varies from a few hours to a few days. The average incubation period is 2–3 days.

For the purpose of international health regulations (IHR) the incubation period is 5 days for quarantine.

Carriers

12

The majority of infections with *V. cholerae* 01 biotype *El Tor* or *V. cholerae* 0139 remain asymptomatic or in more than 90% of cases, cholera is mild and may therefore be difficult to distinguish clinically from other types of acute diarrhoeal disease.

Persons at Risk

Slum dwellers, areas with unsafe water and poor personal hygienic practices with dual water supply system are at risk. Usually in newly affected areas large proportion of cases are in adults. Cholera is mainly a disease of children in the highly endemic areas. Case fatality rate may be very high in untreated cases but do not exceed 1% with prompt treatment.

Typical Case

Presents with sudden onset of profuse, painless and effortless watery diarrhoea (rice water stool) with occasional vomiting, rapid dehydration and circulatory collapse. In addition, patients usually develop base deficit acidosis, hyponatremia and hypokalemia.

Clinical Case Description

- *In an area where disease is not known to be present:* Severe dehydration or death from acute watery diarrhoea in a patient aged 5 years or more.
- *In an area where cholera is endemic:* Acute diarrhoea with or without vomiting in a patient aged 5 years or more.
- *In an area where there is a cholera epidemic:* Acute watery diarrhoea with or without vomiting in any patient.

Case Classification

Suspect case: A case that meets the clinical case definition.

Probable case: Not applicable.

Confirmed: *Vibrio cholerae* 01 or 0139 is isolated from the stool samples of any patient with diarrhoea.

Surveillance and Notification of Cases

Because cholera has the potential of rapid spread leading to acute public health problem, special attention is given to surveillance for early recognition, early response, and reporting of cases. All suspected and presumptive patients aged five years or more who develop severe dehydration from acute watery diarrhoea should be notified to PHC/CHC/district hospital. Early response to prevent and treat dehydration at household level with home available fluids and ORS is important to prevent deaths from cholera. Each state provides weekly notification of confirmed cases to Directorate General of Health Services, New Delhi, with a copy to NICD, Delhi. Under the international health regulations, notification to WHO about cases of cholera is mandatory. National health authorities should report the first suspected case to WHO at the earliest possible moment; laboratory confirmation of cases should also be reported immediately. Thereafter health authorities should report confirmed cases to WHO on weekly basis. Once the presence of cholera in a particular area, has been confirmed, it is unnecessary to confirm all subsequent cases. Moreover, neither the treatment nor the notification of suspected cases of cholera requires laboratory confirmation of the presence of *V. cholerae* 01 (WHO 1993); the decision to initiate anti-epidemic measures must be taken regardless of the causative strain.

Clinical Management

As pointed out in the beginning, the clinical management of cholera is essentially the same as far acute diarrhoea from other causes. Early response and home treatment by home available fluids and oral rehydration therapy (ORT) can reduce the case fatality to less than 1%.

Nearly 95% of patients can be adequately treated with oral rehydration salt (ORS) solution alone, without intravenous therapy and antibiotics. In severely dehydrated patients, ORS should be started as soon as the patients are able to drink; even before initial intravenous therapy has been completed. Drinking fluid should be the first response. Intravenous therapy is required for those with clinically severe form of dehydration and shock. Best I/V fluids is Ringer's lactate solution. Normal saline is less effective but can be used if Ringer lactate solution is not available. *Plain glucose solution is not effective and should not be used.*

In severe cases, antibiotics can reduce the volume and duration of diarrhoea and can shorten the period during which the *Vibrio cholerae* are excreted. Use of antibiotics for mild cases is not recommended; to avoid development of antibiotic resistance. Tetracyclines and norfloxacin are effective antibiotics. Studies done at NICD Delhi, National Institute of Cholera and other Enteric Diseases (NICED), Calcutta and King Institute of Preventive Medicine in Chennai have shown that prevalent *V. cholerae* are resistant to furazolidine, cotrimoxazole, ampicillin, nalidixic acid and streptomycin. Patient should be encouraged to take food such as rice porridge (*Khichri*), curd, cooked and mashed pulses of their liking and plenty of fluids. Breastfeeding of infants and young children should be continued.[4]

Prevention and Control of Outbreaks of Cholera

Control measures for *V. cholerae* 0139 and *V. cholerae* 01 are the same. The cardinal measures include:

- Safe drinking water.
- Sanitary disposal of human excreta (sanitary latrines).
- Improvements in water supply and sanitation can reduce cholera morbidity by 80–100% (WHO 1992).[5–7]
- Hand washing before eating and after defecation.
- Clean food and clean utensil.
- Education of people and involvement of community.

Regular chlorination of water, and ensuring residual chlorine, destroys *Vibrio cholerae* organisms. Sanitary disposal of human excreta prevents contamination of water and food. Hand washing prevents diarrhoeal diseases including cholera.

Recommended chlorine levels in water distribution systems in areas affected by cholera[4]

The minimum levels of free residual chlorine necessary for safe water are:

- At all sampling points in a piped water system......0.5 mg/litre
- At standposts in system with standposts...........1.0 mg/litre
- In tankers trucks, at filling.......................................2.0 mg/litre

Active monitoring is required to ensure that these minimum levels of chlorine are maintained.

Making Water Safe by Chlorination

Make a stock solution of chlorine (1% concentration by weight of available chlorine). Add to 1 litre of water:

Product (percent concentration by weight of available chlorine)	*Amount*
Calcium hypochlorite (70%)	15 g
or	
Bleaching powder or chlorinated lime (30%)	33 g
or	
Sodium hypochlorite (5%)	250 ml
or	
Sodium hypochlorite (10%)	110 ml

Store the stock solution in cool place in a closed container that does not admit light. The stock solution loses effectiveness with time and must be used no later than one month after it has been made.

Use the stock solution to make water safe. Add stock solution to water and ensure proper mixing.

The quantity of stock solution added to water

Stock solution	*Quantity of water*
0.6 ml or 3 drops	1 litre
6 ml	10 litres
60 ml	1000 litres

Allow the chlorinated water to stand for at least 30 minutes before using it.

For Effective Disinfection, there should be a residual concentration of free chlorine of ≥0.5 mg/litres after at least 30 minutes of contact time at pH < 8.0. Chlorine residual should be maintained throughout the distribution system. At the point of delivery the minimum residual concentration of free chlorine should be 0.2 mg/litres.

If the water is turbid (not clear, with a lot of suspended solid matter) then

- Filter it before chlorination or
- Boil it vigorously instead of treating it by chlorination.

Role of Chemoprophylaxis and Vaccination

According to WHO guidelines, chemoprophylaxis, vaccination and *cordon sanitaire,* trade and travel restrictions have been found to be ineffective and are not recommended for the control of an outbreak of cholera or for the prevention of its spread to other areas.

Mass chemoprophylaxis is not only ineffective and inappropriate in preventing the spread of cholera, but it also diverts manpower and resources from delivering other effective measures. In several countries, it has contributed to emergence of antibiotic resistance in the *Vibrio*, depriving severely ill patients from valuable treatment. The value of selective chemotherapy of household contacts is also doubtful. It is not recommended as a routine measure.

Vaccines

- i The currently available cholera vaccines do not have high efficacy, the efficacy is around 50–60%. The protection lasts for 3–6 months only.
- ii Most vaccine producers do not test the vaccine potency and produce vaccine that do not have required potency.
- iii Vaccination does not alter the severity of disease and does not reduce the rate of asymptomatic infections—thus it cannot prevent the introduction of cholera into a country or its spread within an area.[4]
- iv To be effective in a non-endemic area and in children in endemic area, vaccine has to be given in 2 doses at 10–28 days, interval.
- v It generally takes around 8–10 days to induce immunity.
- vi People coming forward to receive vaccine are usually those who are less likely to become ill with cholera.
- vii Vaccine gives a false sense of security to those vaccinated and feeling of accomplishment and complacency to health authorities, who consequently neglect the more effective precautions.
- viii Vaccination campaign even with vaccine obtained free of charge, divert resources, attention and manpower from more useful activities.

Realization of these limitations prompted WHO member states at the 26th World Health Assembly (1973) to abolish the requirement of a certificate of vaccination against cholera in the international health regulations (IHR). Therefore, vaccination campaigns for control of cholera are wasteful of scarce resources which could more profitably be extended in applying more effective measures. Moreover, serum hepatitis is more serious problem, has been found to follow mass vaccination campaign in a number of countries, because of **unsafe injection practices.** Widespread outbreak of cholera occurred in capital city of Delhi (Nand Nagri) in 1988 in urban slums and around 50,000 persons were inoculated and the post-vaccination experience was unpleasant.[8–10]

Trade and Travel

The imposition of restrictions on travel and trade between countries or different areas of one country cannot prevent the introduction of cholera as it is extremely difficult, even with enormous efforts to detain all infected persons. Such an imposition encourages the suppression of information of occurrence of cholera, which impedes bilateral and international collaboration and preparatory effort in cholera control in neighbouring countries. The use of check posts at borders to detect infected person by laboratory examination has proved to be an ineffective exercise.

Management of Outbreak

It is best managed locally by rapid response of nearby facility or by people themselves with the help of area Anganwadi workers, health workers and professionals at PHC and CHC set-up. Ensuring adequate intake of home available fluids, and ORS to prevent dehydration in cholera saves life. Chlorination of drinking water prevents spread of cholera. Education of people to encourage washing hands with soap and water prevents cholera and other diarrhoeal diseases. Surveillance of diarrhoeal diseases and dehydration in children 5 years or older leads to detection of suspected cases and their notification along with rapid response at local level. Similarly-monitoring of water quality for coliform organisms (faecal contamination) should be built into the system. Special attention should be given to high-risk pockets in the pre-monsoon season.

Epidemic Disease Act, 1897

The Act provides powers to health authorities to close ice factories prohibit sale and storage of ice candies and cut vegetables. These measures seldom control outbreak/ epidemic of cholera. This Act is being replaced by Public Health (prevention, control and management of epidemics, bioterrorism and diseases). Bill of 2005, which is most comprehensive and stringent.

Laboratory Investigations

Treatment of cholera does not depend on the results of laboratory examination. However, laboratory examination of stool specimens from the first 10 suspected cases, in an outbreak situation, need to be collected to confirm diagnosis and to determine the characteristics of organism including antibiotic sensitivity. Once the presence of cholera is confirmed, it is not necessary to examine specimens from all cases or contacts. Stool specimens or rectal swabs should be collected before the patient has received any antibiotics. Although *V. cholerae* can be cultured and identified in any district level laboratory, more complicated procedures such as phage typing and toxin testing are undertaken by national reference laboratory at NICD, Delhi and National Institute of Cholera and other Enteric Diseases, Calcutta.

Instructions for sample collection:

- Collect the stool sample before the patient receives an antibiotic.
- Use a clean cotton tipped swab and introduce well into the rectum. When this is done well, the swab will become moist and may be faecally stained.

- Alternatively, collect freshly passed liquid stool in a bottle or a cotton tipped swab.
- Send the sample to the laboratory in a tightly sealed screw capped sterile bottle if the sample can reach the laboratory within 2 hours.
- Send the sample to the laboratory in a tightly sealed screw capped sterile bottle with Cary-Blair transport medium (or VR medium or alkaline peptone water) if it will take more than 2 hours to reach the laboratory.
- If transport medium is not available, soak strips of blotting paper with liquid stool and send these to the laboratory in carefully sealed plastic bags to prevent drying.
- Send the samples using a cold chain. If this is not possible send at ambient temperature.
- Bottles and plastic bags should be placed in separate plastic bags each to prevent leakage of the potentially contaminated material.
- Each sample should be labelled. Detailed information of the patients should be sent for each sample.

REFERENCES

1 WHO. Guidelines for drinking water quality—Addendum microbiological agents in drinking water. 2nd ed. 2002. Geneva: WHO.

2 NICD. Cholera: Need for a constant and continuous vigil. CD Alert monthly newsletter Jan 2000; 4(1).

3 CBHI. Health Information of India, 2003. New Delhi: CBHI MOH and FW, GOI; 2003 and 2008 (National Health Profile).

4 WHO. Guidelines for cholera control. Geneva; WHO; 1993.

5 NICD. Cholera: A continuing challenge to Public Health CD Alert April–June 2008; 12(2) NICD, Delhi.

6 Esrey SA, Potash JB, Roberts L, Shift C. Effects of improved water supply and sanitation on ascariasis, diarrhoea, dracunculiasis, hookworm infection, Shistosomiasis and trachoma. Bulletin of WHO, 1991; 69 (5): 609–21.

7 Curtis V and Cairncross S. Effect of washing hands with soap on diarrhoea risk in community: 'a systematic review', the lancet infectious diseases 2003; 3: 275–81.

8 WHO. Guidelines for cholera control. CDD/SER 1986; 80(4) Rev 1: 14.

9 WHO. Annual WHO Statistical Reports 1991–2015. Geneva: WHO.

10 Krishna S. Health. The Times of India. 1988 Aug. 1; p.3.

VIRAL HEPATITIS

Viral hepatitis is an immense public health problem in India. Acute infection with a hepatitis virus may result in conditions ranging from sub-clinical disease to self-limited symptomatic disease to fulminant hepatic failure. Adults with hepatitis A or B are usually symptomatic. Persons with acute hepatitis C may be either symptomatic or asymptomatic.

Causative Organisms

The "Hepatitis viruses" are diverse group of viruses and affect "Liver" the target organ and give rise to hepatitis or inflammation of the liver.

Case Definition

Suspect

Viral hepatitis is an acute illness which causes yellow colouring of eyes and skin, and dark urine.

Presumptive/Clinically Confirmed

Acute onset, fever of short duration followed by jaundice, malaise, anorexia, hepatomegaly and abdominal tenderness in the right upper quadrant. Increase in ALT >2.5 times and serum bilirubin >2 mg% and epidemiological link or outbreak in the area of residence of a case.

Laboratory Confirmed

Serological tests are necessary to identify the type of the virus.

Classification of Hepatitis Viruses[1]

Enteric Transmitted

Hepatitis A Virus (HAV)

Family Picornaviridae: No chronic infection or carrier state, vaccine available, distributed worldwide, low mortality.

Hepatitis E Virus (HEV)

Family Caliciviridae: No chronic infection or carrier state, no vaccine available, restricted geography, causes high mortality in pregnant women.

Hepatitis F Virus (HFV)

The existence of HFV has not yet been conclusively proven (unclassified). No chronic infection or carrier state, no vaccine available, apparently restricted geography and low mortality.

Parenterally Transmitted

Hepatitis B Virus (HBV)

Family Hepadnaviridae: Sometimes chronic carrier state, vaccine available, distributed worldwide, sometimes leads to fatal liver cancer and chronic hepatitis.

Hepatitis C Virus (HCV)

Family Flaviviridae: Chronic infection in >50% of cases, no vaccine available, worldwide distributed.

Hepatitis D Virus (HDV)

Classified as subviral agent: Often chronic infection, no specific vaccine available, restricted geography, defective virus dependent on HBV, extremely difficult to eradicate.

Hepatitis G Virus (HGV)

Family Flaviviridae: Often chronic infection, no vaccine available worldwide distribution (Table 12.36).

Table 12.36: Characteristic features of hepatitis viruses

Parameters	*HAV*	*HBV*	*HCV*	*HDV*	*HEV*	*HGV*
Transmission	Ent.	Par.	Par.	Par.	Ent.	Par.
Incubation period (days)	28–30	60–90	45–60	15–50	25–45	?
Homologous immunity	Yes	Yes	?	Yes	?	?
Chronic carrier	No	Yes	Yes	Yes	No	?
Liver cirrhosis/ cancer	No	Yes	Yes	Yes	No	?

Ent (enteric), Par (parenteral)

HEPATITIS A

Transmission

Hepatitis A and E are widely distributed. Enteric hepatitis viruses are transmitted primarily by faecal-oral route: explosive epidemics of HAV and particularly of HEV usually result from faecal contamination of drinking water or food.

Occurrence

Hepatitis A and E occur in endemic and epidemic fashion. Endemicity means sporadic cases continue to occur throughout the year in cities/areas where water supply is unsafe and continues to be contaminated with faecal matter. Epidemics occur when water supply becomes too bad and large number of cases are reported and clustering of cases in a locality or an area is a common feature.

Distribution

Hepatitis A has the highest global burden at over 5.5 billion. Worldwide, the global public health impact of enteric hepatitis virus infections is immense. Approximately 15 million cases of clinical hepatitis are reported each year. In USA, 57,929 cases of viral hepatitis (25.3/1,00,000 population) were reported in 1981 of which 45% were hepatitis A, and 31,441 cases in 1990, while 31,582 cases were reported in 1995 (American Academy of Paediatrics, Committee on infectious diseases 1996). HAV is the most common of the acute hepatitis in United States. In Shinghai (China), 3,00,000 cases of hepatitis A and 32 deaths (attack rate of 4083/1,00,000 population) were reported in 1988 as shell-fish associated outbreak.

In developing countries, subclinical infection in childhood years may be universal.

Problem in India

12

It is highly endemic in India. Around 1–1.5 lakh cases of viral hepatitis per annum are being reported in India. Different studies in India have shown HAV sero-prevalence to be between 38 and 92% in different age groups. The actual occurrence or incidence may be much higher because of under-reporting and poor surveillance system in the country (Table 12.37).

Table 12.37: Reported cases and deaths due to all viral hepatitis in India[1]

Year	*No. of cases*	*No. of deaths*	*CFR(%)*
1990	1,24,531	1793	1.4
1992	98,047	1268	1.3
1993	1,17,789	1267	1.1
1995	1,10,012	976	0.9
1996	1,31,808	903	0.7
1998	1,11,210	937	0.8
2001	1,49,262	1147	0.7
2003	1,51,287	1006	0.7
2004	2,36,493	–	–
2005	1,81,621	651	0.35
2006	1,52,623	694	0.45
2007	1,52,623	694	0.50
2009	1,24,085	600	0.50
2010	89,150	430	0.50
2011	99,402	520	0.55
2013	1,10,125	574	0.30
2014 (P)	1,39,662	407	0.30

Of the three enteric hepatitis viruses currently recognized, HAV has the longest and best known history. Initially HAV was known as the "infectious" or "epidemic" hepatitis virus because of its typical association with epidemics caused by contaminated water and food worldwide.

Like many picornaviruses, HAV tends to cause infection that are mild or without clinical symptoms in *children*. The incidence of infection is closely linked with hygiene and sanitation conditions and most people in India and other developing countries contract infection during early childhood period. Typical clinical symptoms of infection are seen in *adults*. Most *adults* show signs and symptoms.

Morbidity

Patient feel ill and confined to bed up to 6 weeks or so and severity of illness depends upon nutritional status and immunodeficiencies and the general state of health. In India general health and nutritional status is low hence severity of illness is more in poor people.

Mortality

Mortality is generally less than 1%.

Immunity

One attack confers lifelong immunity. In adult population in developing countries and communities, immunity to HAV may exceed 95% in contrast to developed countries where level of immunity may be less than 50%.

Resistance

The HAV is highly infectious and can cause explosive epidemics when present in water and food. In addition, it is relatively resistant to unfavourable environmental conditions, including water treatment and disinfection process. Normal doses of chlorination do not destroy HAV. 0.5 mg/litre of residual chlorine ensures safety against HAV.

Incubation Period and Household Infection

Incubation period of hepatitis A may vary from 15 to 45 days with a mean of 30 days. The virus is present in the blood in relatively low number for about 7–14 days with a peak before the onset of clinical symptoms. Faecal-oral transmission of HAV is the result of personal contact or consumption of faecally polluted water or food. If one member of a household contracts an infection from contaminated water or food or from contact with an infected individual outside the home, can infect other members of household by **personal contacts.** Household infection rate of up to 95% have been recorded.

Vaccine Against HAV

WHO considers that in countries where hepatitis A is highly endemic exposure to HAV is almost universal before the age of 10 years, in such countries clinical hepatitis is usually a minor public health problem and large scale immunization efforts against this disease may not be undertaken. Hence, universal immunization of hepatitis A is not recommended as yet. More epidemiological data is required to ascertain the benefit of vaccine. Currently, 4 inactivated vaccines against HAV are internationally available. All 4 vaccines are safe and effective with long lasting protection. None of the vaccines are licensed for children less than 1 year of age. The HAV vaccines are given parenterally as two doses series 6–18 months apart. The dose and schedule should be as indicated by manufacturer.

The HAV vaccines may be used to protect individuals with high-risk situations but the principal barriers to transmission of enteric hepatitis virus are safe drinking water supplies and good standards of sanitation and of personal and food hygiene. Safe water supplies and sanitation will remove or eliminate other dangerous diseases/infections as well (like typhoid fever, cholera and diarrhoeal diseases).

HEPATITIS E

This virus was confirmed in 1970s and early 1980. Infection with this virus was initially referred to as enterically transmitted (or epidemic) non-A, non-B hepatitis (NANB). It eventually transpired that HEV had for many years been mistaken for HAV because the two viruses share same basic clinical and epidemiological properties.

Transmission

Primarily by the faecal-oral route and often associated with water-borne and food-borne outbreaks. However, HEV tends to occur more often in young adults, many of whom are already immune to HAV. **Person-to-person** transmissions is uncommon.

Incubation Period

It ranges from 2 weeks to 2 months; mean incubation period is 40 days.

The clinical course of hepatitis E is similar to that of hepatitis A. More than 50% of HEV infections remain anicteric. In moderate to severe cases, the onset is usually sudden with fever, loss of appetite, feeling of general ill health and abdominal discomfort, followed within a few days, by jaundice. Fever usually disappears by the time jaundice appears. Liver function tests include a rise in ALT > 2.5 times of upper limit and serum bilirubin to more than 2 mg%.

Animal Reservoir

HEV is zoonotic member. Virus has been detected in animal excreta (cows, pigs, goats and even in rodents). *Animals serve* as *reservoir* of HEV and many human infections may originate from water sources polluted by animal waste. This underlines the need to protect water resources and supplies from pollution by *animal wastes.* In the past the animal wastes were not considered to be of particular importance with regard to viruses.

Distribution

Both HAV and HEV are associated with poor standards of hygiene and sanitation. However, geographical distribution of HEV is distinct and restricted. Clinical infections and outbreaks of HEV have been recorded predominantly in countries such as Afghanistan, China, India, Mynamar, Nepal and Pakistan, on the Island of Borneo and in parts of central Asia; in Mexico and in parts of Africa such as Algeria, Côt d'ivoire, Egypt, Ethiopia, Somalia and Sudan.[1]

Mortality

In contrast to hepatitis A, which rarely causes complications and mortality rate of less than 1%, HEV causes fulminant hepatitis and high fatality in pregnant women (case fatality as high as 20–40%).

Outbreaks of Hepatitis E in India

The HEV is most common cause of acute fulminant hepatitis in adults in parts of India, other parts of Asia and in Africa. Most of the outbreaks of viral hepatitis in India are caused by hepatitis E virus hence there are limitation of use of hepatitis A vaccine. Large outbreaks associated with sewage contaminated drinking water include one in 1954 involving approximately 40,000 cases in Delhi, India. One in 1986–1988 with more than 1,00,000 cases in the Xinjian Uighar region of China and one in 1991 with 79,000 cases in Kanpur, India.[2] Several outbreaks between 1989 and 1999 in Andhra Pradesh, Madhya Pradesh, Delhi, Ahmedabad, Rajasthan have been investigated by NICD and all these were due to HEV.[3,4] All these outbreaks occurred in areas having evidence of contaminated pipe water supply irrespective of presence or absence of sewer lines. Only single case occurred in most of the affected households. The majority of cases (80%) were 15 years and above. Males contributed almost three-fourths of cases. Outbreaks occurred mostly in rainy season. Outbreaks subsided in a few weeks once the leakages were identified and corrected.

Prevention and Control

Since transmission of hepatitis A and E is faecal-oral, the measures of personal hygiene and environmental sanitation that apply to control of enteric infections are the basis for control of hepatitis A and E.[3,4]

Ensure safe water supply. Hepatitis A and E viruses are not destroyed by chlorination in usual doses. Ensuring high level of residual chlorine at least 0.5 ppm in the system is effective against viruses. The virus is killed by boiling of water. This is temporary alternate arrangement of safe water supply during the outbreaks; till such time the source of contamination is removed.

Vaccine: Heptitis E vaccine is available in China but not in India so for.

Anticipatory Actions

- Ensure water quality monitoring on regular basis in addition to sanitary surveys and inspections by health agencies and suppliers.
- Disease surveillance through health facilities and institutions. Surveillance data on acute diarrhoeal diseases, typhoid fever and jaundice can provide clue of impending outbreaks well in advance for appropriate and timely actions.
- People participation and education of community on all aspects of prevention of hepatitis by their own action is essential. Multiple channels should be used to disseminate messages.

HEPATITIS F

The existence of HFV has not yet been conclusively proven. The name was proposed following reports of hepatitis cases associated with water-borne transmission of a virus distinguishable from HAV and HEV. Indications are that HFV is associated with sporadic cases in certain geographical areas and not with outbreaks or epidemics. Cases have been reported in India, Italy, the United Kingdom and the USA.

HEPATITIS B

Hepatitis B is a disease of the liver caused by virus—the hepatitis B virus (HBV); it used to be called as serum hepatitis virus in the past. Globally over 400 million people are infected with hepatitis B. Hepatitis B is a silent killer, taking the lives of 500,000 to 700,000 people each year globally.[5,6] Annually around 205,286 deaths related to chronic hepatitis occur in India.

Carrier State in Viral Hepatitis

Over 95% of the people are able to clear the virus from their blood. In those who have mild disease with hepatitis B, some patients do not get rid of virus after acute infection. They become lifelong carriers of hepatitis B virus. Those who are infected when young may carry infection for the rest of their life; often without knowing it. About 10% of infants and up to 30% of adults infected by HBV, develop a short term illness (acute hepatitis B). In contrast, 90% of infants, 30% of children of 1–5 years and about 6% of adults infected with HBV develop chronic infection. Persistence of hepatitis B for more than **six months** is defined as **chronic hepatitis B**. Chronic carriers can infect others and are themselves at risks of serious liver disease in life including cirrhosis and liver cancer. It is estimated that in about 15–25% of such carriers, there is a risk of liver cirrhosis or cancer, 20 years or more after the primary infection. Most of the carriers are those who become infected in early childhood as children have very mild form of illness. In India, the available data indicate that the country has intermediate endemicity of hepatitis B, with prevalence of hepatitis B surface antigen (HBsAg) between 2 and 10%. Around 43 million carriers of hepatitis B exist in India. Of 26 million infant born every year in India one million run the lifetime risk of developing chronic HBV infection.[6] The hepatitis B vaccine, as part of the universal immunization programme would prevent these chronic infections.

The chronic carrier rate of HB virus in adults varies widely in different parts of the country and among different sections of society, from less than 1% to over 15%. On an average, the carrier rate in pregnant women is 2–4%. Annually 26 million babies are born in India. Thus, about half to one million infants are born to women who are chronic virus carriers. The probability of vertical transmission is only about 30%. In other words, some 1,66,000–3,33,000 neonates are likely to be infected. Among them about 90% are likely to become chronic carriers, thus adding 1,49,000 to 2,99,000 to the carrier pool annually. Therefore, prevention of MTCT is an essential component of HB vaccination in National Immunization Programme.

Detection of Carriers

A simple blood test called Australia antigen test (HbsAg) will help determine whether one is infected with hepatitis B virus or not.

Problem

Hepatitis B is a major public health problem, worldwide.

- Highly endemic areas are those where hepatitis B surface antigen (HBsAg) prevalence is >10%.
- Medium endemicity means prevalence between 2 and 10%. India falls in this zone of prevalence.
- Low endemicity means prevalence less than 2%.

Incubation Period

Incubation period is 6 weeks to 6 months, median incubation period is lower than 100 days.

Mode of Transmission

The virus is found in infected blood and other body fluids such as semen, vaginal secretions, wound exudates, etc. Man is the only known reservoir of this virus. The virus is transmitted from one person to another by infected blood or body fluids by unsafe blood transfusion, **unsafe** injections and unsafe sexual intercourse with sexual partners. There are four major routes of transmission:

Parenteral/percutaneous: During transfusion of infected blood and through infected needles.

Horizontal: Between person-to-person (accidental contact with infected blood and other body fluids) by needle stick injuries or other injuries.

Vertical: From infected mother to child at birth.

Sexual: Between sexual partners.

In fact, hepatitis B virus is 100 times more infectious than HIV/AIDS virus and only 0.00004 ml of contaminated blood is sufficient to transmit this virus. Unlike HIV, HBV is able to remain active on surfaces (e.g. table tops, razor blades blood stains, etc.) for about a week without losing infectivity.

At risk individuals: Persons who indulge in unsafe sex and have multiple sex partners, infants born to hepatitis B infected mothers, professional blood donors, persons who receive repeated blood transfusion (thalassaemics and haemophilics) injecting drug users and persons exposed to needle stick injuries like doctors, dentists, nurses and paramedicals.

Majority of infants and children infected with hepatitis B do not show any sign and symptoms of hepatitis B infection. These asymptomatic children can transmit the hepatitis B virus to other healthy children and at later age the asymptomatic child may develop liver cirrhosis and liver cancer. In case of adults, a small number of individuals may not show any sign and symptoms. The others develop initially flu-like symptoms such as loss of appetite, tiredness, chills and mild fever, bodyache and later jaundice (yellowness of eyes, skin, dark urine).

Mortality

Case fatality rate ranges from 16 to 41%.

Outbreaks

Reported outbreaks due to hepatitis B are rare and have been linked to unsafe injections by use of unsterilized needles and one needle and syringe is used for multiple injections. NICD investigated outbreaks of hepatitis B in Mehsana (Maharashtra), Sirsa (Haryana) and Sri-Ganganagar (Rajasthan) in the year 1997. These outbreaks were due to use of unsterilized needles and syringes by private practitioners. Outbreak of hepatitis B in January 2009 in Modasa town in district Sabarkantha of Gujarat State affected 500 persons resulting in 93 deaths—case fatality rate of 18.6%, due to **unsafe injections.** Thus, there is an imperative need of **safe injection.**[7,8]

Prevention by Hepatitis B Vaccine

A safe and effective vaccine against hepatitis B has been available since 1982.

WHO recommends that hepatitis B vaccine be included in routine infant immunization programme in all countries. Hepatitis B vaccine which was introduced in 10 states has been expanded in the entire country as part of UIP.

Objective

The primary objective of routine infant hepatitis B immunization is to prevent the early childhood infection which result in chronic liver disease later in life. By preventing chronic HBV infection this strategy also serves to reduce major reservoir for transmission of new infection.

Immunization Strategies[5,9,10]

Routine Infant Immunization

Immunization of all infants as an integral part of the national programme is the highest priority of all the countries. Additional immunization strategies that should be considered depending upon the epidemiology of HBV transmission in a particular country are:

Prevention of perinatal HBV transmission: In order to prevent HBV transmission from mother to infant, the first dose of hepatitis B vaccine needs to be given as soon as possible after birth (preferably within 24 hours after birth). In countries where a high proportion of chronic infections are acquired perinatally (e.g. SE Asia), a birth dose should be given to infants when feasible. It is usually most feasible to give hepatitis B vaccine when infants are born in hospitals. Effort should be made in these countries to give hepatitis B as soon as possible after delivery to infants delivered at home.

National technical advisory group on immunization (NTAGI): In India recommends 1st dose at birth for institutional deliveries followed by dose 2 at 6 weeks and dose 3 at 14 weeks along with DPT.

For those not receiving a birth dose, three doses at 6,10 and 14 weeks along with DPT are given. DPT and hepatitis B will be given on different limbs unless combination vaccine is available.

Catch up immunization: For children and adolescents-3 doses on demand and on payment. Here the ideal schedule is one month between dose 1 and 2 and 3–5 months between dose 2 and 3. Third dose gives protection of 20–25 years.

The global fund for children's vaccine (GFCV) does not provide vaccine for catch up vaccination. In countries with a high endemicity of HBV infection (hepatitis B surface antigen (HBsAg) prevalence ≥8%, catch up immunization is not usually recommended because most chronic infections are acquired among children <5 years of age and thus routine infant vaccination will rapidly reduce HBV transmission. In countries with lower HBV endemicity, a higher proportion of chronic infection may be acquired among older children, adolescents and adults. Catch up immunization for these groups may be considered (WHO).

Vaccination is essential for all students and staff of health care, including medical, nursing, dental, laboratory and related paramedical disciplines in order to prevent nosocomial transmission to and from health care workers.

Administration: Hepatitis B vaccine is given by intramuscular injection in the anterolateral aspect of the thigh (infants) or deltoid muscle (older children). It can safely be given at the same time as other vaccines. Sterile autodisable (AD) injection devices are recommended.

Dose: For infants 0.5 ml (10 mcg of hepatitis B surface antigen protein). For older children and adults 1 ml (20 mcg of hepatitis B surface antigen protein).

The hepatitis B vaccine is the *First vaccine against a cancer* (primary liver cancer).

HEPATITIS C—THE SILENT KILLER

Epidemiology

WHO estimates that 3% of world population is infected with HCV and around 170 million individuals are chronic carriers at risk of developing liver cirrhosis and liver cancer. Over 50% of cases are asymptomatic. HCV is most common cause of chronic hepatitis. India has an HCV prevalence rate of 1.25–1.8%. India has 14 million people infected with HCV.

Route of Transmission

It is transmitted through transfusion of contaminated blood products. About 50% of cases are related to injecting drug users who share needles. Risk of sexual and maternal transmission is low. In developing countries it is estimated that up to 1,60,000 HIV, 4.7 million hepatitis C and 16 million hepatitis B infections each year are attributable to **unsafe injections.**[11] In February 2012 in Ratia block of Fatehabad district of Haryana, 1584 persons tested positive for hepatitis C.

Salient Features of HCV Infection

- Hepatitis C along with hepatitis B and alcohol are the top three global causes of liver cirrhosis and liver cancer.
- 12–25% sporadic cases
- No symptoms in 50% of cases
- Undetected up to 10 years
- 20% fully recover in 6 months
- 20% of all patients of hepatitis C will develop liver cirrhosis and/or liver cancer in 20–30 years.

Prevention

There is no vaccine to prevent HCV infection. Safe blood, safe injection, and safe sex prevents HCV and HBV. Screening of blood for HBV and HCV is essential to prevent hepatitis B and C. Treatment of choice is combination therapy using weekly injection of interferon and tablets ribavirin for 6 months to one year.[12] This has been replaced by all oral therapy with directly acting antivirals (DAAs), but still not available in India.

NATIONAL PROGRAMME ON PREVENTION AND CONTROL OF VIRAL HEPATITIS IN INDIA

ACTIVITIES

- Surveillance of viral hepatitis to measure the exact burden of viral hepatitis ABCDE by network of 10 Laboratories in different geographical locations.
- Prevention, treatment and control guidelines for viral hepatitis in the country.
- Safe injection handbook/guidelines. 81 outbreaks of viral hepatitis were detected in the year 2014 by IDSP programme.

REFERENCES

1 CBHI. Health information of India in 2003. New Delhi: DGHS MOH and FW; 2003, 2005, and 2015 (National Health Profile).

2 WHO. Guidelines for drinking water quality—Addendum microbiological agents in drinking water. 2nd ed. Geneva: WHO; 2002.

3 NICD. Viral Hepatitis. CD Alert Monthly Newsletter on communicable diseases Sept. 1997; (2).

4 NICD. Outbreaks of viral hepatitis—public health system needs to be alert. CD Alert. Monthly Newsletter on communicable diseases Feb. 2000; 4(2).

5 Willet S. Hepatitis B vaccine introduction lessons learned in advocacy, communication and training. Proceedings of GAVI partners meeting Bill and Melinda Gates Children's vaccine programme PATH; Nov. 21, 2000; Netherlands.

6 GOI. Operational Guidelines for Hepatitis B vaccine in the Universal Immunization Programme MOH and FW, GOI, 2009.

7 Singh J, Bhatia R, Gandhi JC, Kaswekai AP, Khare S, Patel SB, et al. Outbreak of viral hepatitis B in a rural community in India linked to inadequately sterilized needles and syringes. Bulletin WHO 1998; 76(1): 93–8.

8 Singh J, Prakash C, Gupta RS, Bora D, Jain DC, Datta KK. Epidemiology of endemic viral hepatitis in an urban area of India: A retrospective community study in Alwar. Bulletin WHO 1997; 75(5): 463.

9 Willet S, Ashton R. Realizing the full potential of childhood immunization—how health professionals can make a difference. Occasional Paper 1; Bill and Melinda Gates Children's Vaccine Program PATH.

10 GOI. Medium term strategic plan for the universal immunization programme 2004–09—NTAGI recommendations. Draft 16 Feb. 2004.

11 GOI. CD Alert. Special issue safe injection practice. Where do we stand. Monthly Newsletter of NICD, DGHS, January—February, 2009.

12 GOI. CD Alert. Monthly Newsletter of NICD, DGHS, January–February 2007; 11:1.

GUINEA WORM DISEASE (ERADICATED FROM INDIA)

Guinea worm or dracunculiasis has been eradicated from India. Guinea worm is caused by the nematode: *Dracunculus medinensis*. Adult worms live in subcutaneous tissues of man. Disease cycle is maintained through intermediate host: cyclops. Cyclops live in water and embryos develop in the body of cyclops. When unsafe water is consumed by human beings, the cyclops are ingested and further stages of worm develop in man. The female adult guinea worm which measures 60–100 cm in length emerges through skin, causing incapacitating chronic swelling and ulcer in lower limbs or back of the body, when these parts come in contact with water the gravid female liberates thousands of embryos in water. Cyclops ingest these embryos and the cycle is maintained. The disease mostly occurs in rural areas with inadequate safe drinking water and peaks are observed during the summer season when there is scarcity of water. The disease causes incapacitation to the individual, who is unable to perform his regular work, resulting in economic and production loss to the patient and family.

National Guinea Worm Eradication Programme (GWEP) was started in 1983–84 as a centrally sponsored programme. The National Institute of Communicable Disease (NICD), Delhi, functioned as the nodal agency for planning, coordination, guidance and evaluation of GWEP in the country. The programme was implemented by the formerly endemic state health directorates through the primary health care system. India was unique in the world to establish eradication programme against guinea worm. Under Rajiv Gandhi National Drinking Water Supply Mission (technology mission), a sub-mission on guinea worm eradication was set-up. The mission objective was to eradicate guinea worm infestation.[1,2]

Strategies

i To provide safe water to geographical areas having guinea worm infestation on priority basis.
ii Surveillance of guinea worm cases through house-to-house search programme.
iii Management of guinea worm cases.
iv Identification of unsafe drinking water sources and their regular chemical treatment by temephos 50% EC in all guinea worm endemic areas.
v Health education and community participation.
vi Training of manpower at various levels of GWEP implementation, viz. PHC, District and State.
vii Research and concurrent evaluation.

Active Surveillance

Every year during the months of April, May/June and November/December, three active search operations were undertaken with a view to identify guinea worm affected villages, detection of guinea worm cases and their management, study the epidemiological situation of guinea worm disease, identify unsafe water sources and study the safe drinking water requirements and the trend of the guinea worm disease.

Vector Control

Temephos was considered as the safest, with long residual effect and was comparatively economical to use against the control of other vector-borne diseases including onchocerciasis, filariasis, dengue fever and malaria. As a cyclopsicide 1% and 2% sand granule formulations of temephos have been extensively evaluated and found to be safe in India. In India, the task force on GWEP decided to use 50% emulcifiable concentrate (EC) temephos in place of 2% sand granule.

Frequency: Temephos eight times a year and use of fine nylonmesh/double layered cloth strainers by the community to filter cyclops in all the affected villages. Initially temephos first application was done in Feb/March and then repeated twice at an interval of 6 weeks. Another application was done in 2nd and 3rd week of September. Subsequently temephos was applied every month.

Provision and Maintenance of Safe Drinking Water Supplies

It was done in mission mode, high priority was given to endemic areas affected with guinea worm disease.

Management of Guinea Worm Patients

No specific drug is available against dracunculiasis, worm extraction is the only remedy to be done at nearest primary health centre or community health centre by trained professionals.

Organization

The NICD Delhi was made responsible for planning, co-ordination, monitoring and evaluation of GWEP activities by Ministry of Health and Family Welfare and Director General of Health Services.

Results

NICD with financial support from WHO deployed epidemiological surveillance teams in endemic states which closely monitored the programme and helped the district/PHC authorities in effective implementation of various GWEP operational components especially surveillance and GW case containment measures. During the year 1984, when the GWEP was launched there were 40,000 cases of guinea worm disease spread over in 12840 villages of 89 districts of 7 endemic states (Rajasthan, Madhya Pradesh, Chhattisgarh, Karnataka, Maharashtra, AP and Gujarat). During 1996, 9 guinea worm cases were recorded in three villages of Jodhpur district (Rajasthan), all of which were adequately contained. Last case was reported from village Aau in July, 1996.[3, 4]

Impressive gains were made over the period of 13 years of implementation of the programme. India reported "Zero" case in 1997. A National Commission for Certification of Guinea Worm Eradication was set-up by the Ministry of Health and Family Welfare in 1998. WHO team for eradication of guinea worm disease, visited the country from 9.11.99 to 25.11.99 to validate the zero guinea worm disease status for eradication in India and hence India was certified for eradication of guinea worm disease in 2000.[5] This could be achieved as a result of integrated approach to environment, intersectoral approach in endemic region including safe water supplies, community mobilization, effective case surveillance and guinea worm extraction, contributed an effective response to an age old scourge. However, WHO recommended routine survei-llance and IEC to be continued till global eradication of the disease.

REFERENCES

1 GOI. Monograph on integrated training on national programmes for mother and child development New Delhi: CTC on health and nutrition Deptt. of Women and Child Development 1990; 47–57.

2 IPHA. Guinea worm eradication programme. Public health update newsletter May–June 1992; 6(3).

3 UNICEF. Rights and opportunities. India country office, New Delhi: UNICEF; 1998.

4 NICD. Eradicating guinea worm disease an Indian scenario. New Delhi: NICD; 1994.

5 CBHI. Health information of India 2003. New Delhi, DGHS, MOH and FW, GOI; 2003.

ENTERIC FEVERS

Enteric fevers of which typhoid fever (caused by *Salmonella enterica* serovar *typhi*), constitutes an overwhelming majority is an old problem that still persists. Paratyphoid fever can be caused by any of three variations or biotypes of *S. enteritidis paratyphi* A, B, C. It is similar in its symptoms to typhoid fever but tends to be milder, with much lower case-fatality rate. Typhoid fever is a major hazard to public health in India and rated as the fifth most common communicable disease in the country. Typhoid fever—a wide spread disease is a *Salmonella typhi* septicemia related to the presence of the capsule Vi antigen. It results in high morbidity and mortality in developing countries. In industrialized countries, 80% of cases of typhoid fever are contracted by persons travelling in endemic zones. The difficult diagnosis and the emergence of strains multi-resistant to antibiotics effectively delay the setting up of effective treatment and increase the number of complications, the mortality rate and the cost of treatment. Typhoid fever is still a serious disease.

Mode of Infection

The reservoir: The reservoir of bacteria is strictly human (man). No animal reservoir is known. The agent responsible can, however, survive several months in soil or water.

Dissemination of bacteria is by infected subject: They are excreted in large quantities in patient's stools, and also in their vomit and urine, or are excreted in a more sporadic way in the stools of **chronic carriers,** veritable reservoirs of the pathogenic agent that can harbour bacteria in their gall bladder for months or even years. These **chronic carriers** are an important source of infection, maintaining the endemic, even epidemic state of certain geographical regions.

Transmission: There is no animal reservoir in typhoid fever. Typhoid fever is an oro-faecally transmitted disease. In 90% of cases, infection is indirect, by ingestion of water or food contaminated with excreta from infected subjects. This mode of transmission plays a major role in the spread of disease in India and other developing countries in which it is highly endemic and where sanitary systems are often inadequate and also where there are many houseflies from defecation ground and kitchen, which act as mechanical vectors for transmission of disease.

Transmission also occurs directly in the family or contacts of a patient or chronic carriers (Fig. 12.15).

Incubation Period

It ranges between 5 and 21 days.

Following ingestion the bacterium may reach reticuloendothelial system and multiply intracellularly within macrophages, a property that seems dependent on the presence of the Vi antigen. After 5–21 days of incubation the patient experience fatigue, headache, abdominal pain

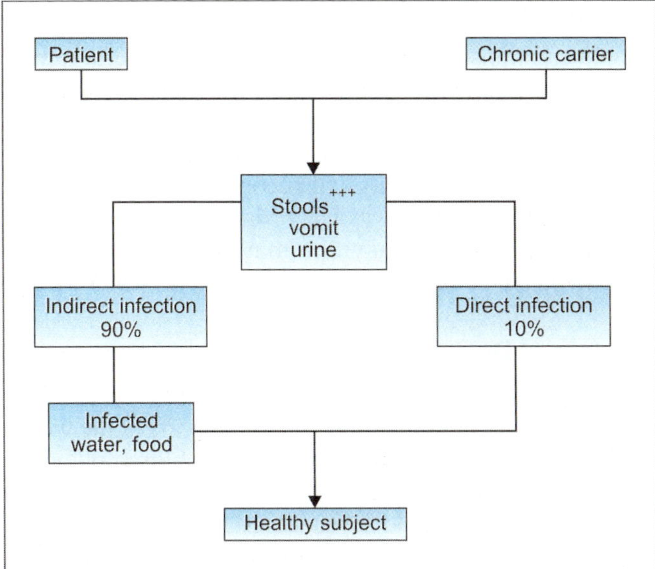

Fig. 12.15: Modes of infection of typhoid fever (enteric fevers)

and fever. Constipation usually occurs in older children and adults, whereas diarrhoea occurs in younger children. Severe form of typhoid fever may entail cerebral dysfunction, delirium, shock, occasional intestinal perforation, and haemorrhages. Immunocompromized individuals suffering from achlorhydria are susceptible to lower infectious doses of *S. typhi* and are at increased risk of severe disease. Regardless of treatment or risk factors, the overall fatality rate is about 4%. Approximately 1–4% of the patients continue to harbour *S. typhi* in their intestinal tract and gallbladder for months or years (chronic carriers). Definitive diagnosis of typhoid fever requires isolation of *S. typhi* from blood, intestinal secretions and bone marrow by culture. Only 50–70% of blood cultures are positive. Chronic carriers show high antibody titre to Vi antigen.

Carrier: If *S.typhi* organisms persist in stools or urine for >1 year after onset of disease, a person is known as **chronic carrier.**

Population Affected

In endemic country like India, young subjects are most affected—children over five, adolescents and young adults with a peak incidence between 8 and 13 years of age. It is an important cause of absenteeism from school or work. In aged subjects, typhoid fever is less frequent but much more severe and the proportion of chronic carriers increases with age. The occurrence of typhoid fever in children under 2 years of age is rare.

Taking into consideration the increasing amount of travel to developing countries, the risk of infection for travellers is becoming greater. 80% of cases of industrialized countries are brought in by travellers.

Military personnel, food sector employees, laboratory and hospital personnel are other populations at risk. Persons in close contact with a chronic carrier are at most risk.

Geographical Distribution

Typhoid fever is widespread and remains a serious disease. Typhoid fever is ubiquitous disease. It is endemic in different regions of the globe (Africa, Asia and Latin America). The exact incidence of typhoid fever is not clear. Notification of the disease to WHO is not compulsory. There is no precise epidemiological data for the countries most affected. Typhoid fever is both a water-borne and food-borne gastrointestinal infection with an estimated global incidence between 16 million and 33 million cases per year with 7,00,000 deaths. WHO conservatively estimates the annual global incidence of typhoid fever at 0.3% corresponding to 16 million cases and 6,00,000 deaths. In some developing countries of Asia and Africa, the annual incidence may reach 1% with case fatality rate as high as 10%. About 70% of all deaths due to typhoid fever occur in Asia.

Problem in India

Disease Burden—Based on Notification

All medical institutions in India are required to report cases and deaths of typhoid (enteric fever) every month to respective state and states report consolidated data to Central Bureau of Health Intelligence (CBHI).

There is inadequate and incomplete information of typhoid fever in India and these reports come from hospitals and dispensaries. Hence it does not depict the true picture of the problem (Table 12.38). Over 10–17 lakh cases per year are being reported.

Study conducted in India in 1997 provides community based prevalence of typhoid in urban slums of Delhi.

Typhoid fever cases were seen in all age groups up to 40 years giving an overall incidence of 9.92 per 1000 person per year. The incidence was 27.28 per thousand in children <5 years of age and 6.63 per thousand in those older than 5 years. The above figures were based

Table 12.38: Reported cases and deaths of typhoid fever in India[1]

Year	*Cases*	*Deaths*
1977	2,52,655	504
1985	2,36,527	549
1987	3,32,281	533
2001	4,90,195	606
2003	5,96,684	839
2005	5,67,638	389
2006	7,89,004	658
2007	8,20,360	452
2008	9,16,161	338
2009	10,99,331	436
2010	10,34,642	379
2011	10,62,446	346
2013	15,37,118	361
2014 (P)	17,07,312	429

Source: (CBHI) Government of India

12

on the culture positive cases of typhoid fever. This may be an underestimate as culture is not positive in all cases (Table 12.39).

Table 12.39: Incidence of culture confirmed typhoid fever in Delhi by active surveillance

Year	Author	Disease incidence per 1000 per year		
		Overall	<5 years	>5 years
1971	Chuttani et al (Delhi slums) 6248 population	9.60	10.49	9.29 (5–17 yrs)
1997	AIIMS study group (Delhi slums) 8000 population	9.92	27.28	6.63 (5–40 yrs)

Source: Water-borne diseases: The continuing challenge Ranbaxy science foundation in India 1997

Paratyphoid fever caused by *S. paratyphi* A constituted almost one-fourth of the total cases of enteric fever. In contrast to typhoid fever, which was more prevalent in children under 5 years, majority of paratyphoid fever cases occurred in those older than 5 years.

There was no change in overall incidence in the last 26 years between 1971 and 1997. It means that the disease is being perpetuated and factors and conditions responsible for it have not changed much over the years.[2, 3]

At this rate, there would be 8.5 million culture positive cases of typhoid in India per year. The actual load may be much higher given that the culture positive cases vary between 50 and 70%. Of these, a guess estimate of 0.73 million cases will need hospitalization and 17000 will die every year.

Problem in Children

There was no disease during the first year of life, the incidence during the second and third year of life was 24.8 and 51.8 per 1000 person years respectively, which has an epidemiological implication of prevention of typhoid with immunization. Incidence in school age groups is not known precisely. Typhoid fever in children below 3 years is not a mild disease.[2–6] But hospital-based studies reveal peak incidence of typhoid between 5 and 12 years of age.

Urban Rural Distribution

It is believed that the incidence of typhoid fever is less in rural areas but there is no scientific evidence. Urban slums are worst affected because of poor sanitation and water contamination. The incidence of diarrhoeal diseases and other water-borne diseases is not less in rural areas as compared to urban areas.

Case Fatality

Case fatality of typhoid fever has been reported as 10%, which can be reduced to 1% with appropriate antibiotic therapy. Case fatality is low in paratyphoid A, B and C fevers.

Communicability

People can transmit the disease as long as bacteria remain in their system. Most people are infectious prior to and during the first week of convalescence. About 10% of untreated patients will discharge bacteria for up to 3 months; 2–5% of untreated patients will become permanent carriers.

One notorious carrier was Mary Mallon or **Typhoid Mary** who was a cook and asymptomatic chronic carrier of *Salmonella typhi*, infected dozens of people in New York city.

Problem of Drug Resistance in Typhoid Fever

Widespread multi-drug resistance in typhoid fever has been reported in India, Bangladesh, and other parts of the world.

The basic drugs (firstline drugs) like chloramphenicol, ampicillin and cotrimoxazole have become blunt and are not effective against typhoid fever. Resistance to the extent of over 80% has been reported by 1991. In Great Britain in 1991, 25% of isolated strains were resistant to chloramphenicol (100%), trimethoprim (87%) and ampicillin (85%).

Even ciprofloxacin is becoming less effective, which at present is the drug of choice for typhoid fever. Amikacin and gentamicin are still very effective against typhoid fever. The cost of treatment is quite high apart from man-days lost due to morbidity.

Prevention

Safe disposal of human excreta and safe water supply and personal hygiene are effective methods of prevention for water-borne diseases including typhoid fever. These measures can reduce morbidity due to typhoid fever by 80–100% (WHO 1992).

Due to growing population, unplanned urbanization and migration to cities, we in India continue to add slum population with deplorable facilities of safe water and excreta disposal. Faeco-oral diseases continue to be rampant and typhoid fever continues to be endemic disease and both incidence and prevalence over the years have not changed much. Under these circumstances, there are no easy solutions for prevention. Slum clearance and planned development with improved quality of life (adequate safe water supply and safe disposal of human excreta) have been the prime responsibility of municipal authorities, but the progress is very slow.

We have the programme of national water supply and sanitation but the coverage is low because of escalating and rising population.

Personal hygiene measures which include washing hands before eating and after defecation with soap and water cuts down the incidence of water-borne diseases to at least one-third. We need water for hand washing. Similarly, eating clean food and safe storage of drinking water should be promoted. Dipping hands into pitcher to draw water is a dangerous practice as it contaminates water. Avoid use of ice and ice candy as also controlling food vendors in schools (avoiding eating exposed food and fruits) and control by parents, and teachers can be helpful measures to cut down the transmission.

Immunization is no substitute or replacement for safe water, sanitation and hygienic practices. It remains an interim measure or intervention to prevent disease in individuals. The efficacy of all vaccines available is limited.

In theory, control of typhoid fever may be achieved by adequate antimicrobial treatment of both clinical cases and asymptomatic faecal excreters of *S. typhi*. This approach requires well-functioning medical services, including access to relevant drugs and reliable diagnostic laboratories, all of which are currently unavailable in the areas of highest endemicity. In addition, rapid development of microbial drug resistance significantly reduces the possibility of containing the spread of the infectious agent. Further, liberal use of antibiotics will accentuate these problems. Hence, until socioeconomic development changes the living conditions of the population most affected, efficacious and affordable vaccines are required as interim measures to control the typhoid fever.

Immunization

Interestingly when India adopted expanded programme of immunization in 1978, typhoid vaccination was included in its programme. It was targeted at 5–6 years children and dose of 0.5 ml in two occasions was given by subcutaneous route. Subsequently, this was discontinued because of severe reactions and low level of efficacy ranging from 50 to 73% and acceptability was low.

Policy Guidelines in India (Recommendations)

1 To make available whole cell Acetone killed and dried typhoid vaccine (Monovalent AKD) to be supplied on demand. This will remain inexpensive choice for wide use and its efficacy has been rated high. Its side effects are not serious and no worse than that of DPT. Moreover, it can be given in infancy.
2 Provide Vi vaccine single dose at an age between 2 and 5 years in all public sector vaccination clinics in all urban communities. Such children may be given one repeat dose after 3–5 years.
3 As part of any typhoid outbreak control, use oral typhoid vaccine in the age group 6–40 years.

Available Vaccines[7–9]

Currently available typhoid vaccines that are licensed in India, includes:

- Heat and phenol killed vaccine (inactivated whole cell vaccine).
- Ty21a vaccine (oral)
- Vi vaccine

Heat and Phenol Killed Vaccine (Inactivated Whole Cell Vaccine)

Heat and phenol inactivated typhoid vaccines are 51–67% effective but their local and systemic effects have limited their use. However, they are the only currently available vaccines for children less than two years of age.

In this category we have:

- **Monovalent Vaccine (Whole Cell Vaccine):** Since typhoid fever is mainly caused by *Salmonella typhi*, the monovalent vaccine is therefore recommended. It is heat killed and phenol preserved vaccine containing 1000 million of *S. typhi* per ml. It can also be prepared with acetone and the vaccine is then known as AKD (Acetone killed and dried) antityphoid vaccine.
- **Bivalent Vaccine:** This contains *S. typhi* and *S. paratyphi* A in the proportion of 1000 million and 500 million organisms per ml. The organisms are killed and preserved by heating at 54°C for one hour and by addition of 0.5% phenol. This vaccine is prepared in India by CRI Kasauli, which also manufactures a paediatric vaccine containing 330 million bacilli of *S. typhi* and 165 million bacilli of paratyphi A. This vaccine can also be prepared by inactivation of organisms with acetone in the dried form (AKD vaccine). CRI Kasauli has the capacity to manufacture AKD vaccine.
- **TAB Vaccine:** This is usually made up of a killed suspension of *S. typhi* 1000 millions, *S. paratyphi* A and *S. paratyphi* B 500 million and 750 million each per ml respectively. WHO has recommended discontinuation of this vaccine.

Primary immunization with this parenteral vaccine consists of two doses given 4 weeks apart. A single booster dose is recommended every 3 years. It is still available in several developing countries and is reasonably priced. Its protective efficacy is 51–67%. This vaccine has been associated with fever, systemic reactions in 9–34% of the recipients and short absence from work or school (2–17%).

Newer Vaccines Against Typhoid

The Vi polysaccharide vaccine: This vaccine is composed of purified polysaccharide from *S. typhi*. It is administered subcutaneously or intramuscularly, dose is 0.5 ml (which contains 25 microgram of Vi antigen). The dose is same for children and adults. There is no contraindication to vaccine except for pregnancy. The vaccine confers immunity after seven days of injection. The vaccine is not effective under two years of age. Vi vaccine offers protection for a period of 3 years. Hence, revaccination is recommended after every 3 years. Efficacy of this vaccine is at least 60% in hyperendemic region, in Nepal trial it was 77%.

This vaccine is poorly immunogenic in children below 2 years of age. Typhoid fever is a severe problem in this age as per Delhi slum study. This vaccine is recommended for children above 5 years of age and adults and other population groups.

Vi polysaccharide vaccine does not protect against paratyphoid fever A and B because the agents responsible (*S. paratyphi* A and B) do not have the Vi antigen. As with many other pure polysaccharide vaccines, no booster effect indicative of an immunological memory is observed. For this reason, protein Vi polysaccharide conjugate vaccines are being developed.

Storage: Temperature +2 to +8°C.

Adverse Reactions

None, because of its purity, mild pain at injection site, redness or local induration in 1% of cases.

Ty21a Vaccine

This is a live attenuated strain of *S. typhi*. It is live oral vaccine against typhoid. This contains 10^9 viable attenuated *Salmonella typhi* organisms strain Ty21a. The vaccine is usually administered orally as enteric-coated capsules and is registered for use from 6 years of age.

Vaccine is indicated for children 6 years and above and adults. One capsule is administered 2 days apart, and 3 doses are recommended on day 1, 3 and 5. When the vaccine is given in 3 doses 2 days apart, protective immunity is achieved 7 days after the last dose.

Protection lasts for a period of 3 years. It has shown protective efficacy of 62% for at least 7 years after the last dose and a trial involving more than 2,00,000 school children in Chile demonstrated the utility of this vaccine. In disease endemic areas, a booster dose is recommended every 3 years. Travellers from non-endemic to disease endemic regions are recommended a booster dose on a yearly basis.

There is no field data to document the efficacy of this vaccine in children under 3 years of age.

A liquid formulation of the Ty21a can be taken by the children as young as 2 years of age and has proved more immunogenic than capsular formulation (WHO). Currently marketed in a small number of countries, it is expected to replace the enteric-coated capsule formulation. In a field trial in Chile among more than 36,000 vaccinees aged 15–19 years, the formulation proved 79% efficacious even up to 5 years after immunization. Ty21a is remarkably well tolerated. The vaccine may be given simultaneously with other vaccines, including live vaccines against polio, measles, mumps and rubella (MMR).

Storage: Temperature +2 to +8°C.

WHO Position on Typhoid Vaccine

The old heat inactivated whole cell vaccine may not be manufactured according to international standards. Because of considerable reactogenicity, the inactivated whole cell vaccine should now be replaced by the less reactogenic and equally efficacious modern vaccines. However, for mainly economic reasons, the old vaccine is still used in some parts of the world.

The current formulations at least the Vi and Ty21a vaccines are moderately efficient (50–70%) in the traditional target groups of children under five years and young adults. In children younger than 3–5 years of age, the corresponding efficacy is insufficiently documented. Although typhoid fever is not considered a public health problem of the first years of life, recent work shows that at least in some disease endemic areas, the highest incidence of typhoid fever is found among children under 5 years of age. Should these findings be confirmed in other areas of high endemicity, vaccination of this age group may become more important than previously appreciated and they will have consequences for future vaccine composition as well as for the vaccination schedule?

Neither the Vi based polysaccharide vaccine nor the Ty21a is licensed for children under 2 years of age. With their current formulation, they are not considered candidates for inclusion into large-scale vaccination programmes in this age group. However, while waiting for improved vaccines against typhoid fever, further assessment of the protective efficacy of the currently licensed vaccine in the youngest age groups seem warranted. National strategies to control typhoid fever should be based on thorough analysis of age specific incidence of typhoid fever and on cost benefit aspects of the planned control measures.

Immunization of school age children and young adults is recommended in areas where typhoid fever in these age groups is a significant public health problem and particularly where antibiotic resistant *S. typhi* strains are prevalent. In those settings, immunization against typhoid fever will be required until socioeconomic improvements finally interrupt transmission of *S. typhi*. Wherever appropriate, the use of typhoid vaccines should be harmonized with the administration of DPT (diphtheria pertussis and tetanus) vaccines.

For the occasional small-scale vaccination in countries of low typhoid endemicity and for individual protection of short-term visitors to areas of high endemicity, either of the two modern vaccines is recommended. It should be noted, however, that the vaccines do not provide complete protection and should not replace hygiene precautions.

As per previous studies and reports, typhoid fever affected mainly children between 5 and 12 years of age and is infrequent in children below three years of age. However, a recent prospective study in low income urban areas of Delhi showed that, 44% of culture positive cases detected were in children below 5 years of age. The incidence rate of typhoid per 1000 person years was 27.3 at 5 years, 11.7 at 5–19 years and 1.1 between 19 and 40 years. Information from rural areas is not available.[2,4]

The National Technical Advisory Group on Immunization (NTAGI) in India recommends:[10, 11]

- Age specific disease burden data be obtained from rural area,
- Cost benefit analysis should be available to facilitate decision making about public use of the vaccine and
- School age pilot programme to assess feasibility and cost of Vi conjugate vaccine when given at the same time as DPT at age 5–6 years.

REFERENCES

1 CBHI. Health Information of India. New Delhi: DGHS, MOH and FW, GOI; 1987–2003.
2 Kumar R, Sazwal S, Sinha A, Sood S, Bhan MK. Typhoid fever. Contemporary issues as related to the disease in India. Proceedings of the second round table conference; 1997 Aug. 1; New Delhi. Ranbaxy Science Foundation.
3 Aggarwal KS, Singh SK, Kumar S, Srivastav R, Raj Kumar R. A Study of Current Trends in Enteric Fever. J. Commun. Disease 1998; 30(3): 171–4.
4 ICDDR, B. Incidence of Typhoid Fever, Dhaka 2001. ICDDR, B. Periodical 2003; 1(3): 249–53.
5 Saha RM, Dutta P. Dutta D. A note on incidence of typhoid fever in diverse age groups in Kolkata, India, J. Infect. Dis. 2003; 56: 121–2.
6 Sinha A, Sazawal S, Kumar R. Typhoid Fever in children less than five years. The Lancet 1998; 354: 734–7.
7 NICD. Fact sheet typhoid. New Delhi: NICD, GOI; 2001.
8 WHO. Typhoid vaccines. WHO position paper weekly epidemiological record 2000; 75: 257–64.
9 Alidac Genetics and Pharmaceuticals. Typhim Vi vaccine against typhoid fever. Ahmedabad (India): Pasteur Merieux/ Alidac Genetics and Pharmaceuticals.
10 Govt. of India. Proceedings of National Technical Advisory Group on Immunization (NTAGI). 2004 Feb. 17th; Nirman Bhawan, New Delhi.
11 GOI. Water-Borne Diseases. CD Alert. Monthly Newsletter of NICD, DGHS. Government of India July–Aug. 2006; 10: 7–8.

ZOONOTIC DISEASES

NATIONAL RABIES CONTROL PROGRAMME (NRCP)

The Government of India has initiated the National Rabies Control Programme in 12th Five Year Plan which has both human and animal components. National centre for disease control is the nodal agency for human component. Ministry of Environment and Forest is the Nodal Ministry for animal component.

Objectives of NRCP

The main objective is to reduce the disease incidence and deaths due to rabies.[1]

The main strategies for control programme are:

i Training of health and veterinary professionals.
ii Implementing use of intradermal route of vaccine.
iii Strengthening of surveillance system.
iv Population survey of dogs.
v Mass vaccination of dogs.
vi Dog population management.
vii IEC activities
viii Strengthening of regional laboratories.

RABIES

It is a zoonotic disease (primarily disease of animals). Rabies is an acute viral disease, which causes fatal encephalomyelitis in virtually all the warm-blooded animals including man.

Rabies is probably the most feared disease of all human diseases. It remains one of the most lethal infectious diseases known, being fatal in virtually 100% of cases. Rabies is a major public health problem in India.

Epidemiology

Rabies is a zoonotic disease, that is, animal infection transmitted to man through contact, most often as a result of a bite, with an animal infected and excreter of the virus. Animal rabies affect most of the world continents.

Distribution

Rabies is widespread throughout the world. Each year more than two million people worldwide are vaccinated after exposure to the virus and inspite of that 50,000 people fall victim to the disease, particularly in developing countries, where infected person cannot always benefit from correct vaccination. The exact number of deaths due to rabies is probably higher as cases of rabies are not always diagnosed. Australia, New Zealand and Japan are free from rabies in human beings. In India an estimated 3 million people are receiving postexposure treatment for animal bites in both public and private sector and many more may be doing so for various reasons.

The disease occurs in all parts of the country in India with the exception of Lakshadweep and Andaman and Nicobar Islands.[2–5]

Causative Organism

It is caused by a virus from Rhabdoviridae family, *Lyssavirus* genus, which are bullet-shaped and which number around 75. The virion is an RNA particle consisting of a central nucleocapsid surrounded by an envelope with spike like projections, which contains what is called the G-protein (glycoprotein) and an antigenic material.[5, 6]

It is with the help of spike like projections, that the virus establishes itself in the cytoplasm of the nerve cells.

The rabies virion is very fragile particle and hence it is readily destroyed by powerful disinfectants like strong alkalis, phenolic compounds, etc. This virus does not exist independently in the environment. In the course of infecting reservoir, host species, it is shed into saliva and is transmitted by bite. Thereafter virus multiplies in muscle cells and spreads further through neural pathways.

Rabies infection has a unique distinction of delivering the virus simultaneously to the brain tissue and the salivary glands. This facilitates the survival and propagation of the virus. Due to involvement of limbic system, the animal displays furious rage and bites, thus depositing the virus in other hosts for further propagation.

Principal Reservoir

Rabies is primarily a disease of animals and almost all warm-blooded animals fall prey to it. Rabies virus can infect all mammals. The main sources of infection in man in cities are first dogs and then cats. Monkey bites are also on the increase.

In India, dog is the principal reservoir of rabies and as many as 97% of the persons undergoing anti-rabies treatment are bitten by dogs, mostly stray dogs. A large population of dogs especially the stray ones and unsatisfactory status of the vaccination in pet dogs make this animal most important reservoir of rabies for man as well as animals. Cats, monkeys, mongooses, jackals, and cattle are other animals to name a few, which are responsible for spread of this disease in India. **Bat rabies** has not been conclusively proved in India. **Bite** by **rodents** (domestic rats, mice, squirrels, hare and rabbits) do not ordinarily require treatment. Bites by all wild animals and bites in forest should be treated as category III exposures.

Epidemiological Cycles

Two epidemiological cycles of rabies are recognized: urban and wild (sylvatic). As many as 99% of human cases in India are due to bites by urban rabid animals, which maintain a cycle amongst themselves. Dog ⇄ Dog ⇄ other animals, and man being an incidental victim and dead end of infection.

The *sylvatic cycle* propagates itself within wild animals who sometimes transmit the infection to urban animals as well as man. Bat rabies has not been conclusively reported from this country. No carrier state has been convincingly demonstrated in dogs and for all practical purposes it is taken as nonexistent.

Infection

Infection in man generally occurs as a result of bite from an animal, whose saliva contains the virus. It can also take place as a result of scratch spattered with an animal's virus laden saliva. Being licked by such an animal can even be enough to transmit rabies, if contact is made with mucous membrane, with a fresh wound or with mere excoriations on a person's skin.

This is quite often the case that children can play with an infected animal, without being aware of the danger or without noticing any suspicious contact.

Endemicity

Rabies is endemic in India. Several factors are responsible for the continued prevalence and endemicity of disease in the country. The most important is the continuing stray dog menace and use of highly reactogenic *Semple vaccine*, which has poor patient compliance due to fear of taking multiple painful injections. Now the production of Semple vaccine has been discontinued in India.

12

Social Factors for Endemicity

In rural and urban slums, street/stray dog keeping is a common practice. In rural areas, every street and home has one or two dogs. Children handle and fondle with dogs most of the times, street dogs are treated as pet animals, and catching is not at all allowed. These street dogs remain unimmunized. Children are worst exposed to the saliva of dogs and dog bites are quite common amongst children. These practices also contribute to the endemicity of rabies in India.

Apart from dogs, monkey population has moved to cities because of widespread deforestation. Monkey bites and monkey menace are on increase, hence chances of exposure increase. Around 17.5 million animal bites occur annually.

Problem of Rabies in India

WHO data indicates that about 30,000 people die of rabies in India. But a recent WHO sponsored Indian rabies survey (2003–04) provided an annual estimate of 20,000 human rabies deaths. Almost two-thirds of the victims of rabies are males and 45% are children less than 14 years of age. 132 and 104 Rabies deaths were reported in 2013 and 2014 respectively.

Pathogenesis—Human to Human Transmission

Compared to other mammals, man is somewhat less susceptible to the rabies virus. It all depends upon virulence of the virus and site of bite. Bite on the face has **contagion index** of almost 100% and that on the body and legs only about 2%. Bite on head, face and hands are more dangerous being proximal to brain or central nervous system. While intact skin protects against infection, infection via mucous membranes of respiratory tract is rare but possible. Inter-human transmission has been reported following cornea transplants obtained from donors who died from encephalitis but whose cause of death due to rabies has not been determined.

Incubation Period

The incubation period varies from 2 weeks to 6 years (average 2–3 months) depending upon the amount of virus in the inoculum and site of inoculation.

On an average it is 30–90 days after contamination, it is shorter in case the bite site is closer to the brain.

The virus multiplies at the site of inoculation, and then penetrates the nerve endings. It then makes its way by the axonal route towards the central nervous tissues, which is the main target organ. It then migrates away from the centre, and is disposed off in the secretory and excretory fluids. Thus, it is found in the salivary glands and the saliva. Target organs are brain and salivary glands.

Symptoms

From 2 to 4 days, before disease takes hold, the affected patient feels pins and needles, itching and pain where the original bite took place, even if it has now healed and this spreads throughout the limb along the nerve tracts. His/her behaviour changes, either becoming disinterested in his/her family or conversely showing excessive affection.

Disease

Rabies can manifest in three different forms: spastic, dementia or paralytic. They all are of equal gravity and end invariably with death of patient.

The Spastic Form: It is characterized by hyperexcitability. Any stimulation of senses (touch, sound, light) causes the patient to suffer contractions, trembling painful spasms or convulsions. Contraction occurring at pharynx, larynx, or the oesophagus is the cause of *hydrophobia*, a characteristic of human rabies. The swallowing of mouthful of water sparks off a very painful and violent spasm, which blocks the upper digestive passages. Mere sight of glass of water or the sound of running water is enough to trigger off a hydrophobic reaction. The patient is distressed and alternates from lying prostrate and having delirious outbursts. He slips into semi-coma gradually and dies 3–5 days after.

The Dementia Form: Hyperexcitability appears very intense. The patient who presents a picture of acute insanity can commit violent acts. But he becomes exhausted very quickly and sinks into coma before dying.

The Paralytic Form: It has a slightly longer development (7–10 days) but one which is equally inevitable. The symptoms are less characteristic and the patient may die before the diagnosis of rabies has been established. The disease begins right away (or after a short period of contractions) with gradual and flaccid Landry's ascending paralysis. Death also occurs once the bulbar nerve centres are affected. Once established rabies is 100% fatal, there is still no treatment available at present. Only vaccination, carried out very soon after the bite enables infected persons to survive.

Rabies in Animals (in Dogs)

Observation of Animal for Rabies

The incubation period is from 10 days to 2 months and sometimes more. In the prodromal phase, dog behaves abnormally—hides in dark corners, shows unusual agitation, or becomes very restless. Reflex excitability is enhanced and there is slight increase in the body temperature. Gradually, dog becomes dangerously aggressive with a tendency to bite objects, animals and man including its own owner and often it will bite itself and inflict serious injuries. Salivation is profuse because animal cannot swallow saliva due to paralysis of muscles of deglutition and the tone of bark changes because of partial paralysis of vocal cords. Generalized convulsions are seen at the terminal phase of illness; followed by muscular incoordination and paralysis of muscles of trunk and extremities. The dumb form of rabies in dogs is characterized by predominantly paralytic clinical features. The excitation phase when present is very short. Progressive paralysis begins with the muscles of head and neck region. Animal has difficulty in swallowing. As a result, owner tries to help the dog, thus, exposing himself to the infection. The course of the disease extends for 5–6 days and death results after general paralysis.

NATIONAL GUIDELINES ON RABIES PROPHYLAXIS (2015)

Because of long incubation period, which is typical of most cases of human rabies, it is possible to institute prophylactic post-exposure treatment. In countries like India, where rabies is endemic, the animal bite management should not depend on laboratory results. The treatment should be started immediately as per recommended guidelines.[6–9]

Approach to Postexposure Prophylaxis (PEP)

The postexposure treatment is a three-pronged approach. All three carry equal importance and should be done simultaneously:

i Management of animal bite wound (s)
ii *Passive immunization:* Rabies immunoglobulins (RIG)
iii *Active immunization:* Anti-rabies vaccine (ARV).

Management of Animal Bite/Wound (s)

Wound (s) Toilet: Since the rabies virus enters the human body through a bite or scratch and virus multiplies locally, it becomes imperative to remove as much saliva, and thereby virus from the wound as is possible by an efficient wound toilet that should not involve additional trauma. Since the rabies virus can persist and even multiply at the site of bite for a long time, *wound toilet* must be performed even if the patient reports late.

1. Prompt and gentle thorough washing with soap or detergent and flushing the wound (s) with running water. If soap and detergent are not available wash with running water. Avoid direct touching of wound with bare hands. Wound washing is crucial step.
2. After thorough washing and drying the wound, any one of the available chemical agents should be applied. Savlon (in appropriate recommended dilution), dettol (in appropriate recommended dilution), povidone-iodine, alcohol, etc. are appropriate.
3. The application of mud soil, chillies, oil, etc. is unnecessary and damaging. In case soil, chillies, oil, etc. have been applied over wound, enough gentle washing with soap or detergent to remove the extraneous material should be done followed by flushing with enough amount of water immediately.
4. Suturing of wound should be avoided as far as possible. If unavoidable, minimum loose sutures should be applied after adequate local treatment along with proper infiltration of anti-rabies serum (RIG).

5 Cauterization of wound is no longer recommended as it leaves a very bad scar; and does not confer any additional advantage over washing the wound with soap and water.
6 Injection tetanus toxoid should be given to the individual. To prevent sepsis suitable antibiotic may be recommended.

Local Infiltration of Rabies Immunoglobulins (RIG)

In category III bites, rabies immunoglobulin is lifesaving. The calculated dose of RIG as anatomically feasible is infiltrated into and around wounds locally to inactivate the virus and any surplus (left over) given by deep intramuscular injection. In immune compromised individuals, RIG should be given in category II and III exposures.

Passive Immunity

Antirabies serum or ERIG: The antirabies serum provides passive immunity in the form of ready made anti-rabies antibody to tide over initial phase of the infection. Antirabies serum (ARS) has the property of binding with the rabies virus thereby resulting in the loss of infectivity of the virus. A purified version of this antirabies serum called as equine rabies immunoglobulin (ERIG) is also now available. It has many side effects.

Human rabies immunoglobulin (HRIG): HRIG is free from side effects encountered in a serum of heterologus origin, and because of their longer half-life, are given in half the dose of equine antirabies serum. The antirabies sera should always be brought to room temperature (20–25°C) before use.

Dose of rabies immunoglobulin: The dose of ERIG is 40 IU per kg body weight of person and is given after testing of sensitivity, up to maximum of 3000 IU. The ERIG produced in India contains 300 IU per ml. The dose of human rabies immunoglobulin (HRIG) is 20 IU per kg body weight (maximum 1500 IU). HRIG does not require any prior sensitivity testing. HRIG preparation is available in concentration of 150 IU per ml.

In category III of animal bites, the antirabies serum after sensitivity test is infiltrated in and around the wound even if the lesion has begun to heal followed by administration of antirabies vaccine. If immunoglobulin was not administered when vaccination was begun, it can be administered up to 7th day after the administration of the first dose of vaccine. Beyond the 7th day, RIG is not indicated since an antibody response to antirabies vaccine is presumed to have occurred. Immunoglobulin should never be administered in the same syringe or at the same anatomical site as vaccine.

Tolerance and Side Effects

With HRIG, there may be transient tenderness at the injection site and brief rise in body temperature, which does not require any treatment.

HRIG must never be given intravenously since this could produce symptoms of shock, especially in patient with antibody deficiency syndromes. With *antisera of equine origin*, in addition, anaphylactic shock may occur and thus sensitivity testing is mandatory before giving ERIG. Skin test may be performed as per the manufacturer's instructions given in the product insert. Otherwise, as a general guideline, the ERIG may be diluted 1:10 in sterile physiological saline and 0.1–0.2 ml may be given intradermally in the forearm. An equivalent intradermal injection of physiological saline solution may be used as a control. The reading made 15 minutes later may be considered to be positive if erythema (>10 mm), local oedema or systemic reaction is observed and the control is negative. A negative skin test must never reassure the physician that no anaphylactic reaction will occur. Those administering ERIG should always be ready to treat early anaphylactic reactions with adrenalin. The dose is 0.5 ml of 0.1% solution (1 in 1000, 1 mg/ml) for adults and 0.01 ml/kg body weight for children, injected subcutaneously or I/M. If patient is sensitive to ERIG, HRIG, should be used.

ERIG carries small risk of anaphylactic reaction (1:150000). ERIG should be given irrespective of the results of skin test.

The total recommended dose of immunoglobulin must not exceed as it may reduce the efficacy of vaccine. If the calculated dose of immunoglobulin is insufficient to cover infiltration in all wounds, sterile saline can be used to dilute 2–3 fold to permit thorough infiltration.

Postexposure Prophylaxis (PEP): Decision to Treat

In rabies endemic country like India where there is sustained dog-to-dog transmission, every animal bite (provoked/unprovoked) is suspected as potentially rabid animal bite, and treatment should be started immediately after exposure. Bite by all warm blooded animals necessitates PEP. As rabies in practically 100% fatal, bites by dogs and cats in particular must be considered as medical "emergency" and the "life-saving" PEP must be provided immediately. Classification of animal bite for PEP has been based upon WHO recommendation (Table 12.40).

Observation of biting dog/cat: The PEP should be started immediately after the bite. The observation period of 10 days is valid for dogs and cats only. The natural history of rabies in mammals other than dogs and cats is not fully understood and therefore the 10-day observation period may not be applicable. The treatment may be modified if dog or cat involved remains healthy throughout the observation period of 10 days by converting PEP to pre-exposure prophylaxis by skipping the vaccine dose on day 14 and administering it on day 28th while using Essen Schedule. While using Intra-dermal administration complete course of vaccination should be given irrespective of status of animal.

Vaccination Status of the biting animal: Although unvaccinated animals are more likely to transmit rabies,

Table 12.40: Type of contact, exposure and recommended post-exposure prophylaxis (PEP) by WHO–TRS 2013

Category	Type of contact	Recommended post-exposure prophylaxis
I	• Touching or feeding of animals • Licks on intact skin • Contact of intact skin with secretions/excretions of rabid animal/human case	• None, if reliable case history is available
II	• Nibbling of uncovered skin • Minor scratches or abrasions without bleeding	• Wound management • Anti-rabies vaccine
III	• Single or multiple transdermal bites or scratches, licks on broken skin • Contamination of mucous membrane with saliva (i.e. licks)	• Wound management • Rabies immunoglobulin • Anti-rabies vaccine

Note: It is re-emphasized that PEP should be started as early as possible after exposure. However, PEP should not be denied to person reporting late for treatment as explained previously. Potentially infected material: consumption of raw milk of rabid animal, contact with saliva and secretions. Bat rabies has not been conclusively proved in India and hence exposure to bats does not warrant PEP.

vaccinated animals can also do so if the vaccination of the biting animal was ineffective for any reason. A history of rabies vaccination in an animal is not always a guarantee that the biting animal is not rabid. Animal vaccine failures may occur because of improper administration or poor quality of the vaccine, poor health status of the animal, and the fact that one vaccine dose does not always provide long lasting protection in dogs. Hence, appropriate documentation of vaccination status of dog/cat and proper history should be elicited before deciding to defer PEP after bite by vaccinated dog/cat.

Anti-Rabies Vaccines for Active Immunization

Neural Tissue Vaccines (NTV)—An Obituary

In the past, BPL inactivated sheep brain vaccine (sample type) was in use. NTVs have been effective, but they contain less antigen, daily injection for 10–14 days followed by boosters are required to produce a protective level of antibody.

WHO has strongly recommended *discontinuation of* the use of reactogenic *nerve tissue derived vaccines* and their complete replacement with safe and potent cell culture vaccines.

Now the production and use of NTV has been discontinued by the Government of India since December, 2004.

Vaccines for Intramuscular (IM) Regimen

1. Cell Culture Vaccines (CCVs)

CCVs available in India:

i Human Diploid Cell Vaccine (HDCV)
ii Purified Chick Embryo Cell Vaccine (PCECV)
iii Purified Verocell Rabies Vaccine (PVRV)

2. Purified Duck Embryo Vaccine (PDEV)

Five-dose Intramuscular Regimen (Essen Regimen)

As recommended by WHO expert committee on rabies (1992), the course of post-exposure prophylaxis should consist of 5 injections (day 0, 3, 7, 14 and 28). Day 0 indicates date of first injection.

PEP for immune-compromised persons requires wound management, local infiltration of RIG followed by complete course of anti-rabies vaccination by intramuscular route in both category II and III exposures and need of additional doses of vaccine after testing anti-rabies antibody.

Dose: 1 ml for HDCV, PCECV, PDEV, and 0.5 ml for PVRV irrespective of age of person. The dose of PVRV by Pasteur Institute of India, Coonoor is 1 ml per injection.

Indications

All cases of animal bites (categories II and III) irrespective of severity of exposure, require the same number of injections and dose per injection. The category III requires administration of rabies immunoglobulins.

Site of Injection

The deltoid region is ideal for the inoculation of these vaccines. Gluteal region is not recommended because the fat present in this region retards the absorption of antigen and hence impairs the generation of optimal immune response. Intramuscular schedule—the most widely used WHO Essen Regimen on day 0, 3, 7, 14 and 28 (1–1–1–1–1).

Abbreviated Multisite IM Regimen

In the abbreviated multisite schedule (Zagreb schedule), the "2–1–1" regimen, one dose [of HDCV or PCECV or PVRV or PDEV] is given in the right arm and one dose in the left arm (IM) on day 0 and one dose given IM in the deltoid region on day 7 and 21. Though this is WHO approved it is not approved by Drug Controller General of India (DCGI) and hence should not be used by medical practitioners in India.[10–12]

Cost of Post-exposure Treatment

Presently many types of cell culture vaccines are available in India. The costs of various CCVs are as given: HDCV costs Rs. 3280, PCEC cost Rs. 1075 and PVRV cost Rs. 1155 if regular five dose intramuscular schedule is followed. Most of these cases also require administration of rabies immunoglobulins, which adds to the cost.

Intradermal (ID) Regimens[12-16]

To reduce the cost of post-exposure treatment with CCVs, WHO has recommended intradermal regimens with CCVs. Based on WHO recommendations, recently the Indian authorities have approved the use of reduced dosage intradermal regimen of PCECV and PVRV initially for use in antirabies centres, which have adequately trained staff and maintain proper cold chain and supplies, and are well versed in management of open vial and safe storage practices. This will be expanded in the country in phased manner. Intradermal regimens are cost-effective and it has been evaluated by WHO and recommended in Thailand. The Thai schedule (Thai Red Cross Schedule) of vaccination as recommended by WHO consists of the ID administration of 0.1 ml at two sites on days 0, 3 and 7, and at one site on days 30 and 90. This schedule (2–2–2–0–1–1) has been recommended by the WHO for use in developing countries. The updated Thai Red Cross schedule (TRC) is ("2-2-2-0-2"): One dose of vaccine in a volume of 0.1 ml is given intradermally at two different lymphatic damage sites, usually the left and right upper arm, on days 0, 3, 7 and 28.

Updated Thai Red Cross schedule (2–2–2–0–2) has been adopted in India.

Eight Site Intradermal Regimen ("8-0-4-0-1-1") Regimen

One dose of 0.1 ml is administered intradermally at 8 different sites (upper arms, lateral thighs, suprascapular region, and lower quadrant of abdomen) on day 0. On day 7, four 0.1 ml injections are administered intradermally into each upper arm (deltoid region) and each lateral thigh. Following these injections, one additional 0.1 ml dose is administered on days 28 and 90. This regimen lowers the cost of vaccination.

Vaccines for intradermal route: Only approved safe and efficacious CCVs are to be used-PVRV (Verorab, Abhayrab, Indirab and Pasteur Institute of Conoor) and PCECV (Rabipur and Vaxirab N).

Storage and Transportation

Though cell culture vaccines are marketed in freeze dried (lyophilized) form, which is more tolerant to higher temperature, yet it is recommended that these vaccines should be kept and transported at a temperature range of +2 to 8°C. Freezing does not damage the vaccine, but there are chances of breaking of ampoule containing the diluent.

Reconstitution

12

The lyophilized vaccine should be reconstituted with the diluent provided with the vaccine immediately prior to use. However, in case of unforeseen delay it should not be used after 6–8 hours of reconstitution.

Potency: The potency is the capacity of the vaccine to induce immune response. For modern vaccine, it is more than 2.5 IU per dose.

Protective Level of Antirabies Antibody

Humoral antibodies are believed to play an important role in protection against rabies and a titre of 0.5 IU/ml or more in serum is considered as protective. This level is achieved in most healthy individuals by day 14 of PEP. Antibody tests, viz. Rapid Fluorescent Focus Inhibition Test (RFFIT), Mouse Neutralization Test (MNT) can be done to know the level of antibody.

Adverse Events Following CCVs

The cell culture vaccines are widely accepted as least reactogenic rabies vaccines available today. The general adverse reaction includes sore arm, headache, malaise, nausea, fever and localized oedema at the site of injection. Only symptomatic treatment is advocated.

Switch Over from One Vaccine to other

Shifting from one brand of CCV to other brand also should not be encouraged as literature supports that good immunity is best achieved with same brand.

Managing Re-exposure Following Post-exposure Treatment with CCVs

If a person is re-exposed who has previously received full pre-exposure/post-exposure prophylaxis (anytime in the past either pre-exposure 3 doses or post-exposure 5 doses) with a potent cell culture vaccine, should be given only two booster doses, intramuscularly or intradermally on days 0 and 3 but no rabies immunoglobulin is necessary in them (WHO 2002).

Managing Exposure Following Pre-exposure Prophylaxis with CCVs

If after recommended pre-exposure prophylaxis, a vaccinated person is exposed to rabies, a proper wound toileting should be done and two IM or ID doses of cell culture vaccine be given on days 0 and 3. Treatment with RIG is not necessary.

Pre-exposure Prophylaxis

It is indicated for high-risk groups—like laboratory staff handling the virus and infected material, clinicians and paramedicals attending to hydrophobia cases, veterinarians, animal handlers and catchers, wild life wardens, quarantine officers, and travellers from rabies free areas to rabies endemic areas.

Pre-exposure immunization should be three full IM or ID doses of CCVs given on days 0, 7 and either day 21 or 28.

Laboratory staff and others at high continuing risk of exposure should have their neutralizing antibody titres checked every 6 months during the initial two years and thereafter every two years. If it is less than 0.5 IU/ml, a booster dose of vaccine should be given. Such individuals on getting exposure to rabies virus after successful pre-exposure immunization require only two booster injections of vaccine given on days 0 and 3 without any antirabies serum (RIG).

Management of Animal Bite Exposure in Pregnant Women and Lactating Mothers

Pregnancy and lactation are no contraindications for rabies vaccination. Post-exposure prophylaxis against rabies takes preference over any other consideration since it is life-saving procedure. Moreover, antirabies vaccine does not have any adverse effect on foetus, mother to be and the course of pregnancy. Hence, complete post-exposure treatment should be given depending upon the category of exposure.

Pre-exposure Immunization in Animals

Pre-exposure immunization of pet animals against rabies is recommended.

Single dose: The vaccine is prepared as 20% suspension of brain from sheep infected with modified rabies virus. The virus in the brain suspension is inactivated with phenol or β-propiolactone (BPL). It is only used for pre-exposure immunization.

Veterinary antirabies vaccine multiple dose: This vaccine is also prepared from sheep brain infected with modified rabies virus. Modern cell line inactivated vaccines in India for animals are available. For dogs and cats, the primary schedule of 2 injections at 2 months age with one month interval and a booster every year is recommended. Oral vaccine for dogs offers a new approach.

NATIONAL PROGRAMME FOR CONTROL OF RABIES IN DOGS

Canine rabies can be eliminated. Canine rabies control programme should incorporate 3 basic elements:

(a) Epidemiological surveillance, (b) mass vaccination and (c) dog population control

a. Epidemiological Surveillance

Rabies should be notifiable disease within national health and veterinary systems. Rabies surveillance is inadequate. Both clinically and laboratory confirmed cases and persons seeking and receiving post-exposure prophylaxis should be regularly reported to capture burden and trends of problem.

b. Canine Mass Parenteral Vaccination Campaigns

i. Mass canine vaccination campaigns have been most effective measure for controlling canine rabies. At least 70% of the dog population in each community should be vaccinated in areas where canine rabies is endemic. Registration and permanent identification of vaccinated dogs is recommended.

ii. *Supplementary measures:* Oral vaccination of dogs. Oral vaccination of dogs offers a new approach that may improve vaccination coverage of stray dogs in rural and urban slum areas.

Although the preferred vaccine for dog immunization shoud be parenteral (inactivated cell culture vaccine), oral vaccine should be used whenever there is higher population of inaccessible dogs.

c. Dog Population Management and Animal Birth Control (ABC) Programmes

Three practical methods of dog population management are recognized—movement restriction, habitat control and reproduction (sterilization of dogs). Attempt to control dog population through culling without alteration of habitat have generally been unsuccessful. Based on 1990 WHO guidelines, ABC programmes have been launched in several countries and the results have been encouraging, with a reported reduction in the size of the street dogs population and the number of human rabies cases.

Since dogs are the major reservoir of rabies transmission in India, hence their population must be controlled. Way back in 1985, the dog population was estimated to be 80 million as per census by Agriculture Ministry. It appears this population might have grown substantially.

The dog destruction used to be one of the pivotal activities at the primary health centre in India. Sanitary inspectors used to destroy dogs in rural areas after obtaining the requisition from village panchayats. Now this has been stopped.

- Sterilization of dogs and monkeys has been attempted to reduce their population.

Various organizations are currently involved in control activities without any intersectoral coordination. Existing rabies control activities are being carried out by Municipal Corporations/Committees, in their respective areas.

Health Education (IEC Activities)

Health education of public on prevention and control of rabies and management of bites and their response to bite at local level is crucial to save lives. This should be attempted through primary health care infrastructure besides mass-media as also formal and non-formal education channels.[17–18]

REFERENCES

1 National centre for disease control (DGHS Nationl Rabies Control Programme. National guidelines on rabies prophylaxis 2015.

2 NICD. Rabies epidemiology—principles of control and treatment. Delhi: NICD; 1992.

12

3 Central Research Institute. Principles and practice of Anti-rabic treatment and control of rabies. Kasauli; CRI; 1971.

4 Singla SL, Kaur M, Lal S. "Monkey Bites"—A public health problem in urban setting. Ind J Pub Health 1997; 41(1): 3–24.

5 Indian Vaccines Corporation Ltd. Verorab—purified rabies vaccine prepared in vero cells. Pasteur Merieux Serum and Vaccines. Alidac Genetics and Pharmaceuticals.

6 Bharucha MR. Rabies: Some questions answered. Bombay (India): Serum Institute of India (P) Ltd.

7 Veera Raghavan N. Rabies and its prevention with detailed instructions for the guidance of medical and veterinary officers responsible for the administration of anti-rabies treatment. Conoor: Pasteur Institute of Southern India; 1972.

8 NICD. Guidelines for management of animal bites. CD Alert Monthly newsletter of NICD, DGHS, GOI March 2002; 6(3).

9 WHO. WHO Expert Committee on rabies. Technical report series. Geneva: WHO; 1992. Report No. 824.

10 APCRI VIII Annual Conference of Association for Prevention and Control of Rabies in India. Souvenir APCRICON-2006 Held at Government Medical College Jammu J & K.

11 Sudarshan MK. Rabies Prevention. A Medical Guidebook. 1st ed. Pune; Serum Institute of India, October 2004.

12 Madhusudana SN, Prem Anand N. Response to Purified chick embryo cell rabies vaccine administered intradermally for post-exposure prophylaxis. National Med J India. 1997; (3): 115–6.

13 Madhusudana SN. Cost effective abbreviated regimen using cell culture rabies vaccine for post-exposure rabies prophylaxis. Journal of Basic and Applied Biomedicine 1996; 4 (2): 5–9.

14 Madhusudana SN, Prem Anand N, Sham Sunder R. Evaluation of two intradermal vaccination regimens using purified chick embryo cell vaccine for post-exposure prophylaxis of rabies. National Med J India 2001; 14(3): 145–7.

15 Madhusudana SN, Saha SM, Sood M, Saxena SN. Multisite Intradermal vaccination using tissue culture vaccine as an economical prophylactic regimen against rabies. Indian J Med Res Jan 1988; 87: 1–4.

16 GOI (2007 and 2013). National Guidelines for Rabies Prophylaxis and Intradermal Administration of Cell Culture Rabies Vaccines—NCDC, DGHS, MOH and FW, GOI; New Delhi.

17 Sandhu TS. Rabies—What we know and what we need to know? Indian J Comm Med Oct–Dec 2004; 29(4): 163–8.

18 GOI. Annual Report 2008–14. MOH and FW, Government of India; New Delhi.

PLAGUE

Plague is primarily a zoonoses, being a disease of rodents and man is affected incidentally.

Plague is an acute communicable disease caused by *Yersinia pestis* and transmitted to man by the bite of infected rat flea. It remains a major life-threatening infection of human beings and animals.

Occurrence

Plague recognized no boundaries and used to occur in pandemic form, in epidemics and it has become endemic in some parts of the world. It has caused millions of deaths. The first pandemic occurred in 543 AD in Egypt during the reign of Emperor Justinian and it killed about 100 million people. The second pandemic started in 1345 and it killed 25 million people and third pandemic started in 1845 and it killed 10.25 million people. More than 12 million people died in India from 1898 to 1950s. The incidence has declined considerably due to improvement in living conditions.[1, 2]

Global Distribution

Plague has been one of the greatest scourge of human race. From time to time, it has swept over the world in relentless waves, in large number of countries especially Europe, Central Asia, Africa, South America, North America and South East Asia exacting a toll of life probably unequalled by that of any other disease. Plague continues to be a threat because of vast areas of persistent wild rodent infection, contact of wild rodents with domestic rats occur frequently in some enzootic areas.

Indian Scenario

Nearly 12.5 million people died in India in the last pandemic which started way back in the year 1894 as recorded deaths in India from 1898 provides this evidence. After 1966 the plague re-emerged in India in 1994 after a gap of 28 years when cases were reported from village Mamla in Maharashtra (Table 12.41).[1]

Table 12.41: The mortality trends of plague in India[1, 2]

Period	Deaths due to plague
1898–1908	60,32,693
1909–1918	42,21,529
1919–1928	17,62,718
1929–1938	4,22,880
1939–1948	3,68,596
1949–1958	59,059
1959–1966	211
1967–1993	0
1994	54
2002	4
2003–2014	0

Natural foci of plague are known to exist in parts of Andhra Pradesh, Gujarat, Himachal Pradesh, Karnataka and Tamil Nadu. The reasons are environmental degrada-tion because of emerging urban slums, deforestation, increase in population of rodents in slums besides rising population. "Char-Minar" at Hyderabad was built to commemorate elimination of plague epidemic.

Outbreak of Plague in 1994

On 30th September 1993, a devastating earthquake struck in parts of Osmanabad and Latur district of Maharashtra. The affected population was rehabilitated in temporary shelters 1–3 km away from affected areas. People of Mamla village in Beed district of Maharashtra abandoned their homes and resettled in temporary shelters. Lots of grains were rushed to the area and probably these environments brought rodents closer to human beings. After a period of one year, the rodent population got built up and cases of bubonic plague were reported from Mamla village. In August 1994, the *R. rattus* population overshot its equilibrium density and eventually led to an epizootic in rats (rat-to-rat transmission of plague by rat flea and leading to death of rats). On 5th August 1994, the inhabitants of village Mamla experienced heavy flea nuisance and rat falls (deaths) were reported. Subsequently, a number of cases clinically resembling bubonic plague were reported from Mamla village and from surrounding villages.[3–5] Afterwards during the third week of September 1994, 876 suspected cases of pneumonic plague were reported and 54 people died in Surat (Gujarat). Recently in 2002, 16 cases and 4 deaths of pneumonic plague were reported from Hat Koti village of Shimla district in Himachal Pradesh. The cases were confirmed by NICD Delhi.[6] *Yersinia pestis* strains were isolated from human and rodent specimens and molecular characterization showed that biotype of the Surat strain was different from the existing 16 biotypes of *Y. pestis*. Three cases of plague occurred in a village in Uttaranchal in 2004.

Epidemiology of Plague in India

Causative Agent

The causative organism of plague is bacteria *Yersinia pestis* which was previously called as *Pasteurella pestis*. It is a small gram-negative, straight oval bacillus of size 1.5 mm × 0.7 mm. The bacillus has rounded ends and convex sides, arranged singly in short chains or in small groups. High degree of pleomorphism is seen in smears from buboes and culture grown on 3% of salt agar. The organism manifests typical bipolar staining (safety pin appearance).

The organism may remain viable for several weeks in water, moist soils and grains. However, it is killed by several hours of exposure to sunlight.

Reservoir

At least 220 species of rodents which inhabit mountains, plains, deserts, cultivated fields and forests both temperate and tropical climate are known to be infected with plague bacillus. The major natural vertebrate reservoir of plague includes field or wild rodents (Tatera indica) including ground squirrels which play an important role as reservoir of *Y. pestis*. Lagomorphs (rabbits and hares), wild carnivores and domestic cats may also be source of infection.

Mode of Transmission

Plague is primarily a disease of rodents in which man is incidentally involved. The principal mode of transmission is bite by infected flea. There are at least 5 basic types of transmission cycles in plague:

1. Commensal rats → rat fleas → man. This is the basic cycle in epidemic bubonic plague.
2. Wild rodents → wild rodent fleas or direct contact → man. The disease is transmitted from rodent to rodent via wild rodent fleas or contaminated soil. Man acquires infection from infectious wild rodent fleas or by direct contact with infected rodents.
3. Wild-rodents, peri-domestic rodents, commensal rodents → wild rodent fleas, peri-domestic rodent fleas, commensal rodent fleas → man. Plague foci impinge upon the habitats of peri-domestic or commensal rodents. Interaction of the rodents and their fleas convey the infection to man.
4. Man → man (through human flea: *Pulex irritans*). This variety may be encountered in certain areas.
5. Man → man (via respiratory route). This results when a primary case of bubonic plague develops secondary pneumonic plague and infects contacts via respiratory route.

Risk Factors

Location of granaries near the vicinity of residential areas attracts rodents. During natural calamities like flood and earthquakes, the temporary shelters are set-up in areas where rat population get attracted due to presence of food grains/food. When human population come in direct contact with rodents or carnivores (such as migrant workers and nomadic population who set-up temporary camps in peri-urban areas, similarly brick kiln workers set-up camps in remote areas; where rats and rodents abound), growing urban slum population and lack of sanitary measures and increase in human population and population of rodents and flea are the predominant risk factors for transmission of rodent diseases to man including plague. The insanitary conditions in slums build up rodent population and the same happened in Surat city in 1994 and after earthquake in Osmanabad and Latur in Maharashtra.

Incubation Period (IP)

Bubonic plague: 2–6 days

Pneumonic plague: 2–4 days or even shorter.

Under International Health Regulations IP is 6 days.

Pathogenesis

Rats (and other rodents) are natural reservoir of plague. The disease is maintained between rodents by the bite of infected fleas. On being bitten by an infected flea, bacteria are introduced into man. The initial response is that of lymphadenitis in those lymph nodes which receive drainage from the site of flea bite. The enlarged lymph node is called bubo and the disease as bubonic plague. If untreated this progresses to septicaemic phase in which the organisms get disseminated to various organs of the body including meninges. Involvement of lungs causes pneumonia which is of special significance since aerosolized droplets of sputum may cause primary pneumonia in another individual.

Bubonic Plague

This is the commonest form characterized by high fever, toxaemia and painful enlargement of lymph glands which are called buboes. Bubo appears on 2nd and 3rd day. Buboes may appear in groin or in the axillary or cervical region depending upon the site of bite and entry of organism. The glands gradually become soft and suppurate and there is marked haemorrhagic tendency with variable septicaemia. Fever usually subsides after 10 days, bubo may burst. Mortality is 25–30% in untreated cases.

Pneumonic Plague

It is due to droplet infection. It is a severe form of disease with high fever and cough with blood tinged tenacious sputum. The disease is highly contagious resulting in explosive outbreaks. Recovery is rare and death occurs in 2–4 days.

Septicaemic Plague

This is a variant of bubonic plague, where there is overwhelming septicemia or over-running the lymph nodes. Consequently, lymph node enlargement is not prominent but the patient is highly toxic. This form also results in very high mortality.

Pestis Minor

It is an ambulant plague, a mild form of disease with fever and buboes which may suppurate. Symptoms are very mild.

Cutaneous Plague

There is pustule, eschar, carbuncle, erythema gangrenosum usually with bubo.

Meningeal Plague

Partially or untreated patients of bubonic plague may progress to meningeal stage, seen commonly in children whose presentation are typical of bacterial meningitis.

Case Fatality

If not treated in time, more than 50% cases of bubonic plague and almost all cases of pneumonic plague die.

WHO Case Definition of Plague

Suspect Plague

Compatible clinical and epidemiological features and suspicious organisms seen or isolated from clinical specimens.

Presumptive Plague (Probable Case)

- *Y. pestis* F1 antigen detected in clinical materials by direct fluorescent antibody testing, or by some other standardized antigen detection method; or
- Isolate from a clinical specimen demonstrates biochemical reactions consistent with *Y. pestis* or PCR positivity; or
- A single serum specimen is found positive for diagnostic levels of antibodies to *Y. pestis* F1 antigen, not explainable on the basis of prior infection or immunization.
- Epidemiological link with a confirmed case.

Confirmed Plague

- Isolate identified as *Y. pestis* by phage lysis or cultures; or
- A significant (equal or more than 4-fold) change in antibody titre to F1 antigen in paired serum specimens.

Prevention and Control

Case Management

The response of plague to antibiotic treatment is dramatic and rapid. The drugs which are effective against plague include tetracycline, chloramphenicol, cotrimoxazole, sulphonamide and streptomycin.

Tetracycline

During first 48 hours, 4–6 g should be administered daily. Intravenous therapy is essential in severely ill-patients as in pneumonic plague. Treatment is to be continued for 10 days or at least 3–4 days after the fever has disappeared in dose of 15 mg/kg body weight every 6 hours. Oral dose for adult is 500 mg every 6 hourly. Tetracycline is contraindicated in children below 7 years, pregnant women and patients with renal failure, in such cases cotrimoxazole should be administered.

Chloramphenicol

Patients with meningitis require a drug that can penetrate the meninges. In such patients, chloramphenicol should be administered intravenously, with a loading dose of 25 mg/kg followed by 60 mg/kg in 4 divided doses daily till patient improves.

Streptomycin

0.5 gm every 4 hours for 2 days followed by 0.5 gm every 6 hours until clinical improvement occurs. This drug is associated with ototoxicity.

Cotrimoxazole

For children less than 5 years of age one teaspoonful of syrup of cotrimoxazole every 12 hours is indicated. children between 5 and 10 years 1 tablet every 12 hours is recommended. Pregnant women require administration of 2 tablets every 12 hours (single strength) and one tablet of double strength every 12 hours. The above mentioned chemotherapeutic agents are effective when given alone. Relapses are exceedingly rare. There is no rationale for using multiple drugs.

Chemoprophylaxis

Chemoprophylaxis is recommended for exposed persons, exposure to bites of rodent fleas during an outbreak or to tissues or fluids of infected animals or coming in contact with suspected case or to pet animal with suspected plague pneumonia.

WHO guidelines for chemoprophylaxis are shown in Table 12.42.

Chemoprophylaxis for general population is not recommended.

During the outbreak of plague at Surat there was large scale exodus of population from Surat to other states (as natives left Surat in panic and migrated to their homes in different states). All people started consuming tetracycline and this drug disappeared from the market. A panic was created and administration wanted to isolate and quarantine the migrants in the camps which appeared to be a futile and unpracticable exercise. People were most comfortable in their homes and were educated to report to nearby facility if they observed any symptom compatible with plague.

Table 12.42: Chemoprophylaxis for plague

Drugs	Dosage	Interval (hours)	Route of administration
Tetracycline			
• Adults	1–2 gm/day	6–12	Orally
• Children	25–50 mg/kg/day	6–12	Orally
Doxycycline			
• Adults	100–200 mg/day	12–24	Orally
• Children ≥9 yrs	100–200 mg/day	12–24	Orally
Sulfamethoxazole/ Trimethoprim			
• Adults	1.6 g/day*	12	Orally
• Children ≥2 mths	100–200 mg/day*	12	Orally

*Sulfamethoxazole component

Sale of masks picked up tremendously and everyone on the roadside was wearing mask particularly in metropolis.

Immunoprophylaxis

A formalin killed plague vaccine is produced in limited quantity by Haffkine Institute, Mumbai. It contains 2000 million organisms per ml.

Dosage

Adult: 0.5 ml given subcutaneously followed by second dose of 1 ml after 7–14 days. Boosters are given every 6 months. Immunity appears after 5–7 days of inoculation and lasts for about 6 months. Repeated boosters induce higher incidence of adverse reactions.

Vaccination is recommended for only high-risk groups of individuals, i.e. medical and public health workers who are dealing with patients of plague or who investigate plague outbreaks and laboratory workers who handle plague cultures or plague infected material. In local outbreaks of plague, vaccination is of no use. Moreover, the vaccinated person who has been exposed to definite risk of infection must be given prophylactic antibiotics, even if his serum is known to contain antibodies against plague bacterium.

All persons exposed to patients with suspected pneumonic plague should receive antibiotics regardless of their immunization status.

Vector Control[7]

The rat fleas are the natural vectors of plague. In India, the most important species involved in disease transmission are *Xenopsylla cheopis*, *X. astia* and *X. brasiliensis*, the most common being *X. cheopis*. Both male and female fleas feed on blood.

Blocked Flea

Yersinia pestis rapidly multiplies in the gut of flea, the speed of multiplication and the enormous number of bacilli may block the lumen of the gut. The blocked flea makes repeated attempts to take the blood meal and each time it attempts to bite, it inoculates large number of plague bacilli in the body of vertebrate host. The extrinsic incubation period of plague bacilli in fleas has been reported to be 5–31 days with an average of 21 days.

Vector Control Measures

Application of insecticidal dusting powder is effective to control the flea population. The rodents pick up the dust on their feet and carry it to their nest and subsequently the insecticide is distributed over its body through constant preening.

Dust Formulation

Five per cent malathion dust powder (1 part of 25% w.p. malathion and 4 parts of chalk powder or inert material).

Insecticidal dust applied on runways and burrows is more effective in controlling fleas. The insecticidal dust should be blown into the opening of burrows and patch of 1 cm thick is left around it. In indoor situations, patches of dust should also be applied to rat runways, which are usually found along the wall. 15–30 cm wide patches of dust should be placed at several points along runways.

Residual Insecticidal Spray

In the absence of insecticide dust formulation, residual insecticide may be sprayed for flea control.

Malathion 25% wp: Malathion suspension is applied @ 2.0 g/m^2 of active ingredient. To get 5% suspension, 2.0 kg of 25% wp. has to be mixed in 10 litres of water. Three rounds of spray may be undertaken annually at an interval of 6–8 weeks.

Synthetic pyrethroids: Only to be used during emergent situation at 10–12 weeks interval. *Example:*

a ***Deltamethrin 2.5% wp:*** The suspension is applied @ 20.0 mg/m^2 of active ingredient. To obtain the desired suspension, 400 g of 2.5% deltamethrin is to be mixed in 10 litres of water.

b ***Cyfluthrin 10% wp:*** The suspension is applied @ 25 mg/m^2. of active ingredient. To obtain the suspension, 125 g of 10% cyfluthrin may be mixed in 10 litres of water.

c ***Lambdacyhalothrin 10% wp:*** The suspension is applied @ 25 mg/m^2. of active ingredient. To obtain the suspension, 125 g of 10% lambdacyhalothrin may be mixed in 10 litres of water.

Residual spray of insecticides may be undertaken in indoor situations up to height of 1.0 meter in the affected areas. The areas used for sleeping by human beings, bedding of animals, under rugs, cracks and crevices in floors and all exterior areas frequented by rodents.

Rodent Control

Mass destruction of rats by baiting, and trapping should be done during inter-epidemic period. During epidemic situation, the rodent control activities should be discouraged because of killing of a large number of rodents may result in large number of fleas leaving their dead hosts and give rise to further increase in plague cases as the flea may attack the human population. Flea control must be done before killing rats.

Chemical Control

Anticoagulants

- Warfarin, fumarin, tomarin, arsenic trioxide, etc. are multiple dose baits, they cause internal haemorrhage and slow death in 4–10 days. They are slow acting, effective and safe rodenticide and marketed as 0.5% concentrate powder.

  Freshly prepared baits (80–100 gm) are tightly wrapped in paper and introduced in active rodent burrows. The rodent will invariably drag it into burrow, feed on it and die. Continuous use leads to development of resistance.
- Zinc phosphide is a single dose effective rodenticide when moist, it slowly releases the phosphine gas, which kills the rats and fleas. Rats are killed within 3 hours. A dosage of 1.0–2.5% is used. About 15 gm bait/rat/burrow is used.

  Aluminium phosphide tablets—2 pellets of 6 g per burrow. After putting the tablets inside the burrow, they are closed with wet mud for killing the rodents. It is highly toxic to human beings and should only be used in killing wild rodents and not in domestic and peri-domestic situations.

Fumigants

Calcium cyanide (cynogas)–Carbon-disulphide, methyl bromide. Cynogas is pumped into the burrow using special foot pump called "cynogas pump". About 56 g dust is pumped into each burrow after closing the exit of burrow and burrow is then sealed promptly with wet mud. On contact with moisture, the cynogas powder gives off hydrogen cyanide which kills the rodents as well as the fleas.

Fumigation of rodent burrows—systemic fumigation of cynogas in rat burrows, grain godowns and market places may be carried out routinely after 3–4 months.

Disposal of Dead Rats

Use mask of double-folded cloth to cover your face. Spray insecticide dust over the dead rat and subsequently bury it in a deep pit. Pick up the dead rat by means of long forceps, long tong, etc. to bury it. The disposable items used should be burnt or buried and other items should be disinfected.

Environmental Control

Improvement in sanitation, proper disposal of waste, proper storage of grains and food stuffs, rat proofing of dwelling units, and plugging of rodent burrows with concrete are useful.

Plague Surveillance

Serosurveillance

i Monitoring the presence of antibodies to plague antigen in wild rodents collected from the identified foci of plague.

ii Monitoring of antibodies to plague antigen in canine is better alternative. Dogs from the villages, considered at potential risk, act as sentinels since they are likely to be exposed to infection, if infected wild rodents and/or fleas have reached human population.

iii Presence of antibodies to plague in humans in the villages at high-risk should be considered a signal for high alert.

Plague antibodies decline rapidly after vaccination or illness and are usually not detectable after a period of 6–8 months.

Warning Signals for High Alert

Commensal rodents are highly susceptible to plague. Rat fall (dead rats found in the village) is a sign of *high alert and trigger* for immediate action/investigation. A system must be in place to receive information about rat fall immediately if this occur. Local people and health workers in high-risk areas identified, should notify rat fall urgently. Health facilities must report immediately any case of fever with painful lymphadenitis (or severe pain in the groin or axilla) for immediate investigation and follow-up.

Geographical areas for surveillance: Erstwhile known foci of plague, rodent serology positive for plague antibody recorded and suspected human case(s) of plague be reported.

Collection of Rat Fleas

Rat fleas are collected to determine the species, rat flea index and susceptibility to insecticides.

The flea index or flea population density is calculated by dividing the number of fleas by the total number of rodents surveyed. For example:

Flea index = No. of fleas/No. of rodents

A flea index of 1 or above should be treated as high-risk factor and an early warning signal of risk of potential outbreak.

Similarly, species index is also calculated, e.g. *Xenopsylla cheopis* index is *X. cheopis* per rat.

Plague Surveillance in India

Central plague laboratory at NICD, Delhi, in close collaboration with Plague Surveillance Unit (PSU), Bangalore and State Plague Control units located in Tamil Nadu, Karnataka, Andhra Pradesh, and Gujarat undertakes plague surveillance in plague endemic states of the country, to detect the evidence of plague antibodies among wild and peri-domestic rodents and to ascertain the current status of sylvatic plague in Chitoor district (Andhra Pradesh), Dharmapuri and the Nilgiris districts (Tamil Nadu), Kolar and Bangalore rural districts (Karnataka), Beed district (Maharashtra) and urban and rural Surat (Gujarat).

Activities: Catching of rodents and examination of serum samples for plague antibodies and organ smears for direct-microscopy for detection of bipolar stained organisms (Table 12.43).

Early warning signals: Positive plague serology in rodents/canines. High flea index, evidence of rat fall and suspected human cases are signals for early action.

Table 12.43: Rodent serology from 1983 to 2001

Year	No. of rodents examined	No. of rodents positive
1983	21,234	0
1984	30,356	0
1990	32,644	0
1991	45,301	50
1992	54,626	135
1993	51,649	21
1994	30,103	30
2000	13,230	0
2001	16,981	0

Occurrence of Plague in Rodents

Sylvatic Plague

The sylvatic plague is maintained in relatively resistant hosts called permanent reservoir hosts. These transmit the infection to less resistant animal host resulting in epizootics. When infection is endemic in sylvatic rodents (jungle rats or *Tatera indica*) it may remain smouldering for a long time before circumstances favour its epidemic spread. During this time, human beings in villages may occasionally contract the disease through handling of an infected animal. The disease does not become epidemic in man unless infection spreads to what sometimes termed as "Liasion rodent" namely a species of rat that comes in contact with man.

Domestic Plague

Domestic plague is intimately associated with rodents living with man. It occurs when infection is picked-up from permanent reservoir host by semi-domestic rodents which in turn transmit it to the commensal rodents and then to man. The rat fall is the harbinger of domestic rodent plague and a sign of imminent outbreak of epidemic bubonic plague in man. Rodents are also known to transmit the infection to remote areas causing pandemics.

Signs in Rodents

In rodents dying of plague, necropsy reveals enlargement of lymph nodes with periglandular inflammation and oedema that is more frequent in cervical lymph nodes due to tendency of rat flea to bite at the neck region. There is pleural effusion, enlargement of spleen with small white areas in the pulp, liver is engorged and mottled, with congestion and haemorrhages under the skin and in internal organs. *Y. pestis* can be demonstrated in material obtained from these organs.

Besides rodents plague can affect other animals too. Domestic animals, rabbits, camels, etc. are all susceptible to infection.

REFERENCES

1 NICD. Plague surveillance and control. CD Alert. Monthly newsletter on communicable diseases Feb. 2002; 6(2).

2 Seal SC. Plague conquest and eradication in India. New Delhi: ICMR; 1987.

3 Saxena VK, Khera AK, Bora D. Earthquake in Maharashtra-Impact Assessment on communicable disease potential. J of Basic and Applied Biomedicine 1994; 2(1): 77.

4 Saxena VK, Verghese T. Observation of urban ecology of Surat and Bubonic Plague transmission in the city. Current Science 1996; 71(10): 803–5.

5 Saxena VK, Verghese T. Ecology of flea transmitted zoonotic infection in village Mamla, Distt. Beed. Current Science Nov. 1996; 71(10): 800–2.

6 GOI. Annual Report 2003–04. New Delhi, MOH and FW GOI; 2004.

7 WHO. Vector control methods for use by individuals and communities. Geneva: WHO; 1997.

BRUCELLOSIS[1]

This is occupational zoonotic disease. This disease seriously affects the live stock of India. Data on this bacterial zoonotic disease among human beings is incomplete. The causative organisms are *Brucella melitensis*, *B. abortus*, *B. suis* and *B. canis*.

Reservoir and Source

The animals that serve as common reservoir include goats, sheep, cattle, buffaloes and swine.

The modes of transmission to man are by ingestion, contact, inhalation and accidental inoculation.

Ingestion

Usual vehicles of infection are:

- Untreated food products or raw milk from infected animals.
- Raw vegetables contaminated by infected animal's urine or faeces.
- Viscera, bone marrow, and lymph nodes and muscle tissue from infected carcasses which may retain brucellae for more than a month after slaughter and much longer in chilled meat.
- Contamination of water supplies by animal excreta.

Contact

Contact with brucellae in vaginal discharges, fetuses, placentae, urine, manure, carcasses and salvaged animals causes a large proportion of human cases. The skin and mucus membranes including the conjunctiva provide the portal of entry. Contact route of transmission is important in veterinarians and farmers.

12

Inhalation

Brucellosis infection can occur by inhalation of infected dried material of animal origin such as dust from sheep wool, railways, trucks, and lorries that have transported infected animals.

Human Brucellosis

Acute and subacute brucellosis is accompanied by fever and bacteraemia. Some patients develop an acute illness of limited duration followed by apparent recovery, others have prolonged fever followed by frequent relapses. Chronic illness may persist for number of years.

Prevention

- Pasteurization of milk (Heating milk at 73°C for 15 seconds and then suddenly chilling it, followed by bottling) or boiling of milk.
- Destruction of diseased animals.
- Safe disposal of animals suffering from brucellosis or their products such as caracasses.
- Personal protection measures in slaughter houses.

REFERENCE

1 NICD. Zoonotic diseases of Public Health Importance. New Delhi: NICD; 2000.

HYDATID DISEASE

Echinococcosis: Echinococcosis is a zoonotic infection caused by adult and larval stages (metacestodes) of the cestode genus *Echinococcus* (Family Taeniidae). The hydatidosis or hydatid disease is restricted to infection with metacestodes, while echinococcosis is applied to both adult and larval infections.

Hosts: Echinococcosis requires two hosts for completion of their life cycles. Definitive host is carnivorous animal usually dog. Sexual cycle is completed in definitive host and eggs are passed in the faeces. Intermediate host is represented by wide range of mammals including man. After their ingestion, cestode eggs hatch to release embryos (oncosphere) in small intestine. Penetration through the mucosa leads to blood-borne distribution to liver, lungs, kidneys, spleen muscles brain and other organs via circulation. These embryos develop into hydatid cyst. Although most primary infection in humans consist of a single cyst, 20–40% of patients may have multiple cysts or multiple organ involvement. The liver is the most common site for hydatid cysts followed by lungs (50%) and less frequently in other organs like brain, kidneys, heart, and bones.

Signs and symptoms depend upon the size and anatomical site of the cyst. Common signs are liver enlargement. Rate of growth of hydatid cysts are highly variable and range from 1 to 5 cm in diameter per year. In humans, the cyst may attain volume of many litres and contain many thousands of protoscolices. Rupture of the cyst may precipitate allergic reactions.

Although disease may not progress or may resolve spontaneously, the risks of anaphylactic reactions, dissemination following rupture, and relentless growth which renders therapy more difficult or impossible provides a strong argument for early therapy. Surgical removal of hydatid cyst remains the most effective treatment. Surgical removal should be followed by injection of a protoscolicidal agent at the site (hypertonic saline or silver nitrate) and complete removal of endocyst.

Diagnosis and surgical removal of intact cysts before the onset of complications result in high cure rates with low surgical mortality (1–4%). In contrast, secondary or recurrent disease often requires repeated surgical intervention with mortality reaching 20%.

If the cyst is at inaccessible site or if it ruptures or if widespread metastasis has occurred treatment with mebendazole or albendazole may be attempted. Liver cysts respond to treatment very well but cysts at other site respond poorly. Mebendazole (50–150 mg/kg of body weight per day, as a single dose for 3 months) or albendazole (10–15 mg/kg per day, in divided oral doses for one month) are recommended, many patients require repeated courses.

Prevention and Control

Preventive measures include personal hygiene, strict dietary regulation of pet dogs to prevent ingestion of sheep offal and avoidance of dogs that are not so regulated. Prophylactic treatment of dogs with praziquantel at intervals just short of *pre-patent period*—before completion of sexual cycle (e.g. 45–50 days) prevents egg excretion in dogs so treated.

The principal objective of control of cystic hydatid disease consists of reducing parasite prevalence in definitive and intermediate hosts to level below those necessary for continued transmission. Essential measures include health education, control of livestock slaughtering in abattoirs and on farms, safe disposal of infected viscera, dog control, and periodic diagnostic testing and mass treatment of dogs with praziquantel. The results achieved by control programme in New Zealand, Tasmania, Cyprus, Falkland, Island, Argentina and Chile have been spectacular. Marked reduction in prevalence of cysts in sheep following the initiation of control methods, as well as in the number of new diagnosed human cases, indicate that the fundamental requirements for effective control are now tried and proved.

TAENIASIS AND CYSTICERCOSIS

Taeniasis and cysticercosis are diseases caused by the adult and larval stages of cestodes or tapeworm parasites, *Taenia saginata* and *Taenia solium* in their definitive host (human) and intermediate hosts (cattle, pigs; humans) both species are meat-borne parasites that localize as adults in the intestines of human host. These intestinal infections, termed taeniasis, normally produce only mild symptoms. Eggs passed in the faeces of human carriers can cause further disease if ingested by cattle pigs or humans. In these intermediate hosts, the eggs develop to the larval (cysticercus) stage and the disease is termed as cysticercosis. The larval stage of *T. saginata* infects cattle, whereas *T. solium* can infect both pigs and humans. Larvae invade mainly skeletal muscles. *T. solium* larvae frequently invade the central nervous system of humans, and is consequently, a serious public health problem (occurrence of epilepsy).

Epidemiology

Transmission

Animals to human: *T. saginata* and *T. solium* are transmitted to humans through the ingestion of raw or inadequately cooked beef or pork.

Human to animals: Human being can contaminate the environments with large number of tapeworm eggs (2,50,000 to > 5,00,000 eggs per day per individual). Indiscriminate open defecation, use of raw sewage for farming can contaminate grazing fields and farms and animals can acquire infections easily. Taenia eggs can survive for long and can survive many sewage treatment processes.

Human to human: Autoinfection of humans can occur with *T. solium* eggs transmitted directly from anus to mouth or transmission can occur between individuals through contaminated hands or food. Humans most commonly become infected like pigs through ingestion of *T. solium* eggs contaminating the environments (i.e. drinking water contaminated by raw or inadequately treated sewage or eating vegetables fertilized with raw sewage).

Diagnosis: By stool examination, by biopsy and by radiology and serology.

Treatment

Taeniasis

Niclosamide (reported efficacy between 85 and 95%); and praziquantel (95% efficacy with single dose of 10 mg. per kg. body weight) are effective for human taeniasis. Praziquantel has the advantage of minimum side effects and it effectively removes scolex.

Cysticercosis

Praziquantel has been shown to be effective in humans for *T. solium* cysticerci. Previously, the only treatment available was the surgical removal of cysts. Traditional supportive therapy includes anti-seizure and steroid medication and decompression for hydrocephalus.

Prevention and Control

Preventive measures consist of:

i Safe disposal of human excreta by sanitary latrines.
ii Treatment of sewage.
iii Proper cooking of meat.
iv Inspection of pork.
v Treatment of infection.
vi Health education.

TOXOPLASMOSIS

Toxoplasmosis is one of the important parasitic zoonoses.

The causative agent is *Toxoplasma gondii*. It is an obligatory intracellular parasite. The organism exists in different forms such as *tachyzoites* which is a rapidly dividing form (which can cross placenta and infect foetus) and *cyst* form.

The life cycle consists of two phases:

- Asexual stages which occur in intermediate and definitive host,
- Sexual stage, which occurs in definitive host.

Epidemiology and Transmission

Toxoplasma infection is widespread globally:

i Congenital infection in person occurs when mother acquires infection during pregnancy and it is transmitted from mother to foetus through placenta.
ii Postnatally toxoplasmosis infection can be acquired by ingestion of food contaminated by mature oocysts present in soil or from under-cooked meat containing tissue cysts (*Toxoplasma* infection being common in many animals like cattle, sheep, rabbits and pigs used for food). Tachyzoites are usually not infective when ingested as these are destroyed by acid in the stomach.
iii In nature, the infection is maintained by members of the felidae when they prey on infected rodents and other infected animals.

Cats and other members of felidae family are the key animals in the epidemiology of postnatal toxoplasmosis. Oocyst formation is greatest in domestic cats. Cats can pass million of oocysts in their stool sample and oocysts can survive in the moist environment for months and even years. Flies and cockroaches can spread oocysts mechanically.

Clinical Features

Infection may lead to abortions and miscarriage or still-birth or birth of baby with manifestations of acute toxoplasmosis. In the benign form, the disease may manifest in infancy, childhood or even adult life. Infection in first trimester are associated with more severe lesions. Two types of congenital infections have been described. In the generalized form anaemia, jaundice, hepatosplenomegaly, lymphadenitis and retinochoroiditis are common. In the neurological form, the tetrad of hydrocephalus, retinochoroiditis, convulsions and intracranial calcification are well recognized.

Acquired infection in man is less severe and can present with varied clinical picture. Lymphadenopathy is the commonest manifestation and may be accompanied with fever, malaise and rash. It is also a common cause of chorioretinitis. Acute generalized toxoplasmosis with involvement of brain may result, especially in persons undergoing immunosuppressive therapy. As many as 70–80% of patients with AIDS have been diagnosed as having toxoplasmic encephalitis.

Laboratory Diagnosis

It is by isolation of organism and by serum antibody test (qualitative and quantitative tests).

TORCH Test

Toxoplasma, others, rubella, cytomegalovirus and herpes (TORCH). This 'acronym' is used to denote an insult to the foetus caused by varied categories of organisms, resulting in multiple organ damage occurring in the same way and presenting as similar manifestations. Earlier only syphilis was considered to fill in the space of "o" (other infections) now many agents are considered to this slot like varicella, tuberculosis, gonococci, parvo-coxsackie, HIV and hepatitis B virus. This test can detect multiple antibodies against organisms mentioned above and is helpful in diagnosis of specific infection in pregnant women for appropriate action.

Treatment

Sulfonamides and pyrimethamines are two drugs widely used for therapy of toxoplasmosis. These drugs have synergistic effect. Spiramycine is used in pregnant women as it does not cross placental barriers.

Prevention and Control

Since man is infected by toxoplasmosis from tissue cysts in meat, the oocysts in soil and tachyzoites transplacentally. The preventive measures include:

i Proper cooking of meat and observing hygienic practices such as washing hands who handle raw meat.
ii Elimination of stray cats. Cats usually get infected by ingestion of raw meat of wild birds, and rodents. Pet cats food should be regulated. Cats shedding oocysts should be treated.
iii Routine serological check-up in antenatal clinics and treatment of infected mothers would be valuable step in protecting the foetus.

PROGRAMME FOR PREVENTION AND CONTROL OF LEPTOSPIROSIS NATIONAL GUIDELINES 2015

Programme on prevention and control of Leptospiroris has been initiated by Government of India with the following objectives:

i Reduction of morbidity and mortality due to leptospirosis.
ii Strengthening diagnostic laboratories.
iii Strengthening patient care management.
iv Development of trained manpower.
v Creating awareness
vi Sensitization of animal husbandry and agriculture personnel.

Leptospirosis is an *emerging* public health problem. Leptospirosis is a zoonotic bacterial disease caused by *Leptospira interrogans* and Leptospira biflexa and clinically manifested by fever of sudden onset, headache, chills, severe myalgia (calfs and thighs) and conjunctival suffusion. Jaundice and haemorrhagic manifestations are present in typical cases. Deaths are predominantly due to hepatic and renal failure; vascular abnormalities with haemorrhage, acute respiratory distress syndrome, or cardiac arrhythmias from myocarditis.

Epidemiology

Causative organism: Leptospirosis is caused by spirochaete *Leptospira interrogans* which has 23 serotypes and more than 200 serovars. It affects the humans and animals.

Reservoir of Infection

Rodents, several domestic (cattle, swine, sheep, and goat) and wild animals (Foxes and rabbits) form reservoir of infection. They excrete leptospires in urine and may contaminate the environment, viz. water, soil, mud, vege-tation, food and fomites. While domestic animals may act as carriers for several months (temporary carrier), rodents usually remain carriers throughout their life (permanent carriers). Leptospires can survive for prolonged period in the environment.

MODE OF TRANSMISSION

Humans contract the infection by direct exposure to the infected animals or to an environment contaminated with urine, blood or tissue of infected animals. The leptospire is transmitted through inflamed or broken skin, intact mucous membrane (buccal cavity, nose) or conjunctiva. Rare cases of congenital infection have been reported.

Period of Communicability

Direct transmission from person to person is absent or extremely rare. Leptospires may be excreted in the urine usually for months following illness, but it has been observed in humans as long as 11 months. In reservoir species, excretion is lifelong.

Distribution

Leptospirosis occurs worldwide but is most common in tropical and subtropical areas with high rainfall. The disease is found mainly wherever humans come in contact with the urine of infected animals or urine polluted environments. In India the outbreaks of leptospirosis have been reported from coastal dustricts of Gujarat, Maharashtra, Kerala, Tamil Nadu, Andhra Pardesh, Karnataka, and Andamans, Goa and Odisha from time to time (NICD and WHO in 2006 and 2015).

Incidence

Precise incidence is not known. According to currently available reports, incidence ranges from approximately 0.1 to 1 per 1,00,000 in humid tropics. During outbreaks, the incidence may reach over 100 per 1,00,000.[1] Data of recent outbreaks investigated by NICD are presented in Table 12.44.

Table 12.44: Recent outbreaks, reported cases, and deaths in Gujarat due to leptospirosis

Year	*No. of cases*	*Deaths*	*CFR%*
1994	158	12	7.6
1995	14	2	14.3
1996	40	9	22.5
1997	657	76	11.6
1998	537	42	7.8
1999	365	31	8.5
2000	112	12	10.7
2011	600	104	17.0

Source: NICD CD Alert 2000

High-risk Groups

Leptospirosis is considered primarily an occupational disease. For example, agriculture, dairy, fish farming, forestry boating, mining, military exercises, working in slaughter house, sewers, laboratories and handling animals increase the risk of infections to leptospires.

Following rains and flood, the incidence increases, moist conditions favour it most besides water logging and salinity.

Incubation period: It ranges from 4 to 19 days.

Age: Most of the cases occur in adults (20–30 years) due to exposure of adults to contaminated materials. Adult males are more exposed than females.

Clinical Manifestation—Two Types of Leptospirosis:

a. **Anicteric Leptospirosis:** While most of the infections (90%) remain subclinical and anicteric, mild or moderate which are not easily recognized as leptospirosis. These patients have fever, headache conjunctival suffusion, myalgia but no jaundice.

b. Icteric Leptospirosis: Illness may be very severe and fatal in some of the cases (5–10%).

The disease has a sudden onset with fever, headache, conjunctival suffusion and myalgia, especially in calf muscles; severe manifestations include hepatic involvement (Jaundice, hepatic failure), renal involvement (oliguria, renal failure), pulmonary involvement (cough, chest pain, breathlessness, haemoptysis), cardiac involvement (myocarditis), meningitis, encephalitis and haemorrhagic manifestations. The more severe form of disease with severe liver and kidney involvement is known as **Weil's syndrome**.

Mortality

Mortality is high (>20%) unless the treatment (antibiotics, penicillin, tetracycline) is started early. Infecting serovars, animal species involved, and general condition of the host determine the severity of illness. The disease is more severe in old and immunocompromised or those having pre-existing liver and kidney problems. More than 90% of deaths are due to pulmonary alveolar haemorrhages.

Diagnosis

Clinical diagnosis is not easy except during the outbreaks. A high degree of suspicion and use of laboratory is essential to diagnose the disease. The typical motility of leptospires in the clinical sample under the dark ground illumination in a clinical compatible case may be helpful for an experienced laboratory person. Diagnosis is confirmed by:

1 Seroconversion or a fourfold or greater rise in titre in paired serum samples in the presence of compatible clinical illness is a major criteria for definitive diagnosis of recent leptospirosis infection.

2 Microscopic agglutination test (MAT) is considered the gold standard or cornerstone of serodiagnosis because of unsurpassed diagnostic specificity in comparison with other currently available tests.[1]

3 Isolation of organism from blood or CSF during the first week of illness and from the urine after the 10th day of illness.

Prevention and Control

Prevalence of leptospires infection in rodents and animals (carriers) and favourable environments make the control of leptospirosis most difficult. Following measures are helpful.[3–7]

1 ***Health education and personal protection:*** The main preventive measure is to create awareness about leptospirosis and its prevention through mass media and inter-personal communication and print material. Hygienic measures such as avoidance of direct and indirect human contact with animal urine, and contaminated water.

2 ***Personal protective measures:*** Protective clothing, boots, gloves and aprons for all people involved in high-risk activities are advisable. Apply betadine ointment on cuts and abrasions before entering fields and affter exit.

3 ***Chemoprophylaxis:*** Doxycycline has been shown to be effective in preventing leptospirosis in exposed personnel when administered 200 mg orally once a week for 6 weeks during the period of high exposure. However, prolonged and mass chemoprophylaxis is not recommended.

4 ***Rodent control:*** Rodents are major reservoir of infection. Rattus rattus (House Rat), Rattus norvegicus (Norway rat) lesser bandicoot and larger bandicoot are reservoirs in India. Rodents are important from both the economic and public health point of view. Denying access to food by proper disposal of garbage and storage of food in rat proof containers and buildings is the most effective way to remove the rodents from the domestic environments.

Trapping and administration of acute and chronic poisons may be useful in some settings. Experts from department of agriculture and animal husbandry should be fully involved to control rodents.

5 ***Control of environment:*** Mapping of water bodies for proper drainage system. Recognize potentially contaminated water and soil and drain such water if possible on regular basis.[6]

6 ***Case management:*** Treatment of cases and supportive therapy with appropriate antibiotic-like—Doxycycline 100 mg twice a day for 7 days, pregnant women and lactating mothers should be given capsule ampicillin 50 mg every 6 hours. Children less than 8 years—30–50 mg per kg per day for 7 days.

7 ***Surveillance:*** A well-established laboratory-based surveillance system supplemented by sero-survey in men and animals to understand the epidemiology of leptospirosis should be in place.

8 ***Vaccination:*** A safe human vaccine, which is effective in field situation for wider use is not available at present. However, immunization of people has been carried out against occupational exposure to specific serovars in Japan, China, Italy, Spain and France, etc. Immunization of farm and pet animals prevents illness but not necessarily infection and renal shedding.

ANTHRAX

Anthrax is an acute infectious disease of herbivorus animals caused by *Bacillus anthracis*. Anthrax is also called malignant pustule, malignant oedema, woolsorter's disease, or Ragpicker's disease. The main source of human infection is direct or indirect contact with an infected animal or contaminated animal product. It is a zoonotic disease.

The causative organism (*Bacillus anthracis*) is a Gram-positive encapsulated, non-motile rod. The organism rapidly grows in sheep blood agar aerobically and is non-haemolytic under these conditions.

Spread

The disease spreads among grazing animals through contaminated soil, feed, and among carnivorous animals through contaminated meat, bone meal and other feeds and in wildlife from feeding on carcasses of animal died of anthrax. Outbreaks of anthrax have been reported from Karnataka (1999 and 2001), Odisha (2003 and 2005 and West Bengal (2000). Human anthrax outbreaks during 2008 were reported from Odisha, Andhra Pradesh and West Bengal (WHO, SEARO).

The spores are resistant to adverse environmental conditions and disinfection, and can remain viable in the contaminated soil for many years.

Mortality

The mortality rate of untreated cutaneous anthrax may be 20% pulmonary and intestinal anthrax results in death in 25 to 60% of cases.

Types of Anthrax[8, 9]

Cutaneous, intestinal, and pulmonary anthrax can occur in human beings.

Cutaneous Anthrax

Cutaneous anthrax occurs when the bacteria enter a cut or abrasion on skin while handling infected animals or their contaminated products such as wool, hides, leather or hair. The incubation period for cutaneous anthrax is usually 1–7 days. The lesion which is on the exposed parts of the body such as face, neck and arms, is first noted as small pruritic papule that resemble an insect bite. Within 1–2 days, it develops into a vesicle.

Occasionally, the papule becomes surrounded by a ring of vesicles, which then coalesce to form a large vesicle around 2–3 cm in diameter. Approximately 5–7 days after the onset, the vesicle ruptures, revealing a painless ulcer with a characteristic black necrotic area in the centre. Effective therapy reduces oedema and systemic symptoms but does not change the evolution of skin lesion.

Occasionally, more severe form of cutaneous anthrax may occur with extensive local oedema, induration and toxaemia. The infection may also spread to bloodstream with overwhelming septicaemia.

Intestinal Anthrax

The intestinal anthrax is characterized by nausea, loss of appetite, vomiting, fever, abdominal pain, vomiting of blood and severe diarrhoea. In severe forms, general toxaemia with shock, sepsis and death may develop. Gastrointestinal anthrax is difficult to diagnose, as the symptoms are nonspecific. However, history of ingesting meat of a sick-animal and cases of cutaneous anthrax in the area may support diagnosis.

Pulmonary Anthrax

The initial symptoms of pulmonary anthrax resemble a common cold, which quickly progresses to severe breathing problems and shock. Diagnosis is difficult but pulmonary anthrax should be suspected if there is history of exposure to aerosol that contains *B. anthracis*. Respiratory secretions may contain the bacilli but these are not present in the sputum.

Antibiotics are effective if the disease is recognized early and the full-recommended dose and course of antibiotic is completed. Death can occur if the antibiotic therapy is discontinued early. Penicillin, erythromycin, tetracycline, chloramphenicol, amoxycillin can be used as oral antibiotics, can be prescribed for mild forms of cutaneous anthrax, for severe cutaneous as well as pulmonary and gastrointestinal anthrax intravenous antibiotics in large doses are necessary.

Laboratory Confirmation

Laboratory confirmation is made by the demonstration of *B. anthracis* from blood, vesicular fluid, cerebrospinal fluid, pleural fluid and peritoneal fluid by direct polychrome methylene blue stained smears or by culture or inoculation of mice, guinea pigs or rabbits. Diagnosis can be confirmed by PCR. NICD must be notified immediately if anthrax is suspected.

Anthrax does not spread from person to person but discharges from lesions and other soiled articles from patients should be disinfected and incinerated. Hypochlorite is sporicidal but other disinfectants can also be used. Spores require steam sterilization, autoclaving or burning to assure complete destruction. The principal disinfecting agents for destruction of anthrax spores are formaldehyde, glutaldehyde (At pH 8.0–8.5), hydrogen peroxide and peracetic acid.

Prevention: If anthrax is suspected in animals the carcass should be immediately buried deep at site if possible, after covering it with anhydrous calcium oxide (quick lime).

Anthrax is important and exploited for *biological warfares* (Bioterrorism) because it is highly fatal and when transmitted through inhalation is almost always fatal. Anthrax spores can remain viable for several decades and it is easy to weaponize and disseminate anthrax as an odourless and invisible aerosol.

REFERENCES

1 NCDC—Programme for prevention and control of Leptospirosis-national guidelines diagnosis, case management and control of Leptospirosis—2015.

2 WHO. Human Leptospirosis. Guidelines for diagnosis surveillance and control. World Health Organization and International Leptospirosis Society 2003.
3 NICD. Leptospirosis gradually spreading to new areas. CD Alert. Monthly Newsletter on Communicable Diseases Nov. 1997; 1(4).
4 Singhal RL, Sood DP. Leptospirosis: Proceedings of the 3rd Round table conference; 1998 Feb. 23; New Delhi Ranbaxy Science Foundation.
5 NICD. Leptospirosis: An emerging public health problem in India. CD Alert. Monthly Newsletter on Communicable Diseases June 2000; 4(6).
6 NICD and WHO (2006). Guidelines for prevention and control of leptospirosis Zoonosis division, NICD (DGHS), 22 Shamnath Marg, Delhi.
7 GOI. Annual Report 2008–09, MOH and FW, Government of India, New Delhi.
8 NICD. Anthrax. CD Alert. Monthly Newsletter on Communicable Diseases Sept 1999; 3(3).
9 NICD and WHO (2006). Guidelines for prevention and control of anthrax, Zoonosis division, NICD (DGHS), 22 Shamnath Marg, Delhi.

Q-FEVER

The causative organism is *Coxiella burnetii*.

Q-fever has been reported from all countries except America.

Mode of Transmission

C. burnetii organisms are generally transmitted when the host inhales infectious aerosols. They enter the host's cells by passive phagocytosis, preferentially infecting histocytes and Kupffer cells.

C. burnetii is carried by many species of tick and although ticks may serve as vector between animals, they probably do not transmit the disease to humans. Humans are usually infected when they inhale aerosols generated by infected live-stocks. Infection occurs most frequently in abattoirs, sheep research facilities, dairies and animal husbandry operations.

Incubation Period

It is 18–21 days.

Symptom and Signs

Most common signs and symptoms are fever, headache, chills, myalgia, skin rashes hepatomegaly and hepatitis.

Laboratory Diagnosis

12

Weil-Felix test is helpful in establishing presumptive diagnosis. Sera of Q-fever fail to agglutinate 0X19, 0X2 and 0XK.

Prevention

Most outbreaks of Q fever in various countries were associated with work-related exposure to sheep and their birth products. Therefore, preventive measures should be directed primarily at:

1 Avoiding exposure in institutions where sheeps are used for research.
2 Educating personnel in agriculture setting about disinfection and disposal of products of conception.
3 Vaccine made from killed organisms provides complete protection to high-risk individuals whose occupation expose them to infected sheep.

Treatment

Effective therapy with tetracycline and chloramphenicol shorten the duration and lessen the severity of the illness.

MAD COW DISEASE AND CREUTZFELDT-JAKOB DISEASE (CJD)[1]

Creutzfeldt-Jakob disease (CJD) is known to affect human beings since 1920s, it caught great public health attention in 1990s when a new variant of CJD (vCJD) emerged in Britain which was etiologically linked to bovine spongiform encephalopathy (BSE), popularly known as mad cow disease. Due to widespread use of cattle and cattle products and their import, the risk of vCJD exists in all parts of the world.

Transmissible Spongiform Encephalopathies (TSEs)

These are group of fatal neurodegenerative disorders which affect humans and certain animal species and produce characteristic neuropathological spongiform changes and deposition of amyloid protein (prion protein) in the grey matter of the brain. The exact nature of aetiological agent is not clear. Most scientists agree that it is self-replicating protein called prion protein and some think agent is virus like.

Creutzfeldt-Jakob Disease (CJD)

The CJD is first human TSE described in early 20s by HG Creutzfeldt and AM Jakob. CJD is a rare and fatal neurodegenerative disease with rapidly progressive dementia, myoclonus and characteristic EEG pattern. It occurs in sporadic, familial and iatrogenic CJD. A new variant of CJD has been described in 1996. The median duration of illness is 4.5 months.

New Variant CJD (vCJD)

A new variant Creutzfeldt-Jakob (vCJD) has been described in the UK and other parts of Europe. The first case was reported in UK in March 1996. Till June 2001, 105 cases of vCJD have been reported. vCJD has been strongly linked to exposure, probably through food, to the BSE.

The fact that the France imported large amount of cattle products from UK perhaps explains the occurrence of cases in that country. In contrast to CJD, vCJD occurs in younger people (average age 29 years vs. 65 years).

CJD in India: A total of 78 cases of CJD have been reported in India from 1968 to 2000.

Bovine Spongiform Encephalopathy (BSE)

BSE is transmissible neurodegenerative and fatal disease of cattle. It is also called as mad cow disease. First case was reported in UK in 1986 and first case outside UK was reported in 1989. A total of 1,80,937 cases of BSE have been reported from UK till 2000. Most cases outside the UK have been reported from countries namely—Portugal, France, Ireland, Germany, Spain, Switzerland and Belgium. Although the original source of BSE agent is not clear, there is strong evidence that the outbreak was amplified by feeding rendered (cooked) bovine meat and bone meal to young calves in UK. There is strong epidemiological and laboratory evidence for a causal association between BSE and vCJD. BSE can be prevented by preventing the use of ruminant tissues in ruminant feed, and by preventing the entry of products of any animal showing signs of TSE into human or animal food chain.

Prevention and Control of CJD and vCJD

- A well-established surveillance system for CJD, vCJD and BSE.
- Ban on import of cattle and cattle products from BSE endemic countries.
- No part of product of any animal which has shown signs of a TSE should enter human or animal food chain.
- Avoid using, tissues, needle electrodes and surgical instruments contaminated by tissues from suspected cases.
- Steam autoclaving (1 hour at 132°C or higher) is highly effective method for disinfection. Chemical agents such as 5% sodium hypochlorite and 1N to 2N sodium hydroxide may not be completely effective. After 1 hour, they are best followed by steam autoclaving. Aldehydes are ineffective.

REFERENCE

1 NICD. Mad Cow Disease and Creutzfeldt-Jakob Disease—Proceedings of an expert group meeting. Monthly Newsletter of NICD, DGHS, Govt. of India Dec. 2001–Jan 2002, Vol 5 No. 12, Vol 6 No. 1.

EPIDEMIOLOGY OF VACCINE PREVENTABLE DISEASES

MEASLES

It is an acute highly contagious viral disease caused by the measles virus.

Measles is such a common communicable disease in India that many communities have accepted it as a normal milestone of growing up.

Occurrence

It is endemic in densely populated areas while periodic outbreaks occur in less populated areas.

Incidence

The WHO estimated that over 40 million cases still occur worldwide each year contributing to approximately 5,30,000 deaths including 1,82,000 in the South East Asia region as reported in 2003. Now measles mortality has been reduced from 7,33,000 in 2000 to 1,64,000 in 2008 (78% reduction). Epidemics occur often every 2 to 3 years and usually last between 2 and 3 months. Many cases of measles are not reported to health institutions. People keep cases confined to their homes and observe varied kind of practices, worshipping Gods and Goddesses. As a result, the incidence and complications that arise due to measles are not known precisely. It was estimated in 1989–90 that in India, every year there were some 20 million cases of measles. Over the years, the reported cases primarily from hospitals, the incidence has declined substantially due to improved coverage of measles immunization.[1–3]

Since the median age of measles infection is around 24 months of age, it is important that children receive measles vaccine at 9 months of age or as soon as possible thereafter and are immunized before they are exposed to the risk of infection. Coverage with measles vaccine has increased from 1.3% in 1985 to 74% in 2009 (coverage evaluation survey 2009–10). The rapid increase in measles immunization coverage levels have saved many lives. However, each year about 15% of the 26 million infants or 3.90 million children remain unimmunized and are potentially at risk of measles infection.

As a result of measles vaccination programme, the reported incidence of measles has declined substantially, as is evident from the reported figures in Table 12.45, however, report tends to be incomplete. Further coverage of measles vaccination is variable in the country.

In India, more than 50% of measles cases are currently reported in children less than five years of age indicating low coverage of measles immunization.

Case Fatality

In spite of case fatality ratio of 1–2% (median case fatality ratio 1.63%), a minimum of 2 lakh, and more likely 5 lakh measles associated deaths occur each year in India.[4] Innumerable children suffer other infections like diarrhoea, acute respiratory infections, malnutrition and vitamin A deficiency as a result of measles. Case fatality is much more in malnourished children. Measles is one of the leading killers in young children.

WHO-UNICEF estimate indicates 1,50,000 measles deaths in India during the year 2006.

Table 12.45: Trends in reported cases of measles

Year	Reported number of cases
1987	2,52,940
1985–1989 annual	1,79,000 average
2000	38,835
1990–93	80,766
2001	51,780
2002	38,927
2003	46,736
2004	51,546
2005	36,711
2007	41,144
2008	48,181
2009	56,188
2010	29,808
2011	33,634
2013	16,479
2014 (P)	23,348

Source: Central Bureau of Health Intelligence (CBHI)

Age of Occurrence

The highest number of cases are observed among children under 2 years of age in the developing countries like India and at school entry in the more affluent countries with the greatest risk of complications and deaths occurring in infants. 90% of cases occur below 10 years of age.[4]

Transmission

Transmission is from person to person by droplet spread from nasal or pharyngeal secretions. Measles is one of the most contagious disease and highly infectious. Cases are infectious even before appearance of rash and up to 7 days after.

Incubation Period

The incubation period is between 7 and 18 days, usually 14 days. Measles is highly infectious and rarely will an unimmunized child escape from getting disease.

Symptoms

Measles is nearly always symptomatic. Diagnosis of measles is easy. The main characteristic features would be a cold, cough, running nose, fever 38°C or more. Eyes are pink or red watery and sensitive to light for 3–7 days followed by generalized rash—a characteristic blotchy rash appears beginning on the face and spreading all over the body, the rash lasts for 4–7 days and often ends with desquamation (peeling of skin). The pigmentation due to rash remains for 2 weeks or even longer. Koplik's spots (greyish white spots with red borders) often appear on the inside of the cheek at about the same time the rash begins. These spots are diagnostic since they occur only in measles.

Post-measles Complications

Measles complications include diarrhoea, pneumonia, otitis media, malnutrition including acute deficiency of vitamin A, which may lead to keratomalacia and blindness. Therefore, measles cases should be given megadose of vitamin A solution as per age (Table 12.46).[5] Occasionally, it may lead to encephalitis. Death strikes the malnourished especially where multiple cases crowd the home. In India, 2 to 3% children die generally following measles but in a measles epidemic, case fatality as high as 30 to 50% is reported. Delayed complications include high-risk of morbidity and mortality.

Table 12.46: Recommended vitamin A schedule for measles cases

Age	Immediately on diagnosis of cases	Next day
< 6 months	50000 1U	50000 1U
6–12 months	100000 1U	100000 1U
12 months plus up to 5 years	200000 1U	200000 1U

Risk Factors

- Measles virus is transmitted through the air by respiratory droplets from infected children even before the rash is seen. Therefore, isolation of a case has no relevance in the control of disease.
- Measles is more rapidly transmitted in large families, crowded homes and urban slums.
- With high density of population, measles is apt to occur year round sometimes with seasonal peaks.
- Without immunization, nearly every child gets measles.
- Measles can occur at any age. In India due to overcrowding and increased contact among young children, effects are mostly seen before the second birthday of the child.
- Secondary cases in home tend to be more severe.
- Measles is severe among infants and malnourished children. Post-measles complications are also more common in these children.

Prevention

Natural disease gives permanent immunity. Infants born of mothers who have had the disease are usually immune for approximately the first 6–8 months. Prevention is by appropriate immunization.

Prevention by Immunization

Being a viral disease measles cannot be cured by antibiotics and therefore prevention is more important. Measles prevention should be priority. Preventing measles by immunization will have the multiple benefits of preventing other diseases, particularly diarrhoea, dysentery, malnutrition, blindness, pneumonia and acute respiratory infections.

Measles Vaccine

It is attenuated live measles virus vaccine. The vaccine stability has improved. Freezed dried live attenuated measles vaccine is available, which can be reconstituted by adding 2.5 ml of diluent. The vaccine is administered by subcutaneous injection in one dose of 0.5 ml at 9 months of age. If the child misses at this age ensure it at 10–12 months of age, i.e. before infancy or first birthday. Unimmunized children beyond age one and up to 5 years can also be given immunization. WHO currently recommend that two doses of measles vaccine should be the standard for all national immunization programmes. As of 2008, 192 of 193 member states of WHO use two doses of measles vaccine in their national immunization programme, India being the only exception.

There are two considerations when determining the minimal age to administer measles vaccine: age distribution of cases and deaths and the immunological response (maternal antibody interference). In India, where disease is common, the vaccine should be given at 9 months of age.

Immunization Strategy for India

- In India, measles vaccine is given through routine immunization—first dose at completed 9–12 months and second dose at 16–24 months of age. In case the child misses this opportunity, the child can be vaccinated at the first available opportunity up to 5 years of age.

Peak response of seroconversion occurs 6–8 weeks after vaccination. Seroconversion rate of measles vaccine varies from 85 to 95%. Outbreaks are generally due to accumulation of measles susceptible persons, including both unvaccinated children and those who were vaccinated but failed to seroconvert. Approximately 15% of children vaccinated at 9 months and 5–10% of those vaccinated at 12 months of age are not protected after vaccination. Previous coverage evaluation surveys have shown that mean national coverage with measles is around 74% with 85% vaccine effectiveness for vaccination at 9 months actual protection was offered to only 63% of annual birth cohorts (74% × 85% = 63%). In other words, 37% remained susceptible to measles. Accordingly, second opportunity for measles immunization is required in order to protect those children who have never been vaccinated as well as those who were vaccinated but did not develop immunity. Immunity conferred by measles vaccine has been shown to persist to at least 20 years and generally thought to be lifelong for most individuals.

Measles Vaccination during Epidemics/Outbreaks

There is no role of measles outbreak response immunization to stop the spread of measles during outbreaks. If children receive vaccine within 72 hours after exposure they may be protected but it is difficult to ensure. In India, mass measles vaccination during epidemics has not been considered useful.

Vaccine Efficacy[6]

The term "vaccine efficacy" refers to the ability of a vaccine to prevent disease when used in routine immunization services.

Efficacy of vaccine is an excellent indicator of the effectiveness of the immunization services.

For example, efficacy of measles vaccine is 85%. If immunization services with measles vaccine shows efficacy of less than 80%, it means there is a problem with the vaccine. This could be due to problem with the cold chain, the injection technique or the age at which the workers are immunizing the children and you should take action to correct it.

To calculate vaccine efficiency you will need to obtain following information from the health records:

$$\text{Attack rate in immunized children} = \frac{\text{Number of cases in immunized children 12–23 months of age}}{\text{Number of immunized children 12–23 months of age}} \times 100$$

$$\text{Attack rate in unimmunized children} = \frac{\text{No. of cases in unimmunized children 12–23 months of age}}{\text{No. of unimmunized children 12–23 months of age}} \times 100$$

$$\text{Efficacy of vaccine} = \frac{\text{Attack rate in unimmunized (–) Attack rate in immunized}}{\text{Attack rate in unimmunized}} \times 100$$

i Size of study population (which is children 12–23 months of age).
ii The coverage of measles vaccine in children 12–23 months of age.
iii The number of cases of measles in immunized children 12–23 months of age.
iv The number of cases of measles in unimmunized children 12–23 months of age.

Efficacy

The vaccine is usually 85% effective if administered at appropriate age and provides long-lasting immunity.[6]

Side Effects

A mild fever and rash lasting 1–3 days may occur in up to 15% of vaccinees, 8 to 12 days after vaccination. Encephalitis has been reported following measles vaccination approximately at the rate of one case per million doses administered.

Storage

Exposure of the vaccine to high temperature and light before or after dilution may inactivate it. Long-term storage should preferably be at –15° to –25°C. Short-term storage should be maintained at 2° to 8°C. The freezed dried vaccine is stable for 1 to 4 weeks at room temperature. To avoid inactivating, the vaccine with hot diluent, the diluent should also be refrigerated at 2° to 8°C. After dilution, the vaccine must be kept at these temperatures and used within 4 hours. Discard the opened vials and left over vaccine after the session and never store or use the opened vials for vaccination in the next session or next day, as it leads to contamination of vaccine.

Toxic Shock Syndrome

If the left over vaccine is stored in the refrigerator or cold box, it may be contaminated with bacteria. Toxic shock syndrome (TSS) results following the administration of contaminated measles vaccine due to the use of unsterile syringes and needles used to draw the vaccine from the vial or reuse of measles vaccine vial for more than one session on the same or subsequent days. TSS occurs when the vial is contaminated with *Staphylococcus aureus*.

The symptoms of TSS are typical. Severe watery diarrhoea, vomiting and high fever are reported within a few hours of measles vaccine administration. There are usually more than one case as all children vaccinated from the contaminated vial will be affected. The disease progresses to hypotensive shock and death within 48 hours. Case fatality rates are high.

TSS is an emergency and no time should be lost in taking the child to district hospital, which can look after the severely ill children and provide supportive care.

If a child is brought first to PHC give ORS/home available fluids give broad-spectrum antibiotics, IV fluids, anti-pyretics, steroids and supportive therapy.

Coverage Levels

Coverage levels in the states and districts of the country are variable. The current coverage level of measles immunization is 74% (CES–2009). Out of 27 million infants in the year 2006, around 11.3 million infants were not fully immunized in the country.[7] Unimmunized infants stand to the risk of getting measles and its complications.

Future Measures

Measles is next candidate fit for *eradication*. After polio eradication, measles eradication would be taken up. UNICEF in India has started urban project on measles immunization covering all children between 9 months and 5 years of age.

12

MEASLES MORTALITY REDUCTION—INDIA'S MULTI-YEAR-STRATEGIC PLAN 2010–2017

Goals and Objectives

1. Reduce 90% measles mortality by 2013 when compared to 2000 estimates.
2. Achieving at least 90% coverage with measles vaccine.
3. Collection of good quality epidemiological data through active surveillance—integrated disease surveillance programme (IDSP) and outbreak investigation and to use this information to guide further action.
4. **Elimination** of measles by 2020 in India

Key Strategies for Measles Mortality Reduction

- ***Strengthening of routine immunization:*** Achieving and maintaining high coverage (>90%) with first dose of measles vaccination in *every district*. Achieve high routine measles vaccination coverage of infants at 9–12 months of age, provide measles vaccine to children who missed routine immunization during infancy at the earliest contact until they are five years old.
- ***Surveillance of measles:*** Establish effective measles surveillance that provides information about number of cases and deaths by month, age and vaccination status of cases and deaths and conduct outbreak investigation supported by laboratory confirmation. The surveillance system for identification of measles outbreaks can be linked to AFP surveillance system.
- ***Case management:*** Improving management of measles cases, including vitamin A supplementation and adequate treatment of cases by integrated management of neonatal and childhood illness (IMNCI) strategy.
- ***Second opportunity:*** Based on evaluated measles immunization coverage and surveillance data, providing a second opportunity for measles immunization to appropriate age group of children either through a second routine dose of measles vaccine or through supplementary immunization activities (SIA).

Government of India has introduced a second dose of measles vaccine in the national immunization programme per below state specific strategies.

Measles Catch up Campaigns

India has conducted measles catch up campaigns: (A one time event targeting multiple cohorts in which susceptible children have accumulated) as part of global effort to reduce measles mortality and morbidity. Target group for this campaign was *9 months* to <*10 year* children irrespective of their previous measles vaccination status or measles infection. Estimated 134 million children were immunized in 14 states where coverage level of measles immunization was less than 80%. Viz. Arunachal, Assam, Bihar, Tripura, Chhattisgarh, Gujarat, Haryana, Jharkhand, Odisha, MP, Manipur, Meghalaya, Rajasthan and UP are being covered through Supplementary Immunization Activity (SIA). Measles catch up campaigns are a one time activity and therefore coverage must be near 100% in the target age group to impact on disease transmission.

Measles follow-up campaign: A periodic event (every 3–5 years according to the accumulation of susceptibles) targeting children born after catch up campaign to maintain low level of susceptibility. The periodicity depends upon routine immunization coverage. The target age group for immunization in these campaign should include all children aged over 9 months who were born after the previous mass immunization.

Measles Containing Vaccine (MCV)

MCV2 delivery strategies for 17 states with sustained high MCV1 coverage (> = 80%): Both measles – rubella (MR) and mumps–measles–rubella (MMR) vaccines should be considered through routine immunization schedule for children between 16 and 24 months of age. Four states/ UTs have already introduced second dose (as MMR) for 1–2 years old children. Based on cost considerations, the ministry will take a final decision on the vaccine to be introduced through Universal Immunization Programme (UIP) in these states. Government of India has now introduced second dose of measles across the country in 2011.

Surveillance

The surveillance of Vaccine Preventable diseases (VPD) including measles will be strengthened. The epidemiological data thus collected will be reviewed for effective and rapid response to improve the programme. From 2006 to 2007 the Government of India has initiated an outbreak based laboratory supported measles rubella surveillance in six states (AP, Karnataka, Kerala, Gujarat, Tamil Nadu and West Bengal). The system is built on sensitive AFP surveillance system already in place in India since 1997. This provides essential information needed to define the basic epidemiology of measles in India. As measles cases often do not report to the hospital, active involvement of clinicians and public health practitioners in case reporting is critical to the success of surveillance system in identifying measles outbreaks.[8,9] Reporting units include government or private health facilities which are engaged in treating a large number of patients below 15 years. Around 10,000 reporting units and 15,000 informer units set up under the AFP surveillance network will be used for measles surveillance as well.

For operational purposes, presence of measles outbreak should be verified if five or more than five clinically diagnosed cases of measles are identified in a block in a weak, or five or more than five clinically diagnosed cases of measles occur in an area bordering several blocks in a weak; or one or more than one death due to clinically diagnosed measles occurs in a block in a weak.

In 2008, 153 suspected measles outbreaks were investigated across six states. Of these, 93 were caused by measles virus, 23 by rubella virus, 26 were due to both measles and rubella virus, 11 were negative for either virus and 14 were pending classification. For the same year, 84% of measles cases from laboratory confirmed outbreaks were less than 10 years old.

Initiative of measles elimination and control was undertaken from 1998 to 2002 by UNICEF in urban areas by giving one additional dose of measles vaccine to all children between 9 months and 5 years regardless of prior vaccination status in campaign mode.

Global Measles Eradication Initiative

This initiative has been supported by WHO, UNICEF and American Red Cross by adopting following strategies:

1. Catch up campaigns: To cover susceptible children with second dose of measles vaccine to achieve high coverage level of 90% or more with meticulous planning.
2. Follow-up campaign after 2–4 years in the areas covered by catch up campaign to cover susceptible cohort.

Proportion of one year old immunized against measles has been used as an indicator to reduce child mortality.

RUBELLA

Most clinicians regarded it as milder form of measles and hence it was also known as German measles.

Causative organism: Rubella virus belongs to genus *Rubella* virus and family Togaviridae. Rubella virus is an RNA virus. Rubella occurs in two forms:

- Acquired rubella, and
- Congenital rubella syndrome (CRS).

Acquired Rubella

It is widely distributed worldwide. The reservoir of infection is a case of rubella (clinical and subclinical cases) and there is no carrier stage. Majority of infections are asymptomatic. After an incubation period of 2–3 weeks the clinical symptoms/signs develop which include; coryza, sore throat, low grade fever and rash and lymphadenopathy. Acquired rubella is a mild disease and seldom leads to complications and encephalitis is very rare. Rubella virus has been suggested to be possible cause of chronic inflammatory joint disease. Natural infection is followed by a very high order of protection from reinfection.

Age

It is mainly a disease of children. Common age group affected is 3–10 years. Because of widespread vaccination programme in developed countries there is shift in age of occurrence beyond childhood period.

Transmission

It is a droplet infection, transmitted from person to person through droplets by coughing and sneezing.

Congenital Rubella Syndrome (CRS)

Rubella infection during pregnancy can lead to congenital malformation of foetus and child may be born with several congenital malformations; premature birth and low birth weights or even abortions. Infection during first trimester is more dangerous. The clinical features of congenital rubella include microcephaly, retinopathy, cataract, deafness, ductus arteriosus, ventricular septal defect, cryptorchidism, inguinal hernia, diabetes mellitus, hepatosplenomegaly, congenital cardiopathies, etc. These defects occur either as singly or multiple and the condition is described as "congenital rubella syndrome" (CRS). The exact incidence is not known. It is estimated that 2 lakh babies are born with CRS each year in India.

Prevention: Introduction of Rubella Vaccine

Rubella can be prevented by vaccination against rubella. MMR (measles, mumps and rubella) vaccine is effective to prevent rubella and congenital rubella infection.

Women during child bearing age (pre-pregnancy period) can be protected against rubella by MMR vaccine. Vaccination during pregnancy is contraindicated. MMR routine child immunization is a preferred strategy. Before introducing MMR in India, we need reasonably reliable data on the presence of CRS in different parts of the country and on mumps and its sequelae. In addition, it needs to be demonstrated that MMR given at 9 months of age will have efficacy equal to the dose given at 12–15 months.

The **Rubella vaccine** in proposed to be introduced in the UIP in India in 2016, as measles rubella campaign targeting 9 months to 15 years age group.

MUMPS

Mumps virus belongs to family Paramyxoviridae. It is acute contagious disease of children and young adults. The reservoir of infection is always a case (clinical or sub-clinical). It spreads by droplet infection. The usual incubation period is 16–18 days. After entering the host, the virus multiplies and viraemia results.

The virus has affinity with several organs and it settles and multiplies in salivary glands especially parotid glands, testis, pancreas, ovaries, thyroid and meninges.

Age Group

It affects primarily children between 5 and 10 years age group. Approximately 85% of infections occur below 15 years of age. In developed countries because of massive MMR vaccination, the infection rate among 10–14 years and above has increased (shift in age of infection due to vaccination).

Clinical Features

It mainly affects salivary glands (parotid, submaxillary and sublingual glands). Bilateral painful swelling of parotid gland along with fever is common. The illness usually subsides after about 10 days time. The mortality rates are insignificant. Most infections subside. The mumps may lead to complications like orchitis, atrophy of affected testicle, sterility, oophoritis, pancreatitis, arthritis, myocarditis and renal dysfunction. Infection during pregnancy in first trimester may cause abortion. Most of the complications are not serious and precise incidence remain unknown.

The incidence of mumps and its complications is precisely not known in India. The mortality effects are probably more if mumps occur beyond 40 years of age. One attack confers lifelong immunity in 95% of individuals. Secondary attack rate in mumps is very high.

Prevention

Mumps can be prevented by MMR vaccine. The vaccine is prepared from Jery Lynn strain or from Leiningard or Urabe or Rubini strain. The efficacy of vaccine is very high, 93–97%.

CHICKENPOX (VARICELLA)

Chickenpox is a communicable disease caused by Varicella-zoster virus which is also responsible for herpes zoster. It is transmitted from person to person by direct contact through droplet infection. The disease is highly contagious with high secondary attack rate of over 90%.

Incubation period: Ranges from 10 to 21 days.

Epidemiology

Who get affected? It affects almost everyone. Children below 10 years of age are more susceptible. Crowded localities are most affected. Rashes appear on the first day of fever. The leisons occur in crops. Distribution of rash is centripetal. A single attack confers lifelong immunity. 31600 cases and 63 deaths were reported in India during 2013 and 34447 cases and 57 deats in 2014.

Prevention

Live attenuated *varicella vaccine* is available. It is indicated against varicella in healthy subjects. From age 12 months to 12 years, a single dose of 0.5 ml by subcutaneous route, from 13 years and above, 2 doses with an interval of 6–10 weeks are given.

It is contraindicated in pregnant women. Varicella vaccine has not been introduced into the national immunization programme in India. The vaccine is very expensive but it is safe and effective. We need more epidemiological data on case fatality and complications and sequelae due to varicella in India.

PERTUSSIS (WHOOPING COUGH)

It is an acute disease involving tracheobronchial tract. The disease is caused by bacterium *Bordetella pertussis*. Seasonal incidence does not have a consistent pattern in tropical climates.

Case Fatality Rate

CFR is approximately 1–3% in children under one year of age but may be higher in some areas. Mortality is especially high in infants under 6 months of age.[10,11]

Transmission

It spreads primarily by droplet infection. Source of infection is a case of whooping cough. It is highly contagious during the early catarrhal stage, becoming negligible in about 3 weeks after the onset of paroxysmal stage.

Incubation Period

Range is 6–12 days and on an average incubation period is 7 days.

Clinical Signs

The catarrhal stage lasts for one to two weeks and is characterized by coryza, sneezing, fever and persistent cough. This is followed by the paroxysmal stage with repeated bouts of coughs that are succeeded by prolonged, sudden and inspiratory whoops. This stage lasts for 4–8 weeks. The whoop is rarely present in young infants.

The child vomits after severe bouts of coughing. Infectivity or communicability is very high during the early stages of the disease.

Complications

These include pneumonia, malnutrition and convulsions.

Disease Incidence

Every year in India, around 30,000 cases are being reported. The reporting of cases is incomplete because of weak surveillance programme. 38,493 cases were reported in the year 2010 against 60,385 cases in 2009 while 39,091 cases were reported in 2011. Similarly 37011 cases and 7 deaths were reported in 2013 and 61417 cases and one death in 2014.

Susceptibles

It is estimated that around 80% of the children in an unimmunized population will contract the disease and 1–3% can die of disease or from its complications.

Prevention

Natural disease generally confers immunity. Effective prevention is through immunization against whooping cough.

Pertussis Vaccine

It is killed vaccine which consists of killed *Bordetella pertussis* bacteria and is usually available combined with tetanus and diphtheria toxoids adsorbed on aluminium phosphate. It is sensitive to freezing.

Administration

It is administered together with diphtheria and tetanus toxoid as a triple vaccine known as DPT. The DPT vaccine can be administered simultaneously with oral polio vaccine.

Immunization Schedule

Infant should have 3 doses prior to 12 months of age. The recommended age for first dose is 6 weeks. The minimum interval between two doses is 4 weeks.

Efficacy

The vaccine is 60–90% effective after 3 doses. There is marked fall-off in immunity 4 to 7 years after vaccination.

Side Effects

Fever, pain, swelling, redness, tenderness at local site are common. These subside after giving paracetamol. These must be explained to parents. In some cases, these are severe, such as convulsions, screaming attack, collapse and very exceptionally brain damage. Newer vaccines with fewer side effects are undergoing field trials.

Storage

The vaccine should be stored at 2° to 8°C and it should not be frozen.

TETANUS

Tetanus is an acute neurological disease caused by toxins of the tetanus bacillus (*Clostridium tetani*). The spores of *Clostridium tetani* are present in animal excreta, which is indiscriminately disposed and it leads to widespread contamination of soil and dust. Tetanus is therefore common in agricultural regions.

Tetanus can occur in all age groups who are unprotected. It is epidemiologically important to distinguish neonatal tetanus in infants under 28 days from tetanus in all other age groups.

Mortality

Untreated neonatal tetanus may have nearly 100% fatality rate with adequate treatment the case fatality may be reduced to 50%. Thus, the case fatality is very high in tetanus neonatorum.

Transmission

The infection occurs when the wound gets contaminated with soil containing spores of *Clostridium tetani*. Neonatal tetanus occurs when the delivery is septic or cord gets contaminated with dust or soil rich in tetanus spores. Post-delivery practices in some areas were bad as application of cow dung over cord or covering the cord with dirty linen makes the neonate vulnerable to tetanus. Aseptic delivery practices can prevent tetanus neonatorum.

Wound cleaning and aseptic dressing can also prevent occurrence of tetanus.

Incubation Period

The average incubation period is 7 days but it may range from 4 to 21 days.

TETANUS VACCINE

Tetanus toxoid is prepared from *Clostridium tetani* toxin. The toxoid comes in 3 formulations—Tetanus toxoid (TT), DT with diphtheria toxoid or with pertussis and diphtheria (DPT). Adsorbed tetanus toxoid is better than plain tetanus toxoid. Vaccine is sensitive to freezing.

Administration

The vaccine may be administered simultaneously with polio vaccine as triple antigen (DPT). Pregnant women should be given two doses of TT, first dose early in pregnancy as early as possible and second dose 4 weaks after 1st dose. Children can have DPT at 6 weeks. Tetanus neonatorum can be prevented by immunizing all pregnant women.

Immunization Schedule for Pregnant Women

In India, since tetanus is common, it is necessary that women of reproductive age group and adolescent girls and boys are immunized with TT. Pregnant women should be immunized as early as possible during pregnancy. Two doses are given with a minimum interval of four weeks. A third dose in subsequent pregnancy or the following year offers protection for newborns for at least five additional years and a fourth dose protects for 10 years (UNICEF). If pregnant women have received 2 doses of TT within last three years, then only one booster dose is given. Ideally TT_2 or booster dose should be given before 36 weeks of pregnancy, however, it may be given even if more than 36 weeks have passed.

Efficacy

The vaccine is highly effective and provides lasting protection.

Storage

The vaccine should not be frozen and should be stored at 2° to 8°C. Direct contact with ice should be avoided to avoid freezing.

MATERNAL AND NEONATAL TETANUS ELIMINATED (MNTE)—WHAT IS ELIMINATION?

The definition of Neonatal Tetanus (NNT) elimination is a rate of less than one case per 10,000 live births in every district. Globally year 2010 was set as target year for NNT elimination. Since the tetanus spores are widespread in the environment. TT immunization and clean delivery practices must be continued indefinitely.[12]

The strategies for elimination of NNT.

i ***Coverage:*** Ensure coverage of all pregnant women with two doses of TT and achieve high level of coverage over 90% through routine immunizations.

ii ***Safe deliveries:*** Ensure safe deliveries. 100% of deliveries should be attended by trained personnel and increase the proportion of institutional deliveries to the level of 80% and above from the current level of 73%. Intensify Training of skilled birth attendants.

iii ***Supply DDK and train dais:*** Supply disposable delivery kits to ensure clean practices for domiciliary deliveries.

iv ***Neonatal care:*** Implement essential newborn care, including cord care to reduce risks of neonatal tetanus.

v ***Strengthen service delivery:*** TT is offered at all antenatal sessions and routine immunization sessions. Provide two doses of TT during first pregnancy and further doses according to national schedule.

vi Cover adolescent girls in school and out of schools for TT immunization at age 10 and at age 16 to build up immunity against tetanus, this will ensure elimination of tetanus to a great degree, however priority of TT under the programme are pregnant women.

vii ***Surveillance:*** Increase reporting and appropriate action. Ensure surveillance of occurrence of NNT and establish NNT as reportable disease. NNT will be included with weekly AFP in active surveillance and zero reporting. Targeted action will be taken around reported and investigated cases by improving and promoting TT immunization for pregnant women and safe and clean deliveries in the community.

viii ***Private sector:*** Involve private sector to promote institutional deliveries and TT immunization to pregnant women.

ix ***Milestones:*** National focal point for NNT is created in all the states by 2005 and 50% of districts to achieve over 90% coverage, by 2007, 50% of states have eliminated tetanus, and progressively 100% districts have coverage of TT over 90% and eliminated NNT by 2009. **Maternal and neonatal tetanus elimination** (MNTE) **has been validated** in India in **May 2015 by WHO**; however the immunization will continue.

x ***Intensify IEC activity.***

DIPHTHERIA (A RE-EMERGING THREAT)

It is an acute communicable disease caused by *Corynebacterium diphtheriae*. The target organs of this disease are tonsils, pharynx, nose, and occasionally other mucus membranes and skin. The bacteria forms membrane over these sites and releases powerful toxins, which may lead to muscular and sensory nerve paralysis and myocarditis.

Epidemiology: Humans are the only reservoir of infection.

Case Fatality Rate

It is 5–25%.

Age Group Affected

Diphtheria mainly affects the unimmunized. Though all age groups stand to the risk of diphtheria, but predominantly children below the age of 15 years are most commonly affected.

Problem

The incidence of diphtheria and its severity has declined over the years but still cases are being reported and some of them are fatal even. Nearly 5000 cases per annum are being reported in India. The reporting is inadequate because of poor surveillance. 5826 cases and 68 deaths were reported during the year 2005 and similarly 3343 cases and 177 deaths were reported in the year 2010 and 4233 cases and 99 deaths were reported in 2011, 4310 cases and 67 deaths were reported in 2013, and 4071 cases and 104 deaths in 2014.

Outbreaks: The last two decades have seen a resurgence of diphtheria in both developed and developing countries. where it was previously well controlled. Due to good vaccine coverage worldwide a shift in age incidence has been observed from pre-school to school age (5–15 years) with more and more cases being reported even in adults. Outbreaks in India were reported in Kolkata (1977), Delhi in 2000 and J & K in 2002–03.

Transmission

The infection is transmitted through contact with a patient or carrier by droplet infection or even by contact. Without adequate treatment, the period of communicability can extend up to 4 weeks from the onset of the disease, otherwise it lasts for 24–48 hours after the initiation of treatment.

Incubation Period

It ranges between 2 and 5 days.

Clinical Features

It leads to formation of patches of greyish membrane with a surrounding dull red inflammatory zone, which may cause pharyngeal obstruction. Swelling and oedema of neck occurs in severe cases. Laryngeal diphtheria is a serious condition. There may be neurological complications and myocarditis. The illness may last for 10–21 days but it depends upon the promptness of treatment and stage of illness when reported for treatment. Administration of diphtheria antitoxin at the earliest is the most important element in treatment of diphtheria. The antitoxin should be given either by intramuscular or intravenous route in doses ranging from 10,000 to 1,00,000 units or more after sensitivity test. Erythromycine or procaine penicillin are the drugs of choice.

Prevention

Clinical attack or subclinical infection does not provide lasting immunity. Active immunity should be initiated against diphtheria at the time of discharge. Maternal antibodies provide immunity for the first 6 months of life.

DIPHTHERIA VACCINE

Diphtheria vaccine is available in the form of diphtheria toxoid and adsorbed toxoid is better and more efficient for immunity. It should be stored at 2° to 8°C and not to be forzen.

Administration

Diphtheria toxoid is routinely administered in combination with tetanus toxoid or additionally with pertussis vaccine. It is administered with oral polio vaccine as per recommended schedule.

Immunization Schedule

An infant should receive 3 doses of DPT prior to 12 months of age. The recommended age for the first dose is 6 weeks and minimum interval between 2 doses is 4 weeks. A booster dose is given at 16–24 months of age and another booster dose of DPT at school entry (5–6 years age) is recommended. DPT can be given till 7 years of age.

Efficacy

The vaccine is highly effective and provides long lasting immunity after 3 doses. Clinical efficacy is 97%. Immunization does not prevent the carrier state.

Side Effects

Local reactions at the site such as swelling, tenderness and redness with fever.

TUBERCULOSIS

It is a communicable disease of public health significance.

Causative organism: The disease is caused by *Mycobacterium tuberculosis* in human beings *M. bovis* causes intestinal tuberculosis.

The disease is distributed widely. It is highly prevalent in India. The urban and rural prevalence is almost equal. Urban slums show higher prevalence rates.

Transmission

Sputum positive cases can transmit infection to other healthy persons through fine droplets. Close contacts are at highest risk of tuberculosis infection. After infection, the subsequent risk of development of progressive pulmonary or extrapulmonary tuberculosis is maximum within a year or two. 30% of people are infected with tubercle bacilli in India, while only 10% of infected persons develop TB disease in life time.

The tuberculosis is killer number one in adults in India. Problem of multi-drug resistant tuberculosis is emerging. HIV and tuberculosis have strong nexus.

Clinical Signs

Clinical signs are pulmonary or extrapulmonary with prolonged morbidity. The initial infection goes unnoticed.

Prevention

Prevention of tuberculosis is difficult. Severe forms of tuberculosis (miliary and meningeal) can be prevented by BCG vaccination.

BCG Vaccine

The vaccine is freeze dried preparation made from attenuation of *Mycobacterium tuberculosis* (*Bacillus Calmette-Guérin*). BCG vaccine is now available in 10 dose vial. Reconstituted BCG vaccine should be used within 4 hours.

Administration

BCG is given intradermally and can be administered concurrently with other vaccines. Dose is 0.1 ml. The dose for children below one month is 0.05 ml.

Immunization Schedule

BCG can be given soon after birth or at any time thereafter till one year of age. It can be combined with first dose of DPT at 6 weeks of age. It is safe.

Efficacy

Variable from 0 to 80% as reported by different trials. Subsequent trials done by WHO indicated that BCG has efficacy between 50 and 60% and offers protection against childhood tuberculosis. It prevents severe forms of (miliary and meningeal) tuberculosis in children hence it is recommended in India. It does not prevent the occurrence of pulmonary tuberculosis. The incidence and prevalence of tuberculosis has not much declined after the introduction of BCG vaccination since 1962 in India. For diagnosing childhood tuberculosis, WHO has recommended scoring system.

Side Effects

At the site of BCG injection, a small red tender nodule appears after about 2 weeks, which might develop into ulcer, which heals by itself leaving behind a scar at the site. This is a normal reaction. Sometimes it might develop into an abscess or sinus, which takes very long time to heal, and may cause swelling of lymph glands in the axilla.

EPIDEMIOLOGY OF POLIOMYELITIS

Poliomyelitis is an acute viral infection caused by 3 antigenic types of polioviruses (1, 2 and 3).

The poliovirus is an enterovirus. There are 3 serotypes: types 1, 2 and 3. All three can cause paralysis, although type 1 causes paralysis most often, type 3 less frequently and type 2 rarely. Most epidemics are due to type 1, cases of paralysis associated with vaccine are usually caused by types 3 and 2. During eradication, the first serotype to disappear is type 2 due to better oral polio vaccine (OPV) take rates followed by serotypes 3 and 1. Type 1 polio virus has propensity to cause huge outbreaks and travel long distances. Wild polio virus 1 accounted for 95% of polio cases in India between 2000 and 2006.

Types of Cases—Clinical Course

- Inapparent infection account for 90–95% of cases.
- Abortive polio occurs in 4–8% of cases.
- Nonparalytic aseptic meningitis occurs in 1–2% of infections.
- Share of paralytic cases is 0.5–1%.

Thus, for every one paralytic case, there are 200 inapparent infections in the community for type 1 and 1000 inapparent infections for type 3 respectively. These inapparent cases continue to excrete wild poliovirus in their faeces.

Social Significance

The cases who develop paralytic manifestation may develop permanent, partial or total disability which lasts lifelong. Thus, polio is disabling disease.

Acute attack may cause death in 2–10% of cases.

Distribution

As of now, most countries in the world have achieved eradication and have been certified. Polio is endemic in just three countries—Pakistan, Afghanistan and Nigeria. India is polio-free since 14th January 2011.

Seasonal Variation

The incidence increases during July to September coinciding with the rainy season.

Age of Occurrence

Median age of occurrence of poliomyelitis was 18 months. Bulk of cases occurred in late infancy and early childhood period.

In endemic areas, polio is now a disease of very young children. In 2006, in western UP, more than 85% of cases were in children less than 3 years of age and 73% were less than 2 years old. Thus, wild poliovirus (WPV) transmission was surviving largely in children under the age of 3 in endemic areas. The survival of transmission in this age group is because, insufficient young children are immune to stop viral transmission and the poorer immunization status of younger children compared to older children. Surveillance data shows that younger children; under 2 years of age have received less doses of oral polio vaccine (OPV) than older age groups.

Transmission

Transmission is primarily person to person via the faecal oral route. Poliovirus multiplies in the intestine and is spread through the faeces. The virus is intermittently excreted for up to 2 months or more after infection, with maximum excretion occurring just before paralysis and during the first two weeks (14 days) after onset of paralysis.

Incubation Period

Average incubation period is between 7 and 10 days but the range is from 4 to 35 days.

Reservoir

Man is the only reservoir and the infection is spread from person to person. Given the large number of inapparent infections it is difficult to find the source of infection. The half-life of excreted virus in the sewage in warm climate is only 48 hours. Detection of wild polio P1 virus in sewage in Delhi continuously in 2010 was a point of worry. Monitoring wild poliovirus in sewage is a continuous activity and is being continued in polio free India.

Communicability

Polio virus is highly communicable. The cases are most infectious one weeks before and two weeks after the onset of paralysis. An infected individual will probably infect all other persons in household and close contacts, especially where sanitation is poor.

Immunity

Immunity obtained through infection with wild virus/or through immunization: Immunity following natural infection or by immunization with oral polio vaccine (OPV) results in both humoral and local intestinal cellular responses. Such immunity persists for many years and can serve to block infection with subsequent wild viruses. Vaccination with inactivated polio vaccine (IPV) confers humoral immunity, but relatively less intestinal immunity.

Clinical Features

In non-paralytic infections, the manifestations are fever, sore throat, headache, nausea, diarrhoea, vomiting and rigidity of neck and back lasting for 2–10 days. In paralytic cases, these manifestations are accompanied by a sudden onset of paralysis of the muscles of the limb, face or the chest/respiratory muscles, with maximum recovery within 6 months. Hence, 6 months follow-up of cases is mandatory if the residual paralysis persists beyond 6 months it is due to poliomyelitis. Paralytic poliomyelitis could be spinal paralytic poliomyelitis (80%) Bulbar polio (2%) and Bulbospinal polio (20%).

Hot Cases

Any case that in the opinion of DIO/SMO looks clinically like polio, based on examination are labeled as "Hot cases". Common characteristics in polio cases are: age less than 5 years + history of fever at onset of paralysis + asymmetrical proximal paralysis or patchy paralysis or age less than 5 years with rapidly progressive paralysis leading to bulbar involvement and death. All "Hot cases" must be notified immediately.

Prevention

Maternal antibodies provide temporary immunity to infants for 2 to 3 months through passive immunity.

Infection with wild virus can provide immunity against specific type and not against all types 1, 2 and 3, hence the administration of polio vaccine to paralytic cases is justified.

Eradication: It is possible and achievable because:

1 Potent vaccine is available against poliomyelitis. OPV is proven vaccine to prevent polio.
2 The man is the only reservoir of infection. There is no animal reservoir of poliomyelitis.
3 Incidence is restricted to few geographical areas.
4 The half-life of excreted virus in the sewage in warm climate is only 48 hours and spread of infection through sewage can only occur during this period.
5 Adequate infrastructure has been developed and available for outbreak response.

NATIONAL POLIO ERADICATION PROGRAMME

During May 1988, World Health Assembly passed a resolution to achieve the Polio eradication by the year 2000.[12] The Government of India launched Polio Eradication Programme in the year 1995.[13,14] The goal to eradicate poliomyelitis by the year 2000 adopted under the UIP could not be achieved. *India* is now *polio free* with effect from *14th January* 2011.

Goal of Eradication

The polio eradication is defined as no case of clinical poliomyelitis associated with wild poliovirus, and no wild poliovirus found despite intensive efforts to do so.

Stages of Polio Eradication

Endemic: When the incidence is more than 1 per 1,00,000 and coverage of OPV is less than 85% and surveillance system not reliable.

Control: When the incidence of polio is less than 1 per 1,00,000 and coverage of OPV is more than 85% and surveillance is adequate.

Elimination: When the incidence is zero for one year and coverage of OPV is more than 85 to 100% and surveillance system is reliable.

Eradication: No indigenous case for 3 consecutive years and coverage of OPV is more than 85 to 100% and surveillance system is reliable.[15]

Key Strategies of National Polio Eradication Programme

1 *Routine immunization:* Achieve and maintain high level of coverage for oral polio vaccine—85% and above through routine immunization in infants. India achieved over 90% of OPV coverage among infants through routine immunization but this was not uniform, in all the states and districts.

2 *Pulse-polio immunization (PPI):* By observing national immunization days (NIDs) and sub-national immunization days (SNIDs) every year.[16–18]

3 *Acute flaccid paralysis (AFP) surveillance:* To recognize; report AFP cases at the earliest and ensure rapid response (outbreak response immunization).

4 *Mopping up round:* As and when wild poliovirus is detected mass supplementary immunization activities (SIAs) are organized by immunizing all 0–5 years old children covering 2–5 million children under this age group with type specific monovalent or bivalent vaccine.

5 *Protection of high-risk population:* Migrant population, urban slums, construction sites and brick kilns workers.

1. Strategy of High Coverage of OPV

Achieve the highest coverage levels possible through the administration of vaccines in routine immunization programme through fixed centres and outreach sessions. Through UIP within 10 years, India achieved over 90% coverage of routine OPV and the cases decreased by 80% from 26,226 in 1984 to 4793 in 1994. Highest coverage levels of 90% achieved but polio cases continued to occur with reduced incidence, *thus routine immunization alone could not interrupt the transmission of wild poliovirus and allow India to achieve the goal of polio eradication.*

2. Strategy of PPI—National Immunization Days (NIDs)

From 1995 onwards, India is implementing nationwide mass immunization campaigns. (NIDs) India conducted its first Pulse Polio Immunization (PPI) on 9th December, 1995 and 20th January, 1996 and more than 75 million children under 3 years throughout the country received two extra doses of OPV on these days. Since then PPIs are being repeated yearly. The target age group in these PPI was increased to cover all children under 5 years of age.[16–18]

WHAT IS PPI?

It means extra doses of Trivalent OPV administered to all children below 5 years on the two fixed dates (*National Immunization days in the country*), at the interval of 4–6 weeks. The term "pulse" has been used to describe this sudden, simultaneous, mass administration of OPV on a single day to all children 0–5 years of age which constitute 13% of total population. During each NID 130 million children less than 5 years were given polio drops and during each SNID around 70 million children are being covered.

Objective

Objective of PPI strategy is to interrupt transmission of wild poliovirus in the community. PPI is primarily an eradication strategy—tested all over the world.

Essentials of PPI

To cover all children of age group 0–5 years and irrespective of their previous immunization status ensuring two extra doses of OPV; achieving close to 100% coverage throughout the country. These two extra doses supplement and do not replace the doses received during routine immunization services.

Epidemiological Basis of PPI

The intention of PPI is to replace "wild poliovirus" by "vaccine virus" in the community. PPI replaces harmful wild poliovirus and thereby eradicates polio in the community.

- December and January are chosen as National Immunization Days (NIDs) as it is the lowest transmission season of wild polioviruses, their population is low and lowest level of circulation during these months. During these months, efficacy of vaccine is much more due to favourable temperature.
- In addition to NIDs, sub-National Immunization Days (SNIDs) are also being organized for endemic states and high-risk states which continue to report more cases of polio (these states were—UP, MP, West Bengal, Bihar, Rajasthan, Assam, Gujarat and Odisha).

In addition, rapid and large scale mop up vaccination rounds, using type specific monovalent oral polio vaccine are being carried out in response to all P1 cases and all P3 cases outside the endemic states as per the India Expert Advisory Group (IEAG) recommendations and WHO resolution. Bivalent OPV was used in India in 2010.

PPI Booths

Pulse polio immunization booth in urban/rural area are set up to cover around 250–300 children of 0–5 years, it roughly covers 2000 population. Booth is established at easily accessible place. A PPI booth is managed by four workers (Health worker, Anganwadi worker, school teacher/community volunteers and NGO volunteer). Booths are also set-up at railway stations and bus terminals and it is ensured to cover migrant population as well.

Planning

Since PPI is intensive and extensive effort, the operations are well planned. Microplans are prepared at PHC and district level well before the activity. The list of 0–5 years children is prepared well in advance with the help of Anganwadi workers and village Panchayats and traditional birth attendants. In Urban areas and non-ICDS areas, the estimates of 0–5 years children are worked out area-wise, as there is absence of system of tracking or registration of complete births area-wise. People are well-informed through mass-media and interpersonal communication and through publicity. It is a big social mobilization as on a single day 130 million children of 0–5 years age group are targeted for 100% coverage. In high-risk areas maps are also prepared so as to ensure 100% coverage.

Intensive pulse polio immunization (IPPI) means covering all 0–5 year children by booth based activity on first day followed by house to house activities on following two days.

3. Surveillance of Acute Flaccid Paralysis (AFP)

A suspect case of poliomyelitis is—a "Syndromic" case of AFP—fever with abrupt onset of paralysis of leg or arm.

Aim of surveillance is to reliably detect circulation of wild poliovirus in areas where polio transmission is occurring or likely to occur. This is achieved by reporting all cases of acute flaccid paralysis. Investigate these cases and above all ensure rapid response on occurrence of AFP in the locality, to contain the spread and interrupt the transmission. The AFP surveillance system for polio-eradication was started in India in the year 1997. For this, National Polio Surveillance Project (NPSP) was established by collaboration of WHO and GOI.[18–22] Initially 57 surveillance medical officers were recruited throughout the country.

Objectives

- The objective of AFP surveillance is to recognize and report AFP cases at the earliest and to ensure prompt outbreak immunization response with OPV.
- The second objective is to confirm the cases of wild poliovirus through isolation of virus in the stool samples. The samples are sent to various laboratories (Central Research Institute—Kasauli or NICD).
- The third objective is to measure the impact of routine immunization and PPI in India.

What is AFP?

Acute flaccid paralysis is defined as sudden onset of weakness and floppiness in any part is the body in a child <15 years of age or paralysis in a person of any age in whom polio is suspected. It should be stressed that surveillance is carried out for all cases of acute flaccid paralysis (AFP) and not just for poliomyelitis. AFP cases include:

- GB syndrome
- Transverse myelitis
- Traumatic neuritis
- Polio case
- Post diphtheric polyneuritis
- Paraplegia, quadriplegia
- Isolated bulbar palsy
- Post viral neuritis

Therefore, all AFP cases should be reported, regardless of final diagnosis to maintain high level of sensitivity of surveillance. Because paralytic poliomyelitis is just one cause of AFP, maintaining a high *sensitivity* of AFP reporting will ensure that all cases of paralytic poliomyelitis are detected, reported and investigated resulting in preventive control measures to interrupt transmission of disease.

Focus: AFP surveillance must focus on children under 15 years. All AFP cases should be reported.

Expected AFP Rate

The goal in India is to have all districts reporting AFP cases, AFP rates of at least one case per 1,00,000 population of children below 15 years of age per year should be achieved by each district. This is an important indicator of adequacy and quality of AFP surveillance. If the rate is less than one, it is poor quality of surveillance.

Response to an AFP case

a Immediately inform and report the outbreak to DIO/SMO.
b Collect two stool samples.
c Case investigation.
d Active case search in the community.
e Outbreak response immunization (ORI).
f Include the case in weekly report of surveillance.
g Sensitize health facilities that have missed the case.

INFORMATION OF THE CASE

a **Information of the case:** Case/Outbreak should be immediately reported by fastest means preferably telephonically or personal messenger to SMO/DIO, nodal officer or nodal person. Immediate reporting is important so that the child is traced, investigated and stool specimen collection is done at the earliest. Complete address of the case should be recorded.

b **Collection of stool samples:** Collect two stool samples at least 24 hrs apart from reported AFP case, within 2 weeks after the onset of paralysis. Stools samples have the maximum chance of yielding a positive result if collected within 2 weeks after paralysis onset. Maximum limit is up to 2 months of onset of paralysis. Therefore, all efforts must be made to collect stool specimens of 8 g or thumb sized amount in clean vial within 2 weeks of paralysis onset. Special vials are provided for stool samples collection. Stool samples should be transported by maintaining proper cold chain system (Reverse cold chain) to the designated laboratory. District immunization officer (DIO) is responsible for transportation of stool samples to the laboratory. Before collection of stool the sample should have the information of date of collection, case identification data, full address, to whom the report should be sent, clinical information, date of paralysis onset, OPV history, date of last OPV dose and correct identification on the specimen container. A minimum of 28 days are required to isolate and identify poliovirus and hence laboratory results become available after 28 days only. If stool samples from "Hot" case are inadequate or could not be collected, then one stool sample each has to be collected from 5 other 0–5 years old children living in or around index case's house.

Target: Eighty per cent of stool samples should be adequate. An adequate stool sample is one where two stool samples 24–48 hours apart measuring thumb size (8 g) are obtained within 14 days of onset of paralysis and are transported to laboratory by maintaining cold chain.

c **AFP case investigation:** Each reported AFP case should be investigated within 48 hours by DIO and his/her team/SMO or by designated medical officer. Case investigation form (CIF) be filled completely for all reported cases of AFP. CIF should be sent to SMO/DIO within 24 hours of investigation.

d **Active case search in the community:** During the outbreak, effort should be made to visit the area, contact the local influential persons, and visit door to door to confirm other cases of AFP in the area.

e **Outbreak response immunization (ORI):** Outbreak response immunization should cover the entire village in rural areas and the municipal ward in urban area where the AFP case has occurred. Before initiating immunization, stool specimen collection as a part of case investigation should be done first. If the AFP case has travelled or had close contact with individuals from other areas of the state/country/district within 40 days prior to the onset of paralysis, the state EPI officer should be informed immediately.

Response

Outbreak containment measures must be started within 48 hours of onset of paralysis and completed within 2 weeks. This consists of ensuring one dose of OPV to all children below 5 years. At least 500 children under 5 years are covered if the locality is small cover all the children with one additional dose of OPV. Outbreak response is meant to prevent the spread of occurrence of poliomyelitis.

AFP Case Classification Scheme (Fig. 12.16)

Within 90 days of paralysis onset all the AFP cases are classified by obtaining results of stool samples from laboratories.

i ***Confirmed case of polio:*** Cases of acute flaccid paralysis are confirmed as polio if wild virus has been detected in stool sample.

ii ***Compatible case:*** Cases having residual paralysis after 60 days of onset but no wild virus reported in stool samples; died before follow-up or lost to follow-up and either stool samples were inadequate and on neurological investigation some deficiency is detected. Such cases are screened by review committee.

iii ***Discarded (non-polio AFP):*** No wild virus is detected and the stool samples were adequate. Despite being discarded as not being polio, all non-polio AFP cases must be reported with their final diagnosis, such as Guillain-Barré syndrome (GBS), transverse myelitis, tumour or traumatic neuritis and AFP due to non-polio other enteroviruses (NPEV): This is important to document the background AFP reporting rate, which indirectly monitors the sensitivity of the surveillance system. Experience in other parts of the world indicates that at least one case of AFP occurs every 1,00,000 population of children aged less than 15 years per year. This is referred to as

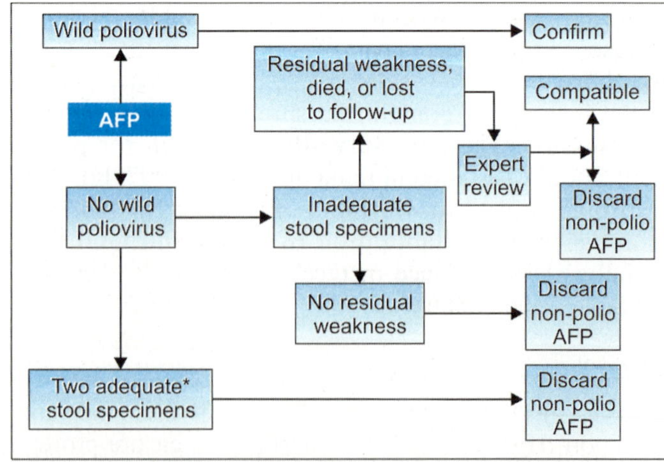

Fig. 12.16: Virological classification scheme

*2 specimens, at least 24 hours apart and within 14 days of paralytic onset: Each specimen must be of adequate volume (8–10 g) and arrive at laboratory in good condition, i.e. no desiccation, no leakage, adequate documentation and evidence that the reverse cold chain was maintained.

12

"background" rate of AFP among children. The other non-polio causes of AFP such as Guillain-Barré syndrome (GBS), transverse myelitis, traumatic neuritis, account for this background rate; regardless of whether acute poliomyelitis exists in the community.

Environmental surveillance: Environmental surveillance involves isolation of polio viruses from sewage samples. It is being carried out in Mumbai, Delhi, Patna and Kolkatta.

4. Mopping Up Rounds/Operations

Mopping up is aimed at stopping transmission in a defined area. It is an end game strategy to ensure PPI at booth and intensive/aggressive efforts to cover all 0–5 years children.

Speed of response: Within two weeks from confirmation of the case of polio.

Extent of mop ups: At least 3 large scale house to house rounds using a short interval approach of 4 weeks and immunization with mOPV or bOPV. Mop up should cover at least 2–5 million children below 5 years per round (5 million is appropriate target as recommended by IEAG).

5. Protecting High-risk Population

The programme is focusing on the migrant population which often escapes and remains unprotected. Maximum number of Type 1 polio cases outside the endemic states in India in 2008 to 2010 were in migrants or children living in proximity to them. The most vulnerable population is urban slums, construction sites, project sites, brick kilns and mobile population. These populations are at higher risk because they are usually missed during polio campaign and during routine immunization. Mobile and transit teams are covering these populations.

CURRENT SITUATION OF POLIOMYELITIS IN INDIA—POLIO ELIMINATED

The polio eradication in India has made major progress since its inception in 1995. Before 1979, when OPV was introduced in the National EPI Programme (1978); an estimated 1,50,000 polio cases occurred annually in the country. As a result of introduction of OPV under the National EPI Programme, polio incidence declined and the estimated number of cases in 1994 dropped to 5000 only. Since the inception of AFP surveillance in 1997–98 more accurate data on incidence of polio cases became available. Since 1998, when 1934 polio cases were confirmed, a consistent decline in incidence has been registered over the years. The number of cases reached an all time low in 2010 with only 42 cases reported against the background of the most *sensitive* AFP surveillance system and geographical spread confined to only a few districts in Western UP, Bihar, West Bengal, Jharkhand and Maharashtra.

During 2006, a marked increase in the number of wild poliovirus cases occurred. As on 30th March 2007, a total of 676 cases were confirmed, including 28 cases due to wild polio type 3 maximum of 548 cases (81%) occurred in UP, 61 in Bihar (9%) and 67 cases (10%) in 14 other states/ union territories of the country. There have been years of resurgence in the year 2002, and 2006, with 1600 and 676 cases respectively (Table 12.47).[23–29] During 2007, in India 874 cases were reported, however, wild poliovirus type 1 (WPV 1) transmission was at an unprecedented low level signaling the high likelihood of eradication of polio from the country.[30] This has been achieved due to accelerated immunization rounds using monovalent oral polio vaccine type 1.

India is *polio-free*. India eradicated type 2 polioviruses in 1999. *No case of polio has been reported after 13th January 2011, thus India is polio free for the third consecutive year. WHO certified of polio free India on 27th march 2014.*

Potential Causes for Resurgence of Polio in 2006–2007

Operational

- Significant decline in supplementary immunization activities (SIAs) performance in later half of 2005.
- Increased percentage of missed houses and decreased coverage of susceptible children (young children).

Environmental

- High population density facilitating child to child transmission. Very poor sanitary conditions facilitating virus transmission.
- High non-polio enteroviruses rate indicating high incidence of other enteroviruses or bacterial infections

Table 12.47: Trends of poliomyelitis in India

Year	*No. of confirmed cases for wild poliovirus*	*No. of districts affected*
1978	1,50,000	All
1994	4793	All
1998	1934	314
1999	1126	192
2000	0265	089
2001	0268	63
2002	1600	159
2003	0225	087
2004	134	43
2005	66	35
2006	676	114
2007	874	99
2008	559	90
2009	741	53
2010	42	17
2011 Jan 13th	1	1
2012	0	0
2013	0	0
2014 (27th March) Wild poliovirus eradicated from India.		

Table 12.18: Trends of P1 wild and P3 wild poliovirus cases in India from 1999–2014

Year	P1 cases	P3 cases	Total cases
1999	730	394	1126
2005	62	4	66
2006	648	28	676
2007	83	794	874*
2008	75	484	559
2009	80	662	741*
2010	18	24	42
2011	1	0	1
2012	0	0	0
2013	0	0	0
2014 (27th March) Wild poliovirus eradicated from India.			

*Mixture of P1 and P3 wild in some cases.

leading to higher incidence of diarrhoea and possibly lesser uptake of OPV.

Sociological

Vaccine avoidance behaviour in minority community (overt and covert) facilitating sustenance of virus circulation and contributes to disproportionately higher incidence of polio in this community.

Useful indicators:[31]

- Number of wild polio cases in India.
- Number of AFP cases per lac per district per annum.
- Non-polio AFP rate per 1,00,000 under 15 years children target is ≥1 per annum per lac. Operational target for India >2/1,00,000.
- Reported AFP cases investigated within 48 hours of notification (target is ≥ 80%).
- Timeliness and completeness of weekly reporting (target >90%). This has been achieved in India in 2011–12.
- Reported AFP cases with adequate stool specimen collection (target 80%).
- India has maintained the global targets of performance (non-polio AFP rate of 11.81 and stool sample rate of 86%).

Post-elimination Policy

Future Strategies after Eradication of WPV

- Zero wild poliovirus (WPV) status in India, this has been achieved in India in 2011.
- On 27th March 2014, India as a part of South-East Asia Region of WHO has been certified polio free by Regional Certification Commission for polio eradication.
- **Decision on use of OPV versus IPV:** It is dependant on global certification of polio eradication. Greatest challenge is to maintain zero incidence in coming years by prevention of entry of wild virus from endemic countries (Afghanistan, Pakistan and Nigeria).[7]
- India has eradicated wild poliovirus and is posed for final elimination of all vaccine associated and vaccine derived polioviruses by introduction of inactivated poliovirus vaccine (IPV), for meeting polio eradication goals and sequential discontinuation of oral polio vaccine.

The possibility of virus importation in polio-free India remains from outside India. To prevent/deal with, such as situation following strategies are being adopted in India.

1. *Maintain high level of population immunity*: Through routine immunizations and conducting regular supplementary immunization activities (SIAs) and NIDs with tOPV.
2. Maintain the quality and effectiveness of the existing surveillance and laboratory systems to detect and respond to any outbreaks. High level of vigilance will be maintained till global certification of eradication and through to cessation of use of oral poliovirus vaccines. All detected vaccine derived polio viruses (VDPVs) would continue to thoroughly investigated to determine any risk of circulation and appropriate action taken based on investigation findings.
3. *National and state emergency preparedness response plan and maintain a rolling stock of bOPV and tOPV*: Rapid Response Teams (RRT) are in place to deal with any importation of wild polio virus in India. Government of India to ensure a rolling stock of 40 million doses of bOPV and10 million doses of tOPV to enable response to any wild poliovirus or vaccine derived poliovirus detection.
4. *Reduce risk of polio importation from neighbouring countries based on WHO recommendations for travelers*: Immunization of travelers at land border crossing points from negihbouring countries is the most significant risk reduction strategy and will continue until there is no longer an epidemiological risk. Ensure effective coverage of border population with SIAs and routine immunization.
5. Conduct periodic sero-surveillance studies in high-risk areas of UP, Bihar and other regions.

Poliomyelitis Vaccines

There are two types of vaccines available:

i. ***Oral polio vaccine (OPV):*** Widely used in India. It is live attenuated, trivalent oral polio vaccine (OPV), containing all three types of polioviruses.
ii. Monovalent oral polio vaccine–mOPV1 and mOPV3 and bivalent polio vaccine (P1 and P3).
iii. ***Inactivated poliovirus vaccine (IPV)*** to be given by intramuscular injection at mid thigh.

Administration

OPV is given orally: The vaccine can be administered along with DPT vaccine. It protects about 99, 98 and 91% of children from type 1, 2, and 3 respectively.

Immunization Schedule

Infants should receive at least 3 doses of OPV at minimum interval of 4 weeks within the first 9 months of age. In endemic areas, the extra dose of OPV (zero dose) should be given soon after birth (up to 15 days after birth). This can be ensured for institutional deliveries.

In non-endemic areas, the first dose of OPV can be started at 6 weeks of age.

Efficacy

OPV produces both circulatory antibodies as well as provides local gut/intestinal resistance. The OPV has been successfully used to eliminate and eradicate poliomyelitis, but some developing countries have reported poor serological response to OPV.

IPV induces circulatory antibodies but does not prevent intestinal infection.

Both IPV and OPV provide long-lasting immunity. Efficacy is 95% for fully immunized children.

Storage

OPV should be stored below –15°C where it can maintain its shelf-life for 2 years, at 0° to +8°C for one year. It can withstand only one day at +37°C.

Risks Associated with the use of Oral Polio Vaccine (OPV) Adverse Effects

Although OPV is the vaccine of choice for polio eradication as it provides both humoral and intestinal immunity. The major concern about OPV is that it is live attenuated virus vaccine and has ability to revert to a form that can cause paralysis called as **Vaccine Associated Paralytical Poliomyelitis** (VAPP). It is associated with a single dose of OPV given to a child or can occur in a close unvaccinated or non immune contact of the vaccine recipient who is excreting the mutated virus. It is estimated that OPV may cause VAPP in one in 2.7 million doses of OPV given (with 25–30 cases per year in India).

Vaccine Derived Poliovirus (VDPV)

When a child is vaccinated with live OPV the virus replicates in the intestine and gets genetically altered during replication. Like wild polio virus the child excretes the altered vaccine virus for a period of six to eight weeks. This is called Vaccine Derived Poliovirus (VDPV). Amongst the three types of VDPV, the circulating vaccine derived poliovirus (cVDPV) may cause paralysis in areas with low routine immunization coverage (low immunity areas). Due to the risk of cVDPVs, OPV must be phased out to secure a lasting polio free world. Type 2 component contained in trivalent OPV accounts for 90% of all cVDPVs cases. 43 cases of paralysis due to VDPVs have occured in India and 40 were due to type 2 VDPVs Since 2009.

THE POLIO ERADICATION ENDGAME STRATEGY 2013–18: THREE STEPS

1 **Introduction of IPV in routine immunization by october 2015:** By the end of 2015 introduce at least 1 dose of IPV into all routine immunization systems at least 6 months before the switch from tOPV to bOPV (containing poliovirus types 1 and 3).

2 **tOPV–bOPV switch by April 2016:** From 2016 switch from tOPV to bOPV (which does not contain type 2 Sabin virus) in routine immunization and polio campaigns.

3. **Widhdrawal of routine OPV use:** Plan for the eventual widhdrawal of OPV in routine use by 2019–2020.

Introduction of Inactivated Polio Vaccine (IPV)

IPV consists of inactivated (killed) poliovirus strains of all three poliovirus types (Poliovirus types 1, 2 and 3). IPV is given intramuscularly at mid thigh. The IPV produces antibodies in the blood to all three types of poliovirus. It is highly effective in preventing paralytic disease caused by all three types of polioviruses. When IPV is given after a few doses of OPV, the IPV not only enhances protection against paralytic disease but also boosts intestinal immunity. Thus combining IPV with OPV provides strong intestinal immunity and antibody protection against all three serotypes. IPV carries no risk of VAPP and VDPV, hence IPV is one of the safest vaccines in use.

IPV has been introduced across all over India in November 2015 along with third dose of OPV in routine immunization at 14 weeks as single dose of 0.5 ml intramuscularly. IPV is heat and freeze sensitive vaccine, can be given up to one year of age.

IPV should not be frozen. It should be stored at 0° to + 8°C. At this temperature it has shelf-life of 12–18 months. It can withstand four weeks at 37°C. IPV is heat sensitive vaccine.

Rationale for Introduction of IPV into Routine Immunization Programme

The primary purpose of introducing IPV into routine immunization is to boost population immunity against type 2 poliovirus during and after the planned global widhdrawal of OPV2 and switch from tOPV to bOPV. The vaccine will also facilitate the interruption of transmission with the use of monovalent OPV type 2 in case of outbreaks, hasten eradication by boosting immunity to poliovirus type 1 and 3, and mitigate the risk of emergence and transmission of cVDPV2.

Evidence indicates that one dose of IPV may reduce risk by protecting individuals against paralytic polio should they be exposed to cVDPV2 or WPV2.

Withdrawal of Type 2 Component of Oral Polio Vaccines (OPVs): Switch from Trivalent OPV (tOPV) to Bivalent OPV (bOPV)

The **endgame strategy** plan mandates that all countries must eventually stop use of OPV beginning with removal of the type 2 component of tOPV through a globally synchronized **switch to bOPV** (containing only types 1 and 3) for routine immunization and all supplementary immunization activities. The global tOPV-bOPV switch, expected to occur in **April 2016** has to be globally coordinated process because any use of tOPV after April 2016 could jeopardize polio eradication by generating circulating vaccine-derived polioviruses from the type 2 component of the vaccine.

Although no wild poliovirus type 2 has been recorded over the past years, the risk of paralytic polio diseases due to the type 2 component of OPV now outweighs its benefits. This switch is necessary because replacing tOPV with bOPV is the key to ensuring the eradication of type 2 polio Sabin virus, which in turn will reduce the risk of new cVDPV type 2 outbreaks after OPV type 2 cessation, if a cVDPV2 appears.

Once the switch is made, tOPV will no longer be used anywhere in the world, and manufacturers will no longer supply tOPV. Selected high risk countries will conduct SIAs with tOPV in the months leading up to the switch.

What is VVM (Vaccine Vial Monitor)?

The VVM is a small square made of heat sensitive material and placed on the outer coloured circle printed on the label of the OPV vial. Combined effect of time and temperature cause the VVM to change colour gradually from light at the starting point and become darker with exposure to heat. The darkening process is irreversible. The outer coloured circle is used as reference to compare the colour of VVM.

VVM does not directly measure vaccine potency but it does give information about heat exposure over a period of time, which affects potency. The VVM, however, does not measure exposure to freezing that contributes to the degeneration of freeze sensitive vaccines.

How to Read VVM?

Start point	□	Square lighter than circle. If the expiry date has not passed, use the vaccine
End Point		Square matches the circle. Do not use the vaccine
End point exceeded	■	Square darker than the circle. Do not use the vaccine

VACCINE PREVENTABLE DISEASES

These are diseases, which can be prevented by vaccination and immunizations. Disease burden due to these diseases is high. These diseases cause premature deaths, disability and malnutrition in young children.

DISEASE BURDEN DUE TO VACCINE PREVENTABLE DISEASES (VPD)

The disease burden due to vaccine preventable diseases in India was very high in 1974–79, i.e. before the start of expanded programme of immunization in 1978. Nearly 6 lakh cases were reported due to VPD and this has declined to 89408 cases of all VPD in the year 2014. Infant mortality rate has declined from 104 in 1984 to 40 in the year 2013. Thus over the last 40 years there has been general decline in the reported number of cases of VPD. However, reporting and surveillance for cases of VPD except polio is incomplete and inadequate in the country as these diseases are seldom reported from field levels or in rural settings. The actual number of cases might be much more. In spite of limitations, the declining trend of VPD is obvious from 1979 to 2014 (Table 12.49).[30, 31]

UNIVERSAL IMMUNIZATION PROGRAMME IN INDIA

Edward Jenner discovered smallpox vaccine in the year 1796. The practice of vaccine existed in India since early 1900s; especially against smallpox and later against typhoid fever. BCG vaccine was introduced in the National Tuberculosis Control Programme in the year 1962. Smallpox eradication was achieved in 1978 through successful vaccination and surveillance programme.

Now the programme of immunization in India is one of the largest in the world. The programme started as expanded programme of immunization (EPI) in 1978; with an objective to reduce morbidity and mortality in under-five children caused by six vaccine preventable diseases (VPD): diphtheria, pertussis, tetanus, polio, typhoid and childhood tuberculosis.

After gaining experience, the Universal Immunization Programme (UIP) was launched in the year 1985. Typhoid vaccine was dropped and measles vaccine was added in the programme in the year 1985. UIP was implemented in phased manner in the districts with the objectives of rapidly increasing immunization coverage; improving the quality of services and achieving self sufficiency in vaccine production, besides establishing a reliable cold chain system up to the level of health delivery system and introducing district-wise monitoring of the performance. UIP was given the status of National

Table 12.49: Average annual reported number of cases of VPD (CBHI)

Years	Diphtheria	Pertussis	Tetanus	Polio	Measles	VPD Total
1974–79	26,855	3,37,930	54,219	15,132	1,37,782	5,71,918
1980–84	22,714	2,71,565	38,929	26,226	1,56,561	5,15,995
1985–89	13,137	1,60,840	30,229	2174	1,79,276	3,85,656
1990–92	9697	83,081	16,553	8368	86,552	2,04,251
2000	5125	31,431	3287*	265	38,835	91,228
			8997			
2001	5472	34,703	1718*	268	51,780	1,00,805
			5764			
2003	4237	34,240	5764	225	46,736	93,116
			1765*			
2004	—	—	3846	134	51,546	55,526
2005	5826	31,122	2981	66	36,711	78,135
			821*			
2009	3529	60,385	898*	741	56,188	1,21,741
2010	3129	38,493	373*	42	29,808	71,845
2013	4310	37011	535	0	16479	58,335
2014 (P)	4071	61467	572	0	23348	89408

*Tetanus neonatorum cases. *Source:* CBHI From year 2000 onwards confirmed cases of Polio Reported

Technology Mission in 1986, which became operational in all the districts of the country during 1989–90. It subsequently became a part of Child Survival and Safe Motherhood Programme in 1992 (UIP + programme) and from 1997 onwards being implemented as a part of Reproductive and Child Health Programme. Focus of UIP is to cover all infants, young children, pregnant women and adolescents.

UIP is one of the interventions for protection of children from life threatening illnesses which are preventable. Now under the UIP programme vaccination is carried out to prevent nine vaccine preventable diseases, i.e. diphtheria, pertusis, tetanus, polio, measles, severe form of childhood tuberculosis, hepatitis B, and Hib Disease. Since 2006 SA–14–14–2 JE vaccine has been introduced in routine immunization in high burden districts.

Multi-year Strategic Plan 2013–17 (cMYP) on Universal Immunization Programme (UIP). UIP is a component of Reproductive, Maternal, Newborn, Child and Adolescent Health (RMNCH + A) strategy in India.

Goal of UIP is to reduce mortality, morbidity and disability due to vaccine preventable diseases through high quality immunization services.

Key objectives of strategic plan

1. Improve programme service delivery
2. Increase demand by effective behaviour change communication and social mobilization
3. Strengthen health system for immunization
4. Strengthen and maintain surveillance system
5. Introduction of new vaccines
6. Contribute to global Polio-eradication, measles, maternal and neonatal tetanus elimination.

National Immunization Schedule (NIS) 2014

The national immunization schedule (NIS) has been evolved on the basis of epidemiology of disease occurrence as also to satisfy the needs of people to get service delivery by minimum contacts. The national immunization schedule is flexible and emphasizes completion of primary immunization within infancy.[33] If the interval between two doses increases, you need not to start afresh, and the first dose is to be taken into account to complete the schedule by administering remaining doses (Table 12.50)[32].

Changes in NIS: 2010–16

- DT Booster has been replaced by DPT Booster at 5–6 years of age.
- Govt. of India has introduced second dose of measles to be given with DPT Booster at 16–24 months
- Inactivated polio vaccine (IPV) has been introduced in UIP along with 3rd OPV.
- Rotavirus vaccine has also been introduced in UIP in March 2016

Prevention of Hib disease by Pentavalent Vaccine

Haemophillus influenza type B Disease (Hib) is a leading cause of meningitis and pneumonia in children under five years of age. About 2.4 to 3.0 million cases of Hib disease occur every year in India with 72000 deaths. Hib vaccine has been introduced in UIP in India as liquid **pentavalent vaccine** (LPV). The vaccine will have 5 antigens (DPT + Hep B + Hib) in a single formulation. Vaccination schedule—Hib containing pentavalent vaccine is indicated

Table 12.50: Vaccination schedule under UIP in India for pregnant women, infants, children and adolescents

Vaccine	When to give	Dose	Route	Site
For pregnant women				
TT-1	Early in pregnancy	0.5 ml	Intramuscular	Upper arm
TT-2	4 weeks after TT-1*	0.5 ml	Intramuscular	Upper arm
TT-Booster	If received 2 TT doses in a pregnancy within the last 3 years	0.5 ml	Intramuscular	Upper arm
For infants				
BCG	At birth or as early as possible till one year of age	0.1 ml (0.05 ml)	Intradermal Unitl 1 month	Left upper arm
Hepatitis B (birth dose)	At birth or as early as possible within 24 hours	0.5 ml	Intramuscular	Antero-lateral side of mid-thigh
OPV (zero dose)	At birth or as early as possible within the first 15 days	2 drops	Oral	Oral
OPV 1, 2 and 3	At 6, 10 and 14 weeks	2 drops	Oral	Oral
IPV one dose	At 14 weeks with OPV3	0.5 ml	Intramuscular	Right mid thigh
DPT 1, 2, and 3	At 6, 10 and 14 weeks	0.5 ml	Intramuscular	Antero-lateral side of mid-thigh
Hepatitis B 1, 2, and 3	Do	0.5 ml	Intramuscular	Anterolateral side of mid-thigh
Rotavirus vaccine	At 6, 10 and 14 weeks	5 drops	Oral	Oral
Pentavalent 1, 2 and 3**	At 6, 10 and 14 weeks	0.5 ml	Intramuscular	Anterolateral side of mid-thigh
Measles 1st dose	9 completed months–12 months (give up to 5 years if not given at 9–12 months age)	0.5 ml	Subcutaneous	Right upper arm
Vitamin A 1st dose	Do	1 ml	Oral	Oral
JE 1st dose***	9 completed months	0.5 ml	Subcutaneous	Left upper arm
For children and adolescents				
DPT 1st booster	16–24 months	0.5 ml	Intra-muscular	Anterolateral side of mid-thigh
OPV booster	16–24 months	2 drops	Oral	Oral
Measles 2nd dose	16–24 months	0.5 ml	Subcutaneous	Right upper arm
JE 2nd dose	16–24 months with DPT/OPV booster	0.5 ml	Subcutaneous	Left upper arm
DPT 2nd booster	5–6 yeasrs	0.5 ml	Intra-muscular	Upper arm
TT	10 years and 16 years	0.5 ml	intra-muscular	Upper arm
Vitamin A	The 2nd to 9th doses of Vitamin A can be administered to children 1–5 years old during biannual rounds, in collaboration with ICDS (Dose 2 ml)			

* Give TT-2 or Booster doses before 36 weeks of pregnancy. However, give these even if more than 36 weeks have passed. Give TT to a woman in labor, if she has not previously received TT.

** Pentavalent vaccine contain a combination of DPT, HepB and HiB. In the states where it has been introduced, it will replace DPT 1, 2 and 3 and Hepatitis B 1, 2 and 3. Hepatitis B birth dose and booster doses of DPT will continue as before. IPV (inactivated poliovirus vaccine) along with 3rd OPV.

*** JE vaccine (SA 14–14–2) is given in select endemic districts, after the campaign is over in that district.

12

in children from the age of 6 weeks up to 12 months. Three doses schedule is followed. The first dose of vaccine is given to children at six weeks of age or older. The vaccine may be given at the same time as DPT, OPV and Hep B vaccines. The dose of Pentavalent vaccine is 0.5 ml by intramuscular injection in the antero-lateral aspect of mid thigh in infants. Children will continue to receive DPT boosters at the age of 16–24 months and 5–6 years of age using DPT vaccine. Similarly, birth dose of Hep B using single antigen Hep B vaccine will continue and must be provided within 24 hours of birth. Pentavalent vaccine is safe and efficacious. They provide 85%–90% protection after completion of schedule. In general, the Hib vaccine provides protection for at least 15years[33–34]. The vaccine is contraindicated in severe allergic reaction and persons with moderate and severe acute illness. The minor illnesses, however, such as upper respiratory infections (URIs) is not a contraindication to vaccination.

1. The Strategies—Improve Programme Service Delivery

The universal immunization programme is an integral part of primary health care and the services are to be provided through existing health infrastructure. The aim is to cover all *"pregnant women, infants, young children and adolscents"* in the area. The programme of services must be sustained and high quality services be provided to the client. Following strategies are being adopted.

Immunization services are being provided through 153655 subcentres, 25308 primary health centres and 5396 community health centres, subdivisional/taluk/speciality hospitals, tertiary hospitals, urban health services provided by municipalities, hospitals and dispensaries run by railways, defence, and public sector undertaking, ESI hospitals and dispensaries. The vast infrastructure is unevenly distributed and some segments of the population may have poor access to services. Pulse polio posts have built massive awareness and enhanced the access to a considerable extent.

In addition to government health infrastructure, the private health sector also provides immunization services. Involving private sector in immunization and other national health programmes is essential to increase the coverage of services/immunization. Sustain high levels of coverage of immunization through fixed sites and outreach sessions.

Fixed Sites

All the facilities/places which provide health services and have cold chain facilities for storage of vaccines such as hospitals, immunization clinics, postpartum centres, district hospitals, medical colleges, community health centres, nursing homes, private practitioner's clinics are designated fixed sites for immunizations under UIP. Immunization services at these fixed sites have been established. Vaccination services should be provided every day or once a week on fixed day. These centres provide quality immunization services, maintain good records, and ensure high level of satisfaction.

Outreach Sessions—Microplanning

Fixed sites mainly provide services in urban areas or bigger villages where the community health centre is located. Fixed sites do not have any area responsibility, i.e. no geographical area or population has been assigned to such centres. People come to fixed centres voluntarily. Hence, the coverage of fixed centres is limited even in the urban set-up. Slum population is left out and fixed sites are not accessible to most rural population. Therefore, it is essential to provide immunization and other services through "outreach sessions" and outreach operations. Under UIP outreach, sessions are being organized on fixed day, fixed time and fixed site. "Wednesday" has been fixed for outreach immunizations in urban slums and rural areas. Health workers organize at least one session per month for every 1000 in rural and 2000 Urban population. In subcentre, area of 5000 population, five sessions per month need to be organized. If a village is very small, a session can be held on alternate month. Outreach session necessitates:

- Adequate planning of outreach sessions by health workers and their supervisors—"Microplanning".
- The beneficiaries must be enumerated (pregnant women and infants) by village or unit-wise. Best option is enumerate beneficiaries Anganwadi-wise (one Anganwadi serves approximately 800 population) on regular basis. Registration of all pregnant women and births in an area of Anganwadi will ensure good planning for outreach session.
- Every month get the number of pregnant women and infants to be immunized from each Anganwadi centre.
- Requirement of vaccines, syringes, needles, etc. must be submitted well in advance.
- Vaccines must be delivered to subcentre ANMs for each session by the medical officer in-charge of PHC or the health supervisors. All this requires the organizational and planning skills of health managers.
- The outreach session can be best held at Anganwadi centre or at any other suitable place conveniently accessible to mothers such as subcentre or school.
- The records of immunization must be maintained on mother and child protection card (MCPC). Every family must have a MCPC. The ANM should fill up the MCPC and must provide adequate information to mothers on immunization and completing the full immunization schedule. The family/mother must insist on having the MCPC and they must insist on the card being filled-up and updated on every occasion.
- Inform and educate mothers that the vaccines will protect their children only if all the doses have been given. Inform them the date/day of next visit and also about expected reactions.

- Reconstituted vaccines (BCG, measles) should be used within 4 hours.

National Open vial policy 2013: Reuse of opened vials in Immunization Programme: This policy does not apply to opened reconstituted vials of Measles, BCG Japanese Encephalitis (JE) vaccines and Rotavirus vaccine. The opened vial policy applies to multi dose vials of the DPT, TT, Hepatitis B, Oral Polio vaccine and Liquid pentavalent vaccine to avoid wastage of vaccines.

Vaccines opened in a fixed or outreach session can be used at more than one immunization session up to 4 weeks provided:

a The expiry date has not passed
b Vaccines are stored at appropriate temperature
c If vaccine vial septum has not been sub-merged in water or contaminated in any way.
d Aseptic techniques has been used to withdraw all doses
e The vaccine vial monitor has not reached the discard point

Discard vaccine vial if there is no label, if vaccine vial is frozen or contains floccules. BCG and Measles must be discarded within 4 hours of reconstitution or at the end of session whichever is earlier.

JE to be discarded after 2 hours of reconstitution or at the end of session whichever is earlier. Date and time of reconstitution must be mentioned on the lable of vial at the begining of session.

Campaigns/Intensive Drives/Mop up Rounds

Campaigns or intensive drives are organized as supplementary effort to boost up coverage. Campaigns and intensive drives are no substitute for regular outreach sessions or fixed centre approach. Campaigns and intensive drives are done to cover most difficult areas or inaccessible areas or these could be in response to an outbreak of vaccine preventable disease. Intensive drives such as pulse polio immunizations or National Immunization days are campaign approaches to cover large number of children. Specific antigen campaigns are also done to enhance coverage such as measles vaccination or special drive for covering pregnant women with tetanus toxoids.

"Mission Indradhanush": A special drive to increase coverage level of immunization has been launched in 2015 to avhieve more than 90% full immunization coverage by 2020.

Scheduling of Vaccination Session

Fix the date and time of vaccination session. This should be predominantly displayed at the fixed centre. In case of outreach operations, the information be displayed at Anganwadi centres and subcentres and advance information must be given to the community.

Ensure adequate supply of vaccines, syringes, needles, trays, forceps, bowls and cards for immunization. Ensure safe injection—one needle, one syringe for one child/injection. Injection safety is essential to avoid untoward reactions, infection and to prevent transmission of diseases from one child to other such as hepatitis B, C and HIV.

Sixty-five percent of **injections** given in India are **unsafe** according to World Bank and Government of India reports. The practice of reusing syringes for injections is rampant in India. Five billion injections are given annually but only 1.5 billion syringes are manufactured in India which shows the reuse of syringes. But for vaccine most other injections are avoidable.

Integration of UIP with RMNCH + A

The Universal Immunization Programme in India is also being used as a vehicle for administration of vitamin A prophylaxis to children and iron and folic acid tablets to pregnant and lactating mothers, apart from combining several activities of maternal and child (growth monitoring, antenatal check-up and promotion of contraceptives) with the immunization session. In essence, the UIP as an element of primary health care has been integrated with maternal and child health services, and family welfare services. It depends entirely on the health workers and supervisors how to make effective use of session on immunization by mobilizing additional resources such as ICDS Anganwadi workers, women groups, adolescents girls ASHAs, and self help groups.

2. Social Mobilization—To Increase Demand

If the immunization programme is to succeed the cooperation and participation of people is a must. This will make the work more interesting and pleasant. Involve women members of village Panchayats, Anganwadi workers, ASHAs, village Panchayats and Nagarpalika elected members and other community leaders, traditional birth attendants, school teachers for building favourable opinion and mobilization of mothers to enhance the acceptance of immunization services and increase demand of immunization services. This would facilitate the work of health workers and it would ensure increased coverage apart from client satisfaction.

Prime Messages for Behaviour Change Communication

- Immunization protects against several dangerous diseases. A child who is not immunized is more likely to become undernourished, to become disabled and to die.
- All primary immunizations should be completed in the first year of child's life.
- It is safe to immunize a sick child.
- Every pregnant woman should be fully immunized against tetanus.
- All adolescent girls at 10 and 16 years of age should get two doses of tetanus toxoid.

Coverage Levels of Primary Immunization

43.5% of children between 12 and 23 months were fully immunized (with BCG 78.2%, three doses of polio 78.2%, three doses of DPT 55.3% and 58.8% of children received measles vaccine) (DLHS3 and NFHS3-2006). UNICEF Survey of 2009 indicated 61% of children fully immunized, coverage for BCG 86.9%, DPT 3rd dose 71.5%, OPV 3rd dose 70.4% and measles 74.1%, Coverage of hepatitis B three doses in sixteen states was 58.9%. Thus the coverage levels of primary immunization need to be improved further through well planned strategy to achieve 90% full coverage (mission Indradhannush).

The major reasons of low coverage in many states are as follows:

- Not a feltneed and lack of knowledge.
- Immunization sessions not held regularly or ill-planned.
- Staff vacancies in the subcentre and lack of training
- Inadequate mobility of staff.
- Problem of delivery of vaccines to outreach sites.
- Inadequate health infrastructure in urban slums.
- Multiple agencies work in urban slum without coordination.

3. Strengthening Health System for Routine Immunization (RIM)

The Government of India under NRHM has taken following steps to strengthen routine immunization:

- Support for alternate vaccine delivery from PHC to subcentres and outreach sessions.
- Deploying retired manpower to carry out immunization activities in urban slums and underserved areas.
- Mobility support to district immunization officer and other officers.
- Review meeting at state level and training of ANMs and staff.
- Support for mobilization of children to outreach sites by accredited social health activisit (ASHA) and women self-help groups.
- Printing of immunization cards and other tools like tickler box, tally sheets, monitoring sheets, cold chain charts and vaccine inventory charts.
- Implementation of routine immunization monitoring system software.
- Introduction of Auto disable syringes for all immunization and replacing the existing glass syringes and needles.
- Downsizing the BCG vial from 20 doses to 10 doses.
- Strengthening of cold chain system in the state.
- Expansion of hepatitis B vaccination under the routine immunization programme in 2009.
- Introduction of HIb vaccine in UIP as pentavalent vaccine

4. Strengthen and Maintain Surveillance of VPD

The surveillance of VPD except for poliomyelitis is almost missing. The health workers must be motivated to report cases of VPD. Standard case definitions in simplified manner have been provided to them so that the cases are suspected by them are recognized, reported for quick response. Similarly community members be motivated to report the occurrence of VPD to the health workers. During the field visit, the workers collect information on occurrence of disease, and death due to any of the vaccine preventable diseases and adverse events following vaccinations. Similarly, the fixed centres can act as sentinel Surveillance stations for VPD. This has now been integrated with IDSP.

Sensivity of vaccines:

- BCG and Measles are sensitive to light.
- BCG, OPV, Measles, DPT are most heat sensitive
- DT TT, Hep.B, JE are least sensitive to heat.
- HepB, DPT, DT and TT are sensitive to freezing.

The Cold Chain System

The cold chain is a system of storing and transporting vaccines at recommended temperature from the point of manufacture to the point of use. The cold chain system ensures maintaining potency of vaccine and thereby its effectiveness. If the vaccines are not stored at desirable temperature, they lose their potency and ensure a false sense of security and we lose face in the community and it brings set back to the programme. The community and the health workers lose faith in the vaccine. Hence, cold chain is essential component of immunization programme in India.

Unnecessary large stocks of vaccines are not to be maintained at the peripheral health facilities and the principle of "first in, first out" (FIFO) to be followed. Follow the "earliest expiry, first out" (EEFO) procedure during distribution.

The cold chain system for the storage, distribution and transportation of vaccines consists of the following equipment:

i Walk-in cold rooms and walk-in freezer rooms at the regional level.
ii Ice-lined refrigerator and deep freezers at the district level.
iii A twin set of ice lined refrigerator/freezer at the PHC level.

From the PHCs, the vaccines are taken in vaccine carriers as no storage of vaccine is done at subcentre or village level.

Walk-in Cold Rooms (WICs)

Walk-in cold rooms (WICs) are used for storing the bulk supply of vaccines received from the manufacturers/

central stores. From the WICs, the vaccines are distributed to the command districts through vaccine delivery vans. Each WIC serves about 4–7 districts. WICs are situated at 113 locations in the country. Each WICs is supplemented with three deep freezers (300 litres each) and 10 cold boxes (22 litres each). The deep freezers are used to store oral polio vaccine and measles vaccine at –20°C. The deep freezers are also used to produce ice packs, which are required for transportation of vaccines in cold boxes from WICs to the districts.

Walk-in Freezer Rooms

Walk-in freezer rooms are located in few selected locations. These are used for the bulk storage of OPV and measles vaccines received direct from the suppliers through the cargo.

ICE-lined Refrigerators (ILRs) Capacity (300 or 240 Litres)

ILRs are top opening refrigerators. The ILRs are lined with pipes of ice packs. These act as buffer in case of power failure and the temperature inside the ice-lined refrigerator does not rise, once cold the ILRs can keep the vaccines within the safe temperature range even with an electricity supply of 8 hours in 24 hours cycle.

The bottom of these refrigerators is the coldest place. Hep B, DPT, DT, TT and BCG vaccines should not be kept directly on the floor of the ILRs as they can freeze and get damaged. Keep Hep B, DPT, TT, DT and BCG in the baskets provided with ILRs. There is no freezer compartment in the ILRs. You cannot freeze ice packs or ice in the ILRs. Maintain a cabinet temperature in ILR between +2° and +8°C. Place a functional dial/stem thermometer in every cold chain equipment to record the daily temperature even if there is an inbuilt thermometer.

The risk of cold chain failure is far less in an ILR than conventional refrigerator specially where there are periodic power failures. Avoid opening of ILRs several times.

Deep Freezer (Capacity 140–300 litres)

It maintains a cabinet temperature between –15° and –25°C to store OPV and measles vaccine besides preparing ice packs at district level. At *Primary Health Centre,* Deep freezer is used for preparation of ice packs and are not to be used for storing UIP vaccines. About 20–25 ice packs can be prepared by a 140 liter Deep freezer in 24 hours with at least 8 hours of continuous electric supply.

Conventional Refrigerator

This is being used less and less these days for stroing vaccines. If you are forced to make use of it then keep measles and polio vaccine on the top shelf near the freezer. These vaccines can also be kept in the freezer.

Keep DPT, TT, DT and BCG on the middle shelf so that they are away from the evaportator.

Keep the diluent (for measles and BCG) in the refrigerator not in the freezer. Keep the plastic bottles of water or spare ice packs on the lower shelf to help the refrigerator maintain low temperature in case of power failure.

Regular temperature checking is important and so is the defrosting. Maintain cabinet temperature between +2° and +8°C.

Cold Boxes

Adequate number of cold boxes have been supplied to all peripheral centres. These are mainly to be used for transportation of vaccines. In emergency, they can also be used to store vaccines. Before the vaccines are placed in the cold boxes, fully frozen ice packs should be placed at the bottom and sides. The vaccine should be placed in cartons or polythene bags and then placed in the cold box. Cover the vaccines with a layer of fully frozen ice packs and close the cold box. The vials of DPT, DT and TT should not be placed in direct contact with the frozen ice packs. The temperature in cold boxes should be +2° to +8°C.

Vaccine Carriers

Vaccine carriers have thick walls and lids. They are made of special material, which do not allow heat to pass through it. Vaccine carriers cannot make vaccine cold. Only a refrigerator or ice can make things cold. But these vaccine carriers can keep ice and vaccines cold for short time, because heat cannot go inside to warm them. Vaccine carriers are very useful for bringing or transporting vaccines from the primary health centre to subcentres for one day use. They will keep the vaccines safe and protect the children you immunize. Vaccine carriers are used to carry small quantities of vaccines (16–20 vials) for outreach sessions. Four fully frozen ice packs are to be used for lining the sides and the lid must be closed tightly. The vials of DPT, DT and TT should not be placed on direct contact with the frozen ice packs. The inside temperature should be maintained between +2° and +8°C.

Day Carriers

Never use day carriers which contain two ice packs or thermos flasks for routine immunization.

ICE Packs

Ice packs are used for lining the walls of the vaccine carriers to keep them cold. They are flat plastic sealed bottles filled with water. The ice packs are frozen by keeping them in the deep freezer. These packs help increase the holdover time.

Conditioning of frozen ice packs: Keep frozen ice packs in open till sound of water can be heard by shaking the ice pack. Wipe the ice packs dry and place the four conditioned ice packs against the side of carrier. Unconditioned icepacks may damage the freeze sensitive vaccines (DPT, TT and Hep B).

ADVERSE EVENTS FOLLOWING IMMUNIZATION (AEFI)

The vaccines introduced in the national programme are safe and effective but some reactions do occur after their administration, which are transient and subside in due course of time. Life-threatening adverse events following immunization can occur but these are extremely rare.

Definition: An adverse event following immunization (AEFI) is defined as a medical incident that takes place after immunization, causes concern and is believed to be caused by immunization.

AEFIs can be classified into five types: (A) vaccine reactions (B) programme errors/human errors (C)-coincidental, (D) injection reaction and (E) unknown.

A. Vaccine Reactions

This can occur due to active component of vaccine or one or the other components of vaccine (e.g. adjuvant, preservative and stabilizer). Types of AEFI can be:

a **Non serious vaccine reactions:** Most vaccine reactions are minor such as pain, swelling and/or redness, fever and systemic symptoms (vomiting, diarrhoea, malaise) can result as part of normal immune response to the vaccine. These reactions settle on their own

b **Rare and serious vaccine reactions:** Serious vaccine reactions are rare and may or may not have long-term sequelae.

- i Anaphylaxis 1–6 per million doses } can result from any vaccine
- ii Anaphylactoid reaction } can result from any vaccine
- iii Vaccine associated paralytic poliomyelitis with OPV up to 0.4 per million doses
- iv Disseminated BCG infections, lymphadenitis (including suppurative lymphadenitis) and osteitis from BCG (100–1000 per million doses)
- v Encephalopathy–From measles and pertussis
- vi Hypotonic, hyporesponsive episode (HHE or Shock collapse)–Mainly DPT
- vii Infection site abscess–from injectable vaccines
- viii Toxic shock syndrome (TSS)–from all injectable vaccines mainly measles. TSS: Abrupt onset of fever, vomiting and watery diarrhoea within a few hours of immunization, offen leading to death within 24–48 hours.
- ix Severe local reaction–from all injectable vaccines
- x Sepsis–From all injectable vaccines
- xi Seizures–All vaccine esspecially pertussis and measles.
- xii Inconsolable continuous crying lasting for 3 hours or longer after DPT, Pertussis vaccine. Adrenaline injection, antihistamine, hydrocortisone should be available at the outreach sessions and at the facility to manage AEFI.

B. Programme Errors (Human Errors)

Non-sterile injections, reconstitution with incorrect diluent, reuse of the reconstitution syringe, use of expired vaccine, inadequate shaking of T-series vaccine, incorrect site (Gluteal region) and route of injection, faulty storage and transportation, use of expired vaccine or diluent, contraindications ignored; use of reconstituted vaccines beyond the stipulated time (4 hours for BCG and measles, 2 hours for JE), and reuse of constituted vaccine at subsequent sessions.

C. Co-incidental Events

In general co-incidental events are clearly unrelated to vaccination for example pneumonia after OPV.

D. Injection Reactions

Some vaccinated children and adults may develop reactions, such as fainting, light headache, dizziness, tingling around mouth and in hands, breath holding in anticipation or as a result of an injection of any kind. Mass hysteria is also possible. Wherever possible the caregiver should be allowed to accompany the child being vaccinated.

E. Unknown

In same cases the cause of AEFI can not be determined.

Isolated AEFI

This is a solitary medical incident that takes place after immunization, causes concern and is believed to be caused by immunization.

Cluster AEFI

A cluster is defined as two or more cases of the same or similar event, which is related in time, and has occured within the same district or geographical unit, or associated with the same vaccine, same batch number or same vaccinator.

Surveillance of AEFI

All serious AEFI are to be immediately notified by the first person who identifies the event, to the nearest government PHC, CHC and/or the DIO by quickest means of communication. Detect, report and respond to AEFI timely and promptly, identify unusual high rates of AEFI, promptly address programmatic error (human errors) and maintain confidence of community and health workers in the UIP and promptly responding to their concerns are the objectives of surveillance of AEFI. Timely investigations and completeness of reporting are critical indicators of a functioning AEFI system.

Community preparation and communication with caregivers is imperative. Support and encourage reporting of AEFI by Health workers/Supervisors and by community.

5. Introduction of Newer Vaccines in UIP and Adult Immunization

The National Immunization Programme (NIP) established in 1978 continues to use the seven original EPI vaccines namely, DPT, BCG, OPV, measles and hepatitis B vaccines even though several newer vaccines with proven efficacy and safety are available and utilized in many countries in the world. We have not introduced any of them for want of the necessary mechanism to evolve policies and provide budget support. Prevention and control of diseases and their outbreaks using vaccination has been proved highly cost-effective. Therefore, the introduction of newer vaccines is likely to achieve cost savings for the national economy. The currently available newer vaccines, already licensed in India are MMR, oral typhoid, Vi typhoid, Hib, JE, Hep A, Varicella vaccines, rotavirus and pneumococcal vaccine besides IPV.j

MMR (MEASLES, MUMPS AND RUBELLA VACCINE)

WHO recommends two approaches for rubella vaccination:

a Prevention of CRS only through immunization of adolescent girls and/or women of childbearing age.
b Elimination of rubella as well as CRS through universal vaccination of infants, and in women of child bearing age as also community surveillance.

Globally most countries use MMR instead of single antigen—measles vaccine. Their intention is to control congenital rubella syndrome (CRS), which is a condition causing serious neurological, cardiac and eye (blindness) handicaps. By controlling the incidence of rubella infections, CRS can be significantly reduced. Routine childhood immunization is a preferred strategy of all such countries. Prevention of mumps is generally considered a bonus in using MMR. Interestingly India is the world's largest manufacturer of MMR vaccine.

Inactivated Polio Vaccine (IPV)—Salk Vaccine

The health goal of polio eradication is to stop wild poliovirus transmissions, but the economic goal is to discontinue vaccination in order to save all expenses on that account. India uses OPV exclusively for the eradication of wild virus. However, the price paid is of vaccine associated paralytic polio (VAPP) that accounts for about 25–30 cases annually. Moreover, the occurrence of reversion of vaccine strain viruses to pathogenic wild form and causing outbreaks of polio has been recognized in different parts of the world. For the above two reasons, all countries who can afford IPV have already abandoned OPV in favour of IPV. IPV has been introduced as an additional dose along with 3rd dose of OPV in Nov 2015 in entire country. While it is inevitable that India has to introduce IPV in the near future, the problem of high cost will remain as a deterrent. IPV or combination vaccine with DPT is licensed for use in India. **IPV** has been introduced as **one additional dose along** with **3rd dose** of **OPV** in **Nov 2015** in the entire country.

Newer Typhoid Vaccines

12

Typhoid fever is highly endemic in the country, predominantly in urban communities but less in rural communities. Urban slums have very high incidence with shift in age to the left and peak prevalence in 4–6 years of age. Although typhoid fever is transmitted via human fecal contamination of water supplies and globally the main control measure is provision of safe potable water, vaccination remains as an interim intervention to prevent disease in individuals. Today the cost of treating typhoid fever has increased enormously on account of drug resistance of the pathogen to standard treatment. Thus, prevention is imperative both as a public health measure and for helping in poverty alleviation. Interestingly when India adopted EPI in 1978 typhoid vaccination was included but later removed because of the perceived side effects of pain and fever. There are two new vaccines that are devoid of such side effects. It is recommended:

- To make available the whole cell killed typhoid vaccines to be supplied on demand. This will remain an inexpensive choice for wide use and its efficacy has been rated high. Its side effects are not serious and no worse than those of DPT. Moreover, it can be given even in infancy.
- Provide Vi vaccine, single dose at ages between two and five years in all public sector vaccination clinics in all urban communities. Such children may be given one repeat dose after an interval of 3–5 years.
- As part of any typhoid outbreak control, use, oral typhoid vaccine in the target age group, viz. 6–40 years.

Japanese Encephalitis Live Vaccine

It is a preparation of live attenuated JE virus (strain SA 14–14–2) grown on monolayer of hamster kidney cell culture. It is freezed dried vaccine, reconstituted by adding 2.5 ml of diluent. It has been manufactured in China. It is stored below 8°C. One injection of 0.5 ml subcutanceously to children between 1 and 15 years provides immunity lasting for more than 10 years. Efficacy of vaccine is between 80 and 99%. It has been given in campaign mode in the month of April–May well before the anticipated epidemic of JE. Following the campaigns in the high risk districts, the vaccine has been integrated into the Universal Immunization Programme (UIP) of the district. Children aged 16 months up to the age of 2 years are being targeted for JE vaccine. **JE vaccine for adults in 21** high endemic districts of India has been introduced in the middle of 2015 in age group 15–65 years.

Haemophilus influenzae Type B Disease (Hib)

Haemophilus influenzae Type B (Hib), a Gram-negative coccobacillus is estimated to cause approximately 8.1 million cases of serious Hib disease, and an estimated 3,71,000 deaths globally. Like Measles, Hib is passed from an infected person to an uninfected via droplets of saliva when an infected person coughs or sneezes. In India, available data on Hib diseases indicates that Hib is a leading cause of meningitis and pneumonia in children aged less than 5 year. The WHO has estimated that annually 2.4 to 3.0 million cases of Hib disease occur in India, with total deaths estimated to be at 72,000 (Watt et al, 2009; NATAGI Subcommittee, 2009). Hospital based studies in India indicate that Hib contributes 40–50% of all meningitis and 25%–30% of all pneumonia cases. Hib is most common cause of Meningitis and second largest cause of Pneumonia (after streptococcal pneumonae) in India. The case fatality ratio for Hib meningitis and pneumonia is in the range of 10–30%. In addition to mortality, Hib causes a substantial morbidity burden with 25–30% of Hib meningitis survivors suffering from long-term neurological sequelae. The introduction of Hib vaccine in UIP in India would prevent the morbidity and mortality associated with Hib disease and will reduce the infant mortality rate (IMR) in India. It has been estimated that control of Hib related diseases will reduce IMR by 4 percentage points. HIb vaccine has been introduced as pentavalent vaccine in India in UIP (2011) in eight states of india (Tamil Nadu, Goa, Kerala, Karnataka, Puducherry, Gujarat, J & K and Haryana).

Hepatitis A Vaccine

Although India is highly endemic for hepatitis A, the epidemiology is shifting towards gradually increasing median age of infection. Where endemicity has declined, adult disease will increase. Thus, we expect increasing prevalence of adult hepatitis A including fatal fulminant disease. The vaccine is safe and effective but very expensive. However, In India most epidemics are due to hepatitis E. Therefore, it is recommended that:

- Regional serological epidemiology be conducted to document the median age of infection in different regions and in different strata of communities. Universal immunization for Hepatitis A is not recommended in India as yet.

Varicella Vaccine

Chickenpox virus infects virtually everyone. Therefore, the annual incidence of infection equals birth rate. However, the age of infection is broad and covers infancy to senior citizens. A proportion of infected persons (about 20%) may have subclinical extremely mild disease. In many places, the disease is seasonal and outbreaks may occur once in a few to several years. Thus the magnitude of disease is recognized, however, case fatality and the frequency of serious complications and sequelae have not been documented. The vaccine is safe and effective but very expensive.

It is, therefore, recommended that:

- A review of published and available unpublished data on chickenpox, its complications, mortality on varicella zoster is undertaken.

Varicella vaccine may be used either at an individual level to protect susceptible adolescents and adults but will not have a significant impact on the epidemiology of the disease on a population basis. Varicella in persons who have received the vaccine ("Break through varicella") is substantially less severe than the disease in unvaccinated individuals. At the present time WHO does not recommend the inclusion of Varicella vaccination into routine immunization programme of developing countries.

Rotavirus vaccine: Govt of India has introduced rotavirus vaccine in UIP in 2016. It is live attenuated, oral liquid vaccine to be given to infants.

Documentation of Vaccination

All institutions or health workers offering vaccination must ensure the provision of institution retained records and clients retained records. This will help preventing unnecessary repetition of vaccine at a later age.

The Government of India has launched Mother and Child Tracking System (MCTS) to improve registration of pregnant women and infants and utilization of Antenatal Care (ANC) and immunization services. All immunizations should be recorded on Mother and Child Protection Card (MCPC) prepared jointly by Ministry of Women and Child Development and Ministry of Health and Family Welfare.

6. Contribute to Global Polio Eradication and Measles, Maternal and Neonatal Tetanus Elimination (*see* polio Eradication)

Adult Immunization Programme

There is sizeable disease burden due to vaccine preventable disease in adults (tetanus, diphtheria, rubella, mumps, hepatitis A and B, papillomavirus, varicella, influenza and meningococcal meningitis). Adult immunization schedule has been recommended by Centre for Disease Control Atlanta (CDC). Respective chapters on these diseases provide indications for adult immunizations.

REFERENCES

1 CBHI. Health information of India 2003. New Delhi: DGHS, MOH and FW, GOI; 2004.

2 GOI. National Child Survival and Safe Motherhood Programme. Programme interventions. Maintaining cold chain. New Delhi: MOH and FW, GOI; 1994.

3 GOI. National child survival and safe motherhood programme. New Delhi: MCH division, MOH and FW; 1994.

4 GOI. An update on measles immunization. New Delhi: GOI; 1990.

5 GOI. Measles Perspectives and Issues. CD Alert. Monthly Newsletter of NICD, DGHS, May 2005; 9:(5) GOI.

6 GOI. National Child survival and safe motherhood programme conduct disease surveillance. New Delhi: MOH and FW, GOI; 1992.

7 GOI. Medium term strategic plan for the universal immunization programme 2004–09. New Delhi: MOH and FW; Feb. 16; 2004.

8 GOI. Field guide for measles surveillance and outbreak investigations, GOI. DH and FW, November 2005.
9 NPSP Measles. Monthly Bulletin, January 2009.
10 GOI. Towards universal immunization. New Delhi: MOH and FW, GOI; 1990.
11 UNICEF. Assignment children—universal child immunization by 1990. Journal Concerned with Children, women and youth in development 1946–86; 69/72.
12 GOI. Basic guide to reproductive and child health programme for use by NGOs, New Delhi: GOI.
13 GOI. Polio eradication—National Programme launched. CSSM review 1995 July; 31.
14 WHO. The initiative for global eradication of poliomyelitis—a guide for clinicians. Geneva: WHO; 1994.
15 School of health sciences, IGNOU. Immunization, growth and development. New Delhi: IGNOU; 2003.
16 GOI. Pulse polio immunization in India—Operational guide. New Delhi: MCH division, MOH and FW; 1996.
17 GOI. Evaluation of pulse polio immunization (National Immunization Days) India 1995–96. New Delhi: MOH and FW, GOI; 1996.
18 GOI. Evaluation of Pulse Polio Immunization in India 1996–97. New Delhi: MOH and FW, GOI; 1997.
19 GOI. Surveillance of acute flaccid paralysis. Field guide and supplementary guidelines for institutional surveillance at district level. New Delhi: MOH and FW; 1997.
20 Anadrus JK, Quadras C, Olive JM, Hull HF. Screening of cases of acute flaccid paralysis—ways to improve specificity. Bulletin of WHO 1992; 70(5): 591–2.
21 GOI/WHO. National Polio Surveillance Project. AFP Alert Sept. 1997; 1(1).
22 Taylor CE, Cutts F, Taylor ME. Ethical dilemmas in current planning for polio eradication. Am J Pub Health June 1997; 87: 922–4.
23 Andrus JK, Banerjee K, Hull BP, Smith JC, Mochny I. Polio eradication in the WHO South East Asia Region by 2000: Midway assessment of progress and future challenges. J. Infect Dis 1997; 175 (Suppl. 1): 586–9.
24 GOI/WHO. National Polio surveillance Project Mapping up: Critical Issues. AFP Alert Feb. 2001; 5(1).
25 GOI/WHO. National Polio Surveillance Project. AFP Alert Nov–Dec 2001; 5(6).
26 GOI/WHO. National Polio Surveillance Project. AFP Alert. Jan–Mar 2004; 8(1).
27 GOI/WHO. National Polio Surveillance Project. AFP Alert. Apr–July 2004; 8(2).
28 GOI/WHO National Polio Surveillance Project. AFP Alert. Jan–March 2007; 11(1).
29 GOI. WHO National Polio Surveillance Project. AFP Alert. June–Sept 2006; 10(2).
30 GOI. Health Information of India. Central Bureau of Health Intelligence. DGHS, MOH and FW, Govt. of India, New Delhi 2003, 2004, and 2014.
31 GOI and WHO. AFP Alert. National Polio surveilance Project Jan-March 2008; 12:1.
32 GOI. Field Guide Surveillance of AFP. Third Edition. September 2005. Child Health Division. Department of Family Welfare. MOH and FW, New Delhi.
33 GOI, MOH and FW 2011: Operational Guidelines. Introduction of *Haemophilus influenzae* B (Hib) as Pentavalent vaccine in UIP in India, GOI, New Delhi.
34. GOI, MOH and FW, NRHM: Year of Intensification of Routine Immunization (2012–13). Ready Reference Guide for Health Workers. GOI, New Delhi.

ACUTE RESPIRATORY INFECTIONS

EPIDEMIOLOGY OF ACUTE RESPIRATORY INFECTIONS

Acute respiratory infections (ARI) in under-five children is one of the main public health problem in India. It is the major cause of morbidity and mortality in infants and young children below age 5. ARI contributes to 15–30% of all under-five deaths in India and most of these deaths are preventable.[1]

Definition

Acute respiratory infections comprise a group of conditions caused by a variety of pathogens including bacteria, viruses and ARI is defined as:

"An episode of acute symptoms and signs resulting from infection of any part of respiratory tract or any related structure, including nose, throat, larynx, trachea, bronchi, bronchioles, lungs, paranasal and middle ear." A new episode is one occurring in an individual, who has been free of symptoms for at least 48 hours.[2, 3]

Major Signs

Cough, difficult breathing, sore throat, runny nose, ear problem and fever.

Age Group

Under-five children are most susceptible to ARI.

Morbidity

Morbidity due to ARI is considerable. Most young children have about 3–5 ARI episodes each year and each episode lasts for 7–14 days. Although the vast majority of ARIs are self-limiting, these cause considerable discomfort; as well as adverse nutritional impact. Annually around 25 million cases of ARI are being reported in India (Table 12.51).

Economic Loss

Huge expenses are incurred by the community with massive expenditure on a wide variety of medications as well as burden on limited hospital facilities. ARI accounts

Table 12.51: Trends of acute respiratory infections (ARIs) in India from 2000 to 2014

Year	Cases Reported (million)
2000	19.65
2001	20.55
2002	22.13
2003	24.25
2004	27.48
2005	25.73
2006	26.15
2007	26.17
2008	25.54
2009	28.24
2010	24.72
2013	33.42
2014 (P)	34.81

Source: National Health Profile 2015 and 2013. CBHI, DGHS, MOH and FW; GOI 2015.

for 30–60% of all out patients visits and 20–40% *paediatric* admissions.[3,4]

Case Fatality

Ten to fifteen per cent of all ARI may progress to disease of moderate to severe intensity pneumonia. Case fatality rate varies from 5 to 10%.

Mortality

ARI contributes to about 20% of mortality in children less than 5 years of age, it is the second most common cause of death in this age group. ICMR multi-centric study shows ARI accounting to 15–30% of childhood deaths. It is estimated that ARIs claim around 6–8 lakh deaths among children each year.

Pneumonia

Around 10–15% of all children suffer from pneumonia each year. *Pneumonia* is by far the major cause of death in ARI.

Etiology

In India around 60% of pneumonia are caused by bacteria, mainly *Streptococcus pneumoniae*, *Haemophilus influenzae*, *Staphylococcus aureus* and *Klebsiella pneumoniae*. Fortunately, cheap and effective anti-microbial drugs are available to control these bacterial infections, and if given timely, selectively and with appropriate dosage schedules can substantially reduce mortality.

Risk Factors

1 Malnutrition (weight for age z score <–2).
2 Low birth weight, lack of exclusive breastfeeding during first 4 months.
3 Urban slum children living in overcrowded localities are much more exposed to the risk of ARI.
4 Lack of measles immunization.
5 Indoor air pollution.
6 Parental smoking.

NATIONAL POLICY ON ARI CONTROL[5–8]

Objective

The main objective of ARI control programme in India is to reduce deaths due to *pneumonia* in children.

Strategies

1 The main strategy is accurate and early detection and standard case management for reduction of mortality and the focus of ARI control is on children under 5 in whom majority of *pneumonia* deaths occur.
2 Continued high coverage of UIP vaccines is the key preventive strategy against measles, whooping cough and diphtheria.

Most of ARIs are self-limiting, but pneumonia needs to be treated. Fortunately, most bacterial pneumonias in Indian children are susceptible to the broad-spectrum antibiotics. However, wide indiscriminate use of antimicrobials can lead to bacterial resistance. Limiting the use of antimicrobial drugs to only those children who need them will have numerous health and economic benefits. The national policy on ARI control therefore emphasizes decreasing the inappropriate use of antibiotics for treatment of ARI, other than *pneumonia* in children. It is recognized that acute upper respiratory infections (AURI) rarely cause death.

Initiation

The ARI control programme was initiated in 14 districts as a pilot project in 1990. More districts were added in 1991. Since 1992, the ARI control strategy became part of CSSM programme which continued into the RCH-1 programme in 1997. Now ARI is part of IMNCI.

Standard Case Management

WHO—protocol/algorithm is widely used. This can be used at home level by mother, family and community and by all health care providers.

The basic criteria for diagnosis of pneumonia is based on the counting of respiratory rate. WHO recommends breathing rate of 60 per minute or more in an infant less than two months of age, 50 or more in an infant 2–12 months of age and 40 or more in children 1–5 years of age as **fast breathing.** In each case, respiratory rate should be carefully counted in resting child for a full one minute.

Management of ARI Infections in Children (Cough or Difficult Breathing[2])

The strategy of integrated management of childhood illness (IMCI) as applied to management of ARI can reduce mortality and prevent morbidity. ARI presents with cough and difficult breathing and most children with cough and difficult breathing have only mild infection such as cold and cough or bronchitis. Children may cough because nasal discharge from cold drips down the back of throat or they have viral infection of bronchi (bronchitis), they are not seriously ill and can be treated at home without antibiotics.

Four steps are applied:

1 Assessing the child by asking—looking, listening and feeling.
2 Classifying the illness of the child.
3 Decision for treatment
4 Follow-up of case (Tables 12.52 and 12.53).

By carefully "asking", "looking" and "listening" the condition of the child can be assessed. A child with cough or difficult breathing could have pneumonia, which is a serious disease that can result in death. However, the cough or difficult breathing can also be caused by common cold, blocked nose, dusty environment, whooping cough (pertussis), measles, tuberculosis and wheezing disorders.

1. Assessing the Child

The assessment is done by "Asking" how old is the child? Is the child coughing or have difficult breathing? For how long?

Age 2 months to 5 years:	Is the child able to drink?
Age less than 2 months:	Has the young child stopped feeding well? For how long? Has the child had convulsion? Has the child had fever?

Look; Listen; and Feel

Child must be calm.

- Count the breaths in one minute
- Look for the chest indrawing
- Look and listen the stridor
- Look and listen the wheeze is it recurrent?
- See if the child is sleepy or difficult to wake
- Feel for fever or low body temperature (or measure temperature)
- Look for severe malnutrition.

Danger Signs

Unable to breastfeed or drink, lethargic or difficult to wake have convulsions and vomits everything, strider in calm child and fever or low body temperature.

2. Classifying the Illness of the Child

12

Classifying illness means making decision about the 'severity' of disease. The purpose of classification is not specific disease diagnosis, its purpose is to make decision about severity of disease and choose line of action or treatment. Classification and categorization is done on the basis of danger signs or other signs and respiratory rate.

Colour Coding

Based on the signs, the child is classified into:

- Very severe disease—Red
- Severe pneumonia—Red
- Pneumonia (not severe)—Yellow
- No pneumonia: Cough or cold—Green

Each disease classification has corresponding treatment plan and should be followed after the child has been classified.

Treatment plan varies in children below 2 months and 2 months to 5 years.

Young infants (less than 2 months) can become sick and die very quickly from serious bacterial infections, are much less likely to cough with pneumonia, and frequently have only non-specific signs such as poor feeding, fever and low body temperature. Further mild chest indrawing is normal in young infants because their chest wall bones are soft.

- Some of the danger sings are different. In a young infant, danger signs include "stopped feeding well" "fever or low body temperature", and "wheezing". The sign "severe malnutrition" is not a danger sign in young infant, although it is in older children.
- Young infant must have severe chest indrawing to be classified as having severe *pneumonia*. A child aged 2 months up to 5 years is classified as having severe pneumonia if there is any chest indrawing that is clearly visible.
- The cut off for **fast breathing** is different.
  A young infant (less than 2 months) has fast breathing when he or she is breathing 60 times per minute or more. The cut-offs for fast breathing are 50 times per minute or more if the children are aged 2 months up to 12 months, or 40 times per minute or more if they are aged 12 months up to 5 years.
- Any pneumonia in young infant is considered to be severe hence should be referred immediately to hospital. Older childern can be classified as having "pneumonia" (which can be treated at home with antibiotic) or "severe pneumonia" (in which case they should be referred urgently to a hospital).

The classification of illness is assigned into three colour-coded columns, these are either red, yellow or green.

Red: Refer urgently to hospital.

Yellow: Give an antibiotic and home care.

Green: Give home care.

The colour of the boxes will help to determine the severity of illness and appropriate treatment plan quickly.

Table 12.52: The young infant age less than 2 months—classify the illness

SIGNS:	• Stopped feeding well, • Convulsions, • Abnormally sleepy or difficult to wake, • Stridor in calm child, • Wheezing, or • Fever or low body temperature	
CLASSIFY AS:	*VERY SEVERE DISEASE*	
TREATMENT:	• Refer URGENTLY to hospital • Keep young infant warm • Give first dose of an antibiotic	

SIGNS:	• Severe chest indrawing, or • Fast breathing (60 per minute or MORE)	• No severe chest indrawing and • No fast breathing (LESS than 60 per minute)
CLASSIFY AS:	SEVERE PNEUMONIA	NO PNEUMONIA COUGH OR COLD
TREATMENT:	• Refer URGENTLY to hospital • Keep young infant warm • Give first dose of an antibiotic (If referral is not feasible, treat with an antibiotic and follow closely)	• Advise mother to give the following home care: – Keep young infant warm – Breastfeed frequently – Clear nose if it interferes with feeding – Return quickly if: • Breathing becomes difficult • Breathing becomes fast • Feeding becomes a problem • The young infant becomes sicker

Source: WHO. Classification of illness and treatment guidelines WHO algorithm.

Young Infants (0–2 months) (Table 12.52)

There are three classifications of illness for a young infant with a cough or difficult breathing: Very severe disease, severe pneumonia and no pneumonia: Cough or Cold.

- ***Very severe disease:*** The presenting features are stopped feeding well, convulsion, abnormally sleepy or difficult to wake, stridor in calm child, wheezing, or fever or feels too cold. In such cases, the scope of treatment is very limited at first level of health facility. After giving first dose of antibiotic, the cases are to be referred to next higher level.
- ***Severe pneumonia:*** This illness is presented with fast breathing (60 or more/minute) and severe chest indrawing. Here also after giving first dose of antibiotic, the case is to be referred.
- ***No pneumonia:*** Cough or cold in this case the child will have a breathing rate of less than 60/minute and there will be no severe chest indrawing. Antibiotic is not needed in this case. Only the mother is to be advised for giving "home care".

In young infants, the pneumonia cases are to be taken as severe and to be referred after giving the first dose of antibiotic.

Children 2 months to <5 years (Table 12.53)

There are four classifications of disease for a child aged 2 months up to 5 years: Very severe disease, severe pneumonia, pneumonia (not severe), and no pneumonia: Cough or Cold.

- ***Very severe disease:*** The presenting features are—not able to drink, convulsion, abnormally sleepy, stridor in calm child, clinically severe malnutrition. Before referring the child (which is a must), first dose of antibiotic is to be given. Moreover, if there is fever, necessary first dose of paracetamol is to be given.

Table 12.53: The child age 2 months up to 5 years—classify the illness

SIGNS:	• Not able to drink, • Convulsions, • Abnormally sleepy or difficult to wake, • Stridor in calm child, or • Severe malnutrition
CLASSIFY AS:	*VERY SEVERE DISEASE*
TREATMENT:	• Refer URGENTLY to hospital • Give first dose of an antibiotic • Treat fever, if present • Treat wheezing, if present, • If cerebral malaria is possible, give an anti-malarial

SIGNS:	• Chest indrawing (if also recurrent wheezing, go directly to treat *wheezing*)	• No chest indrawing, and • Fast breathing (50 per minute or more if child is 2 months up to 12 months; 40 per minute or more if child 12 months up to 5 years	• No chest indrawing and • No fast breathing (less than 50 per minute if child 2 months up to 12 months; (less than 40 per minute if child 12 months up to 5 years)
CLASSIFY AS:	*SEVERE PNEUMONIA*	PNEUMONIA	NO PNEUMONIA: COUGH OR COLD
TREATMENT:	• Refer URGENTLY to hospital • Give first dose of an antibiotic • Treat fever, if present • Treat wheezing, if present (if referral is not feasible, treat with an antibiotic and follow closely)	• Advise mother to give home care, • Give an antibiotic, • Treat fever, if present, • Advise mother to return with child in 2 days for reassessment, or earlier if the child is getting worse	• If coughing more than 30 days, refer for assessment • Assess and treat ear problem or sore throat, if present • Assess and treat other problems • Advise mother to give home care • Treat fever, if present, • Treat wheezing, if present

	Reassess in 2 days a child who is taking an antibiotic for pneumonia:		
SIGNS:	WORSE • Not able to drink, • Has chest indrawing • Has other danger signs	THE SAME	IMPROVING • Breathing slower • Less fever • Eating better
TREATMENT:	• Refer URGENTLY to hospital	• Change antibiotic or Refer	• Finish 5 days of antibiotic

Source: WHO. Classification of illness and treatment guidelines WHO algorithm.

12

- ***Severe pneumonia:*** Here the only presenting feature is chest indrawing. For management, after giving first dose of antibiotic and first dose of Paracetamol for fever (if present), the child is to be referred.
- ***Pneumonia (Not severe):*** There will not be any chest indrawing. But fast breathing will be present (rate is 50 or more) per minute for 2 months to one year age group and 40 or more/minute for one year to <5 years of age group.

  In this category of illness, oral antibiotic (Tab. cotrimoxazole) for 5 days is to be given along with treatment of fever if present. The mother is to be advised for "home care". Reassessment of the condition of the child is to be made after 2 days. If the condition gets worse, the child is to be referred.
- ***No pneumonia:*** The child will come with cough and cold without any fast breathing or chest indrawing. No antibiotic is needed. Only treatment of fever, if present is to be given orally. Mother must be advised to give home care. However, if the cough is there for more than 30 days, the child is to be referred for assessment.

3 and 4. Decision for Treatment and Follow-up First Line Drug—At community Level

Dose schedule of cotrimoxazole (pediatric 20 mg trimethoprim plus 100 mg of sulphamethoxazole):

- 0–2 months–one tab. 12 hourly for 5 days.
- 2 months to 1 year–2 tab 12 hourly for 5 days.
- 1 year to 5 years–3 tab 12 hourly for 5 days.
- Cotrimoxazole is available at sub-centre

In view of increasing resistance of *S. pneumoniae* and H influenzae to cotrimoxazole, amoxycillin is recommended as the first line antibiotic for non-severe pneumonia at both community level and clinic settings. It is important to identify wheezing which can be cause of fast breathing, which may improve with bronchodilators without requiring antibiotics. Children with severe or very severe pneumonia should be admitted and treated with injectable ampicillin and gentamicin and supportive care including oxygen and IV fluids.[9]

When Referral is not Possible

If referral services for needed cases are not available, or if mothers are unwilling or unable to go to PHC/hospital, the above dose schedule has to be followed by the concerned health care providers for respective cases.

Treatment of Fever

Fever: All fever cases in young infants (less than 2 months of age) are to be referred to PHC or hospital.

In case of a child between 2 months and <5 years if the fever is low at 38–39°C, mother is advised to give only more fluids to child and continue breastfeeding and feeding.

But if the fever is more than 39°C Paracetamol tablet, in appropriate dose, at 6 hourly intervals is to be given. Mother has to advised to keep the child lightly clothed.

Home Care and Follow up

At home, mother should keep the child warm, continue breastfeeding and feeding the child and to increase feeding after recovery.

- To clear the nose if it interferes with the feeding.
- Proper dose of antibiotic for 5 days.
- Cough can be relieved by home made decoctions, e.g. ginger and tea.
- To bring back the child after 2 days for reassessment.
- To watch for danger signs, viz. breathing is difficult, child becomes sicker, and in such conditions, the child should be brought back to facility urgently.

Prevention of ARI

- This includes complete immunization against diphtheria whooping cough, measles and Hib as per schedule.
- Adequate diet and exclusive breast feeding.
- Vitamin A supplementation.
- Reduce indoor air pollution by good ventilation.
- Avoid exposure to cold.
- Education of parents and families: In most cases of cold or fever, parents need to do no more than give the child plenty of liquids, continue breastfeeding and keep the child warm and keep the air passages clear, and parents should know the danger signs apart from no smoking by parents.

REFERENCES

1 GOI. Acute Respiratory Infections in children—Policy document. New Delhi: MOH and FW, GOI; 1990.

2 NICD. Acute Respiratory Infections—Epidemiology and control. New Delhi: NICD, DGHS, GOI; 1988.

3 NICD. Acute Respiratory Infections and its control (in under-five children). New Delhi: NICD, DGHS, GOI; 1991.

4 WHO/UNICEF. Basic principles for control of acute Respiratory Infections in children of developing countries. A joint statement. Geneva: WHO/UNICEF; 1986.

5 WHO. The management of Acute Respiratory Infections in children—Practical guidelines for out-patient care. Geneva: WHO; 1995.

6 WHO/UNICEF/CARE. Better Health and Nutrition of children—Guide for Health Workers. New Delhi: WHO/CAH (SEARO); 2001.

7 GOI. RCH-II and family planning programme implementation plan. New Delhi: MOH and FW, GOI; 2004.

8 IGNOU. MME-103—Child health primary paediatric care. Indira Gandhi National Open University, SOHS, New Delhi 2003.

9 Mathew JL, et al. Acute Respiratory Infection and Pneumonia in India: A systematic review of literature for Advocacy and Action. UNICEF—PHFI series on Newborn and Child Health in India. Indian Pediatrics, March 2011; 48.

MENINGOCOCCAL DISEASE

Meningococcal disease is an acute bacterial disease caused by the Meningococcus bacteria (*Neisseria meningitidis*) and manifested by sudden onset of fever, severe headache, nausea and vomiting, stiff-neck and frequently a petechial rash, with pink macules and very rarely vesicles often accompanied by delirium and coma. Occasionally, fulminating cases exhibit severe sudden prostration, ecchymoses and shock at onset. Thirteen subtypes of sero-groups of *N. meningitidis* have been identified and four sero groups (namely A, B, C and W135) are recognized to cause *epidemics*.[1] The other serogroups (X,Y,Z) are less virulent.

Occurrence and Distribution

Meningococcal meningitis occurs globally, it can occur in endemic form, sporadic form and epidemic form. Outbreaks have been reported all over the world. In 1996, Africa experienced the largest recorded outbreak of epidemic meningitis in history, with over 2,50,000 cases and 25,000 deaths registered. Between that crisis and 2002, 2,23,000 new cases of meningococcal meningitis have been reported to the WHO. There is increasing evidence of serogroup W135 being associated with outbreaks of considerable size. In 2000 and 2001, several hundred pilgrims attending the Haj in Saudi Arabia were infected with *N. meningitidis* W135. Then in 2002, W135 emerged in Burkina Faso, striking 1,30,000 people and killing 1500. During 1999, outbreaks were reported from Ethiopia, Central African Republic, Hungary, Angola, Rwanda and Sudan. In Sudan, 22,000 cases and 1600 deaths were reported in 1999 and 10.7 million doses of meningococcal vaccine were distributed to the affected states.[2] In 2009, Nigeria reported outbreak of Group A meningococcal disease accounting for 17,462 cases and 960 deaths[3] while Niger reported 4513 cases and 169 deaths.

Indian Scenario

Major outbreaks in the country were reported since 1883. Major outbreak occurred in the year 1966 in Delhi. The outbreak was due to Meningococcus serogroup A. Another outbreak was reported in Delhi in 1985–86, after a gap of 20 years. During the outbreak (1966), a total number of 6133 pyogenic meningitis cases with 799 deaths were reported with an overall case fatality of 13% as compared to 1731 cases and 569 deaths in the year 1984. From 1986–89, outbreaks were reported in Delhi, Gujarat, Maharashtra, Madhya Pradesh, Andhra Pradesh and Haryana and from 1989–99 sporadic cases were reported from different parts of the country.

The CBHI data do not reflect the true situation of the disease due to under reporting. It is primarily institutional data and many institutes do not report or report irregularly. Another outbreak has been reported in Delhi and Haryana in the year 2005. During 2008 outbreaks was reported in Meghalaya with 2100 cases and 260 deaths and during 2009 Tripura reported 277 cases and 60 deaths. Durng the year 2013 total of 3578 cases and 194 deaths were reported in India (Table 12.54).[4]

Table 12.54: Cases and deaths due to meningococcal meningitis in India from 1984–2013

Year	Cases	Deaths
1984	1731	569 (Delhi only)
1985	10,446	831
1986	20,972	856
1987	10,679	794
1988	16,834	3304
1989	16,749	2291
2000	7857	991
2003	8761	623
2007	5077	307
2008	5924	534
2009	6745	467
2010	6885	367
2011	6629	464
2013 (P)	3821	197

Source: CBHI

EPIDEMIOLOGY

The meningococci most often inhabit the human nasopharyngeal area without causing any symptoms or with only local symptoms. The disease may become invasive with involvement of meninges and presenting as acute purulent meningitis.

Reservoir

Man is the only reservoir no animal reservoir is known. The bacteria can be carried, in the pharynx and sometimes for reasons not fully known, overwhelm the body's defences allowing infection to spread through the blood-stream and to the brain. It is estimated that between 10 and 25% of the population carry *N. meningitidis* at any given time, but of course carriage rate may be much higher in epidemic situation.

Transmission of *N. meningitidis*

From person to person by direct contact including–droplets and discharges from nose and throat of patients and carriers. Infection usually causes only a subclinical mucosal infection. Invasion sufficient to cause systemic disease is comparatively rare. Carrier prevalence rate up to 25% or more may exist without a case of meningitis.

Incubation Period

2–10 days (average 3–4 days) seasonal variation, more in winter months or spring.

Age-group affected: Primarily a disease of young children, occurs commonly in children or young adults. However, no age is exempt. About 50% of total cases occur in children below 5 years and about 80–85% of cases are under 25 years.

Male-female ratio: 2:1 in clinical cases.

Seasonal variation: More in winter months or springs.

Period of Communicability

Until meningococci are no longer present in discharges from nose and mouth. Susceptible meningococci usually disappear from the nasopharynx within 24 hours after institution of specific treatment.

Risk Factors

Younger children are more at risk. Crowded localities as in urban slums are more at risk.

Case Fatality Rate (CFR)

It depends upon how early the cases are detected and accessibility and availability of medical care. The CFR ranges between 5 and 10%. In untreated cases, however, it reaches 50% or more and during epidemics may rise dramatically.

Cyclic Trend

Cyclic trends have been observed. Epidemics occur every 8–12 or more years and lasting 4–6 years; the decline of epidemic takes place slowly.

Notification

Presently the disease is notifiable or reportable in few states/UTs of the country only. Considering the cyclic trend of meningococcal disease and occurrence of outbreaks in 1999 in many parts of the world, which may be due to rapid travel can spread to any country; it becomes mandatory to augment surveillance.

Vaccination

Vaccines against four specific antigens related to serogroups A, C, Y and W 135 are currently available. Two types of vaccines are in use—capsular polysaccharide vaccines and conjugate vaccine. In our country only polysaccharide vaccines are licensed for use. They are distributed in freezed dried form. Route of administration is intramuscular as either bivalent A+C vaccine or quadrivalent A+C+Y+W135 vaccine containing 50 μg of each antigen. Dose of vaccine is 0.5 ml given sub-cutaneously. The group A vaccine is more immunogenic than some other polysaccharide vaccines and it can induce an appreciable antibody concentration even in 3 months old infant. In some countries, recruits are routinely vaccinated with A+C vaccine at the beginning of military service. Duration of immunity is 1–3 years.

Vaccination Policy in the Country

- Haj pilgrims
- High-risk groups
- Routine vaccination of adult population at large is not recommended except during epidemic situation.

Chemoprophylaxis

Chemoprophylaxis has been considered for control of meningococcal disease but it has several limitations and its use should be limited to special circumstances. The aim of chemoprophylaxis is to prevent secondary cases by eliminating nasopharyngeal carriers. Chemoprophylaxis must begin within 48 hours of diagnosis. The chemoprophylaxis with rifampicin, spiramycin, ciprofloxacin and ceftriaxone is recommended. Mass chemoprophylaxis to control/prevent epidemic is not recommended. It is recommended for close contacts of case in the family or contacts in school or nursery classes or room mates, etc.

MENINGOCOCCAL DISEASE AND HAJ PILGRIMS

Visitors from the entire world arriving for the purpose of pilgrimage are required to produce a certificate of vaccination against meningitis issued not more than 3 years and not less than 10 days before arrival in Saudi Arabia.

- Adults and children over the age 2 must be given one dose of quadrivalent vaccine (A + C + Y + W135).
- If necessary children between 3 months and 2 years must be given 2 doses of polysaccharide vaccine with a 3 months interval between 2 doses.

In case of documented outbreak at the Haj site, all the Hajis returning to the country should receive chemoprophylaxis irrespective of their vaccination status.

Travellers Health Information

Travellers to areas affected by meningococcal outbreaks are advised to be vaccinated. For pilgrimage to the Haj and Ramadan Omra, Saudi Arabia requires visitors to obtain a tetravalent vaccine (against A, C, Y and W135) at least 10 days prior to their arrival in the country (Ref. WHO International travel and health. Vaccination requirements and health advice).[5,6]

INVESTIGATION OF AN OUTBREAK OF MENINGITIS

When analysis of observational epidemiology reveals a suspected increase in the number of cases in a given area or when clustering of cases is observed, an investigation should be initiated promptly.

Preparation

Trained epidemiologist should conduct the investigation. Team should carry with them adequate material for obtaining, analyzing and transporting spinal fluid specimens as well as antibiotics and other supplies.

Investigation should involve:

i ***Confirmation of case:*** Confirm that clinical illness is compatible with the bacterial meningitis.
ii ***Search additional cases*** in the community including those that may have been misdiagnosed/undiagnosed.
iii Obtain appropriate clinical specimens and send to the reference laboratory for confirmation and sensitivity testing.
iv Define the extent of outbreak geographically.
v Assure that appropriate therapy is given to the cases.
vi Proper control measures are instituted.
vii Make interim recommendation to local authorities concerning preventive measures.

The investigating team should review the hospital and laboratory records of all hospitals and health posts in suspected area and adjoining areas. Information concerning all suspected cases of meningitis and all examinations of spinal fluid samples should be assembled.

Determine whether or not an outbreak is in progress and define the extent of outbreak and control measures are to be implemented promptly.

There is no role of nasopharyngeal carrier estimation of meningococci in the control of outbreak.

STANDARD CASE DEFINITION OF MENINGOCOCCAL MENINGITIS

1. Suspected Cases of Acute Meningitis

- Sudden onset of fever (>38.5°C rectal or 38.0°C axillary), with
- Stiff neck

In patients under one year of age, a suspected case of meningitis occurs when fever is accompanied by a bulging fontanelle.

2. Probable Case of Bacterial Meningitis

- Suspected case of acute meningitis as defined above, with
- Turbid CSF

3. Probable Case of Meningococcal Meningitis

- Suspected case of either acute bacterial meningitis as defined above, with
- Gram stain showing Gram-negative diplococcus, or
- Ongoing epidemic, or
- Petechial or purpural rash.

4. Confirmed Case

- Suspected or probable case as defined above, with either:
- Positive CSF antigen detection for *N. meningitidis*, or
- Positive culture of CSF or blood with identification of *N. meningitidis*.

This case definition allows the detection of cases of meningococcal septicaemia.

Often the diagnosis can be made in the dispensaries (peripheral level of health care).

Diagnose in health centre where lumbar puncture and CSF examination are feasible (intermediate level).

Diagnose in well-equipped hospital (state or central level) for elaborate tests.

Standard Case Definition of Meningococcaemia

Probable

Sudden onset of fever (>38.5°C rectal or 38.0°C axillary) with or without shock, and one of the following:

- Petechial or purpural rash.
- Gram stain showing Gram-negative diplococcus.

Confirmed

- Probable case, and
- Demonstration of *N. meningitidis* or antigen in blood and/or CSF.

How to Manage Patients with Meningococcal Disease?

Meningococcal disease (either meningitis or septicaemia) is potentially fatal and should always be viewed as a medical emergency.

- Admission to a hospital or health centre is necessary for diagnosis (lumbar puncture and CSF examination) and for treatment.
- Antimicrobial therapy is essential and should be combined with supportive treatment.
- As contagiousness of patients is moderate and disappears quickly following antimicrobial treatment, isolation of the patient is not necessary.

Antimicrobial Therapy

Antimicrobial treatment must be instituted as soon as possible after the lumbur puncture has been carried out. Many antimicrobials are active against meingococci in vitro, but only those that penetrate sufficiently the cerebrospinal space and are affordable should be used. A range of antibiotics used for treatment are—penicillin, ampicillin, chloramphenicol and ceftriaxone. Chloramphenicol is a good and inexpensive alternative. The third generation cephalosporins, ceftriaxone and cefotaxime are also very effective.

Control of Epidemics

Management of Patients

- Prompt management of patient in hospital
- Augmentation of surveillance and
- Epidemiological investigation.

Immunoprophylaxis

It has been documented that mass vaccination campaign, if appropriately carried out is able to halt the epidemic due to serogroups A and C within weeks. However such a decision depends on many other issues, e.g. geographical distribution of cases, age specific attack rates and the resources available. If the number of cases is below the epidemic threshold, mass vaccination is not recommended. Mass vaccination of population may be considered only when attack rate of disease exceeds *10 cases per lac population* in a given area—usually a district. During epidemics vaccination can also be given to health care workers and other close contacts of cases. For the first time in the country, mass vaccination of the entire population (2–50 years age group) of two of the worst affected districts of Meghalaya by meningococcal disease outbreaks, has been carried out using bivalent (A+C) meningococcal polysaccharide vaccine during may 2009.

REFERENCES

1 Verghese T, Kumari S, Ichhpujani RL. Meningococcal meningitis. New Delhi: NICD; 1990.

2 NICD. Meningococcal disease—need to remain alert. CD alert. Monthly Newsletter on communicable diseases Dec 1999; 3(6).

3 NICD. Meningococcal disease—CD Alert. Monthly Newsletter of communicable diseases. October–November 2009; 13(3).

4 GOI. Health information of India 2003–04. New Delhi: CBHI. DGHS, MOH and FW; 2004, 2008 and 2010.

5 WHO. Meningococcal meningitis. Fact sheet N141 revised May 2003. World Health Organization: Geneva.

6 NICD. Meningococcal disease. CD Alert. Monthly Newsletter on communicable diseases. Special issue April 2005; 9(4).

SEVERE ACUTE RESPIRATORY SYNDROME

A new disease called severe acute respiratory syndrome (SARS) emerged in several countries of Asia in epidemic form in the year 2003.

SARS is a newly identified human infection caused by corona virus unlike by any other known human or animal virus in its family.

The disease came into notice when a patient was admitted in Hanoi (Vietnam) on 26th Feb. 2003 with respiratory illness and died on 13th March 2003 and seven workers who cared for this patient also became ill on 5th March 2003 (Nosocomial Infection).[1]

Incubation Period

2–10 days. Once a person is exposed to infection, it may take 2–10 days to develop the illness.

Clinical Features

The illness begins with fever which is sudden in onset and may be accompanied with chills and rigors, headache, general feeling of discomfort, muscular stiffness, body aches, loss of appetite, confusion and diarrhoea. Some people also experience mild respiratory symptoms at the onset. The main symptoms of SARS are high fever more than 38°C or 100.4°F, dry cough, shortness of breath, or difficulty in breathing. Changes in X-ray indicative of pneumonia also occur in 10–20% of cases, disease may become severe enough to require intubation and mechanical ventilation.

Spread and Transmission

The infection spreads through droplets/aerosols. The persons having close contacts with cases especially the health care workers and family members are at higher risk. Transmission mainly occurs from person to person during face-to-face exposure to infected respiratory droplets expelled during coughing or sneezing or following contacts with body fluids during certain medical intervention.

Case Fatality Ratio

The overall case fatality ratio was 11% but with much higher rates among elderly persons.

Case Definition (By WHO)

The patients are classified as suspected or probable based on the following criteria:

Suspect Case

A person presenting after 1st November 2002 with all of the following:

- Sudden onset of high fever (more than 38°C or 100.4°F),
- One or more respiratory symptoms (cough, shortness of breath, difficulty in breathing),
- And one or more of the following:
  - History of visit to SARS affected countries within 10 days of onset of symptoms.
  - History of having cared for, having lived with, having had face-to-face contact with or having had contact with respiratory secretions and body fluids of a person who has been diagnosed with SARS.

Probable Case

A suspect case having X-ray findings of pneumonia, or A suspect case with an unexplained respiratory illness resulting in death, with an autopsy examination demonstrating the pathology of respiratory disease syndrome without identifiable cause.

Occurrence

The disease occurred in epidemic or outbreaks and spread to 30 countries resulting in 8422 cases and 916 deaths up to 7th August 2003 giving case fatality ratio of about 11%. Outbreaks started in China (5327 cases) and Hong Kong and Canada and imported cases were recorded in other countries. It was thus a global phenomenon (pandemic).[2, 3]

12

PREVENTION AND CONTROL

Against SARS there is no vaccine or any specific drug available. The treatment of cases is symptomatic.

Response

The cases were notified to WHO by China and Canada as also by other countries of the world. Prevention and control measures were:

1. Isolation of suspected and probable cases of SARS in hospital or home, preferably in homes.
2. Observance of Universal Precautions by the health care workers and others who are likely to come in contact with SARS cases would prevent the further spread of disease as there is no vaccine or specific drug available for SARS.
3. WHO recommends that international travellers departing from places on the affected list should be screened for possible SARS at the point of departure. Such screening involves answering a few questions only. Travellers with one or more symptoms of SARS and who have history of exposure or who appear acutely ill should be assessed by a clinician and may be advised to postpone their trip until they feel better.
4. Under the international health regulations, all aircrafts pilots and masters of ships are required to provide a general declaration of health to the airport/port authorities and PAHOs/PHOs wherein any sickness on board is declared. This needs to be further strengthened and sensitizing all concerned to remain vigilant.
5. Do not visit hospitals where SARS cases have been isolated to avoid contacts.
6. Persons who come in contact with SARS cases should report to local health authority if they develop the symptoms of SARS within 10 days of exposure.
7. All persons disembarking in India were required to fill-up proforma and any person meeting the criteria of suspected/probable SARS would be referred to hospital for treatment and isolation. Mandatory screening for SARS was introduced in 12 ports and 21 airports in the country for all the persons disembarking in India.

NICD, Delhi and National Institution of Virology, Pune, were identified as nodal agencies for laboratory investigations.

Infection Control Guidance at Hospitals

- All persons requiring assessment for SARS at the hospital should be assessed at a separate area to minimize transmission to others.
- Cases under investigation should be isolated from probable cases.
- All suspected/probable cases to wear N95 mask or three layered surgical facemask or any mask of 0.3 mm filter size.
- Health care staff involved in treatment or cleaning should wear personal protective equipment (disposable masks N95 or triple layer surgical or a 0.3 mm filter size mask).
- *Hand washing* is very important and should be done before and after contact with patient, after activities likely to cause contamination and after removing gloves.
- Alcohol-based skin disinfectants can be used if there is no organic material contamination.
- Cases should be isolated or cohort placement should be done with independent air supply, exhaust system and bathroom facilities.
- Turn off the air conditioners and open windows, if independent air supply is not possible.
- Strict barrier nursing using precautions for air-borne, droplet and contact transmission.
- Movement of patient outside the isolation area should be avoided.
- Non-essential staff should not be allowed in the ward.
- Use disposable equipment wherever possible and dispose appropriately. All devices to be reused should be sterilized properly. Surface should be cleaned with broad-spectrum disinfectants of proven antiviral activity.
- All sharps should be dealt with promptly and safely.

LESSONS LEARNED

i. Early notification of cases and no hiding of cases.
ii. Timely global alert by WHO
iii. Travel recommendation and screening measures introduced in all the countries.
iv. International collaboration was achieved in this outbreak.
v. Weaknesses in the existing health system were identified.
vi. Outbreak was contained swiftly with general measures in the absence of any vaccine or drug against SARS.
vii. SARS will not be the last new disease. We must be prepared to face challenges of new emerging diseases.

REFERENCES

1. NICD. Severe Acute Respiratory Syndrome (SARS). CD Alert. Monthly Newsletter of NICD April 2003; 7(4).
2. WHO. World Health Report 2003—shaping the future. Geneva: WHO; 2003.
3. GOI. Annual Report 2003–04. New Delhi: MOH and FW, GOI; 2004.

INFLUENZA

The influenza is an acute viral respiratory tract infection caused by influenza virus types A, B and C. These are anti-genically distinct and there is no cross-immunity.

It occurs in pandemic and epidemic forms. Most pandemics and epidemics are associated with type A and

B viruses. These have two distinct surface antigens—the haemagglutinin (H) and the neuraminidase (N) antigens. Influenza is one of the oldest and most common disease known to man. It can also be one of the deadliest. The "Spanish flue" pandemic of 1918–19 considered to be the worst disease outbreak in the last century claimed up to 40 million lives and infected half of the world's population. The world could still experience an estimated 2 to 7.4 million deaths (projected from data obtained during the 1957 pandemic). An alarming reminder came again with the emergence of an avian influenza virus known as H5NI in Hong Kong, Special Administrative Region of China, in 1997 when one-third of affected patients died. Fortunately, this outbreak did not develop into a global health emergency.

PANDEMIC INFLUENZA

Influenza pandemics are caused by new influenza viruses. Pandemics are rare events that occur every 10–50 years (Table 12.55). During the 20th century, 3 influenza pandemics occurred[1] and During 2009 H1N1 pandemic occured.

Characteristics of influenza pandemics:

- Occurrence outside the usual season
- Extremely rapid transmission with concurrent outbreaks throughout the globe
- High attack rates in all age groups with high mortality rates even in young adults.

The world may be on the brink of another pandemic. Health experts have been monitoring a new and extremely severe influenza virus—the H5N1 strains. Fortunately, it has not spread easily from one person to another. Very limited human-to-human transmission was documented in health care workers and family contacts. If H5N1 evolves to a form as contagious as normal influenza a pandemic could begin and all countries will be affected leading to widespread illness and large number of deaths apart from economic and social disruption. Medical supplies, vaccines and antiviral drugs will run short. Regular flu shots do not provide any protection against the pandemic influenza viruses that are circulating right now. However, in India, there is no policy for vaccination against seasonal influenza.

Table 12.55: Influenza pandemics and antigenic shifts[1, 2]

Years	Designation	Severity	Death toll
1892	H3N2	Moderate	Not available
1918	H1N1 (Spanish)	Devastating	50–100 million
1957	H2N2 (Asian Flu)	Moderate	1–2 million
1968	H3N2 (Hong Kong Flu)	Moderate	7,00,000
2004–09	H5N1 (Avian Flu)	Mild	262
till date	442 human cases till Sept 2009		
2009	H1N1	Moderate	80,000

Disease Burden

During the most recent influenza outbreak in Madagaskar which began in early June 2002 and lasted until late August, more than 22,000 people were infected and 671 died. The victims were mainly children and had poor nutrition apart from lack of access to care. In the United States in the year 2001 influenza killed an estimated 20,000 people.

Clinical Features

For most healthy people, influenza leads to high fever, headache, coughing and a few days off work or school, followed by complete recovery. For the elderly and chronically ill, however, the disease can mean hospitalization and even death. In developing countries where it is often not perceived as a major public health problem, there is particularly urgent need to assess the impact of influenza and tackle the disease appropriately.

Reservoir

Human cases (clinical and subclinical) are the major reservoir during epidemic/outbreak. During inter-epidemic period, the virus may survive in animal reservoir (birds, poultry, pigs, equines, dogs and cats).

Incubation period is 24–72 hours and the period of infectivity is about 3 days after the illness. It is transmitted through droplet infection and it spreads very rapidly in crowded places.

Incidence and Vulnerability

It is not known how many people are infected and die from influenza, particularly in the developing world; but the elderly, chronically ill and young children are particularly at risk. In addition to death toll, influenza also inflicts a huge toll of suffering, medical consultations, hospitalization, absenteeism and economic loss.

Problem

Effective control of influenza epidemics or individual infection has not yet been achieved. The main reason for this is the continued antigenic variation of the viral surface glycoproteins, particularly of the haemagglutinin (HA), but also of the neuraminidase (NA), giving rise to minor amino acid changes at antigenic sites **(antigenic drift)** or major changes of the HA or NA structure that generate new influenza A virus subtypes **(antigenic shift)**.[2] Because of these problems, every year WHO expert committee meet and decide the composition of influenza vaccine.[3–4]

Vaccine

Each year WHO brings together, international influenza experts to decide the composition of the influenza vaccine for the next year. More than 250 million influenza vaccine doses are then produced and administered globally every year, saving hundreds of thousands of lives and reducing illness. WHO recommends that Governments begin vaccination campaigns prior to the influenza season and ensure that as many vulnerable people as possible are covered before the first case of influenza appear.[3–4]

In the absence of epidemiological surveillance regarding the influenza serotypes in our country, presently the use of influenza vaccine in India is not recommended.

Control of Epidemics

The epidemics are sudden and unpredictable. The influenza vaccine does not help to contain epidemic or its spread.

REFERENCES

1 GOI. CD Alert. Monthly Newsletter of NICD, Delhi. DGHS, May–June 2006; 10:5–6. GOI.
2 WHO (1981). Viral vaccines and antiviral drugs. Tech. Rep Ser No. 693. WHO: Geneva.
3 WHO (2004). WHO Urges an Increase in Influenza Vaccination. Composition for Southern Hemisphere 2003. Season Influenza Vaccine Announced. Press Release WHO/70 26 September 2002.
4 WHO (2005). WHO Recommends Influenza Vaccine Composition for Northern Hemisphere 2005–06. Influenza Season Note for the Media WHO/5–10 February 2005.

AVIAN INFLUENZA AND HUMAN HEALTH (NEW THREAT)

Avian influenza or "bird flue" is a contagious disease of animals caused by viruses that normally infect birds and, less commonly, pigs. Avian influenza viruses are highly species specific but have, on rare occasions crossed the species barrier to infect humans.

Avian influenza viruses cause two main forms of disease. "Low pathogenic" and "highly pathogenic" which has high mortality reaching 100% within 48 hours. Viruses responsible: influenza viruses are grouped into 3 types, designated A, B and C. Influenza A and B viruses are of concern for human health. Only influenza A virus can cause pandemics. The H subtypes are epidemiologically most important, as they govern the ability of the virus to bind to and enter cells, where multiplication of virus then occurs. The N subtypes govern the release of newly formed virus from the cells.

Current Outbreaks in Poultry

The current outbreaks of highly pathogenic avian influenza, which began in South-East Asia in mid-2003 are the largest and most severe on record.[1]

The causative agent, the H5N1 virus has proved to be especially tenacious. Despite the death or destruction of an estimated 150 million birds, the virus is now considered endemic in many parts of Indonesia and Vietnam and some parts of Cambodia, China, Thailand and Lao People's Democratic Republic. The outbreaks in poultry have affected many countries between December 2003 and October 2005: Republic of Korea, Vietnam, Japan, Thailand, Cambodia, Lao People's Democratic Republic, Indonesia, China, Malaysia, Russia, Mongolia, Turkey and Romania. Avian influenza affected India in Feb–March, 2006. West Bengal outbreak of 2008 was more serious than the previous outbreaks in Maharashtra and Manipur. More serious risk factors are associated with this outbreak.[2]

Outbreaks in India were investigated by NICD. No human case has been reported in India up to 2015.

Risk to Human Health

The widespread persistence of H5N1 in poultry population poses two main risks for human health. One: The virus passes from poultry to humans, resulting in very severe disease unlike normal seasonal influenza, where infection causes only mild respiratory symptoms in most people. In the present outbreaks with H5N1, more than half of those infected with virus have died. Most cases have occurred in previously healthy children and adults. A second risk, or even greater concern, is that the virus—if given enough opportunities will change into a form that is highly infectious for humans and spreads easily from person to person. Such a change could mark the start of a global outbreak (a pandemic).

Current Outbreak in Human Population

In the current outbreak, since 1997 more than 100 laboratory confirmed human cases have been reported in four countries: Cambodia, Indonesia, Thailand and Vietnam. Up to Sept. 2009, 442 human cases and 262 deaths have been reported in 48 countries. No human case has been reported in India despite of devastating bird flue.

Transmission

Direct contact with infected poultry or surfaces and objects contaminated by their faeces, is presently considered the main route of human infection. Most human cases have occurred in rural or peri-urban areas where many households keep small poultry flocks, which often roam freely, sometimes entering homes or share outdoor areas where children play.

The poultry products are safe for consumption in areas free of disease, provided these are properly cooked and following hygienic practices. In area experiencing disease outbreaks, poultry products can also be safely consumed provided these items are properly cooked and properly handled during food preparation.

Pandemic Risk

Though more than 400 human cases have occurred in current outbreak, this is small number compared with the huge number of birds affected and the numerous associated opportunities for human exposure especially in areas where backyard flocks are common. A pandemic can start when three conditions have been met: a new influenza virus subtype emerge; it infects humans, causing serious illness, and it spreads easily and sustained among humans. The H5N1 virus amply meets the first two conditions: it is a new virus for humans (H5N1 have never circulated widely among people) and it has affected more than 400 humans, killing over half of them. No one will have immunity should an H5N1 like pandemic virus emerge. All prerequisites for start of a pandemic have therefore been met save one: the establishment of efficient and sustained human-to-human transmission of the virus. Though rare instances of limited human-to-human transmission of H5N1 and other avian influenza viruses have occurred in association with outbreak in poultry and should not a cause of alarm. In no instance has the virus spread beyond a first generation of close contacts or caused illness in the general community. There have been a number of instances of avian influenza infection occurring among close family members. It is often impossible to determine if human-to-human transmission has occurred since the family members are exposed to the same animal and environmental sources as well as to one another. WHO overall assessment of the pandemic risk remains. The virus can improve its transmissibility among humans via two principal mechanisms "reassortment" mechanism and more gradual process of "adaptive mutation".

Other Reservoirs

Domestic ducks can excrete large quantities of highly pathogenic virus without showing signs of illness, and are now acting as a "silent" reservoir of the virus perpetuating transmission to other birds. H5N1 appears to have expanded its host range, infecting and killing mammalian species previously considered resistant to infection with avian influenza viruses.

Vaccine

Vaccines effective against a pandemic virus are yet not available. Vaccines are produced each year for seasonal influenza but will not protect against pandemic influenza.

Drugs

Two drugs (in the neuraminidase inhibitor class), oseltamivir (commercially known as Tamiflu) and zanamivir (commercially known as Relenza) can reduce the severity and duration of illness caused by seasonal influenza. These drugs should be administered within 48 hours after symptoms onset. These drugs involve limited production capacity and prohibitive cost for many countries.

So far most fatal pneumonia seen in cases of H5N1 has resulted from the effects of the virus, and cannot be treated with antibiotics. Nonetheless, since influenza is often complicated by secondary bacterial infection of the lungs, antibiotics could be lifesaving in case of late onset pneumonia. WHO regards it as prudent for countries to ensure adequate supplies of antibiotics in advance.[3]

Prevention

To prevent influenza, we have to eliminate the virus from birds, but it cannot be achieved in near future.

WHO will have a stockpile of antiviral medications sufficient for 3 million treatment courses by early 2006. These drugs could be used prophylactically near the start of pandemic. Despite of advance warning the world is ill-prepared to defend itself during pandemic. 40 countries have developed preparedness plans. India has prepared a contigency plan for management of human cases of Avian influenza.[3] India has stockpiled 10 million doses of Tamiflu.

PANDEMIC INFLUENZA (H1N1) 2009 (SWINE FLU)

The problem—Global problem.

Globally Pandemic influenza A (H1N1) 2009, first caused illness in Mexico and the US in March and April 2009. It continues to spread globally with more than 4,00,000 laboratory confirmed cases and 80,000 deaths reported to WHO.

INDIAN SCENARIO

India reported 19046 cases with 1747 deaths, in 2009 mostly in Maharashtra, Gujarat, with case fatality rate of 9.17%.

Current Pandemic

The current pandemic in humans is associated with influenza A (H1N1) which was earlier referred to as "swine flu" because initial testing showed many of the genes in the virus were similar to influenza viruses normally occurring in North American swine. But further research has shown that the outbreak is due to a reassortment strain of H1N1 not previously reported in pigs.[4]

Influenza type A viruses are divided into subtypes and named on the basis of two proteins on the surface of the virus: haemagglutinin (HA) and neuraminidase (NA). There are 16 known HA subtypes and 9 known NA subtypes. Many different combinations of HA and NA proteins are possible. For example, "H1N1" virus has an HA1 protein and an NA1 protein only. Some influenza A Subtypes (i.e. H1N1, H1N2 and H3N2) are currently in circulation among people.

Epidemiology

i Pandemic influenza 2009 was caused due to emergence of a novel virus to which all individuals are susceptible, i.e. overall population holds no immunity.

ii New virus has been able to replicate and caused disease in humans.

iii New virus is being transmitted efficiently from human to human (H2H)

In late April 2009, WHO, declared H1N1 influenza a "Public Health Emergency of International Concern". On 11 June 2009, WHO declared *Pandemic Phase 6* in response to spread of new influenza A (H1N1) virus. What it means? The same identified virus has caused sustained community level outbreak in at least one or other countries in another WHO region.[4,5] It is not related with severity. At this time WHO considered the overall severity of the influenza Pandemic to be moderate (Table 12.55). Monitoring the evolution of Pandemic virus and sharing information for public health response have been key components of the global response.

Phases

Phase 1: Predominantly animal-to-animal transmission-few human cases.

Phase 2: An animal influenza virus is capable of human infection.

Phase 3: Small outbreaks among close populations.

Phase 4: Sustained human-to-human transmission (H2H)

Phase 5: Spread across two countries or more in one of the WHO regions (continents).

Phase 6: Spread across two countries or more in one of the WHO regions plus spread to another WHO region.

The current WHO phase of pandemic alert is 6. WHO has declared the outbreak as *public health emergency* of *international concern*.

(*Source:* WHO: Pandemic influenza preparedness and response).

Post Peak Period: Levels of pandemic influenza in most countries with adequate surveillance have dropped below peak levels.

Possible New Wave: Levels of pandemic influenza activity in most countries with adequate surveillance rising again.

Post-pandemic Period: Levels of Influenza activity have returned to levels seen for seasonal influenza in most countries with adequate surveillance.

Who declared pandemic to be over in August 2010. In the post-pandemic phase India experienced outbreaks, as presented in Table 12.56.

Table 12.56: Cases and deaths of influenza A H1N1

Year	*Cases*	*Deaths*	*CFR (%)*
2009	19046	1747	9.17
2010	20604	1763	8.55
2011	603	75	12.4
2012	5044	405	8.0
2013	5253	699	11.0
2014	937	238	25.4
2015 (Till 9th march)	25000	1747	5.5

THE AGENT

Novel influenza A (H1N1) virus: The 2009 novel A H1N1 appears to be of swine origin and contains a unique combination of gene segments that has not been identified in the past. Genetic sequencing shows a new sub-type of influenza A (H1N1) with re-assorted segments from four influenza viruses: North American swine, Eurasian swine, North American Avian and Human virus. It has not been previously detected in pigs or humans. The present novel virus has shown sensitivity to oseltamivir but is resistant to both amantadine and rimantadine. It is an enveloped RNA virus and belongs to the family Orthomyxoviridae.

Transmission

It is transmitted from person to person. Influenza virus is present in respiratory secretions of infected persons. As a result, influenza virus can be transmitted through droplets by sneezing and coughing. It also spreads by *touching infected objects* and then touching nose or mouth. The pandemic H1N1 influenza virus can survive on hard and nonporous surfaces, in plastic and stainless steel up to 24 hours, on cloth, paper and tissue for 8–12 hours.

Incubation Period

It ranges from 1–7 days and more likely from one to four days.

Communicability

From one day before to 7 days after the onset of symptoms. If illness persists for more than 7 days chances of communicability may persist till resolution of illness. Childern may spread the virus for a longer period.

Infectivity

H1N1 appears to be more contagious than seasonal influenza. Secondary attack rate of seasonal influenza is 5–15% while secondary attack rate of H1N1 is estimated between 22 and 33%.

Clinical Manifestations

The clinical manifestations of H1N1 influenza A pandemic are fever, cough, sore throat, malaise and headache; vomiting and diarrhoea. Childern are less likely to have the usual influenza signs and symptoms such as fever and cough. Infant may present with fever and lethargy and may not have cough. Symptoms of severe disease in infants and young childern may include apnoea, tachypnoea, dyspnoea, cyanosis, dehydration, altered mental status and extreme irritability.

Outcome

Most people recover from infection without the need for hospitalization or medical care or antiviral drugs. Overall national levels of severe illness from influenza A (H1N1) appear similar to levels seen during local seasonal influenza periods, although high levels of disease have occurred in some local areas and institutions. Overall, hospitals and health care systems in most countries have been able to cope with the number of people seeking care.

High-risk Group (HRG)

HRG for complications of influenza is defined as a person such as:

- Residents of institutions for elderly people and the disabled.
- Elderly people and very young persons.
- People with certain chronic health conditions (chronic heart or lung disease, metabolic or renal disease or immunodeficiencies).

Influenza Surveillance

Surveillance of influenza like illness (ILI) is an essential epidemiological tool to monitor:

- Geographical spread of influenza pandemic.
- To identify high-risk groups
- To know the burden of disease in terms of health and economic impact
- To plan for preventive and other responses to control the pandemic.
  Standard case definitions are essential for comparison between different areas within a country and also between countries.

CASE DEFINITION OF PANDEMIC INFLUENZA IN HUMANS[5]

A Suspected Case

A suspected case of the pandemic influenza A H1N1 virus infection is defined as a person with acute febrile respiratory illness (reported or documented fever and one of the following: cough, sore throat, shortness of breath, difficulty in breathing or chest pain) with onset:

- Within 7 days of close contact with a person who is a probable or confirmed case of the new influenza A (H1N1) infection, or
- Within 7 days of travel to a community internationally where there has been one or more confirmed pandemic influenza A (H1N1) cases or
- Resides in a community where there are one or more confirmed new influenza cases.

A Probable Case

A probable case of pandemic influenza A (H1N1) 2009 virus infection is defined as an individual, with an influenza test that is positive for influenza A, but is unsubtypable by reagents used to detect seasonal influenza virus infection;

or

An individual with a clinically compatible illness or who died of an unexplained acute respiratory illness who is considered to be epidemiologically linked to a probable or confirmed case.

A Confirmed Case

A confirmed case of pandemic influenza A (H1N1) virus infection is defined as an individual with laboratory confirmed new influenza A (H1N1) virus infection by one or more of the following:

- Realtime reverse transcriptase (RT-PCR)
- Viral culture.
- Four-fold rise in new influenza A (H1N1) virus specific neutralizing antibodies.

Chemotherapy of Influenza A H1N1

Oseltamivir is the drug of choice. Dosages are according to body weight and age for 5 days.

Dose shedule of oseltamivir

Body Weight (in kg)	Age in years	Therapeutic dose for 5 days	Prophylaxis dose for 5 days
<=15 kg	1–2	30 mg BD	30 mg OD
15–23 kg	3–5	45 mg BD	45 mg OD
24–40 kg	6–9	60 mg BD	60 mg OD
>40 kg	10–12	75 mg BD	75 mg OD
For infants			
	<3 month	12 mg BD	Not recommended unless situation judged critical
	3–5 month	20 mg BD	20 mg OD
	6–11 month	25 mg BD	25 mg OD

CONTAINMENT STRATEGIES OF MOH AND FW (GOI)[6]

- Early detection, investigation and containment of cases of influenza A H1N1.
- Training and equipping manpower to investigate and contain number of cases.
- Strengthening of health care infrastructure.
- Stockpiling of antiviral drugs, personal protection equipment (gloves, mask, long-sleeved cuffed gowns, cap and plastic apron), N95 and triple layer mask.
- Increasing awareness by information education and communication.
- Management of cases.

- Lab network for influenza A H1N1 surveillance and contact tracing.
- Drug resistance monitoring
- Enhanced surveillance.

Broad Guidelines for Schools and Educational Institutions

1. To reduce the possibility of spread of infection, schools should be advised to avoid any large gathering of students during the course of the day.
2. It should be made mandatory by the school authorities that all class teachers should begin their class with active screening of each student in the class so as to detect any student who is having symptoms of flu (mild fever with cough/sore throat with or without bodyache, headache, diarrhoea and vomiting). If such student is detected, he/she should be referred immediately to the medical facility of the school. He/she should be further advised to stay at home for 7 days and observe strict discipline of home isolation. The onus of observance of discipline of isolation henceforth is shifted to the parents and accordingly the school health authorities should write a letter to the parents.
3. Closure of schools has not been recommended by Centre of Disease Control, Atlanta, USA. Its value in prevention of spread of disease within school is outweighed by the possibility of community spread, which is more likely because the childern will play and mix with public in various places and social gathering and there will be nobody to advise them or prevent such incidents. However, school authorities have to use their own judgment for any type of temporary closure in the event of wide spread H1N1 influenza in school.
4. In case of students staying in hostels, the school authority should monitor the health status of students as well as other ancillary staff in the hostel on regular basis.
5. In case there are suspected cases in the hostel, the authorised local medical authority should be called for examination of all students and school authority should not close the hostel/send the students back to their home.
6. School should discourage excursion of students to the affected countries.
7. However if students go on tour to affected countries, they should be thoroughly examined on return by medical doctor before permitting attendance in the class. If there is one suspect case of H1N1 then the whole group should be kept under isolation at home and their health status regularly watched.
8. All the schools should display and circulate "DO'S and DON'T" for H1N1 infection and frequently asked questions to the students.
9. Students, teachers and other employees working in schools/educational institutions are advised to stay at home if they develop flu like symptoms. They should consult the medical doctor and take treatment as advised including home isolation and drugs for treatment of the symptoms.
10. Students, teachers and other employees working in schools/educational institutions are advised to continue to stay at home for at least 7 days if they are advised by the doctor to take oseltamivir treatment and they should observe home isolation. There should be constant self monitoring and if symptoms deteriorate, it should be reported to health authorities immediately.
11. School authorities should not insist on production of medical certificate from such absentees.
12. Students, teachers and other employees working in schools/educational institutions are advised to *wash their hands frequently* with soap and water as also to observe strict cough/sneeze etiquette, i.e. using tissue while sneezing and coughing. The tissue paper so used should be kept in a separate bag, so that it can be disposed of safely. "Namaste" is better than hand shake to prevent swine flue and is well accepted in Indian culture. Regular cleaning of the area with cleaner is desirable, so that all the droplets and shreddings from mildly infected students are taken care of.

Guidelines for sample collection and handling of human clinical samples for laboratory diagnosis of H1N1 influenza:

Whom to test—Individuals with an acute febrile respiratory illness (a measured temperature of 100°F or higher and recent onset of at least one of the following: rhinorrhea, nasal congestion, sore throat, or cough).

Priority of testing should be given to:

Those who require hospitalization and those who are at high risk of severe complications.

To establish the diagnosis of pandemic H1N1 influenza A, an upper respiratory sample (nasopharyngeal swab, nasal swab, throat swab, combined oropharyngeal/nasopharyngeal swab, or nasal aspirate) should be collected. In intubated patients, an endotracheal aspirate should also be taken. Specimens should be placed in viral transport media and placed on ice (4°C) or refrigerated immediately for transportation to designated laboratory. Sample should be collected as soon as possible after symptoms begin, before antiviral medication.

Recommended tests: Real time reverse transcriptase (RT-PCR) in designated laboratories. Virus isolation should be carried out only by those laboratories which have BSL3 facility.

Management of Suspected Patients of Influenza A H1N1

Category A

Patients with **mild fever + cough/sore** throat with or without bodyache, headache, diarrhoea and vomiting. They **do not require** oseltamivir and should be treated for the symptoms mentioned above. The patients should be monitored for their progress and reassessed after 24–48 hours by the doctor. **No testing of patient for H1N1 is required**. Patients should confine themselves at home and avoid mixing with public and high risk members in the family.

Category B

i Category A + if the patient has high grade fever and severe sore throat – home isolation + oseltamivir;

ii Category A + one or more of the following high risk conditions shall be treated with oseltamivir:

Childern under five, pregnant women, those above 65 years, those with lung diseases, heart disease, liver disease, kidney disease, blood disorders, diabetes, neurological disorders, cancer and HIV/AIDS; and patients on long-term cortisone therapy. All patients of category B(I) and (II) should confine themselves at home and avoid mixing with the public and high risk members in the family. **No Tests for H1N1 are required for category B (I) and (II).**

Category C

Categories A and B + if the patient has one or more of the following: breathlessness, chest pain, drowsiness, fall in blood pressure, sputum mixed with blood, bluish discolouration of nails, irritability among small children, refusal to accept feed, worsening of underlying chronic conditions. Such patients require **testing, immediate hospitalization and treatment** with oseltamivir.

Guidelines for screening centres and isolation facilities in hospitals should be strictly observed.

Influenza A H1N1 Vaccine

Pandemic vaccine have their greatest impact as a preventive strategy when administered before or near the peak incidence of cases in an outbreak. In response to current influenza H1 N1 pandemic, the WHO strategic advisory group of experts (SAGE) have recommended use of influenza vaccine for health care workers as a first priority. The Government of India has taken the initiative to fast track the indigenous production of the H1N1 vaccine in the country. Target group for vaccine include pregnant women, people who live with or care for childern younger than 6 months of age, health care and emergency medical services personnel, persons between ages 6 months and 24 years old, and people aged 25 to 64 years of age who are at higher risk because of chronic disease or compromised immune systems. The US Food and Drug Administration (FDA) has approved the use of one dose of 2009 H1N1 flu vaccine for persons 10 years of age and older and two doses for children 9 years of age and younger. India launched a monovalent H1N1 indigenous produced vaccine on 4th June, 2010 meant for people aged 18–60 years.

REFERENCES

1 http://www.who.int/csr/disease/avian influenza/avian faqs/en/index.html. Retrieved on 23 Jan., 2006.

2 WHO. Bird flu outbreak worst so far WHO, Hindustan Times Friday, January 18, 2008, New Delhi, Chandigarh Metro.

3 GOI 2005, Contingency plan for management of human cases of Avian Influenza, DGHS, MOH and FW, Nirman Bhawan, New Delhi.

4 WHO weekly epidemiological record 4 September 2009, 84th year No 36, 2009, 84, 31-372 http: 11www. WHO.int/wer.

5 Government of India. CD Alert. Pandemic Influenza H1N1 2009, National Centre for Disease Control, DGHS. Aug–Sept 2009; 13:2.

6 GOI: CD Alert. Special issue: Human Swine Influenza: a Pandemic threat. Monthly newsletter of National Centre for Disease Control, DGHS. March–April 2009; 12:8.

MIDDLE EAST RESPIRATORY SYNDROME-CORONA VIRUS (MERS-COV)—GLOBAL ALERT AND RESPONSE (GAR)

It is a novel corona virus. The virus is believed to circulate among bats and camels. It has been around since 2012—for over a year, so it has been persistent in Middle East and continues to cause cases. It has been quite severe in those that it has infected; the case fatality has been about 50%. The tally of laboratory confirmed cases reported was 114 cases including 54 deaths up to 7th Sept 2013. MERS has spread to South Korea in 2015 where 87 cases and 7 deaths were reported till June 7th 2015.

While it is transmissible in health care settings. It is not that easily transmissible outside of that. There is no specific medicines right now. Firstly, observe general measures such as hand washing, hand hygiene as it turns out to be an extremely important way to prevent yourself from getting infected. Secondly, if respiratory symptoms become severe—high fever and troubled breathing you must seek care. Thirdly, cough and sneeze into tissue papers or perhaps into sleeves of your shirt. Ensure systematic implementation of infection control measures in hospitals. WHO is monitoring the situation very closely and so far it has not been declared as Public Health Emergency of concern under IHR. Health care providers are advised to maintain vigilance and continue their surveillance for severe acute respiratory infection (SARI).

Ebola Virus Disease (EVD)

The world Health Organization declared EVD outbreak in West Africa as a public health emergency of international concern on 8.8.2014 and issued detailed advisories for countries to prevent their citizens from risk.

Epidemiology and Surveillance of EVD

Ebola virus has been named after a river in Congo, where disease was first recognised in 1976. EVD is severe, often fatal illness, with case fatality rate of up to 90%. It is one of the word's most virulent diseases.

Transmission

Ebola is introduced into human population through close contact with the blood, secretions, organs or other body fluids of infected animals. In Africa infection has been documented through handling of infected chempanzees, gorillas, fruit bats, monkeys, forest antelopes and procupines found ill or dead in rainforest. Ebola then spreads in the community through human to human transmission, with infection resulting from direct contact (through broken skin or mucous membranes) with the blood, secretions, organs and other body fluids of infected people and indirect contact with environments contaminated with such fluids.

People are infectious as long as their blood and secretions contain the virus. Ebola virus was isolated from semen 61 days after onset of illness in a man infected in laboratory.

Incubation Period

Incubation period is 2–21 days (Time interval from infection to onset of symptoms)

Distribution of EVD: 1711 cases of EVD and 932 deaths (case fatality rate of 54%) have been reported from Guinea, Liberia, Nigeria and Siera Leone up to 4th August 2014.

Symptoms

Sudden onset of fever, intense weakness, muscle pain, headache, sore throat, vomiting, diarrhoea, impaired kidney and liver function and in some cases internal and external bleeding. Laboratory findings include low white blood cell and platelet counts and elevated liver enzymes.

Diagnosis

Other diseases should be ruled out before the diagnosis of EVD be made include: malaria, typhoid fever, shigellosis, cholera, leptospirosis, plague, rickettsiosis relapsing fever, hepatitis and other viral haemorrhagic fevers. Lab tests include ELISA (antibody capture enzyme-linked immunosorbent assay), antigen detection test, reverse transcriptase polymerase chain reaction (RT-PCR) assay, electron microscopy and virus isolation by cell culture.

Management of Cases and Prevention of EVD

This includes isolation and quarantine measures and symptomatic treatment as there is no vaccine or specific drug against the virus. Standard precautions are to be observed to reduce the risk of transmission of bloodborne and other pathogens. These include the basic level of infection control–hand hygiene, use of personal protective equipment to avoid direct contact with blood and body fluids, prevention of needle stick injuries from other sharp instruments, and a set of environmental controlls.

In India advisories to state disease surveillance units for early detection and management have been issued by Ministry of Health, and all Air ports have designated facilities to manage travellers manifesting with Ebola symptoms.

The disease (EVD) has killed 4922 till 26.10.2014 people in West Africa with no sign of Abating. Number of confirmed, Probable and suspected cases has risen to 10141.

A spanish nurse: Teresa Romeo, this is the first person to have contracted Ebola outside of Africa as also a nurse in USA. One UN health worker died in Germany. WHO says there could be upto 10000 new cases of Ebola per week within two months if the response to the Ebola crisis is not stepped up within 60 days (isolation of 70% cases within two months to reverse the outbreak).

REFERENCE

1 WHO Global Alert and Response (GAR). Ebola virus disease update–West Africa Disease outbreak news 4th August 2014.

YAWS AND ITS ERADICATION PROGRAMME (YEP)

Yaws is disfiguring, disabilitating, non-venereal treponemal infection. It is a contagious disease transmitted by direct (person-to-person) contact with infectious yaws lesions. The disease can be cured and prevented by a single injection of long-acting benzathine benzyl penicillin. Yaws is amenable to eradication.

Causative Organism

The organism responsible for Yaws is *Treponema pallidum* subspecies *pertenue*. It is morphologically and immunologically identical to *T. pallidum* (the organism that causes venereal syphilis).

Lesions

Early or Infectious Yaws

Yaws is characterized by skin lesion with exudates which may dry up to form scabs and yellow crusted granulomatus eruptions on the skin. The lesions may appear as papillomata, ulceropapilloma; crab yaws appear on plantar surface causing limping in gait; hyperkeratosis on palmar and plantar surface, nodules, polydactylitis due to inflammation of interphalangeal joints, osteoperiostitis and hypertrophic osteitis.

The initial lesions may persist for 3–6 months and heal spontaneously, often leaving a scar.

Late Yaws

Usually after 5 years of onset of illness, destructive and often deforming lesions of skin and bone may appear. The late lesions are non-infectious. The late lesions consist of gummas of skin and subcutaneous tissues, hyperkeratosis, chronic ulcers of skin and subcutaneous tissues, scars, multiple pathological fractures and ulcerated nodules.

Reservoir

Man is the only reservoir of infection. The early cases of yaws are infectious and serve as source of infection.

Incubation period: 9–90 days (average 21 days).

Mode of transmission: Yaws is transmitted by direct (person-to-person) contact with exudates or serum from infectious yaws lesions. Abrasions, scratches and injuries to skin facilitate penetration of *Treponema*. Infection through intact skin is doubtful.

Person affected: Early yaws is primarily a disease of children and adolescents in the endemic areas.

Seasonal variation: Because of humid environments during rainy season, transmission of infection increases and the incidence of eruption of lesions in latent cases result in high prevalence.

Geographic distribution: It is endemic in several countries. Due to the efforts of WHO and UNICEF in launching of Treponema control programme (TCP), the Prevalence was reduced by more than 95% in 46 countries. Subsequently, the TCP became the part of primary health care.

India

Yaws has been endemic in India. The disease has been reported from the communities living in hilly and forested areas in the tribals inhabited belt, affecting 51 districts of 10 states namely—Andhra Pradesh, Assam, Chhattisgarh, Gujarat, Jharkhand, Madhya Pradesh, Maharashtra, Odisha, Tamil Nadu and Uttar Pradesh. Yaws begins where road ends in these areas.

Problem

It affects the tribal areas. It is disabling disease and has social relevance. During the acute infection, the patient is highly infectious, but it is the chronicity of the infection that gradually destroys the bones and cartilages leading to permanent crippling and disfiguring of individual.

Latent cases are 5–10 times more than clinical cases. In India, the disease is mostly known by the name of the tribe affected. For example in Bastar district, the disease is called "Madia Roga" and in Maharashtra in Sironcha area it is called "Gandi Roga" and in Andhra Pradesh it is called "Koya Rogam".

Due to mass campaign launched in 1950 by WHO and UNICEF, the disease prevalence has been brought down from 14.0% to below 0.1% in many areas. Following dramatic decline in transmission, the active anti-yaws activities were abandoned in endemic area and consequently there was resurgence of yaws in 1977. NICD, Delhi was made nodal agency by the Government of India for planning, guidance, coordination, monitoring and evaluation of the programme.

Laboratory Diagnosis

Commonly used tests are venereal disease research laboratory (VDRL) test and the rapid plasma reagin (RPR) test. Both these tests are inexpensive.

Treatment

Injection Benzathine pencillin is the drug of choice. Alternate drugs are tetracycline and erythromycin (Table 12.57).

Tetracycline is not given to pregnant and lactating women and children below 8 years of age.

YAWS ERADICATION PROGRAMME

The disease is a significant public health problem in tribal areas. Yaw is not a killer disease but it is crippling and disabling disease affecting tribal people who are poor, unreached and susceptible. A simple, affordable and acceptable treatment is available for eradicating the disease. WHO expert committee on venereal disease and treponematoses has also stressed that from technical considerations, eradication is feasible.

The Government of India launched eradication programme on Yaws as Pilot Project in Koraput district of Odisha in 1996–97. Subsequently, the scheme was expanded to the states of Andhra Pradesh, Gujarat, Madhya Pradesh and Maharashtra. The programme was extended to all endemic areas in 1999. Currently, the programme is operational in 51 districts of 10 states; which are endemic.[1,2]

Programme Objectives

The yaws eradication programme aims to interrupt the transmission of yaws infection in the country (i.e. no

Table 12.57: Dosages of drugs used in Yaws eradication programme

Age	*Drug*	*Dose*	*Route*	*Duration*
<10 years	Benzathine benzyl penicillin	0.6 million units	IM	Single dose
>10 years	-do-	1.2 million units	IM	Single dose
<8 years	Erythromycin	30 mg/kg body wt. in 4 divided doses	Oral	15 days
8–15 years	Tetracycline or erythromycin	250 mg four times daily	Oral	15 days
>15 years	Tetracycline or erythromycin	500 mg four times daily	Oral	15 days

infectious cases) and ultimately achieving the goal of yaws eradication (i.e. no sero-reactivity to RPR/VDRL in 1–5 years old children). National health policy has set the goal to eradicate yaws by 2005.[3]

Programme Management

NICD has been identified as nodal agency by the Government of India for planning, guidance, coordination monitoring and evaluation of the programme. The programme is being implemented by the states as integral to part of primary health care delivery system in collaboration with the department of Tribal Welfare and other related institutions.

Programme Strategies

To achieve the stated objectives, following strategies are being adopted:

- Manpower development by in-service training.
- Case finding—by active surveillance, by making house-to-house visit, by trained paramedical workers and community level functionaries at frequent intervals. The active searches are required to be carried out every year of which one should be in post-monsoon season for better yield of cases,[4] besides passive surveillance and rumour reporting.
- Treatment of cases and contacts simultaneously.
- Information, education and communication activities.
- Multisectoral—coordinated approach.

Yaws "Eliminated" in India

India declared Yaws elimination on 19th September 2006. However monthly surveillance, active search operations, verification of rumour reports, health eduction and sero-survey in 1–5 years children are being undertaken as per international requirement to eradicate the disease. One of the criteria for eradication has been to establish "NIL" Yaws transmission by proving 'NIL' Sero-reactivity to RPR/VDRL/TPHA among 1–5 years old children.[5,6]

Desired sample size of children 1–5 years from yaws affected villages and yaws non-affected villages will be collected by random sample method. Sero-surveys shall be carried out once a year coinciding with active searches.

Impact (Table 12.58)

Reports received from 1996 to 2015 from various states confirm zero incidence of new infectious cases from 2004–15, based on the evidence of search and lab tests.

Problems

Physical inaccessibility in tribal areas, poverty, ignorance, illiteracy poses problems in coverage and search activities. Ensuring effective coordination between tribal welfare, health sector, Anganwadi workers, schools, local tribal community leaders will ensure better outcomes.

REFERENCES

1 Government of India, NICD. Yaws surveillance and Eradication. A tool to reach the unreached tribal areas. CD Alert; Vol 6(6): 2002. Monthly Newsletter of NICD, DGHS; Govt. of India.

2 Government of India, NICD. Yaws: Diseases of antiquity, challenge for future CD Alert; Vol. 1 (1): 1997. Monthly Newsletter of Communicable disease. NICD, Delhi.

3 Government of India. National Health Policy-2002. Govt. of India.

4 Government of India. Annual Report 2003–04. Ministry of Health and Family Welfare, Govt. of India, New Delhi.

Table 12.58: Reported cases of Yaws from 1996–2015

States	1996	1997	1998	1999	2000	2001	2002	2003	2004–2015
Andhra Pradesh	223	249	338	339	442	152	135	6	0
Chhattisgarh	NA	71	170	40	38	12	0	0	0
Odisha	3348	379	111	82	124	137	145	40	0
Maharashtra	NA	0	48	0	1	0	0	0	0
Gujarat	NA	36	0	2	17	8	0	0	0
Tamil Nadu	NA	0	0	0	34	0	0	0	0
Assam	NA	NA	NA	4	7	4	1	0	0
MP and Jharkhand	NA	NA	NA	NA	0	0	0	0	0
UP	NA	0	0	0	1	0	0	0	0
Total	3751	735	667	467	664	313	281	46	0

12

5 GOI and WHO. Yaws elimination in India. A step towards eradication. NICD. New Delhi, Sept 2006.
6 GOI. NICD. Yaws Eradication, CD Alert. Monthly Newsletter of NICD, DGHS, August 2008; 12: (4).

NATIONAL PROGRAMME FOR CONTAINMENT OF ANTIMICROBIAL RESISTANCE IN 12TH PLAN AT NCDC

Activities

- Surveillance for containment of antimicrobial resistance in various geographical regions.
- Rational use of drugs.
- Development and implementation of national infection control guidelines.
- Training and capacity building of professionals.
- Information education and Communication activities to build awareness.
- A common unified national treatment guidelines for treatment of different infectious diseases.
- Development of national repository of bacterial strains/ cultures.

ZIKA VIRUS INFECTION/DISEASE

In may 2015 Brazil reported first case of zika since then the disease has spread to 28 countries. The diseases is commanding worldwide attention becauses of an alarming link with severe birth defects (microcephaly) and Guillain barre syndrome. The disease is transmitted by aedes aegyti mosquito. Common symptoms and signs are fever, rash, joint pains and conjunctivitis. There is no vaccine or specific medicine against the virus. Zika virus outbreak has been declared by WHO as a Global Public Health Emergency of International concern on Feb 01, 2016. About 3 million cases were estimated in Latin American countries hardest hit was Brazil with 1.5 million cases.

CHAPTER

13

Epidemiology of Non-communicable Diseases and Related National Health Programmes

Disease burden: India is faced with double burden of communicable and non-communicable diseases (NCDs). It was estimated that in the year 2008, NCDs accounted for 54,66,000 (53%) of all deaths (1,03,62,000) in India.[1, 2] 10% of deaths were due to injuries while communicable diseases accounted for 37% of deaths. WHO 2009 report indicated that 43% of DALYs losses in India were due to non-communicable diseases, 44% due to communicable diseases and 13% due to injuries. As per the NCD country profile 2014, overall mortality due to NCDs was 60%. The disease specific share was as follows: Cardiovascular diseases-26%, cancer 7%, diabetes 2%, COPD 13%, and other NCDs 12% (Table 13.1).

Overall non-communicable diseases are the leading causes of deaths in the country, constituting 42% of all deaths. Communicable, maternal and perinatal and nutritional conditions constitute another 38% of deaths. Injuries and ill-defined causes constitute 10% of deaths each (SRS in 2003). Overall disease burden due to NCD in India is 51% (including 11.8% injuries).

Rising burden of NCDs is due to rise in expectancy of life, unhealthy lifestyles and exposure to environmental risk factors and use of tobacco and alcohol.

- Data of 52nd round of NSSO indicated that tobacco and alcohol use were higher in the poorest 20% of the income quantile and hence the prevalence of tobacco related NCDs is likely to be high in this group.
- It is estimated that there are 2.8 million of cancer cases in the country and this would double over the next two decades.
- The prevalence of coronary heart disease (CHD) is now reported to be 1.6 to 7.4% in rural areas and 6.5 to 13.2% in urban areas in adults. Based on these data, it is estimated that there were approximately 29.8 million patients with CHD in 2003. Nearly 1.5 million people die due to CHD every year.[1, 2]
- 25% of urban and 10% of rural adult population suffer from hypertension.

Table 13.1: Non-communicable diseases (NCDs) country profile (mortality) in adults published by WHO, 2014

NCDs	*Mortality (%)*	*Prevalence (burden) of NCDs (%)*	*Rural*	*Urban*
Overall mortality due to NCDs	60	Coronary heart disease	1.6–7.4	6.5–13.2
(a) Cardiovascular diseases	26	Hypertension	10	25
(b) Cancer	7	Diabetes	2–5	5–15
(c) Diabetes	2	Obesity	10	25
(d) COPD*	13	*COPD	3.3–5.4	3.7–5.4
(e) Other NCDs	12	Cancers (Rural + Urban)	2.8 million	
		Overall burden of NCDs 39.1% + 11.8% injuries		

*COPD: Chronic obstructive pulmonary disease.

- The estimated prevalence of rheumatic heart disease (which constitutes 20–30% hospital admissions due to cardiovascular diseases) in India, is 5–7 per 1000 in the 5–15 age group.
- A record study carried out in 6 cities in India showed age standardized prevalence of diabetes and impaired glucose tolerance of 12.1% and 14% respectively with no gender difference in adults.

During 10th five-year plan and onward, major thrusts would be:

- A well-structured IEC for primary and secondary prevention of NCD.
- Reorientation and skill upgradation of health care providers in diagnosis and management of NCD at different levels.
- Establishment of referral linkages between primary, secondary and tertiary institutions.
- Development of institutions for rehabilitation of disabled persons, teaching persons to live with their disability.
- Development of hospices for care of terminally ill people who cannot have home-based care.
- Creation of an epidemiological database on NCD especially cavdiovascular diseases (CVDs), strokes and diabetes.

NCDs require lifetime continued care and lifelong medicines intake after diagnosis. Cost of treatment is very high, hence prevention should be the mainstay.

The National Programmes on non-communicable diseases include, National Trauma Control Programme, National Programme for Control of Blindness, National Mental Health Proggramme and National Programme on Control of Iodine Deficiency Disordess, Fluorosis Control and National Oral Health Programme besides National Programme for the health care of elderly and National Programme for Prevention and Control of cancer, diabetes, CVD and strokes as also drug deaddiction programme.

CARDIOVASCULAR DISEASES (UNHEALTHY LIFESTYLE DISEASES)

Cardiovascular diseases—ischaemic heart disease (IHD) and stroke (cerebrovascular disease) are two of the three leading causes of burden of disease in adults in India (Tables 13.2 and 13.3).[3]

In today's world, most deaths are attributable to non-communicable diseases (38 million) and just over 46% of these (17.5 million) are the result of CVDs. More than one-third of these deaths occur in middle-aged adults. In developed countries, heart diseases and strokes are the first and second leading causes of death for adult men and women. In developing countries also, the CVD is emerging as public health problem and trend is rising. Number of estimated cases of coronary heart disease in India during 2000 and 2010 were 2,70,40,912 and 4,69,68,695 respectively. Cardiovascular disease prevalence in India has risen four fold in the past 4 decades and is expected to be leading

Table 13.2: Disease burden of NCD in India—2008 estimated deaths by cause

Diseases	*Percentages*
A Communicable diseases	37
B Non-communicable diseases	53
C Injuries	10
1 Infectious and parasitic diseases	22
2 Peri-natal conditions	7
3 Respiratory infection	7
4 Maternal conditions	0.6
5 Nutritional deficiencies	0.5
6 Cardiovascular diseases	24
7 Respiratory diseases	11
8 Malignant cancers	6
9 Digestive diseases	5
10 Genitourinary diseases	2
11 Diabetes mellitus	2
12 Neuropsychiatric conditions	1.4
13 Congenital anamolies	0.7
14 Unintentional injuries	7
15 Intentional injuries	3
16 Others	0.9

Table 13.3: Disability adjusted life years in India, 2009 (estimated % of DALY loss by cause

Causes (diseases)	*DALYs (%)*
1 Infectious and parasitic diseases	19.28
2 Perinatal conditions	11.62
3 Respiratory infections	7.11
4 Nutritional deficiencies	3.23
5 Maternal conditions	2.69
6 neuropsychiatric conditions	9.49
7 Unintentional injuries	10.50
8 Intentional injuries	2.53
9 Sense organ diseases	6.30
10 Respiratory diseases	3.67
11 Digestive diseases	2.85
12 malignant anamolies	1.88
13 Musculoskeletal diseases	1.49
14 Genito-urinary diseases	0.54
15 Diabetes mellitus	0.54
16 Skin diseases	0.21
17 Endocrine disorders	0.10
18 Other neoplasms	0.08

cause of death and disability by 2020. CVD already causes 29 percent of all deaths (33% in urban and 23% in rural areas) in the country. "Indians are succumbing to heart diseases and strokes in the most productive years of their lives, about a decade earlier than their Western counterparts" (Dr. K. S. Reddy). Cause of concern in developing countries is relatively early age of CVD deaths. One in two of CVD-related deaths in India occur below the age of 70, compared with one in five in economically well-developed nations. In India, the risk factors for CVD are fast emerging because of unhealthy lifestyles like: overeating—fast-foods, physical inactivity and obesity in urban middle and high class, it has not spared the urban slum dwellers as well.

World Health Report 2002 points out that world faces some common large and certain risks to health. India falls in-group of high mortality countries and risk factors like tobacco use, high cholesterol and high blood pressure are fast emerging.[4]

The world is living dangerously, either because it has little choice or because it is making wrong choices. Today there are more than 7 billion people co-existing on this fragile planet on one side who are dangerously short of food, water and security they need to live. Developing countries still face the burden of poverty, undernutrition, unsafe sex, unsafe water, unsafe excreta disposal, poor sanitation and hygiene, micronutrient deficiency, indoor smoke from biomass fuels. On the other side, lies unhealthy consumption, particularly of tobacco and alcohol. The risks from blood pressure, and cholesterol strongly linked to heart attacks and strokes are also closely related to excessive consumption of fatty, sugary and salty foods. They become even more dangerous when combined with the deadly forces of tobacco and excessive alcohol consumption.[1]

Obesity, a result of unhealthy consumption coupled with *lack of physical activity*, is itself a serious health risk. All of these risk factors—blood pressure, cholesterol, tobacco, alcohol and obesity and the diseases linked to them are known to wealthy societies. The real worry is that they are now also increasingly dominating in low mortality developing countries where they create a double burden on top of infectious diseases that always have affected poorer countries. They are even becoming more prevalent in high mortality developing countries.

The Framingham study, the best known study, and a model for many others launched in 1950s developed the concept of coronary risk factors. The study brought out the classic *consistent risk factors* such as cigarette smoking, blood pressure and total cholesterol. Others were less common (diabetes mellitus), less consistent (obesity and exercise) or less readily measured (diet, alcohol and psychological factors). Subsequently, many other studies were conducted and the world's largest study of heart diseases, strokes, risk factors and population trends was undertaken by MONICA project (Multinational monitoring of trends and determinants in cardiovascular disease) from 1979–2002.[5]

In summary, the major CVD risk factors of tobacco use, inappropriate diet and physical inactivity (primarily expressed through unfavourable lipid concentrations, high body mass index, and raised blood pressure) explain at least 75–85% of new cases of coronary heart disease.[1] In the absence of elevation of these risk factors, coronary heart disease is a rare cause of death.

Only about 5% of adult men and women in wealthy countries are at low-risk with optimal risk factor levels. There are only a very few poor countries in which these factors have not yet emerged as major public health problem. The basic underlying conditions and **risk factors** for CVD are:

1. Tobacco use
2. High blood pressure >140/90
3. High total cholesterol >200 mg/dl
4. (a) Obesity, (b) BMI $\geq$30 kg/m^2
5. Physical inactivity—sedentary lifestyle
6. Low intakes of fruits and vegetables
7. Diabetes mellitus
8. Harmful use of alcohol
9. Stress
10. Hereditary and genetics

PRIMORDIAL PREVENTION

It begins during childhood period, i.e. shaping lifestyles during early years of life. Primordial prevention in CVD consists of prevention of development of coronary risk factors in population/community. This measure is directed to healthy community or total population. *Generally primordial prevention should begin during childhood continue through adolescents, and youth and later years of life.*

Since the clinical manifestations of CVD appear in fourth or subsequent decades of life, the pathological process begins much earlier during childhood period.

Primordial prevention focuses on prevention of emergence and establishment of known risk factors or unhealthy lifestyles in *population*.

Actions

- The government should have comprehensive *policy* to discourage tobacco use, ban on tobacco production, sale and consumption. **Smoking** at public places is banned in India and similarly sale of cigarette to minor is an offence in India; however, comprehensive ban is lacking.
- *National policy* and *programmes* on **nutrition** involving the agriculture sector, the food industry, and food import/export sector to curb excessive use of **saturated fats,** transfats and "fast-foods" through food 'giants' and regulating *salt* in processed foods and encourage production of **fruits and vegetables** and to promote healthy eating practices in population by regulating food prices/industries.

- Shaping personality and healthy lifestyles such as "no smoking", avoid eating excess of "junk foods", "fast-foods" and promoting healthy eating to avoid overweight and obesity begins in family and home first. Unfortunately, the high fat fast foods are much cheaper than fruits, vegetables, whole grains and pulses today. This coupled with aggressive marketing in the media promotes unhealthy eating habits which increases cholesterol levels and obesity. "The food Industry is driving nutrition off the natural path."Promoting **physical activities** in childhood and adolescent period prevents obesity. Development of **healthy lifestyles** begins at home and parents and family lay down foundations of these lifestyles. Dietary patterns, smoking habits are family-based and transmitted from parents to children and conditioned by environments in later life where peer groups play important role. Similarly, preschool education programmes and school teachers leave permanent impression on the mind of child and have great influence in shaping healthy lifestyles and personality development. Teachers are good role models and can have positive influence on children and adolescents. Similarly, peer group education can make difference.

PRIMARY PREVENTION

Once the risk factors have been established or have appeared in the population, attempt is made to prevent the development of CVD in persons having risk factors.

Purpose

Purpose of primary prevention is to *limit the incidence* of CVD by controlling risk factors and causes or by modification of risk factors.

There are two approaches in primary prevention:

i Whole population

ii High risk approach.

Focus on Whole Population—Population-based Approach

Population-based primary prevention strategies are much more beneficial, cost effective, make high impact, here effort is made to focus on total population. Population—wide risk factors modification such as reduction in tobacco use/salt, saturated fats and sugar intake, control of factors which can give rise to hypertension and diabetes mellitus, regular physical exercises, diet rich in dietary fibre (containing lot of green leafy vegetables, whole grain cereals, mixed cereal diets, fresh fruits and vegetables, dried beans, peas) maintenance of ideal body weight and avoidance of stress (relaxation techniques like yoga and meditation) could prevent a large proportion of disease events in the whole population. It aims at community adoption of *healthy lifestyles*; by health promotion and behaviour change communication strategies.

Preventive Measures and Strategies

Mean blood pressure of a population accurately predicts the number of hypertensive individuals and mean body weight predicts the number of obese subjects. Rose identified that the prevalence of a high-risk state (hypercholesterolaemia, hypertension, obesity, etc.) is largely a reflection of the *lifestyles* and *attitudes* of the masses. Population wide approach corrects the *underlying cause* of the epidemic and is safer, cheaper and more cost-effective than the high-risk corrective approach.[6, 7]

Epidemiological studies have identified that many traditional coronary risk factors are important in Indians. Adopting *healthier lifestyles* as *norms* for the entire population can change most of these factors. Following lifestyle changes as applicable especially to urban Indians are appropriate:[6–8]

- Tobacco control requires a variety of measures including, but not limited to, restrictions on smoking in the workplace and in public, enhanced community education programmes and physician supervised counselling on smoking cessation and quiting smoking/tobacco use.
- Reduction of salt, alcohol and calorie intake, regular exercise, stress management and greater intake of calcium, potassium, magnesium and fibre can prevent hypertension.
- Control of hypercholesterolaemia and decrease in mean LDL cholesterol levels can be achieved by reducing intake of saturated fats, meat and dairy products and greater intake of polyunsaturated fats and fibre.
- Low HDL cholesterol levels can be influenced by greater intake of monounsaturated and polyunsaturated fats, fruits, green vegetables and exercise.
- Truncal obesity and insulin resistance can be reduced by regular exercise.

Behavioural and environmental changes in the whole population that are relevant to these risk factors are: changes in eating patterns, drinking and smoking, increased physical activity and modulation of psychosocial factors.

High-risk Approach

Here attempt is made to screen out high-risk individuals by **periodical medical check-up** at regular intervals measuring of risk factors such as blood pressure, weight and cholesterol level. Those individuals who show abnormal values are prescribed individualized programme directed at modifying or reducing or eliminating the risk factors and thus preventing the CVD and delaying the development of CVD.

Screening of risk factors is a costly proposition.

The relationship between risk factor and disease events is continuous and most events of CVD occur in people in middle range of the risk factor distribution, who are not normally judged high-risk. The effort spent in measuring risk factors in individuals is therefore questionable.

SECONDARY PREVENTION

This level of prevention is applied to persons who have developed CVD. In CVD, secondary prevention aims to cure patients of CVD and reduce more serious complications through early diagnosis and prompt treatment. It also aims at reducing morbidity and mortality and *reduces the prevalence* of CVD. Apart from prompt treatment, the measures include avoiding smoking, promoting physical exercise, lowering lipids, controlling obesity, hypertension and diabetes by diets, drugs and exercise regimen. Low doses of aspirin and use of β blockers are popular regimen. Treatment is lifelong.[9]

TERTIARY PREVENTION IN CVD

This consists of disability limitation and rehabilitation by advanced treatment and surgical interventions like angioplasty and coronary bypass. It treats the complications and sequelae of CVD. *Rehabilitation* of patients of myocardial infarction and strokes in the *community* and at *home* by physical, emotional and psychological rehabilitation by yoga and biofeedback. The aim is to enable the individual to take part in daily social life.

Modifiable risk factors of CVD are being explained in details here under.

Smoking and Second-hand Smoke (SHS)

Tobacco is the second major cause of death in the world. Use of tobacco is harmful to health and heart. Tobacco use in any form is harmful to heart, it increases the atherosclerosis, raises the level of cholesterol besides producing lung cancer. Tobacco kills 5.4 million people every year in the world mostly in poor countries and poor population. Controlling tobacco is primordial prevention. Governments of various countries have various forms of bans on use of tobacco, but these are not sufficient. Tobacco consumption is still prevalent. Second-hand smoke (SHS) or environmental tobacco smoke (ETS) exposure among the population in general and women and children in particular at home, at public places and at work places is alarming. 40.3% of students are exposed to SHS in India by cigarette in public places.

In India, more than 0.8 million people die due to tobacco consumption. India is second largest consumer of tobacco in the world.

Recognizing the grave problem of tobacco use, WHO evolved Framework Convention on Tobacco Control (FCTC) adopted by 192 member states. This constitutes a major turning point in control of tobacco in the world to tackle major "global killer". It signals a new era in global and national tobacco control activities. Tobacco control begins at family, school and work place and with peers. It requires to be curbed at family level by parents and school teachers who can become role models and similarly NSS units and universities can play a pivotal role. Quitting smoking is beneficial at any stage to prevent heart disease and cancers.

Smoking cessation by health workers and in patients with clinical CVD is essential to avoid miseries of CVD. Ultimate objective is to develop smoke free societies in India.[10]

Hypertension

A subject (adult) is called hypertensive if the blood pressure level is >140/90 mmHg. Blood pressure control helps prevent development of CVD. Goal is to keep blood pressure less than <140/90 mmHg. Adopt **healthy lifestyles right from early childhood** period to control eating and body weights and to achieve normotensive level.

High blood pressure adversely affects the heart and blood vessels. Elevated blood pressure levels produce a variety of structural changes in the arteries that supply blood to the brain, heart, kidneys, eyes and elsewhere. High blood pressure increases the work of heart and produces hypertrophy of left ventricle. An increase in bulk means increased oxygen demand for the heart muscle. Since at the same time, blood flow is facing an obstruction, the heart does not get enough oxygen. This is how the blood pressure increases the risk of heart attacks. High blood pressure does not produce symptoms as such, therefore, it is called "silent killer".[11]

In recent decades, it has become increasingly clear that the risks of strokes and ischaemic heart disease, renal failure and other diseases are not confined to population with particular high levels (hypertension), but rather continue among those with average and even below average blood pressure. Worldwide high blood pressure is estimated to cause 7.1 million of deaths.

Regular blood pressure check-up after the age of 30 has been recommended. Any one with pressure higher than 140/90 mmHg needs treatment. The main modifiable causes of high blood pressure are diet, especially salt intake, levels of exercise, obesity, tobacco and harmful use of alcohol. As a result of cumulative effects of these factors, blood pressure usually rises steadily with age, except in societies where salt intakes are low and physical activity is high and obesity absent. Most adults have blood pressure levels that are suboptimal for health. This is true for economically developing and developed countries. Globally, it is estimated that about 62% of cerebrovascular disease and 49% of ischaemic heart disease are attributable to suboptimal blood pressure (systolic >115 mmHg) with little variations by sex.

Objective is to achieve optimal mean levels of blood pressure in population. Therefore, population-based primordial and primary prevention is the best strategy by reducing the salt contents of manufactured food. For each decline of 1 mmHg in diastolic pressure, the risk of heart attack is reduced by 2–3% in population.[6]

National strategies on diet and physical activity are essential to get over the problem of obesity and hypertension and to reduce CVD in the community. Population-based strategies help and are most cost-effective and feasible.

High Cholesterol Level

Cholesterol is key component in the development of atherosclerosis—the accumulation of fatty deposits on the inner lining of the arteries. High cholesterol is estimated to cause 18% of global cerebrovascular disease and 56% of global ischaemic heart disease. Overall, this amounts to 4.4 million deaths. Normal level of cholesterol is 150–250. Safe level is 200 mg/100 ml or less. Hyper-cholesterolaemia is a risk factor in CVD.

There are two sources of cholesterol in body. Food cholesterol (exogenous source) and endogenous source synthesized by body tissues such as liver. The dietary cholesterol is derived from animal products and no plant food has it. The richest sources are egg yolk, whole milk dairy products and organ meat. Cholesterol is carried as lipoprotein molecules in plasma. There are 3 classes of lipoproteins, high density lipoprotein (HDL), low density lipoproteins (LDL), very low density lipoproteins (VLDL) and chylomicron.

HDL (α-lipoprotein) is protective and friendly to heart it contains 20% of cholesterol. LDL (β-lipoprotein) contains 45% of cholesterol and is not good for heart. VLDL contains 60% of triglycerides and is not good for heart. Chylomicron contains 90% of triglycerides and again not good for heart.

High consumption of animal fats, eggs, organ meat and saturated fats raises the level of cholesterol and increases the level of harmful lipoproteins (LDL, VLDL and chylomicron). Monounsaturated fatty acids (MUFAs), and polyunsaturated fatty acids (PUFAs) lower the cholesterol level in the body. A blend of rice bran oil with palm oil in the proportion of 3:1 can yield a blend with ideal ratio of saturated fatty acids (SFAs), MUFAs and PUFAs (1.0: 1.5:1.0) which can be good for prevention of heart disease according to American Heart Association and Japanese Ministry of Health and Welfare.

Indian diets are vegetarian primarily hence fats come through vegetable oils and some are derived from milk and milk products.

Visible fats are consumed through coconut, vanaspati, groundnut and red palm; these are all saturated fats and provide SFAs (Saturated fatty acids). Unsaturated fatty acids are derived from soyabean, sunflower, safflower, sesame oils and mustard oil. These oils provide unsaturated fatty acids like MUFA (Monounsaturated fatty acid), linoleic acid (LA) and alpha-linolenic acid (ALA).

In Indian diet, 25–40 g of visible fat as oil is recommended per adult person per day and children should have at least 25–30 g per day and pregnant women 30 g per day.[8]

Invisible Fats (IFs)

In Indian diet IF come through cereals, millets, pulses and adequate intakes of these can provide 8–10 g of invisible fats. Invisible fats of plant are known good sources of oleic acid, linoleic (LA) and alpha-linolenic acid (ALA). Pulses and green leafy vegetables and spices contain high proportion of ALA.

Most of vegetable oils contain LA predominantly. However, oils extracted from soya bean, rapeseed, mustard and rice bran contain both LA and ALA, further human body can synthesise n-3 PUFA from ALA. Mixed use of groundnut oil, rice bran, sesame, safflower, sunflower, cotton seed oil can provide adequate amount of ALA. This will also balance the overall intake of erucic acid (present in mustard oil) which is undesirable. Besides fatty acids, the vegetable oils contain various tocols (tocopherols and tocotrienols). These tocols have hypocholesterolemic, antioxidant, antithrombotic and anticarcinogenic properties.

Right proportion of PUFA-SFA and LA/ALA can reduce the cholesterol levels in the body. Therefore, Indian vegetarian diets, which are cereal-based with adequate quantity of legumes, fruits, green vegetables and oils can reduce the level of cholesterol in the body and are good for heart. Excess consumption of saturated fats (derived from eggs, meat and dairy products); "junk foods" and "fast-foods" and "transfats" can be harmful and raise the level of harmful cholesterol. Vegetarian diets promote the level of good cholesterol (HDL). Dietary fibre, which are insoluble and soluble fibres. Insoluble fibres are cellulose, hemicellulose and lignin. These are present in plant cell wall. Soluble fibres may reduce LDL level by 5–15%. The soluble fibres are psylium, pectins, gums and mucilages. Sources of soluble fibres are fresh fruits, dry fruits, pulses, legumes, coarse cereals and isabgol. These foods lower the level of harmful cholesterol and hence should be encouraged. Refined carbohydrates as in white flour, white bread, polished rice, sugar are poor sources of fibre and are harmful. Natural antioxidants in food like vitamin E and C, β-carotene and selenium are present in green leafy vegetables, yellow fruits, nuts, garlic and onion and are good for heart. No more than 20–30% of calories should come from fats in daily diet.

Obesity, Overweight and High Body Mass Index

The prevalence of overweight and obesity is commonly measured by using body mass index (BMI), weight in kg/height in m^2 which has a strong correlation to body fat content. WHO criteria define *overweight* as a BMI of at least 25 kg/m^2 and *obesity* as a BMI of at least 30 kg/m^2. These markers provide common benchmark for assessment, but risks of disease in all populations increase progressively from BMI levels of 20–22 kg/m^2. NIN has revised the normal range of BMI as 18.5 to 23.

Excessive consumption of free sugar (refined carbohydrates), saturated fats and harmful consumption of alcohol combined with reduced physical activity lead to obesity and obesity rates are on increase in prosperous people. Urban middle class, rich and higher economic status people, have more tendency to develop obesity.

Overweight and obesity lead to adverse metabolic effects on blood pressure, cholesterol, triglycerides and insulin resistance. Risks of coronary heart disease, ischaemic strokes and type 2 diabetes increase steadily with increasing BMI. Type 2 diabetes mellitus confined to older adults for most of the 20th century—now affects obese children before puberty.

Raised BMI also increases the risk of cancer of breast, colon, prostate, endometrium, kidney and gallbladder. Similarly, chronic overweight and obesity contributed significantly to osteoarthritis, a major cause of disability in adults.

58% of diabetes mellitus, 21% of ischaemic heart diseases globally are attributable to BMI above 21 kg/m^2.

One in ten adolescents and young adult in Delhi (India), is clinically obese and 5% have high blood pressure. The reason: over 80% are inactive "we are sitting on twin epidemics of diabetes and heart diseases" (Anoop Misra). Current dietary trends combined with inactivity will expose this generation to hypertension, heart disease and diabetes by middle age.[12]

Physical Inactivity

The world health survey found that overall, 29% of the population had inadequate physical activity.

Overall, physical inactivity was estimated to cause more than 2 million deaths. Physical inactivity is estimated to cause globally 10–16% of cases each of breast cancer, colon and rectal cancers and diabetes mellitus and about 22% of ischaemic heart disease.[2]

Physical activity reduces the risk of cardiovascular disease; some cancers and type 2 diabetes. In general, physical activity improves glucose metabolism, reduces body fat and lowers blood pressure. These are the main ways in which it is thought to reduce the risk of cardiovascular diseases and diabetes. Physical activity also reduces risk of colon cancer by effects on prostaglandin, reduced intestinal transit time and higher antioxidant level. Besides, this, physical activity can improve the musculoskeletal health, control body weight and reduce symptoms of depression, stress and reduced risk of breast cancer and prostate cancer.

Urgent population wide measures are required to change the scenario of physical inactivity and it is worthwhile to emulate targets set by the US National Institute of Health:

- All individuals should engage in regular physical activity appropriate to their capacity needs and interest. Non-occupational, travel-related, and occupational physical activity levels should be increased.
- At least 30 minutes of moderate intensity physical activity on most of the weekdays is recommended.
- 3–4 times per week (walking, jogging, cycling and other aerobic activity).

For those with known cardiovascular disease, physical activity should be combined with a comprehensive risk-reduction programme. Physical activity should begin sooner rather than later in one's lifespan. Parents, schools and community organizations should provide a supportive environment.

When you walk briskly, play, skate, clean house or climb stairs, you are moving for health. Any amount of physical activity will make you feel better. The minimum amount of physical activity required for prevention of disease is at least 30 minutes of moderate activity everyday.[13, 14]

Low Fruit and Vegetable Intake in India

Adequate consumption of fruits and vegetables prevents CVD and certain cancers principally of digestive system. There are several mechanisms by which these protective effects may be mediated, involving antioxidants and other micronutrients such as flavinoids, carotenoids, vitamin C and folic acids as well as dietary fibres. These and other substances block or suppress the action of carcinogen, and as antioxidants, prevent oxidative DNA damage. In India, fruits and vegetable intake is low. Horticulture and agriculture policies can increase their consumption. One should encourage the consumptions of fruits and vegetables to control weight and reduce CVD apart from reduction of risk of cancers.

Diabetes Mellitus

Normal fasting blood sugar level of healthy adult varies between 80 and 100 mg/100 ml. Diabetes accentuates the risk of CVD by 2–3 times in men and 3–7 times in women. Reduction in the risk of CVD with well-controlled diabetes is well established. But this requires a control of other risk factors too. Diabetic must ensure that blood pressure and cholesterol levels are normal. They should avoid smoking, control their weight and exercise regularly. Excessive alcohol consumption is harmful to health and heart.

Stress

Stress does exert adverse effects on heart and blood vessels. It results in release of hormones, which damage the inner lining of blood vessels. Such an injury promotes cholesterol deposition to produce atheroma. Stress hormones also damage the heart muscle and can change the properties of platelets and help in formation of clots. Hence, there is indirect evidence of the value of stress control for prevention of ischaemic heart disease.

Type A behaviours are more prone to the effect of stress and consequences of stress (Table 13.4).

Hostility and anger are probable independent risk factors to CVD, both letting out anger and suppressing produce negative emotions, which increase the risk to CVD.

Stress Management

Number of stress management/prevention techniques are available and are useful to cope stress and prevent stress.

- Relaxation technique
- Biofeedback

Table 13.4: Characteristic behaviour patterns of type A and type B personalities[9]

Type A behaviours	*Type B behaviours*
• Hurried speech • Constant rapid movement/eating • Open impatience with the rate at which things occur and how others operate • Chronic sense of time urgency • Thinking and performing several things at once • An active attempt to dominate the conversation, to determine the topics and to remain preoccupied with one's own thoughts when others are talking • Vague guilty feelings during period of relaxation when doing nothing • Over concern with getting things worth having no time to become the things worth being • No compassion for others • Characteristic nervous gestures—tics, clench fist and jaw, pound on table, grind teeth	• Complete freedom from all type A traits • No sense of time urgency • No free-floating hostility • No felt need to display or discuss one's achievements and accomplishments unless the situation demands it • An ability to relax without guilt and to work without agitation

- Thought stopping
- Cognitive behaviour modification
- Yoga and meditation.

Relaxation Techniques

Stress encountered by the individual produces state of muscular tension which disrupts the adaptive functions of various body systems. Relaxation techniques are helpful in altering certain physiological parameters associated with CVD like blood pressure and anxiety. Various techniques have been used for releasing muscular tension. Jacobsonian technique has been used widely; deep-breathing and physical massage are other techniques.

Biofeedback

It is a technique of achieving voluntary control over autonomic function by constant feedback of visual, auditory or graphic signals through instrumental conditioning like controlling heart rate, body temperature and so on. This helps to control anxiety, reduction of muscle tension and is helpful in treatment of cardiac arrhythmia and angina pectoris, hypertension and type A behaviour.

Thought Stopping

Negative thoughts like thoughts about succeeding, being a failure, if left unchecked lower down one's self-esteem, self-control, and builds-up physical tension and lead to stress. Counselling techniques and family support can stop these negative thoughts.

Cognitive Behaviour Modification

Individual can be trained to learn positive self-enhancing rational thinking by variety of procedures to inculcate positive beliefs and thinking.

Yoga and Meditation

Practice of yoga and meditation relieves tension, improves psychological functions and lowers heart rate, respiratory rate and blood pressure. Yoga and meditation under guidance are helpful to reduce stress. Beginning should be made in schools, continued during adolescents and in later life.

Heredity and Genetic Factors

There is strong likelihood that Indians have genetic predisposition to CVD mediated by Lp(a) a form of LDL cholesterol with an additional protein called Apo(a). It binds with other components in blood to form plaques, which deposit inside the arterial wall. Lp(a) also promotes intravascular clotting and prevents clot lysis as its structure is homologous to plasminogen.

Lp(a) is 10 times more atherogenic than LDL and 15 times more deadly than total cholesterol.

Individual with high Lp(a) levels should be targeted for rigorous lifestyle modifications to minimize the risk of CVD.

Surveillance of Risk Factors

To achieve 25% reduction in mortality Epidemiological surveillance of risk factors of CVD is appropriate; to monitor the trends, to evaluate the risk reduction strategies and to improve the implementation of strategies in a region or country as also to draw comparison of prevalence between different regions.[15] Surveillance can be part of integrated surveillance of communicable and non-communicable diseases. Surveillance operations involve, substantial cost and these should be taken up with definite objective or policy in mind. Academic surveillance is of little use. Parameters of risk assessment can be simplified to be used at field level by paramedical workers and by people themselves such as weight and height records, smoking status, family history of CVD, past history of disease, diets, physical activity, etc.

REFERENCES

1 GOI. MOH and FW, Annual Report 2006–07, NRHM; GOI, New Delhi.

2 WHO. Subodh Verma India has largest pool of Patients (WHO). Times of India, 3rd April 2007, 'Nation' Chandigarh Edition.
3 World Health Organization. The World Health Report shaping the future. Geneva: WHO; 2003.
4 World Health Organization. The World Health Report—Reducing risks, promoting life. Geneva: WHO; 2002.
5 World Health Organization. MONICA. Monograph and multimedia source book. World's largest study of heart disease, and stroke. WHO; 2005.
6 Beaglehole R. Global cardiovascular disease prevention—time to get serious. Lancet; 2001 358: 661–3.
7 Yusuf S, et al. Global burden of cardiovascular diseases. Part I : General considerations, the epidemiologic transition, risk factors and impact of urbanization. Circulation 2001; 104: 2746–53.
8 C, Gopalan: Fatty acids in India—Current research and Government Policies. NFI Bulletin 2003; 24(1).
9 Siddiqui MA. An overview of risk factors for coronary heart disease and prevention strategies. Ind Journal of Com. Health 1997; 9(2): 4–6.
10 GOI. Annual Report 2003–04, MOH and FW. New Delhi: GOI; 2004.
11 NIPHC—ESCORTS. Seminar on preventive cardiology. Proceedings: NIPHC Health Care Promotion Trust, New Delhi; Nov. 1996.
12 Hindustan Times. Sanchita Sharma: Gen x eating dangerously. Hindustan Times: New Delhi; Sept. 25, 2004.
13 WHO. Rajeev Gupta. Role of physical activity in primary prevention of cardiovascular diseases. A South-East Asian Perspectives—Move for health. Geneva: WHO; April 7, 2002.
14 Gupta R, Prakash C, Dedwania, MR Soangra: Prevention of Coronary Heart Disease in India: An epidemiological perspective. IJCM 2002; 27(4).
15 WHO. Global Status Report on non-communicable diseases 2014; "Attaining the nine global noncommunicable diseaes targets; a shared responsibility".

OBESITY (AN EPIDEMIC IN INDIA)

Lifestyle Diseases

Globalization has brought in lot of changes in the food habits of children and adolescents because of availability, accessibility and affordability of fast foods—junk foods.

Less than 20% of Delhi adolescents took on to any physical exercise like walking and participating in sports. Over the last 3 decades, there have been substantial changes in the socioeconomic status of people, some increases in the dietary intake of men and women, especially of the affluent segments, in rural and urban areas, ready availability of fast-foods, ice creams and other energy rich food items at affordable costs have resulted in increased energy consumption. About 48% of households consumed more than adequate amount of both proteins and calories, while 20% of households consumed inadequate amount of calories (NNMB 96–97).[1] With increasing access to cooking gas, piped water supply, power and electricity, transport, etc. have been useful labour saving devices and consequently there has been substantial reduction in physical activity pattern and energy expenditure especially among the middle and upper income groups. Data from NNMB repeat surveys indicate that there has been some reduction in undernutrition and some increase in obesity over the last 2 decades (Fig. 13.1).[1]

Data from NFHS-2, 3, and 4 confirm that currently both undernutrition and overnutrition are problems in women aged 15–49. There are significant interstate differences. The percentage of women with undernutrition varies from 16.4% in Arunachal Pradesh to 41% in Odisha and those who are overweight from 4.6% in Bihar to 26.4% in Delhi, 30% in Punjab and 16.6% in Haryana. In Delhi and Punjab, which are more prosperous over 9% of women of 15–49 years were clinically obese having BMI of over 30.

According to NFHS-3 data, 29.9% of women in Punjab were overweight or obese. The percentage of men obese in Punjab was 22.2%, making Punjab as the heaviest state in India.

Defining Obesity

The obesity can be defined simply as the disease in which excess body fat has accumulated to such an extent that health may be adversely affected. However, the amount of excess fat, its distribution within the body and associated health consequences vary considerably between obese individuals.

Measuring Obesity

Skin Fold Thickness

Measuring skin fold thickness indicates deposition of fat and indirectly measures the level of obesity in a person. Triceps skin fold and subscapular skin fold thickness is measured commonly. Harpenden calipers are used for this purpose. The standards have to be fixed locally.

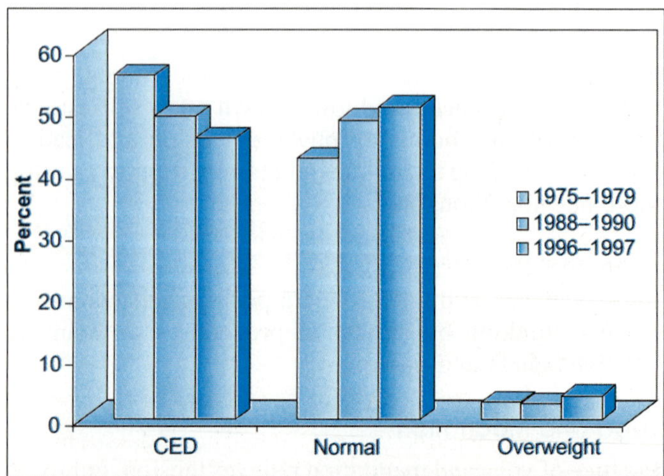

Fig. 13.1: Nutritional status of adult males (NNMB-1999)

Waist Circumference and Waist Hip Ratio (WHR)

This has been used to measure central or abdominal obesity. A waist hip ratio exceeding 0.85 in female and 0.95 in male is indicative of abdominal obesity. To maintain appropriate waist hip ratio is most desirable. It is measured at a midpoint between the lower border of rib cage and iliac crest in cm and may provide more practical correlate of abdominal fat distribution and associated ill-health.

Body Weight

Obesity has been measured by using weight of an individual for his/her height. It has been suggested that if the weight-for-height exceeds 120% of standard weight-for-height than the subject should be labelled as an obese. Excess weight is most likely due to excess deposition of fat in the body but it may also be due to excess muscle mass and other tissues as well. Body weight alone is thus insufficient measure of obesity.

Body Mass Index (BMI)

BMI is now used as an indicator of choice to diagnose obesity in adults. Garrow's earlier classification of obesity has been replaced by the International Obesity Task Force criteria developed and endorsed by the WHO 2000, and 2004 (Table 13.5).[2, 3] NIN new guidelines on range of normal BMI is—18.5 to 23 keeping BMI in the range of 21–23 is good for health.

WHO definition of overweight for South Asians is:

(BMI > = 23 compred to BMI > = 25 for other regions)

BMI is most useful tool in estimating the prevalence of obesity and chronic undernutrition or chronic energy deficiency (CED) in adults. A person with BMI of 25 and above is overweight, BMI between 25 to 29.9 is pre-obese and BMI of 30 and above is obese. A person with BMI of 40 and above is called "morbid obese".

Other Methods

Techniques of body fat assessment are more sophisticated and costlier.

Global Problem

Obesity is a global public health problem. On an estimate, nearly 1.4 billion adults worldwide are obese.

In Europe, the trends of obesity are on rising side from 6–8% in 1980 to 15% in 1991. WHO MONICA Project provides most comprehensive data on prevalence of obesity worldwide in European population. Between 50% and 75% of adults aged 35–64 were either overweight or obese during the period 1983 and 1986.

Epidemic of obesity is unfolding in Asia (Table 13.6).[4]

Cut-off levels: Cutt-off levels for BMI in Indian studies have been >25, which includes overweight and obese both, hence over estimated prevalence rates in India.

Table 13.5: International classification of adult overweight and obesity according to BMI

Classification	*BMI kg/m² principal cut-off points*	*Additional cut-off points*
Normal range	**18.50–24.99**	**18.50–22.99** **23.00–24.99**
Overweight	**≥25.00**	**≥25.00**
Pre-obese	25.00–29.99	25.00–27.49 27.50–29.99
Obese	**≥30.00**	**≥30.00**
Class I	30.00–34.99	30.00–32.49 32.50–34.99
Class II	35.00–39.99	35.00–37.49 37.50–39.99
Class III	≥40.00	≥40.00

Source: Adapted from WHO 1995, WHO 2000 and WHO 2004.

These BMI values are age independent and the same for both sexes. However, BMI may not correspond to the same degree of fatness in different populations due, in part, to differences in body proportions. The health risks associated with increasing BMI are continuous and graded and begin at a BMI below 25. The interpretation of BMI gradings in relation to risk may differ for different populations. The WHO Expert Consultation concluded that the proportion of Asian people with a high risk of type 2 diabetes and cardiovascular disease is substantial at BMI's lower than the existing WHO cut-off point for overweight (= 25 kg/m²). However, the cut-off point for observed risk varies from 22 to 25 kg/m² in different Asian populations and for high-risk, it varies from 26 to 31 kg/m². The Consultation, therefore, recommended that the current WHO BMI cut-off points (Table 13.5) should be retained as the international classification. But the cut-off points of 23, 27.5, 32.5 and 37.5 kg/m² are to be added as points for public health action.

Obese grades of BMI are on the rising side-up from 3.4% in 1975–79 to 11.6% in 93–94 and NFHS-3 and 4 data shows 12.6% of women and 9.3% men had BMI over 25—who were overweight or obese (Tables 13.7 and 13.8).[5] Currently, India is in nutrition transition with 10% of rural adults and 25% of urban adults are suffering from overnutrition.

Epidemiology

Obesity is an *emerging epidemic* in India. Adult male and female are equally affected. High prevalence of obesity in adult women has been reported in some states. One-fourth (25%) of Indian children above the age of eight in urban India are obese and overweight as per new national survey on physical fitness. (The Tribune Sept 11, 2010.) These children have poor endurance, based on indicators of BMI, aerobic (walking and running) and anaerobic (sprinting) capacities, muscle strength, endurance and flexibility.

Developed and Developing Countries

The belief that obesity or overnutrition was the problem of developed countries alone is no longer true. Affluent sections in India and urban middle class and higher classes are affected much more hence India is one of the developing country along with other countries showing emerging and rising trends as indicated by NNMB surveys in adult women.

Table 13.6: Prevalence of obesity in India and other South-East Asian countries[4]

Name of the country	Overweight (%)	Obese (%)
The Republic of Korea, 1995	20.5	1.5
Thailand	16.0	4
Malaysia	–	4.7 (men), 7.7 (women), 16.7 (Indian women)
China, 1992	–	2 (men and women)
Japan, 1990–94	24.3 (men), 20.2 (women)	3.0
Bombay—India	–	10.7 to 53.1* (young adult males)
Delhi—India	–	27.8*
Kashmir—India	–	15.0*

* Cut-off of BMI >25
Source: Prakash Shetty, NFI 2(3) 2003.

Table 13.7: Nutritional status of evermarried women 15–49 NFHS-2 and NFHS-3

Areas	BMI < 18.5 (kg/m^2)		BMI > 25 (kg/m^2)	
	NFHS-2	NFHS-3	NFHS-2	NFHS-3
All India (pooled data)	35.8	35.6	12.8	12.6
Delhi	12.0	14.8	33.8	26.4
Punjab	16.9	18.9	39.3	29.9
Haryana	25.9	31.3	20.5	17.4

Figures in percentage.

Table 13.8: Trends in body mass index of adult women (15–49) in India

Surveys years	CED (%) BMI <18.5	Normal (%) BMI 18.5–25.0	Obese (%) BMI >25
NNMB 75–79	51.8	44.8	3.4
88–90	49.3	46.8	4.1
1994	47.1	46.3	6.1
NNMB 93–94 (slum)	36.7	51.7	11.6
NFHS-2 98–99	35.8	51.4	12.8
India nut. profile 1998	32.9	62.5	4.5
NFHS-3–2006	35.6	51.8	12.6
NFHS-4–2015–16	6.4 ot 30.4	–	11.7–36.7

Source: HPS Sachdev, NFI 24(2) 2003 and India Nutrition Profile 1998, NFHS-3, and NFHS-4 (in 15 states).

Urban Rural Differences

In India, the available information indicates the urban affluents are more at risk and have high prevalence of obesity because of sedentary lifestyles, consumption of junk foods rich in calories and lack of exercise. There are more obese women in Urban Punjab (45.4%) as compared to rural areas (32.9%). Similarly 34.1% men in urban Punjab and 27.4% in villages were obese (NFHS-3).[6] Approximately 30–65% of urban adults are overweight/obese.

Socioeconomic Status

Upper socioeconomic classes and affluents are more affected as compared to urban poor; however, it all depends on lifestyles of eating and exercise. NNMB data observed high obesity levels in urban slums indicating that obesity is now affecting urban poor.

Ethnicity

People of Indian origin living in USA, UK and Malaysia have high incidence and prevalence of obesity as compared to local people.

Physical Inactivity

With increase in prosperity, the lifestyles have changed because of urbanization, industrialization and mechanization. The lifestyles have changed and physical activity much reduced due to use of automobiles, long hours of watching of television and playing computer games and load of books which confines the children, adolescents and adults in homes. The energy spending is less and energy consumption is much higher with higher use of junk foods (refined carbohydrates). Eating junk foods and television watching go together, due to excessive use of mobile telephones, the mobility is further reduced and this has led to physical inactivity and all these are highly associated with development of obesity. Urban surveys from Indian cities have revealed low level of physical activities in 61–66% of men and 51–75% of women.

Risk Factors

Physical inactivity, unhealthy eating, overweight and harmful consumption of alcohol are the risk factors in obesity.

New Trend

Obesity is emerging as a problem of younger age groups, i.e. younger children in urban affluent areas have the tendency towards overweight due to more amenities and less of physical activities as also overeating tendencies.

A study of 4000 Indian children in 15 cities indicated that 25% of children in 5–14 year age bracket in urban schools being overweight, while nearly 11% kids were obese. While malnutrition continues to be a major health concern in many parts of the world, excess of food consumption and sedentary lifestyles are leading to an epidemic of obesity and chronic non-communicable diseases (NCDs).

Obesity is strongly linked to low physical activity and a major cause for insulin resistance. Insulin resistance is a characteristic feature of Asian Indians even with non-obese body mass index. A genotype which provided metabolic defence at times of famine has probably placed the present generation at a higher risk of developing metabolic disorders when exposed to constant overnutrition and physical inactivity.

In the United States, obesity causes 3,00,000 deaths annually, a number exceeded only by the tobacco-related deaths. A high rate of obesity is found in many countries of Latin America, the Middle East and Asia. Some Island nations of Western Pacific have especially high rates of obesity. In China, an estimated 200 million people could become obese in the next 10 years.

Hitherto, our concern remained on undernutrition in young children. Long-standing malnutrition in India exposes these children during adulthood period to the consequence of degenerative metabolic disorders even at low BMI when they indulge in overeating and physical inactivity. Currently, the *dietary transition* (of overeating and physical inactivity) has affected the urban rich and adults; however, obesity and metabolic disorders have affected the urban poor as well as rich in India. India is currently fighting against undernutrition as well as impending outbreak of overweight and obesity.

Consequences of Obesity

Overweight and obesity is a risk factor for development of various non-communicable diseases (NCD), over the years epidemiological data has proved that obesity and overweight leads to increased mortality and increased risk of chronic diseases like cardiovascular diseases, diabetes, hypertension, osteoarthritis, osteoporosis, gallbladder diseases, gallstones and certain cancers like breast and uterine and infertility. Obesity is a major risk factor for non-insulin dependent diabetes mellitus also apart from non-alcoholic fatty liver disease. Diabetes and obesity is often referred as *diabesity*.

Prevention and Control of Obesity

Since overweight and obesity is an emerging epidemic and significant public health problem, its prevention and control strategies are important. Following strategies can be applied.

Primordial Prevention

It involves prevention of development of obesity risk factors in population/persons not known to have the risk factors of the disease. The aim is to avoid emergence and establishment of the social, economic and cultural pattern of "lifestyles" that are known to contribute to an increased risk of obesity. In obesity, primordial prevention consists of physical activity and regulating dietary pattern. WHO says obesity cannot be prevented or managed or physical activity promoted, solely at the level of individual governments. The *food industry*, *International agencies*, the media and the community all need to work together to modify the environments so that it is less conducive to weight gain.

Lifestyles such as eating pattern, overweight and taking on to physical activity begins early in life during childhood period. Hence, the *primordial prevention* of *obesity begins during childhood period*. Developing healthy lifestyles is the responsibility of parents, school teachers, media, industrial establishment and the government (regulating town planning and eating establishments). Let us give our future generation a healthy start. During this *transition period* when we are faced with undernutrition on one hand and overnutrition on the other, we have to strike a balance.

Habit of regular physical exercises can be inculcated during childhood at home by parents, in schools by school teachers and at work place by peers and the management. Any amount of physical activity helps at any age. The minimum amount of physical activity required for prevention of obesity is at least 30 minutes of moderate activity every day or to spend 150 calories or energy per day. Therefore, 30 minutes of moderate activity every day is helpful. Half an hour is a minimum recommendation, of course, more time you spend moving for health, the more you gain. Walking 2.34 km in 30 minutes; or walking 3.12 km in 30 minutes, basketball game for 15 minutes, cycling, gardening, dancing fast for 30 minutes and washing a car or motorcycle, etc. help and keep away obesity. Exercise to your capacity. Everybody above 2 years of age should undertake for a cumulative duration of 30 minutes moderate physical activity. Persons with medical problems should consult a physician and take medical advice before starting a vigorous exercise. Avoid extremes and inappropriate or excessive physical activities. One can have interrupted physical activity of 10 minutes session or two sessions of 15 minutes each.[7, 8]

Diet—Curb on "Junk Foods"

Improve nutrition knowledge of people and eating sensibly and avoiding excess of eating. Caloric excess and physical inactivity lead to obesity. Avoidance of eating junk foods helps to reduce calories. Curb sale of junk foods in the vicinity of schools. Eating more of protective foods like green leafy vegetables and fruits in place of sweets is beneficial. Have only 20 g of visible fats in the food and right proportion of saturated, monosaturated and poly-unsaturated fatty acids in diets to maintain optimum level of HDL in the blood. Derive 60–65% of energy from carbohydrates with emphasis on complex carbohydrates of cereals which are good sources of fibre. Sugar should provide less than 10% of total energy. 10 15% of energy should be obtained from proteins and 20–30% from fats. Vegetarian diets based on complex carbohydrates, edible oil such as groundnut oil, sesame oil with moderate level of linoleic acid and GLV (green leafy vegetables) and fruits are helpful and better than animal foods. Fish and lean meat are good.

Primary Prevention

Primary prevention in obesity involves preventing the development of obesity in those who are overweight. Know your weight by checking your weight periodically at home or at workplace. Regular weighing at an interval of 1 to 3 months helps screening of persons for risk factor of overweight. If a person is overweight, regular programme of diets and physical activity can be chalked out and results can be monitored by the individual himself.

Secondary Prevention

If one has developed obesity, attempts are made to avoid further progression of obesity to morbid obesity and its complications. Graduating physical activity and dietary regimens can still be useful. Physical activity reduces stress and promotes active life.

Tertiary Prevention

It involves treating of advanced obesity and associated illnesses with obesity to reduce mortality and morbidity by advocating combination of drugs, physical activity, diet regulation, avoidance of tobacco, alcohol and weight loss bariatric surgery procedures for "morbid obesity".

Different strategies have to be adopted in rural and urban areas in the light of National Nutritional Policy and action plan on nutrition.

REFERENCES

1 GOI. Nutrition and food security Tenth Five-Year Plan 2002–07. New Delhi: GOI; 2002.

2 WHO. Obesity prevention and managing the global epidemic. Technical Report Series 894. Geneva: WHO; 2000.

3 Shetty PS. Body mass index: Is it the ideal universal weight for height index? NFI 2002 Oct; 23(4).

4 Shetty PS. Obesity: an emerging public health problem in Asia. NFI 2003 July; 24(3).

5 Sachdev HPS. Recent transition in anthropometric profile of Indian Children—Clinical and public health implications. NFI Bulletin 2003 Apr; 24(2).

6 IIPS-2006, NFHS-2 and NFHS-3, IIPS, Mumbai, India.

7 WHO. World health day 2002: Move for health. Regional office for South East Asia, New Delhi: WHO; 2002.

8 Shetty PS. Obesity and physical activity. NFI Bulletin 1997 Apr; 18(2).

DIABETES

World Health Day 7th April 2016—"Halt the rise beat diabetes". Diabetes as a non-communicable disease is significant public health problem. The prevalence rate all the world over is rising.

Diabetes mellitus is characterized by hyperglycaemia and disturbance of carbohydrate, fat and protein metabolism that are associated with absolute or relative deficiency of insulin action and/or insulin secretion. Therefore although diabetes is an endocrine disease in origin its major manifestations are those of metabolic diseases (WHO).

"Cut-off" level for diabetes (Table 13.9).[1]

These "cut-off" levels help in making decisions to manage diabetes and also help in determining the disease burden and prevalence level of diabetes in population.

Criteria for the Diagnosis of Diabetes Mellitus[2]

1 Symptoms of diabetes plus casual plasma glucose concentration ≥200 mg/dl (11.1 mmol/l). Casual is defined as any time of day without regard to time since

Table 13.9: World Health Organization recommendations for the diagnostic criteria for diabetes and intermediate hyperglycaemia

Diabetes should be diagnosed if one or more of the following criteria are met:

- Fasting plasma glucose ≥7.0 mmol/l (126 mg/dl)
- Two-hour plasma glucose ≥11.1 mmol/l (200 mg/dl) following a 75 g oral glucose load

Impaired glucose tolerance (IGT) should be diagnosed if **both** of the following criteria are met:

- Fasting plasma glucose <7.0 mmol/l (126 mg/dl)
- Two-hour plasma glucose 7.8–11.1 mmol/L (140–200 mg/dl) following a 75 g oral glucose load

Impaired fasting glucose (IFG) should be diagnosed if **both** of the following criteria are met:

- Fasting plasma glucose 6.1–6.9 mmol/L (110–125 mg/dl)
- Two-hour plasma glucose <7.8 mmol/L (140 mg/dl) following a 75 g oral glucose load

last meal. The classic symptoms of diabetes include polyuria, polydipsia, and unexplained weight loss. OR

2 Fasting plasma glucose (FPG) ≥126 mg/dl (7.0 mmol/L). Fasting is defined as no caloric intake for at least 8 hours. OR

3 Two hours post-load glucose ≥200 mg/dl (11.1 mmol/L) during an OGTT. The test should be performed as described by WHO, using a glucose load containing the equivalent of 75 g anhydrous glucose dissolved in water.

In the absence of unequivocal hyperglycaemia, these criteria should be confirmed by repeat testing on a different day. The third measure-oral glucose tolerance test (OGTT) is not recommended for routine clinical use.

Types of Diabetes

Type I

Formerly known as insulin-dependent diabetes mellitus (IDDM). Proportion of IDDM is less than 15% mostly in children and below 30 years.

Type II

Formerly known as non-insulin-dependent diabetes (NIDDM). Proportion of NIDDM is over 85% mostly above 40 years of age.

This is the predominant type of diabetes in India. This classification has significance because etiology and management of these 2 types of diabetes are different. In type I, the definite risk factors are obscure while in type II, the environmental risk factors are known and therefore these can be minimized or reduced to control the prevalence and incidence of diabetes. Most preventive programmes are against type II diabetes.

Type II is much more prevalent as compared to type I. Prevalence and incidence of type II has risen all the world over.

Gestational diabetes mellitus (GDM): It is defined as diabetes first recognized during pregnancy. The degree and severity of hyperglycaemia in this form of diabetes vary considerably. Following delivery, some women revert to normal glucose tolerance. About 3% of pregnant women have GDM.

Impaired glucose tolerance test (IGT) and impaired fasting glucose (IFG): Fasting Plasma Glucose (FPG) 110–125 mg is called Impaired Fasting Glucose (IFG) and 2 hours post-load glucose 140–199 mg/dl is called Impaired Glucose Tolerance (IGT). IFG and IGT are associated with the metabolic syndrome.

Malnutrition-related diabetes: This develops in young persons who were low birth weight babies and infants who were malnourished, and when they grow as adults they develop insulin resistant diabetes. Such adults are below 30 years with body mass index less than 18.5. Such adults are prone to develop metabolic disorders.

Prevalence

World over the prevalence of adult diabetes was around 4.7% in the year 1980 and has risen to 8.5% in 2014.

In India, prevalence is estimated to be 4.0% in 2000 and projected figure for 2025 was 6% in adults, indicating that diabetes was a major public health problem and epidemic of non-communicable diseases (Table 13.10). Number of estimated cases of diabetes in India during 2000 and 2010 were 2,58,14,117 and 3,76,71,965 respectively (National health profile 2010). In 2008, a survey conducted in both urban and rural areas reported a 5.9% prevalence of diabetes in India. Sub-centres screening data of 53341686 persons, of 30+ age indicates 6.05% as suspected diabetes in year 2014.

Table 13.10: Estimated prevalence of diabetes in adults (18 + years) in WHO regions[2, 3]

WHO regions	*Prevalence (%)*	
	1980	*2014*
African region	3.1	7.1
Region of the Americas	5.0	8.3
Eastern Mediterranean region	5.9	13.7
European region	5.3	7.3
South East Asian region	4.1	8.6
Western Pacific region	4.4	8.4
India	**4.1**	**7.8**
World	4.7	8.5

Global Burden

Globally, an estimated 422 million adults were living with diabetes in 2014, compared to 108 million in 1980. The global prevalence (age-standardized) of diabetes has nearly doubled since 1980, rising from 4.7% to 8.5% in the adult population. This reflects an increase in associated risk factors such as being overweight or obese. Over the past decade, diabetes prevalence has risen faster in low- and middle-income countries than in high-income countries.

With the current rates of prevalence, it is projected that India along with China and US will be "top three" countries to have most diabetics in terms of numbers. Thus most of the burden will fall on developing countries and India would be home to 123.5 million cases of diabetes (Table 13.11).[4] Currently 69 million Indians are living with diabetes (year 2014).

The number of people with diabetes is mounting due to rapid population growth, ageing, urbanization and increasing prevalence of obesity and physical inactivity.

Table 13.11: Top ten countries for number of adults (20–79 years) with diabetes—2015–40		
Country	Number of people with diabetes (million) 2015	2040
China	109.6	150.7
India	69.2	123.5
USA	29.3	35.1
Brazil	14.3	23.3
Russian Federation	12.1	12.4
Mexico	11.5	20.6
Indonesia	10.0	16.2
Egypt	7.8	15.1
Japan	7.2	–
Bangladesh	17.1	13.6

Source: IDF diabetes atlas, 7th edition, 2015

Deaths due to Diabetes

In India, 60% of all deaths were due to non-communicable diseases. During the base year of 1998 mortality due to Diabetes was to the extent of 0.2% which has now risen ten folds in the year 2014 (Table 13.12).

Risk factors: **Physical inactivity, overweight, obesity, family history** of diabetes are important risk factors of diabetes.

Age

The prevalence increases as the age advances. The type I diabetes which is more severe diabetes occurs mostly in younger people while type II diabetes prevalence is much more in middle and old age group. As the life expectancy is increasing, the people above the age group 60 and 65 will have to bear the brunt of diabetes. Data on diabetes in younger age group below 20 and above 65 is limited. In developing countries, the majority of people with diabetes are in 45–64 years age range while in developed countries most people have diabetes above the age of 64.

Sex

The prevalence of diabetes is higher in men than women.

Rural and Urban Distribution

For most developing countries in rural areas, the prevalence is assumed to be one-half that of urban areas. Urbanization leads to increased risk of diabetes because of altered diet, obesity and physical inactivity and other factors such as stress. In India, the prevalence of diabetes in rural area was 1.6% against 2.4% of urban areas in the year 2000. Studies/Surveys conducted in 2007 indicate increasing prevalence of DM in urban and rural India with figures varying from 5 to 15% in urban and 2 to 5% in rural areas.

Economic Status

Diabetes is more prevalent in higher income brackets, because of unhealthy lifestyles and physical inactivity leading to problem of overweight and obesity.

Family History of Diabetes

It is a strong risk factor and indicates genetic predisposition. Person who has family history of diabetes needs to observe precaution and undergo regular check-ups.

Nutritional Status

Low birth weight babies and severely and moderately malnourished children, when they grow-up as adults suffer from *metabolic disorders* including insulin resistant diabetes. These persons when they develop diabetes have BMI less than 18.5 and require large doses of insulin for glycaemic control. In Indian context, this is quite significant in view of widespread childhood malnutrition.

Prevention of Diabetes

Primordial prevention: It consists of prevention of emergence and establishment of risk factors (physical inactivity, overweight and obesity). Initiate actions to prevent people becoming overweight and obese begining **before birth** and in **early childhood**. Promote breast-feeding and consumption of healthy foods and discourage the consumption of unhealthy foods, such as sugary sodas and promote physical activity.

Table 13.12: Share of deaths (%) due to CCDs and NCDs in the world and India WHO (2014)[5]

Causes of death	Proportion of global deaths under the age 70 years by cause 2012	India 1998	India 2014
Communicable, maternal, perinatal and nutritional condition	34	68	30
Injuries	14	8.7	10
Non-communicable diseases	52	32	60
• Cardiovascular diseases	24.02	13.0	26
• Malignant neoplasm	11.8	3.4	7
Chronic respiratory diseases	5.56	6.7	13
• Diabetes	2.08	0.2	2
• Other NCDs	9.15	–	12

Primary Prevention

Adoption of healthy lifestyles (dietary modification and physical activity) are the corner stones of both primordial and primary prevention of diabetes. These are beneficial for the total population, hence the focus should be on total population. Healthy lifestyles are not only beneficial for diabetes alone but are generally good for prevention of other non-communicable diseases like obesity, coronary heart disease, strokes, hypertension and some cancers. Hence, integrated preventive programmes for non-communicable diseases are called for because most of the risk factors are common.[6, 7]

Prevention of Type I Diabetes

It occurs much less frequently and it results form autoimmune destruction of the β cells of the pancreas. Though the environmental and genetic factors appear to be involved, but there is no convincing evidence of role for lifestyle factors which can be modified to reduce the risk. The primordial and primary prevention for type I diabetes, is not practical for want of evidence.

Prevention of Type II Diabetes

Type II diabetes results from an interaction between genetic and environmental factors, however, the environmental factors play a major role and are the main risk factors. Overweight and obesity are associated with an increased risk of type II diabetes and the evidence is convincing. Increased BMI and increased waist HIP ratio and obesity are important determinant of insulin resistance which is the underlying abnormality in most cases of type II diabetes.

Overweight and Obesity

Voluntary weight reduction improves insulin sensitivity maintaining optimum BMI, i.e. striving for BMI at the lower end of normal range. For adult population, this means keeping BMI in the range of 21–23 kg/m^2 and maintaining waist hip ratio of less than 0.9 is good for health. It is more important for Indians because abdominal/central obesity is predominant obesity in India and they are more susceptible to develop insulin resistant diabetes and **syndrome X** (insulin resistance syndrome).[8] **Syndrome X** consists of abdominal obesity, insulin resistance, hypertriglyceridaemia, hyperinsulinaemia and hypertension.

Syndrome X and insulin resistance syndrome have been renamed by WHO in 1998 as "Metabolic syndrome". The modified adult treatment panel (ATP) III and third report of National Cholesterol Education Programme criteria works better for the diagnosis of metabolic syndrome in Indians.[9]

Physical Activity

Increased physical activity which has a major beneficial effect on insulin sensitivity independent of its effect on weight. People have adopted sedentary life and have become inactive and have put on weight on account of excessive consumption of food. For hours, people watch TV, are busy with computers and use vehicles and contact people on telephones and mobile phones and thereby they have become inactive. Physical inactivity has added a new dimension of iatrogenic problem or self-created problem of obesity and diabetes. Rapid urbanization and reduced playground space and excessive load of books and reading have reduced physical activities of children. Moderate level of physical activity of half an hour brisk walking, cycling or jogging or running, jumping, dancing or intense physical activity depending upon one's physical capacity is good for maintaining appropriate weight and helps reduction of weight. Physical activity should be done on regular basis and on most days per week. Physical activity means you move for your health. Moderate to intense physical exercise enhances insulin sensitivity.

Voluntary weight loss in overweight and obese people decreases the risk of diabetes because of improved insulin sensitivity.

Diets

High-saturated fat intake and excess of refined carbohydrates has been associated with a higher risk of impaired glucose tolerance, higher fasting glucose, insulin levels, and risk of type II diabetes. Consumption of unsaturated fatty acids and polyunsaturated fatty acids from vegetable sources are associated with reduced risk of type II diabetes. MUFA and PUFA increase the insulin sensitivity and improve glucose tolerance. Total visible fat intake should not exceed 20 g per day and not more than 20–30% of total calories or energy be derived from fats, lesser the better.[10, 11]

Dietary Fibre (DF)

Dietary fibre or complex carbohydrates have beneficial effect on weight reduction. Adequate intake of dietary fibre prevents obesity. Achieving adequate intakes of DF by regular consumption of whole grain cereals, legumes, pulses, fruits and vegetables (particularly green leafy vegetables) are most probably helpful in prevention of development of type II diabetes.[9, 10] Indian diets which are predominantly cereal-based provide adequate quantities of dietary fibre. We need to promote intakes of green leafy vegetables, fruits and pulses by adopting dietary and agriculture policies to be saved from type II diabetes. Recommended intake of DF is 20–35 g per day.

Fenugreek seeds (Methi seeds) which have high level of Insoluble dietary Fibre (48.6%) and Soluble dietary Fibre (20%) is very effective in reducing blood glucose and cholesterol levels.

Secondary Prevention

This involves early diagnosis and prompt treatment of type II diabetes, to prolong life or to live full life. Make essential medicines such as **human insulin** available and affordable to all who need them

The primary purpose of secondary prevention is early detection or identification of individuals without symptoms who either already have a disease or are clearly at high-risk of developing it, through screening programme.

Screening programme have two approaches: Population-based screening programme for type II diabetes remains controversial, it involves high cost and is not feasible for whole population. However, it is done for epidemiological research purposes to determine prevalence and trends of diabetes for the purpose of planning and measuring the impact. Population-based screening is not recommended to screen children and young adults for NIDDM.

Selective screening: This is feasible and undertaken for high-risk individuals. The possible high-risk groups are:

- Those with a strong family history of diabetes.
- Migrant Asians and Indians, other ethnic groups who show high prevalence and those changing traditional to westernized lifestyles.
- Obese and overweight persons and women with history of Gestational Diabetes Mellitus (GDM) or high birth weight babies.
- Those with other elements of chronic metabolic syndrome, e.g. hypertension, obesity, dyslipoproteinaemia.
- Persons above the age of 30 years at the point of primary contact with health facility.

Opportunistic screening: This is most practical way, when high-risk people present themselves to health care facility, they are screened for diabetes and hypertension. This is highly cost-effective and no extra resources are used to organize the screening programme.

Sereening of TB in diabetes and diabetes in TB has been initiated in 2015 for integrated management of diabetes, TB and HIV/AIDS.

Screening strategies include testing of casual blood glucose, measurement of blood pressure, BMI, physical activity, tobacco and alcohol use.

Screening for diabetes and hypertension as on December, 2012: 1,32,59,143 persons have been screened for diabetes and hypertension. 7.47% found suspected to be diabetes and 6.80% found suspected to be hypertension.

Tertiary Prevention

When the diabetes is established; all attempts should be made to keep it under control. Aim here is to prevent complications such as blindness, kidney failure, foot ulceration which may lead to gangrene and subsequent amputation, increased risk of infection, coronary heart disease and stroke. Education of individual to observe practice of personal hygiene to prevent infection and trauma and seek early treatment of infection and trauma. Life can be prolonged and full life despite diabetes is possible. Life-threatening complications can be avoided by effective treatment. Diet regulation, physical exercise and regular drugs including cheaper human insulin ensure effective control of diabetes.

Main lifestyle changes that reduce insulin resistance and prevent NIDDM:

- Increased physical activity
- Voluntary weight reduction
- Correction and prevention of obesity
- Limit fat intake and saturated fats
- Increase PUFA and MUFA in diet
- Encourage dietary fibre.

National diabetes control programme was launched as pilot programme in the 7th Five-Year Plan. The project was initiated in two districts in Tamil Nadu and one district in Jammu and Kashmir.

Now the national programme for prevention and control of cancer, diabetes, CVD and strokes has been launched in India.

REFERENCES

1 WHO (2016). Global report on diabetes.

2 IDF diabetes atlas seventh edition 2015.

3 King H, Aubert RE, Herman WH. Global burden of diabetes, 1995–2025. Prevalence, numerical estimates and projection. Diabetes Care 1998; 21: 4–31.

4 Wild SH, Roglic G, Green A, Sicree R, King H. Global prevalence of diabetes: Estimates for the year 2000 and projections for 2030. Diabetes care 2004; 27: 1047–53.

5 WHO (2002). Non-communicable diseases in SEAR 2002. India Country report of surveillance of major non-communicable disease. WHO/SEARO, New Delhi.

6 WHO (1994). Prevention of diabetes mellitus. WHO Technical Report Series 844. WHO; Geneva.

7 WHO (2003). Recommendations for preventing diabetes. WHO Technical Report Series 916.

8 Yajnik CS. Diabetes and Insulin resistance syndrome in Indians. NFI Bulletin July 1995; 16(3).

9 Adult treatment panel III. Third Report of the National Cholesterol Education Programme (NCEP). Expert panel on Detection, Evaluation and Treatment of High Blood Cholestrol in adults. Final report Circulation 2002;106: 3143–421.

10 Mohan V. Experience with dietary management in diabetes mellitus in South Indians. NFI Bulletin July 2003; 24(3).

11 Vishwanath M, Mohan V. Dietary management of Indian Vegetarian diabetics. NFI Bulletin 1991; 12(2).

HYPERTENSION (A Silent Killer)

"High blood pressure" was chosen as Theme of World Health Day 7th April 2013. Hypertension is a "silent killer". Hypertension is a complex public health problem. The higher the blood pressure in the community, the higher is the prevalence of cardiovascular diseases, strokes and renal diseases. Hypertension constitutes an important risk factor for coronary heart disease, stroke, eye and renal complications.

RULES OF HALVES IN HYPERTENSION

Majority of the persons suffering from hypertension are unaware of the disease. In accordance with the "rules of Halves", 50% of persons do not know about their higher blood pressure; only 50% of cases who are aware of the disease are on medication. These patients who are being treated, 50% are on proper antihypertensive therapy with their BP regularly monitored. It is, therefore, estimated that BP of only 10–12% hypertensive is controlled with appropriate treatment. Cardiology society of India reports —33% of adults tested had high blood pressure, over 60% had no clue of having high BP, while 42 % had controlled BP. In developed and developing countries with low mortality, higher blood pressure is the second most important risk factor in terms of DALYs losses. Over 11% of DALYs lost in developed countries are attributable to high blood pressure.[1] In developing countries, 2.5% of DALYs are lost due to high blood pressure (Table 13.13).

At least, 30% of all disease burden in high mortality developing counties such as sub-Saharan Africa and South East Asia is due to just 5 factors: underweight, unsafe sex, micronutrient deficiency, unsafe water and indoor smoke. In low mortality developing countries such as people's republic of China and most countries in Central and South America, the top 5 risk factors (tobacco, blood pressure, alcohol, cholesterol and overweight) cause at least one-sixth of their total disease burden. The population of these countries face double burden of risks, as these countries already face many of the same risks as faced by industrialized countries—tobacco and high blood pressure.

In developed countries of North America, Europe and Asian Pacific at least one-third of disease burden is attributable to tobacco, alcohol, blood pressure, cholesterol and obesity.

Tobacco burden alone kills 2.4 million people every year in industrialized countries. In addition, suboptimal blood pressure causes 7.1 million of deaths annually worldwide.

Hypertension is a risk factor for coronary heart disease and stroke and is three times more prevalent in urban areas as compared to rural, this may be because of different lifestyles in two populations.[2] But hypertension level of >140/90 is almost equal in two populations indicating low prevalence of risk factors in majority population of rural areas. These studies were done in 1990s in various parts of the country (Table 13.14). Epidemiological survey by Chadha, et al. showed prevalence rate of 12.75% in adult population (25–64 years) of urban area in Delhi in the year (1989–1992).[3]

Table 13.13: Leading selected risk factors as percentage of disease burden measured in terms of DALYs losses (%)

Risk factor	*Developing countries*		*Developed countries*
	High mortality	*Low mortality*	
1. Underweight	14.9	3.1–2.7*	7.4*
2. Unsafe sex	10.2	–	0.8
3. Unsafe water sanitation and hygiene	5.5	1.8	–
4. Indoor smoke from fuels	3.6	1.9	–
5. Zinc deficiency	3.2	–	–
6. Iron deficiency	3.1	1.8	0.7
7. Vitamin A deficiency	3.0	–	–
8. **Blood pressure**	2.5	5.0	10.9
9. Tobacco	2.0	4.0	12.0
10. Cholesterol	1.9	2.1	7.6
11. Low fruit and vegetable intake	–	1.9	3.9
12. Physical inactivity	–	–	3.3
13. Illicit drugs	–	–	1.8

*Overweight

Source: World Health Report, 2002

Results of several community-based studies in India reveal prevalence of hypertension in 25% of urban and 10% of rural population. Sub-centres screening data of 5,45,79,996 persons above 30 years of age in the year 2014 indicates prevalence of 4.97%. NFHS-4 data reported hypertension prevalence ranging from 5.9 to 27.3% in 15 states of India.

What Constitutes Hypertension?

The distribution of blood pressure values differ considerably among various populations. For example, the 90th percentile of systolic blood pressure varies between 146 and 176 mmHg resulting in wide differences in the proportion of people having "hypertension" in various parts of world. The worldwide projects like MONICA, INTERSALT and INTERHEALTH have contributed on the subject of hypertension substantially. The question is—What is most appropriate level at which the treatment should begin? This "cut-off" level determines the burden of hypertension in the community. Level of >140/90 has been chosen as "cut-off" point for classifying person into hypertensive and normal. Classification of blood pressure into various categories such as normal, prehypertension, stage 1 and stage 2 hypertension is depicted in Table 13.15.

The risk of blood pressure with adverse outcome of disease operate on "continuum" rising progressively over a range of systolic (upper) and diastolic (lower) blood pressure. It is desirable that the resting blood pressure in

Table 13.14: Prevalence of various risk factors for non-communicable disease in India[2]

Risk factor	Cut-off level	Prevalence (%)	
		Urban area	Rural area
1. Hypertension	≥160/95 mmHg	10–15 (4)	3–8 (4)
2. Hypertension	≥140/90 mmHg	20–30 (6)	15–25 (4)
3. Overweight	BMI ≥25	20–40 (2)	10 (1)
4. Hypercholesterolemia	≥220 mg/dl	20 (1)	10 (1)
5. Sedentary (physical inactivity)	Varied	50–60 (6)	8–30 (3)

Source: WHO; Non-communicable disease in SEAR 2002; Figures in brackets show the number of studies

Table 13.15: Classification and management of blood pressure for adults[4]

BP classification	SBP mmHg	DBP mmHg	Lifestyle modification
Normal	<120	and <80	Encourage
Prehypertension	120–139	or 80–89	Yes
Stage 1 hypertension	140–159	or 90–99	Yes
Stage 2 hypertension	≥160	or ≥100	Yes

DBP: Diastolic blood pressure; SBP: Systolic blood pressure
Source: Joint National Committee on Cardiovascular Diseases, 2003 (JNC-VII).

adults should not exceed 120 mmHg systolic and 80 mmHg diastolic since the risk of complications associated with blood pressure are minimal at such levels. However, the range up to 140 mmHg systolic and 90 mmHg diastolic is considered within normal range and does not qualify for the label of "hypertension" but are classified as "prehypertensives". In this intermediate range (120–139 mmHg systolic and 80–89 mmHg diastolic), it is advisable that persons should attempt to lower the pressure to desired level or at least avoid its rise into hypertensive range through lifestyle measures like regular physical exercise, reduced salt intake, avoidance of obesity, daily intake of adequate amount of fresh fruits and vegetables rich in potassium and management of stress through individual, family and community mechanisms.

Interventional levels: Blood pressure in the range starting with 140 mmHg systolic or 90 mmHg diastolic are at higher risk of blood pressure related complications and need effective intervention to lower blood pressure. Such interventions necessarily include all of the lifestyle measures listed above and may also require drug therapy.

Goal: The goal of therapy is to lower the blood pressure to values lower than 140/90 mmHg and then attempt progressively to bring it closer to desirable level, if such reductions are well tolerated. Much depends on initial blood pressure.

13

Diagnosing Hypertension

WHO recommends use of affordable and reliable electronic devices. Blood pressure measurement need to be recorded for several days before diagnosis of hypertension is made. BP is recorded twice daily, ideally in the morning and evening. Two consecutive readings are undertaken, at least a minute apart and with the person seated. Average value of all measurements is taken to confirm hypertension.

Natural History of Hypertension

"Natural history of hypertension presents us with continuum not a dichotomy." Use of dichotomy label such as "hypertensive" and "normotensive" are therefore not a description of natural order or natural history. However, the risks associated with hypertension operate on a continuum (Flowchart 13.1).

Stages

Desirable level → high initial blood pressure → border line hypertension → hypertension.

High initial blood pressure is the strongest, but still a weak predictor of future hypertension. Predictive value increases if more readings are taken.

Risk Factors for Hypertension

Environmental (Behavioural Risk Factors)

Body weight and obesity: Obesity is risk factor for hypertension thus putting on excess weight during childhood,

Flowchart 13.1: Natural history of hypertension

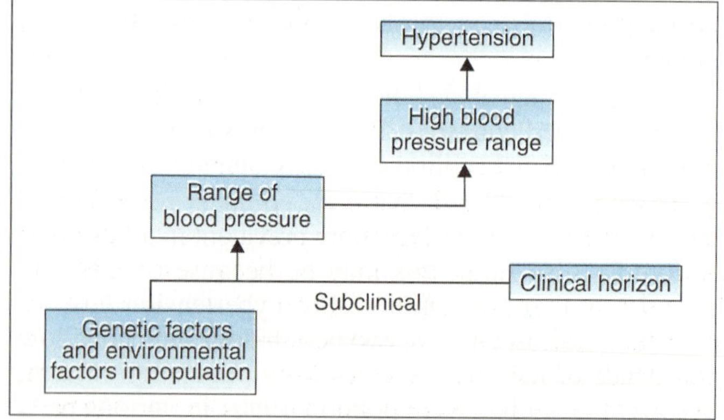

adolescence and youth period is undesirable. Weight control should result in decreased prevalence of hypertension, i.e. favourable weight control in a population can reduce the prevalence of hypertension by as much as 25%.

Salt and other Dietary Factors

Excessive salt intake particularly in those who have family history of hypertension can be in injurious. Communities where salt consumption is low have low blood pressure but other dietary factors are important such as excess of saturated fats and excess of energy or calories and low consumption of fruits and vegetables. Reduction of salt intake helps in control of hypertension.

Sodium intake, potassium intake and other dietary factors may have important influences on blood pressure regulation in individuals with different backgrounds. The decrease of sodium intake and/or an increase in potassium are potentially important primary prevention measures. It is desirable that diets of young children and adults limit the salt consumption of 5 g per day. It is advantageous in population where the prevalence of hypertension is high and salt intakes are also high. NIN (ICMR) recommends 6 g of salt intake per day per person.

Alcohol: Harmful use of alcohol and **tobacco** use are injurious and a potential risk factors in hypertension.

Physical Inactivity

Physical inactivity and lack of excercise leads to metabolic disturbance—obesity, raised blood lipids, impaired glucose tolerance and higher fasting insulin levels compared with normal is seen in hypertensive patients. Physical activity reduces the level of obesity and improves sensitivity towards insulin and prevents increased blood pressure.

Psychological and Social Influences

Acute stress situation like anxiety and worry elevates blood pressure through increased central sympathetic outflow. Sustained stress may have deleterious effects on blood pressure. Modifications of psychological influences may be an important approach in primary prevention of hypertension. Reduction of stress and modification of individual response to stress may be useful in primary prevention. Stress management is an important area in modern world to reduce its impact on untoward outcomes.

Social Factors/Determinants

The role of social factors/determinants such as globalization of unhealthy lifestyles, urbanization, economic conditions, social status, rural and urban distribution needs to be evaluated carefully in conjunction with levels of obesity, alcohol consumption, sodium and potassium intake, psychological stresses and various kinds of other lifestyles and habits. Some other factors have been implicated for hypertension such as noise pollution, air pollution and water quality. Noise pollution and air pollution may have a bearing on the primary prevention of essential hypertension.

Other Factors

Age

Average blood pressure increases with age and in many individuals it may rise little after adolescence, but in others it may increase progressively as the age advances.

Genetic Factors

Blood pressure levels are determined partly by genetic factors, but environmental factors play a major role. The detailed mode and mechanism of heredity in hypertension has not yet been conclusively analyzed. It is possible to identify and modify the environmental factors, causing progressive risk of blood pressure, to prevent "essential hypertension".

Primary Prevention[5]

Primary prevention of hypertension means to reduce the incidence of essential hypertension in the population by reducing the risk of onset. Primary prevention of essential hypertension has two approaches:

1. ***Population-based strategies:*** *Reducing salt and trans fats contents of manufactured foods:* Reduction in mean population blood pressure values has been achieved in the USA by reducing the salt content of manufactured food. Manufacturers have to mention the salt content of food item under law. Following NIN recommendation, the Food Safety and Standards Authority of India (FSSAI) has asked the packaged food manufacturers to use less salt in their products and display sodium level on their packaging. Dietary intake of sodium from all sources influences blood pressure level in population and should be limited so as to reduce the coronary artery disease and strokes both. Salt intake should be restricted to less than 5 g per day; it is beneficial in reducing blood pressure.

Reduction in mean population blood pressure values averts millions of deaths in population. This can be achieved by policies on salt restriction in food and diets, promoting physical activity, reduction of obesity and cholesterol level and cessation of smoking and tobacco use and avoiding harmful use of alcohol.

Information and education: Community education on salt intakes, diet control, healthy diets through multimedia channels and interpersonal communications can build a favourable environment and raise the level of awareness on the subject of hypertension in the population beginning at home, schools, colleges and workplace wellness programmes.

Physical Activity

The promotion of physical activity is a public health priority especially in the context of nutritional abundance and to counter the pandemic of obesity, serious consideration should be given to the environmental determinant of obesity and physical inactivity. Regulating the diets of *infants*, *young children* and *adolescents* and promoting physical activity helps prevention of obesity and thereby hypertension along with other lifestyle diseases. WHO recommends physical activity for at least 30 minutes a day—five times a week.

Diets

Reduce saturated and trans fats intake. Adequate dietary intake of potassium lowers blood pressure and is protective against stroke and cardiac arrhythmias. Potassium intake should be at a level which will keep the sodium to potassium ratio close to 1:1, i.e. daily potassium intake level of 50 mmol per day. This may be achieved through adequate consumption of fruits and vegetables.

Dietary fibre: Fibre is protective against coronary heart disease and has also been used to lower blood pressure. Adequate intake of 25–35 g per day may be achieved through fruits, vegetables and whole grain cereals as also pulses.

Tobacco

Stopping tobacco use and exposure to tobacco products.

Stress

Management of stress through individual, family and community mechanism by yoga and meditation. It eases tension and helps in maintaining normal blood pressure. Adequate sleep of 8 hours helps reduce blood pressure.

2 *High-risk approach:* The relations between high blood pressure and disease events such as cardiovascular disease is continuous and most events occur in people in the middle range of high blood pressure, who are not normally judged as hypertensive. Hypertensives who are considered to be high-risk are only part of risk continuum, rather than a distinct group. Preventive strategy focusing on the high-risk individuals will deal with only margin of the problem. This approach does not alter the underlying cause of hypertension. People with slightly raised blood pressure suffer more from cardiovascular events then hypertensive minority. While high-risk approach is more appropriate to individuals and their physicians but it has little impact at population level. High-risk approach requires continued and expensive screening for few high-risk individuals.[1]

Secondary Prevention

It aims at reduction of prevalence of essential hypertension in the community. Early diagnosis and prompt treatment necessitates opportunistic screening programmes, i.e. measuring blood pressures of adult population (30 years and above) who come in contact with health facility.

Prompt and continued treatment with modification of lifestyle will keep the blood pressure to desired level and will prevent the complications of hypertension.[6] Opportunistic screening programme can be encouraged through self-examination of blood pressure. Training to record correct blood pressure is essential—heath workers have not been trained and they lack this skill. The instruments for measuring blood pressure have not been standardized/calibrated and available instruments are in bad shape. New component of control of non communicable diseases has been added in the job description of health workers.

Tertiary Prevention—Limiting Disability and Rehabilitation

It means to limit the disability in persons who have developed complications due to hypertension, by treating the complications (coronary heart disease, retinal haemorrhages, cerebral haemorrhages/strokes) and sequelae of hypertension. Family-based rehabilitation is advisable.

National Programme

World Hypertension League strongly advocates for national health programme on non-communicable diseases including all diseases related to unhealthy lifestyle. Comprehensive programme for all non-communicable diseases such as CVD, diabetes, obesity, hypertension and cancer is imperative in view of emergence of an epidemic of non-communicable diseases.[6, 7]

REFERENCES

1 WHO (2002). The World Health Report 2002. Reducing risks, promoting healthy life. Geneva: WHO; 2002.
2 WHO Non-communicable disease in South East Asia region. New Delhi: South East Asia regional office, WHO; 2002.
3 Preventive cardiology—Health care—Clinical care. The J Applied Primary Health Care 1991 Apr-Sept, 3(4).
4 WHO. Diet, Nutrition and Prevention of Chronic Diseases. Tech Report Series No. 916. Geneva: WHO.
5 WHO. Primary prevention of essential hypertension. Tech Report Series No. 686, Geneva: WHO; 1983.
6 NIPHC—Escorts. Proceedings of seminar on preventive cardiology 1996 Nov. New Friends Colony, New Delhi: Health Care Promotion Trust, Regd.
7 WHO. A global brief on Hypertension, Silent Killer, global Public Health Crisis World Health day 2013.

RHEUMATIC HEART DISEASE (RHD)

Rheumatic heart disease (RHD) continues to be a major cardiac problem in India. Chronic RHD is a consequence of episodes of acute rheumatic fever. Recurrent episodes of acute rheumatic fever (ARF) increase the severity of cardiac lesion and consequently increase morbidity and mortality of RHD.

ACUTE RHEUMATIC FEVER

Acute rheumatic fever (ARF) is caused by group A haemolytic streptococcal infection. It causes repeated attacks of sore throat. Only 0.3 to 3% of children with streptococcal sore throat develop ARF. Susceptible individuals mount an exaggerated immune response to streptococcal throat infection. Antigen, antibody reaction affects the connective tissue of heart and joints mainly. ARF "Licks the joints and bites the heart", ARF leads to RHD. The RHD is a chronic disabling heart disease, which may require frequent hospitalization and cause physical disabilities, growth retardation and premature death.

Problem in India

Rheumatic heart disease in India accounts for 20–30% of hospital admissions due to all cardiovascular diseases (CVDs). In India, estimated prevalence is 5–7 per 1000 in the age group 5–15 years.[1]

Nature of Problem

RHD is a chronic heart disease which reduces growth, physical work capacity and leads to disability and premature death. It affects young children and adolescents.

Socioeconomic Factors

It is primarily a disease of poor socioeconomic groups—who live in crowded urban slums in Sub-human conditions. Rheumatic fever and RHD are typically associated with poverty, in particular with poor housing, overcrowding both of which favour the spread of streptococcal upper respiratory infection. The disease has almost disappeared from economically developed countries because of improvement in standards of living. Over-population, urbanization and industrialization lead to unplanned development and slums. Nearly 50% of urban population live in slum areas with Sub-human conditions which increase the susceptibility to all infections including streptococcal sore throat.

Pathogenicity

The association between group A beta haemolytic streptococcal upper respiratory tract infection and subsequent development of acute rheumatic fever is well established.

The absence of rheumatic fever in young children suggests that repeated exposure of the human host to the group A *Streptococcus* may be required to precipitate the illness. The clinical syndrome of rheumatic fever and carditis might be the result of an autoimmune mechanism.[2]

Criteria for Diagnosis of Rheumatic Fever

The Jones criteria were introduced in 1944 as a set of clinical guidelines for the diagnosis of rheumatic fever (RF) and carditis. The clinical features of RF were divided into major and minor categories based on the prevalence and specificity of manifestations. Major manifestations were least likely to lead to an improper diagnosis and included carditis, joint symptoms, subcutaneous nodules, and chorea. A history of RF or pre-existing rheumatic heart disease (RHD) was considered to be a major criterion since RF tends to recur. Minor manifestations were considered to be suggestive, but not sufficient, for a diagnosis of RF. The minor manifestations comprised clinical findings (such as fever and erythema marginatum, abdominal pain, epistaxis and pulmonary findings), and laboratory markers of acute inflammation, such as leukocytosis (WBC), and elevated erythrocyte sedimentation rate (ESR) or C-reactive protein (CRP) (Table 13.16). It was proposed that the presence of two major, or one major and two minor, manifestations offered reasonable clinical evidence of rheumatic activity. Since a previous history of definite RF or RHD was considered a major criterion, diagnosis of a recurrence of RF did not require strict application of these guidelines, and minor manifestations were considered sufficient for the diagnosis.

The importance of the Jones criteria was soon realized, especially as objective guidelines that allowed RF to be diagnosed uniformly in multicentre studies of RF. The Jones criteria were subsequently reviewed by the American Heart Association (AHA) and the World Health Organization (WHO) and were modified to encompass vexing clinical issues and to improve the specificity (Table 13.16). Although the Jones criteria have been revised repeatedly, the modifications were often made without prospective studies and were based on the perceived effects of previous revision(s).

The importance of a preceding streptococcal infection has been emphasized in subsequent revisions of the Jones criteria, in which a diagnosis of RF required the demonstration of streptococcal etiology. Although the inclusion of this criterion helped to improve diagnostic specificity, it impaired sensitivity when evidence of antecedent streptococcal infection had already subsided (such as with insidious and chronic carditis), or if manifestations of RF were delayed (such as with chorea). Therefore, late manifestations of RF were subsequently exempted from the requirement to demonstrate streptococcal etiology.

WHO Criteria for Diagnosis of Rheumatic Fever and Rheumatic Heart Disease (based on Revised Jones Criteria), 2002–2003

These revised WHO criteria (Table 13.16) facilitate the diagnosis of:

- A primary episode of RF
- Recurrent attacks of RF in patients without RHD
- Recurrent attacks of RF in patients with RHD
- Rheumatic chorea
- Insidious onset rheumatic carditis
- Chronic RHD.

Table 13.16: WHO 2002–03 criteria for the diagnosis of rheumatic fever and rheumatic heart disease (based on the revised Jones criteria)[2]

Diagnostic categories	*Criteria*
• Primary episode of rheumatic fever (RF)[a]	Two major* or one major and two minor** manifestations **plus** evidence of a preceding group A streptococcal infection***
• Recurrent attack of RF in a patient **without** established RHD[b]	Two major or one major and two minor manifestations **plus** evidence of a preceding group A streptococcal infection
• Recurrent attack of RF in a patient **with** established RHD	Two minor manifestations **plus** evidence of a preceding group A streptococcal infection[c]
• Rheumatic chorea Insidious onset rheumatic carditis[b]	Other major manifestations or evidence of group A streptococcal infection not required
• Chronic valve lesion of RHD (patients presenting for the first time with pure mitral stenosis or mixed mitral valve disease and/or aortic valve disease)[d]	Do not require any other criteria to be diagnosed as having rheumatic heart disease
*Major manifestations	• Carditis • Polyarthritis • Chorea • Erythema marginatum • Subcutaneous nodules
**Minor manifestations	• *Clinical:* Fever, polyarthralgia • *Laboratory:* Elevated acute phase reactants (erythrocyte sedimentation rate or leukocyte count)
***Supporting evidence of a preceding streptococcal infection within the last 45 days	• Electrocardiogram: Prolonged P-R interval • Elevated or rising antistreptolysin-O other streptococcal antibody, or • A positive throat culture, or • Rapid antigen test for group A streptococci, or • Recent scarlet fever

[a]Patients may present with polyarthritis (or with only polyarthralgia or monoarthritis) and with several (3 or more) other minor manifestations, together with evidence of recent group A streptococcal infection. Some of these cases may later turnout to be rheumatic fever. It is prudent to consider them as cases of "Probable rheumatic fever" (once other diagnosis are excluded) and advise regular secondary prophylaxis. Such patients require close follow-up and regular examination of the heart. This cautious approach is particularly suitable for patients in vulnerable age groups in high incidence settings.

[b]Infective endocarditis should be excluded.

[c]Some patients with recurrent attacks may not fulfill these criteria.

[d]Congenital heart disease should be excluded.

For the diagnosis of a primary episode of RF, it is recommended that the major and minor clinical manifestations of RF, the laboratory manifestations, and evidence of a preceding streptococcal infection should all continue according to the 1988 WHO recommendations. In the context of a preceding streptococcal infection, two major manifestations, or a combination of one major and two minor manifestations, provide reasonable evidence for a diagnosis of RF, WHO has continued to maintain that a diagnosis of a recurrence of RF in a patient with established RHD should be permitted on the basis of minor manifestations plus evidence of a recent streptococcal infection.

Physicians should use their clinical judgment to diagnose carditis in an episode of RF, especially during a recurrence of RF, and should use the above recommendations as guidelines for the diagnosis.

Prevention of Rheumatic Fever and RHD

Primary Prophylaxis (Primary Prevention)

13

This is ideal but hard to achieve. Primary prophylaxis is the identification and treatment of upper respiratory tract infection due to group A streptococci to prevent initial attack of acute rheumatic fever (ARF). If group A streptococcal infection could be eradicated, rheumatic fever would disappear and RHD would not occur. Prevention of rheumatic fever is possible by early and effective treatment of upper respiratory tract infections caused by group A streptococci. This makes rheumatic heart disease one of the most readily preventable cardiovascular disease. Where facilities for throat culture are not available, clinical criteria like yellow exudates on the throat, presence of anterior cervical lymph nodes are quite suggestive of streptococcal infection.

Primary prophylaxis is effective in preventing rheumatic fever and is strongly recommended for the individual patient with streptococcal pharyngitis, however, the concept of broad-based primary prophylaxis at the community level is more controversial while various approaches to community primary prophylaxis programmes have been tried (e.g. seasonal prophylaxis, school-based programmes), these programmes are difficult to implement.

The infection can be eradicated by single intramuscular injection of benzathine benzylpenicillin or by 10 days treatment with oral penicillin. Other bactericidal antibiotics, e.g. erythromycin have also been shown to be

Table 13.17: Recommended treatment for streptococcal pharyngitis[3, 4]

Antibiotic	Mode of administration	Dose
Benzathine benzylpenicillin	Intramuscular	• 12,00,000 units for adults and children weighing more than 30 kg. • 6,00,000–9,00,000 for children weighing less than 30 kg. (given as a single injection)
Phenoxymethyl penicillin	Oral	250 mg 4 times daily for 10 days very small children (weighing less than 20 kg) may be given 125 mg 4 times daily

effective in eradicating group A streptococci, but penicillin remains a drug of choice because it is safe, effective and inexpensive (Table 13.17).

For patient allergic to penicillin, oral erythromycin is accepted alternative.

Secondary Prophylaxis

Secondary prophylaxis is regular administration of an antibiotic (usually penicillin) to a patient who has had rheumatic fever, in order to prevent colonization and/or infection of the upper respiratory tract with group A streptococci and subsequent development of recurrent attacks of rheumatic fever. Secondary prophylaxis has been shown to reduce recurrences. Additional data are available to show that, in about 70% of patients who have suffered an initial attack of rheumatic carditis, heart murmurs will disappear, if effective secondary prophylaxis is given. Secondary prophylaxis programmes are cost-effective in reducing morbidity and mortality due to rheumatic fever.

Two main methods of prophylaxis are available: monthly (or in special circumstances 3 weekly) intramuscular injections of benzathine benzylpenicillin, or daily administration of antibiotics orally (either penicillin, sulfadiazine or rarely erythromycin).

The duration of secondary prophylaxis must be adapted to the individual but some general principles can be stated. Patients without carditis in a previous attack should have prophylaxis for a minimum of 5 years after the last attack of ARF and at least until age 18 and sometimes longer. Patients with cardiac involvement in the initial attack should continue prophylaxis at least until the age of 25 years and longer if environmental conditions or other risk factors warrant it.

For patients with chronic valvular RHD, secondary prophylaxis for prolonged periods even for life has sometimes been recommended (Table 13.18).

Tertiary Prevention

The valve replacement is extremely expensive and it may cost Rs. 90,000 or more and few may be able to afford this.

Table 13.18: Antibiotic regimens for secondary (continuous) prophylaxis for RF/RHD[3, 4]

Mode of Administration	Penicillin	Sulfadiazine
Intramuscular	• Benzathine benzyl-penicillin • Single injection once a month* • For children <30 kg 6,00,000 units • For children >30 kg and adults 12,00,000 units	
Oral**	Phenoxymethyl penicillin 250 mg twice daily	For children <30 kg 0.5 g daily ≥30 kg and adults 1 g daily

* In special circumstances or for high-risk patients one injection may be given every 3 weeks.

** For patient allergic to penicillin and sulfonamide erythromycin 250 mg twice daily is suggested.

Improvement of Socioeconomic Factors

Poor socioeconomic conditions are associated with high-risk of rheumatic fever and RHD. An increased risk may also be associated with the overcrowding that frequently accompanies mass migration from rural to urban areas. Improvement in socioeconomic conditions (particularly better housing) will in the long run reduce the incidence of rheumatic fever.

Health Education

Since the attacks of ARF occur primarily in children (as opposed to the morbidity and mortality from RHD which is common in adult life) education of parents regarding the importance of recognizing and treating streptococcal sore throats to prevent RHD is necessary. However, ARF primarily affects the poor who are often illiterate or semiliterate and difficult to reach.

Health education should be done through primary health care infrastructure and through mass media or through school teachers. Teacher's training and training of health workers on communication, recognition and treatment of streptococcal sore throat is important.

NATIONAL PROGRAMME FOR PREVENTION AND CONTROL OF CANCER, DIABETES, CARDIOVASCULAR DISEASES AND STROKES (NPCDCS)

GLOBAL BURDEN OF NCDs

A total of 56 million deaths occurred worldwide during 2012 of these, 38 million were due to NCDs; principally cardiovascular diseases, cancers and chronic respiratory diseases. Nearly three quarters of these (28 million) occurred in low middle income countries.[5]

DISEASE BURDEN DUE TO (NCDs) IN INDIA

According to WHO in India (2008 data), 53% of total deaths were caused by non-communicable diseases (NCDs) 37% of deaths were caused by communicable diseases (CCDs) and the rest 10% deaths were as a result of accidents and injuries. In sharp contrast to the situation in industrialized economies of Europe for instance 6% of all deaths were caused by communicable diseases, while a whooping 86% were due to metabolic disorders and the remaining were due to other causes. India is worst of both the worlds. India is thus faced with double disease burden (NCD and CCD). The public health policy has to address both types (Table 13.19).

Table 13.19: Global burden of NCD deaths in 2005 WHO

Region	*Comm. diseases (%)*	*NCD (%)*
Europe	6	86
China	15	68
India	47	44
Africa	70	22

Non-communicable diseases (NCDs) are emerging as the leading causes of deaths in India accounting for over 42% of all deaths (RGI—2006): NCDs cause significant morbidy and mortality both in urban and rural population, with considerable loss in potentially productive years (aged 35–64 years) of life.

It is estimated that overall prevalence of diabetes, hypertension, ischaemic heart diseases (IHDs) and strokes is 62.47, 159.46, 37.00 and 1.54 respectively per 1000 adult population in India. There are 2.8 million cancer cases in India at any point of time. The leading sites of cancer are oral cavity, lungs, oesophagus and stomach among men and cervix, breast and oral cavity amongst women. NCDs especially cardiovascular diseases, cancers, chronic respiratory diseases and diabetes caused 57% of all deaths in 2008. Total deaths from NCD are projected to increase by a further 17% over the next 10 years. These diseases are largely preventable by *modifying* the four common *risk factors*, tobacco use, unhealthy diet, physical inactivity and harmful use of alcohol.

To address problem of NCD National Programme for Prevention and Control of Cancers, Diabetes, Cardiovascular Diseases and Strokes (NPCDCS) has been Launched in 2010–11 after integrating the National Cancer Control Programme.[6]

The NPCDCS has two components, viz. (i) Cancer and (ii) Diabetes, CVDs and strokes. These two components have been integrated at different levels.

Premature mortality Global Target[5] (Sustainable Development Goal). The premature mortality target is, a 25% reduction in overall mortality from cardiovascular diseases, cancers, diabetes and chronic respiratory diseases by 2025 (referred to as "25 × 25") between the age 30 and 70 years from base year of 2015.

13

Major Objectives of NPCDCS

- Prevention and control of NCDs
- Provide early diagnosis and treatment
- Train human resources for NCDs
- Identification of major risk factors.

STRATEGIES

The strategies to achieve the objectives

i Promotion of healthy life styles—by education.
ii Early diagnosis by opportunistic screening of persons above 30 years.
iii NCD clinics at CHC and District level for treatment.
iv Development of trained manpower.
v Strengthening of tertiary level facilities.
vi Monitoring, evaluation and surveillance of risk factors of NCDs as also morbidity and mortality.

NCD: Risk Factors Surveillance

The key to control of epidemic of NCDs is **primordial** and **primary prevention.** The basis of prevention of NCDs are:

a Prevention of emergence of risk factors by promoting healthy lifestyles.
b Identification of risk factors by screening programmes and modification of these risk factors (Fig. 13.2).

1. Prevention through behaviour change: The major risk factors of cancer, hypertension, obesity, diabetes and cardiovascular diseases are—unhealthy diet, physical inactivity, stress and consumption of tobacco and alcohol. Attempts are being made to prevent emergence of these risk factors by creating general awareness about the non-communicable diseases (NCDs) and promotion of healthy lifestyle habits right from carly childhood period. Such interventions will be done through the peripheral health functionaries and NGOs. The various approaches such as mass media, community education and interpersonal communication will be used for behavior change focusing on the following five messages:

1 Increased intake of healthy foods.
2 Increased physical activity through sports, and exercise.

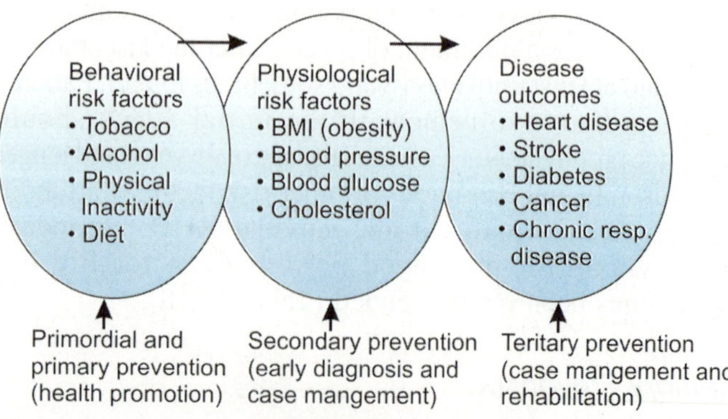

Fig. 13.2: Risk factors (RF) and level of NCD prevention and management

3 Avoidance of tobacco and alcohol.
4 Stress management by Yoga and Meditation.
5 Warning signs of cancer, etc.

Interpersonal communication will be carried out through ASHAs/AWWs/SHGs/Youth clubs, Panchayat members, etc. for which education material will be developed at Central/State level to facilitate IEC/BCC activities. These workers/groups will also help in social mobilization for diagnostic camps. Targeted intervention programmes will be designed to bring awareness in **schools, workplaces,** and **community**. The health Promotion for behaviour change will be carried out by National, State, and district level **Multi-Sectoral Action Plans**.

2. Early diagnosis—opportunistic screening: Strategy for early diagnosis of chronic non-communicable diseases consists of opportunistic screening of persons above the age of 30 years at the point of primary contact with any health care facility, be it the village, CHC, District hospital, tertiary care hospital, etc. Opportunistic screening will have in built components of mass awareness generation, self-screening and by trained health care providers.

Such screening involves risk assessment by simple clinical history comprising of relevant questions and easily conducted physical measurements (such as history of tobacco and alcohol consumption, physical activity and measurement of blood pressure and blood sugar, weight and height (body mass index), etc. to identify those individuals who are at a high risk of developing diabetes and CVD, warranting further investigation and action. Actions include counseling and lifestyle modification. The investigations which may not be carried out in the health facilities can be outsourced. District NCD clinic also screens women of age group 30–69 years approaching to the hospital for early detection of cervix cancer and breast cancer.

3. Treatment: NCD clinic at Community Health Centre: Under NPCDCS 364 districts have been selected for programme implementation. All selected CHCs shall establish a 'NCD clinic' for comprehensive examination of patients referred by the health workers as well as reporting directly to rule out complications or advanced stages of common NCDs. The clinic shall run on all working days of the week. Screening, diagnosis and management (including diet counselling, lifestyle management) and home-based care will be the key functions. For providing effective comprehensive care the following staff shall be appointed on contract basis by the state government—Doctor 1, Nurses 2, Counsellor 1, Data Entry Operator 1.

Medical officer and a nurse shall impart health education during the OPD as well as to the inpatients if any. Counsellor appointed under the programme shall counsel on diet, nutrition and tobacco, alcohol, and warning signs of cancer, etc.

Diagnosis and management: The unit of NCD clinic at CHC which involves doctor and paramedical personnel will do the diagnosis, management and **stabilization of common CVD,** diabetes and stroke cases (outpatient as well as inpatients.)

Laboratory investigations: CHC shall do the required investigations/tests for comprehensive examination for NCDs like blood sugar measurement, lipid profile, ultrasound, X-ray, ECG, etc. In case there is no facility for particular investigations/tests it may be referred to District Hospital. Provision of outsourcing of required investigations to some extent can be done where investigations are not available at the hospital.

Home-based care: One of the nurses appointed under the programme shall undertake home visits for bedridden cases, supervise the work of health workers and attend monthly clinics being held in the villages on a random basis. She shall visit one village per week for home visits and advise the bedridden patient with diabetes, stroke, etc. about the care and will refer the case to the CHC/District Hospital if required. In total she shall visit 4 times in a month.

Referral: Complicated cases of diabetes, high blood pressure, etc. shall be referred from CHC to the District Hospital for further investigations and management on the prescribed format.

Data recording and reporting: "NCD clinic" at CHC shall maintain individual diagnosis, treatment and referral records on the patient chronic disease card, with verbal and pictorial advice for the patient. This record shall be sent monthly to the District NCD Cell set up under NPCDCS.

NCD clinic at district level: The selected district shall provide the full complement of preventive, supportive and curative services for cancer, diabetes, hypertension and cardiovascular diseases including stroke through the selected District Hospital. Following services will be provided by district hospital.

District shall identify a district hospital to be strengthened under NPCDCS for providing NCD services. The hospital shall have an ICU and basic laboratory facilities available attached to it. A 'NCD clinic' will be established at the identified district hospital to provide emergency care and management of cancer, diabetes, hypertension and acute cardiovascular diseases. The clinic shall run on **all working** days of the week. ICU of the district hospital will be upgraded/strengthened with a cardiac care unit (2–4 beds) with ventilator and other necessary pieces of equipment.

District NCD clinic shall also screen women of the age group 30–69 years approaching to the hospital for early detection of cervix cancer and breast cancer. District hospital would be assisted to purchase the required pieces of equipments like colposcope, mammography, etc.

Human Resources at District Hospital

Following additional staff will be recruited on contract basis by the State Government to manage NCD clinic and to provide acute and chronic care services:

a. Doctor (specialist in diabetology/cardiology/MD physician)
b. Medical oncologist, cytopathologist
c. Cytopathologist technician, nurses, physiotherapist, counsellor, data entry operator and coordinator.

4. Capacity building of human resource: Health personnel at various levels will be trained for health promotion, prevention, early detection and management by a team of trainers at identified training institutes/centres. These training institutes/centres will be identified by the state in consultation with the centre.

5. Supervision, monitoring and evaluation: Regular monitoring and review of the scheme will be conducted at the District, State and Central levels through monitoring formats and periodic visits and review meetings. For the purpose, NCD cell at different levels (at National, State and District levels) are envisaged to supervise and monitor the programme as also other NCD programmes. The NCD cell at various levels will ensure implementation and supervision of the programme activities related to health promotion, early diagnosis, treatment and referrals and further facilitates partnerships with laboratories for early diagnosis in the private sector. The NCD cell would ensure convergence with the ongoing activities of National Health Mission, National Tobacco Control Programme and National Programme for Health Care of Elderly. The evaluation is the integral part of the programme and will be carried out concurrently and periodically, as and when required.

Package of services: In the programme, it is envisaged providing preventive, promotive, curative and supportive services (core and integrated services) in cancer, diabetes, cardiovascular diseases (CVDs) and stroke at various government health facilities.

The package of services would depend on the level of health facility and may vary from facility to facility. The range of services will include health promotion, psycho-social counseling, management (out- and inpatient), day care services, home-based care and palliative care as well as referral for specialized services as needed. Linkages of District Hospitals to private laboratories and NGOs will help to provide the additional components of continuum of care and support for outreach services. The district will be linked to tertiary cancer care health facilities for providing comprehensive care.

The non-communicable diseases are expensive to treat. National strategies have to focus on prevention and health promotion as key to reduce disease burden. Health education programme that promotes exercise, weight reduction, early diagnosis, and screening are some of the key interventions that need to be promoted at various levels of health facilities.

Package of services at various levels of health systems

Health facility	*Package of services*
Sub-centre	• Health promotion for behavior change and counselling • 'Opportunistic' screening using BP measurement and blood glucose by glucostrip method • Identification of early warning signals of common cancers and referral • Referral of suspected cases to CHC/nearby health facility
PHC	• All above + clinical diagnosis and treatment of simple cases of hypertension and diabetes
CHC/FRU	• Prevention and health promotion including counselling • Early diagnosis through clinical and laboratory investigations • (Common lab investigations: Blood sugar, lipid profile, ECG, ultrasound, X-ray, etc. if not available, may be outsourced) • Management of common CVD, diabetes and stroke cases • 'Opportunistic' screening of common cancers (oral, breast, cervix and prostate) • Referral of difficult cases to District Hospital/ higher health care facility
District Hospital	• Early diagnosis of diabetes, CVDs and cancer • Investigations: Blood sugar, lipid profile, kidney function tests • (KFT), liver function test (LFT), ECG, ultrasound, X-ray, mammography, etc. if not available, will be outsourced. • Medical management of cases (outpatient, inpatient and intensive care) • 'Opportunistic' screening of common cancers (oral, breast, cervix and prostate) • Referral of difficult cases to higher health care facility • Health promotion for behavior change and counselling • Follow-up chemotherapy in cancer cases • Rehabilitation and physiotherapy services
Medical college	• Mentoring of district hospital • Early diagnosis and management of diabetes, CVDs and other associated illnesses • Training of health personnel • Operational research
Tertiary cancer centre	• Mentoring of District Hospital and outreach activities • Comprehensive cancer care including prevention, early detection, diagnosis, treatment, minimal access surgery, aftercare, palliative care and rehabilitation, training of health personnel, operational research

The services under the programme would be integrated below district level and will be integral part of existing primary health care delivery system and vertical at district and above as more specialized health care are needed both for cancer component and diabetes, CVD, and stroke. In the 12th Five-Year Plan NPCDCS is being implemented in the 35 states/UTs in 364 districts. NPCDCS has now been brought under the umbrella of NHM in Programme Implementation Plan (PIP) Mode. Interventions up to district level and below have been integrated under the mission and funds provided through NCD Flexipool.

Cancer Component under NPCDCS Services

- Provision of common diagnostic services, basic surgery, chemotherapy and palliative care for cancer patients.
- Each district is being supported with ₹ 1.66 crore per annum for chemotherapy drugs for 100 pateints, day care chemotherapy, facility for laboratory investigations including mammography, home based palliative care, and contractual manpower (medical oncologist, cytopathologist technician and two nurses).

Tertiary cancer centre: Provides comprehensive cancer care including early detection, diagnosis, treatment, minimal access surgery after care, palliative care and rehabilitation services, training and operational research.

NCD Risk Factors Survey (Assessment of Prevalence of Risk Factors)

The following risk factors prevalence were measured by periodic sample surveys conducted once in five years under IDSP. The target population of 15–64 years has been covered. WHO step-wise approach to NCD has been followed (*see* chapter of Epidemiology). Risk factors included: Tobacco use, alcohol consumption, raised blood pressure, obesity, diet, physical inactivity, diabetes mellitus and high serum cholesterol.

Periodic survey in 15–64 years of age by WHO step-wise approach has been completed in seven states under IDSP—to provide data on the risk factors.[7, 8] These data will help the state administrators to plan strategies for the control of NCD. The first phase of the survey included seven states (Andhra, Kerala, Madhya Pradesh Maharashtra, Mizoram, Tamil Nadu and Uttarakhand) covering 22,008 persons.

Urban Health Check-up for Diabetes and High Blood Pressure

On the World Diabetes day on 14th November 2010 an Urban Health Check-up Scheme for Diabetes and High Blood Pressure in urban slums was launched in New Delhi. In the first phase the scheme was initiated in seven metros, viz. Delhi, Bengaluru, Hyderabad, Kolkata, Mumbai, Chennai and Ahmedabad with the objective of:

1 Screening urban slum population for diabetes and high blood pressure.
2 To create database for prevalence of diabetes and high blood pressure.
3 To sensitize the urban slum population about healthy lifestyles.

The blood sugar and blood pressure will be checked for all persons ≥30 years and all pregnant women of all age groups.

WHO Global Action Plan and Monitoring Framework for Prevention and Control of Non-communicable Diseases

The action plan provides road map to attain **nine** voluntary global targets to be achieved by 2025 including 25 indicators for prevention and control of non-communicable diseases.

Targets

1 25% relative reduction of premature mortality from cardiovascular diseases, cancer, diabetes and chronic respiratory diseases by 2025 (*Referred to as 25 × 25*).
2 At least 10% relative reduction in the harmful use of alcohol
3 10% relative reduction in prevalence of physical inactivity
4 A 30% relative reduction of mean population intake of salt/sodium
5 A 30% relative reduction in prevalence of current tobacco use in person aged 15+ years
6 A 25% relative reduction in the prevalence of raised blood pressure or contain the prevalence of raised blood pressure
7 Halt the rise in diabetes and obesity
8 At least 50% eligible people receive drug therapy and counselling (including glycaemic control) to prevent heart attacks and strokes
9 An 80% availability of affordable basic technologies and essential medicines

REFERENCES

1 Planning Commission. Tenth Five-Year Plan (2002–07). Vol II. Sectoral policies and programmes. New Delhi: Planning Commission GOI; 2002.
2 WHO. Technical Report Series 923. Geneva: WHO; 2004.
3 WHO. Community prevention and control of cardiovascular diseases—report of WHO expert committee. Tech Rep Ser 732. Geneva: WHO; 1986.
4 WHO. Rheumatic fever and rheumatic heart disease. Tech Rep Ser 764. Geneva: WHO; 1988.
5 WHO. Global status reprt on noncommunicable disease 2014. "Attaining the nine alobal goals NCDs target; a shared responsibility".

6 GOI. MOH and FW, Annual Report 2007–14. National Programme for Prevention and Control of Cancer, Diabetes, Cardiovascular Diseases and Strokes. GOI; New Delhi.
7 WHO. WHO STEPS Surveillance Manual. The WHO STEP wise approach to chromic disease risk factors Surveillance. Geneva, World Health Organization, 2005.
8 GOI. IDSP—Risk Factors Survey Fact Sheet—India Phase 1—States, 2010–11. MOH and FW. GOI; New Delhi.

ACCIDENTS AND INJURIES

PANDEMIC OF ROAD TRAFFIC ACCIDENTS (RTA)

Increasing mechanization in agriculture and industry, induction of semiskilled and skilled workers in various operations and rapid increase in vehicular traffic have resulted in morbidity, mortality and disability due to accident and trauma. Overcrowding due to rise in population and lack of awareness and poor implementation of essential safety precautions result in an increasing number of accidents. Apart from accidents, the vehicular traffic causes air pollution, which adds to the woe of respiratory and heart diseases and deaths which may outnumber accidental deaths. Noise pollution is another hazards of road traffic. Road traffic accidents are "hidden epidemic" which though a priority, has received much less attention.

Spectrum of Accidents

1 Road traffic accidents (RTA)
2 Industrial accidents
3 Domestic and peridomestic
4 Railway accidents
5 Agriculture accidents
6 Intentional or suicidal injuries.

The spectrum may not cover the total range of accidents; but for the purpose of management and prevention of accidents this may be helpful. Road traffic injuries are leading cause of morbidity and mortality the world over.

Epidemiology of RTA

Human beings, the **vehicles** and environment make 3 components of the **epidemiological triad** within which safety is shared responsibility.

Problem

Accidents and injuries are global problem. These are common in developed and developing countries. Injuries represent 12% of global burden of disease, the third most common cause of overall mortality and the main cause of death amongst 1–40 years old. More than 20 million people are severely injured and 1.2 million get killed on the world's roads each year.[1]

Mortality

According to WHO data for 2002, road traffic injuries accounted for 2.1% of all global deaths and ranked as 11th leading cause of death. WHO data shows that in 2002 nearly 1.2 million people died as a result of road traffic injuries. This represents an average of 3242 persons dying each day around the world due to road traffic accidents. In addition to these deaths, between 20 and 50 million people globally are estimated to be injured or disabled each year due to RTA.[2]

Mortality Rate

Global road traffic injury mortality rate was 19.0/1,00,000 population.

Accidents Burden

Overall injuries accounted for 14% of adults disease burden in the world during 2002.

Rank

Road traffic accidents are 4th leading cause of mortality and disease burden worldwide (next to HIV/AIDS, IHD and tuberculosis) in 15–59 years age group. By 2020, RTA would be 3rd leading cause of DALYs losses or disease burden (Table 13.20).[1]

Distribution

90% of road traffic accidents were in low and middle income countries and only 10% of road traffic accidents occurred in high income countries.

Age, Sex and Road Traffic Accidents

Over 50–60% of road traffic accident deaths occur in age bracket 15–44 years. It kills young people in their prime of life, costing significant economic losses to country. In 10–24 years (young people), RTA has become number one killer in the world which accounts for 10% of deaths in this age bracket. Deaths due to RTA outnumber in men as compared to women, because of use of vehicle and road, exceeds for men. According to WHO estimate of 2002

Table 13.20: Leading causes of mortality and disease burden (DALYs) among adults (15–59) worldwide 2002

	Cause of mortality	Deaths (000)	DALYs (000)
1.	HIV/AIDS	2279	68661
2.	Ischaemic heart disease	1332	26155
3.	Tuberculosis	1036	28380
4.	Road traffic accidents	814	27264
5.	Cerebrovascular disease	783	18749
6.	Self-inflicted injuries	672	18962
7.	Violence	473	19567
8.	Unipolar depression	–	57843

Source: World Health Report (2003)[1]

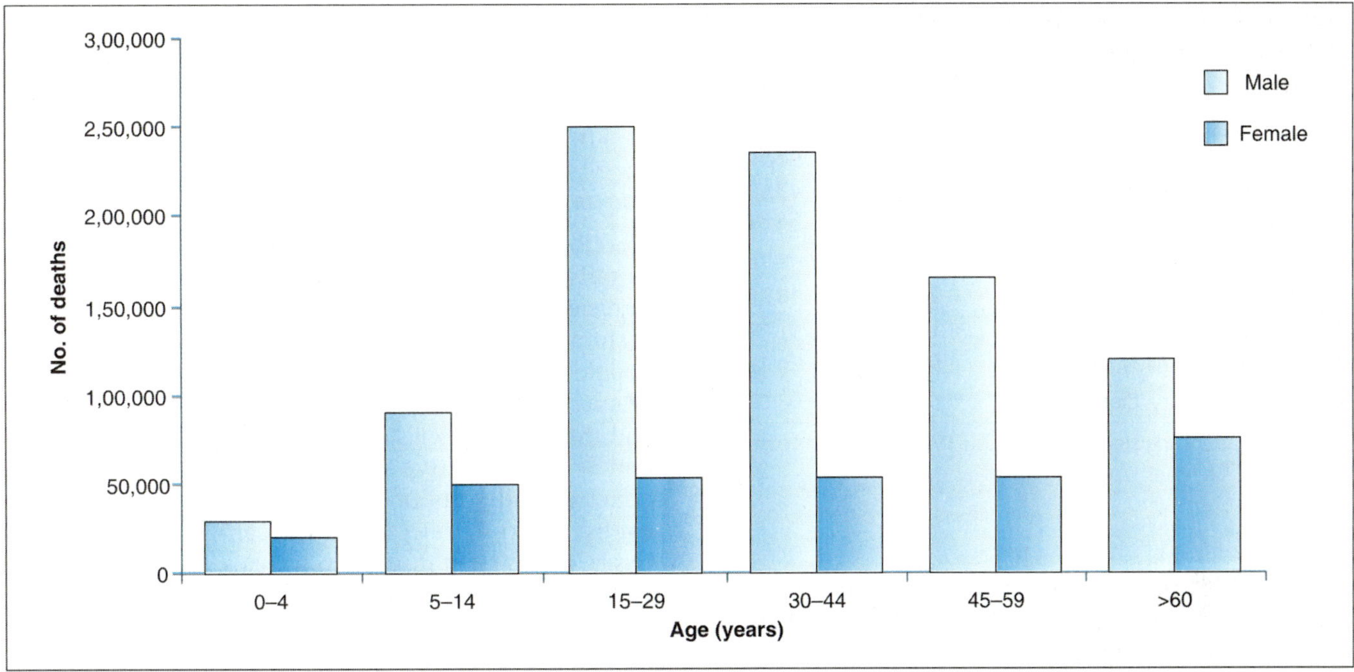

Fig. 13.3: Road traffic deaths by sex and age group in the world (2002). *Source:* World Bank Report, 2004

around 1,80,500 children were killed as a result of road crashes (Fig. 13.3).[2]

Using epidemiological evidence from national studies, conservative estimates can be made of ratio between road deaths, injuries requiring hospitalization treatment, and minor injuries as being 1:15:70 respectively in most countries.

Economic Loss

The trauma due to RTA is enormous and besides loss of human life it requires economic expenditure to manage trauma emergencies. One-third or even more beds in emergency may be occupied due to trauma and injuries and much of the scarce resources get spent to manage trauma emergencies.

RTA in India

Data on road accidents in India is limited. As per National Crime Records Bureau Ministry of Home Affairs 1,44,587 to 1,66,506 deaths due to RTA have been reported per annum (Table 13.21).[3]

Overall mortality due to RTA in India in one block (rural area) was 2.80% in the year 1996 and it is expected much more in urban areas.[4]

Non-communicable disease and injuries would increase in India much more by the year 2020 (Fig. 13.4).[5]

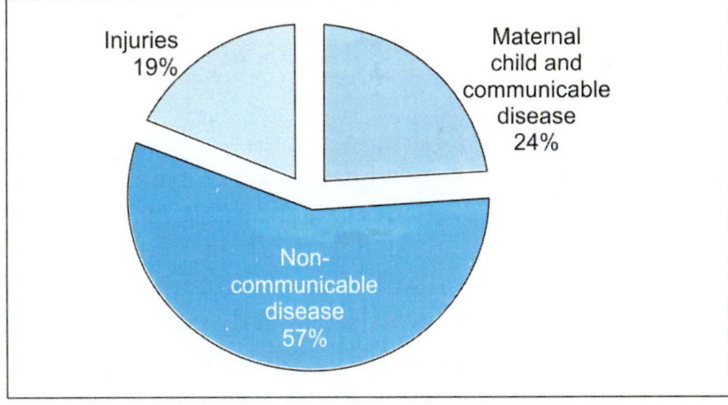

Fig. 13.4: Disease burden estimate in India (2020). Source: WHO, 1996

Table 13.21: RTA deaths in India[3]

Year	*Total accidental deaths*	*RTA deaths*	*Percentage of RTA to total deaths*
2008	342309	144587	24.3
2009	356353	122689	24.0
2010	384649	161731	24.0
2011	390884	165072	24.4
2012	394982	168301	25.0
2013	400517	166506	25.0

Burden of Injuries in India

World development report 1993 estimated DALYs losses due to injuries over 9% and this has increased further to the level of 13% in 2009 (Table 13.22). WHO estimates rise of traffic fatality rates in India by 79% in 2002 against the base year of 1981. It is attributable to growth of population, urbanization, mobility and growing number of vehicles. In Delhi alone, the population of vehicles has grown tremendously. By 2020, the road traffic deaths in India will increase by 147%.

Table 13.22: Distribution of percent DALYs* loss by cause in India in 1990 and 2009

Cause	India 1990	India 2009
Communicable diseases	50.5	43.94
Non-communicable diseases	40.4	43.02
Injuries	9.1	13.04
Cancer	4.1	2.78
Nutritional deficiency	6.2	3.23
Neuropsychiatric disease	6.1	11.79
Cerebrovascular disease	4.9	9.49
Chronic respiratory diseases	0.6	3.67

*DALY: (Disability adjusted life years). One DALY loss means one year loss of healthy life.

Who gets Killed in RTA?

In India pedestrian, bicycle, and motorized two wheelers account for much greater proportion of road traffic deaths. Over 78% of pedestrian in Bombay, 53% in New Delhi were killed in RTA (WHO 2004). These groups are most vulnerable to RTA deaths and it is clear indication that policies and programmes must focus/ target these groups (Table 13.23).

Risk Factors

Motor Vehicles

Growing number of motor vehicles—number of cars, buses, trucks and two wheelers have tremendously increased over the years. Overpopulation of motor vehicles is posing a great risk factor in RTA. In USA, 779 vehicles are available per 1000 persons against 34 in India. Motor vehicles are heavily concentrated on city roads which have limited space. In addition, non-motorized traffic has also increased (like cycles and carts). Pedestrian and cyclist population have increased at an alarming rate in developing countries including India. In India, the vehicle traffic is going to escalate with rise in income level and improvement of economic status. However, predominant modes of travel remains walking, cycling and use of public transport. The needs of pedestrian and cyclists have to prevail over the needs of others because of their vulnerability.

Table 13.23: Proportion of road users killed at different locations in India (figures in %) WHO, 2004

Type of road users	Mumbai	New Delhi	Highways
Lorry	2	2	14
Bus	1	5	3
Car	2	3	15
TSR	4	3	–
MTW	7	21	24
HAPV	0	3	1
Bicycle	6	10	11
Pedestrian	78	53	32
Total	**100**	**100**	**100**

TSR: Three wheeled scooter; MTW: Motorized two wheelers; HAPV: Human powered vehicles; a statistical summary of 11 locations not representative for whole country (tractor fatalities not included).

Roads Network

Development of network of roads or other form of transport as railways is a challenge. Roads have been constructed in residential areas and if all sorts of traffic flow through residential areas it has profound effect on health of people-like accidents, air pollution and noise pollution. Planning and construction of road for different purposes and different vehicles is in the process of development and it is imperative need. At present in developing countries, all sorts of traffic are mixed-up (pedestrian, cyclists, two-wheelers, bullock carts, other carts, cars, buses, trucks) and result into a chaos. Better planning of roads and land use led to efficient flow of traffic on major routes bye-passing urban residential areas, and with built-in safety measures has reduced RTA.

Road Users

In low income countries young people are predominantly involved in road crashes. Older people will be dependent on public transport or will walk. Providing safer and shorter pedestrian routes and safe and convenient public transport can reduce RTA.

Crash Risk Factors of RTA

Drivers and Road Users

Speed: Speed thrills but it kills. Rash driving on road by young people predispose them to RTA. Speed limits fixed by the authorities must be observed. Cameras on main crossing have been installed to check the speed. Speed means loss of control, improper overtaking and misjudgment leading to fatal accidents. Risk between speed and crash has been well established. Super-bikes and stunts and race on road can lead to fatal accidents.

Pedestrian and Cyclists

They get mixed with high speed vehicles and they are unprotected and exposed to risk of accidents. Road safety rules are generally poorly observed by pedestrian and the alcohol use impairs the judgement.

Age

Young drivers and riders run more risk of crash accidents. Young often tend to be over-confident, less experienced, run with high speed and use of alcohol makes the worse combination of risks.

Alcohol

Alcohol and driving should never be mixed. Increased use of alcohol and other drugs in drivers expose them to the risk of accidents as the judgement gets impaired and control over vehicle is lost due to the effect of alcohol and other drugs. National maximum legal blood alcohol concentration is 30 mg/100 ml.

Fatigue

Long distance driving and inadequate sleep leads to fatigue. Driving while feeling sleepy is risky.

Mobile Telephones

Driving with hand held mobile telephones has become a fashion, it is risky and misuse of mobile telephones. It affects the reaction time and maintenance of lane hence more risk of RTA. In many countries, use of hand held mobile phones have been banned.

Habit of use of Safety Belts and Helmets

Use of safety belts is picking-up but many drivers and occupants of vehicles do not use seat belts. Seat belt use reduces the impact of accident. Similarly, motorized two-wheelers do not use crash helmets and non-use of bicycle helmet adds to the risk of fatal head injuries. The use of light during day time by two-wheeled vehicle reduces chances of accidents.

Travel

Travel if you must. Unnecessary travel and joy ride and choice of less safe travel modes is a habit with adolescents. Teenagers below the age of eligible age of licence, drive two-wheelers and cars and risk their lives as also lives of others on road. Parents have to curb this habit.

Vehicle Condition

The pedestrians are most at risk of accidental deaths. Cycles and motorized two-wheelers are mostly involved in accidents and are most risky and unstable vehicles. Public transport system vehicles are in bad conditions because of poor maintenance and poor upkeep. Road worthiness (lighting, breaking, handling and speed management) of vehicles must be ensured to prevent RTA. Old vehicles are being phased out. The new vehicles (cars) must confirm the standards adopted by advanced countries to prevent accidents and to prevent the menance of air pollution.

Environment

Visibility

Poor visibility due to foggy conditions or smog of vehicles or dust storms decreases the visibility. At night, driving needs extra-precautions as vision is seriously affected by head lights. Pedestrians, cyclists and mixed traffics like bullock carts or camel carts, tractors often get hit by motor vehicles as they do not observe the rules and often these have no lights/indicators.

Poor Road Conditions

Uncovered sewer and flooding of roads, breaches and pits make the road conditions worse and may result in severe accidents. Speed breakers and bumps are meant for cutting speed preventing accidents, but poor marking and visibility of speed bumps and breakers result into severe accidents and injuries to occupants in particular. At many places speed breakers are car breakers and vehicle breakers. Crossings and intersection of highways, with poor demarcation and absence of indicators and lights result in severe and serious accidents. Sharp bends and blind turns and unfamiliar routes are other risky conditions. At times, roadside objects such as trees, poles and other rigid objects such as road signs tend to be safety problems. The design of roads and road network is a critical factor in RTA.

Intentional Injuries (Suicide)

RTA deaths account for 25% of all injury deaths worldwide and share of suicidal death is next only to RTA. Intentional injuries-group that include self-inflicted injuries and suicide, violence and war account for an increasing share of burden, especially among economically productive young adults.

Nationwide data on intentional injuries is not available, such injuries are reflected and mixed with total injuries. Suicide rate is one of the indicators of mental health status of a territory. In a limited study done in one rural community development block in Haryana, the proportion of suicidal deaths to total deaths was 6.67% and it ranked as 6th leading cause of mortality. It speaks of level of unrest, unemployment, unhappy married life and other social problems. Suicidal deaths were due to use of poisoning predominantly celphos tablets (aluminium phosphide), burns, hanging and railway accidents, drowning, etc. Over 1.35 lakh suicide deaths were reported in 2013 (National Health Profile India 2015). WHO in 2012 reported 258075 suicidal deaths in India.

Home Accidents

Children are at risk in and around the home and on the roads. Home injuries include burns and scalds, cuts, choking by swallowing small objects, poisoning, falls, drowning, animal bites and injuries due to unsafe playing. It necessitates safe environments for young children in home and in the vicinity of home, safe play and safe toys and keeping medicines and harmful substances out of reach of young children. Similarly, in preschool activities safe play methods and safe toys be used to prevent accidents.[7]

Prevention of Accidents

Education and Awareness

It is the first step in the direction of bringing behaviour change through effective communication on road safety measures. This should be ongoing activity in schools, colleges and should form integral part of formal and non-formal education programmes. Awareness generation on safety of RTA in masses by organized programme through network of television, radio and press is in place but it needs to be strengthened. Road safety rules and habits of their observance should be inculcated during childhood period in the family and in schools.

WHO recognized road injuries as a global epidemic and devoted world health day 7th April, 2004 to theme "road safety is no accident" and in collaboration with World Bank launched the World report on "road traffic injury prevention" to help nations to develop their national plans on road safety and prevention of RTA accidents. Through this effort WHO, focused on building awareness and building a suitable climate on prevention of RTA.

Regulations

Government has responsibility to regulate the behaviour of road users. Human beings are human beings, their behaviour needs to be controlled through education and by regulation through Road Safety Motor Vehicle Act: Licensing for driving should be strictly regulated, driving tests, medical fitness to drive, enforcing speed limits, enforcing use of safety belts, helmets and regular inspection of vehicles and to prevent alcohol impaired driving. Regulations are most often defined than observed. Self-regulation of behaviour is fundamental to save oneself and save others on the road. Government should set and enforce uniform vehicle safety standards.

Improving Public Transport System

To decrease the number of vehicles on the road, the safe, efficient and affordable public transport system must be developed by the Government. Improving public transport system is under way through provision of adequate roadworthy transport and developing metro-railways in metropolitan cities. Government alone will not be able to provide fleet of adequate and efficient transport system. Privatization is partial answer to the problem. If people develop confidence in public transport system, they will avoid use of personal vehicles. Other innovative and user-friendly methods to reduce the vehicle population on the road should be developed. Developing habits of walking and encouraging cycling is an opportunity to lose weight and prevent obesity, however, safe lanes for pedestrian and cyclist are essential. Human population and population of vehicles need to be controlled and stabilized; it is a dire necessity/need.

Pedestrians

Since pedestrian, cyclists, and motorized two-wheelers are affected maximally, their needs should have prime focus to prevent RTA. To prevent crash from happening, separating pedestrian from cars and trucks, by creating barriers and fences, building guard rails, widening shoulders and eliminating "black spots". Shortest routes, subways and overbridges for pedestrian to cross road safely helps prevention of accidents. Behaviour of pedestrian is important and this can be modified through mass campaigns.

Personal Behaviour

Wearing helmets and seat belts saves life. One should develop habit of safety. Driving without alcohol and with safe limit of speed for self and others on the road, prevents accidents.

Vehicles

Technological improvements in car include impact absorbing front ends, collapsible steering column, seat belts, integral head rests, air bags and child seats. Crash resistant vehicles can be built. World will witness many more advance technologies. One worry is to control vehicular population or traffic on road and use safe fuels to prevent air pollution and noise pollution. Air pollution in the long run may lead to more deaths than trauma due to increased morbidity of respiratory illness and heart diseases.

Safe Roads

Roads are always risky. Risks can be reduced by having safe roads and smooth movement of traffic. In the first instance, the vehicular traffic should be regulated during peak hours and risky hours. Many developments have ensured this—such as adequate traffic lights at crossings, placing barriers between traffic moving in opposite direction, broadening of roads, four lanes highways, one-way traffic and to eliminate highway intersections and marking safety lines and providing warning signals, etc. have helped to reduce RTA. Building flyovers and bye-pass roads and developing national highways are positive in many ways but growing population needs to be controlled.

Management of Accidents

To a large extent, RTA are preventable. Premature deaths and morbidity are avoidable to a great degree. The epidemic of RTA in India and other developing countries is still at an early stage and we can learn lessons from the developed countries and from within our own country.

Trauma Management

Accidents can be minimized but cannot be eliminated altogether. Trauma on road will occur due to human errors and to some extent failure of vehicle. Trauma management is essential component of saving lives and limbs and preventing disabilities.

Self-help and Local Help

Self-help during trauma and help of local persons or co-passengers is the first response. First-aid measures, such as dressing for bleeding and safe and prompt transportation of injured to nearby health facility can save lives.

TRAUMA CENTRES (NATIONAL TRAUMA CONTROL PROGRAMME)

Trauma services in big cities in State Government Hospitals located on national highways have been developed. Police assistance on highways has been developed for rapid response. Trauma centres on national highways have come up but much remains to be done. Fleet of ambulance services have been added but it needs to be augmented further. However, comprehensive trauma care services need to be developed by the central and state Governments at tertiary care centres.

A conceptual model for Delhi has been prepared which emphasizes:

- On site resuscitation of trauma victims.
- First-aid and transport to nearest tertiary care hospital by fully equipped ambulances with all life-saving measures.
- Networking of institutions for manpower, material and communication. Apart from communication networking the apex centre would be utilized for human resources development and computerized data base.

Developing network of 140 trauma centers along the golden quadrilateral covering 5,846 km connecting Delhi–Kolkata, Chenai, Mumbai–Delhi, North South and East–West Corridors covering 7,716 km connecting Kashmir to Kanyakumari and Silchar to Porbandar respectively on the national highways have been set-up. Another 160 trauma centres will be set-up in 12th plan period connecting capital cities and major cities, ports and major cities as also industrial cities. The scheme provides for 3 categories of trauma care centers, viz. L-III, L-II and L-I. The level-III trauma center is designed to stabilize the patients and to manage the trauma victim and refer the trauma victim to level-II and level-I centers as per requirement for further management. The level-II would provide definite care to severe trauma victims while the level-I would provide the highest level of definite and comprehensive care to patients with complex injuries. Financial assistance of Rs. 4.8–16 crores has been provided to strengthen the manpower, building, equipment, communication network, legal services and data entry operator in existing State Govt Hospitals. One advance life support ambulance is augmented by Ministry of Surface Transport at each of trauma care centers, while National Highway Authority of India (NHAI) is providing one basic life support ambulance at a distance of every 50 km of the national highways.

Research

Data on RTA and impact of safety measures need to be generated. Police and Bureau of Crime under Ministry of Home Affairs should collect data, analyze and generate adequate information to improve the system of road safety. It is a multisector endeavour. Data collection on physical circumstances of accidents, features of vehicles involved and their movement, characteristic of road users, such as use of alcohol or drug, nature of initial injuries sustained and their subsequent evolution. Police officials and officers need to be trained to collect such data and disseminate it on regular basis to effect improvement. Health sector can collect regular information on nature and extent of trauma necessitating development of improved trauma centres and services at various levels.

The Transportation Research and Injury Prevention Programme at the Institute of Technology in New Delhi has contributed much to a better understanding of the road injury problems of vulnerable road users and to identify possible intervention in low income and middle income countries. District, state and national data help for better planning for prevention of RTA.[8]

REFERENCES

1 WHO. The World Health Report 2003. Shaping the future. Geneva: WHO; 2003.

2 WHO/World Bank. World report on road traffic injury prevention. Geneva: WHO; 2004.

3 GOI Accidental deaths and suicides in India 2012 National Crime Records Bureau Ministry of Home Affairs RK Puram New Delhi.

4 Kumar V. Causes of mortality in rural community development block Lakhanmajra (dissertation). Rohtak: Maharshi Dayanand University, 1999.

5 Planning Commission. Tenth Five-Year Plan 2002–07. Vol II, New Delhi, GOI; 2002.

6 World Bank. World Development Report 1993. New York: World Bank; 1993.

7 Charistian Medical Association of India. Accidents and injuries, action at community level. Health dialogue 1999 Dec; 19.

8. WHO “Global Status Report on Road Safety 2013”.

MENTAL DISORDERS

What is mental health? “It is a state of well-being in which the individual realizes his or her own abilities, can cope with the normal stresses of life, can work productively and fruitfully and is able to make a contribution to his or her community” (WHO).[1]

DISEASE BURDEN

Mental disorders are on the increase because of increasing stress. *One in four people* in the world will be affected by mental or neurological disorders at some point in their lives. Globally around 450 million people currently suffer from such conditions, placing mental disorders among the leading causes of ill-health and disability worldwide. Depressive disorders are already the fourth leading cause of the global disease burden (WHO); they are expected to rank second by 2020, behind ischaemic heart disease.[2]

The year 2001 was a landmark in the development of mental health services. Since the problem of mentally challenged is a global problem, WHO chose the theme: "Mental Health: Stop exclusion—Dare to Care" during the year 2001 to focus worldwide attention on the issues related to mental health. The most common mental disorders which need focused attention are given below.[2]

Depression

An estimated 121 million people currently suffer from depression. An estimated 5.8 % of men and 9.5% of women will experience a depressive episode in any given year, these figures can, however, vary across different populations.

Schizophrenia

24 million people worldwide suffer from schizophrenia. The disorder is found equally in men and women. With modern drug advances, half of the sufferers can expect full recovery.

Alzheimer's Disease

Alzheimer's disease is a degenerative brain syndrome characterized by the progressive decline in memory, thinking, comprehension, calculation, language, learning capacity and judgement. An estimated 37 million people worldwide live with dementia—with Alzheimer's disease causing the majority of cases. About 5% of men and 6% of women over 60 years of age are affected with Alzheimer's disease with the ageing of population; this is likely to increase rapidly over next 20 years.[3] There is no cure.

Epilepsy

Epilepsy is most common of brain disorders. It is characterized by repeated seizures or "fits" which range from the shortest lapse in attention to severe, frequent convulsion. An estimated 50 million people of all ages around the world are affected by epilepsy. Up to 70% of newly diagnosed people with epilepsy can be seizure free if treated with antiepileptic drugs.

Mental Retardation

It is a condition of arrested or incomplete development of the mind characterized by impairment of skills and overall intelligence in areas such as cognition, language, motor and social abilities. Prevalence is between 1 and 3%. It is more common in developing countries.[3]

Substance-abuse Disorders

These disorders result from use of psychoactive substances such as alcohol, opioids such as opium or heroin, cannabinoids such as marijuana, sedatives and hypnotics, cocaine, other stimulants hallucinogens, tobacco and volatile solvents. Around 1.2 billion use tobacco, 70 million people have alcohol use disorders and 5 million people worldwide inject illicit drugs.

Suicide (intentional injuries): See accidents and injuries.

Disorders of Childhood and Adolescence

Mental and behavioural disorders are common during childhood and adolescence. An estimated 10–20% of children have one or more mental or behavioural problems. These include disorders of psychological development, e.g. dyslexia or autism and behavioural and emotional, e.g. attention deficit hyperactivity disorders (ADHD) or conduct disorders.

Against the massive burden of mental disorders: 40% of countries have no mental health policies and 25% have no legislation in the field of mental health (WHO April, 2002). Community care facilities are yet to be developed. Of the total number of psychiatric beds, 65% are still in mental hospitals. The availability of mental health professionals in large areas of the world is extremely poor. More than 680 million people, the majority of whom are in Africa and Asia, have access to less than one psychiatrist per million population.

Burden of Mental Disorders in India

Disease burden due to neuropsychiatric diseases in India in terms of DALYs losses was 6.1% as per world development report 1993.[4] This will rise substantially by 2020. Mental disorders are not fatal but are responsible for great loss of healthy life. In India, joint family system support continues to absorb many ill effects of disease and provides stable environments for shaping and developing lifestyles and personality traits. This support is gradually diminishing due to urbanization and industrialization and migration of young people to urban areas. Because of stress and strain of life, unemployed youth, and disturbed sex ratio; the mental disorders are on the rise.

Prevalence

Meta-analysis of various epidemiological studies on psychiatric morbidity in India was done in 1998 and 2000. According to these studies, mental disorders prevalence was arrived at 58.2 and 73 per thousand population respectively (Table 13.24).[5, 6]

Available data of meta-analysis, ICMR studies and NIMHANS indicated that there were 15 million people suffering from severe mental disorders (psychoses) in India (point prevalence).

Analysis of Present Situation

According to most of surveys, about 10–20 per thousand of population are affected by severe mental disorders at

Table 13.24: Nature of mental disorders in India

Mental disorders		Prevalence rate/1000 (Venkataswamy, 1998)		Prevalence rate/1000 (Ganguli, 2000)
Organic psychoses	Severe mental disorders	0.4	15.4	–
Schizophrenia		2.7		2.5
Affective disorders		12.3		34
Mental retardation		6.9		5.3
Epilepsy		4.4		–
Neuroses		20.7		16.5
Alcohol/drug addiction		6.9		–
Miscellaneous		3.9		14.7*
All disorders		58.2		73

*It includes 3.3% of hysteria.

any point in time (point prevalence). The figures for neuroses and psychosomatic disorders are about two to three times higher, thus indicating 30–45 million people may require our attention. Mental retardation is estimated at 0.5 to 1.0% of all children, while alcohol and drug dependence rates though still low as compared to world scene, reveal a disturbing rising trend in some parts or regions. Injectable drug use rate is high in North-Eastern states while alcohol consumption is very high in Punjab. Prevalence of mental disorders as per world health report 2001 is around 10% and is predicted that burden of disorders is likely to rise by 15% by 2020. According to various community based surveys prevalence of mental disorders in India is 6–7% for common mental disorders and 1–2% for severe mental disorders. ICMR reported severe mental morbidity ranging from 4.6 to 14.1 per 1000.[7]

With such a magnitude of mental disorders it becomes necessary to promote mental health services for the well-being of general population, in addition to provide treatment of mental illness.

Rural/Urban Distribution

Prevalence rates are significantly higher in urban areas as compared to rural areas except for epilepsy and hysteria which were more in rural area.

Gender-wise Distribution

The prevalence rates for female were higher as compared with men. Mental disorders are more prevalent in nuclear family members. 35–44 years age group was most affected. Lower socioeconomic status suffered most. More community database and evidence is required in India to know the distribution of mental disorders in relation to various known risk factors or attributes.

Social Stigma

Treatment is available but nearly two-thirds of people, with a known mental disorders, never seek help from the health facility or institution or health professionals. Stigma, discrimination and neglect comes in the way of treatment. Social stigma and discrimination in mental disorders is widespread in India. People tend to hide and seldom disclose the mental disorders even to most near and dear ones till these become unmanageable.

Existing Mental Health Services

Currently, 50% of the medical colleges have a psychiatry department. It is estimated that there is one psychiatry bed per 30,000 population. There are 20,000 beds in mental hospitals and 2,000 to 3,000 psychiatric beds in general and teaching hospitals. 50% of beds are occupied by patients undergoing long-term treatment. Only 10% of mentally ill persons have access to appropriate care. Prevention of mental illness and promotion of mental health remains a distant dream. Less than one psychiatrist is available for every three lakh population in India and one per million in rural area.

Utilization of Mental Health Services (Treatment Gap)

The treatment is available but not being used. Treatment gap even in severe mental disorders is 50% and in case of common mental disorders is over 90%. Even the available services for mental disorders are being poorly utilized. Nearly two-thirds of persons with known mental disorders never seek help from health professionals and most clients utilize the services of other agencies and resort to harmful practices and keep on visiting faith healers and delay the treatment till the condition deteriorates which compels them to seek the treatment from established government institutions. Stigma, discrimination and neglect prevents care and treatment reaching people. 'Mental health literacy' needs to be built-up strongly in the community to scale up the utilization of available mental health services and to reduce treatment gap.

Beliefs—Attitudes and Practices in Relation to Mental Disorders

Common beliefs held by masses: By and large, literate and illiterate, rich and poor people from all walks of life think that mental disorders are due to 'evil spirits' or being possessed by some spirit or intrusion of Ghosts in the body or external divine forces. Accordingly, they resort to drive away Ghosts from body of the mentally challenged person by adopting harmful practices such as beating by ex'orcist or priest, application of hot iron on body parts and several other harmful practices varying from region to region. Wearing charms and amulets is a common feature to ward off spirits.[8]

Most often the treatment for mental disorders is sought through "Faith healers" or magico-religious practitioners. The author observed that a 'prodigy child' thought to be *Awtar* (incarnation) of some religious Guru became a centre of attraction in Haryana and started pulling huge crowd from all over India and especially from the state of Punjab, J&K, Uttar Pradesh, Himachal, West Bengal, Maharashtra and even from United Kingdom. Daily influx of client varied from 5000 to 20,000 and these clients included cases of chronic ailments including 15.5% clients with schizophrenia, affective disorders and psychoses (severe mental illness) who were brought chained or tied with ropes. After getting "Jhhara" (miraculous healing/blessings) from Babaji (prodigy child), the chains and ropes were removed and hung on tree nearby. The relatives had confidence for a moment and believed that miraculous blessings have been showered and they returned home with all kinds of stories to tell. Such like 'prodigy child' or *Awtars* keep on appearing from time to time to attract people. In sum, large part of the community still looks forward with tremendous faith in magico-religious practitioners to get their suffering ameliorated. Religious factors, worshipping and deriving satisfaction through blessings hold firm ground in the course of natural history of chronic diseases.[8]

NATIONAL MENTAL HEALTH PROGRAMME (NMHP)

National Mental Health Programme was launched in India in 1982 with the following objectives:[9]

i To ensure availability and accessibility of minimum mental health care for all in foreseeable future; particularly to the most vulnerable and underprivileged section of population.
ii To encourage application of mental health knowledge in general health care and in social development.
iii To promote community participation in the mental health services development and to stimulate efforts towards self-help in the community.

Approaches

i Integrating mental health services with the existing primary health care set-up to increase the access and availability of mental health services.
ii To utilize existing infrastructure of health services and also to deliver minimum mental health services.
iii To link mental health services with existing community development programme like ICDS and education.
iv To provide appropriate task oriented training to the existing health staff.

Components of National Mental Health Programme

There are 5 components of the programme, namely.

1 Treatment
2 Rehabilitation
3 Prevention
4 Training
5 Research (operational and applied research of district mental health services).

1. Treatment

The treatment programme has been planned keeping the primary health care approach as the sheet-anchor. At the same time, it consists of the creation of an appropriate referral system at various levels. It is proposed that the specialized psychiatric services should be made available at the district level.

The mental hospitals, medical colleges, teaching institutions and mental institutes shall also be linked together into the national grid for the mental health care particularly in the field of education and research.

- Strengthening and modernization of mental hospitals to support referral services is in progress.

2. Rehabilitation Sub-programme

Community or family based rehabilitation of psychiatric patient will be the mainstay of the programme. The counselling regarding principles of rehabilitation would be provided by medical officer at primary health centre and at village level by health workers and volunteers. Wherever practical, the rehabilitation centres would be developed at the district level as well as at the higher referral centres.

3. Prevention Sub-programme

This component of service programme will be community-based with only limited involvement of health service personnel. The main focus in its initial phase will be prevention of alcohol-related problems. However, it would expand its concern to cover problem like addiction, juvenile delinquency, acute-adjustment problem (e.g. suicidal attempts) and to an ability to articulate community mental health needs from the citizens point of view. The main carriers of this subprogramme will be the medical officers and community leaders at the primary health centre level.

4. Mental Health Training

Since specialist like psychiatrists would be in short supply the health personnel of general health services or primary health care services (medical officers, supervisors and health workers and health volunteers) will be imparted short-term training on basic skills in psychiatry to provide minimum mental health care services to all. Under district mental health programme in—service training of health workers, health supervisors and medical officers is the key component. Training guidelines have been prepared by NIMHANS.

Secondly, the training of undergraduate (MBBS students) will have to improve in quality and contents for minimum mental health services. Besides this basic training of health workers and nurses must have strong components of mental health services (at least essentials of mental health).[10]

India was one of the first countries in the world to formulate a National Mental Health Programme (NMHP) in 1982. However, the budgetary allocation for implementing the NMHP was made in 1996–97. Implementation of DMHP has been quite tardy and slow.

DISTRICT MENTAL HEALTH PROGRAMME (DMHP)

Based on the experience and learning from various community health initiatives in particular the "Bellary model in Karnataka State" DMHP was launched in 1996 initially in four districts and subsequently expanded to 241 districts in the country. 350 new districts would be taken up in phased manner to reduce treatment gap. DMHP aims at decentralized community based mental health care through the existing Primary Health Care System. In most cases the departments of psychiatry of medical colleges were identified to implement DMHP.

Objectives of District Mental Health Programme (DMHP)

1 Providing sustainable basic mental health services to the community and integrate these services with general health services.
2 Early detection and treatment of patients within the community itself.
3 Taking pressure away from mental hospitals.
4 Reducing stigma attached to mental illnesses through changes in attitude and public education.
5 Treatment and rehabilitation of mentally ill patients discharged from the mental hospital within the community
6 Continuing education (mental health literacy).

DMHP Team

A five member technical team consisting of a psychiatrist/trained medical officer will act as programme officer mental health (POMH) at district level, a clinical psychologist/trained psychologist, a psychiatric social worker/trained social worker a psychiatric community nurse or a trained community nurse, a record keeper and two member managerial team consisting of a community nurse and an assistant for coordination and implementation of activities in each district. The programme manager would establish linkages for referral and programme implementation with the District Health Society under NRHM. The training of medical officers and other categories of staff will be for four and three months respectively and nurses would be trained for one month at identified institutions.

A district mental health team is expected to provide services to mentally ill patients and their families by:
- Conducting daily outpatient service.
- Providing 10 beds indoor facilities.
- Referral services.
- Liaising with primary health centres.
- Follow-up services.
- Undertaking community survey, if feasible.

Necessary medicines, equipment, vehicles and other infrastructure are also made available to support the programme. It also has IEC and training components.

Based on the series of national consultations and findings from the independent evaluation of NMHP during 2009, the implementation plan for DMHP was revised during XIth plan period.

New Components of DMHP/Revised DMHP

In addition to existing components of DMHP, which mainly focused on severely mentally ill, DMHP has now incorporated promotive and preventive activities for positive mental health. New components like suicide prevention, workplace stress management, adolescent mental health and college counseling services, aimed at addressing mental health needs in a comprehensive manner forms the part of the DMHP from XIth plan onward. Activities covered by DMHP now include.

i. Service Delivery for Mental Health

a ***Early Detection and Treatment:*** Detection of common mental health ailments by trained physicians/health workers/community volunteers and referring of patients to nearest PHCs/appropriate centre. Commonly used drugs have been made available at the PHC level. Simple record keeping for monthly reporting would be observed. The DMHP team would provide supervision and referral support to the mental health services at the CHC/PHC level. DMHP team will also provide in-service training to peripheral staff.

b ***School Mental Health Services Life Skills Training and Counseling in Schools:*** There is growing evidence of increased rate of adolescent behavioral problems and suicides, crime, violence, sexual permissiveness, drug abuse, academic competition and school dropouts are on the rise among youth. Life skill approach (LSA): WHO: "Life skill" education curriculum, promotes empowerment of school children/adolescents. This would address the mental health needs of school children/adolescents, so as to enable them to lead a healthy life by coping with emotional stress during special circumstances. The training will be imparted by master trainers/counselors and trained school teachers using standard manuals.

c ***Counseling Services in College:*** A significant proportion of college students have mental disorders in the form of depression, anxiety, somatoform disorders, adjustment disorders, personality disorders and alcohol and drug abuse as also emotional disturbances. Under DMHP counseling services will be provided by supporting infrastructure for counseling center.

d *Workplace Stress Management:* Workshops for stress management would be conducted at identified workplaces by DMHP team/NGOs by using standard manuals for formal and informal sector including farmers and women, etc.

e *Suicide Prevention Services:* The District Counseling and Crisis Center would aim at providing round the clock helpline support, sensitization workshops and by counseling center at district, level besides IEC activities.

f *Role of NGO:* Active collaboration of NGOs is imperative in all the activities of DMHP for all the targeted interventions.

ii. Training Most Important Input

All medical officers and health staff of the district have been trained in basic mental health care at nodal institute. Training in mental health has been integrated in the training modules of health staff and grass root health workers.

It was envisaged that decentralized district training on essential mental health care will be provided to all health professionals so that psychiatric care will be provided in all health care facilities. The departments of psychiatry or mental hospitals have been identified as nodal institutes and they have organized training of district medical officers and health supervisors at the institutional level for a period of 2 weeks. Five days training was organized at district level for Anganwadi workers and health workers. Training manuals/modules prepared by NIMHANS in local languages were used for health professionals. The departments of psychiatry of respective medical colleges supported the development of services at district hospitals. The district mental health programme (DMHP) is a model of community-based mental health services on sustainable basis.[11, 12]

iii. IEC Activities

IEC/BCC (Behavior Change Communication) activities using local/folk media and interpersonal communication would focus on early identification of mental illness, availability of treatment and reduction in stigma associated with mental disorders. Very few districts hve utilized funds allocated for raising community awareness.

Integration of NMHP with NRHM

To further mainstream NMHP and mental health in general health system, steps have been taken to integrate NMHP with NRHM/NHM. This will also ensure a sustained flow of funds and a regular monitoring of programme implementation plans (PIPs).

Expansion: District Mental Health Programme will be further expanded to cover more districts in 12th Five-Year Plan as stated before.

Present Status of NMHP

Areas or Concern/Programme Weakness

Most of the mentally ill (90% or more) remain untreated. Poor awareness, myths and stigma related to illness, lack of services, lack of knowledge on treatment availability and potential benefits of seeking treatment are important causes for the *high treatment gap of 90 percent.*

Increasing Community Awareness and the Demand for Mental Health Services

The treatment gap for mental health services may be minimized by improving the demand for utilization of mental health services by the community, through aggressive (i) mental health literacy (ii) by involving NGO and the private sector, (iii) by community mobilization and participation besides and (iv) augmenting human resources is key to scaling up of mental health services.

The major challenges for reduction of treatment gap for mental disorders are:

i Lack of mental health services to vast majority of population.

ii Stigma, lack of awareness on mental disorders and availability of treatment/services amongst patients and their care givers.

iii Lack of coordination between medical colleges and state health departments in implementation of DMHP.

iv Lack of involvement of community, NGOs, civil society and specialists from private sector.

Mental Health Act, 1987

The derogatory Indian Lunacy Act of 1912 which was based on earlier English Lunacy Act of 1890 has been replaced by 1987 Mental Health Act with a focus to improve the quality of services/care and protect the rights of mentally ill. Mental Health Act has been a very important milestone in the development of modern psychiatric services in the country, hopefully, the Act is made patient-friendly. The state Governments took a long lead time to establish mental health authority and to implement this Act. The Mental Health Care Bill 2013 is a replacement of Mental Health Act, 1987 and it is likely to become Act soon.

Past of Mental Health Services

The year 2001 was a landmark in the development of mental health services. Since the problem of mentally challenged is a global problem, WHO has chosen the theme: "Mental Health: Stop exclusion—Dare to Care" during the year 2001, to focus worldwide attention on the issues related to mental health.[13] The past, in the history of mental health services has been gloomy, but nevertheless it has taught us many lessons. Past experience of mental health built a strong myth and perception in the community. The common man perceived mental illness as stigma, admission in asylum or mental hospital, electric shocks and confinement in institution with subhuman conditions. The picture has changed drastically and the modern mental health care goes far beyond the institutions and in a way it is trying to restore and build the lost confidence of common man by changing his/her perception through educational programme. Mass media continues to focus on miserable conditions of asylums and mental hospitals and subhuman conditions of these hospitals, to draw the attention of authorities for improving these conditions. Directives of Hon'ble Supreme Court have made substantial contribution in the area of mental health programme.

Future of Mental Health Services

In the first instance, the services and infrastructure for mental health services in public sector are inadequate and mostly confined to bigger cities and hospitals. Distt. programme of mental health services has just taken off, primary health care infrastructure on the other hand is reasonably well developed and is almost universally accessible to rural areas. Minimum package of mental health services for all can be best delivered through primary health care system. Preventive and promotive programme along with awareness generation can be undertaken on sustainable basis through this infrastructure.

The institution of Anganwadis has been recognized as sheet anchor in personality development of young children. This is one of the finest examples of development of positive mental health, international programme developed by WHO to stimulate mother-child interaction has much more chances for success if pursued actively in the family through ICDS system. This system involves families in total child development through integrated services of nutrition, health and education and relies on intersectoral coordination.

NIMHANS has rightly picked-up ICDS system to involve them in National Mental Health Programme through district mental health services. They are being imparted 5 days training programme at district level. Their training would be critical, as these workers will serve as link workers between community and the formal health services system. Since Anganwadi workers are locally resident voluntary workers, deeply rooted in the community they can be most effective in dissemination of knowledge of mental health programme besides identification of clients at the earliest stage of morbidity because of their continuous contact with families. Strengthening of this institution can be most rewarding and will have high payoff/effects in the long run. National Population Policy envisages enlarging the sphere of ICDS to cover school going children up to the age of 9. Continuous on the job training of Anganwadi workers through supervisory support can further enrich the non-formal education programme. The in-service training on mental health should be undertaken by supervisors or trained child development programme officers and it should focus on child development, personality development and learning by play way activities.[14]

Adolescent boys and girls who are the future parents need greater degree of mental health services to develop value based learning and balanced personality.

School Mental Health Programme/Services

Teachers training programme for balanced development of physical, mental and social faculties of school going children is essential for healthy lifestyles. Teachers along with parents can shape balanced personality. District mental health services programme must entrust the responsibility of teacher's training to district health teams. Though the teachers are trained during their teachers training programme on child psychology but they need continuous education on balanced personality development of child. District mental health programme should not miss the opportunity, as it would be a real investment in preventive, promotive and positive mental health or extended community mental health. The outreach district mental health services should embody this component of the programme on sustainable basis. WHO's "Life Skills" education curriculum which attempts learning of wide range of skills amongst school children to improve their psychosocial competency through problem solving, critical thinking, communication, equity, tolerance, interpersonal skills, empathy and methods to cope with emotions can be made effective through school teachers and parents teachers interaction on continuous basis and much more through "child friendly schools". Children with special learning disability, behavioural, emotional, scholastic and personality disorders can be identified for *counselling* and special services.

Community Care in Mental Health

There is shift in approach of mental health care services. From hospital-based care (institutional) the approach now is towards providing community-based mental health care, as majority of mental disorders do not require hospitalization and can be managed at community level.

It is widely acclaimed that community care is more effective as well as more humane than inpatient stay in mental hospitals. It is, therefore, essential to develop mental health services in the community settings as an integral part of primary health care; to root out stigma, myths and misconceptions and discrimination against mental disorders. The World Health Report 2001 advocates community-based mental health programmes and active involvement of families, givers care, persons living with mental illness, consumers, and community.[15]

Key recommendations of World Health Report 2001 are: (i) Integrate mental health care into primary health care, (ii) make psychotropic medicines available, (iii) give care in the community, (iv) educate people, (v) involve

13

communities, families and consumers, (vi) develop human resources, (vii) link with other sector, (viii) monitor community mental health, (ix) support more research.[16]

FAMILY SUPPORT

People are the biggest resources available in India. Many of the problems in the area of mental health can be effectively dealt with by the people and within resources available to them. Large scale dissemination of knowledge and simple skills to people and health volunteers should be addressed through primary health care. 70–80% of persons with mental disorders in India live with their families. Capacity of family must be built and primary health care infrastructure should support the family to build their capacity to prevent and manage the mental health problems within the available means. What people do with their lives and those of their children affects their health far more than anything that government does. Building knowledge and awareness of families can make the real difference. Health guides, ASHAs, Anganwadi workers and health workers as also Non-Governmental Organizations (NGOs) should raise the level of awareness of people on sound mind in sound body and attainment of positive mental health, through their own actions and practices as also utilization of available services to reduce *treatment gap*.

5. Research

Operational research studies on community-based mental health services are called for. We have just two models evolved long back at Chandigarh (Raipur Rani) and Bangalore (Sakalwara) in 1975–76 which are indeed insufficient. These two models limited their approach to curative services at the community level through primary health care. District Mental Health Programme was initiated at Bellary (Karnataka). Success of operations in programme conditions at the ground level needs to be documented further. Outcome and impact of district training programme in terms of coverage of mental health services and awareness level of community needs to be explored through operational research studies. The task can be undertaken by nodal agency or independent institution can be entrusted this task. Built in system of monitoring and evolving parameters of mental health in the community could be another area of interest. Similarly, longitudinal follow-up of preschool children and school children for personality development could be another worthwhile area of research. Many more interventional studies can be evaluated in adolescents in and out of schools in community settings. Delineation of role of NGOs, Panchayati Raj Institutions and partnership of public and private sector in delivery of mental health services can be thought of as an area of exploration. Working of drug de-addiction centres, their cost benefit ratio and impact should form part of community-based operational research.

13

NEW PATHWAYS NEW HOPE[17] NATIONAL MENTAL HEALTH POLICY OF INDIA (OCTOBER 2014)

Vision

The vision of National Mental Health Policy (NMHP) is to promote mental health, prevent mental illness, enable recovery from mental illness and reduce stigma and segregation and ensure socioeconomic inclusion of persons affected by mental illness by providing accessible, affordable and quality health and social care to all persons through their lifespan within a right-based framework.

Goals and Obbjective

Goals

i To reduce distress, disability, exclusion, morbidity and premature mortality associated with mental health problems across lifespan of a person.

ii To enhance understanding of mental health in the country.

iii To strengthen the leadership in the mental health sector at the National, State and District levels.

Objectives

i To provide universal access to mental health care.

ii To increase access to and utilization of comprehensive mental health services (preventive, curative, care and support services) to persons with mental health problem.

iii To increase access to mental health services for vulnerable groups (homeless persons, persons in remote areas, difficult terrains, deprived sections).

iv To reduce prevalence and impact of risk factors associated with mental health problems (poverty, homelessness, illiteracy and borken families, etc.).

v To reduce risk and incidence of suicide and attempted suicide.

vi To ensure respect for rights and protection from harm of persons with mental health problems.

vii To reduce stigma associated with mental health problems.

viii To enhance availability and equitable distribution of skilled human resources for mental health.

ix Adequate financial allocations and its progressive enhancement and improved utilization.

x To identify and address the social, biological and psychological determinants of mental health problems and to provide appropriate interventions.

Strategic Areas for Action

a. Effective Governance and Accountability for Mental Health

i Develop relevant policies, programmes, laws and regulations within relevant sectors in line with Mental

Health Policy, with associated implementation and monitoring mechanisms.

ii Adequate budget for implementation of evidence-based mental health plans and actions.

b. Promotion of Mental Health

i Redesign Anganwadi centres to cater to the early child care developmental and emotional needs of children below 6 years with priority to under 3 years of age. Introduce mother–child session on parenting skills in ICDS programme

ii Train Anganwadi workers

iii Life skill educaton (LSE) should be offered to school-children and adolescents.

iv Train school teachers in mental health promotion.

c. Prevention of Mental Illness and Reduction of Suicide and Attempted Suicide

i Address stigma, discrimination and exclusion

ii Enable access to tratment and to other care giving facilities to promote early recovery.

- Implement programmes to address drug abuse and alcohol as also tobacco.
- Implement suicide reduction programmes to reduce the likelihood of suicide and attempted suicide.
- Set up crisis intervention centres and helplines as part of District Mental Health Programme.

d. Universal Access to Mental Health Services

Mental Health Services should be provided within the existing health care system using the Primary Health Care approach. Comprehensive services for mental health problems should be made universally accessible. A continuum of such services should be available across facility, community and family as also across lifespan. Promote community-based programmes to support families and caregivers. Involve private sector and NGO to increase access to mental health services.

e. Improve Availability of Adequtely Trained Human Resources to Address Mental Health Needs

To reduce the treatment gap provide adequate trained manpower such as psychiatrists, psychiatric nurses, psychologists, counsellors, medical psychiatric, social workers, trained nurses and auxiliaries.

f. Community Participation for Mental Health

Involve users, families, communities VHSNC, RKS, NGOs and other sectors in NMHP for planning, implementing, monitoring and evaluation and advocacy.

g. Research

Develop and implement a comprehensive research agenda for mental **health** including epidemiological, clinical and health systems research together with sociological, ethnographic and other multidisciplinary methods including participatory research methods. Adequate funds should be provided for this component.

SUBSTANCE USE DISORDERS (DRUG ABUSE)

The abuse of drugs and alcohol is an international problem which affects almost every country in the world both developed and underdeveloped. The World Health Report (2002) identifies tobacco, alcohol and illicit drug use as 3 risk factors among the list of leading 20 selected risk factors.

Drug addiction in *India* has of late emerged as a matter of great concern both due to the social and economic burden caused by substance use and due to established linkage with HIV/AIDS. Problem of substance use takes its roots during adolescent period and it becomes much more worse during youth and advancing age if left unattended. Besides adolescent and youth, the drug abuse is also visible amongst middle and old age. The adverse outcome of substance use costs the individual in terms of his bad health (increased morbidity and mortality) to the family and to the community and the nation).[18]

Common substances which are used for instant high are:

Cocaine: By injection, by inhalation (shorting) and smoking also known as **crack.** It is central nervous system stimulant.

Heroin: Highly addictive white or brown powder, processed from morphine, also known as smack–chitta or white powder.

Marijuana: It is mixture of flowers and leaves of cannabis also known as pot.

"MDMA" or Ectasy or love drug: Synthetic psychoactive drug with stimulant and hallusinogenic effect.

Methamphetamine: It is referred to as speed, meth or chalk. Meth-hydrochloride or crystals resembling ice is referred to as ice, crystals and glass.

Opium (Bhua or Kalmai): It has capacity to relieve pain and produce a sense of well-being.

Solvents: Paint, thinner, gasoline, glues, cough syrups, anti-spasmodic, iodex with bread, correction fluid, etc. are used to get an instant high.

National Household Survey (2002) indicated that tobacco, alcohol, cannabis and opiates were the substances most commonly abused in India (Table 13.25). Similar observations were made by drug abuse monitoring system. Between 17 and 26% of users were dependent users (using ICD-10 criteria, WHO, 1992). 65–80% of everusers were current users.[19–21]

Table 13.25: The extent and pattern of drug abuse in India (National household survey 2002) in 12–60 years of age

Major drugs of abuse	*Percentages*	*Estimated users in India (million)*	*Drug abuse monitoring system (%)*
Tobacco	55.8	180.2	—
Alcohol	21.4	10.5	43.9
Cannabis	3.0	2.3	11.6
Opiates	0.4		8.6
Heroin	0.2	0.5	11.1
Other opiates	0.1		3.7

ADVERSE OUTCOME

Adverse outcome of substance use disorders can be classified into two categories:

- Health problems
- Behavioural and social problems.

Health Problems

Injecting drug users (IDUs) run the risk of HIV/AIDS, hepatitis B, hepatitis C and excess morbidity and mortality due to overdose of the substance.

Social and Behavioural Problems

Increased rate of suicide, accidents and trauma, absenteeism and delinquency are linked with drug abuse.

Social Problems

Personality changes, serious effect on overall development and economy of community besides political instability and threat. Illicit drug use in India is most commonly visible in North-Eastern states because of heavy drug trafficking across the international borders with Myanmar, Thailand and Laos (Golden Triangle). Punjab is also important corridor and international route of illicit drug trafficking from Iran, Afghanistan, and Pakistan to Amritsar in Punjab (Golden Crescent). 60% of illicit drugs come in India through this route. Anngarh locality of Amritsar in Punjab is known as retail mandi of all geners of drugs and intoxicants. 'Maqboolpura' in Amritsar is called "Locality of widows". Around 40–50% of young people between 15 and 35 years are hooked to subsance abuse in Punjab and many of them are injecting drug users. Injecting drug use also occurs, although to a lesser extent in many Indian cities such as Kolkata, Mumbai, Delhi and Chennai. The sharing of contaminated injecting equipment without cleaning has contributed to explosive increase in HIV prevalence rates among IDUs (IBBS, 2015).

Causes

13

Overpopulation, illiteracy, industrialization, urban migration, urban slums, unemployment, problem families, broken homes and inability to cope with stress have been the root causes of social problems including substance abuse. New lifestyles has given birth to substance abuse. Drug abusers have multiple risky lifestyles and behaviours such as multiple sexual partners, unsafe sex, promiscuity, smoking, drinking alcohol and many other antisocial behaviours.

Adolescents and youth experiment and indulge into risk taking behaviour. To begin with, it is fun in company with friends and subsequently peer pressure grows on and it becomes a habit with them. Unemployed and restless youth indulge in antisocial behaviour, more so in urban slums and university culture.

Primary Prevention (Supply Reduction)

It attempts to reduce the incidence of substance use by "Supply reduction".

Primary and Primordial Prevention (Supply Reduction)

Primary and primordial prevention in substance abuse consists of control of drug production, supply, availability and its sale through regulatory mechanism: Enforcing laws related to drug industry. This comes under the Ministry of Home Affairs. Prohibitions and partial restriction are difficult to enforce in practice. Apart from legislations, awareness generation and personality development in schools/colleges and work place plays pivotal role.

Secondary Prevention (Demand Reduction)

The demand reduction activities focus on awareness building, treatment and rehabilitation. It attempts to reduce the prevalence of substance use by "Demand reduction". By education and counselling the abusers, the prevalence can be reduced. Religious organizations, Non-Governmental Organization and mass media can have popular appeal for *demand reduction*. Family and parents can lead their offspring as good role model. Educational campaigns in schools and colleges through good role models can have a positive influence on the lifestyles of adolescents and youth. MOH and FW is responsible for demand reduction.

National Drug De-addiction Programme

To provide effective and acceptable de-addiction services to 3 million drug users excluding alcohol dependent is a herculean task. The basic role of Ministry of Health and Family Welfare in the area of drug de-addiction is "*demand reduction*" by way of providing treatment services including preventive health and after care. The drug de-addiction programme of the ministry was started in 1987–88 first as pilot projects at AIIMS, Smt. S.K. Hospital, RML Hospital and LHMC, New Delhi, JIPMER, Pondicherry, PGI, Chandigarh, NIMHANS, Bangalore and subsequently the programme was expanded to cover all states. National nodal centre the "National Drug Dependance Centre" has been established under AIIMS, New Delhi located at Ghaziabad. NIMHANS,

Bangalore and PGI, Chandigarh has also been upgraded by the Ministry of Health and FW.

Drug De-addiction Centres (DDCs)

Drug de-addiction centres (DDCs) or harm reduction centres have been established in most of the states/ districts in India to reduce the prevalence of drug abuse through treatment and counselling focused on client and family. Under the drug de-addiction programme, 122 drug de-addiction centres have been established in various states. Out of 122 DDCs 43 have been established in North-Eastern region. DDCs provide the facilities of indoor admission, treatment, counselling and rehabilitation services.

Opioid substitution therapy (OST) under NACP: "It is also called harm reduction treatment. Though not ideal, it is one of the approaches to the treatment of addicts. The patient substitutes one drug with another less harmful one. Buprenorphine is the main component of opioid substitution therapy. OST helps treatment of injecting drug users (IDUs) to curb the prevalence of HIV".

Tertiary Prevention

It consists of advance treatment and rehabilitation at well-established mental health institutes which deal with such problems. Family remains the sheet anchor for rehabilitation in India after stabilization of cases. *Community-based rehabilitation* is the answer. Currently 50% or more beds in mental hospitals are occupied with chronic mental illness including substance users.

Alcohol and Substance Demand Reduction

Nation has worked out an integrated approach to supply and demand reduction for curbing the growing problems of alcoholism and drug abuse in the country by:

1 **Restriction/reduction** in the production of alcohol within the country and strict enforcement of legislation such as prevention of illicit traffic in Narcotic Drug and Psychotropic Substance Act (NDPSA), 1988 to prevent the flow of drugs into the country and for detention of persons trafficking in drugs.

2 **Awareness generation:** To reduce the demand for alcohol and drugs, the existing comprehensive community-based programme for awareness generation and preventive education, counselling, treatment, de-addiction and rehabilitation of addicts are specially strengthened and expanded to reach needy areas and groups especially in rural sector and in North East region.

3 **Research:** To enable nationwide identification of thrust areas and groups and suggest appropriate strategies, a national programme for demand reduction will be formulated using a database of the national survey on drug abuse (Table 13.24).

4 **High-risk groups** such as school and college students, street children, transport workers, occupational groups, and sex workers are being targeted for special intervention like awareness generation, counselling, treatment and rehabilitation. The nexus between injecting drug and HIV infection particularly in North East region, geat priority.

Mainstreaming of Addicts

Use of self-help groups, therapeutic communities, half-way homes, non-governmental organizations, religious congregation and alternate system of medicine for awareness generation and mainstreaming of addicts, can make a real difference besides the network of PHCs, hospitals and charitable organizations and de-addiction centres.

Training

Training component of control of alcohol and drug abuse in medical and nursing professionals, social workers, prison officers, police, etc. are being constantly updated to deal with newly emerging variations of substance abuse.

National centre for drug abuse prevention (NCDAP) was set-up in 1998 at Ghaziabad (UP); its 5 regional resource training centres one each at Chennai, Pune, Bengaluru and two in Kolkata have developed training manuals in 13 specific areas on rehabilitation and relapse prevention and management of drug abuse and HIV/AIDS, etc.[22]

TOBACCO PANDEMIC

Tobacco is the biggest killer, much bigger in dimension than all other forms of pollution. Children are the most vulnerable. Habits start in youth. Nicotine—the main pharmacological agent in tobacco is one of the most addictive substances known to mankind. The consumption of tobacco has reached the proportion of global epidemic. In the 20th century, the tobacco epidemic killed 100 million people worldwide, currently 5.4 million deaths every year are tobacco related globally (WHO, 2008).[23] In India, more than 8 lakh die due to Tobacco consumption. Nearly 30% cancers in Inida are related to tobacco use. The majority of cardiovascular diseases, cancers and lung disorders are directly attributable to tobacco use. Staggering economic cost of ₹ 1,04,500 crores is attributed to tobacco use, which is 1.16% of GDP and is 12% more than combined state and central government expenditure on halth in 2011–12.

Problem in India: Global Adult Tobacco Survey (GATS) October 2010

GATS was carried out in all 29 states and two union territories of India. The major objectives were:

- To estimate prevalence of tobacco use (smoking and smokeless tobacco).

13

- To estimate exposure to second-hand smoke (SHS), cessation, exposure to media, and economics of tobacco as also knowledge and perception towards tobacco.

Major Findings (Table 13.26)

- Current tobacco use in any form: 34.6% of adults; 47.9% of males and 20.3% of females use tobacco.
- Current tobacco smokers: 14% of adults; 24.3% of males and 2.9% of females.
- Current users of smokeless tobacco: 25.9% of adults; 32.9% males and 18.4% of females.
- Average age of initiation of tobacco use was 17.8.
- The risk of smokeless tobacco use is alarming as 90% of oral cancers in India are linked to it. Around 5.7% of adults smoked cigarettes against 9.2% of bidis (Table 13.26).
- Among minors (age 15–17 years), 9.6% consumed tobacco in some from and most of them were able to purchase tobacco products. Five in ten current smokers (46.6%) and users of smokeless tobacco (45.2%) planned to quit or at least thought of quitting. Among smokers and users of smokeless tobacco who visited a health care provider, 46.3% of smokers and 26.7% of users of smokeless tobacco were advised to quit by a health care provider. About five in ten adults (52.3%) were exposed to second-hand smoke at home and 29.0% at public places (mainly in public transport and restaurants). About two in three adults (64.5%) noticed advertisement or promotion of tobacco products. Three in five current tobacco users (61.1%) noticed the health warning on tobacco packages and one in three current tobacco users (31.5%) thought of quitting tobacco because of the warning label (Table 13.26).

The Global Youth Tobacco Survey (GYTS), 2009 for India also indicates that approximately 14.6% children in age group 13–15 years were tobacco users.

Types of Tobacco use

Over 15 billion cigarettes are smoked worldwide everyday. In India, 7 bidis are sold for every one cigarette. In Mumbai (India), 56% of women chew tobacco and some snuff tobacco.

Tobacco is also used in a wide variety of smokeless form (chewing tobacco as plug, loose leaf and twist, pan masala, or betel quid which consists of tobacco, areca-nuts and slaked lime wrapped in betel leaf.)

Table 13.26: Prevalence of tobacco use (%)[24, 25]

Users	Males	Females	Adults
Tobacco users	47.9	20.3	34.6
Smokers	24.3	2.9	14.0
Users of smokeless tobacco	32.9	18.4	25.9
Current cigarette smokers	10.3	0.8	5.7
Current bidi smokers	16.0	1.9	9.2

Source: GATS in India 2009–10.

India has 275 million tobacco users, out of which 206 million (75%) use smokeless tobacco: Khaini, Gutkha and Pan Masala. Health Ministry has notified ban on use of tobacco and nicotine in any food product (since 5th August 2011) including Gutkha, Khaini, and Pan Masala.

The water pipe or hukkah smoking (hubble-bubble) is common in rural areas of Northern India. The practice of cheroot (Chutta) smoking in reverse manner is prevalent in Andhra Pradesh and Odisha.

- By far the most popular way to smoke tobacco is the "Bidi". Bidis consist of small amount of tobacco, hand wrapped in dried Temburni leaf and tied with string. Despite their small size their tar and carbon monoxide derivatives can be higher than cigarettes. The 'bidis' is poor man's smoke; as such it is exempted from increases in excise duty. A designated sin tax to finance a part of the health budget can lead to reduced consumption of tobacco and alcohol.

People start smoking due to many wrong reasons

- The youth feel that smoking makes them more wanted.
- It makes them to feel grown ups.
- They feel that smoking gives them feeling of relaxation.
- They smoke for 'kick' and also to defy authority at home and school/college.
- They also think smoking helps them to concentrate and stimulates thinking, releases tension. Young people smoke to imitate adults.
- Many believe that it improves digestion and helps get rid of gas or wind problem and also helps in the act of defecation. But these are all false notions. Smoking is a socially acceptable practice in rural and urban areas and group smoking is a common practice in rural areas.[26]

Industry

Tobacco is a big industry all over the world. India produces 7,01,000, metric tonnes of tobacco and is the second largest producer in the world after China which produces 26,61,000 metric tonnes of tobacco per year. Nearly 0.23% of land area or 4,63,200 hectares of land area are used for growing tobacco in India.

Health Risks

Smokers have markedly increased risk of multiple cancers, particularly lung cancer, oral cancers in India, and are at greater risk of heart diseases, strokes, and emphysema. Smoking is responsible for 90% of all lung cancers, 75% of chronic bronchitis and emphysema, 31% of cases of ischaemic heart diseases,[27] Strokes and vascular diseases 21%, smoking affects almost every system besides accidents like fires. Nearly 30% of cancers in India are related to tobacco use. Nearly 8–9 lakh people die every year in India due to diseases related to tobacco use.

WHO report: Two in five deaths among adults aged 30 years and above in India are caused from the use of smokeless tobacco.

Every cigarette takes 7 minutes of your life. Harmful substances present in tobacco are—nicotine, carbon monoxide and tar. Nicotine causes increased heart rate, blood pressure, raised serum cholesterol, serum triglycerides and free fatty acids. Carbon monoxide combines with hemoglobin and converts it into carboxyhemoglobin and thus reduces oxygen supply to tissues, and heart muscle.

Other Harmful Substances

Tobacco smoke includes acetone, ammonia, arsenic, butane, cadmium, carbon monoxide, DDT, hydrogen cyanide, methanol, naphthalene, toluene, vinyl chloride. Tobacco smoke contains over 4000 chemicals which have marked irritant properties and some 60% are known or suspected carcinogens.

Passive Smoking (Second-hand Smoke) or Environmental Tobacco Smoke (ETS)

Smoker is source of risk to other family members. Non-smokers in the family are exposed to the risk of smoke. As a passive smoker, the non-smoker breathes "sidestream" smoke from the burning tip of the cigarette and "mainstream" smoke that has been inhaled and exhaled by the smoker. Passive smokers are exposed to the similar health risks.

Deaths: 10–15% of total deaths in adults over 35 years of age are attributable to tobacco use.

Tobacco Control

The tobacco menace can be controlled by education drive through mass media, extension education and through curriculum, besides legislation.

As a result of WHO initiative against tobacco, many countries of the world have passed legislations against tobacco. Doctors, school teachers and parents can play significant role in tobacco control by being good role models and advocates.

Quiting smoking at any stage is beneficial to health. There are many techniques to assist those who want to quit smoking. These techniques include social support, clinics, quitlines, internet sites, skills training, nicotine replacement therapy and other pharmaceutical treatments. Intervention against tobacco should have focus on both, prevention of initiation and cessation of *smoking/chewing tobacco*.

Nodal Ministry

The Ministry of Social Justice and Empowerment is the nodal agency for implementation of programme of de-addiction and substance abuse. It coordinates between various sectors to deal with the problem.[28]

Tobacco Control Legislation in India

A comprehensive tobacco control legislation titled "*The cigarettes and other tobacco products* (prohibition of advertisement and regulation of trade and commerce, production, supply and distribution) Act (COTPA), 2003", was passed by the Parliament in April, 2003 and received the assent of the President of India on 18th May, 2003. This was notified in the official gazette on 19th May, 2003. The Act is applicable to the whole of India and covers all types of tobacco products. The important provisions of the Act are as follows:

- Ban on smoking in public places (from 2nd Oct, 2008).
- Regulation of smoking scenes in movies.
- Ban on direct and indirect advertisement of cigarette and other tobacco products.
- Ban on sale of cigarette and other tobacco products to a person below the age of 18.
- Ban on sale of tobacco products within 100 yards of education institutions.
- Ban on tobacco in Gutkha, Pan Masala and Khaini and any food product.
- Mandatory depiction of statutory warnings (including graphic or pictorial warning) on tobacco packs: "Smoking kills, Tobacco kills" "and tobacco causes cancer". At least 85% of area on both sides of tobacco pack to be covered with health warning (60% for picture and 25% for text).
- Mandatory depiction of tar and nicotine contents along with maximum permissible limits on tobacco packs.
- Testing of tobacco products for tar and nicotine.

The Food Safety and Standards Authority of India laid down that tobacco and nicotine can not be used as an ingredient in any food product. India has been a forerunner in the WHO Framework Convention on Tobacco Control (FCTC) negotiations in Geneva since its inception. India signed the said convention on 10th September, 2003 and later on ratified the same on 5th February, 2004. India has already translated a number of provisions of the FCTC into domestic law by enactment of above legislation.

Proposed amendments include: Enhancing legal age for tobacco consumption from 18 to 21 years, ban on sale of loose cigarettes and raising penality.

NATIONAL TOBACCO CONTROL PROGRAMME (NTCP)

The Government of India has launched a pilot phase of NTCP in 2007–08 in 18 districts of 9 states and upscaled to cover 53 districts of 29 states during the year 2013 under National Health Mission (NHM).

Objectives: The main objectives are to implement anti-tobacco laws and bring about greater awareness and take "Tobacco control initiatives" to the community level.

Components: The main components of the programme are:

1. Public awareness building and behavioural change–through mass media anti-tobacco campaign.
2. Establishing tobacco product testing labs as required under COTPA, 2003.
3. Capacity building at state and district level by setting up dedicated State Tobacco Control Cell and District Tobacco Control Cell.
4. Providing alternate livelihood to tobacco farmers, and workers: Ministry of Health and Family Welfare has also released grant in-aid to Central Tobacco Research Institute (CTRI), Rajahmundry (AP), for pilot studies on alternate cropping to tobacco and alternate vocations to bidi rollers.
5. Monitoring and evaluation including surveillance, e.g.

   Global Adult Tobacco Survey (GATS), India: In India, it has been conducted with the technical assistance from WHO and CDC, Atlanta. The main aim of GATS is to establish the state wise prevalence of tobacco use, ascertain level of awareness/knowledge about the ill effects of tobacco products. The survey has provided baseline data to states on tobacco control initiatives.
6. Mainstreaming the programme components as part of the health delivery mechanism under the National Health Mission framework.

Tobacco control cells at National, State, District have been set up along with coordination committees at district, bock and village level for implementation of programme. Toll free National Helpline (24 × 7) (1800-110-456) has been established to report violations of prohibitions of smoking in public places.[29]

Dedicated component will be integrated with NHM activities for implementation of provisions under the law. To undertake tobacco control initiatives, e.g. school programmes, trainings of health and social workers, and school teachers setting up cessation facilities (Tobacco Cessation Centres), and monitoring tobacco laws.

The global tobacco control fraternity is now focusing on END GAME, i.e. reducing tobacco use prevalence to less than 5% in the country.

Main Challenges Facing Tobacco Control

- Low level of awareness regarding harmful effects of tobacco consumption.
- Availability of large number of tobacco products.
- Low age of initiation of tobacco use.
- Limited capacity of states to implement laws.
- Low priority to tobacco control.
- Limited availability of tobacco cessation facilities.
- Challenge of providing alternate livelihood to large workforce in tobacco farming.
- Lack of coordination among stakeholder departments.

REFERENCES

1. WHO. Strengthening mental health promotion. Fact sheet 220. Geneva: WHO; Revised 2001.
2. WHO. The World health report—Mental disorders affect one in four people. Press release WHO/42. Geneva.
3. WHO. Mental and neurological disorders. Fact sheet 265. Geneva: WHO; 2001.
4. World Bank. World Development Report 1993. New York: World Bank; 1993.
5. Ganguli HC. Epidemiological findings on prevalence of mental disorders in India. Ind J. Psychiatr 2000;42(1): 14–20.
6. Reddy VM, Chandra Shekhar CR. Indian J Psychiatr 1998; 40(2): 149–57.
7. Issac MK. Severe Mental Morbidity. ICMR Bulletin 1988 Dec; 18(12).
8. Lal S, Vasudeva YL. Morbidity pattern of clients and patients visiting Navan Baba (Faith healer). Ind J Prev Soc Med 1976; 7: 47–49.
9. Government of India. National mental health programme for India. New Delhi: Central Council of Health and Family Welfare; 1982.
10. Trivedi S, Srinivasa DK. Proceeding of National Workshop on undergraduate medical education in mental health (Sponsored by WHO) 1985 Dec 22–24: JIPMER, Pondicherry, India.
11. NIMHANS. Mental Health Mannual for Health Workers. Bangalore: Centre for advanced research. NIMHANS; 1990.
12. NIMHANS. Features of Mental Disorders—A Folder. Bangalore: ICMR centre for advanced research. NIMHANS; 1987.
13. Kumar N. Development in Mental Health Scenario: Need to stop exclusion—Dare to Care. ICMR Bulletin 2001 April; 31(4).
14. Lal S, Vashisht BM. Moving away from mental institutions— towards community mental health care. Ind J Comm Med 2002 Oct-Dec; 27(4): 147–50.
15. WHO. The world health report. Mental health—new understanding, new hope. Geneva: WHO; 2001.
16. WHO. The Mental health. Policy and service guidance package. The Mental Health Context. WHO, 2003.
17. Ministry of health and family welfare. New pathways new hope national mental health policy oct, 2014.
18. Gossop M, Grant M. Preventing and controlling drug abuse. Geneva: WHO; 1990.
19. UNODC (2004). Ministry of Social Justice and Empowerment Government of India. The extent, pattern and trends of Drug Abuse in India, National Survey.
20. UNODC. Ministry of Social Justice and Empowerment, Government of India (2002). Drug Abuse Monitoring system. A profile of treatment seekers.
21. UNDCP (ROSA), MOSJE, GOI (2002), Rapid assessment survey of Drug Abuse in India.

22 GOI. Annual Report 2008–09. MOH and FW, GOI; New Delhi.
23 WHO: WHO Report on the Global Epidemic, 2008.
24 Global Adult Tobacco Survey India 2009–10. CDC, WHO, IIPS. MOH and FW, Government of India.
25 GOI. NFHS-3, 2005–06.
26 Gupta PC, Sinha DN. Tobacco research in India. Editorial—Indian Journal of Public Health 48: (3) July-Sept 2004.
27 WHO. "Smoking or Health the Choice is Yours" Theme of World Health Day, 7 April 1980. Backgrounder WHO.
28 Planning commission. Tenth Five-Year Plan 2002–07, Vol II. New Delhi, GOI; 2002.
29 GOI. and HRIDAY—SHAN Tobacco Control Laws—A Resource Manual, MOH and FW, New Delhi (India) January 7, 2008.

MENTAL RETARDATION

"Mental retardation is a condition of arrested or incomplete development of the mind characterized by impairment of skills and overall intelligence in areas such as cognition, language, motor and social abilities." Also referred to as intellectual disability or handicap, mental retardation can occur with or without any other physical or mental disorder. In addition to genetic factors, injuries at birth and brain infections, a common cause of mental retardation is *iodine deficiency* which is the *single largest cause of preventable brain damage* and severe mental retardation (*cretinism*).[1]

Prevalence

It is estimated that overall prevalence of mental retardation is between 1 and 3%. It is more common in developing countries because of higher incidence of injuries and deprivation of oxygen at birth and early childhood brain infections, all of which cause retardation.[1]

According to WHO 1989 estimate, 3% of people have intelligence quotient (IQ) falling below 2 standard deviation.

Definition

The American Association on Mental Deficiency (AAMD) 1961 developed the following definition:

"Mental retardation refers to sub-average general intellectual functioning which originates during the development period and is associated with impairment in adaptive behaviour".[2]

It is evident from the above given definition that 3 things need to be borne in mind:

i Intelligence should be significantly sub-average, i.e. IQ is less than 70.
ii This should have occurred in developmental period, i.e. up to 18 years of age.
iii Behaviour should be significantly inappropriate.

Persons having IQ between 70 and 89 are put in the category of borderline functioning and those between 90 and 109 are of average intelligence while person with IQ of 130 and above is called genius.

Mild Mental Retardation

Mild mental retardation includes the following

- Feeble-mindedness
- Mild mental subnormality
- Mild oligophrenia
- Moron

Diagnostic Guidelines

If the proper standardized IQ tests are used, the range 50–69 is indicative of mild retardation (Table 13.27). Understanding and use of language tend to be delayed to a varying degree and executive speech problems that interfere with the development of independence may persist into adult life.

Moderate Mental Retardation

Moderate mental retardation includes the following

- Imbecility
- Moderate mental subnormality
- Moderate oligophrenia

Individuals in this category are slow in developing comprehension and use of language, and their eventual achievement in this area is limited. Achievement of self-care and motor skills is also retarded, and some need supervision throughout life. Progress in school work is limited, but a proportion of these individuals learn the basic skills needed for reading, writing, and counting. Educational programmes can provide opportunities for them to develop their limited potential and to acquire some basic skills; such programmes are appropriate for slow learners with a low ceiling of achievement.

Diagnostic Guidelines

The IQ is usually in the range 35–49 (Table 13.27). Discrepant profiles of abilities are common in this group, with some individuals achieving higher levels in visuo-spatial skills than in tasks dependent on language, while

Table 13.27: Degree of mental retardation[3,4]

Severity	*IQ range*	
	APA	ICD-10
1. Mild mental retardation	50–55 to appx. 70	50–69
2. Moderate mental retardation	35–40 to 50–55	35–49
3. Severe mental retardation	20–25 to 35–40	20–34
4. Profound mental retardation	Below 20–25	Under 20

APA (American Psychiatric Association); ICD-10 international classification of diseases others are markedly clumsy but enjoy social interaction and simple conversation.

Severe Mental Retardation

Severe mental retardation includes
- Severe mental subnormality
- Severe oligophrenia

This category is broadly similar to that of moderate mental retardation in terms of the clinical picture, the presence of an organic etiology, and the associated conditions. The lower levels of achievement mentioned under moderate mental retardation are also the most common in this group. Most people in this category suffer from a marked degree of motor impairment or other associated deficits, indicating the presence of clinically significant damage to or maldevelopment of the central nervous system.

Diagnostic Guidelines

The IQ is usually in the range 20–34 (Table 13.27).

Profound Mental Retardation (Table 13.27)

Profound mental retardation includes
- Idiocy
- Profound mental subnormality
- Profound oligophrenia

The IQ in this category is estimated to be under 20, which means in practice that affected individuals are severely limited in their ability to understand or comply with requests or instructions. Most of such individuals are immobile or severely restricted in mobility, incontinent, and capable at the most of only very rudimentary forms of nonverbal communication. They possess little or no ability to care for their own basic needs, and require constant help and supervision.

Other Mental Retardation

This category should be used only when assessment of the degree of intellectual retardation by means of the usual procedures is rendered particularly difficult or impossible by associated sensory or physical impairments, as in blind, deaf-mute, and severely behaviourally disturbed or physically disabled people.

Causes of Mental Retardation

i ***Deficiency of iodine*** in mother during pregnancy or iodine deficiency disorders leading to cretinism.

ii ***Genetic causation:*** Either due to single mutant gene abnormalities of chromosomes and multifactorial inheritance. These disorders include phenylketonuria (PKU), galactosemia, cretinism, chromosomal abnormalities, consanguineous marriages.

iii ***Congenital malformation***, microcephaly and hydrocephalus.

iv ***Prenatal*** inadequate nutrition, infection due to Rubella or German measles during pregnancy, blood incompatibility (Rh incompatibility between maternal and foetal blood), radioactivity, exposure to toxic agents like lead, nicotine, and alcohol.

v ***During labour:*** Prolonged difficult labour and traumatic birth injury and asphyxia.

vi ***Prematurity:*** Low birth weight.

vii ***Postnatal causes:*** Head injuries, postnatal infections, encephalitis and meningitis, measles in particular and other viral and bacterial encephalitis, malnutrition in babies, lead poisoning, etc.

Prevention

Mental retardation can be prevented. Actions to prevent retardation include:

i Adequate diet during pregnancy and prevention of low birth weights. Iodization of salt to prevent iodine deficiency and mental retardation (cretinism).
ii Vaccination against Rubella, measles and whooping cough.
iii Blood testing screening for Rh group during pregnancy.
iv Abstinence from alcohol by pregnant women to avoid foetal alcohol syndrome.
v Dietary control to prevent mental retardation in people with phenylketonuria.
vi Safe delivery avoiding trauma and asphyxia. Environmental control to prevent mental retardation due to poisoning from heavy metals such as lead.
vii Prenatal genetic testing to detect certain forms of mental retardation such as Down syndrome.

Treatment Goals

- Early recognition and optimal utilization of intellectual capacities of the individual by training, family education and support.
- Vocational training and opportunities for work in protected environments.
- Training of parents to act as teachers and trainers of daily life skills.
- Support groups for parents.

Legislation

The persons with disabilities (equal opportunity, protection of rights and full participation) Act, 1995. The Act gives fundamental rights to all disabled people in the country for the equal opportunity.

INTELLIGENCE

According to concise definition of intelligence "it is global or aggregate capacity of the individual to think rationally, deal effectively and act purposefully with his environment".

Intelligence tests were introduced in 1908 in United States by Goddard. Goddard developed the classification of mental retardation into "idiots", "imbeciles", and "morons". These terms have become derogatory and are unacceptable. Terman developed the concept of IQ: The ratio between mental and chronological age.

Intelligence Quotient (IQ)

This is the ratio of mental age and chronological age expressed in percentage.[5]

$$IQ = \frac{\text{Mental age}}{\text{Chronological age}} \times 100$$

The mental age of a child is ascertained by administering a standard psychological test. For example, if the chronological age of a child is 12 and his mental age by standard psychological test is 6 then the IQ is $^{6}/_{12} \times 100 = 50$. A child who has mental age equal to chronological age, his IQ level is 100 and if the mental age is 6 years and chronological age is 5 then the IQ is 120. A normal child should have IQ more than 90.

The concept of mental maturity raises interesting problem. Thus, a child of 15 years old with mental age of 15 years, clearly his IQ is 100 or normal. What happens five years later when he is 20 years old? Since he is mentally mature, his mental age is still presumably 15. Therefore, if we stick to this formula his IQ has sunk to $^{15}/_{20} \times 100$ or 75 which is decidedly inferior. This cannot be true. In order to compute adult IQ, we must take the denominator age as 15.

For infants, a clinical judgment of significantly sub-average intellectual functioning is to be done since available intelligence tests do not yield numerical IQ values.

IQ tests except for persons with significant retardation are not predictive of adaptive functioning and many mildly retarded persons function as well as non-retarded persons once they are out of school. As a result of these findings, the criterion of social adaptation was added to the definition of mental retardation.

Several psychological tests/intelligence tests are available to measure the level of intelligence. These tests are to measure the level of development or maturation (Bayley infant scale, Gassell's developmental schedule, National Institute for Mentally Handicapped Development Assessment Schedule); verbal tests (Binet Kamat test, Binet Kulshrestha test, Binet Shukla test and Malin's Intelligence scale for Indian children—verbal scale), nonverbal tests (developmental screening test, Raven's progressive matrices-coloured), performance tests (Seguin Form Board test, Gessell's drawing tests, draw a man test, and Malin's Intelligence Scale for Indian Children-Performance Scale); adaptive behaviour scales (Vineland social maturity scale, American Association on Mental Retardation Adaptive Behaviour Scale); and tests for specific abilities (attention, concentration, and tests for perception).[6, 7]

JUVENILE DELINQUENCY (JD)

Antisocial behaviour in young children below the age of 16 in boys and below 18 in girls is known as juvenile delinquency. The common antisocial behaviours are—stealing, cruelty, crimes, lying, gambling, substance abuse, sexual offences and destructiveness or simply delinquent juvenile means a juvenile who has committed an offence.

Who is Juvenile?

The Juvenile Justice Act, 1986 defines a "juvenile" as a boy who has not attained the age of 16, and a girl who has not attained the age of 18. JD includes not only "juvenile offence" but all other antisocial unacceptable behaviours and practices.[8]

Causes of JD

i Increasing population (with too many children), urbanization, urban slums, poverty, broken families and illiteracy compel these children to adopt antisocial activities.

ii There may be some genetic predisposition, but primarily these are environmental influences.

Such children are not well adjusted in the family. A substantial proportion of 37 million children living in urban poverty are living in informal (illegal) settlements or other temporary constructions, which include living along railway lines, drainage canals and fringe areas of the city. Large number of them become rag pickers, work in restaurants, start begging and such children indulge in offences. Under the **Juvenile Justice Act of 1986,** the police send them to remand homes meant for juveniles.

Protection

It is the responsibility of the state to look into the problems of juvenile social maladjustment and make all special efforts to mobilize all possible resources of the family, community and social organization for rehabilitation and betterment of juvenile future.

Any juvenile who is likely to be abused, exploited and induced into criminogenic life is in need of legal support to be appropriately rehabilitated.

Apart from prohibiting the confinement of the juvenile in a police lock-up or jail, his contact with the police has been reduced to minimum. Inquiry of this case should be completed within a period of 3 months from the date of commencement. Such juvenile should be produced before the Juvenile Welfare Board; and the delinquent are to be dealt with the Juvenile Court. Criteria for admission in juvenile homes, local observation homes (Borstal Jail), special homes, have been defined in the Act.

Prevention includes limiting the size of family, formal and non-formal education, management of street children and involvement of non-Governmental organization.

STREET CHILDREN

An estimated 4,14,700 children scattered over urban areas live in difficulty. These children run away from home in a village to the big city they have dreamed about or their family abandon them on the streets or they find themselves alone in the urban jungle, after the man-made or natural calamity. These children struggle for their survival. The problems of street children have grown with urbanization and grow as the city grows. While earning money for themselves or their families, street children serve several needs of the city. Large number of them become rag-pickers. Often this is the first job a child on the street learns to do. Some of them start begging and some are forced into theft, crime or sexual abuse. Even if a child is not directly exploited by the local mafia, he/she has to pay their part of earnings and live in constant fear of abuse. Children have to face brutality from antisocial elements apart from police. Police usually picks them and book them under Juvenile Justice Act, 1986.

Children on the street have no access to education or health facilities. These children live in precarious conditions, unhealthy environments, shelter, inadequate and unsafe water.[9]

Problems

These children are at risk of exploitation, sexual abuse, drug trafficking and other antisocial activities. They are most vulnerable to STD and HIV and other epidemic prone diseases due to lack of basic amenities.

The study on Child Abuse, 2007, was Commissioned by Ministry of Women and Child Development in Children age group 5–12 years. Two out of every three children were physically abused. Around 53% reported having faced one or more forms of sexual abuse and every second child reported emotional abuse (neglect of girl child).

The Government in all the major metropolis is undertaking slum clearance and settlement programme. The existing government programmes of education, health, nutrition, vocational training, self-employment should be encouraged for street children. At the government policy level, as for the other major child-related problems of the child labour, and prostitution, the problems of street children will end as education has been made compulsory, rural initiatives are taken to provide meaningful employment to adults and stop urban migration.

Role of NGOs

In all the major cities, many NGOs are working towards improving life for the street children. They provide night shelters, non-formal education and some provide vocational training. NGOs can make critical intervention in a street child's life. But so far they have been able to reach only a small percentage of any city's street children. For reaching more children initiative can come from local citizen's groups or even government bodies after being sensitized to the situation of the street children.

Police station should be child-friendly and help these children sympathetically. Compulsory education and vocational training helps for gainful employment.

CHILD LABOUR

Children are abused as child labour. Under the Child Labour (Prohibition and Regulation) Act, 1986, "child" means any person who has not completed his 14th year of age and under Factories Act, 1948 no child who has not completed his 14th year shall be required or allowed to work in any factory. The number of child workers in India vary from 11.3 to 44 million.

Child labour appears to be widespread in India. Children work as bonded labourers in the glass industry, bidi industry, in matchmaking, carpet weaving, slate pencil making, mining, handlooms and agriculture. Sometimes entire family is bonded to the employer. It is reported that in the final polishing of gems with oxides, the entire labour force consists of children. Many of the young children work in hazardous jobs such as in brass making furnace. In cities, child workers contribute to city's economy as waste recyclers, dish washers, cleaners, truck loaders, waiters, and coolies. Yet besides being exploitive, their job environments are unhealthy and hazardous.

Abolishing child labour would directly and indirectly raise wage costs. The Government has not imposed total ban on child labour because they feel survival of the poor depends on it. Many argue that if child labour is removed from traditional trades than the traditional craft will die out and children who have not been trained since early childhood will not be able to make vocation out of traditional craft.

The Supreme Court in a landmark judgment in December 1996 called for urgent measures to eliminate hazardous child labour and imposed fine on employers as well as an implementation mechanism with reporting back to the court. There are other legislations but enforcement is a big problem.

But removing children from the horrors of child labour is possible, though often costly. Many NGOs have succeeded partially through setting-up of night schools and education camps and educating parents and youths. MV Foundation in Andhra Pradesh has been successful in liberating bonded labour.[8]

CHILD PROSTITUTION

Prostitution is illegal in India but is widely prevalent. The central advisory committee on child prostitution gives aid to only six metropolitan cities in India—Mumbai, Delhi, Kolkata, Chennai, Hyderabad and Bengaluru, where there are about 100,000 prostitutes. Out of these, 15% are below 15 years of age and 24% are between 16 and 18 years of age.

Unofficial estimates say that India has 2 million prostitutes of which 20% are below 15 years of age. But almost all of them become victims of exploitation when they are children less than 15 years old.

Reasons

Because of poverty and economic reasons the girls are forced to adopt profession and many of them end-up as commercial sex workers. Many sex traffickers take advantage of the tradition bound groups and exploit other victims through their poverty stricken background.

Consequences

The spread of HIV/AIDS and STDs is related to widespread unprotected sexual activity through commercial sex workers and bridge population. 40% of all new HIV infections are in youth group. The problem of child prostitutes must be tackled urgently to control the spread of HIV/AIDS by educating people and especially youth and school children. Strategies towards ending prostitution need to have large preventive component. As a direct and immediate measure, this means working in an area which is known for selling their children, changing attitudes and creating other choices. It means mobilizing youth themselves to protect each other from illegal marriages or open sale by group action and public exposure. Panchayati Raj Institutions and women groups can take the lead. Rescue and rehabilitation of prostitutes is another strategy. Enforcement of existing laws against child marriage and education for all is the answer to this problem.

CHILD MARRIAGE

The Child Marriage Restraint Act of 1976 raised the legal age of marriage for girls from 15 to 18 years and for boys from 18 to 21 years. The aim of this legislation is to prevent child marriages. Child marriage is violation of child rights. In practice, 30% of marriages in India occur below the age of 18 which exposes them to teenage pregnancies and high maternal morbidity and mortality, besides illegal abortions and complications thereof. Though the incidence of marriages below 18 is declining still it is a major problem in some states like Rajasthan, Bihar, Uttar Pradesh and Madhya Pradesh. Besides high morbidity and mortality, it leads to high reproduction and large-sized families and increase in population.

Universal elementary education, vocational training and promoting education for girls can prevent teenage marriages and pregnancies.

DISABLED CHILDREN

Disabled children face discrimination and neglect. A striking feature of Indian society is to treat such children as "handicapped" and set-up separate facilities for them. There is very little public consciousness of the need to integrate such children into the mainstream.

What is most urgently needed is first and foremost to prevent avoidable disability among children. Vitamin A to prevent blindness, iodized salt to prevent mental retardation, polio vaccination to eliminate paralysis from polio, prenatal and obstetric care to prevent birth injury. But even then, disability of one form or another affect 5% to as much as 10% of children.

Disabled children should get the same treatment as other children. They have a right to health care, to be dealt with like others in primary school, ensure dignity, self-reliance and active participation in the community. Government needs to provide special support services for these groups of children besides integrating them in the mainstream of community.

Under International Classification of Functioning (ICF) Disability and Health, the term disability serves as an umbrella term for impairments, activity limitation and participation restriction. The term handicap has been dropped altogether.

CHILD GUIDANCE CLINIC/CENTRE (CGC)

"The child guidance centre/clinic is a service agency that addresses itself to needs of children with learning behaviour or development problems through comprehensive, bio-psychosocial assessments, counselling and therapeutic services. In addition, the service agency may choose to extend itself to organize primary and/or secondary level services for children as well."

Behavioural problems amongst children and adolescents are very common. The scholastically backward (poor performance in schools) and learning disabilities are problems of great magnitude in children below 14 years.

An epidemiological study of child and adolescents psychiatric disorders in urban and rural areas conducted by ICMR (2001) indicated the overall prevalence of mental and behavioural disorders in children to be 12.8%. According to World Health Report (2001), 15% have emotional disturbances. The severity of problem can be assessed by the fact that 3500 children below 14 years kill themselves annually (Thomas, 2003).[10, 11]

Child and adolescent mental health, which is future of our country, is given inadequate attention. Changing structure of the family, modernization, westernization, industrialization, globalization, urbanization and competition in academics has negatively influenced child and adolescent mental health. Incidence of mental health problems is on increase (278% increase in pedophilia). Depression and suicides have increased to three to four-folds in large number of states in India.

In view of multitudes of behavioural problems in children and adolescents, child guidance clinics (CGC) were initiated in India way back in 1937 and till date 164 of such clinics have been located by NIPCCD survey (2003).

Objectives of CGCs

i To offer skilled diagnosis, assessment and treatment for children having any behaviour, emotional and personal disorders (guidance and counselling services to children).
ii To guide parents and teachers in promoting the mental health of the children.
iii To work towards preventing behaviour and emotional problems and promoting mental health of children by raising awareness at the community level.

Beneficiaries

Children and adolescents in the age group 0–18 years which has been now extended till 20 years.

Staff of Clinic

Child guidance and counselling requires multidisciplinary interventions and team work at CGC ideally consists of psychiatric social workers, a psychiatrist, a clinical psychologist and speech therapist.

Mode of Function

i CGCs carries out comprehensive assessment of the behavioural problems of the child.
ii Therapeutic interventions are worked out in relation to assessed problem.

Services

This covers: Assessment and therapeutic services to children with behavioural, emotional, scholastic and personality disorders. A wide variety of psychological problems are seen and treated by various treatment modalities like individual counselling, play therapy, behaviour therapy, different psychotherapeutic approaches, parental counselling, family therapy, and vocational guidance, etc. Children with special learning disability are covered and some clinics cover sexually abused children and adolescents. Therapeutic group work with both children, adolescents and parents is a regular feature.

Referrals

The sources of referrals to these CGCs are hospitals and health agencies, medical practitioners and paramedical staff, schools, welfare organizations and institutions, social workers, parents, guardians and relatives and parents of past clients.

Historically, child guidance clinics/centres (CGCs) has been the oldest mental health agency to address the mental health concerns of children and their families. Since their inception, these CGCs are confined to urban areas in big cities and towns and do not cover rural children and adolescents. 164 CGCs cover part of urban population only in big towns. Further the staff component of many of the CGCs happen to be inadequate/deficient. Rarely CGCs were found to be functioning as independent units. Most of them were administratively a part of big institutions or organizations. The CGCs are functioning through hospitals, or through disability or mental health programmes, through welfare programmes for children and through technical institutions.

New Thrust Activities of CGCs

All CGCs were undertaking tertiary level clinical activities. The new client groups are being reached through by many CGCs which include:

- Street and working children
- Sexually abused children
- Children committed under JJ Act (Juvenile Justice Act)
- Neonates and high-risk babies
- Developmentally delayed children
- Physically handicapped children
- Children with multiple disabilities
- Children with autism or Autism Spectrum Disorders (ASD): It results in impaired social interaction and communication as also restricted and repetitive behaviour. Some may not even develop speech.
- Some rarely use language to communicate
- Children with learning disabilities
- Preschool children

Future

It is proposed to expand CGCs horizontally to serve as base of mental health for children and adolescents of the country. We need to establish at least 10,000 CGCs at the rate of 1:100,000. Even if the country plans for urban population alone, India would require 566 CGCs.

The present CGCs are facing the problem of lack of professionally qualified staff, which negatively affects the quality of their services.

Medical Social Worker

These workers are specially trained in social case work. These workers are helpful in identifying relevant social, psychological/emotional and economic factors related to health/disease by interviewing and counseling. Medical social worker can work directly with the family or at clinic to provide social work services. Medical social worker's functions are:

i To assess the need for social work services of individual, family and community.
ii Arrange or provide social work services.
iii Participate in overall planning and evaluation of social work services.

Example: Social case work is significant in chronic diseases, mental disorders, HIV/AIDS, leprosy, tuberculosis, Cancer, behavioural problems of children, etc. Services consist of counseling, psychotherapy, rehabilitation (physical, social and occupational) prevention of disease/ disability, etc.

REFERENCES

1 WHO. Mental and neurological disorders. Fact Sheet 265; 2001.

2 Rehabilitation Council of India. Manual for Training of PHC Medical Officers. New Delhi: Rehabilitation Council of India; 2000.

3 American Psychiatric Association. Diagnostic and Statistical Manual of Mental Disorders (DSM-IV TM). First Indian edn, New Delhi: Jaypee Brothers Medical Publishers (P) Ltd; 1995.

4 WHO. International classification of diseases. Tenth Revision. Geneva; WHO; 1993.

5 Sterling AP, Gill HS. Psychology made simple. London: WH Allen and Company; 1967.

6 GOI. Mental Retardation—a manual for psychologists. Secunderabad: National Institute of the Mentally Handicapped; 1989.

7 Dogra R, Sindhu B, Vohra AK. Psychological Assessment, Haryana Medical Journal 2002 May-June; 22(2).

8 The Gazette of India. The Juvenile Justice Act, 1986 [Act No. 53 of 1986].

9 UNICEF (1998). Rights and opportunities—the situation of children and women in India. New Delhi: UNICEF, India Country Office; 1998.

10 NIPCCD. National consultation meet on Upscaling Child Guidance Services in the country—a report. New Delhi: NIPCCD; 2004.

11 NIPPCD. Scholastic Backwardness: Analysis of children coming to the child guidance centre. Research Study. New Delhi: NIPCCD; 2004.

BLINDNESS

WHO defines blindness as "visual acuity of less than 3/60 (Snellen) or its equivalent" and for lay persons, it is further simplified as "inability to count fingers in daylight at a distance of 3 metres". The latter definition can be used by health workers, Anganwadi workers and health guides to *screen* the cases of *blindness* at the village level for rapid diagnosis of blindness and referral thereof to nearest health facility. This helps reaching blinds and enhances coverage.

Global Prevalence

The blindness is a global problem. Recent estimates of World Health Organization suggest that there are 40 million people, who are blind worldwide and that more than 90% of them live in developing countries. Nearly one-fifth of them are in India.[1]

Blindness in India

Using a visual acuity cut-off of <6/60 in the better eye (the definition used by national programme for control of blindness in India), the number of blinds increased to the level of 13 million in India. Prevalence varies from region to region (Table 13.28).

Definition of Blindness in India under National Programme for Control of Blindness (NPCB)

Inability of a person to count fingers from a distance of 6 meters or 20 feet.

Technical Definition

Blindness	**Low vision**
• Presenting visual acuity less than 6/60 in the better eye	• Presenting visual acuity better than 6/60 but less than 6/18 in the better eye

Every year we add on 2 million blinds in the total pool of blindness, which is the incidence rate of blindness in India.[2] Three-fourths of these blinds in India live in rural areas needing restoration of their vision. How to reach rural blinds remains an important issue? Alternate strategies like "camp approach" was used to reach rural blinds. Rural blinds can be reached through primary health care set up. Therefore, the blindness control programme has to be an integral part of primary health care.[3]

Causes of Blindness in India

Cataract, Refractive Errors and Glaucoma

Cataract (62.6%) continued to be the major cause of curable blindness in India. Uncorrected refractive errors were responsible for 19.7% of the blindness. Other important causes of blindness include glaucoma (5.8%), posterior segment pathology (4.7%), corneal opacities 0.9% and others 5.1% (Table 13.29).[4, 5] Estimated childhood blindness/ low vision at 0.8/1000.

Table 13.28: Prevalence of blindness (visual acuity <6/60) 2001–04

Category	*Prevalence (%)*	*States*
Low	Less than 1	Tamil Nadu, Maharashtra, Kerala, Himachal Pradesh, Uttranchal, UP, Bihar, Sikkim, Meghalaya, Mizoram, Tripura
Moderate	1 to 1.49	Gujarat, Punjab, MP, Andhra Pradesh, Odisha and West Bengal
High	1.5 to 1.99	Jharkhand, Chhattisgarh, Manipur, Nagaland, J & K, Haryana, Rajasthan, Karnataka
Very high	2 and above	Assam, Arunachal Pradesh

Table 13.29: Causes of blindness in India		
Causes	*Years of survey*	
	1986–89 (%)	*2001–02* (%)
Cataract	81	62.6
Refractive errors	7	19.7
Corneal opacities	3	0.9
Trachoma	0.20	NA
Glaucoma	2.0	5.8
Posterior segment pathology	NA	4.7
Surgical complications	NA	1.2
Vit. A deficiency	0.04	NA
Others	6.76	5.1
Total	**100**	**100**

Source: Reference 4 and 5

Trends of Blindness

Blindness in India is declining (Table 13.30).

Between 1974 and 1989, the prevalence of blindness remained unchanged.

The results of 2001–02, national survey in 15 districts indicate declining trends of blindness but we are far away from the goal of 0.3%. *Prevalence* of blindness declined to 1.12% by 2002 and it further declined to 1.0% as per rapid survey of avoidable blindness conducted under NPCB during 2006–07. The goal of 0.3% was to be achieved by 2000 AD under 'Health for All' strategy. Now we have revised this goal and the goal to be achieved is 0.3% level by 2020. India has made tremendous efforts to clear the backlog and reduce the level of blindness but the goal is far away. Ever increasing population of aged and increased life expectancy eludes us. We have 8.3% of population above the age of 60 and it has gone up to 9% in 2016.[8]

Incidence of Blindness

Every year we add on 2 million blinds in the total pool of blinds.

Types of Blindness

a. Preventable Blindness

Blindness due to smallpox infection has been eradicated. A blinding malnutrition due to vitamin A deficiency has been significantly reduced and nearly eliminated but problem of vitamin A deficiency still exists in certain pockets. Vitamin A prophylaxis programme as a part of primary health care continues to eliminate blindness due to vitamin A deficiency. Keratomalacia has almost disappeared in India and bitot spots declined to the level of 0.7% in the year 2001 in children below 6 years of age.[9] Infection like, trachoma has been controlled in the country due to improved socioeconomic conditions and access to primary health care. Programme of trachoma control has been made an integral part of blindness control programme since 1976.

Table 13.30: Trends of blindness in general population in India[6,7]	
Years of survey	*Prevalence of blindness (%)*
1971–74 ICMR	1.38
1986–89 NPCB	1.49
2001–02	1.12
2006–07	1.0
Childhood blindness/ low vision	0.8 per 1000
Goal by 2010	0.5
Goal by 2020	0.3

b. Curable Blindness

Cataract is an example of curable blindness and its prevalence is very high in India. Cataract is major cause of social and economic blindness in India.

c. Avoidable Blindness

It is the sum total of preventable and curable blindness. In India, 85–90% of blindness is avoidable.

Blindness in Persons above 50 Years National Survey 2001-02

The overall prevalence of blindness as per NPCB definition (presenting vision <6/60 in the better eye) is 8.5%. High prevalence was observed in Gulbarga, Rajnanadgaon, Bharatpur, Prakasam and Dhankanal (more than 10%).

Following criteria have been used to categorize a person having social and economic blindness[5] (Table 13.31):

The prevalence of *social blindness* in this age group (vision <3/60 in the better eye, which corresponds to the WHO definition of blindness) is around 5.3%. The inability to count fingers at a distance of 3 meters (with the better eye) with best correction is used to define social blindness. Since this level of visual impairment curtails the day-to-day movement of an individual and prevents social interaction with family and peer groups it is also referred as WALK VISION. There are wide inter-district variations in the prevalence of both social and economic blindness.

The overall prevalence of *economic blindness* is 3.2% (one eye <6/60–3/60, fellow eye <6/60 NPL).[5] Since this level

Table 13.31: Classification of blindness under the NPCB	
Near normal (NN)	One eye >=6/18; fellow eye >=6/60
Low vision (LV)	One eye <6/18–6/60; fellow eye <6/18–NPL
Unilateral blind (UL)	One eye <6/60; fellow eye =>6/18
Economic blind (EB)	One eye <6/60–3/60; fellow eye <6/60–NPL
Social blind (SB)	Both eyes <3/60–NPL
Bilateral blind	Both eyes <6/60–NPL

NPL (No perception to light)

of vision prevents a person from earning his wages, it is also referred to as WORK VISION (presenting vision <6/60).

Sex

Females have higher prevalence of both social and economic blindness as well as low vision as compared to males. This is because of more exposure of females to indoor air pollution.

Urban Rural Distribution

Urban areas have low prevalence of economic and social blindness as compared to rural areas. Prevalence is higher in poor and illiterate.

Age

Prevalence of blindness of all types increases with advancing age.

Literacy

Persons educated beyond high school have lower prevalence of blindness as compared to illiterate.

Cataract Surgery

Blindness is a big social problem in India, besides being an economic problem. Restoration of sight increases self-reliance and increases longevity and productiveness. In view of the high prevalence of blindness in India and its social relevance, the Government of India initiated Blindness Control Programme in India in 1976.

NATIONAL PROGRAMME FOR CONTROL OF BLINDNESS (NPCB)

National Programme for Control of Blindness (NPCB) was launched in the year 1976 as a 100% centrally sponsored scheme. The control of blindness was accorded high priority and included in the Prime Minister's 20-point programme; emphasis on camp approach was one of the highlight of this programme.

Problem: High prevalence of blindness in India 1.38–1.49% in 1974 and 1986 respectively and in 2001–2002 it declined to 1.12% and it further declined to the level of 1.0% in 2006–2007.

Goal: The goal of blindness control programme was to reduce the prevalence of blindness from 1.4% (1974) to 0.3% by 2020 AD. The goal has not been achieved, as level of blindness in the country is 1.0% as per prevalence survey of 2006–2007.

Target for 10th Five-Year Plan and beyond: To reduce the prevalence of blindness to 0.8% by 2007 and to reduce this further 0.5% by 2010[10] and 0.3% by 2020.

Objective of NPCB

The objectives of the programme are:

- To reduce the backlog of avoidable blindness through identification and treatment of curable blinds at primary, secondary and tertiary levels.
- "Eye Health for All" and prevention of visual impairment through provision of comprehensive universal quality eye care services.
- Strengthen and upgradation of regional institutes of ophthalmology (RIO) to centres of excellence.
- To develop additional human resources for providing high quality comprehensive eye care in all districts of the country.
- To improve quality of service delivery.
- To secure participation of voluntary organizations, and private practitioners in delivering eye care and to enhance community awareness on eye care and lay stress on preventive measures.
- Control of corneal blindness including establishment of eye banks.
- Increase and expand research for prevention of blindness and visual impairment.

Reduction of Backlog of Curable Blindness

By two approaches: *Eye camps* and *fixed facility* for *eye surgery*.

Implementation of Programme

National Programme for Control of Blindness (NPCB) was launched in the year 1976 as 100% centrally sponsored programme. The activities under this programme included upgradation of Medical Colleges and District Hospitals, development of mobile eye units, recruitment of required ophthalmic manpower and provision of various ophthalmic services.

Eye Camps (Reach Out Strategy)

Eye camp approach has been used to cover inaccessible rural, tribal and difficult areas. Mobile eye clinics were added in various states to augment eye care services primarily to focus on cataract surgery. Eye camps have been very popular and India has longest and largest experience of eye camps. Eye camps were organized by voluntary agencies in a big way. Lions clubs, Rotary clubs and many Non-Government Organizations (NGOs) organized eye camps to cover the backlog of cataract surgery. Support of NGOs, voluntary organizations and private practitioners has been significant as over 80% of backlog was covered by these agencies and Government sector could reach only to 20% of needy blinds. Blindness programme has achieved strong public–private partnership. All the voluntary agencies and NGOs were provided funds by the Government at fixed rate of ₹ 150 per case.

Camp surgery has its limitation, over the years, it served the compelling needs and trend has now shifted to fixed centre approach. Dependence on eye camps has now been reduced except in remote and tribal areas.

Fixed Centres (Reach in Strategy)

The Government has given substantial financial help to upgrade the eye services at the district, sub-district and medical college hospitals, besides hospitals of non-Governmental organizations. The country is now self sufficient to tackle the problem of blindness.

A national survey was conducted in 1986–89 to evaluate the programme, which revealed a prevalence rate of 1.49%, hence there was no decline and prevalence levels remained unaltered from 1976 to 1989.[5] Revised strategy was evolved but still progress of the programme was very slow. In 1994, World Bank assistance for NPCB was obtained for states (Andhra Pradesh, MP, Maharashtra, Odisha, Rajasthan, Tamil Nadu, Uttar Pradesh and J & K), which performed poorly.

DISTRICT BLINDNESS CONTROL PROGRAMME (DBCP)

DBCP was revamped in 1994 to give it a new push. District blindness control societies (DBCS) were established in each district and funds were directly provided to DBCS by the central Government. Since the launch of national rural health mission (NRHM) DBCS have merged with district health mission.

The main objectives of DBCP are:

1. To achieve the goal of 0.3% level of prevalence of blindness.
2. To achieve excellence in eye care services resting on high quality patient care.

The primary purpose of DBCS is to plan, implement and monitor all the blindness control activities in the district under the overall guidance of the state/central organization for the NPCB.

Composition of DBCS

District collector/magistrate is the chairman of the DBCS and the chief medical officer is the vice chairman. District programme manager is the coordinator and member secretary and chief ophthalmic surgeon or head of ophthalmology of medical college is the technical advisor. The medical superintendent, district education officer, project director DRDA, ophthalmic surgeon of mobile eye unit, president indian medical association and 3 representatives of NGOs, district mass media officer and practising ophthalmic surgeons are the members. There should be at least one women and one SC/ST member in the DBCS. The membership of non-officials should be for one year only.[11]

Expenditure

The total expenditure on drugs and consumables should not exceed ₹150 × number of cataract operations performed in the Government sector. Standard lists of consumables have been evolved.

Key Functions of DBCS

1. To assess the magnitude and spread of blindness in the district by means of active case finding village-wise to be recorded and maintained in blindness registers.
2. To review periodically and monitor the implementation of the district action plan.
3. To prepare a list of voluntary agencies and private hospitals/practitioners and actively involve them in the programme. DBCS should coordinate activities of the Government, non-Governmental and private sectors in the field of eye care in the district.
4. To motivate people to pledge their eyes for donation by utilizing all available media.

Microplanning at District Level

Each district should evolve a microplanning for preparing a district action plan through resource mapping by following steps.[11–14]

Line listing of blind persons by active screening (50+ years) in each village of the district. Screening can be done by trained health staff, involvement of NGOs, Panchayat and volunteers (after one day training). This would lead to village-wise registers of blind persons.

Mapping of eye care infrastructure: By plotting all fixed facilities and eye surgeons in Government, voluntary and private sector available within the district to know available trained manpower in the district to undertake cataract surgery (ICCE or IOL).

Allocate targets: Each eye surgeon should be given 700 cataract operations per year.

Considering the objective of clearing the backlog of cataract blind persons now the minimum target is to achieve 400 cataract surgeries per 100,000 populations per year.

Technical targets: It is expected that minimum of 30% of operations should be performed by IOL surgery and 70% of the total by conventional surgery but this will depend on demand of the clients.

Social targets: As there is higher prevalence of cataract amongst women, it is expected that more than 50% of all operations shall be for women.

Social class: On the basis of census population percentages of operations performed on SC/ST and minorities should match with the proportion of these population groups. In fact there is an evidence that prevalence of blindness is higher in such classes.

Economic criteria: As defined by DRDA percentages of people living below poverty line should invariably be covered with free cataract surgery. There is an evidence to show that the prevalence is higher in such classes and programme must reach poorest people.

It is advisable to have equitable distribution of services to each community development block and each primary health centre. Assign targets to each PHC and each block.

Targets by eye care facilities: Various norms have been fixed on the basis of eye beds, eye surgeons. These are minimum norms and efforts should be made to enhance the output. Operation per surgeon per year 700, operations per bed per year 50 operations.

Emphasis is on quality of eye surgery. Better options are using operation theatres constructed and maintained as per specifications to avoid infections and postoperative complications. Therefore, the current trend of conducting surgeries in camp conditions has been reversed. Now most surgeries are performed in hospitals. Camps should only be held if it is must or area is difficult. Camps should have conditions for safe surgery.

Reach in strategy: It is suggested that 75–80% of total target must be achieved through institutions and hospitals to ensure quality of service. Patient should be referred to identified hospital as per geographical access. *Reach out strategy* (camps) should be meant for remote and inaccessible or difficult areas without compromising quality aspect.

Major Performance Indicators

Against the target of 6 to 7 million per annum 5.8 to 6.3 million cataract operations have been performed per annum, thus achieving 90–96% of target from year 2009 to 2013. Over 5 to 7 lakh children in schools have been provided free spectacles per year against the target of 9 lakh.

Achievements

Percentage of cataract surgeries where IOL was implanted increased from 20% in 1997–98 and to 95% in 2012–13. Minimum target for cataract surgery rate per lakh population was set at 400 per year. The states of Gujarat, Punjab, Tamil Nadu, Andhra Pradesh, Maharashtra, Delhi and UT of Pondicherry have attained the rate of 400 operations per lakh population. Bihar and Assam were the lowest performing states.

School Screening Programme for Refractive Errors

Around 6–7% of children aged 10–14 years have problems with their eyesight affecting their participation and learning at school. Children are first screened by teachers and later on confirmed by ophthalmic assistants. The teachers can use the 6/9 optotype ('E' card with "4E". The size of 'E' in the card is equal to 6/9 optotype of Snellen's chart) to categorize the normal and abnormal children. All children unable to pick up the 6/9 optotype with either eye are then referred to nearby PHC/CHC. School teachers are able to identify 80–90% of children with poor vision by this method. Corrective spectacles are prescribed or provided free of cost to the poor. School eye screening programme is very weak and is done in the absence of parents and mostly by ophthalmic assistants who are trained for eye work for one year after plus two and are posted at community health centre.[14]

Development of Infrastructure

Construction of eye wards, operation theatres, dark rooms was undertaken during the 9th plan in the states covered under the World Bank assisted Cataract Control Blindness Project to enhance capacity of eye care in public sector. State-of-the-art equipment were also provided under the project.

Training

Since 1996–97, training of eye surgeons in IOL surgery was taken up. 100 faculty members of medical colleges were trained as trainers. This was followed by training of district eye surgeons in IOL surgery. So far, 1525 eye surgeons have been trained in the country. Training of nurses, ophthalmic assistants and teachers is also supported.

IEC Activities

Special campaigns for mass awareness were undertaken during eye donation fortnight and World Sight Day (2nd Thursday of October). IEC material and training manuals are produced centrally and disseminated to the states. Currently 5–7 Lakh donated eyes are collected per annum in India. Eye banks have been established and hospital retrieval programme is the main strategy for collection of donated eyes, which envisages motivation of relatives of patients and accident victims.

Support to Voluntary Organizations

Since voluntary organizations play key role in NPCB, the DBCS were established all over the country. Till date 575 DBCS have been set-up. Decentralized mechanism is working through DBCS. Many of the eye units with NGOs have been upgraded besides establishing eye banks.

Sentinel Surveillance Units (SSUs)

25 SSUs have been established under NPCB in various medical colleges with the objective to study the cataract outcome by review of cataract surgical records (CSRs) and to conduct survey and monitor the pattern of eye morbidity in the hospital and in the community. These units have generated useful information, which has been fed back to NPCB for improving the quality of services.

Vision 2020: The Right to Sight[15]

- "***Vision 2020:*** The Right to Sight" is a global initiative launched by the World Health Organization and a task force of International Non-Governmental organizations to combat the gigantic problem of blindness in the world. It was launched in the year 1999.

- ***The right to sight initiative:*** A global initiative has been launched to control avoidable (preventable plus curable) blindness by the year 2020. India is committed to this initiative. Plan of action for the country has been developed in line with Global initiative with following main features:
- ***Target diseases:*** Cataract, refractive errors, childhood blindness, corneal blindness, glaucoma, diabetic retinopathy and trachoma to combat blindness.
- ***Human resource development:*** Augmenting middle level ophthalmic personnel and increasing the capacity and skills of available human resource in various areas of ophthalmology besides development of professional eye care managers, etc. One eye surgeon for every 5 CHCs has been proposed under NRHM.
- ***Infrastructure development:*** Proposed four-tier structure includes centre of excellence (20), training centres (200), service centres (2000) and vision centres (20,000).

Target in 10th Plan and Beyond

- Increase cataract surgery rate to 450 operations per lakh population with a view to clear the backlog.
- Improvement in visual outcome of cataract surgery by performing IOL implantation in >80% by 2007.
- Development of 50 paediatric ophthalmology units.
- Facilities for early diagnosis of glaucoma and diabetic retinopathy and screening of all 35 years and above for glaucoma.
- Setting-up of 20,000 vision centres in rural areas.
- Developing 25 fully functional eye banks.
- Training of personnel and supply of equipment and grants in aids to NGO.
- To reduce prevalence of blindness to 0.8%.

Trachoma Elimination by 2020—Global Trachoma Mapping Project has been Initiated in 29 Countries

An estimated 146 million people have the active infection with the microorganism *Chlamydia trachomatis*, for which antibiotic treatment is indicated. There are approximately 10.6 million adults with in-turned eye lashes (trichiasis/entropion) for which eyelid surgery is needed to prevent blindness. An estimated 5.9 million adults are blind from corneal scarring due to trachoma. Trachoma is a second most common cause of blindness in sub-Saharan Africa, China and Middle-Eastern countries. Trachoma is to be controlled through implementation of **SAFE** strategy integrated into primary health care.

S: Surgery by trained paramedical staff for trichiasis.

A: Antibiotic treatment (either tetracycline eye ointment or oral azithromycin) for children with active disease.

F: Facial cleanliness promotion—to reduce transmission.

E: Environmental improvement, including personal hygiene: To increase access to clean water and improved sanitation as part of primary health care.

Refractive Errors

In India, this is the second most common cause of blindness.

The provision of refractive services and low vision care for patient by:

1. ***Screening:*** Identification of individuals with poor vision which can be improved by spectacles or other special devices.
2. ***Refraction:*** Evaluation of the patient to determine what spectacles or device may be required.

Vitamin A prophylaxis programme is there to prevent blindness due to vitamin A deficiency. Mega dose of vitamin A given to children between 9 months and 5 years of age has reduced the blindness due to vitamin A to a significant extent. Similarly, immunization against measles prevents blindness. Ophthalmia neonatorum is preventable.[16]

New Initiatives During 12th Five-Year Plan

- Provision of setting up of 400 multipurpose district mobile ophthalmic units.
- Provision for distribution of 10 lakh spectacles at ₹ 100 per spectacle to old persons suffering from presbyopia.

REFERENCES

1. NPCB. World Bank assisted cataract blindness control project. Cataract blindness and surgical outcomes survey. Bharatpur, Rajasthan. New Delhi: AIIMS; 1999.
2. Planning Commission. Ninth Five-Year Plan 1997–2002, Volume II. Thematic issues and sectoral programmes. New Delhi: GOI; 1997.
3. WHO. Management of cataract in primary health care services. Geneva: WHO; 1990.
4. GOI. Present status of national programme for control of blindness (NPCB). New Delhi: Ophthalmology section DGHS, MOH and FW, GOI; 1993.
5. GOI. National Survey on blindness 2001–02. NPCB Quarterly Newsletter 2002; 1(2).
6. GOI. Annual Report 2003–04. New Delhi: MOH and FW GOI; 2004.
7. All India Ophthalmological Society. Vision 2020—the right to sight. CME Series; 9.
8. Planning Commission. National Population Policy 2000. New Delhi: GOI; 2000.
9. ICMR. District Nutrition Project. Report of ICMR Task Force, 2001.

10 Planning Commission. Tenth Five-Year Plan 2002–07, Vol II. Sectoral policies and programmes. New Delhi: GOI; 2002.

11 GOI. National programme for control of blindness highlights. Guidelines for district blindness control society. New Delhi: Ophthalmology division DGHS, MOH and FW; 1994.

12 GOI. A manual for Medical officers. Community Ophthalmology Practice at Primary care level. DGHS, MOH and FW, Government of India; October 2004.

13 GOI. National Programme for control of Blindness in India DGHS, MOH and FW, GOI; October 2004.

14 GOI. GVS Murthy, Sanjeev K Gupta, Damodar Bachani. The principles and Practice of Community Opthalmology National Programme for Control of Blindness, GOI. New Delhi, 2002.

15 GOI. National Programme for Control of Blindness in India. The right to sight plan of action DGHS, MOH and FW, GOI; New Delhi.

16 Comm. Ophthal. Unit and ORBIS India. Community based intervention for control of childhood blindness and visual impairment. A manual for district level Ophthalmologist, New Delhi, 2007.

CANCERS AND TOBACCO CONTROL

Demographic transition in India has resulted in rise in life expectancy. During the year 2013, the life expectancy in India was 66 years (RGI): The proportion of aged above 60 years has risen from 7.4% in 2001 to 9% by 2016.[1]

Non-communicable diseases are bound to rise in India because of change in lifestyles and longevity. Cancer is one of the non-communicable disease, will emerge as a leading morbidity (disease) in the future. Right now, India has one of the lowest rates of cancer in the World.[2]

Problem of Cancer in India

Cancer is an important public health problem in India. It is estimated that disease burden due to cancer is around 2–2.5 million cases in India. On an estimate 7,00,000–9,00,000 new cases are being detected every year. Over 9.8 lakh new cancer cases were detected in 2010. Of these, two-thirds of the cases are detected in advanced stages when the chances of cure are minimal. Around 40% of cancer cases in the country are related to tobacco use. Around 5,56,400 cancer patients die every year.[3] (Million death study 2010.) Tobacco related cancers represented 42% of male and 18.3% of female cancer deaths among 30–69 years.

Hopes

Around 40% of all cancers in India are *preventable*. These cancers are attributable to tobacco consumption by chewing and smoking. If tobacco consumption is totally stopped, 40% of cancer load can be reduced.[4,5] It is a question of changing lifestyle or behaviour through effective education and communication. Nearly 30% of cancers in India are *curable* by early detection and prompt treatment or intervention. Early detection of cervical cancers, breast cancer and oral cancer offers a good chance of cure. Thus, with modern technological advances, cancers can be detected at an early stage and high cure rate can be achieved. Common man perceives cancers as sure way to death and all hopes lost but scientific evidence suggests that 30% of cancers are *curable*, 40% are *preventable* and rest of 30% of cancers are left for palliative care which are in advanced stages needing effective pain relief measures.

Patients with all sort of chronic diseases thought to be 'cancers' by majority of people of district Bathinda and adjoining areas (in Punjab) board Bikaner Express train popularly known as "cancer express train" by local people for treatment of their illnesses at Bikaner medical college and return by the same train next day. This practice is prevalent since long.

Early Detection and Prompt Treatment of Cancer at Stage I or State A and 5-Year Survival in Common Cancers

Cancer of breast	75%
Cancer of cervix	90%
Cancer of vocal cords	90%
Cancer of rectum	85%

Common Cancers in India

The most common cancer in India or *Indian cancer* is oral cancers (oral cavity, pharynx, tongue and lips) attributable to tobacco consumption.[3,6,7]

Cervical cancer is the commonest cancer among females followed by breast cancer. These two cancers account for 38 to 52% of cancers in females (Table 13.32).[5]

An Atlas of Cancer in India

ICMR has prepared Atlas of cancer in India which maps the cancer in India—highlighting that mouth, tongue, pharynx and nasopharynx cancers are the world's highest cancers in India related to tobacco (Fig. 13.5).[8]

Since National Cancer Registry Programme data emanates from selected urban areas and only one rural registry that covers part of one district, it would be difficult to provide valid estimates of burden of cancer in the entire country, where over 69% of population lives in rural areas.

Incidence Rate

On an average, about one in 15 men or one in about 12 women in the urban areas could develop cancer in their

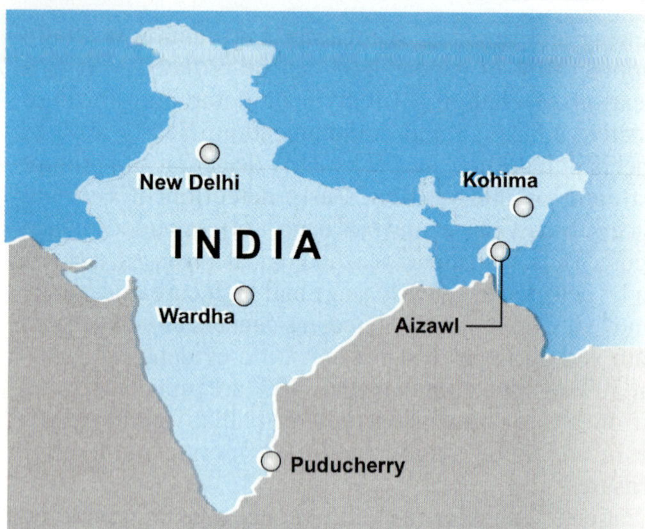

Fig. 13.5: An atlas of cancer. Aizawl has world's highest incidence of lower pharyngeal and tongue cancers in men. New Delhi has world's highest incidence of gallbladder cancer in women. Wardha has world's highest incidence of mouth cancer. Puducherry has among the world's highest incidence of mouth and tongue cancers among men. Kohima has one of the world's highest incidence of nasopharyngeal cancer

life time. Estimated number of new cancers diagnosed in India every year are between 7,00,000 and 9,00,000 (Table 13.32). Cancer incidence rate is generally expressed as age adjusted or age standardized (according to world standard population) incidence rate per 1,00,000 persons. For all anatomical sites, the rate varies from 97.8 (in Bangalore) to 121.9 (in Bhopal) in urban males. In urban females, the rate varies from 92.2 (in Bhopal) to 135.3 (in Delhi). Incidence rate in rural registry of Barshi is lower (46.2 and 57.7 per 1,00,000 in males and females respectively). The urban incidence rates are similar in Indians in Singapore (105.5 and 122.7 per 1,00,000 males and females respectively) but lower than the rates observed in the registries of developed countries in the west and Oceania or Japan.

Table 13.32: Estimated incidence of cancer in India, 2001

Types	Males		Females
Lips and oral cavity	39,000		31,000
Pharynx and larynx	53,000		14,000
Oesophagus	31,000		26,000
Stomach	35,000		16,000
Trachea, bronchus and lungs	34,000		7000
Breast	–		80,000
Cervix uteri	–		1,00,000
Others	2,01,000		1,39,000
Total	**3,93,000**	+	**4,13,000 = 8,06,000**
Projected in 2020	**6,22,203**	+	**6,98,725 = 13,20,928**

Cancer incidence can also be expressed as crude rates, age adjusted rate and truncated rate. Crude incidence rate is the total number of new cancer cases in a particular year per 1,00,000 population in the defined geographical area. Crude rates represent the actual burden of illness in the country and changes in it over time. In the urban registries, this varies from 72.1 per 1,00,000 (in Bhopal) to 107.6 (in Chennai) among males, and 77.5 (in Bhopal) to 117.6 (in Chennai) among female in 2009–11. Highest crude rate of 168.2 was observed in Aizwal district.

Truncated age adjusted incidence rate (TR): This is similar to age adjusted rate except that it is calculated for the truncated age group 35–64 years of age. Over 60% of cancers occur in this age bracket.

Leading Sites of Cancer in India

Tobacco-related Cancers (TRCs)

Sites of cancer that have been associated with use of tobacco (tobacco-related cancers—TRCs) include oral cavity, pharynx (including oropharynx and hypopharynx, oesophagus, larynx, lung and urinary bladder).

Overall, among males, cancer of sites associated with use of tobacco are the most frequent. Cancer of the lung is numerically the number one cancer. It is the leading site in Delhi, Mumbai and Bhopal, wherein it constituted around 10% of cancer of all sites. It is the second and third leading site among males in Bengaluru and Chennai, respectively.

Based on currently available data, in registries in all continents, males in Bhopal have the highest age adjusted incidence rate (8.8 per 1,00,000) of cancer of tongue. Similarly, the rates of cancer of the oral cavity in both males and females in all urban registries are among the highest in the World.

The total proportion of TRCs relative to all sites in males varies from 35.6% in Bengaluru to 50% in Bhopal, whereas in females Bengaluru has the highest proportion of TRCs (17.3%). In males among the TRC sites, pharynx and lung are the common sites and in females oesophagus and oral cavity are the commoner sites. These two sites together account for 80% of all TRCs in females.[3,8]

In women, cancers of the cervix and breast together account for over 40% of cancers in urban women and over 65% of cancers in the rural registry in Barshi. The age adjusted incidence rate (8.9 per 1,00,000) of cancers of the gallbladder in Delhi, women is one of the highest in the world. The reasons are being investigated and most probable reasons are **obesity,** and excess of fats in diet and consumption of **Junk foods.**

Though India has one of the lowest rates of cancers in the world, the current projection suggest that the total cancer burden in India for all sites will double by 2026 because of increasing longevity, greater exposure to environmental carcinogens due to industrialization, use of fossil fuels, the use of wide variety of chemical agents in industry and agriculture and the continued use of tobacco.[9]

- The most frequent cancers among Indian males are those of mouth/oropharynx, oesophagus, stomach and lower respiratory tract. In women, cancers of cervix, breast, mouth/oropharynx and oesophagus are common.
- Tobacco-related cancers (especially cancer of oral cavity, lung) and cancer cervix form more than 50% of the overall cancer burden in the country.

An increase in tobacco smoking instead of chewing might lead to rise in incidence of lung cancer, which is more difficult to detect and treat.

Causes and Risk Factors in Oral Cancer

The chief cause implicated in oral cancer is prolonged chewing of tobacco, zarda, pan and pan masala. In India and other parts of South East Asia, chewing of tobacco mixed with pan is believed to be the cause of high rate of mouth cancers. Heavy smoking and drinking, apart from poor oral hygiene and jagged teeth and ill fitting dentures have been incriminated for a continuous injuries and oral cancers. In some parts of India, teeth are cleansed with toothpastes containing tobacco. Thus, oral cancers are related to behaviour of smoking by adopting unhealthy lifestyle of chewing tobacco plus smoking and drinking. Human papillomavirus (HPV) is associated with >95% of cervical cancers which is second most common cancer in India.

Risk Factors in Cervical Cancers

There is strong etiological association between human papillomavirus (HPV) and cervical cancer. Persistent infection with oncogenic HPV is necessary cause for cervical cancer. Almost 7.9% of women in general population are estimated to harbour cervical human papillomavirus (HPV) at any given point in time, 82.5% of invasive cervical cancers are attributed to this virus. The four common oncogenic HPV types: HPV 16, 18, 31 and 45 are responsible for cervial cancer.

1. Early marriages, early childbirth and too many births.
2. Promiscuity in her or her partner and having multiple sex partners.
3. Poor hygienic practices.
4. Reproductive tract infection/sexually transmitted infections. HPV infection is one of the most common sexually transmitted infections.

Risk factors in *breast cancer* include unmarried women, delayed marriages, low fertility, obesity, high fat diet, lack of exercise, high oestrogenic status and family history of breast cancer. However, breastfeeding is protective against breast cancer. Breast cancer in urban females is on rise due to late marriages and obesity.

NATIONAL CANCER CONTROL PROGRAMME (NCCP) IN INDIA

The Cancer Control Programme was initiated in 1975–1976 as a central sector project. Based on the baseline information of cancer registries, it was modified and renamed as National Cancer Control Programme (NCCP) in 1985 and further revised in 2004. National Cancer Control Programme has been now integrated with diabetes, cardiovascular diseases and strokes in the year 2011. The objectives of NCCP were:

1. Primary prevention of tobacco-related cancers (TRCs), by health education through Government and non-Governmental organizations and legislation against tobacco.
2. Early detection and diagnosis of cancers especially oropharyngeal, cancer cervix, and breast cancers.
3. Developing and strengthening of existing cancer treatment facilities through regional cancer centres, medical and dental colleges.
4. Increasing access to palliative care in the terminal stage of cancer.
5. Training of manpower.[10]

Strategies

1. For Primary Prevention and Primordial Prevention, Focus is on Total Population or Targeting Most Vulnerables—School Children and Adolescents

These measures include **prevention of establishment of tobacco habits/culture (smoking, chewing and snuffing)** in the community. Educating young children in the family through role model of parents in the family and continuing the educational activities in preschool, school and college level. Tobacco free society should be aimed at. School teachers should become ideal role models in the schools. Similarly, mass media and child to child programme and school health programme can play effective part in health education. Celebration of no tobacco day on 31st May every year can reinforce the drive against tobacco use. Mass media and indigenous media apart from counselling in hospitals and clinics and interpersonal communication can help build mass movement against tobacco use.

The World Health Organization's (WHO) Tobacco Free Initiative (TFI) is being conducted from headquarters in Geneva and the regional and national offices around the world. There is now a WHO focal point on "Tobacco or Health" in all countries, and the TFI is supported by number of other international agencies such as UNICEF, the World Bank, IARC and UN Foundation.

Tobacco Control

"Tobacco is a killer, we need a broad alliance against tobacco, calling on a wide range of partners to halt the relentless increase in global tobacco consumption (pandemic of tobacco)". Dr. Gro Harlem Brundtland Director General, WHO, 1998. So far 12 World Conferences on "Tobacco or Health" have been held in different countries. 171 member states of the World Health Organization (WHO) have finalized a ground-breaking Public Health treaty to control tobacco supply and consumption. They agreed on a final text for a WHO Framework Convention on Tobacco Control (FCTC), governing—tobacco taxation, smoking prevention and treatment, illicit trade, advertising, sponsorship and promotion and product regulation.[11–13] It is a milestone in the history of global public health. India ranks second only to China to produce 7,01,000 metric tonnes of tobacco every year. In India, we have legislation: Smoking in public places and offices is banned to protect the health of non-smokers as also cessation of tobacco habits. Similarly, sale of cigarettes and bidis is banned on railway stations. We have legislation which bans tobacco advertising and health warning appears on each pack "Smoking is injurious to health". Basically, it requires adoption of healthy lifestyles. Indian Government passed a comprehensive Cigarettes and Other Tobacco Products Act (COTPA) in 2003. Parts of the Act have been enforced from May 1, 2004. These parts deal with a complete ban on advertisement of all tobacco products in all media, ban on smoking in public places and ban on sale of tobacco products to persons below the age of 18.[14–17]

Specific Protection

There is no specific protection against cancer, except hepatitis B vaccine (which prevents liver cancer), avoiding sunrays can prevent skin cancers and avoidance of carcinogens can prevent cancer. Similarly, human papillomavirus (HPV) vaccine is available against cervical cancer and cervical pre-cancers. Bivalent (HPV 16 and 18) and quadrivalent vaccines are available which are safe and effective but not yet introduced in the programme in India. Three doses of vaccine (0, 1 and 6 months) via intramuscular injection into deltoid area are given. The best immune response is observed in younger age groups (9–13 years) before the onset sexual debut. However, since all sexually active women continue to remain at risk of acquiring an HPV infection hence all women in 10–45 years can benefit from vaccination. Screening for cervical cancers should be continued in spite of HPV vaccination.

Encouraging green leafy vegetables, fruits and dietary fibre provide protection against cancers. Consumption of junk foods and harmful use of alcohol leads to **obesity**—a risk factor in cancer.

13

2. Early Detection Strategies

The objective is to detect pre-cancerous lesions. The secondary prevention is directed towards those persons who have been exposed to risk factors and have developed the pre-cancer and cancer lesions. Self-help is best help. People are being educated to suspect cancer themselves and report to the nearest facility of their own. Fortunately oral cancers, breast cancers and cervical cancers are easier to diagnose by visual examinations, speculum examination, and self-examination of breast. The people should be aware of warning signals like:

- Any lump or swelling in the body
- Persistent non-healing ulcer of more than 2 weeks
- A white or red raised patch in the mouth
- Restriction in mouth opening
- A lump or growth in the mouth
- Change in the size or texture of a wart or mole
- Excessive discharge or bleeding per vaginum
- Difficulty in chewing and swallowing or indigestion
- Any lump in the breast or elsewhere
- Unexpected weight loss
- Unusual bleeding or secretion
- Change in urinary or bowel habits
- Persistent jaundice + loss of weight
- Nagging cough or hoarseness of voice.

Self-examination of breast and oral cavity helps early reporting of cases. "3 minutes, three fingers once in 30 days" can help women to detect breast cancer herself. Early diagnosis measures include "Pap smear" test for precancerous lesions of cervix, mammography for breast cancer, X-rays, ultrasonography and CT scan for lung cancer and endoscopies plus FNAC for other sites besides study of markers of tumours.

The NCCP envisages Pap smear test for all women above 35 years of age at least once in 3 years. These facilities are available in most medical colleges. Oncology wing is fast developing in most medical colleges to encourage early detection of cancers besides developing outreach services and training of health workers in the districts and states. Papanicolaou (Pap) test is common in industrial countries, but attempt to replicate those efforts in developing countries have rarely been successful. Such programmes could, however, be made cost-effective by the use of simplified design that targets women over 35, screens only every 5 to 10 years and uses inexpensive outpatient treatment (such as freezing abnormal cells) for severe pre-cancerous conditions. When backed-up with good follow-up services such interventions are cost-effective.[14]

An alternate to Pap smear screening test—a combination of visual inspection with acetic acid (VIA) and lugol iodine (VILI) is acceptable in rural settings.

Pilot projects for early detection of cancers and raising the level of awareness in rural communities were launched in 2001–2002 and medical colleges undertook the activity in their field practice areas. Results of these limited experience was quite rewarding. Encouraged with these results, nationwide campaign on awareness generation on cancer was mounted in all the 543 parliamentary constituencies of the country in 2004 through camp mode wherein stalls on non-communicable diseases (NCDs): primarily cancer stalls were set-up as part of "Health Melas". These cancer stalls were funded by NCCP and each stall was authorised to spend ₹ 30,000. Varied kinds of activities (exhibition, distribution of educational material on cancers, video-films, CD on computer) of early detection and counselling on cancer were undertaken in all the districts.

3. Developing and Strengthening of Facilities for Early Detection and Treatment[18]

Regional cancer centres: The programme has provided funds to 27 regional cancer centres (RCCs). The RCCs are centres for diagnosis, treatment and follow-up of cancer patients. These centres undertake surveys on mortality and morbidity due to cancer, training of medical and paramedical personnel in cancer care and preventive measures with emphasis on health education and research. NCCP provides funds for the purchase of equipment (Cobalt unit, mammography unit) and for development of oncology wings in Government medical colleges/voluntary organizations.

It is envisaged that these centres would set-up cancer registry in their respective region by coordinating their efforts with the medical colleges and district hospitals and private nursing homes and practitioners in the area. An amount of ₹ 50 million one time grant is given to RCC. The 11th and 12th Five-Year Plan will establish new regional cancer centres and upgrade the existing RCCs.

District Cancer Control Programme (DCCP)

Under the health care delivery system, the district is unit for planning, organizing and implementation of health services. Under secondary prevention of NCCP, the Government of India has launched a district cancer control programme in which financial assistance is being provided for complete 5 years in the identified districts. The programme was launched in 1990–91. The district cancer centre aims at:

1 Promoting health education
2 Early detection of cancer
3 Pain relief and palliative treatment
4 Training of medical and paramedical personnels
5 Intersectoral coordination and monitoring of activities.

The district programme has been linked with respective regional cancer control centres (RCCs). District cancer society has been set-up in these districts for optimal functions and fund flow mechanisms.

Further each RCC has been involved to train paramedical/health workers of two districts in their region. These trained health workers will initiate early detection of cancer besides generating awareness on cancer in community. The progress in ongoing efforts for cancer prevention, early detection and management has been very slow in district cancer control programme.

India needs a rural community-based NCCP. Unless there is a good community oriented programme to detect early stage curable cancer cases and refer them promptly to such centres, these centres (RCC) will continue to provide less optimal services and care for the more advanced cancer cases at a terrible cost.

The homes and family could take responsibilities of developing healthy lifestyles in their off-springs, use of clean linen during menstruation, hygiene of cervix, right age of marriage as also limiting size of family and have only one faithful sexual partner and seek treatment of excessive vaginal and cervical discharges (treatment of STI/RTI). Women should be educated about self-examination of breast and similarly self-examination of oral cavity for early lesion and seeking consultation from nearby facility. Families and community have to be partners in prevention and early detection of cancers as also management of terminal stages of cancer (palliative care).

Cancer awareness if properly pursued could reverse the present trend of 20–25% cases being detected early as against 75–80% detected in advanced state.

National Cancer Registry Programme (NCRP)

The National Cancer Registry Programme was initiated by the ICMR in 1981–82 to generate information on cancer for better planning and evaluation of NCCP.[3]

Objectives

1 To generate data on cancer incidence and trends over a period of time or disease burden due to cancers.
2 To know geographical variation of cancer incidence in the country and the associated risk factors for effective control measures specific to a region.
3 To evaluate the effectiveness of cancer control strategies in the country.
4 Epidemiology and operational research activities can be based on evidence-based data generated through cancer registry.

Mechanism

A **Hospital-based registries** are located within identified hospitals. Under NCCP, these have been set-up at Dibrugarh, Thiruvananthapuram, Chennai, Mumbai, Bengaluru and Chandigarh. Hospital-based cancer registries (HBCR) have no denominator of population at risk. Incidence rate cannot be derived from such data. However, cancer extent, stages, therapy and survival rate information are more reliable from such data.

B **Population-based cancer registries:** Under the NCCP these registries have been set-up at Madras, Mumbai,

Delhi, Bengaluru, Bhopal, Ahmedabad and at one rural site at Barshi in Maharashtra.

It covers mainly urban population which is 12.8% and coverage of rural population is 0.06%. The total coverage of population is 3.3% only.

The fourteen population-based registries provide valuable epidemiological data on incidence of cancer in the population, crude incidence rate for all ages, age adjusted standardized incidence rates, annual age adjusted (world population) incidence rates, etc. Truncated incidence rate is age adjusted rate based on age specific rates in age group 35–64 and adjusted to world population. More than 60% of cancer cases in the registries are in this age group.

These registries (27 cancer registries) provide information on common cancers in India and geographical variation of occurrence of cancers and nature of cancers for effective control measures.[18]

Evaluation of National Cancer Control Programme

Monitoring and concurrent assessment of the activities of any programme are prerequisites for their successful implementation. In respect of the NCCP, the evaluation process would include an assessment of primary prevention, secondary prevention and cancer treatment.

a Assessment of primary prevention activities would include:
   - i Monitoring of tobacco habits.
   - ii Monitoring of tobacco consumption
   - iii Knowledge/attitude/practice (KAP) surveys
   - iv Reduction in incidence (particularly of tobacco-related cancers)
   - v Reduction in mortality (particularly of tobacco-related cancers)

b Assessment of secondary prevention (early detection) activities would include:
   - i Number of cases detected, the clinical stage and histological grade of the disease at the time of initial diagnosis and follow-up when relevant.
   - ii Reduction in incidence
   - iii Reduction in mortality.

c Assessment of treatment activities would include:
   - i Calculation of survival rates
   - ii Quality of life after treatment
   - iii Pain relief measures.

The above evaluation strategy would provide both short-term and long-term information, the former being a basis for mid-course alteration in strategies and the latter providing a base for assessing the impact of the programme as a whole.

Role of Medical Colleges

It is realized that regional cancer research and treatment centres alone would not be able to handle the entire load of cancer prevention, detection, diagnosis, treatment and rehabilitation.

The second line of attack on the cancer problem will be through medical colleges in country which handle considerable volume of cancer cases. Under NCCP, the goal is to provide radiotherapy and other minimum facilities for cancer treatment to all the medical colleges. These medical colleges will form an important link between the regional cancer centre on the one hand and the more peripheral health infrastructure (District Hospital, Taluka Hospital, CHC and Primary Health Centre) on the other hand.

Further *oncology wing* in each medical college would be developed which would provide services as envisaged above. Medical college would provide palliative care for all cancers and full range of services of diagnosis and management of cancers of the uterine cervix and oral cavity. Besides this, medical colleges would provide training in oncology to undergraduates, postgraduates as also to paramedicals apart from outreach services in their field practice areas on educating people on awareness building on cancer. Operational research and applied research activities in the field of cancer will also be undertaken by medical colleges. Similarly, dental colleges will also have an important role to play in cancer control programme of oral cavity and cessation of smoking. Dental colleges will be part of oncology wing of medical colleges.

4. Increasing Access to Palliative Care

Three goals of cancer control programme are prevention, early detection and diagnosis, and prompt treatment and the fourth goal is palliative care. Palliative care is "prevention and treatment of suffering". The focus here is quality of life. WHO defines palliative care as the "active total care of patients whose disease is not responsive to curative treatment".

There comes a time, despite our best efforts and all of modern advances in medicine, we have to admit that we have nothing more to offer to patients with advanced and terminal cancer to control their disease. These unfortunate individuals have lost their battle against cancer, but still living human beings broken in body, mind and soul. Where we send them to die? At home, in hospital or hospice! **Hospice** is specialized intensive care unit and has a trained team where each patient is special, right to the very end and hence best place for terminal care of cancer patients. Principles of palliative care include:

- Relieve the patient of pain and fear of pain.
- Management of other symptoms specific to the cancer.
- Management of psychological problems in a patient with cancer.
- Management of social problems and family problems.
- Management of spiritual problem.

This is a support system to help families cope during illness and death.[5]

Palliative care is being provided through the hospices in India (Shanti Avedna Ashram, Mumbai). Terminal care to cancer patients could be at home, hospital or hospice. When treating physician feels that no further active treatment of cancer is going to help to control the disease, he must shift over to palliative care, which is humanitarian service free of cost, relieving pain and agony and providing emotional support till the sufferer dies. Selfless care is provided away from hospitals at institutions called as hospices.

5. Training of Manpower

During the 10th Five-Year Plan, a major effort was made to sensitize and upgrade the skills of health care providers in the primary, secondary and tertiary institutions so that they could take the responsibility of:[2]

- Health education for cancer prevention
- Early diagnosis and management according to standard treatment protocols at appropriate institution
- Referral of cancer patients with complications
- 12th plan will further strengthen the training activities.

REFERENCES

1 GOI. National Population Policy 2000. New Delhi: MOH and FW, GOI; 2000.

2 Planning Commission. Tenth Five-Year Plan 2002–07. Sectoral policies and programmes. Vol. II, New Delhi: GOI; 2002.

3 ICMR. National cancer registry programme—an overview 1981–2001. New Delhi: ICMR; 2001.

4 ICMR. Cancer registry abstract. National cancer registry programme newsletter 2003 Oct; 10(1).

5 NIPHC. Cancer home care management, comprehensive cancer care—a total commitment. New Delhi: NIPHC Seminar; 1995.

6 Prakash H, Shah N. National oral health care programme implementation strategies. New Delhi: DGHS, MOH and FW; 2001.

7 GOI. Oral health training manual for health workers. National Oral health care programme. New Delhi: DGHS, MOH and FW; 2001.

8 ICMR: Development of an Atlas of Cancer in India. A project of the National Cancer Registry Programme. First all India Report 2001–2004, mapping patterns of cancer sponsored by WHO 2006.

9 ICMR. National cancer registry programme—consolidated report of population-based cancer registries 1990–96. New Delhi: ICMR; 1996.

10 GOI. National cancer control programme for India. New Delhi: DGHS, MOH and FW, July 1984.

11 WHO. Agreement reached on global framework for the tobacco control—major step forward for the health of people and nations. Geneva: WHO Press release 21; 2003.

12 NIPHC. Tobacco use health implications—statement of World Medical Association on health hazards of tobacco products. NIPHC Publication 1995; 5 (7):15.

13 Mackay J, Erikson M. The Tobacco Atlas. Geneva: WHO; 2002.

14 ICMR (2003). Estrogen Breast Cancer. ICMR Bulletin 33(2) Feb. 2003, New Delhi.

15 GOI (2003–04). Annual Report, MOH and FW, Government of India, New Delhi.

16 World Bank (1993). World Development Report Investing in Health World Development Indicators. Washington DC; USA.

17 WHO (2002). The World Health Report, reducing risks promoting healthy life, Geneva: WHO; 2002.

18 GOI. Annual Report 2009–10. Department and Health and Family welfare MOH and FW, New Delhi.

NATIONAL ORAL HEALTH PROGRAMME (NOHP) 2012–17

Problem (Oral Disease Burden)

The prevalence of oral diseases is very high to the tune of 90% at the age above 35 years. The major oral health problems in India are dental caries (decay), gum diseases (periodontitis), malocclusion and oral cancers.

1 ***Dental decay (dental caries):*** In India, dental caries has been consistently increasing in both prevalence and severity over the past five decades. This can be attributed to shift in dietary pattern towards more refined foods (fast-foods and junk foods) and poor oral hygiene. About 80% of children and 60% of adults suffer from dental caries. The prevalence of dental caries varies from 52 to 80% in India.[1] The average number of decayed, missing and filled teeth (DMFT) per child at the age of 16 is about 4 in rural areas and 5 in urban areas, with almost no dental restorative help available particularly in the rural and deprived areas.

2 ***Gum and periodontal diseases:*** These are most prevalent oral disease affecting almost 90% of the population and also most frequent cause of tooth loss. The main cause is plaque due to poor hygiene and lack of brushing. Initially it is painless, in the long-run it becomes chronic, self-destructive, leading to gradual tooth loss and mostly people accept it as the disease of old age. A large segment of adult population is toothless due to crippling nature of dental diseases.

3 ***Oral cancer:*** Oral cancer is the most common cancer in India, hence oral cancer is called Indian cancer; as

35–40% of all body cancers diagnosed are oral cancers. The major culprit is tobacco chewing and smoking. Oral cancer is preventable cancer.

4 ***Malocclusion:*** About 30% of children suffer from malalligned teeth and jaws affecting proper functioning of dentofacial apparatus and aesthetics.

5 Prevalence of *dental fluorosis* in children (at 12 and 15 years) is 6%.

Majority of population in the country lack knowledge about dental diseases and its relation to general health.

Over 80% of dentists are clustered in urban areas catering to 31% of population. About 69% population, which lives in rural areas has been neglected. There is no dental surgeon posted at the primary health centres (PHCs) in most of the states. There is acute shortage of manpower and equipment at community health centres (CHCs) and even at district level hospital.

Preventive and promotive oral health care is more relevant to rural areas, it will save economic burden.

Large number of dental problems: Dental caries, periodontal diseases, malocclusions and oral cancers are preventable by simple actions by the people themselves by adopting healthy lifestyles and practices right from early childhood period and to maintain these practices as part of life to enjoy sound status of oral health and better smile.

National Oral Health Programme (NOHP) was initiated in project mode in 1998 and department of dental surgery, AIIMS was chosen as nodal agency to implement it.

The aim of NOHP: To improve the oral health of the masses and to prevent/reduce burden of oral diseases in the country.

Long-term Goals[2]

- 50% of 5–6 year olds to be free of dental caries.
- To bring down the DMFT (decayed, missing and filled teeth) in school children (between 6 and 12 years) to less than 2.
- 85% should retain all their teeth up to the age of 18.
- Reduction of high prevalence of periodontal diseases to lower prevalence level of 40% from existing prevalence of 90%.
- To achieve 50% reduction in levels of edentulousness between the age of 35 and 44.
- To achieve 25% reduction in levels of edentulousness at the age of 65 and above.
- To achieve 50% reduction in the present level of malocclusion caused by oral habits in children.
- To reduce the number of new cases of oral cancers and precancerous lesions from the existing level of 9 per lakh.
- Finally to provide oral health care for all.
- To establish database monitoring system on oral health.

New Initiative

Government of India has taken a new initiative in 12th Five Year Plan to launch National Oral Health Programme in 200 districts (50 districts per year) with the following objectives:

- Improvement in the determinants of oral health, e.g. healthy diet and oral hygiene.
- Reduce disparity in oral health accessibility in rural and urban population.
- Reduce morbidity from oral diseases
- Strengthening of existing health care delivery system in India at primary and secondary level.
- Integrate oral health promotion and preventive services with general health care system and other sectors that influence oral health.

Strategies for Implementation

a Oral health education to masses through mass media and information, education and communication channels, for behaviour change communication.

Oral health education to school children and school dental health programme.

b Training of teachers, health staff, Anganwadi workers and dental surgeons on the strategies of oral health programme.

c To strengthen oral health services set-up at various levels (Human Resources).

d Logistical support.

e Comprehensive programme management.

f Monitoring and evaluation.

g Legislation against tobacco.

a. Oral Health Education

This is the major strategy under NOHP. This would cover:

- General population
- Targeted population of school children.

Approaches

i For general population to disseminate information/messages and action by people themselves on oral health through mass media like television, radio, print and folk media and through education material.

ii The information, education and communication material (IEC) on oral health have been produced by AIIMS and Central Health Education Bureau and distributed in an organized manner to masses through the system of health care (PHCs, CHCs and urban health set up). An education film on oral health "*Kirpaya Muskuraiye*" has been produced by nodal agency (AIIMS, New Delhi).

iii The school children have been specifically targeted for oral health promotion programmes like demonstration of regular brushing and rinsing techniques, regular dental check-ups and atraumatic restorative techniques for treatment, adequate diet and avoidance of cariogenic food (fast-foods or junk foods). In addition, chapters on oral health has been included in school textbooks of primary school children.

b. Training

General oral heath training to all the health care staff and special training to nodal officer on oral health programme. The short-term in-service training of teachers, health workers, health supervisors has been undertaken and the area assigned to them for launching of educational activities in schools and community and refer cases for further investigation and treatment. Anganwadi workers will inculcate brushing habits by involving parents in her Anganwadi set-up as part of non-formal preschool education activities. AIIMS has prepared oral health training manuals for teachers and health workers for their training and orientation.

The dental surgeons in the district were trained to impart training to health workers and teachers for organizing oral health activities in their respective areas.

c. Human Resources

Hire dental surgeons, dental hygienist and dental assistants on contract basis to supplement the efforts of State/UTs.

d. Logistical Support

One dental chair with supportive pieces of equipments and consumables.

e. Comprehensive Programme Management

At national, state and district oral health cells, and at periphery levels by coordination and linkages with various stakeholders.

f. Monitoring, Supervision and Evaluation

The NOHP shall be monitored at all the levels from district to the central level utilizing the existing Human Resource support of non-communicable diseases (NCDs) cell under the programme.

Strengthening Oral Health Services

Proposed Oral Health Services Set up

- One dental surgeon for PHC or 30,000 population.
- One dental surgeon for 50,000 school children.
- One health assistant/hygienist to cover population of 20,000.
- 3–4 mobile dental clinics for 4.5–5 lakh population.

1. At least one dental clinic for every 30,000 population in rural areas at the PHC level be established in a phased manner.
2. District and subdivisional level clinics should be strengthened in respect of dental manpower and dental equipment.
3. Existing dental clinics at various levels to be equipped with latest dental equipment and material as per established norms.
4. Local practitioners should be involved on contractual basis for imparting oral health education and to perform interceptive treatment like ART (atraumatic restorative treatment).
5. Every dental college/institution can adopt one district/rural centre/slum in their areas so as to provide the preventive oral (dental) health services to the community of the district by interns/ postgraduates under supervision of their teachers and should also impart oral health education and undertake interceptive and basic curative and emergency treatment for two months on rotational basis. The department of community dentistry should be strengthened to organize such activities.
6. Intensive dental health care programme for the school children need to be implemented. School teachers, medical and paramedical personnel, Anganwadi workers and opinion leaders of the community should be trained in giving oral health education. Post-graduate students of community dentistry should provide leadership to community health workers in initiating and implementing oral health care activities at the grass root level.
7. Intensive dental health care programme for the public in the form of free dental check ups and special oral health campaigns be organized frequently. Dental marathons, long marches, smiles and healthy teeth competitions should be organized.
8. Fully equipped dental clinics to provide on the spot diagnostic, preventive, interceptive and curative services to the people and school children in far-flung rural areas of the state be established.
9. In house training of dental doctors at Government dental colleges and other institutions recommended by the Ministry of Health should be provided to impart oral health education and to provide preventive, interceptive and curative treatment at the community level.

g. Legislation

Indian Government has passed a comprehensive Cigarettes and Other Tobacco Products Act (COTPA) in 2003, which has been discussed under tobacco control programme.

Strategies in Urban Areas

- Involving and reorienting dentists, teaching staff posted in the dental colleges, hospitals as well as private practitioners for 2 weeks refresher courses for primary prevention of oral diseases. This can be started after the training of dentists from various states for the implementation of the NOHP in the rural areas is completed.

- The dentists of school health schemes are operative in large number of urban areas; this could serve as good nucleus, after training, for services in urban areas.
- Motivation and involvement of school/college teachers of urban area.
- Involving voluntary organizations (Rotary and Lion Clubs, etc.).

WHO Strategy on Oral Health

WHO strategies and approaches for better Oral Health in 21st century focus on modifiable risk factors such as tobacco use, cariogenic diets (excessive use of sugar, fast and junk foods, carbonated drinks), abuse of alcohol, oral hygiene and use of Oral Health Services. The approach integrates oral health promotion with prevention and control programmes of non-communicable diseases in Primary Health Care.[3]

Reorientation of Dental Education in India

Community dentistry component in all of 305 dental colleges can be made more dynamic, active and viable. From the Planning Commission, special funds can be allocated to each dental college for adopting one district to implement oral health care programmes, but these programmes would have to be standardized, monitored, evaluated and accountable. Basic dental curriculum need to be preventive and community need-based.

Training of trainer is essential on oral health policy and 2 teachers from each dental college would be imparted training on strategies under National Oral Health Programme. These doctors would be responsible to organize reorientation programmes in their own colleges.

At the moment, the services for rural areas and urban slums are almost negligible. Community dentistry departments also do not exist in most of dental colleges. A few departments of community dentistry, which exist in the country, undertake minimum preventive programmes, which are not sustainable, and no impact is visible, as there is no continuity of service or programme. Over the years, evidence-based "information" on oral health has accumulated in the country but this is largely confined to dental clinics, hospitals, dental colleges/institutions, libraries, with dentists and a few schools. The challenge is to communicate the present knowledge and information to all schools, families, homes and community for appropriate actions. The information, which can promote/improve the oral health of millions of young children, school children, adolescent and youth, pregnant women and older people, is the information which must become available to all school children, families and communities for appropriate action. Therefore, the biggest challenge before us is to accept the challenge of communication of "facts on oral health" to all, in rural, tribal and remote areas. Nodal agency has imparted training but the status of implementation and monitoring reports indicating progress of action is wanted till now. Nevertheless, NOHP lays down firm foundations for future activities and it is a challenge for dentist community to accept and excel.[4] The 12th Five-Year Plan focuses on neglected area of oral health services as one of the thrust area. DCI has commissioned a nation wide survey on dental health manpower and pattern of diseases to help policy formulation.

Developing Surveillance System in Oral Health

The STEP wise approach developed by WHO can be followed to capture modifiable risk factors such as unhealthy lifestyles—use of tobacco, excessive intake of sugar, fast foods, oral hygiene practices and use of oral health services as also source of drinking water on regular basis for appropriate actions. These risk factors can be gathered by questionnaire method (Step 1).[5] Oral diseases were officially included in a recent United Nations Declaration (Sept 2011) in the list of non-communicable diseases.

NATIONAL PROGRAMME FOR PREVENTION AND CONTROL OF DEAFNESS

Hearing loss is most common sensory impairment in human today. World over it is second leading cause for years lived with disability (YLD) after depression; responsible for 24.9 million YLD globally.

In India, there are approximately 63 million people who are suffering from significant auditory impairment as per WHO estimates.

Problem in India

- NSSO estimated (2001) prevalence of severe to profound hearing loss of 291 per lakh of population.
- Estimated prevalence of hearing loss was 6.3% in Indian population as per WHO estimates (2003).
- The estimated burden of hearing loss in school going age group in India is 26.4 million at the prevalence level of 6.3%.

Over 50% causes of hearing impairment are *preventable* including hearing loss caused by infection of the ear (ASOM and CSOM), secretory otitis media, traumatic and Rubella deafness, noise-induced hearing loss and ototoxicity. Common causes of all degrees of hearing loss in India are given in Table 13.33.

Objectives

1. To *prevent* the avoidable hearing loss on account of disease or injury.

Table 13.33: Common causes of all degrees of hearing loss in India

Causes	*Prevalence %*
Ear-wax	15.9
Chronic suppurative otitis media (CSOM)	5.2
Serous otitis media	3.0
Dry perforation	0.5
Congenital deafness	0.2
Non-infectious and other unknown causes	10.3

2 Early identification, diagnosis and treatment of ear problems responsible for hearing loss and deafness.
3 To medically rehabilitate persons of all age groups suffering from deafness.
4 To strengthen intersectoral linkages for continuity and rehabilitation programme.
5 To develop institutional capacity for ear care services by providing equipment, material and training of personnels.
6 Creation of *district level data base* for the programme.
7 To facilitate *need-based research.*

Long-term Objective

To reduce the total deafness burden by 25% of existing burden by the end of 12th Five Year Plan.

Strategies

1 To strengthen the service delivery for ear care
2 To develop human resource for ear care services by training of grassroot workers.
3 To promote public awareness through appropriate and effective IEC strategies with special emphasis on prevention of deafness.
4 To develop institutional capacity of the district hospital, community health centres and primary health centres in respect of ENT/audiology infrastructure.

These strategies were piloted in 25 districts of 10 states and one UT to begin with. The programme is being implemented through existing primary health care delivery system with adequate referral support developed at district level. At present it covers 281 districts in 27 states and 3 UTs, 200 more districts are proposed to be covered in 12th Five-Year Plan.

Capacity of 83 district disability rehabilitation centres at district level will be utilized for speech therapy and rehabilitation.

As a part of strategy one audiometric assistant and one instructor/lecturer will be deployed in each district.

The levels of prevention of hearing loss would include:

***Primary prevention*:** This includes health education, immunization against measles, mumps and rubella, protection against noise and prevention of acute respiratory infections.

***Secondary prevention*:** Screening for early detection and prompt treatment, management of acute respiratory infection by standard treatment protocols besides surgical interventions.

***Tertiary prevention*:** Provision of hearing aids and rehabilitation (speech and hearing therapy)[6].

NATIONAL PROGRAMME FOR PREVENTION AND MANAGEMENT OF BURN INJURIES (NPPMBI)

"Burn" is a major public health problem all the world over. In India alone, every year around 7 million people suffer from burn injuries, out of which 7 lakh need hospitalization and 2.4 lakh become disabled. Approximately 1.4 lakh people die of burn injuries every year.

Objectives of the programme

i To reduce incidence, mortality and morbidity due to burn injuries.
ii To improve awareness among general masses and vulnerable groups especially the women, children, industrial and hazardous occupational workers.
iii To establish adequate infrastructural facilities for behaviour change communication, burn management and rehabilitation interventions.
iv To carry out research for assessing behavioural, social and other determinants of burn injuries for planning, monitoring and evaluation.

***Components*:** The programme consists of two major components, i.e. establishing dedicated burn units at 70 medical colleges and 25 burn wards at district hospitals. During 12th plan district hospital component will be implemented through NRHM division whereas; medical college component will be part of "Human resource in Health and Medical Eduction Scheme". Fund sharing between centre and states is 60:40.

The main components are

- Prevention programme (IEC)
- Treatment and rehabilitation
- Training
- Monitoring and evaluation
- Research.

NATIONAL ORGAN TRANSPLANT PROGRAMME (NOTP)

NOTP scheme has been approved in 12th Five-Year Plan for carrying out the activities as per transplantation of human organs and tissues Act.

OBJECTIVES

- The main objective of the programme is to organize a system of deceased organ and tissues procurement and distribution for transplantation.
- To promote deceased organ and tissue donation and prevent organ trafficking.

Components

Under the programme national organ and tissue transplant organization (NOTTO) we have:

- Component of National Networking.
- National Registery
- National biomaterial centre and facility of cadaver and tissue retrieval being set up at Safdarjung hospital. Similar networking system and tissue banks are proposed to be developed on regional basis at Mumbai, Chennai, Kolkata and Chandigarh.

REFERENCES

1 GOI. National Oral Health Survey and Fluoride Mapping 2002–2003. New Delhi: Dental Council of India, MOH and FW; 2004.

2 http://www.nophcaiims.org/primstrategies.htm Retrieved on 11/9/2003.

3 Peterson PE. The World Oral Health Report 2003: Continuous improvement of oral health in 21st century—the approach of the WHO Global Oral Health Programme. Community Dent Oral Epidemiol 2003; 31 (Suppl 1): 3–24.

4 Lal S, Paul D, Pankaj, Vikas, Vashisht BM. National Oral Health Care Programme. Implementation Strategies. Indian Journal of Community Medicine, 2004 Jan-Mar; 29(1): 3–10.

5 Peterson EP, Bourgeois D, Bratthall D, Ogawa H. Oral health information system—towards measuring progress in oral health promotion and disease prevention. Bulletin of World Health Organization 2005; 83: 686–93.

6 GOI. National Programme for Prevention and Control of Deafness. Resource material for use by primary Level Doctors. DGHS, MOH and FW, GOI, New Delhi 2007.

CHAPTER

14

Geriatrics—"Add Life to the Years"

World Health Day 7th April 2012 – Theme – "Ageing and Health"

"May the man live for a hundred years,
may he be a centenarian with
all senses intact till the end"
Yajurveda

According to Vedic and ancient Indian concept, the human life cycle has been divided into four 'Ashramas' each consisting of 25 years span, i.e.

1. **Brahmcharya:** The quarter ascribed to educational and religious training,
2. **Grihastha:** The quarter ascribed to worldly enjoyment and emotional fulfilment,
3. **Vanprastha:** The quarter assigned for preparing towards service of humanity at large, and
4. **Sanyasa:** Complete absolvement from individual or social responsibility as also dedicating one's remaining life towards spreading one's own experience.

The term "Greying of Nations", "Ageing of Nations" and demographic transition of "Pyramid to Pillar" are the concerns voiced all the world over.

Gerontology is the science, which studies the process of ageing and it describes physiological, biochemical and psychological changes during the process of ageing.

The word 'geriatrics' was coined by Nascher in 1914 and is derived from Greek words *gerus* and *iatrea*, which means old age and treatment respectively.

Butterworths Medical Dictionary has given the following definition: "of clinical study and treatment of old age and its manifestation". Geriatrics or geriatric medicine is now a well-recognized medical discipline in developed countries and also in India by Medical Council of India.

Senescence means process of ageing (Webster's Medical Dictionary). Due to all round socioeconomic development in India, the life expectancy has increased to 66 years (2012) from 37 years (1951). Thus, we have added 29 years to longevity of life and it is going to increase further in coming years.[1]

Demographic changes in India have resulted in change in structure of population, the population of 60 years and above which was 8.3% in the year, 2011has risen to 9% by the year 2016. In absolute number, the population of persons above 60 years was around 100 million in 2011, will rise to nearly 198 million by 2030 and 326 million by 2050.[1, 2]

What is Old Age?

What we understand by old age or aged person? The word "aged" is relative depending upon the society, its culture, the time and the prevalent conditions. For standardization, the United Nations have defined an aged person as one who is 60 years and above. Generally, people above the age of 60 years are considered as senior citizens in India. People between 60 and 74 years are categorized as "young old" between 75 and 84 as "middle old" and people above the age of 85 are classified as "oldest old" or infirm. There is marked difference in the health needs of these age groups.[3]

Distribution

Nearly 69% of elderly live in *rural areas* and half of these are below poverty line. The remaining 31% of elderly live in *urban areas*. Further, about 90% of old persons in India are from *unorganized sector*, which means they do not have regular source of income.[3] Elderly population of unorganized sector includes large industrial workforce, labour force, the agriculture labour and the daily wage earners, etc. with no benefit from their employers or from the government. About 13% of elderly belong to *organized sector* who have access to some distinct benefits like service pensions and health care facilities in the shape of CGHS, etc. these are the elderly who have retired as defence services personnel, the central and state government employees, others from corporate sectors, etc.

Thus, the elderly people belong to several categories like-rural, urban, elderly women, single elderly, the healthy, the sick and differently abled, distressed and disadvantaged elderly, the poor, middle class and the elite elderly.

The implication of ageing population is—to earmark lot of budget to deal with their needs and problems. It also adds on to dependent population in India.

1 40% of older people live below poverty line and another 33% are just marginally over it.[4]
2 69% live in rural areas.
3 73% are illiterate and can only be engaged in physical labour.
4 55% of 60+ women are widows many of them with no support whatsoever.
5 There were 1,50,000 centenarians in India in 1991 and increased to nearly 6,05,449 by 2011.
6 Old age dependency ratio in 1991 was 118 and it rose to 131 per 1000 in the year 2001 and during 2004 it was 119.[5]
7 Female sex ratio of old persons as per census 2001 was 1029 and NSS 2004 reported 999.

Problems of Elderly[6]

Ageing in humans refers to multidimensional process of physical, psychological and social change in a person over time. Some dimensions of ageing grow and expand over time, while others decline. Reaction time, for example may slow down with age, while knowledge of world events and wisdom expand. Research shows that even in late life, potential exists for physical, mental and social growth and development.

Ageing is a biological process and not a disease or curse, and during the biological process significant changes occur in human body. However, ageing is inevitable, irreversible and progressive. Prevention of disability and loneliness can help elderly to live happy and longer life.

There are 4 basic problems:

1 Multiple illnesses, multiple therapy and iatrogenic diseases.
2 Diminished vision, hearing, mobility and activity.
3 Social isolation, and underemployment.
4 Psychological (mental stress, loneliness, and depression).

Tata Institute of Social Sciences carried out a survey in 1972 to capture the problems of the elderly:

Financial	40.88%
Lack of occupation	27.35%
Health	10.29%
Family and future worries	10.28%
Dependence and isolation	7.06%
Accommodation (housing)	3.25%

14

National Surveys in India

In 1986 87 (NSS 42nd round), countrywide health survey was conducted by the NSSO on individuals aged 60 years and above. The main objective was to study the socioeconomic status of the elderly. Fifty thousand households in 8312 villages and 4546 urban blocks were surveyed. 39.5 million rural and 8.74 million urban population was covered.

Chronic illness was reported in 45% of males and 44.8% of females. Chronic illness included problems of the joints and other disabilities, heart diseases and blood pressure, cough, urinary problems and piles. The most common problems were problems in the joints (35–50%), followed by cough (22–35%). Hypertension; heart diseases and diabetes were reported more by the urban population. With increasing age, employment and economic independence declined in both men and women.

The available data on older persons indicate that half of the older persons above the age of 60 have one or the other ailment at any point of time. In rural settings in community-based study, 66% of aged person manifested one or the other ailment (Table 14.1).[7, 8] Report No 507 of 60th round of NSS survey in year 2004 estimated the state of self perceived health status of older people. As high as 55 to 63% of aged with sickness felt that they were in good or fair condition of health. The proportion among the aged without sickness was 77–78%. About 16–21% of the aged who were not even sick considered themselves as having a 'poor' state of health. Possibly they considered their sickness as a part of "usual/ normal ageing".

This observation has a lot of significance as self-perceived health status as an important indicator of health services utilization and compliance to treatment/interventions.

About 8% of the aged were either confined to their home or bed.[5,9] NSS results show that about 57% of the aged were living with their spouses, and another 32% were living without their spouses but with their children, while 4–5% were living with other relations. Nevertheless 4–5% were living alone. Of the economically dependent aged a majority—76–78% had to depend on their children and 13–15% on their spouses for economic support.

The *social* and *economic* problems of elderly people are much more than *medical/health problems*; hence the priority needs of the elderly people are other than health problems. In essence, the prime needs of elderly are emotional security and care, love and affection at family level besides *financial security*.[10]

The leading causes of mortality in aged persons are—heart diseases, cerebrovascular diseases and cancers. Alzheimer's disease is probably 4th leading cause of death chiefly affecting persons above 65 years of age.

Indicators of Old Age

Age is a state of mind. One is as old as one feels.

- **Physical signs:** Stooping, unsteady gait, cautious steps, wrinkles, loose skin, grey head, prominent temple vessels, tremors, edentulous and dementia.

Table 14.1: Community-based studies on problems of older persons[6,7] (Figures in percentages)

Problems	ICMR (rural areas) 1981–84 Age group 60+	NIPHC Rohtak (rural) 1997 Age group 65+	NIPHC (urban South Delhi) 1997 Age group 65+
Visual handicap	65	61	36
Pain in joints	34	53	47
Vague body pain	15	–	–
Giddiness	15	–	–
Cough (respiratory problems)	10	45	11
Sleeplessness	8	–	–
Hearing deficit	6	20	6
GI tract problems	–	8	36
Psychological	–	8	23
Heart problems	–	2	43
Neurological	–	1.65	3
Urinary	–	1.52	21
Diabetes	–	0.28	6

- **Physiological:** Ageing is a natural process in which cardiac reserve decreases, senile emphysema develops, respiratory functions diminish, arteries are thickened, resulting in reduced blood flow, nephrons and neurons are decreased, endocrines involute, defensive mechanisms get reduced. At times, the degenerative physiology may progress to pathological processes.

An old person is usually quiet, apathetic, insecure and depressed. The lack of confidence in near and dear ones may result in severe depression. Some may be euphoric, exuding confidence, are jolly, repetitive, boastful and even ambitious.

CARE OF ELDERLY PEOPLE

Self-care

Old age does not come suddenly it has long process. Healthy lifestyles established during childhood practiced during adolescence and youth age and continued in later life are helpful in delaying the ageing process and maintain quality of life. This is the predominant principle of active ageing advocated by WHO. The goal of care of elderly people is "add life to the years" and not merely the "years to life". Self-care addresses to adoption of healthy lifestyles by individual, family and the community, which are discussed under primordial prevention.[6–10]

Risk Factors for Older Persons

- Physical inactivity
- Obesity, smoking, harmful use of alcohol, drug abuse
- Diabetes mellitus
- Hypertension
- Cardiovascular diseases
- Visual impairment
- Hearing loss
- Accidents (falls and trauma)
- Breakdown of family support, death of spouse.

Primordial Prevention

It begins during childhood period, i.e. shaping healthy lifestyles during early years of life. Primordial prevention focuses on prevention of emergence and establishment of above mentioned risk factors by intervention of education and legislation measures.

WHO has promoted the concept of "*active ageing* makes the difference". Year 1999 was designated by United Nation as the International year of older person. The WHO has taken a worldwide lead in promoting active ageing by choosing the theme for WHO day as "Active Ageing Makes the Difference".[11,12]

The main concept of this principle of active ageing is to promote better health and well-being of older people.

Active ageing means "Elderly people continue to participate in social, economic, cultural, spiritual and civic affairs in addition to being physically active and have economic independence." Active ageing is linked to all phases of life cycle.

Information about 'healthy lifestyles' needs to be promoted to add quality of life to remaining years of life. Importance of balanced healthy diet, adequate exercise, avoidance of smoking and excessive alcohol consumption, avoiding stress by relaxation techniques is essential for active ageing. These principles of active ageing can help to maintain health and creativity throughout the lifespan and especially in the later years.

Lifestyle and Ageing (Table 14.2)[4]

The capacity of our biological systems (e.g. muscular strength, cardiac capacity) increases during the early years

Table 14.2: Action towards active ageing

Factors	*Individual action*	*Policy action*
Foetal environment	• Ensure balanced nutrition in girls and pregnant or lactating women • Avoid smoking during pregnancy	• Focus health promotion activities on girls and women • Increase awareness about importance of balanced nutrition for girls and women
Childhood environment	• Breastfeed babies for at least 6 months • Ensure balanced nutrition and adequate physical exercise for your children • Have your child immunized and observe good hand and food hygiene to prevent infection	• Promote breastfeeding, legislate against advertising for milk powder and baby foods in areas of malnutrition • Ensure access to immunization programmes • Improve sanitation and housing and reduce domestic overcrowding
Smoking	• Stop smoking—cessation is beneficial at any age • Educate your children about the ill effects of smoking	• Ban tobacco advertising • Ban sale of tobacco to children • Provide health education in schools and workplace
Alcohol	• Maintain moderate drinking limits • Seek professional help if you think you may drink excessively	• Ban sale of alcohol to children
Physical activity	• Exercise regularly from the earliest years through to older ages walking, climbing stairs, and housework are effective forms of exercise	• Incorporate exercise into school curricula • Create workplace, which provides exercise facilities • Encourage sports for seniors
Diet	• Consume a diet high in fibre and low in animal fat and salt • Reduce your weight if you are overweight and maintain normal body weight	• Increase consumer awareness about direct links between good nutrition and health
Adult diseases	• Make above listed lifestyle adjustments • Make use of available prevention programmes (screening and vaccination) • See your doctor at regular intervals	• Implement evaluated prevention programmes • Ensure access to safe maternity services • Provide accessible and affordable health care for all and reduce environmental threats
Social integration	• Stay involved in your family, your community, a club, or a religious organization • Be aware of and speak out against ageism • Continue to evaluate yourself and all your children	• Support activities that foster social cohesion • Provide access to lifelong learning • Promote solidarity among the generations
Gender	• Be aware of and speak out against gender discrimination and prejudice • Educate boys and girls to avoid gender stereotyping	• Implement legislation against gender discrimination in education, jobs, health care, property rights, marriage and inheritance laws • Promote health education on the dangers of high-risk lifestyles by targeting population groups that are particularly at risk • Integrate gender analysis in health research and health care programmes
Income security	• Be informed about public and private measures intended to protect income security over the life course	• Promote income security and access to appropriate health care for older persons • Fight age discrimination in the workplace

Source: Ageing exploding the Myths; WHO/HSC/AHE/99.1

of life, reaches its peak in early childhood and declines thereafter. How fast it declines, is largely determined by external factors relating to adult lifestyle, including smoking, alcohol consumption, diet and social class. The natural decline in cardiac function, for example, can be accelerated by smoking, leaving the individual with lower functional capacity than would normally be expected for his/her age. The gradient of decline may become so steep as to result in disability. However, the acceleration in decline caused by external factors may be reversible at any age. Smoking cessation and small increases in the level of physical fitness, reduces the risk of developing coronary heart disease in later life and it also reduces progression of disability. Many chronic diseases, which reduce functional capacity, are as a result of an unhealthy lifestyle.

Primary Prevention

Once the risk factors have been established and have appeared in population attempt is made to prevent development of chronic diseases in old persons by modification of risk factors.

Lifestyles

Lifestyles have become unhealthy in modern society. Tobacco, alcohol, and drug abuse, physical inactivity and faulty diets lead on to many lifestyle diseases. Healthy lifestyles like regular exercise and good diet improves health.

Tobacco

Tobacco cessation is beneficial at any age. Tobacco use and smoking should be discouraged at all costs, by education, by legislation and peer pressures and by controlling production, sale and consumption of tobacco. Smoking or tobacco consumption in any form contributes to diseases of lung, oral cavity, heart diseases, cancer and diseases of peripheral blood vessels. Over 60–80% of older people in Haryana and many other states (rural areas) continue smoking Hooka (Hubble-bubble) and it has become a socially acceptable behaviour which needs to be curbed by strong drives and self motivation or by providing alternate means of leisure in village Chaupal (community centre).

Alcohol

Alcohol is also injurious to health. Intake of alcohol should be restricted to 60 ml/day better to avoid it and switch over to vegetable soup drink/lime drink. Lonely, elderly and particularly well to do elderly indulge in excessive use of alcohol and they pay the heavy price of life.

Physical Inactivity

Physical inactivity brings in many diseases in elderly. Regular exercise keeps away many diseases. 'Move for health', keeps the elderly fit, improves their physical capacities and removes free radicals from the body, keeps elderly mobile, prevents osteoporosis, improves cardiorespiratory functions, controls BP and improves sense of well-being and self-esteems. Apart form this it generates self-reliance and increases socialization in groups and company.

Exercise includes both physical and yogic exercise. Unless contraindicated due to presence of certain problems like heart disease exercise is very useful. Moderate increase in physical activity such as walking 30–60 minutes every day even in older ages can reduce significantly the risk of heart diseases. Exercise improves circulation to all parts, prevents constipation, bone loss and fracture, promotes good sleep, helps reducing weight, cholesterol, blood pressure and lower blood sugar levels in diabetics besides reducing stress, anxiety and depression.[13]

Breathing Exercises

Deep breathing helps to achieve relaxation and relieves stress. *The technique of deep breathing:* Lie flat on hard bed or floor with palm of the hand often facing the roof. Leave your body free of tension. Take a deep breath without expanding your chest, stomach should be drawn out, or expanded as if filling a balloon. Inhale and exhale through the nostrils gradually. With each inhalation, say the world "relax" or "calm" fairly loudly for producing autosuggestion. Repeat the whole process 10 times.

Physical Relaxation

Physical relaxation can be performed anywhere by sitting quietly in comfortable position. Relax your muscles; begin with the feet and progress up to your face. Breathe through your nose easily and naturally. Try to be aware of your breathing. As you breathe out, say the world "one" silently to yourself. Repeat the pattern, breathe in and breathe out, and say "one" for 10–15 minutes. One can learn to relax by experience. Relaxation should be performed in peaceful atmosphere.[4]

Diet and Nutrition

Requirement of calories for elderly persons is 25% less than those of normal adults doing sedentary work. The caloric requirement of the elderly male is 1800 kcal and for elderly female 1400 kcal (ICMR RDA 1995). Malnutrition in elderly is common because of loss of teeth, appetite and lack of care. Calories restriction is an anti-ageing measure. Protein intake of 50–60 G per day is recommended for female and male respectively. Cooking fat should not be more than 15–20 G per day (visible fat). One should strike a balance between PUFA, MUFA and SFA. Choose a variety of vegetable oils. Mix 2 or more oils of different composition—a good choice is an equal mixture of PUFA rich sunflower, safflower or corn oil, with MUFA rich groundnut oil. Mustard oil is not a good choice as sole cooking medium. Sesame (Til) oil is also good as it contains nearly equal amount of PUFA and MUFA. Encourage whole cereals, fruits, vegetables, salads and spices (onion, turmeric, olive, tea), consumption of dietary fibre to avoid constipation and to use these as cholesterol lowering agents. Vegetarian diets are proven to be good.

The following is the brief account of several nutrients, their role and benefits in ageing process.[5]

Nutrient	*Physiological role*	*Specific role in ageing process*
Iron	Immuno-competence	Preventing vulnerability to infectious diseases in old age
Iron/folate	Prevention of anaemia	Maintaining appropriate level of activity in old age
Calcium	Bone calcification	Preventing osteoporosis and fractures in old age through falls and other types of accidents
Selenium	Antioxidant	Preventing free radical damage in biological process of ageing
Vit. A; β-carotene ascorbic acid, vitamin E, lycopene	Antioxidants	Preventing free radical damage in old age, e.g. atherosclerosis, cataract, prevention of malignancies and controlling free radical damage on other tissues and enzyme system

Vaccines

Currently there is no programme of immunization for older persons. Elderly are vulnerable to diphtheria, tetanus, zoster, pneumococcal, meningococcal, hepatitis A and hepatitis B infections.

Secondary Prevention

When the emergence of risk factors cannot be prevented, the attempt is made to detect the disease process in older people at the earliest and ensure prompt treatment. This can be achieved by screening of elderly or periodical check-ups of older people. Several attempts have been made by professional bodies (IMA) and voluntary organization to organize free check-ups or screening camps for non-communicable diseases like diabetes, hypertension, heart diseases and cancer. National Cancer Control Programme helps raising the level of awareness of prevention of cancers as also screening of cancers by trained paramedical personnel in rural and urban setting. Detection of cervical cancer through Pap smears and self-examination of breast helps early detection of cancer. Elderly themselves can organize for regular check up. Cataract surgery is boon for the older people. The National programme on prevention of blindness provides free operation facilities in many institutions and through organized camps, free IOL and glasses are provided. Screening programmes for early detection of cataract by paramedical workers helps to seek early treatment of cataract.

Free sputum examination and treatment facilities are made available for tuberculosis under the National Tuberculosis Control Programme.

Accidents

Falls in elderly people are common. Because of advancing age, osteoporosis is quite common and bones become fragile. Slipping and falling in home environments most commonly leads to fracture neck femur or fracture of other bones.

These accidents can be avoided by using nonslip tiles/mats on floors, by adequate lighting and using proper toilets (elevated seat with grab bars) and having bed height 18" from top mattress to floor and chair height 14"–16".

Oral Health

Many of the older persons have poor oral health and hygiene. 19% of older persons above the age of 65 were edentulous, 80% had partial, 3% had intact teeth, and only 1.5% were using dentures. The objective of the National oral health policy seeks to reduce the prevalence of edentulousness to 50% above the age of 65 years; thus, it is a big challenge.

ALZHEIMER'S DISEASE (AD)

Alzheimer's disease is also called primary degenerative dementia or as previously called pre-senile dementia. In 1907, Dr. Alois Alzheimer, a famous German neuropathologist described the disease first of all.

In age bracket 65–69, between 2 and 3% of older people have Alzheimer's disease (AD) while 4–8% have AD between age group 70 and 80 and above 80 around 20–25% manifest AD. As the age advances, the prevalence increases. Exact etiology is not known.

In India it is projected that 4 million people are affected with AD; however 10% of these affected get diagnosed.

Risk Factors for AD

In relation to dementia common term in practice is "use it or loose it". Research evidence indicates beneficial effect of intellectually stimulation activities on brain.

Common risk factors for dementia are—tobacco use, heavy drinking, physical inactivity and lack of social engagement, midlife hypertension and unhealthy diet.

Warning Signs

i Forgetfulness of recently acquired information
ii Disorientation of time, place and person
iii Poor self-care and inappropriate dressing up
iv Problem with logical thinking and reasoning
v Difficulty in performing routine tasks
vi Difficulty in speech and written lannguage recognition
vii Misplacement of objects
viii Loss of initiatives and social withdrawal.

What Happens to Patients?

AD leads to loss of cognition. Patients with AD are extremely disabled in function, they get lost in their own house; they forget that they have just eaten food and continuously ask for food and they even cannot recognize their children or their spouses. Thus, memory is severely impaired. The patient becomes worse after sunset.

Treatment

There is yet no known cure for disease but we can reduce the risk. No specific treatment or drug is available; therefore, the treatment is symptomatic. Family members have to ensure adequate nutrition, personal hygiene, nursing care and prevent accidents and fluid maintenance. Family members can be trained to provide care.

Tertiary Prevention

This is applicable to ensure rehabilitation and use of the remaining capacities of the elderly. The family is sheet anchor for rehabilitation of elderly people. Most of the elders (85%) between 60 and 75 years tend to be active and only 15% have some physical disabilities, most of these get managed at family level and with self-support and support of primary and secondary health care institutions. Rehabilitation may be required for 1–2% of severe disabilities. Most elderly people are physically active and can perform activities of daily living (ADL) or self-care activities, i.e. bathing, dressing, toileting transferring from one position to another one and eating, besides working in the surroundings. Hardly 1% had grade four severe disabilities.

In essence, the residual capacity of elderly should be harnessed through a number of measures such as working in development programme, e.g. health education, literacy drive, child welfare and development and mass education and other national building activities. Elders are wisdom banks as they have life experiences, which can be used for the benefit of society and community.

As over 86% of elderly persons in rural and urban areas are staying with the joint families, therefore, the cherished institution of family happens to be "pivotal" institution for the care of elderly. Therefore, the government and all non-governmental organizations should support the family system for sustainability. The elders have played a pride role as "home makers" have made a pride place and dignity for themselves in the family environments. Family needs them and they need the support of family and this way it is a symbiotic and mutual support, self-fulfilment and co-existence.[14]

Family ensures social security, economic security, and emotional security and ensures most congenial environments. The most important security is emotional security. It is important that the family support system continues to be functional and the ability of the family to discharge its obligatory caring responsibilities; continue. The National Policy for aged recognizes the value of family institution and gives primacy to promote family values and sensitize the younger on necessity and desirability of inter-generational bonding and continuity. State policies will encourage children to co-reside with their parents by providing tax relief, allowing rebates for medical expenses and giving preference in the allotment of houses.

Institution of joint family system is shrinking because of nuclear families and only one or two children being born to family the stress is likely to be more in coming years.[14] One hears the news of ill-treatment of parents by sons and daughters-in-law on the issue of property, but these are rare instances and speak of imbalanced personality. Some case studies of happy adjusted aged are presented below.

A YOUNG MAN OF HUNDRED YEARS (1997)

In this large world, chosen few are those who get a large number of years to tread on and fewer are those who really enjoy it. Jaagar is one of them. He is resident of village Ghironthi. He was born in the family of carpenters. His mother was a housewife. His parents left him in childhood for their heavenly abode. He had 6 sisters, 3 elder and 3 younger. Being a lone boy, he successfully undertook the responsibility of getting his sisters married. He was married to a young girl in his early adolescence. She gave him 4 sons and left him 2 years before independence. He recalls his contribution to the struggle for independence. He made indigenous guns for freedom fighters.

Out of his 4 sons, one was mentally ill and died in early age. Second died while serving the army. Third, one lives with him and the fourth one is in the Navy. He has been a true patriot, no doubt giving his sons to the nation.

As one approaches Jaagar, a shadow with stick comes out of a dark room. His head shakes as if he is welcoming you. The wrinkles on his face stand out prominently as if each tells a story of the years gone by.

The years have taken in toll on to him, as he is hard of hearing. He cannot see clearly with both eyes, which he got operated for cataract. He was operated for enlarged prostate 15 years back. He used to smoke *Hookka* but left 10 years back. He could play cards with his peer group but left as his vision diminished. He has read Ramayana and Mahabharata. He is a short-tempered person. He often refuses food if it is given 10–15 minutes late. He takes two meals a day and gets ₹ 100 as old age pension from Haryana Government. He has no land of his own. He left working as carpenter 25 years back.

He has no grudges against his family. He wishes Government could increase the old age pension from ₹ 100/- to 300/-.

Jaagar is a respectable father figure and considered to be god man to the village. No marriage is complete without him. He is consulted for all important matters. The villagers respect him and he cares for them.

The story of Jaagar compels me to think about the present set-up in society. There are a few Jaagars, who have seen generations come and generations go. Seen many droughts and floods and still survived to tell the tales of years gone by and guide the people for years to come.

Jaagar is self-reliant and confident. As a master craftsman (carpenter) he earned his name and fame in the village community. He feels proud to demonstrate his creative art, craft and carvings on door panels in many of the dwellings in village Ghironthi.

He earned respect because of his craft and good deeds. One makes his place in the society by his own attributes and skills.

VILLAGE CHAUPAL—THE DAY CARE CENTRE (1997)

"Villages are the heart of India and Chaupal the Soul." No village is complete without the Chaupal (community centre).

As one approaches village Ghironthi, one sees from a distance a group of old people sitting together. One thinks it could be a kind of conference going on but on coming nearer, one sees that they are playing cards and enjoying group smoking.

One of them is Jogiram, a 65-year-old man, widower since 30 years, he has a son and a daughter. Son is married and stays with him. Jogiram has 16 acre of land and works on it. He is illiterate and does not get pension. Asking about the Chaupal, he says it is his lifetime. He cannot live without it. He comes here after taking care of cattle and stays there till the sunset.

In the Chaupal, he likes playing cards and smoking Hookka. He gossips about everything and anything. There is a Hookka culture and they smoke Hookka only among their caste group. This Chaupal is called Jatwali Chaupal. In the Chaupal, he consults with his peer group about every important decision in life, like marrying his grandson and daughter, farming techniques and day-to-day happenings. He often borrows money from them when in need and they oblige him with the same. For the elderly he wants that the younger generation should respect elders and take care of them.

The Chaupal is the only place to beat the boredom of the evening of life. It is exclusive only to villages of India. The Government should look into the set-up of these Chaupals and help establish them to strengthen this set-up further to serve as day care centre for elderly.

ROLE OF COMMUNITY

The Panchayati Raj institutions (PRIs) and Nagarpalikas have a special role to play for care of elderly people. These institutions will be encouraged to participate in the implementation of National Policy.[15]

In village setting, village community centres (village Chaupals) have been established by the communities. Apart from social functions (meetings and marriages) the village Chaupals are used by older people. They come here and spend most of their daytime and in a way, it is a "day care centre" for the elderly. Elderly exchange all sorts of information and have made social groups for smoking, reading newspaper, playing cards, exchange information and solving problems. Similarly, municipal parks in cities are used by older people who get together as social groups, indulge in-group discussion, share the problems with each other, and discover their solution.

The Government and NGOs can play useful role in supporting these institutions by organizing information, recreational material, reading material and using it as a day care centre for elderly with a view to enhance the self-esteem of elderly. PRIs can organize camps for elderly and support the transport.

ROLE OF NGOs/International Organizations

Several NGOs are playing useful role in India for the cause of elderly. The notable NGOs in the field of care of older people are:

i Helpage India and Helpage International
ii Age-care-India
iii Elder home society
iv Care of the elderly—Age care centre for Retired Airforce Personnel
v International Medical Sciences Academy (USA)

Helpage India has been an instrument for getting the National Policy for the older person in place.

Functions

1. These organizations play the role of advocacy for older persons.
2. To create an awareness and understanding amongst masses about the problems of older persons.
3. To raise funds.
4. To organize relief measures for elderly persons in the form of mobile medical programmes, cataract operation camps, day centres, day hospitals, geriatric centres, vocational rehabilitation, domiciliary care, meals on wheels programme, to set-up elder homes and hospitals.

These organizations are playing useful role and supplement the efforts of the government.

International Efforts

Several international efforts such as Madrid Plan of actions and United Nations Principles for senior citizens adopted by UN General Assembly in 2002, Shanghai Plan of Action 2007 and Macau outcome document 2007 form the basis for the global policy guidelines. The government of India is signatory to all these documents.

HOMES FOR ELDERLY

These have been set-up for destitute elderly persons.

In Western world, more and more elderly people stay in such homes.

Objectives are to provide residential facilities/accommodation, to serve as alternate to home care, to ensure social and financial stability and to provide rehabilitation through social contacts, recreation and vocational facilities.

Services

These include educational, vocational, medical and health, recreational, food and domiciliary services through social workers. These homes are linked with specialist care and doctors are available on call. The person has to pay heavily and for poor these are subsidized.

But, these homes are homes away from home and it is a sort of solitary confinement in a palace. There is no emotional security or support of family members in these homes. Elders have to support themselves. Relatives or near and dear seldom visit older person, only the God is near to them and human beings are far away from them.[16,17]

ROLE OF GOVERNMENT

The Government has formulated National Policy for older persons. National Policy seeks to assure older persons that their concerns are national concerns and they will not be unprotected, ignored or marginalized. The goal of the National policy is well-being of the elderly. It aims to strengthen their legitimate place in the society and help older persons to live the last stage of their lives with purpose dignity and peace.

The Government has supported the elderly by:

i Old age pensions
ii Houses and shelter
iii Welfare measures
iv Health and nutrition through primary health care set-up supported by secondary and tertiary level of care and specialized services of medical colleges
v Government has supported NGOs financially to take up and organize services for the older people.

It is now up to older people and community how best they are able to utilize these services and relief measures.

Geriatric medicine as a speciality has yet to develop. The faculty of medical colleges all over the country needs to be oriented on the policy guidelines for elderly in order to focus on priority problems of the elderly. The curriculum of UGs and PGs should have adequate contents of geriatric medicine. The present model of four days course of sensitization of some professors of medicine at AIIMS, New Delhi, covering different medical colleges in the country is insufficient. The experience of such in-service courses has not been encouraging as very few reported for such courses. Madras Medical College at Madras offers Postgraduate Course in Geriatrics, it has geriatric ward of 35 beds, which is cited as an example in the country, but the problems of aged can be tackled within the existing system. The elderly need "more care" than cure. IGNOU has started distance learning diploma course on geriatrics and WHO has prepared modules for training of paramedical workers; hopefully it gets implemented at primary health care level.

War against smoking, improving food habits, promoting regular exercises and other healthy behaviours should become important component of health care from now onwards, with focus on young children, adolescent and youth to have or develop active and healthy ageing.

NATIONAL POLICY ON OLDER PERSONS (1999)

National Policy for older persons (NPOP) was formulated in January 1999 to fulfil the long-standing demand and need of the elderly in India. The Union Ministry of Social Justice and Empowerment is the nodal agency for implementation of the policy, which contains a series of good intentions and proposals that are sacrosanct. Overall, it is a very comprehensive document and covers all the aspects, which directly affect the older persons. NPOP has been revised as National Policy on Senior Citizens 2011 (draft to be approved).

Key Features of Policy

a ***Financial security:*** Through expanded old age pension scheme to include the private sector and regulatory authority to monitor pension funds.

b ***Taxation:*** Increased standard tax deduction for senior citizens.

c ***Legislation:*** On parents right to be supported by their children.

d ***Health care and nutrition:*** Subsidized health care network with private sector involvement.

e ***Shelter security:*** Easy access to housing loans.

f ***Life security:*** Special provision in Indian Penal Code for Protection of older persons.

The central theme of this policy is to achieve integration between *young and old* and develop a support system, formal as well as informal, to increase the potential of the families to take care of the old persons. Mainstream senior citizens especially older women. The policy also focuses on the significance of tapping human resources among the elderly. This will serve as a dual purpose the society will benefit tremendously from their expertise and experience and older persons will lead an active life with healthy outlook.[18,19]

National Council for Older Persons (NCOP) has been constituted and approved by Prime Minister to review the policies and programmes for ageing population.

a. FINANCIAL SECURITY

A great anxiety in old age relates to financial insecurity. The financial situation of two-thirds of 60+ tends to be fragile and many live below poverty line.

- For elderly below poverty line old age pension provides some financial support. The scheme of old age pension which was started in 1977 will be expanded to cover all older persons below poverty line in rural and urban areas. The national scheme provides for Rs. 200 pension per month for the uncared old above 65 years of age and widows above 50 years of age and disabled having inadequate income. Some states are supplementing the pension amount provided by the Central Government and have also relaxed the age criteria to extend coverage.
- The base of pension coverage needs to be expanded considerably. It would be necessary to facilitate the establishment of pension schemes both in the private and in the public sector for self-employed and salaried person in non-Governmental employment, with provision for employers also to contribute. Pension funds will function under regulatory authority.
- It will be ensured that settlement of pension, provident fund, gratuity and other retirement benefits is made promptly to avoid hardships to retired persons.

b. TAXATION

- Higher standard deduction to tax payer elderly has been implemented. Standard annual rebate for medical treatment whether domiciliary or hospital, where the retired persons do not get medical coverage from their erstwhile employers, will be considered.
- Interest rate on long-term savings will be reasonably enhanced.
- Pre-retirement counselling programmes will be promoted and assisted.
- Employment in income generating activities after retirement should be choice of individual. Organizations, which provide guidance, training and orientation and support services, will be assisted.

Programmes of Non-Governmental Organizations for generating income of old persons will be encouraged.

c. LEGISLATION

Considering the growing number of elderly population accompanied by changes in the society of economy and its impact on morbidity pattern, Government of India enacted "The maintenance and welfare of parents and senior citizen's Act, 2007". The rights of parents without any means to be supported by their children having sufficient means have been recognized by this law. Many states have passed legislations.

d. HEALTH CARE AND NUTRITION—SECURITY

The older people face multiple diseases/ailments and many of these are long-term chronic ailments necessitating long-term or lifelong treatment.

1 Under the policy, health care needs of older persons will be given high priority. The goal should be good affordable health services, very heavily subsidized for the poor and graded system of user charges for others.

   The policy envisages having a reasonable mix of public health services, health insurance, and health services provided not for profit organizations including trusts, charitable and private medical care.

2 The primary health care system will be the basic structure of public health care. WHO supports "Towards age friendly primary health care". It will be strengthened and oriented to be able to meet the health care needs of older persons as well as public health services, preventive, curative, restorative and rehabilitative care will be considerably expanded and strengthened and geriatric care facilities will be provided at secondary and tertiary levels. This will imply much larger public outlays.

3 The development of health insurance will be given high priority.

4 Trusts, charitable societies and voluntary agencies will be promoted, encouraged to provide free beds, medicines and treatment to the very poor elder citizens and reasonable user charges for the rest of the population.

5 Private medical care system and general practitioners will be extended opportunities for orientation in geriatric care.

6 Public hospitals will be directed to ensure that elderly patients are not subjected to long waits and visits to different counters for medical tests and treatment. Separate counters for elderly will be provided. Geriatrics wards will be set up.

7 Medical and paramedical personnel in primary, secondary and tertiary health care facilities will be given training and orientation in health care of the elderly. Facilities for specialization in geriatric medicine will be provided in the medical colleges.

8 Mobile services and special camps for elderly will be promoted to increase access to services.

9 For the old people who are chronically ill and are deprived of family support, hospitals supported or assisted by the state, public charity, and voluntary organizations will be necessary.

10 Assistance will be given to geriatric care societies for production, and distribution of instructional material on self-care by the older persons.

11 Concept of healthy ageing will be promoted. It is necessary to educate older persons and their families that diseases are not a corollary of advancing age nor is a particular chronological age, the starting point for decline in health status.

12 Health education programme will be strengthened by making use of mass media, folk media and other channels of communication, which reach out to different segments of population. The capacity to cope with illness and manage domiciliary care will be strengthened. Programmes will also be developed targeting younger and middle age groups to inform them how lifestyles during early years affect health status in later years. Messages on how to stay healthy for the entire lifespan will be given.

13 Mental health services will be expanded and strengthened.

14 Non-Governmental Organizations will be encouraged and assisted through grants for providing ambulatory services, day care, and health care to complement the efforts of the state.

e. SHELTER—SECURITY

Shelter is a basic human need. Housing schemes for urban and rural lower income segment will earmark 10% of houses/house sites for allotment to older persons. This will include Indira Awas Yojna and other schemes of Government.

Older people will be given easy access to housing loans. Group housing for older persons comprising flatlets with common service facilities such as meals, laundry, common room rest rooms, will be encouraged.

Education

Education, training and information needs of older persons will be met. These have virtually received no attention in the post. Information and education material specially relevant to the lives of elderly people will be developed and widely disseminated, using mass media and non-formal education channels.

- Schools will be encouraged and assisted to develop outreach programmes for interacting with older persons on regular basis, participate in the running of senior citizens centres and develop activities in them.
- Educational curriculum will incorporate material to strengthen inter-generational bonds and mutually

supporting relationships. Older people with professional qualifications and knowledge in science and art could interact with children and young persons.

- Individuals of all ages, families and communities will be provided with information about the ageing process and the changing roles, responsibilities and relationships at different stages of the life cycle. The contributions of older persons inside the household and outside will be highlighted.

Welfare

The main thrust of welfare will be to identify the more vulnerable among older persons such as the poor, the differently-abled, the infirm and chronically sick and those without family support and provide welfare services to them on priority basis. The policy will consider institutional care as last resort when personal circumstances are such that stay in old age homes becomes absolutely necessary.

Welfare activities under the policy comprise non-institutional services by voluntary organizations, construction and maintenance of old age homes, subsidized heavily for poor, day care, multi-service citizens centres, reach out services, supply of disability related aids and appliances, besides help line telephones.

A welfare fund for older persons will be set-up, and contribution to the fund will be given tax relief.

f. PROTECTION OF LIFE AND PROPERTY

Older people become soft targets for criminal elements. The government, NGOs and police will provide necessary safeguard to protect the life and property of older persons as also their exploitation.

The potential of 60+ will be harnessed and realized fully as important human resource. The institution of family in India is unique in care of elderly and this shall be supported adequately by the Government and the NGOs. No other institution can replace family.

The action plans will be developed by each state to implement the policy in letter and spirit.

WHO (2007) and Helpage International advocate an integrated planning where care is included in overall development strategy. WHO global guide advocates age friendly cities initiative to harness the potentials of aged.[20]

NATIONAL PROGRAMME FOR HEALTH CARE OF ELDERLY (NPHCE)

As a follow-up measure of National Policy on older persons the NPHCE has been launched in May, 2010 in 100 districts of 21 states and will be expanded in 12th Five-Year Plan to cover 225 more districts in phased manner.[21]

Objectives

- The main objective of the programme is to provide an easy access to comprehensive health care (Promotive, Preventive, Curative and Rehabilitative) services to elderly people through community based primary health care approach.
- To promote the concept of active ageing and healthy ageing.
- *Other objectives are*—strengthen referral system, to develop specialized manpower by training and to promote research in geriatrics and gerontology.

OPERATIONAL GUIDELINES

Core strategies to achieve the objectives of the programme are:

- Community based primary health care approach including domiciliary visits by trained health care workers.
- Dedicated services at PHC/CHC level including provision of machinery, equipment, training, and additional human resources at CHC, as also IEC, etc.
- Dedicated facilities at District Hospital with 10 bedded ward, additional human resources, machinery and equipment, consumables and drugs, training and IEC.
- Strengthening of 8 Regional Medical Institutes (RMI) to provide dedicated tertiary level medical facilities for the elderly (setting up of geriartic department), introducing PG courses in Geriatric Medicine, and in-service training of health personnel at all levels. 12 more RMI would be added in 12th plan.
- In addition two National Institutes of Ageing (NIA) care also being established at AIIMS, New Delhi and Madras Medical College, Chennai.
- Information, Education and Communication (IEC) using mass media, folk media and other communication channels to reach out to the target community.
- Continuous monitoring and independent evaluation of the programme and research in geriatrics and implementation of NPHCE.

Supplementary strategies include:

- Promotion of public private partnerships in Geriatric Health Care.
- Mainstreaming AYUSH—revitalizing local health tradition, and convergence with programmes of Ministry of Social Justice and Empowerment in the field of geriatrics.
- Reorienting medical education to support geriatric issues, including geriatric care in the syllabus of medical courses including nurses courses.

Pakage of Services

The services under the programme would be integrated below district level and shall be integral part of the existing

Package of services available at different levels under NPHCE[22]

Health facility	Package of services
Sub-centre (SC)	• Health education related to healthy ageing • Domiciliary visits for attention and care to home bound/bedridden elderly persons and provide training to the family care providers in looking after the disabled elderly persons • Arrange for suitable calipers and supportive devices from the PHC to the elderly disabled persons to make them ambulatory • Linkage with other support groups and day care centres, etc. operational in the area
Primary health centre (PHC)	• Weekly geriatric clinic run by a trained medical officer • Maintain record of the elderly using standard format during their first visit • Conducting a routine health assessment of the elderly persons based on simple clinical examination relating to eye, BP, blood sugar, etc. • Provision of medicines and proper advice on chronic ailments of lungs, heart, and diabetes • Public awareness on promotional, preventive and rehabilitative aspects of geriatrics during health and village sanitation day/camps • Referral for diseases needing further investigation and treatment, to Community Health Centre or the District Hospital as per need
Community health centre (CHC)	• CHC will be First Referral Unit (FRU) for the Elderly patients from PHC and SC • Geriatric Clinic for the elderly persons twice a week • Rehabilitation Unit for physiotherapy and counselling • Domiciliary visits by the rehabilitation worker for bed ridden elderly and counselling of the family members on their home-based care • Health promotion and prevention • Referral of difficult cases to District Hospital/ higher health care facility
District Hospital	• Daily Geriatric Clinic for regular dedicated OPD services to the elderly • Facilities for laboratory investigations for diagnosis and provision of medicines for geriatric medical and health problems • Ten-bedded Geriatric Ward for in-patient care of the elderly • Existing specialities like General Medicine; Orthopaedics, Ophthalmology; ENT, etc. will provide services needed by elderly patients • Provide services for the elderly patients referred by the CHCs/PHCs, etc. • Conducting camps for Geriatric Services in PHCs/ CHCs and other sites • Referral services for severe cases to tertiary level hospitals
Regional geriatric centre or Depatment of Geriatric	• Geriatric Clinic (specialized OPD for the elderly) • 30-bedded Geriatric Ward for inpatient care • Tertiary health care to the cases referred from medical colleges, district hospitals and below • Developing treatment protocols, training modules and research on specific elderly diseases/geriatrics

health care delivery system and vertical at district and above as more specialized care is needed for the elderly at these levels.

Monitoring of the programme will be done by the common non-communicable disease cell established at various levels under national Programme of Cancer, Diabetes, Cardiovascular Diseases and Strokes.[21]

REFERENCES

1 GOI. National Population Policy-2000. New Delhi: MOH and FW, GOI; 2001.
2 IIPS/ORC. Macro. National Family Health Survey I (1992–1993). Introductory Report. Mumbai: IIPS; 1994.
3 NIPHC. Proceedings of NIPHC/HCPT seminar on services for the aged—a national commitment; 1996 Oct: New Delhi.
4 Bhatla PC. Lecture Series in Geriatrics. New Delhi: Health Care Promotion Trust NIPHC; 2000.
5 GOI. Morbidity, Health Care and condition of the aged. National Sample Survey 60th round (January to June 2004) Government of India, March 2006; pp. 54–65.
6 Bhatla PC. Community Geriatrics—Care of the elderly. Issues, Status, Solutions. New Delhi: NIPHC; 1993.
7 ICMR. Health care of the elderly. ICMR Bulletin 1996; 26(5).
8 Lal S, Vashisht BM, Punia MS. Health and Social Status of Senior Citizen in rural areas. Ind J Comm. Health 1997 Sept–Dec; 19(3).
9 GOI. XIth Five-Year Plan Thrust areas, MOH and FW, GOI, New Delhi.
10 Lal S. Adding life to years. Ind J Comm Med 1999 Oct–Dec; 24(4):143–6.
11 Helpage India. Annual Report 1998–99. New Delhi: Helpage India; 1999.
12 Christian Medical Association of India. Yearning for Love. Health Dialogue 2002 Apr–June; 29.
13 WHO. World Heart Federation, global movement for active ageing "Active Ageing: Moving Hearts for Health" press release WHO/72, 27 September 2002.
14 Helpage India. Research and Development Journal 1997 Feb; 3(2).
15 Shah B. Public Health Implication of Ageing in India. ICMR Bulletin 1993 March; 23(3).
16 Kusum. Lonely at eventide. Hindustan Times. 1998 March 27; 13.
17 WHO. The third age. World Health 1979 April.
18 Soneja S. Out at last. Helpage India Research and Development Journal 1999;5(3): 3.
19 Helpage India. National Policy for Older Persons. Helpage India's Efforts Materialize 1999;14(2).
20 Hindustan Times, Chandigarh, November 19, 2007—Vipul Mudgal 'Research'. Too old to work, too young to die.
21 Govt of India, MOH and FW Annual Report 2010–2014.
22 GOI. MOH and FW. National Programme for the Health Care of the Elderly-Operational Guidelines 2013.

CHAPTER

15

Health Management

HEALTH CARE DELIVERY SYSTEMS IN INDIA

"Health" in India is the responsibility of State Government. Under the constitution, state government is responsible to provide health services to its people.

The health care delivery systems in India comprise mix of public and private providers of health services.

VARIOUS HEALTH CARE SYSTEMS

1 Government run services and municipal health services (Municipal Corporation) in urban areas.
2 Private health sector.
3 Industrial-organizations-corporate sector, Employees State Insurance (ESI) Scheme–Health Insurance.
4 Central Government Health Services (CGHS) Scheme.
5 Railway health services.
6 Armed forces health services.
7 Indian system of medicine (AYUSH).
8 Non-Governmental Organizations (NGOs) and Philanthropic Organizations (Charitable).

GOVERNMENT HEALTH SERVICES

This system consists of Sub-centres, PHCs, CHCs, sub-district hospitals, district hospitals, medical college and hospitals, municipal corporation hospitals, dispensaries and hospitals of Indian system of medicine (ISM).

The Government health system provides almost, 95%, of preventive and promotive health services apart from curative services free of cost or at very low cost. The hospital care of government set-up is cheaper and accessible to rich and poor people. Government sector alone cannot provide total health services.[1] The health care delivery in India has been envisaged at 3 levels namely—primary, seconday and tertiary level.

'Health for All' through Primary Health Care

The Bhore Committee made one of the most outstanding contribution in health services planning in the country way back in 1943–46. It recommended three-tier system of primary health centre, subdistrict hospital and district level health set-up, i.e. primary, secondary and tertiary health care services. The Committee recommended establishment of one primary health centre (PHC) for 40,000 population in short-term and achieve the goal of one PHC for 10,000 to 20,000 in the long run. The foundation of primary health care in India was laid in independent India in 1952. The movement of integrated all round development programme was launched in the country in 1952, one primary health centre for each community development block (CDB) in rural areas was established. The functions of PHCs consisted of medical care, control of communicable diseases, maternal and child health, nutrition, health education, school health, environmental sanitation and collection of vital statistics.

The work on building up of PHC infrastructure in India started through 5-year plans and various health committees were constituted to review the health planning in India. We built our own model of primary health care in India after independence, it has the strong base of "community development", and "health" was considered and perceived as *development function* and overall part of socio-economic development of the country. Thus, health in India was integral part of community development.[2,3]

Era of 'Health for All'

- ***Alma-Ata Declaration (1978):*** Joint declaration was made in 1978 in Alma-Ata, USSR, in September 1978 on "Health for All" by 2000 AD through "primary health care". Most nations of the world (134 countries and 67 NGOs) including India signed this historical declaration and committed themselves to achieve health for all by 2000 AD.[4,5]

National Health Policy (NHP) in India was formulated in 1983 with the broad objective to provide "Health for all" "through universal primary health care" by 2000 AD.

- ***What is health for all (HFA)?*** "The attainment by all citizens of the world by the year 2000 a level of health, that will permit them to lead a socially and economically productive life".

The level or standard of health will be determined by each country following the principles laid down by WHO. HFA is a global strategy, formulated in 1981.

PRIMARY HEALTH CARE (PHC)

"Primary health care is an essential health care, based on practical, scientifically sound and socially acceptable methods and technology, made universally accessible to individuals and families in the community, through their full participation and at a cost that the community and the country can afford ....". It forms an integral part both of country's health system of which it is the central function and main focus and of overall social and economic development of the community.[6, 7] It is the first level of contact of individuals, the family and community with the national health system bringing health care as close as possible to where people live and work and constitutes the first element of a continuing health care process. Thus, primary health care is not an inferior health care. It is based on sound scientific methods. The hallmarks of PHC are universal *availability*, *accessibility*, *acceptability* and *affordability* and community participation.

Primary health care addresses the main health problems in the community providing promotive, preventive, curative and rehabilitative services. Accordingly, it attempts to intervene at all levels of the natural history of disease.

India has played a leading role in planning and establishing primary health care system in the country ever since health survey and development committee (Bhore Committee) submitted its report in 1943–46.

Principles of Primary Health Care

1. ***Equitable distribution*** of health services to all sections with priority to weaker sections. Achieve equity between rural–urban, rich–poor and gender—male and female.
2. ***Active community participation:*** People must be part of planning, programming, implementation, management and evaluation of health services.
3. ***Multi-sectoral approach:*** Health is not only the function of health sector alone but much more health comes through many other sectors like water supply and sanitation, literacy and education, nutrition and agricultural development, etc. hence health is a multisectoral subject.
4. ***Appropriate scientifically sound technology:*** Which is socially acceptable and directed against relevant health problem, e.g. Growth monitoring, ORS, breast feeding, immunization, family planning, female literacy and food supplements—Vit A, iodized salt and IFA (GOBIFFF as advocated by UNICEF).

Basic Elements of Primary Health Care

The PHC gives primacy to following essential elements:

i. *Education* concerning prevailing health problems and the methods of preventing and controlling them.
ii. Promotion of *food* supply and *adequate nutrition*.
iii. An adequate supply of safe water and basic sanitation.
iv. *Maternal and child health* care including family planning.
v. *Immunization* against the major infectious diseases.
vi. Prevention and control of locally *endemic diseases*.
vii. Appropriate treatment of *common diseases* and injuries.
viii. Provision of *essential drugs*.

It reflects clearly that goal of health for all is to be achieved through 8 components, which belong to not just one sector but to many inter-related sectors, and sectors other than health sector. It necessitates achieving inter-and intra-sectoral coordination. Health cannot be attained by health sector alone.

Supportive Activities for Primary Health Care

These include following in order to successfully implement primary health care. WHO has identified the following supportive activities:

1. Community involvement and participation.
2. Intra-and inter-sectoral coordination.
3. Provision of effective referral support.
4. Development and mobilization of resources.
5. Managerial processes (Policy, goals and objectives).
6. Medical and health services research, including innovative approaches.
7. Development and application of appropriate technology
8. Health manpower development.

India had a rich experience in the field of primary health care and has been a world leader in developing primary health care strategies. Most significant strategy was to initiate movement of community development since 1952 onward of which health was an integral part. India established network of primary health centres in rural areas one in each of the smallest administrative unit, i.e. community development block of 1,00,000 population.

The global strategy of health for all was formulated in 1981 and global targets were set.

Global Targets

1 All persons in every country will have ready access at least to essential health care and to first level referral facilities.

2 All people will be actively involved in caring for themselves and their families as far as they can and in community action for health.

3 Communities throughout the world will share, with governments, responsibility for the health care of their members.

4 All governments will assume overall responsibility for the health of their people.

5 Safe drinking water and sanitation will be available to all people.

6 All people will be adequately nourished.

7 All children will be immunized against the major infectious diseases of the childhood.

8 Communicable diseases in the developing countries will be of no greater public health significance in the year 2000.

9 All possible ways will be applied to prevent and control non-communicable diseases and promote mental health through influencing lifestyles and controlling the physical and psychosocial environment.

10 Essential drugs will be available to all.

The declaration on primary health care was not binding. The Primary Health Care gave way to more affordable model of "selective health care" which targeted specific diseases and conditions.

In October 2008, the commitment to the principles to primary health care was renewed to strengthen health system by 65 countries of the world. The Alma-Ata agenda of comprehensive primary health care is perhaps as pertinent today as it was in 1978. Ottawa chapter of Health promotion of 1986, Jakarata declaration of 1997 and RIO Declaration of 2011 reiterates the concept of health promotion.

"Moving Towards Universal Health Coverage" in 12th plan period—"Ensuring equitable access for all Indian citizens in any part of the country, regardless of income level, social status, gender, caste or religion, to affordable, accountable and appropriate, assured quality health services (promotive, preventive, curative and rehabilitative) as well as services addressing wider determinants of health delivered to individuals and populations, with the government being the guarantor and enabler, although not necessarily the only provider of health and related services" (*See* National Health Mission).

Rodmap for Universal Health Coverage (UHC)

- Health services will be delivered with seamless integration between primary, secondary and tertiary levels
- The primary Health care will be strengthened to deliver both, preventive, public health and curative services
- Government and private sector mix to deliver Essential Health Package (EHP) services
- No fee of any kind levied on primary health care services
- UHC model—cashless delivery of essential health package (EHP) to all (Free Services for all National Health Programmes).

PRIMARY HEALTH CARE SYSTEM IN RURAL AREAS

The primary health care system infrastructure has been developed as a *three-tier system* (consisting of sub-centre, primary health centre, and community health centre—being the three Pillars of Primary Health Care System) based on the population norms. The norms for tribal areas are different.[8,9]

Over 69% of population of India lives in rural areas. Health care of rural India has been reorganized ever since the launch of National Health Policy, 1983. The primary health care has been universalized in the country to realize the goal of health for all in India. Over the years, India has established the vast public health infrastructure in the country which includes 153655 sub-centres, 25308 primary health centres and 5396 community health centres to provide health services to 69% of the country's population living in rural areas. The primary health care organization at various levels is depicted in Table 15.1.

PRIMARY HEALTH CARE ORGANIZATION

At Village Level—VHSNC

At village level, we have trained birth attendants, Anganwadi workers and health volunteers (*Village health guide*) at the rate of 1:1000 population and now accredited social health activist (ASHA) has been introduced by National Rural Health Mission (NRHM). A village health sanitation and nutrition committee (VHSNC) (consisting of PRI, ANM, AWW, ASHA, Teacher and

Table 15.1: Primary health care organization*

Level	*Population size*	*Functionaries*
Village	1000	• Health volunteers or health guides (Female) • Anganwadi workers • Trained birth attendants • Accredited social health activist (ASHA)
Sub-centre	5000	Multipurpose health workers (Male and female)
PHC	30,000	Health professionals (Doctors)
CHC	1,20,000	Specialists

* People themselves are the biggest resource of health organization

15

NGOs) has been constituted under NRHM for village health action plan and its implementation with untied money of ₹ 10,000 per annum. Over 5.12 lacs village health and sanitation committees have been established. *Village Health Nutrition and Sanitation Day* is organized every month at the Anganwadi centre in each village for RCH (Reproductive and child health) services.

Village Health Guide (VHG)

The health guide scheme was started on 2nd October 1977 in all the states except in Arunanchal Pradesh, J&K, Kerala and Tamil Nadu. The scheme was made 100% centrally sponsored scheme in 1981. According to the scheme the village community selects a volunteer as village health guide (VHG), who after training acts as link between the community and the Government health system. About 3.18 lakh VHG were reported to be working in 1985. Each VHG was paid an honorarium of ₹ 50 per month. The scheme of male VHG has been discontinued in 1986.

The purpose of VHG was to elicit community participation in primary health care and VHG were recruited to mobilize community for self-reliance in health promotive activities, such as village sanitation, safe water and promotion of nutrition and acceptance of contraception to limit the size of family and space children on voluntary basis. They were given medicines for minor ailments and first aid. One VHG was assigned 1000 population. ASHAs are now being used as health guides at village level under NRHM.

Traditional Birth Attendant (TBA)

Traditional birth attendants were trained and one trained birth attendant has been provided for 1000 population or for each village. Over 6,00,000 trained birth attendants are in place. They are voluntary persons and not Government servants who work for safe home deliveries, help in early registration of pregnancy, births, deaths, and help sub-centre workers on voluntary basis. Better linkages should be established between TBAs and sub-centre. TBAs from now on are being trained as *Skilled Birth Attendants.*

Anganwadi Workers (AWWs)

Anganwadi workers are honorary village based locally resident workers under-integrated child development services scheme (ICDS), chosen by village people. One AWW works for 400–800 population in plain area and for 300–800 in tribal and difficult areas. AWW guides ASHA in organizing health day at Anganwadi once a month and other activities at village level.

Mahila Swasthya Sangh (MSS) and ASHAs

At present, 79,512 MSS are working at village level. ASHAs (Accredited social health activists) at village level (One per 1000 population) have been introduced under NRHM. Over 9 Lakhs ASHAs have been trained so far.[10]

15

SUB-CENTRE (SC)—FIRST TIER OF PHC

Under the three-tier system of Primary health care delivery sub-centre is community based first level of Primary health care system in rural area. A sub-centre provides interface with the community at grass root level providing *basic primary health care services.* The Ministry of Health and Family welfare is providing 100% central assistance to all sub-centres in the country.

Manpower at Sub-centre

The sub-centre is the most vital peripheral contact point between the primary health care system and the community. It is the first formal ladder of primary health care system. It is manned by one multipurpose health worker (female) and one multipurpose health worker (male), who are skilled paramedical trained workers, having undergone one year (male worker) and one and a half year training (female worker). One more multipurpose health worker female on contract basis has been added at sub-centre under National Rural Health Mission (NRHM) besides one voluntary worker (optional) preferably a trained birth attendant (TBA) and be paid Rs. 200 per month (with equal contribution by GOI and concerned state).

Population of Sub-centre

The SC is established for every 5000 population in plain area and 3000 in tribal, hilly and desert area. This population may be located in 2–5 villages and may not be in one village. On an average, the village size has been estimated to be of 1000 population but there are many hamlets of small habitations, scattered widely and inaccessible. Sub-centre is located in one of the village. It is desirable that the location of SC should be central to population it serves. Some SCs need to be relocated. Every panchayat and urban municipal ward should have at least one sub-centre

Coverage

The sub-centre is expected to cover 5000 population but it may not be covering the entire population, the access may be difficult. Most often, it covers the population of the village where it is located. Selected services like immunizations are provided to all children. Additional ANMs now known as multipurpose workers (female) were provided under NRHM and RCH programme on contract basis to cover the difficult and remote villages.

Buildings

The sub-centre buildings, about 66% have been built by the Government under Family Welfare Budget, but 34% of sub-centres run in rented buildings or buildings given by village Panchayats which may be in bad condition.

Delivery Huts Under RCH-2

Delivery huts have been set-up in selected sub-centres to promote institutional deliveries. Delivery huts provide facility of running water, electricity and clean physical facilities apart from necessary equipment and material.

Majority of the female and male workers do not stay at the sub-centre and they commute from nearby town, hence not available to conduct deliveries or provide postnatal and neonatal care.

Drugs, Equipment and Materials

Drug kit A and B have been provided at the level of sub-centre. Two kits were provided per annum under CSSM programme. Contents of drug kits A and B are elaborated in Table 15.2.[11]

Table 15.2: Content of drug kits A and B

Name of item	Quantity
Contents of drug kit A	
Oral rehydration salt	150 Packets
Tablets IFA (large)	15000 Tabs.
Tablets IFA (small)	13000 Tabs.
Vitamin A solution	12 Bottles of 100 ml each
Tablet cotrimoxazole	1000 Tabs.
Contents of drug kit B	
Tablets chlorpheniramine	400
Tablets methylergometrine	500
Tablets paracetamol (500 mg)	500
Injection methylergometrine maleate 1 ml ampoule for IM use	5
Tablet mebendazole 100 mg	300
Tablets dicyclomine hydrochloride (10 mg)	250
Chloramphenicol eye ointment 1% w/w in applicaps	500
Ointment povidone iodine 5%	5 Tubes
Cetrimide powder	5 packets of 125 g each
Absorbant cotton	1 Roll
Cotton bandage 4 × 4 cm	120 Rolls

In addition, a midwifery kit for safe delivery and equipment kit for IUD insertion, blood pressure apparatus stethoscope, and weighing machine are available at sub-centre level. The cost of these kits is born by central Government. Pressure cookers for autoclaving and auto-disable syringes are also available.

The vaccines to sub-centre and contraceptives are made available from primary health centre besides *drugs for different national disease control programmes.*

Strengthening of Sub-centres under NRHM

Under NRHM sub-centres have been strengthened by provision of one additional ANM on contractual basis and Untied fund of Rs. 10,000 per annum for local health actions. This fund is jointly operated by the MPHW (F) and Mahila Panch/Sarpanch. Additional sub-centres have been opened up to meet the population norms. Ensure that one ANM out of two stays at sub-centre.

Annual maintenance grant of Rs. 10,000 per annum has been made available to every sub-centre for undertaking repairs and maintenance of facility besides funds for *Janani Suraksha Yojna* (JSY) and incentive money for ASHA.

In order to provide quality care in the sub-centres, Indian Public Health Standards (IPHS) have been prescribed to provide *basic primary health care services* to the community and achieve and maintain an acceptable standard of quality of care.

The sub-centres are envisaged to be under the management of the local Panchayat to increase community ownership and control.

Expenditure per annum for existing sub-centres

Item	Amount
Salary of ANM and LHVS	As per state Govt pay scale
Rent	Rs. 3000
Medicines	To be supplied under RCH
Contingency	Rs. 3200
Voluntary worker	Rs. 1200 as honorarium

Govt of India bears the salary of ANM and LHV besides rent liability and contingency as also drugs and equipments, whereas the salary of the male health worker is borne by state government.

Functions/Services at Sub-centre

The sub-centre provides following promotive, preventive and curative health services in the community of 5000 in plain areas and 3000 in tribal hilly/desert areas, at sub-centre *clinic* or by *outreach* activity.

1. Maternal and Child Health Services

- Early registration of pregnancies, antenatal care, natal care, postnatal care (essential obstetric care), promotion of institutional deliveries, identification and referral of RTI/STI cases to PHC.
- Identification of cases for referral services (high-risk pregnancies, neonates, sick children and for MTP).
- Essential newborn care, exclusive breastfeeding, immunization, vitamin A prophylaxis, iron and folic acid for prophylaxis and treatment of anaemia in pregnant women, children and adolescent girls.
- Treatment and control of diarrhoeal diseases and acute respiratory infection, fever, malnutrition by integrated management of neonatal and childhood illness strategy.
- Contraception services to eligible couples—spacing methods and motivation of couples for sterilization (tubectomy and vasectomy).
- Treatment of common ailments.

- Malaria surveillance at sub-centre (passive surveillance) and prevention and control of vector borne diseases
- Organization of *Mahila Swasthya Sanghs* and their meetings and village health and nutrition day (VHND) at Anganwadis at least once a month.
- Outreach immunization session for young children and school children (DPT, TT10 and TT16).
- Pulse polio immunization and surveillance of AFP.
- Health check-up of 0–6 years children at Anganwadi and other functions at Anganwadi centres.
- Registration of births, deaths, marriages, and pregnancies.
- Integrated diseases surveillance besides outbreak reporting and response and monitoring of water quality.
- Training of traditional birth attendants and ASHAs.
- Health and nutrition, education (behaviour change communication)/counselling.
- Inter-sectoral coordination with school teachers, Anganwadi workers, Gramsevikas and Panchayati Raj Institutions (PRIs) for community needs assessment under RCH and preparation of sub-centre action plans.
- Periodical activities like—intensive drives for family health awareness campaigns, special surveys, observe universal precautions to prevent infections.
- Preparation of monthly progress reports and holding sector meeting with AWW once a month.
- Promotion of sanitation and use of toilets and water quality monitoring.
- Establish DOT Centre and services for other National Health Programmes.
- Record keeping and reporting.

With the introduction of RCH programme and community needs assessment approach (CNAA), the functions and spectrum of services at sub-centre have been enlarged. Newer areas like adolescent health, RTI/STI including HIV/AIDS, universal practices, safe injections are additional components of services. More emphasis is now on quality of services and client satisfaction.

2. Other Services

Adolescent health and counselling, referral of suspected TB cases and cataract cases to PHC/CHC, besides opportunistic screening and education about prevention of cancers and other non-communicable diseases. 153655 sub-centres were functioning as on March, 2015 against the requirement of 179240 (20% short fall). As the population has increased, we require additional sub-centres.

Work Plan at Sub-centre

The MPHW(F) prepares her fixed work schedule for covering total population of sub-centre and to hold clinics at subcertre and outreach activities (home visits schedule) for contacting eligible beneficiaries for services, surveillance of diseases and community need assessment besides preparation of sub-centre action plan (see sub-centre action plan).

Sub-centre Team

The sub centre team consists of health workers (male and female), trained birth attendants, Anganwadi workers, health guides, voluntary worker and one female link worker (ASHA) in each village besides one more ANM under NRHM. In addition, village Chowkidar who collects events of births and deaths is also helpful to sub-centre team.

There are large number of vacancies (over 63%) in the posts of male multipurpose health workers (MPHW) whose salaries are borne by the State Government. Only 56464 male health workers are available against the required strength of 151684 (63% shortfall).

The functioning of sub-centres is critical component in delivery of primary health care services at the village level. The success of *all national health programmes depend largely on the well-functioning sub-centres providing services* of *acceptable standards to the people*. The NRHM has laid down "Indian public health standards for sub-centres" (IPHS) in terms of assured services, buildings, equipment, material, drugs and job functions to enhance the quality of maternal and child health services in rural areas.

Supervision and Support

The sub-centre health workers (male and female) are supervised by health assistant male and female. One supervisor provides supportive supervision to 6 sub-centres. The major role of supervisor is to ensure supplies—vaccines, contraceptives and drug kits (A and B), support service delivery and helps worker to plan and implement the work schedule and on the job training to improve the skills of workers. Medical officer of PHC is also required to supervise the sub-centre team at least once a month, to ensure preparation of sub-centre action plan and community consultation and coverage of area for services.

Even though the sub-centre/population norms at the national level have been met, there are wide-inter-state variations. States with poor health indices do not have the required number of sub-centres especially in remote areas. The Government of India has decided to fund (pay salary of all the ANMs lady health visitors, and supply drug kits, equipment and contingency) all the 1.45 lakh sub-centres in the country from 1.4.2002 onwards. The state will in return take over the funding of the staff of rural family welfare and postpartum centres.

Sub-centre report: Monthly report on single reporting format plus IDSP report on form 'S' are sent to PHC.

PRIMARY HEALTH CENTRE (PHC) TWO-TIER OF PRIMARY HEALTH CARE

Health survey and development committee popularly known as Bhore committee gave the concept of Primary Health Centre (PHC) way back in 1946. One PHC was recommended for 40,000 rural population in short-term perspective and for 10,000 to 20,000 population in the long run. PHCs were designed to provide **comprehensive primary health care**—including promotive, preventive and curative health services to rural population. Now each PHC covers 30,000 population in plain rural area and 20,000 in tribal, hilly, desert and difficult areas. The PHC and Sub-centre should not be set up on rigid population norms, it should be accessible using "time to care" approach, within 30 minutes of travel time. At this level of primary health care—services of professionally qualified medical officer, male and/or lady medical officer are available. These PHCs are established and maintained by the state governments under the minimum needs programme (MNP), and basic minimum service programme (BMSP). PHCs are primarily state funded. One PHC acts as a referral unit for 6 sub-centres. Each PHC has 4–6 indoor observation beds, it has operation theatre complex and a labour room.[8] The staff of new primary health centre is as under; besides additional staff under NRHM to improve quality of services and 24 hours services.

Organization: Staffing Pattern PHCs Come Under CHC for Supervision

PHCs are manned by medical officers nursing professionals, pharmacist and other support staff. The staffing pattern of the existing PHC and as recommended under NRHM, (Indian Public Health Standards) is shown in Table 15.3.

Buildings, Equipment and Essential Drugs

The state government is responsible for buildings of PHCs and most of the PHCs (90%) are in Government buildings. The medical officer and the staff seldom stay at PHC hence not available for emergency care and emergency obstetric care or deliveries. The vehicle at new PHCs is not available which becomes a limiting factor for mobility and to carry out effective supervision of sub-centres and to provide essential support at village level. The drugs and equipment supplied to PHCs are minimal which compels people to utilize private sector for medical care. National Rural Health Mission (2005) intends to supply essential drugs and equipment to all the PHCs in phased manner with focus on 18 states.

Table 15.3: Staffing pattern of new PHC

Category	*Existing*	*Recommended under NRHM 2007 (IPHS)***
Medical officer	1	3*
AYUSH practitioner	0	1
Accounts manager	0	1
Health assistant male	1	1
Health assistant female (LHV)	1	1
Health educator	1	1
Health worker female	1	1
Nurse midwives (staff nurses)	1+2 (on contract basis)	5
Pharmacists	1	2
Lab. technician	1	2
Clerks (information assistant)	2	2
Driver	1	1
Class IV	4	4
Total staff (excluding contractual)	15	25

* At least one lady medical officer; ** Indian Public Health Standards.

Functions of PHC

PHCs are cornerstone of rural health services—a first port of call to a qualified doctor of public health sector in rural areas for the sick and those who directly report or referred from sub-centres for curative, preventive and promotive health care. Functions of PHC are given below.

A. Technical Functions (Clinical Functions)

1. Medical care: Medical care consists of curative services through routine outdoor, indoor and 24 hours emergency services for patient. Outdoor services—4 hours in the morning and 2 hours in the evening/afternoon with minimum OPD attendance of 40 patients per day. PHC provides referral medical care services to all its sub-centres.
2. Monitoring and supervision of sub-centres.
3. Arrange referral transport
4. Maternal and Child Health services including family planning—essential obstetric and initial emergency obstetric services and 24-hour delivery services both normal and assisted.
5. MTP (Medical Termination of Pregnancy).
6. Management of Reproductive Tract/Sexually Transmitted Infection (RTI and STI).
7. Essential newborn care
8. Integrated management of Neonatal and Childhood Illness (IMNCI).
9. Specific nutrients to women and children.
10. School health
11. Adolescent health
12. Promotion of safe drinking water and basic sanitation.
13. Prevention and control of locally endemic diseases like malaria, kala-azar and Japanese encephalitis.
14. Integrated diseases surveillance and control of epidemics/outbreaks.
15. Collection and reporting of vital events.
16. Behaviour Change Com-munication to Promote Healthy Behaviour.
17. Training and continuing education of staff
18. Dental health services in some states.
19. Services for all National Health Programmes of Communicable and Non-communicable Diseases.
20. Basic laboratory services
21. Mainstreaming AYUSH services as per local people preference.

B. Managerial Functions

Medical officer is the leader of health team at the PHC. He is responsible for *planning* (sub-centre action plans and PHCs plans), *organizing*, *implementation*, *coordination, decision making monitoring* and *supervision* as also evaluation of services, *personnel management*, reaching material and supply to *sub-centres*, *training* and *continuing education* of *health teams*, *financial management* and *ensuring inter-* and *intra-sectoral coordination* and also *reporting* the performance to higher level, i.e. community health centre. Holding staff meetings to get information and give information to staff and also to solve their problems. Planning of work in sector or monthly meeting with AWWs and health workers and their supervisors is also an essential function. Thus, the medical officer is not only a doctor to provide curative, preventive and promotive services, but he is a manager as well to perform essential managerial tasks as listed above apart from leadership role. Above all, challenging management task under NRHM is to utilize the budget for improving quality of services and functions of PHC. *Functioning of PHC is critical to implement all the national health programmes in rural areas* as also to support referral services.

Against the requirement of 29337 PHCs, by 2015 March, 25308 PHCs have been set up (shortfall of 23%).[12,13] There are no functional PHCs in many remote areas in dire need of health care. As of now 90% of the PHCs are running in government buildings. Majority of PHCs lack essential infrastructure and inputs. *Essential drugs* for the treatment of common ailments are not available in majority of PHCs. No more than one-third of PHCs provided delivery services in them and on an average 26 deliveries occurred in the last 3 months. Thus, the PHCs are functioning suboptimally.

Every PHC now have a *Rogi Kalyan Samiti*/Primary Health Centre's Management Committee for improvement of the management and service provision at the PHC. This committee have the power to generate its own funds and utilize the same for service improvement of the PHC besides monitoring the functions of PHC.

Strengthening of PHCs under NRHM

i PHCs have been strengthened by regular supplies of essential drugs and equipment.

ii Round the clock services (24 × 7) in all PHCs of the country, in phased manner.

iii Upgrading single doctor PHC to 3 doctors PHC by posting AYUSH practitioners at PHC level and 3 staff nurses.

iv Observing standard treatment protocols and Indian Public Health Standards (IPHS).

v Untied grant of Rs. 25,000 for local health planning and action and maintenance grant of Rs. 50,000 per annum has been provided to support essential services and programmes, as also physical infrastructure.

vi PHCs are proposed to be transfered to the local elected Panchayati Raj institutions for management and control. *Rogi Klyan Samiti* (RKS) has been constituted at each PHC to increase community control and participation.

vii Citizen charterat PHC—services and rights of citizens.

COMMUNITY HEALTH CENTRE (CHC) THREE-TIER OF PHC

The Primary Health Care infrastructure has been developed as three tier system with Sub-centre, Primary Health Centre (PHC) and Community Health Centre (CHC) being three pillars of Primary Health Care system.

The CHCs were established and maintained by the State Government under minimum needs programme/basic minimum service programme for rural population.

The CHC were designed to **provide referral health care** for cases from primary health centres level and for cases in need of **specialist care approaching** the centre directly. A CHC is referral centre for four Primary Health Centres. A CHC is responsible, for 1,20,000 population in plain and 80,000 in tribal area. Generally it covers the population of One Community Development Block geographical area. By March 2015 nation could establish 5396 CHCs against the requirement of 7322 (shortfall of 32%). CHC is a 30 beded hospital providing specialist care in Medicine, Obstetrics and Gynaecology, Surgery and Pediatrics. It has facility of labour room, operation theatre, X-ray and laboratory. It provides **emergency obstetric care** besides specialist services.

Manpower: Trained and competent human capital is the foundation of an effective health system. Each CHC is manned by four Qualified or specially trained medical specialists namely—surgeon, physician, obstetrician and gynecologist, pediatrician, supported by paramedical and other staff.

Indian Public Health Standards (IPHS) lays down that a CHC is to be managed by six Medical Specialists, including one anesthetist and one Public Health Manager on contract basis. One eye specialist for five CHCs has been provided, besides general duty medical officers and additional staff nurses (Table 15.4).[12, 13]

The seniormost specialist has been designated as Block Health Officer and made responsible for overall administration/management of CHC. The National Rural Health Mission (NRHM) envisages bringing up the CHC services to the level of Indian Public Health Standards (IPHS) to achieve and maintain acceptable standard of quality of care and to provide optimal specialist care to community. Accordingly the standards for manpower, equipments, drugs and buildings have been prescribed for assured services. These standards would help monitor and improve the functioning of CHCs.

The revised manpower for CHC as per IPHS is depicted in Table 15.4. Standard treatment protocols for all national health programmes and locally common diseases have been made available at all CHCs. Standard Treatment Protocols is the "Heart" of quality and cost of care. All the support services (Lab, Transport, Nursing, Diet, CSSD, Laundry and Blood Storage) have been strengthened at the CHC level. The IPHS for CHC have been projected on the basis of assumption that there will be average bed occupancy of 60%. The strength may be further increased if the occupancy increases. Distressingly there is considerable shortfall (81.2%) of specialists at the level of CHCs in India and occupancy of beds is low in most situations. Some of the CHCs have been upgraded to the level of first referral units (FRUs) by providing blood transfusion service and a part time/on contract basis services of an anesthetist. A majority of the CHCs do not function as FRUs because they either do not have any specialist or the posted specialists are not from the specified specialities.

- To fill the gap of specialists, multiskilling of doctors by offering short courses to doctors in lifesaving anaesthetic skills, and obstetric skills are being offered. Due to shortage of manpower at CHC, doctors of primary health centres are being located at CHCs on shift duties after attending to routine OPD duties at primary health centre, in order to provide round the clock clinical services.
- A microscopy centre has been established at each CHC for diagnosis of sputum smear positive cases of tuberculosis.
- *Citizen's Charter for CHCs:* All CHCs now have the Charter of Citizen's Health Rights and entitlements prominently displayed at the entrance. It enables the citizens to know the availability of services at CHC, their rights and entitlement.

Assured Services/Functions of CHC—Clinical Functions

- All "Assured Services" as envisaged in the CHC should be available, which include—routine and emergency care in Surgery, Medicine, Obstetrics and Gynaecology and Pediatrics, in addition to services for the National Health Programmes.
- To provide specialist services and referral services to four Primary Health Centres area.
- 24-hour delivery services (normal and assisted delivery).
- Provides essential and emergency obstetric care including caesarean section.
- Full range of family planning services including laparoscopic service and no scalpel vasectomy.
- RTI/STI services and ICTC for HIV/AIDS.
- Medical Termination of pregnancy (safe abortion services).

Table 15.4: Staffing pattern of CHC

Category	*Existing*	*As Per IPHS (NRHM) 2007*
Medical specialists	4*	Specialists—6 (General Surgeon, Physician, Obstetrician and Gynaecologist, Pediatrician, Anaesthetist and Public Health Manager)
Dental Surgeon	0	1
Eye Surgeon	0	1 For every 5 CHCs
General Duty Medical Officers	0	6 (with at least 2 lady MOs)
Specialist of AYUSH	0	1
GDMO of AYUSH	0	1
Nurse Midwives (Staff Nurses)	7	19 (Staff Nurses)**
Public Health Nurse (LHV)	0	1
ANM	0	1
Block Extension Educator	1	0
Pharmacist	1	3
Radiographer	1	2
Pharmacist AYUSH	0	1
Lab Technician	1	3
Ophthalmic Assistant	0	1
Dressers	1	2
Accountant	1	1
Registration Clerks	0	2
Computer/Statistical /Oblique/information Asst	1	2
OT. Technician	0	1
Driver	1	1
Others (Ward boy, Dhobi, Sweepers, etc.)	10	25

* Either qualified or especially trained to work as surgeon, obstetrician, physician, paediatrician. One of the existing medical officers similarly, should be either qualified or specially trained in public health.

** For providing round the clock service at operation theatre, labour room, casualty, male and female ward and provision of leave reserve.

- Newborn care (Newborn Care Stabilizing Unit)
- Routine and emergency care of sick children
- School health services/Adolescent health.
- Referral transport services—Round the clock
- Cold chain maintenance for vaccines
- Designated microscopy centre for TB.
- Essential laboratory and X-ray services
- Indoor (admission) services
- Dental health services
- Blood storage facility
- Training and continuing education of health teams
- Integrated disease surveillance and control of outbreaks
- Ensure inter-sectoral convergence
- To elicit community participation
- To enhance public–private partnership
- Services for National Health Programmes

Strengthening of CHCs under NRHM

- National Rural Health Mission (NRHM) aims at operationalization of all existing CHCs as 24 hours first referral units (FRUs).
- Opening up of additional CHCs to meet population norms.
- Two specialists namely anaesthetist and public health programme manger have been provided on contractual basis.
- Provision of Untied money ₹ 50,000 per annum for local health actions.
- Provision of maintenance grant of Rs. 1 lakh per year.
- Adoption of Indian Public Health Standard for CHCs. Initial funds of ₹ 20 lakh per CHC provided for its upgradation to achieve Indian Public Health Standards.
- *Rogi Kalyan Samiti* for every CHC for accountability ownership and monitoring of functions of CHC.
- Multiskilling of Doctors to close specialists gap.
- Public–private partnership to close specialists gap.

First Referral Unit (FRU) or Comprehensive Emergency Obstetric and Neonatal Care Centre

Essential requirement of fully operational first referral unit (FRU) are:

An existing facility (CHC, or sub-district hospital) can be declared a fully operational FRU only if it is equipped to provide round the clock services for comprehensive emergency obstetric and newborn care **(CEmONC)**, in addition to all following:

- 24 hours delivery services including normal and assisted deliveries.
- Emergency obstetric care including surgical interventions like caesarean sections* and other medical interventions
- Newborn care* (Newborn Care Stabilization Unit).
- Emergency care of sick children.
- Full range of family planning services including laparoscopic services.
- Safe abortion services.
- Treatment of STI/RTI.
- Blood storage facility*.
- Essential laboratory services.
- Referral transport services.

The foundation of FRUs was laid in the country by Child Survival and Safe Motherhood Programme (CSSM).

*Critical determinants of functionality.

Purpose: Purpose of FRU is to reduce/prevent maternal and neonatal deaths.

Managerial Functions at CHC

CHC, which is responsible for 1,20,000 population, has 40–60 skilled and trained technical staff in 20–25 rural sub-centres, in addition to health guides, trained birth attendants, ASHAs and over 100 Anganwadi workers and their supervisors under ICDS programme, who are responsible for women and child development. Thus, the senior medical officer I/C of CHC is endowed with large resources of manpower at CHC, besides funds from NRHM.

His job functions and responsibilities fall into the broad areas of curative, preventive, promotive and managerial tasks.

1 He is first and foremost ***manager*** of extensive resources available at his command; both manpower and material, which is a major means of reaching 1,20,000 population under his care. The managerial tasks consist of providing effective leadership to health teams, planning of health services (community needs assessment) of all Sub-centres, PHCs and the CHC, organizing, finding out community resources, implementation action plans, decision making supervision, monitoring, coordination of teams, inter-sectoral coordination, and eliciting community participation.
2 ***Trainer for continuing education:*** In view of large number of para-professional personnel under his control/charge, he is responsible for continuing education and training, monitoring, motivation and progressive improvement of technical skills of his teams, in order to improve the quality of services and client satisfaction.
3 ***Clinical care:*** He is a clinician whose decision is critical in the care of sick/patients and the decision in their management, either by him or his delegates.
4 He is responsible to the ***communities*** (1,20,000 people). In short, the SMO of CHC is a leader of large team of personnel and is responsible both to his team and to the communities they serve.

It is widely recognized that the managerial functions of the CHC and PHC are badly neglected and doctors are generally not adequately prepared and are seldom interested in management functions.

Thus, medical doctors (SMO and MO) are key facilitating figures in the national strategy of 'Health in all'. The health system is adequately designed to provide comprehensive, high coverage of promotive, preventive and curative services throughout India. A large trained staff of workers with tasks appropriately defined to meet the major public health needs of the rural poor is in place. There remains a question of motivated *leadership* of each health team their continued education, supervision, motivation is essential if the potential is to be fulfilled. Most medical officers are unwilling to assume this role. Wherever this *leadership* is good, the results are dramatic in improvement in health of poor rural population in India.

Supervision and Support to CHC

The CHCs are linked to district health organization for supportive supervision and referral services. CHCs refer cases to district hospitals and district health organization helps support mass camps and campaigns at CHC level including training activities. District programme officers periodically visit CHC for supervision and support. Each CHC reports its performance to Chief Medical Officer.

Accessibility of Primary Health Care

Instead of population norms "time to care" approach should be followed. A travel time of 30 minutes to reach a primary health care facility and a total of 2 hours to reach FRU could be a reasonable goal or secondary care should be distributed such that within what is known as the golden hour—a secondary care facility can be accessed.

National Mobile Medical Units/Health Camps

With the objective to take health care to the door step of the public in the rural areas, especially in under-served areas, national mobile medical units (MMMUs) have been provided, one per district under NMMUs. The states can adopt more suitable and sustainable model for the MMU to suit their local requirements.

Two kinds of MMUs are envisaged, one with diagnostic facility for the states other than North-East states, Himachal Pradesh and J & K. In addition, for the North-East states, Himachal Pradesh and J & K, specialized facilities and services such as X-ray, ECG and ultrasound are provided in MMMUs due to their difficult hilly terrain. District health society will decide the operation of MMUs locally.

Functioning of Primary Health Care System—(SCs, PHCs and CHCs)

- The system of primary health care functions at sub-optimal level because of poor leadership and poor management.
- Absence of health care providers particularly of doctors and other care givers (43 percent).
- Poor accessibility of facilities to difficult areas and underserved poor people.
- Utilization of facilities is poor—no more than 20–30% of people utilize the primary health care system and many turn to private practitioners.
- Equipment and medicines are in short supply.
- *Panchayati Raj* institutions have been marginally involved in the system. Community participation lacks.
- Most of CHCs do not function as first referral units.
- Lack of integration of services.
- Referral support system is very poor.
- Indoor beds at PHCs and CHCs remain under-utilized (occupancy rate is low).

URBAN PRIMARY HEALTH CARE SERVICES

Nearly 31% of India's population lives in urban areas and half of this population lives in urban slums, which have subhuman living conditions.

Over 75% of dispensaries, 60% of hospitals, 80% of doctors and para-professionals are in urban areas. Urban population is most aware and has ready access to health care. Data from SRS, NFHS and other surveys indicate that the health indices of urban areas are better than those in rural population. A large number of private practitioners, nursing homes, hospitals, specialists and super-specialists are available in urban areas, besides NGOs and religious organizations, yet the urban poor have poor access to health care. Thus, there is "Poverty in Plenty" in urban slums in terms of primary health care. WHO Choice of Theme of World Health Day on 7th April 2010: "Urban Health Matters" was most timely.

Migration

Migration has resulted in rapid unplanned growth of urban slums. The slum population faces greater health hazards due to overcrowding, poor sanitation, lack of access to safe drinking water and environmental pollution. Health indices of urban slums dwellers in some areas are worse than those of rural population.

Unlike the *three-tier rural health services* there have been no efforts to provide well-planned and organized primary, secondary and tertiary care services in geographically delineated urban slum areas. As a result in many areas, primary health care facilities are not available.

Urban Family Welfare Centres (UFWC)

The scheme of UFWC was launched during the first Five-Year Plan and subsequently expanded and established in a phased manner. At present 1083 UFWC are functioning in various states and providing outreach services, primary health care, Maternal and Child Health Services and distribution of contraceptives. There are three types of

UFWC, i.e. I, II and III, depending on the population size covered by these centres, i.e. Type I covers a population of 10,000 to 25,000, Type II covers 25,000 to 50,000 and Type III covers 50,000 or more population. Type I and Type II centres are manned by 2 and 4 paramedical staff respectively and Type III centres are manned by one Medical Officer (Preferably Female) and 4 paramedical staff (LHV, ANM, Family Planning field worker and a storekeeper-cum clerk). The service delivery in these centres tends to be irregular and patchy and most of these centres are not located in slum areas.

In order to remedy existing situation and to improve the outreach of Primary Health Care, Family Planning and Maternal and Child Heath Services in urban slums, the urban Revamping Scheme for Family Welfare was evolved by Krishnan Committee in 1983. This committee recommended that no new UFWC are to be set up. The existing centres shall be reorganized into Urban Health Posts gradually as and when these cities are considered for revamping. The committee recommended four types of health posts for urban slums as elaborated below:

Urban-Revamping—Urban Health Posts (UHPs)

The health posts are to be located mainly in slum areas or in their vicinity. The services provided are mainly outreach RCH services, first aid and referral services. These UHPs are of four types—A, B, C and D depending upon the population size to be covered.

Type A covers less than 5,000 population with one Nurse Midwife.

Type B covers 5,000–10,000 population with two health workers.

Type C covers 10,000–25,000 with four health workers.

Type D covers 25,000–50,000 slum population with one lady doctor, 6–8 health workers, 2 support staff and one voluntary woman for 2,000 population. If population of the area is more than 50,000 then it is to be divided into sectors of 50,000 populations and health posts provided.

Types A to C health posts were attached to a hospital for referral and supervisory services. Type D health post was to be attached to a hospital for sterilization, MTP and referral services. At present 871 UHPs are functioning. Evaluation of Health Posts conducted by NIHFW indicated that many of these posts were not located in urban slums.

Functions: Their main function is to provide integrated maternal and child health services in addition to primary health care to the assigned population. Services include—education, family planning, immunization, antenatal care, postnatal and infant care, services for national health and disease control programmes, contraceptives, and limited curative services. For the purpose of providing MTP and sterilization services the cases will be referred to adjacent hospital.[14,15]

NATIONAL URBAN HEALTH MISSION (NUHM)

Rapid urbanization has led to rapid increase in number of urban poor-population; majority of them live in slums. The need for improving the health care for the urban poor has been recognized as "thrust area" by the National Health Policy (2002), the National Population Policy (2000), Eleventh Five-Year Plan and RCH-2. Urban poor have been recognized as "vulnerable and underserved communities" in RCH-2. The challenges: These are—rapid urbanization, degraded environmental conditions, poor health indicators of urban poor population, inadequate and sub-optimal functioning of urban primary health infrastructure, overcrowding at secondary level, multiplicity of service providers with weak or almost missing coordination, sub-optimal utilization of the strength of private and charitable service providers and weak community capacity. All these indicate imperative need of different strategies.[16]

NUHM was set up in January 2008. The NUHM aims to address essential primary health care needs of urban poor in 779 cities with population of 50000 and above in all the districts and state headquarters with active involvement of Urban Local Bodies (ULB). The NUHM would be covering 375 million urban population with a special focus on 76.6 million urban poor living in slums and beyond spread over in 779 cities.

The existing Urban Health Posts and Urban Family Welfare Centres, Urban RCH centres, etc. will be strengthened and upgraded as Urban Primary Health Centres (U-PHCs).

Focus of National Urban Health Mission (NUHM-2013): The NUHM would have high focus on:

- Urban poor population living in listed and unlisted slums
- All other vulnerable population as homeless, rag pickers, street children, rikshaw pullers, construction and brick and lime kiln workers, sex workers and other temporary migrants
- Public health thrust on sanitation, clean drinking water and vector control
- Strengthening of public health capacities of urban local bodies (Municipal Corporations, Municipalities, Notified area committees.

Aim

The NUHM aims to improve the health status of urban population in general, but particularly of the poor and other disadvantaged sections.

Service Delivery System Core Strategies

i **Public–Private partnerships** i.e. with private service providers or with NGOs or faith based organizations

ii **Through public-public partnership** i.e. partnership with Railways Hospitals, Employee State Insurance Corporations and Public sector companies Hospitals.

An optimal mix of these strategies is desirable. With the launch of NUHM the existing urban health posts/urban family weafare centres/dispensaries would cease to exist and these will be strengthened and revamped into an "Urban Primary Health Centre". The National Urban Health service delivery model would make a concerted effort to rationalize and strengthen the existing public health system through various partnerships as per core strategies. The components for urban health service delivery model is shown in Fig. 15.1.

URBAN PRIMARY HEALTH CENTRE (UPHC) MODEL

The urban health delivery model basically comprises an Urban Primary Health Centre for provision of primiary health care with outreach and referral linkages as described below.

Components of Urban PHC Model

Community Level

i Each slum/community would have frontline community worker called Urban Accredited Social Health Activist (U-ASHA) similar to ASHA under NRHM, covering about 1000 to 2500 population, of 200–500 househlds based on spatial considerations preferably co-located at the Anganwadi Centre functional at the slum level. U-ASHA will be a link between the UPHC and the urban slum community to generate demand for services and behaviour change communication to promote healthy practices and help ANMs in delivering outreach services. ASHAs will be provided with photo ID cards to boost her self esteem. U-ASHA will be entitled for performance based incentive fixed by states. U-ASHA will perform 5 major activities–Home visits up to 2 hours per day, attend monthly Health Sanitation and Nutrition day, Accompany pregnant women and children to urban health centre, holding ward level meeting and record keeping.

ii Mahila Arogya Samiti (MAS): MAS is a women's health committee of 10–12 members for 50–100 urban slum household having population between 250 and 500. The MAS acts as a community group, gets involved in generating community awareness through interpersonal communication, undertakes community based monitoring and promotes linkage with services and referrals. MAS elects its chairperson and a treasure, supported by an U-ASHA to manage revolving fund. Annual grant of ₹ 5000 to each MAS every year will be provided for conducting fortnightly/monthly meetings of MAS. Capacity of MAS would be built by orientation workshops.

iii Outreach session by ANM for slum dwellers vulnerable population:

a The purpose of outreach session is to provide preventive, promotive healthcare services at houshold level by regular visits and outreach sessions. Each ANM will organize minimum of one routine otureach session in her area every month (monthly health, sanitation and nutrition day).

b Special outreach sessions (for slum and other vulnerable population) once a weak in partnership with other health professionals (doctors/pharmcist/technician/nurses—government or private) at the community level.

It will include screening and follow up, basic lab investigations, drug dispensing and counseling. For

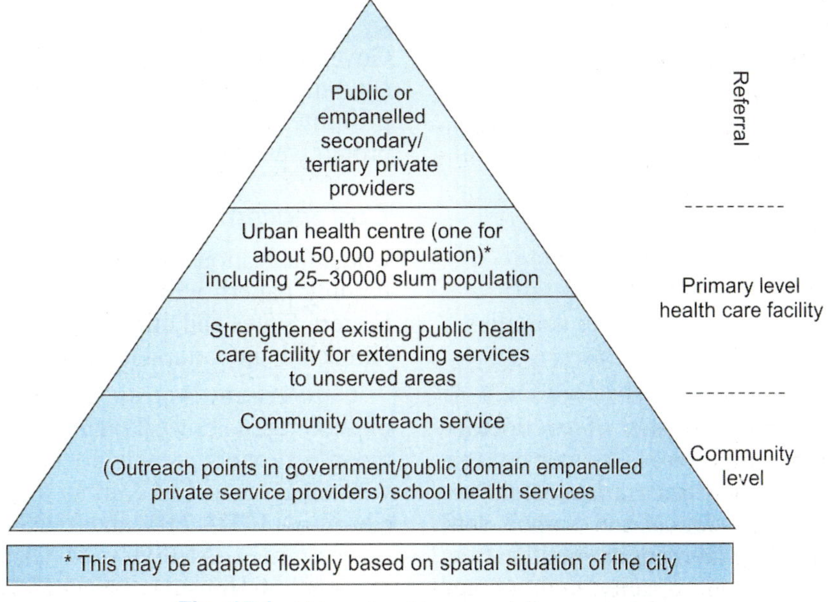

Fig. 15.1: Urban health care delivery model

15

improving routine outreach services ANM will be provided with mobility support of ₹ 500 per month. 4–5 ANMs are posted in one U-PHC and each ANM covers around 10,000 population.

Population covered by UPHC: Each U-PHC functions for a population of 50000–60000, located preferably within a slum or near a slum within half kilometer radius, catering to slum population of approximately 25000–30000 with provision for OPD from 12 noon to 8 pm in the evening. The cities based upon the local situation may establish a U-PHC for 75000 for areas with very high density and can also establish one for around 5000–10000 slum population for isolated slum clusters. Unlike rural areas, sub-centres have not been established in urban areas. U-PHC will be located in Govt. building.

Beneficiaries of U-PHCs: Primary health care through U-PHCs and Urban CHCs will be universally available to all citizens residing in urban areas; whereas the outreach services will be targeted for slum dwellers and other vulnerable population. Targeting is needed especially for secondary and tertiary care to all. It can be provided free only to those who cannot afford it otherwise. Urban poor will be indentified by household surveys conducted through community organizations/NGOs under supervision of ULB (Urban Local Bodies).

Services

At the UPHC level the services provided will include OPD (consultantion), basic laboratory diagnosis, drugs/ contraceptives apart from distribution of health education material and counseling for all communicable and non-communicable diseases.

In order to improve access to urban slum population at convenient timings, the UPHC may provide services from 12 noon to 8 pm in the evening. It will not include in-patient care. Broadly the services include:

- Medical care: OPD services
- Services prescribed under RCH-II
- National health programmes services
- Collection and reporting of vital events and IDSP
- Referral services
- Basic Laboratory services
- Counseling services
- Services for non-communicable diseases
- Social mobilization and community level activities

Staffing Pattern

UPHC will be staffed by contractual staff of two doctors, one regular and one on part-time basis. Apart from that there will be 3 staff nurses, 1 pharmacist, 1 lab technician, 1 LHV and 4–5 ANMs as also clerical and support staff and one manager for supporting community mobilization; behaviour change communication, capacity building and strengthening of referrals.

To further strengthen the delivery of services, UPHC can also engage the services of specialist doctors to provide services periodically at U-PHC based on needs on re-imbursement basis.

The government facilities strengthened as U-PHC will also be provided annual financial support in the form of Rogi Kalyan Samiti/Hospital Management Committee Fund of ₹ 50,000 per U-PHC per year. The recurrent cost support provided to U-PHCs of ₹ 20 lakh per year would include cost of all contractual staff.

Referral Unit

Urban Community Health Centre (U-CHC) may be set up as a satellite hospital for every 4–5 U-PHCs to support UPHC for referral specialist services. The U-CHC would cover a population of 250000. It would provide inpatient services and would be 30–50 beded facility. U-CHCs would ;be set up in cities with a population of above 5 lakhs wherever required. These facilities would be in addition to the existing health facilities (District hospital and Sub-district hospital).

For metro cities, the U-CHCs may be established for every 5 lakh population with 100 beds. Indian Public Health Standards will be observed for UPHCs and U-CHCs.

Referral Linkages

The existing hospitals including urban local body maternity homes, state government hospitals and medical colleges, apart from private hospitals will be empanelled/accredited to act as referral points for different types of health, diabetes, trauma care, orthopaedic, dental surgeries, mental health, critical illness, deafness control, cancer management, tobacco counseling, cessation, etc.

School Health Services (SHS)

In urban areas, the scheme of SHS would cover Government and Private schools located in slums (U-PHC catchment area) or government schools near slums to promote healthy lifestyles and other preventive and promotive services.

Cost Sharing

Under the National Urban Health Mission the Centre-State funding pattern will be 60:40 for all states except North Eastern States and other special category States of J & K, Himachal and Uttarakhand where it would be 90:10.

Convergent Action in Urban Areas: Beacuse of multiple agencies working in urban areas, the convergence (coordination) is essential for better outcome. Convergence with other sectors like urban local bodies, department of education, ICDS, HIV and AIDS control, National Health programmes, Ministry of Urban Development and Ministry of Housing, Jawaharlal Nehru National Urban Renewal Mission, Basic services for urban poor, water and sanitation (public health); Rajiv Awas Yojna, Women and Child Development and other stake holders is essential.

Community Participation

The NUHM encourages effective participation of the community in planning and management of health care services. It promotes a community health volunteer: Urban ASHA, or link worker in urban poor settlements, creation of community based institutions like *Mahila Arogya Samiti* (MAS) and *Rogi Kalyan Samitis*.

Planning Process

The urban local bodies become the units of planning with its own approved norms. The District Health Society will function as the coordinating body at the district level for urban health also. NUHM will be implemented through the Health Department in the urban local bodies except in very large Municipal Corporations, which will receive funds from state Health Society.

PRIMARY HEALTH CARE IN TRIBAL AREAS

Tribal people (about 106 million) in India are considered to be socioeconomically the most disadvantaged group. They constitute 8.2% of the country's total population.

National Health Policy 1983, 9th Plan as well as National Population Policy (2000) and RCH-2 have given primacy to tribal areas for primary health care services.

Some of the problems of accessibility and utilization of health services unique to tribal areas are because of difficult terrain and sparsely distributed population in forest and hilly regions. There are locational disadvantage of sub-centres, PHCs and CHCs, non-availability of service providers due to vacant posts and lack of residential facilities, lack of suitable transport facilities for quick referral of emergency cases. Lack of appropriate human resources development and policies to encourage/motivate the service providers to work in tribal areas, inadequate mobilization of NGOs, and lack of integration with other health programmes. IEC activities are not tuned to the tribal vocabulary, beliefs and practices, services not being client-friendly in terms of timings and cultural barriers and non-involvement of local traditional faith healers.

Tribal areas are most vulnerable to falciparum malaria, with problem of drug resistance, tuberculosis, yaws, sickle cell anaemia, thalassaemia and G6PD deficiency. Infant mortality rate is higher in tribal population and only 26% of children receive all vaccines. Sex ratio is better in tribal areas.

The norms for population coverage have been relaxed for tribal areas (Table 15.5). Tribal areas need special attention.

Most of the centrally sponsored disease control programmes have a focus on the tribal areas. Under the National Anti-Malaria Programme (NAMP), 100 identified predominantly tribal districts in Andhra Pradesh, Bihar, Gujarat, Madhya Pradesh, Maharashtra, Odisha and Rajasthan are covered. In spite of all these, the access to and utilization of health care remains suboptimal and health and nutrition indices in the tribal population continue to be poor.

Table 15.5: Norms for tribal areas for primary health care[8]

Institution	*Population covered*
One sub-centre	3000
One PHC	20,000
One CHC	80,000

Some Experiments for Tribal Health

- ***Andhra Pradesh:*** Committed Government functionaries are running health facilities in tribal areas.
- ***Odisha:*** Additional central assistance is provided for mobile health units.
- ***Karnataka and Maharashtra:*** NGOs have adopted and are running PHCs in tribal areas.

The success of all these experiments is mainly due to commitment of individuals and credibility of NGOs which is difficult to replicate.

Essential Drugs and Medicines and Rational use of Drugs

Currently, non-governmental service providers are treating large number of patients at the primary level for major diseases. However, the treatment regimens followed are diverse and not scientifically optimal, leading to an increase in the **incidence of drug resistance.** Such practices need to be curbed by training and by providing adequate information to private practitioners on drug regimens to be followed under national health programmes for major endemic diseases.

Drugs and medicines form a substantial portion (almost 72%) of the out of pocket spending on health by households. Components of drugs and medicines form 10% of the overall health budget. Share of drug expenditure to total household health expenditure is 69%. Over 60,000–80,000 brands of medicines are available in India but only 350 are considered essential or required to meet the needs of majority of population. WHO has its essential list of drugs known as "Model List" of 312 medicines of 2003 has been revised and released in 2011. The Government of India plans to open *Jan Aushadhi*—a country wide chain of 3000 medical stores to make quality generic and other drugs available at reasonable prices. Most states have adopted an essential drugs list for public health system selected from Model List of WHO. Availability of essential drugs in every PHC and CHC will increase people's confidence in public health system and increase utilization of services. The states are promoting:

- Use of generic drugs.
- Rational use of drugs by adopting standard treatment guidelines and prescription audit.
- Use of **Standard Treatment Guidelines:** These have been adopted in the country for National Programmes on Malaria, Tuberculosis, STI/RTI, IMNCI, ARI, AIDS and diarrhoeal diseases control programme. Standard case management protocols are available. Now the central Drug Authority of India has been set-up.

Essential drugs at sub-centres are provided by primary health centre kit A and B. Essentially there are—ORS, cotrimoxazole vit A, IFA tablets, vaccines, contraceptives, mebendazole, chloroquine, paracetomol, methylergometrine and chlorine tablets. National Rural Health Mission supports provision of essential drugs and equipment to all PHCs of 18 high focus states.

Under the National Health Mission—Free Drug Service initiative and free diagnostic service initiative, substantial funding is being provided to state that implement these initiatives.

Cost-Effective Treatment Rules for 40 killer Diseases

With affordable health care out of bounds for commoners the government has decided to issue guidelines on cost effective treatments for top killer diseases. The move involves publishing standard treatment guidelines and best technologies for the management of priority diseases on the line of UK's National Institute for Health and Care Excellence. Fifteen top priority diseases identified include—cancers, cardiovascular diseases, diabetes, TB, malaria, mental disorders, suicides and substance use, diarrhoeal diseases, neurological diseases (including epilepsy, dementia, schizophrenia, HIV/AIDS, dengue and other vector borne diseases, hepatitis, snake and scorpion bites and malnutrition. Patients will be able to make choices about the treatment technologies. Affordable medicines and reliable implants for treatment (AMRIT) stores have been set up.

SECONDARY HEALTH CARE

Health care delivery in India has been envisaged at 3 levels, namely primary, secondary and tertiary levels. The secondary level of health care essentially includes community health centres (CHCs) constituting the first referral units (FRUs) and private hospitals and nursing homes.

The secondary health care is available in FRUs, sub-divisional/sub-district, district hospitals and urban hospitals in government as also in private sector. Strengthening of the sub-divisional/sub-district, and district hospital is an approved activity under NRHM.

The secondary health care infrastructure at the CHC and district hospital, today functions both as primary health care infrastructure for taking care of the needs of the population in the city/town in which it is located and also as secondary care centre. This dual role dilutes its effectiveness.

Purpose of secondary care at district level is to support referral services by establishing linkages between PHC-CHC and district hospitals. There should be two-way flow of patients, specialists, services and records but unfortunately, the referral linkage is absent or very poor. Strengthening of secondary care services was identified as priority area in 9th plan period. In addition to state Government funding, 7 states have taken World Bank loan to initiate projects to build up FRUs/district hospitals.

During the 10th plan period, efforts were made to strengthen the physical infrastructure, functional improvement in terms of patient care, organization of referral linkages between CHCs, district hospitals and tertiary care institutions; improvement in different components of care such as hospital waste management, disease surveillance and rapid response and health management information system and these would continue in 12th plan period and beyond.

Cost

Since the cost of secondary care is going high, operationalization of cost recovery through user charges from people above poverty line has been started. Public–private partnership has also begun. Most of secondary care is made available in district through private sector, which includes nursing homes, private hospitals and private practitioners, charitable hospitals, dispensaries and Non-Governmental Organizations.

District Health Plan and District Health Organization

Under National Rural Health Mission (NRHM), district becomes core unit of planning, budgeting and implementation of health services. All vertical health and family welfare programmes at the district and state level merge into common "district health mission" at the district level and the "state health mission" at state level. Progressively the district health mission to move towards paying hospital for services by way of reimbursement, on the principle of "money follows the patient". The services will be standardized as per Indian public health standards. Hospital Management Committee/*Rogi Kalyan Samiti* for community management of public hospitals has been setup. Public–private partnership for secondary and tertiary care have been promoted. Annual health survey data of 2010–11 can be used for district planning.

National Rural Health Mission has allocated grant to upgrade district hospital services as per Indian public health standards. Besides efficient ambulance services, this step will improve secondary health care at district level.

District Health Organization

Civil Surgeon/Chief Medical officer is the leader of health organization at districl level. Several programme officers/

health programme managers work under him for implementation of various national health programmes in the district. Rapid response teams (RRT) for outbreak investigation and rapid response exist at district level.

TERTIARY HEALTH CARE

Tertiary care is available through medical college hospitals, super-speciality institutions and bigger hospitals set-up by private organizations.

Many state governments are facing resource crunch and have not been able to obtain funds for equipment, maintenance, supply of consumables and upgrading the infrastructure to meet the rapidly growing demand for complex diagnostic and treatment modalities. Therefore, private organizations have taken a lead to set-up big hospitals, in most of metropolitan cities there are reputed institutes providing quality tertiary care at cost beyond the reach of many. The government intends to open up regional institutes on the pattern of All India Institute of Medical Sciences, Delhi, in various parts of the country; these would strengthen the tertiary care services.

User charges from people above poverty line have been the mechanism to recover cost and retain it locally to upgrade the services and infrastructure and to sustain the system of tertiary care.

Some states have provided land, water and electricity at lower cost to private organizations. The private organizations in return hold the responsibility to provide free care to certain proportion of people below poverty line as per agreement with the state Governments (30% inpatient facilities and 40% of the out-patient/diagnostic services).

Tertiary health care services are being strengthened under *Pradhan Mantri Swasthya Suraksha Yojna* (PMSSY). The PMSSY comprises establishment of 6 new AIIMS like institutions and upgradation of 13 medical colleges to the level of AIIMS to correct regional imbalances.

REFERRAL SYSTEM

The referral system is poorly developed in India. Primary health care is three-tier system. It is expected that patients from sub-centres are referred to PHCs and from PHCs to CHCs and from CHCs to district hospital and district hospital to tertiary level of care. It is free for all affair, any one can walk into secondary and tertiary levels of care directly and that increases the load of patients at these levels. The diseases/ailments which can be dealt with at primary health care level are being treated at district and even at higher level of care. An ideal referral system means regionalization of health services (accepting responsibility for health care for a **defined geographical area** and **population**), developing strong linkages between SCs and PHCs; CHCs, district and tertiary level of care, two-way flow of patients, two-way flow of specialists, two-way flow of records, two-way flow of services to avoid duplication of efforts and resources. First referral units (FRUs) have been developed for emergency obstetric and newborn care services but most of FRUs are not functioning well. Referral system needs to be strengthened to support primary health care. Success of integrated management of neonatal and childhood illness (IMNCI) and Integrated Disease Surveillance Project (IDSP) will largely depend upon strong support of referral system. A good referral system could reduce the patient load at secondary and tertiary care levels, apart from saving precious lives. It would also reduce cost and avoid duplication of efforts and time.

The referrals should not be automatic to the next higher level, instead the referring institution should be free to refer the cases to the institution, which in their opinion has the necessary facilities for providing competent services, required by the case (Fig. 15.2).

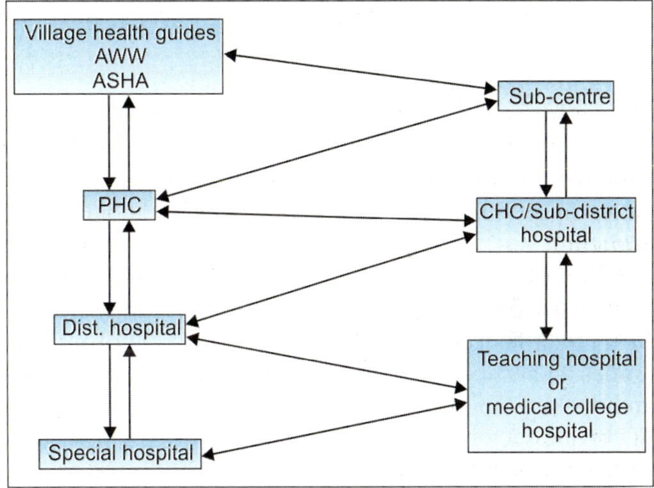

Fig. 15.2: Referral system

PRIVATE HEALTH SECTOR

Over 80% of doctors, 26% of nurses and 49% of beds are available in private sector. The private sector accounts for nearly 80% health expenditure in India. It consists of private practitioners, solo-practitioners, polyclinics, nursing homes, general and speciality hospitals of allopathy system and Indian system of medicine, mostly in urban areas and some in rural areas. Many unqualified practitioners (compounders, RMPs, traditional healers, herbalists faith healers, dais, etc.) are also available in rural and urban areas. The curative services provided by them are of variable quality. Private sector provides around 78% of ambulatory outdoor services and around 60% of indoor patient care.[1] Both rich and poor people seek services from private sector.

Private sector is the dominant provider of curative health care services with substantial share of outpatient treatment and inpatient care, but the quality of care is variable. The regulatory mechanism by the Government can lay standard for service and charges and can involve the private sector in secondary and tertiary care. The private sector/ practitioners can be paid for the services rendered by them. Tertiary care can largely be left to private sector after the regulatory mechanism.

Similarly, private sector can be involved in national health care programmes and primary health care in urban slums on the basis of payment for service by the government, to fill the gap of urban primary health care.

The rural and urban poor of India have limited resources to meet their health needs despite the big network of primary health care services. Most often they have to bear out of pocket expenses (OOP) for various unforeseen situations. These put them into the never ending debt trap. The problem is further aggravated as they resort to medical treatment only when faced with loss of wages due to illness. The preventive and promotive health care is almost nonexistent for them because of their preoccupation in field/labour for daily wage during the working hours of health institutions in the public sector.

Ongoing Partnership between Private and Public Sector[1]—Public-Private Partnership (PPP)

Contracting is the predominant model for PPP in India. Accordingly under this the States are trying contract in, contract out, outsourcing of diagnostic services, management of hospitals facilities by leading NGOs, hiring staff, service delivery including family planning services, MTP, treatment of STI/RTI, etc. Accreditation of nursing homes and hospitals for institutional deliveries under JSY and opening up of new medical colleges with partnership of private sector.

- In most states, Government doctors are allowed private practice and they provide care to patients.
- Contractual appointment of health care personnel and hiring of private-practitioners for providing services in the PHCs; however, the response has been poor.
- Part time hiring of general doctors and specialists to visit and provide health care in PHCs/CHCs in under-served areas. Limited success has been reported in this experiment. Anaesthetists and lady doctors were used on part time basis in FRUs. Involving NGOs and private sector practitioners in the national programmes like leprosy, blindness and HIV/AIDS control programme has been quite encouraging. Indian Medical Association is supporting "Vande Mataram" scheme to provide maternal health services to reduce maternal mortality.
- Private sector—individuals/institutions/industries, e.g. Tata Steel Company, have adopted population for providing services in defined geographical area.
- Private sector—super-speciality, tertiary/secondary care hospitals are given land, water and electricity, etc. at a concessional rate and permission for duty free import of equipment, tax holiday, with the understanding that they will provide 30% of inpatient and 40% of outpatient services to poor patients free of charge.
- Private practitioners provide information for disease surveillance and were involved in pulse polio immunization in a big way.
- State and central Governments, and public service units, reimburse cost of medical services provided by recognized private hospitals.

In the absence of an effective Public Health System most people in India turn first to the private sector for curative care and even poor people are prepared to pay substantial sums for it. Private sector limitations are that it primarily focuses on curative services because that is what the clients are prepared to pay for, that a poorest person cannot always afford services, that quality of services as in the public sector is variable. The private sector accounts for three-quarters of all health expenditure in India. Around 87% of expenditure on health tends to be out of pocket expenditure in India.

Direct consumer education on quality care and cost information could help patients when they seek providers. The public sector should take responsibility to guide private providers on standard regimens of diagnosis and treatment through training programmes to improve their practices. Regulatory mechanism for private sector as proposed in NHP 2002 may be difficult to implement on the ground situation—public–private partnership (PPP) within these limitations can be mobilized for enhancing access to health care. NRHM tries to ensure that more than 70% of the resources are spent through bodies that are managed by people's organizations and at least 10% of resources are spent through grant in—aids to NGOs.

HEALTH INSURANCE

Over the last two decades, several health insurance schemes have been introduced. These are individual, family and group insurance schemes for health care, senior citizens' insurance and insurance for specific disease. Some of the currently operationalized schemes include Mediclaim, Group Medical Insurance Scheme, Group Health Insurance Scheme, *Bhavishya Arogya* (insurance for senior citizens), senior citizen unit plan, Carrier Insurance, *Ashadeep* and *Jan Arogya Bima* Policy.

Development of health care system through health insurance has been in operation in several countries of the world with different mix-ups and results. In India, very recently Insurance Regulatory and Development Authority (IRDA) has been set-up with a stipulation that authority still offers priority to those insurance companies, which take up the health insurance as an exclusive operation. Licences have been given to 15 private companies by now with the condition that these companies will have to market viable health care products. Most of these schemes of insurance subscribe to limited approach of limiting reimbursement of hospitalization charges for medical interventions. The hope and expectations are that the health insurance would lead on to development of "health care system" which provides cover for preventive and public health services besides curative services. The Government has so far covered workers under ESI and central Government employees under CGHS. The health benefits under these schemes are limited to small segment of workforce and Government employees and moreover, these services enjoy heavy Government subsidies. Health insurance system appears to be a shrewd business with heavy investment; the coverage may be limited to urban elites only, who may have abilities to pay premium. The coverage of rural population by insurance is not foreseeable in near future. People in rural area use public health system or private sector with distinct line of choices. Government have opened up avenues for social insurance schemes for urban poor and below poverty line people on experimental basis in few selected districts to begin with (NHP-2002). Private health insurance system has its potential for group coverage and initiate competitions amongst private companies. The Government is to ensure that consumer's interests are protected and premia are regulated and effective monitoring is ensured to regulate quality of services.

Community-based health insurance (CBHI) is emerging as promising concept and existing experience in different states has shown that well-managed pre-payment systems with risk pooling are effective in protecting the poor from impoverishments due to high medical cost during **catastrophic** health events.

Government was able to cover around 12% urban and 13% of rural population under health protection coverage through RSBY or similar plan while 12% of upper class Urban HH were covered by private providers.

Employees State Insurance Scheme (ESIS)

Health insurance means you pay a premium out of your salary or income and get agreed upon services. The Government of India passed Employees State Insurance (ESI) Act in 1948. Under this Act, the employer–employee and the state and central Government contribute and provide specified medical and health care besides social security to the employee.

Focus

The focus of the programme is "employee" and his family. The employees of factories are covered in the scheme and it is primarily urban-based scheme where the factories are located.

Coverage

It covers those factories or institutions, which employ 20 or more persons for wages and 10–19 employees if power is used to run the factory. Under the Act, various factories and institutions are covered.

Benefits

The medical benefits include medical care (outdoor, indoor and emergency services) as also maternity benefits, preventive and promotive and rehabilitative services including family planning services to employees and their families.

Establishment

The ESIS provides services through dispensaries, ESI hospitals and through arrangements of beds in hospitals and services of private practitioners. It has the provision of reimbursing the cost of treatment or provides free medical and health services against the contribution and eligibility of employees.

Rashtriya Swasthya Bima Yojna (RSBY)—Renamed as *Rashtriya Swasthya Suraksha Yojna*

We have a huge working population of about 400 million. Almost 93% of this workforce is in the unorganized sector. RSBY covers unorganized sector.

RSBY introduced in 2007 was designed to meet the health insurance needs of the poor. The RSBY provides "cashless" inpatient treatment for eligible beneficiaries through an insurance based system. Without any bar on age and pre-existing conditions. The RSBY provides for cashless smart card based health insurance cover of ₹ 30,000 per annum to each enrolled family comprising up to five individuals. The beneficiary family pays only ₹ 30 per annum as registration/renewal fee. The scheme covers hospitalization expenditures (outpatient expenses are not covered) including maternity benefit and for enlisted diseases. A transportation cost of ₹ 100/- per visit is also paid. The premium payable to insurance agencies is funded by central and state governments in a 75:25 ratio which is relaxed to 90:10 for the North East region and J & K. The maximum premium is capped at ₹ 750/- per insured family per year.

The RSBY was originally limited to below poverty line (BPL) families but was extended to building and other construction workers, MGNREGA beneficiaries, street vendors, beedi workers and domestic workers. The scheme is being currently implemented in 24 States/UTs. K.ey features of RSBY is that it provides for private health services providers, to be included in the system, if they meet certain standards and agree to provide cashless treatment which is reimbursed to the insurance company. This has the advantage of giving patients a choice between alternative service providers where such alternative are available. Employee State Insurance (ESI) scheme is the nodal agency of RSBY. It is possible to expand the package of services under RSBY into an Essential Health Package (EHP) of Universal Health Coverage (UHC) as proposed under 12th plan period. Criticism of RSBY is that it does not cover outpatient expenses which forms major component of out of pocket expenditure on health by poor people.

Coverage: Government was able to cover around 12% urban and 13% of rural population under health protection coverage through RSBY or similar plan while 12% upper class households were covered by private provides.

A general problem with any "Fee for service" payment system financed by insurance mechanism is that it creates an incentive for unnecessary treatment which raises the cost and premium. The shortcomings of RSBY—lack of coverage of primary health and outpatient care apart from high transport cost. RSBY has been shifted to the Ministry of Health and Family Welfare under NHM.

New Health Protection Scheme 2016

Central government will launch a new scheme to provide ₹ 1 lakh insurance cover to BPL household as 'family floater plan. This scheme may replace RSBY ultimately.

Ex-servicemen Contributory Health Scheme (ECHS)

This scheme is meant for ex-army personnel. They have to contribute as per laid out norms and they are entitled for specified services in lieu of contributions. ECHS was launched with effect from April 1, 2003, with an objective to provide quality medicare to its members and their authorized dependents through 227 ECHS polyclinics (106 in military stations and 121 in non-military stations) across the country and a network of empanelled hospitals/nursing homes and diagnostic centres. The scheme covers 20 lakh ex-servicemen and around 10 million beneficiaries.

Community-based Health Insurance (CBHI)

CBHI is "any not for profit insurance scheme that is aimed primarily at the informal sector and formed on the basis of a collective pooling of health risks and the members participating in its management". Pooling of resources/risk refers to the accumulation of prepaid funds (before the event of illness occurs, allowing the individual to draw out funds as and when the need arises) on behalf of a population. What distinguishes these schemes from public or private for profit insurance scheme is that the targeted community is involved in defining the contribution amount and collection mechanism, content of benefit package, and allocating the scheme financial resources. CBHI schemes in India are very diverse in nature in terms of design, management and size of targeted population. ACCORD, BAIF Karuna Trust, Self Employment Women Association (SEWA), DHAN Foundation and VHS are some examples. During Eleventh Plan, CBHI schemes through the public system and by accredited private providers were encouraged.

CENTRAL GOVERNMENT HEALTH SERVICES (CGHS) SCHEME

15

It is a contributory health scheme. The CGHS was started in 1954 with the objective of providing comprehensive medical care facilities to the central Government employees and their family members. Now besides central Government employees, the scheme also provides services to members and ex-members of parliament, judges of supreme court, high court (sitting and retired), freedom fighters (free of cost); central Government prisoners, employees of certain autonomous bodies/semi Government organizations, accredited journalists and ex-Governors and ex-Vice Presidents of India. The scheme was initially started in Delhi and now extended to 25 cities.

Set-up under CGHS

274 Allopathic dispensaries (now named as wellness centres), 85 AYUSH dispensaries, 34 homeopathic and 9 Unani, 2 Siddha and 3 Yoga dispensaries have been set-up in different parts of the country. In addition to above, 19 polyclinics, 73 laboratories, 74 dental clinics, 2 geriatric clinics and 4 hospitals and 19 postal dispensaries were functioning under CGHS.[16]

Facilities

The facilities of outpatient care and emergency inpatient care, free supply of drugs, lab and radiological investigations, domiciliary visit to seriously ill patients and specialists consultation are being provided to beneficiaries, through the above set up. Recognized private hospitals and diagnostic centres provide specialized treatment and investigation facilities.

There are special facilities for the convenience of pensioners and senior citizens entitled to CGHS. Pensioners can obtain a 'whole life' CGHS card by paying 10 years subscription. Recognized hospitals also provide credit facilities to valid card holder.

Beneficiaries

There are 11.12 lakh card holders and 3.88 million beneficiaries of CGHS. Each beneficiary has to contribute part of pay on regular basis.

RAILWAY HEALTH SERVICES

The organization of railways maintain, 613 dispensaries, health centres and 125 hospitals with 13702 beds for their employees to provide primary, secondary and tertiary level of care. There is comprehensive networking of services.

ARMED FORCES HEALTH SERVICES

Armed forces run well-organized comprehensive health care for their personnel during peace and war situation. The services include preventive, promotive, curative and rehabilitation services through network of military hospitals, military and specialized centres. Military hospitals provide wide range of services for army personnel and their dependents. Well-organized rehabilitation services are in place to provide artificial limbs besides provision of vocational and occupational rehabilitation services.

INDIAN SYSTEM OF MEDICINE OR AYUSH

AYUSH (Ayurveda, Yoga and Naturopathy, Unani, Sidha and Homeopathy). There are over 736538 practitioners of AYUSH all over India. They are also important source of medical care to vast majority of population in rural and urban areas. These Indian systems have established institutions, hospitals and dispensaries for health services. People have faith in concepts and practices of indigenous system of medicine. AYUSH system has been involved in national health care programmes like family planning, malaria; and tuberculosis. They have the potentials to support primary health care in rural and urban slum areas. The Government intends mainstreaming of AYUSH for reproductive and child health programme. This is an additional resource of trained medical manpower in India to support medical care. This potential resource can be used at PHC for 24 hours service as envisaged under National Rural Health Mission 2005. Under NRHM, AYUSH practitioners are co-located in 40% of PHCs, 65% of CHCs and 69% of District Hospitals. International Yoga Day of United Nations was celebrated in India on 21st June 2015 to popularise Yoga in the world. Department of AYUSH has been made ministry of AYUSH.

OTHER SECTORS

NON-GOVERNMENTAL ORGANIZATIONS (NGOs) AND VOLUNTARY SECTOR/AGENCIES

This sector provides services on non-profit basis. They supplement the efforts of Governmental health services. They work in difficult and underserved and unserved areas with voluntary zeal.

Apart from purely private providers of health care, the NGOs and voluntary sector have been providing health care services to community both in urban, rural and tribal areas. It is estimated that more than 7,000 voluntary agencies are involved in health-related activities.

A wide inter-state differential exists in the coverage of villages by NGOs. NGOs providing a variety of services are relatively, unevenly distributed across and within states and have limited area of operation. Some implement Government programmes of the department of family welfare and health, others run integrated or basic health services programme or provide special care/rehabilitation to people suffering from specific diseases, e.g. leprosy patients; blinds and handicapped. Health care activities are also carried out by agencies like the Red-Cross, Industrial establishments, Lion's Club, Helpage India, etc.

The National Rural Health Mission seeks to build greater ownership of the programme among the community through involvement of Non-Governmental Organizations. Promotion of public–private partnership for achieving public health goals is one of the strategy initiated by the department in this regard. This partnership will reinforce the strategy of involvement of NGOs already spelt out in the National Population Policy, 2000.

The Government of India is committed to voluntary and informed choice in family planning, reproductive and child health care services. Towards this end, the government, the corporate sector, voluntary and non-voluntary sector are expected to work together in partnership. The professional bodies like Indian Medical Association, Federation of Obstetricians and Gynaecologists are also involved in the partnership to achieve the desired goal.

PARTNERSHIP WITH NON-GOVERNMENTAL ORGANIZATIONS

The Government of India envisages collaboration with NGOs through enhanced participation by the State Governments also. Under RCH II, the ownership of the program has been decentralized to the State Governments. The planning process now starts from the district level. The scheme has been included in the State PIP for NRHM under RCH II.

NGOs in particular, have been assigned supplementary or complementary role to that of the government health care delivery, thus aiding them in reaching the masses meaningfully. They have a comparative advantage of flexibility in procedures, rapport building with communities and are at the cutting edge of programme implementation. NGOs have been involved in ASHAs' training, activities relating to National Disease Control Programmes, PNDT Act and service delivery in addition to health education and awareness programmes.

New Guidelines

According to the revised guidelines of NGO scheme, the states have been given an important role in selection/approval of the NGOs and overseeing implementation of the projects undertaken by them.

Key Features

These are:

- Decentralization of the schemes to the State and District level.
- Integration with NRHM.
- Training of ASHA.
- Activities relating to various National Disease Control Programmes.
- Awareness relating activities concerning PNDT Act.
- Shift from exclusive IEC and awareness generation to Service Delivery.
- Delivery of RCH services by NGOs in unserved and underserved areas.
- Clearly defined eligibility criteria for Registration, Experience, Assets and Jurisdiction.
- Rationalization of the jurisdiction area serviced by the NGO to provide in-depth service and optimize resources.
- Mainstreaming gender issues in all intervention areas.

- Enhanced male participation and involvement in delivery of all RCH services.
- Emphasis on measurable, qualitative and quantitative performance indicators.
- Selection, approval, funding and monitoring of MNGO/SNGO projects by state and district RCH committees.
- Increased interface of NGOs with local government bodies.

MOTHER NGO (MNGO) SCHEME

The underlying philosophy of the Mother NGO (MNGO) Scheme is one of nurturing and capacity building through partnership. In accordance with the National Population Policy-2000, National Health Policy (NHP)-2002 and 10th plan document that places emphasis on decentralization of program management and RCH service delivery using a gender sensitive approach, the NGO guidelines were revised in accordance with the RCH II approach.

The objectives of the MNGO scheme are to improve RCH indicators in the underserved and unserved areas, with specific focus on MCH, FP, Immunization, Institutional delivery, RTI/STI and adolescent reproductive health care. It is expected that the gender concerns and male involvement will be addressed across all the interventions. Currently, 338 MNGO are working in 450 districts.

The unserved areas specifically include hilly, desert and mountainous regions, SC/ST habitats, urban slums and areas where the government infrastructures are functioning sub-optimally. Under the revised mode, NGOs are expected to facilitate RCH service delivery in addition to addressing the awareness, education and advocacy requirement.

The overall approach has shifted from a *project* to a *program mode* (from one year cycle to 3–5 year cycle). Rationalization of NGO jurisdiction (reducing coverage form 5–8 districts or more to 1–2 only), and each MNGO to work with only 3–4 Field NGOs (FNGOs) from each district, encouraging each MNGO to identify the un-served and underserved pockets within the district, in consultation with District Health Officials, identification of FNGOs from the same pockets to serve population covering 1–2 subcenters in the provision of RCH service delivery related to NRHM, FP, Immunization, MCH and access to institutional delivery. RTI/STI, adolescent reproductive health care implementation are the salient features.

Service NGO (SNGO) Scheme

The Service NGOs (SNGOs) are, those NGOs, which are expected to provide clinical services and other specialized aspects, such as Dai training, MTP, male involvement, covering 1,00,000 population and contributing to achieving the RCH objectives.

NGOs with an establishment of institutional and infrastructure for service delivery are encouraged to complement the public health care delivery system in achieving the goals of RCH II program. These SNGOs will cover an area co-terminus to that of a CHC/block PHC with approximately 1,00,000 population or around 100 villages. Service NGOs are expected to provide a range of clinical services, directly to the community, as an integrated package of RCH II services. Some of the services expected to be provided by SNGOs include safe deliveries, neonatal care, treatment of diarrhoea and ARI, abortion and IUD services, RTI/STI, etc.

Institutional Framework for Programme Management

The programme management under the revised scheme is decentralized to the State RCH Society, which has the responsibility for the overall management of the scheme. The State NGO committee will be responsible for MNGO selection, recommendation of project for MNGO selection, recommendation of projects for Govt. of India approval, fund disbursement, capacity building, monitoring and evaluation. The District RCH society is responsible for all the operational aspects of the program management at the district level. The district NGO committee holds the responsibility for recommendation of MNGO composite proposals to State RCH Society, facilitating the signing of MOU with the MNGO and passes it on for fund release to state RCH society, undertakes review meetings and periodic monitoring in the field for assessing FNGO/ MNGO performance.

State NGO Coordinators (SNGOCs)

The SNGOCs are responsible for monitoring the implementation, facilitates timely submission of NGO reports to the state government, providing government feed-back to NGOs, communicating government policies and programmes, and facilitating NGO dialogue with district health system. At present there are 13 SNGOCs in position and other states are in active process of positioning them soon.

Institutional Framework for NGO Capacity Building

The Regional Resource Centres (RRCs) and the Best Practice Centres (BPC), are the two institutional mechanisms available to support this programme. As on date there are 10 functional RRCs. NGOs with expertise and experience in RCH and having national level stature, are identified as RRCs.

The RRCs are playing role to be a catalyst, advocacy and net-working with State Governments, strengthen managerial and technical competencies of the MNGOs, supports and oversee FNGO training, document and disseminate best practices, collect and disseminate RCH policies, laws, and programme from the respective states, where they work, and maintenance of database on technical and human resources related to RCH.

Human Resources in Health (Health Manpower in India): Total number of allopathic doctors registered up to 2014 were 938861 (1:1319 population), 736538 Ayush doctors (1:1682 population), 120897 dental surgeons

(1: 10120 population), total number of ANM were 786061, and registered nurses and midwives were 1780006. Nurse population ratio was 1:482. Human resources in Health Consume over 50–70% of the budget hence their role in the system of Health Care delivery is critical at all the levels.[17]

HEALTH CARE UTILIZATION

Despite a steady increase in public health care infrastructure, utilization of public health facilities by population for outpatient and inpatient care has not improved. The NSSO (1996–2014) data clearly show a major decline in utilization of public health facilities for inpatient care and corresponding increase in utilization of same from private health care providers in both rural and urban areas.

In rural areas 42% hospitalization took place in public hospitals and 58% in private hospitals the corresponding figures in urban India were 32% and 68% respectively.

With the exception of a few states there has been a very low utilization of outpatient care as well (22%). Despite higher costs in private sector, this shift shows the people's growing lack of trust in the public system. Reasons for low utilization—critical shortage of health personnel, inadequate incentives, poor working conditions, absenteeism, long wait, inconvenient clinic hours, poor outreach, insensitivity to local needs, inadequate planning, management and monitoring of service/facilities were the main reasons, besides poor quality of services.

REFERENCES

1 Planning Commission—Health Division Report of the Steering Committee on Health for the 12th Five-Year Plan February 2012.
2 NIHFW. Management Training Modules for Medical Officers. Primary Health Centre. New Delhi: NIHFW; 1987.
3 Handbook for the delivery of care to mothers and children in a community development Block. Ed., FJW Miller. Designed for the use of Medical Officers and to assist the training and education of undergraduate medical students and interns.
4 World Health Organization. Formulating strategies for Health for all by the year 2000. Geneva: WHO; 1979.
5 NIHAE. Health for All by 2000 AD. Problems, approaches and challenges. Technical Paper. New Delhi: NIHFW; 1983.
6 NIHFW. Primary Health Care in India. New Delhi: NIHFW; 1986.
7 WHO. Implementation of the Global Strategy for "Health for All" by the year 2000. Second evaluation. Eighth report on the World Health Situation, Vol I, global review. Geneva; WHO; 1993.
8 GOI. Rural Health Statistics in India. New Delhi: MOH and FW, GOI; 2013.
9 GOI. Report of working group on "Health for All" by 2000 AD. New Delhi: MOH and FW, GOI; 1981.
10 GOI. Annual Report 2006–07 MOH and FW. NRHM, pp 104, GOI; New Delhi.
11 GOI. Reproductive and child health programme schemes for implementation. New Delhi: MOH and FW, GOI; 1997.
12 Government of India. Bulletin on Rural Health Statistics in India, 2007–13. Infrastructure division, Dept. of Family Welfare, MOH and FW, Government of India.
13 GOI. Indian Public Health Standards (IPHS) for sub-centre, PHC and CHC. DGHS, MOH and FW, Government of India Feb 2007.
14 Lal S and Mathur SC. "Poverty in plenty". Editorial, IJCM, April–June 1998; 23:(2).
15 GOI. National Health Policy: MOH and FW, New Delhi 2002.
16 GOI. Annual report 2008–2014. MOH and FW, GOI; New Delhi.
17 National Health Profile 2013–Human Resources in Health Sector.

MINIMUM NEEDS PROGRAMME AND 20-POINT PROGRAMME

FOCUS ON DETERMINANTS OF HEALTH AND CONVERGENCE

India continued to pursue the development programmes through Five-Year Plans; however, the results of planned development did not trickle down the rural poor and disadvantaged sections of the society. The measures for providing larger employment and income to these sections were, therefore, considered necessary for bringing them up to at least certain minimum nationally acceptable standards. Therefore, minimum needs programme (MNP) was initiated in 1974, with the objective of establishing a network of basic minimum services including education, health, nutrition and drinking water and housing, etc. The programme was designed to improve the standard of living of those belonging to the rural areas, and urban slums and whose consumption levels were below poverty line. Important needs identified during 5th plan period consisted of:

- Elementary education
- Rural health
- Rural water supply
- Rural roads
- Rural housing
- Rural electrification
- Nutrition
- Adult education
- Environments
- Improvement of urban slums

Subsequently rural sanitation and public distribution system were also included under MNP during 7th plan period.

The minimum needs programme in health sector consisted of:

- Safe water supply and rural sanitation.
- Establishment of one sub-centre for 5,000 in the plains and 3,000 in tribal and hilly area.

- One PHC for 30,000 population in plain and 20,000 in tribal and hilly areas by 2,000.
- ₹ 2,000/- medicines for a sub-centre and ₹ 12,000/- worth medicines for PHC per annum.

Nutrition

Minimum needs programme aimed at expansion of *ICDS projects*, consolidation of *mid-day meal* programme and linking it with *health, potable water* and *sanitation* in rural area to improve the nutritional status of women and children.

Among the basic minimum needs, the priority has been given to primary health care, primary education and safe drinking water and it was resolved in 1996 to achieve all these in a time bound manner.

20-POINT PROGRAMME IN 1986 (Table 15.6)

The nation launched 20-point programme in 1975 to promote social justice and growth. Many of the points included under minimum needs programme were also included under 20-point programme. While formulating the National Health Policy 1983 it took into consideration the national 20-point programme. This programme was revised in 1986. The schemes under 20-point programme are being implemented by the concerned department of the state. Performance of the district is monitored at the state level by the planning department on the basis of criterion adopted by Ministry of Planning and Programme implementation, Government of India and accordingly, ranking of districts is decided by the state. On the basis of the ranking, incentives are given to the districts, based on their performance in selected programmes and on the basis of sample survey of selected programmes. Maharashtra has done a commendable job. Sometimes, there is over-reporting of performance to achieve the target. Many of

Table 15.6: 20-point programme—components

Components
1. Attack on rural poverty
2. Strategy for rain fed agriculture
3. Better use of irrigation water
4. Bigger harvests
5. Enforcement of land reforms
6. Special programme for rural labour
7. Clean drinking water
8. Health for all
9. Two child norms
10. Expansion for women
11. Justice for S. caste and S. tribes
12. Equality for women
13. New opportunities for youth
14. Housing for the people
15. Improvement of slums
16. New strategy for forestry
17. Protection of the environments
18. Concern for the consumer
19. Energy for the villages
20. A responsive administration

Table 15.7: Health-related sustainable development goals laid by United Nations 2015

Targets	*Level to be reached by 2030*
• Stunting and wasting in children under 5 years of age	• By 2025 end all forms of malnutrition
• Under-five mortality rate	• 25 per 1000 live births
• Neonatal mortality	• 12 per 1000 live births
• Maternal mortality ratio	• 70 per lakh
• Halve the number of deaths and injuries due to road traffic accidents	• By 2020
• Tuberculosis malaria and HIV/AIDS combat hepatitis, water borne and other communicable diseases	• End the epidemics of TB, malaia and HIV and other communicable diseases
• Water and sanitation for all—end open defecation	• Universal access to safe drinking water and sanitation for all
• Premature mortality due to non-communicable diseases	• Reduce by one-third
• Promote mental health—prevention and treatment of substance abuse	By 2030
• Universal health coverage, affordable essential medicines and vaccines for all	Do
• Ensure universal access to sexual and reproductive health care services	Do
• Reduce number of deaths and diseases due to air, water and soil pollution	Do
• Substantially increase health financing and workforce	Do
• Strengthen the implementation of tobacco control (FCTC)	Do

the points relate directly to health sector and others have indirect bearing.

MILLENNIUM DEVELOPMENT GOALS (MDGs)[3]

1 Eradicate poverty and hunger.
2 Achieve universal primary education.
3 Promote gender equality and empower women.
4 Reduce child mortality.
 • Under-five mortality rate, and infant mortality rate
5 Improve material health.
 • 5B: Universal access to reproductive health.
6 Combat HIV/AIDS, malaria and other major diseases.
7 Ensure environmental sustainability.
8 Develop a global partnership for development.

These goals have been evolved as a result of several global summits that took place in 1990s. The MDGs place health at the heart of development and represent commitments by Governments throughout the world to do more to reduce poverty and hunger and to tackle ill-health, gender inequality, lack of education, access to clean water and environmental degradation. Three of the eight goals are directly health related, all the others have important indirect effects on health.[1]

The revised Millennium Development Goals framework agreed by the United Nations General Assembly at the 2005 World Summit, effective from 15th Jan 2008 included specific target on reproductive health: MD Goal 5, Target B, which seeks to "Achieve, by 2015, universal access to reproductive health". This new target falls within the goal of "improving maternal health". The new indicators have been evolved for monitoring.

Further most of the objectives/indicators relate to reproductive and child health (RCH) framework. The programmes to attain MDG are already in hands through RCH and other national health programmes as also National Population Policy 2000 (immediate and medium term goals) and Revised National Health Policy 2002 apart from National Rural Health Mission (NRHM).

Countdown to 2015 was formed in 2005 by a group of scientists, policymakers, activists and institutions to track progress toward Millennium Development Goal 4. New official list of indicators and of key maternal, newborn and child health policies have been stressed.[2]

Progress of MDGs in India so far (2015)

Base Year 1990

India could reduce its IMR to the level of 40 under-five mortality from 123 to the level of 48 per thousand live births—a good progress indeed. Nearly 81% of deliveries were safe in India and the MDG 5, has made the least progress and India's maternal mortality of 167 stays at high level. Similarly, adolescent birth rate stays at high level of 39. Nearly 33% of the under-three-children are

Sustainable development goals[3]	
Goal 1	**End poverty** in all its forms everywhere
Goal 2	**End hunger,** achieve food security and improved nutrition and promote sustainable agriculture
Goal 3	Ensure **healthy lives** and promote well-being for all at all ages
Goal 4	Ensure inclusive and equitable quality **education** and promote lifelong learning opportunities for all.
Goal 5	Achieve **gender** equality and empower all women and girls
Goal 6	Ensure availability of **water** and **sanitation** for all
Goal 7	Ensure access to affordable, reliable, sustainable modern **energy** for all
Goal 8	Full and productive employment and decent **work** for all
Goal 9	Build resilient infrastructure, promote inclusive and sustainable industrialization and foster innovation
Goal 10	Reduce inequality within and among countries
Goal 11	Make cities and human settlements inclusive, safe, resilient and sustainable
Goal 12	Ensure sustainable consumption and production patterns
Goal 13	Take urgent action to combat climate change and its impacts
Goal 14	Conserve and sustainable use of the oceans, seas and marine resources for sustainable development
Goal 15	Protect, restore and promote sustainable use of terrestrial ecosystems
Goal 16	Promote peaceful and inclusive societies
Goal 17	Global partnership for sustainable development

underweight. Nearly 90% of population use improved drinking water source but only 40% of population use improved sanitation facilities (2015). HIV prevalence in adult population is stable at low level of 0.26% and DOTS programme is making rapid progress as high cure rate of over 85% is being achieved. Tuberculosis prevalence, and incidence has come down to the level of 195 and 167 per lakh population and mortality reduced to 17 per lakh. Vector-borne diseases including malaria continues as high morbidity, and pose continuous threat of outbreaks and epidemics in different parts of the country.

Sustainable Development Goals (SDGs) of UNs

The MDGs have been reframed as "sustainable development goals". The 17 sustainable development goals and 169 targets and 200 indicators seek to build on the millennium development goals and cmplete what they did not achieve, by 2030 (Table 15.7). The SDGs have been based on five core principles—the 5 Ps **p**eople, **p**lanet, **p**artnership **p**rosperity and **p**eace. The SDGs provide a framework to shape policies and agenda for next 15 years.

REFERENCES

1 WHO (2003). Shaping the future. The World Health Report.
2 UNICEF. The state of the world's Children 2009.
3 MDGs, India country report 2015 New Delhi central statistical organization 2015.
4 United Nations—Tranforming our world: The 2030 Agenda for sustainable development September 2015.

HEALTH MANAGEMENT FUNCTIONS

The simplest definition of management is "getting things done". The health management is defined as "purposeful and efficient use of health resources" to achieve predetermined goals/goal. The senior medical officers and medical officers have to perform essential managerial functions besides technical functions.[1,2]

Technical Functions (Clinical Functions)

Technical functions include diagnosis and treatment of patients, their follow-up and referrals besides, preventive and promotive services. These functions are most satisfying to doctor, much more rewarding and results can be achieved within short period. In most situations, doctor works alone and has one-to-one relations with his patient and client. Public health needs qualified *managers* and not merely *clinicans*.

Essential Management Functions of Medical Officer and their use in Decision Making

15

The important management functions of medical officer are as under:

P: *Planning,* organizing, implementing and evaluating the health activities (what needs to be done and methods of doing).

O: *Organizing resources* (men, money and material) and assignment of tasks and responsibility.

S: *Staffing:* Training and continuing education of staff and their supervision, besides recruitment of staff.

Delegation: transferring work/responsibility and authority downwards to subordinates.

D: *Directing:* Day-to-day direction to subordinates—making decisions and issuing specific orders and instructions.

Co: *Coordination* of work of health teams and other health-related sectors like ICDS, school teachers and village Panchayats.

R: *Reporting:* Submission of regular reports of performance to higher level.

B: *Budgeting:* Spending contingencies and maintenance of accounts and preparation of budget.

C: *Controlling:* Through annual performance reports, regular supervision, sanction of leaves, rewards and punishment.

I: *Innovation:* New work methods and eliciting community support.

R: *Representation:* Representing the organization at various levels.

The acronym to reproduce these components is **POSD CORB-CIR**.

Management functions are required at each level but at lower levels more of technical functions as also human relations and less of managerial functions, but higher an officer's position in a health organization, the greater is the need for managerial skills and the lesser need for technical skills. One has to strike a balance between technical and managerial functions. Management functions have been neglected or are poorly performed because of lack of training in management functions during undergraduate medical education or lack of interest or both. The management functions are more important in Indian settings because of scarce resources. The best health manager is one who is able to achieve maximum within limited resources.

Most management responsibilities are seldom taken and enjoyed by doctors and they attach low value to these functions and have seldom been trained to perform these functions.

Medical officer is responsible to *plan* and *organize* the health activities for 30,000 population of defined geographical area. His concern is total community of 30,000 people (sick and healthy both). This is one of the important job function of medical officer. "*People themselves are important resources.*" The job of medical officer is to organize people and use people's organization

(Panchayati Raj Institutions) and their resources and plan health activities with them and involve them in village health activities and consult them periodically to have their opinions and reactions to improve the services. The plan of work must start from the bottom, i.e. from people, who are the most important resources and users of health services. Community mobilization and ensuring its participation is heavy responsibility and a challenging task.

Doctor is *responsible to "community"* and his job is to ensure health to all people; 30,000 population under his charge. This is the community, he serves and he must organize "community health care" for this much population. He alone cannot look after such a large community and essentially he will use health auxiliaries or health workers to do the job in the community. The doctor must *delegate* the work responsibilities to health workers. In order that these health workers do the job well and provide quality services, they must have appropriate "skills" and doctor is responsible to *upgrade their skills* from time to time and support them to do their job. He continuously undertakes management needs assessment (MNA). Management needs assessment is critical function.

The health manager is a *leader of the health team* in a primary health centre and community health centre, he is responsible to plan and organize the health work with health teams, *motivate them, impart skill training*; delegate the work, supervise and coordinate their work, assess their performance, improve their work performance, develop health team, involve community in promoting health functions and report the activities to higher levels on regular basis, evaluate the performance of health centre and keep on innovating the things at local level and come out with new model/models of health care delivery in his area and learn from people and health teams to solve their problems.[3]

In short, the performance of health centre depends upon the health work done by the health teams at sub-centre and village level volunteers/honorary workers. Therefore, the health teams must perform well and plan their activities meticulously to ensure high level of coverage and quality of services.

Medical officer is also "*responsible for patient care*" and his decisions are vital to save lives. Management functions in relation to patient care include organization of outdoor, indoor and emergency care, referral arrangement, laboratory services, indenting drugs including essential drugs, maintenance of equipment, material management besides control and prevention of outbreaks, notification of diseases, keeping records of vital statistics, etc. Quality of medical care will depend upon quality of management functions related to such care.

Health is a state subject in India, meaning thereby that state Government is responsible to provide health services to its people. Article 21 of the constitution requires the state to ensure the health and nutritional well-being of all people. The role of central Government is to give financial support to states to implement National Health Programmes including reproductive and child health programme. Broad policies on health and population are laid by the central Government, which are adopted by the state Governments for implementation. It is the state health infrastructure, which translates the policy into actions at various levels.

DIFFERENT LEVELS OF MANAGEMENT

The **Goal** is "Health for All" through primary health care. National population policy, Health Policy 2002, and Universal Health Coverage have laid down measurable objectives/indicators to be achieved by 2017 and beyond.[4,5]

Base of Pyramid—Health System Organization

The organization (structure) of health system is pyramidal in nature (Fig. 15.3). The organization is the structure or anatomy, while the management is the physiology of the system of health services/care.

People are the most important resource in India. People themselves and large number of auxiliaries and health volunteers with lesser skills form the base of pyramidal organization, who work in the community and are accessible to people for primary health care. These auxiliaries and Anganwadi workers besides health guides and ASHA constitute strong community-based human resources to respond to the preventive, promotive and curative health needs of people (Fig. 15.3).

We have 1,53,665 sub-centres, 2,36,034 MPHWs (female) and 56,464 male health workers besides 13 lakhs Anganwadi workers, traditional birth attendants and over 8.9 lakhs ASHAs, which form the strong base of pyramid.[6,7] The effectiveness of services in India largely depends upon the auxiliaries and their skills and competence. Their basic training and continuing education will determine their skills and competence and quality of service they render in the community. Health care functions of community health centre and primary health centre rest on the shoulders of health auxiliaries.

First Level Managers

They are called supervisors. These managers function at the lowest level of the organization and are in contact with the workers whom they supervise. No other managerial personnel are placed below them. The health supervisor male and female supervise the work of health workers male and female who are operating workers providing or delivering services. Such supervisors are often called first line managers.

Middle Level of Pyramid

This is constituted by health professionals who hold the responsibility of health team leaders/managers. At this

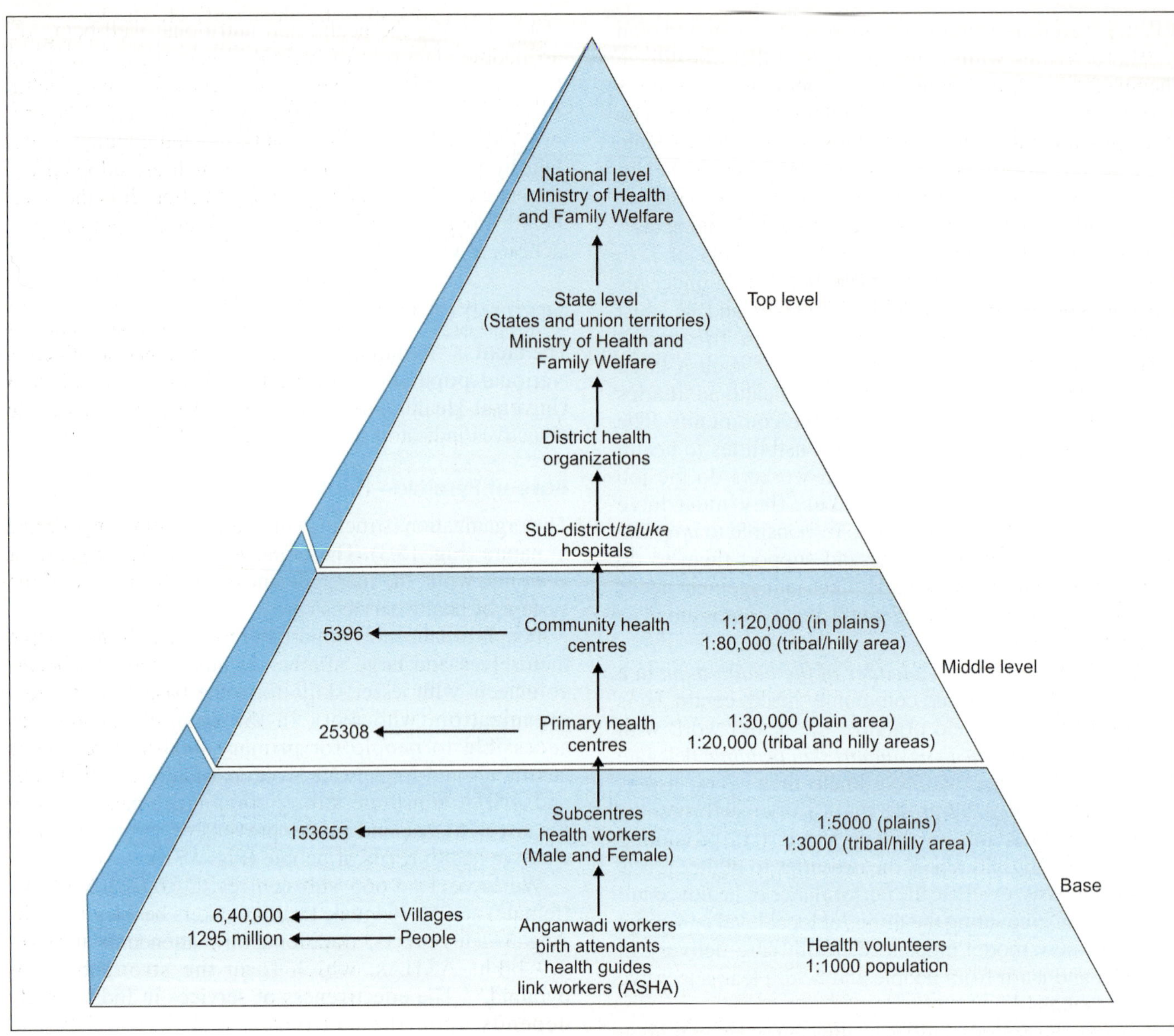

Fig. 15.3: Health system organization
Source: Rural Health Statistics in India, and National Health Profile 2015

level, we have primary health centres, community health centres to provide referral services to sub-centres. Apart from referral support, this level is responsible for planning, programming, implementation, monitoring and supervision, continuing education, coordination, and evaluation of health services and health programmes in the assigned community of 1,20,000 for each CHC. The challenging task is to attain reasonable and acceptable level of health status for whole community and their success is measured not by number of patient cured or treated but how much the disease rate, death rate and disability rate have been reduced. The impact indicators of performance of these health centres and CHCs are reduction in fertility rate, infant mortality rate, maternal mortality rate, reduction of disease rate (diarrhoea, respiratory infection, malaria, tuberculosis). The ultimate goal remains to eradicate diseases and achieve health for all. At this level of the organization, the medical officers and senior medical officers have to devote 50–60% of their total time for health management functions and to ensure achievement of the goals of organization: "Health for/in all".

Middle Level Managers

These groups of managers comprise a few levels. They supervise other managers and operating workers. They look after the activities necessary for implementation of organizational plans for achievement of its goals. The medical officers and district programme officers are middle level managers who supervise the first line managers and managers of PHC and CHC respectively and can also supervise the operating workers in the field.

Top of Pyramid

At the top level of the organization, the senior level managers are entrusted with the function of directing, monitoring and control of the health services and health programmes. District and State level programme officers supervise the assigned area, besides coordinating the health activities and ensure that plans of work are prepared and implemented at various levels. This level is also responsible to arrange for in-service training of various cadres, besides sending progress reports to higher formation and represent their organization at district, state and central levels. It also controls the budget, posting, promotion and transfers of employees.[1,3] This level continuously undertakes management needs assessment (MNA) to improve the services/system.

Top Level Managers

These managers are at the highest level of hierarchy and are in overall charge of the organization. The district civil surgeon and director health services may be called as top level managers (Fig. 15.3).

Top level manager spends more time in planning and organizing than a lower level manager. Higher the level of management greater is the need for managerial skills and lesser is the need for technical skills. Lower the level of management more of the technical and human relations skills are required than managerial skills (Fig. 15.4).

The general policies, plan and the guidance of Indian health system have been laid down by National Population Policy (2000) and National Health Policy (2002) and more recently by National Health Mission (2013). Objectives and plan of national disease control programme have been defined by the Ministry of Health and Family Welfare. The role of primary health centre/community health centre, doctors, health supervisors and workers is to interpret policies at local level, plan their implementation and see that these are implemented.

PRINCIPLES OF HEALTH MANAGEMENT

Hierarchy: Whenever a group of people are involved in the accomplishment of a task, some form of organization emerges and hierarchy develops. Hierarchy means a ranking system ordered according to status or authority. (Who is responsible to whom?) Hierarcy describes relationship and responsibility within an organization. Hierarchy consists of levels of responsibility, chain of command, recognition and span of control (number of subordinates who can be supervised effectively) and respecting authority, not supersede authority, upward, downward and lateral relationships in an organization.

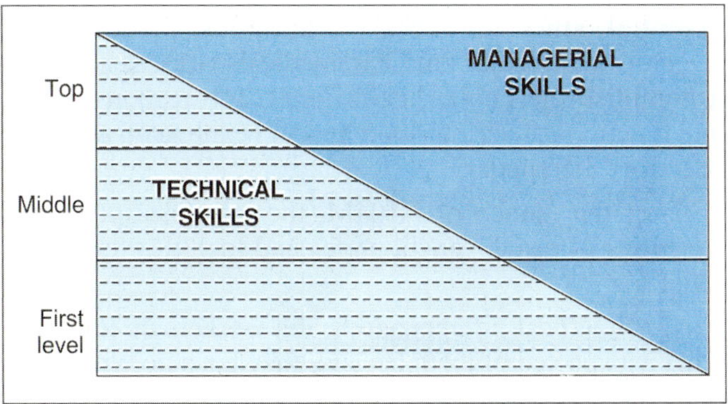

Fig. 15.4: Levels of management and skill required

Delegation: It means downward transfer of work/functions, responsibility and authority for decision making and problem solving to subordinates. Delegation does not release the delegator from the final responsibility for outcomes. It results in additional relationship between functionaries and responsibilities, authority and accountability.

Most of the functions of health centre have been *delegated* to auxiliaries (health workers and their supervisors). However, the support system and supportive supervision and referral support is a weak link. Most of the investments in medical education have been made on doctors, whereas training and continuing education of health auxiliaries have been neglected. Therefore, it is most essential to invest in these auxiliaries and support them adequately to enhance coverage and quality of health services. Since 69% of population lives in rural areas, the capacity of auxiliaries needs to be strengthened. Recently, it has been clearly stated in the National Population Policy that health services and planning should begin from below, i.e. from people. All sub-centre action plans should be evolved in consultation with the people; however, this has not taken off well and needs to be done on emergency basis. Here comes the role of health manager to perceive the needs of training and support to health auxiliaries.

Decentralization

Devolution of authority (powers) and responsibility to local levels—Panchayati Raj Institutions and Nagarpalikas, in rural and urban areas respectively. Under constitutional provision "States" have the primary responsibility to provide health care to its people. However the health care delivery system in many states remain largely centralized at the departmental level in spite of strong and effective presence of institutions of local self government at village, block and district levels. **Decentralized Management** of health institutions especially those at primary level through Panchayati Raj Institutions (PRIs) has been strongly—advocated by National Heath Policy. The 73rd and 74th Constitutional Amendment Act, 1992, made **health family welfare** and **eduction** a responsibility of Village Panchayats and Nagarpalikas respectively. Local self governments are an important means of furthering decentralized planning and programme implementation. However in order to realize their potentials, they need strengthening by further delegation of administrative and financial powers including powers of resource mobilization. Decentralized programme management should also be reinforced by convergence of all vertical Public Health Programmes at the district level and below. This would avoid duplication of efforts in areas like information, eduction and communication, training and supervision.

Examples of Decentralization of Planning and Programme Implementation

National Health Mission (NRHM and NUHM) under its umbrella integrates all related and stand alone health programmes in health sector.

- Funds, functions and functionaries have been transfered to Panchayati Raj Institutions like untied funds to Village Health Sanitation and Nutrition Committees, for local action and planning, increased role of PRIs in ASHA programme, Constitution of *Rogi Kalyan Samitis*/hospital development committee, district health society for decentralized district, CHC, PHC, SC and village health planning with PRIs and people, community monitoring system and greater space for NGOs participation.
- Provision of untied funds at every level and contractual appointment route to immediately fill human resource gaps as well as ensuring locally resident health staff/ workers are other examples of decentralization.
- Village health plans, sub-centre, PHCs, CHCs and district action plans are examples of decentralized participatory planning.[8, 9]

Convergence

Convergence means working together or coming together or coordinating two or more sectors to produce a combined effect greater than the sum of their separate effects. Indicators of health depend as much on drinking water, sanitation, nutrition, female literacy, early childhood development, women empowerment, etc. as they do on hospitals and functional health systems. Realising the importance of wider determinants of health, coordination and convergence between health sector and other sectors such as ICDS, water and sanitation (Total Sanitation Campaign), Eduction, Nutrition, PRIs and Rural and Urban Development sectors is an imperative need. Anganwadi centres and school system at the village level are the principal hubs for health and development actions. Village is the first level of convergence of programmes of all the Ministries.

Methods of Convergence

At Village Level

- Colocation of Anganwadi Centres with Sub-centres/ in schools—**a best management practice.**
- Joint home visits by AWWs, ANMs and ASHAs. and Joint household surveys—**a best practice**
- Immunization outreach sessions with AWWs at Anganwadi Centre—**a best practics**
- Village Health Nutrition and Sanitation day at Anganwadi centre once a month.
- Sharing of information between ANM, AWW and school teachers and development functionaries

At sector level: Geographical area coterminus for supervision between health supervisors and ICDS supervisors, Joint touring, and preparation and sharing of monthly monitoring/progress reports and planning of work and review of work together at sector level meeting besides problem-solving and continuing eduction of ICDS and health teams and their development.

At block level: Joint planning by Medical officer, CDPO and Block Samiti and Block Development and Panchayat offices and Block eduction officer.

Supplementary nutrition will have little effect if diarrhoeal diseases in children remain unchecked. Provision of safe water and sanitation at Anganwadi centre/at village in convergence with total sanitation campaign makes more sense/impact. Hence, convergence actions with other sectors are essential to reduce morbidity and mortality and improvement of nutritional status as also to achieve high coverage level of all services.

All national health programmes—school health programme, adolescent health, national anaemia control programme, mental health programme, *Rashtriya Bal Swasthya Karyakram*, national tobacco control and national oral health programme are being implemented by convergence with eduction department and district early intervention centre.

At District Level

District Action Plans, Block, PHC, sub-centre and village health action plans are important means to enhance intersectoral and intrasectoral convergence.

HEALTH TEAM (PUBLIC HEALTH TEAM)

To deliver health services to community "Teamwork" is essential, since the work is enormous. Professionals (Doctors and Nurses) and Paramedicals work as a team to accomplish the public health goals. Job responsibilities and functions of various members of health team are being described hereunder.

After the launch of NRHM, the job description and functions of health functionaries and facilities have been redefined.

Most medical officers and health workers do not know what is expected of them because they have no written job descriptions, or guidelines are out of date, or supervisors donot tell providers what they should do.

JOB RESPONSIBILITIES OF MEDICAL OFFICER, PRIMARY HEALTH CENTRE[10]

The medical officer of primary health centre (PHC) is responsible for implementing all activities grouped under health and family welfare delivery system in PHC area. He/she is responsible in his individual capacity, as well as overall incharge. It is not possible to enumerate all his tasks. However, by virtue of his designation, it is implied that he will be solely responsible for the proper functioning of the PHC, and activities in relation to RCH, NRHM and other national health programmes. The detailed job functions of medical officer working in the PHC are as follows:

1. Curative Work

- MO will plan organize, and provide outpatient, indoor, emergency and referral services besides dental and laboratory services. He will provide curative services at sub-centre once a fortnight/month and organize "Health day" at Anganwadi once a month and coordinate with other institutions providing medical care in his area.

2. Preventive and Promotive Work

- He/she will prepare operational plans and ensure effective implementation of various National Health and Family Welfare Programmes including National Rural Health Mission by *deploying the health teams* under his control.
- The MO will promote institutional deliveries and all maternal and child health services and ensure that PHC becomes 24 × 7 service station.
- MO will coordinate and facilitate the functioning of AYUSH doctor in the PHC.
- With the help of health teams and people he will organize, manage and implement the various National Health Programmes (as per guidelines) which are—Reproductive and Child Health Programme, Family Planning, Universal Immunization Programme (UIP), National Vector-borne Disease Control Programme (Malaria, kala-azar, Japanese encephalitis, filariasis and dengue fever and outbreak of these disease), Control of Communicable Diseases (outbreak epidemics) and Integrated Disease Surveillance Programme, National Leprosy Eradication Programme, Revised National Tuberculosis Control Programme, Sexually Transmitted Disease, School Health, National Programme for Prevention of Visual Impairment and Control of Blindness, National HIV/AIDS Control Programme and National Programmes of Non-communicable Diseases.

3. Training and Continuing Education of Staff

He/she will organize training programme including continuing education for the staff of PHC and under the guidance of district health authorities. He will also make arrangement/provide guidance to the health assistant male and female in organizing training programmes for indigenous dais and ASHAs.

4. Administrative Work

- Supportive **Supervision** guidance and directions to ANMs, Health Assistants (Male and Female) ASHAs, Anganwadi Workers, and Health Guides.
- Help PRIs in Preparing Village Health and Sanitation **Plan,** Community Needs Assessment, Help Preparation of sub-centre Action Plan, and PHC Plan of work every year.
- Regular **Monitoring** of all programmes and preparation of records of all services and submission of monthly progress/monitoring reports to higher level.
- Holding monthly **meetings** of staff.
- Arrange/indent **drugs, equipment, vaccines,** contraceptives and materials as per requirement and ensure maintenance of equipment and buildings of PHC and sub-centres.
- **Financial management** of untied money, maintenance grant, users fee and other budget under his control.
- **Management** of vehicle/referral **transport** service.
- Attend monthly meetings at CHC and District level.
- Every PHC should have a *Citizen's Charter* and *Rogi Kalyan Samiti* to monitor the functioning of the PHCs and have ownership of the programmes and functions.

In essence Medical Officer provides **leadership, guides** and **motivates** health teams and accountable to community he/she serves.

He/she will keep close liaison with block development officer and his/her staff, community leaders and various social welfare agencies in his/her area and involve them to the best advantage in the promotion of health programmes in the area.

Wherever possible, the MO will conduct field investigations to delineate local health and management problems for planning, and changes in the strategy of the effective delivery of health and family welfare services.

JOB RESPONSIBILITIES OF HEALTH EDUCATOR

Working Relationship

The health educator will function under the technical supervision and guidance of the block extension educator. However, he/she will be under the immediate administrative control of the PHC medical officer. He/she will be responsible for providing support to all health and family welfare programmes in the block.

Job Responsibilities of Health Educator

His/her main responsibilities are:

- Develop, plan, organize, implement and evaluate Health Education Activities/Behaviour Change

Communication (BCC) Activities in PHC area, under the guidance of MO and Block Extension Educator.

- Maintain **record** of the activities of BCC and send regular **report** every month to MO.
- **Conduct/Assist** MO for **training** of Health Workers, Health Supervisors, ASHAs, AWWs in the area of BCC.
- Organize orientation training of health and family welfare workers, opinion leaders, local medical practitioners, school teachers, dais and others involved in health and family welfare work.
- **Supply** education material on health and family welfare to health workers and supervisors and maintain audio-visual equipment.
- Organize population education and health education sessions in schools and for out of school youths, organize mass communication programmes like film shows, exhibition, lectures and dramas and celebration of health days with the help of District Mass Education Officer.
- Supervise and verify entries in Eligible Couple Registers and meet prominent acceptors of family planning methods and opinion leaders and involve them in the promotion of health and family welfare programmes.
- Supervise the depot holders of Conventional Contraceptives and motivate resistant cases and drop outs in the health and family welfare programmes.
- Communication needs assessment (CNA) of clients and segmentation of clients for education and formulate annual action plan of BCC in PHC area and to implement and evaluate these plans regularly.

JOB RESPONSIBILITIES OF HEALTH ASSISTANT FEMALE (LHV—LADY HEALTH VISITOR) (FEMALE SUPERVISOR)

Under the multipurpose workers scheme, a health assistant female is expected to cover a population of 30,000 (20,000 in tribal and hilly areas) in which there are 6 sub-centres, each with the health worker female. The health assistant female will carry out the following duties.

Supportive Supervision and Guidance

- Visit each sub-centre at least once a week on fixed day to provide supportive supervision and guidance to health workers female, birth attendants and ASHAs and cover all the six sub-centres in a month. Use checklist system for supervision.
- On the job continued education to upgrade the deficient skills and knowledge of health workers.
- Carry out supervisory home visits—on sample basis to assess the service delivery and satisfaction of clients and quality of records.
- Ensure adequate supplies, equipment, drugs, midwifery kit, IUD kit and Dai kit at sub-centre. In collaboration with health assistant (male) check at regular intervals the stores available at sub-centres and ensure that equipment is functional.
- Conduct weekly Maternal and Child Health and Family Planning Clinics at each sub-centre with the help of health worker female.
- Provide information on availability of services of Medical Termination of Pregnancy (MTP) and for sterilization. Refer suitable cases for MTP to the approved institutions.
- Training: Carryout training needs assessment (TNA) of health workers, organize and conduct training for Health Workers, Dais, Skilled Birth Attendants and ASHAs at sub-centre with the assistance of health worker female as also assist the MO in conducting training programmes.
- Conduct deliveries when required at PHC level and provide domiciliary and midwifery services.
- Records and Reports: Help and improve the quality of records of health workers and collect reports from health workers every month and compile these reports and submit report to MO of PHC.
- Conduct regular staff meetings with health workers and attend staff meetings at PHC.
- Coordinate the activities with health assistant (male) and other health personnel besides coordinating the health activities with other sectors (ICDS) Education, Rural Development, Panchayati Raj Institutions.
- Where kala-azar, lymphatic filaria, Japanese encephalitis and leprosy is endemic: She will supervise the work of health worker (female) during concurrent visit and check sample of 10% of the houses in village to assess the performance of the health worker and her quality of work. In collaboration with health assistant male she will ensure complete treatment of kala-azar and leprosy patients in the area and Mass Drug Administration to filaria cases to achieve coverage level of more than 80% besides undertaking health education activities.
- She will help and support the workers in Organizing Outreach Session of Universal Immunization Programme in her area.
- Help MO in School Health Services, ensure referrals of malnourished children, treat common ailments and carry out health education activities related to national health programmes of communicable and non-communicable diseases by arranging group meetings with leaders, women groups, *Mahila Mandals,* Teachers, AWWs and other Women/self help groups.
- Recognize, report, and respond to epidemics/outbreaks.

JOB RESPONSIBILITIES OF HEALTH ASSISTANT (MALE SUPERVISOR)

Under the Multipurpose Workers Scheme, a health assistant (male) is expected to cover six sub-centres, each with one health worker (male). The health assistant (male) will carry out following duties.

Supportive Supervision and Guidance

- Provide supportive supervision and guidance to all health workers (males) by visiting each health worker at least once a week on fixed day. Health assistant male can use a check list system for supportive supervision.
- Carry out supervisory home visits on sample basis in the area of health worker (male) to assess the performance of health worker and his quality of work.
- Help and guide the health worker (male) in planning and organizing his programmes of activities.
- Training and continuing education—help improving deficient skills and knowledge by on the job training and continuing education sessions.
- Ensure supplies, drugs, contraceptives, equipment and maintenance of sub-centres. In collaboration with the health assistant (female), check at regular intervals the stores/stocks available at sub-centre and ensure that these are adequate, available and functional.
- He will be responsible for prompt radical treatment to positive cases of malaria and prepare thick and thin smear of cases he encounters during his visit and ensure full treatment as per guidelines.
- He will plan supervise Indoor Insecticides spraying operation along with health worker.
- He will supervise the beat programme of the health worker for active case detection of malaria (surveillance) by concurrent visits, besides checking 10% of the houses to assess the quality of work performed and records maintained.
- Where kala-azar, Japanese encephalitis and lymphatic filariasis are endemic he will supervise the work of health worker (male) during concurrent visit and check minimum of 10% of households to assess the quality of work of male worker.
- Recognize and report outbreaks of communicable disease and take all possible remedial measures.
- Ensure that all cases of leprosy, tuberculosis under treatment are taking regular and complete treatment. Motivate defaulters for regular treatment.
- Environmental sanitation—help and educate community on safe water, construction of soakage pits, kitchen gardens, manure pits, compost pits and sanitary latrines, smokeless chullah and supervise the chlorination of water sources including wells.
- Universal Immunization Programme: Conduct immunization of all schoolchildren with the help of health workers (males).
- Family Planning: Personally motivate resistant cases for family planning. Guide health workers (males) in establishing (male) depot holders. Provide information on the availability of services for Medical Termination of Pregnancy (MTP) and refer MTP cases besides follow-up of cases of vasectomy, tubectomy, IUD and other family planning acceptors.
- Help-educate community on risk factors of non-communicable diseases.

JOB FUNCTIONS OF HEALTH WORKER (FEMALE) OR AUXILIARY NURSE MIDWIFE (ANM)

Under the Multipurpose Workers Scheme, a health worker (female) is available at sub-centre covering 5,000 population or five Anganwadis areas in plain and 3,000 population in hilly/tribal/desert and difficult areas. She is supervised by Health Assistant (female). Her job functions are as under:

1. **Maternal and Child Health Services**
   a. This includes essential obstetrical care services in allocated 5,000 population. Services include early recognition and registration of all pregnancies, antenatal care—4 check-ups, safe delivery services at sub-centre or supervised home deliveries and promote institutional deliveries and provide post-natal care. She refers cases of Medical Termination of Pregnancy (MTP) to appropriate facility. Other maternal services include management of Reproductive and sexually transmitted infections and Implementation of *Janani Suraksha Yojna* (JSY) in her area as per guidelines, with the help of ASHA.
   b. Child health services include newborn care, integrated management of neonatal and childhood Illness, immunization, growth monitoring, identify cases of malnutrition among infants and young children, vitamin A prophylaxis and iron and folic acid tablets to control anaemia, school health services and services for adolescent girls.
2. ***Family planning services:*** This includes identification, registration and motivation of all eligible couples in her area and providing conventional contraceptives (copper T, condoms and oral pills) and refer cases of sterilization to PHC/CHC, or district hospital. She also helps and guides couples who have infertility.
3. Training and continuing education to Dais and ASHAs and organize **village health** and **nutrition** day at Anganwadi centre once a month.
4. ***Communicable diseases:*** Implement Integrated Diseases Surveillance Programme (IDSP) in her area and notify regularly occurrence of diseases (fever with or without rash, jaundice, fever with altered consciousness, diarrhoeas/cholera, acute flaccid paralysis, sputum smear positive TB cases) to Medical Officer. Any abnormal increase in cases (outbreaks) should be notified immediately and ensure control measures at local level till such time help comes from higher level. Monitor the quality of drinking water by H_2S strip and orthotoluidine test, besides promotion of sanitation by use of toilet and manure pits.

5 ***National health programmes:*** Services for all national health/disease control programmes (NVBD, tuberculosis, blindness, HIV/AIDS, IDDs, leprosy and Universal Immunization Programme).

6 Treatment of common ailments and health education.

7 *Vital events:* Regularly record and report pregnancies, births and deaths in her area.

8 ***Records and reports:*** Maintain essential records and prepare and submit performance report every month.

9 ***Team activities:*** Coordinate the work with Health worker (male), Anganwadi workers, ASHAs, Block development functionaries, Panchayati Raj Institutions, School teachers, self help groups and NGOs.

10 To undertake community needs assessment for workload assessment and prepare sub-centre action plan with the help of PRIs, ASHAs and AWWs.

11 Prevention and control of non-communicable diseases. (health promotion and opportunistic screening).

Role of ANM as Facilitator of ASHA and AWW

ANM holds monthly/fortnight meeting with ASHA and AWW, acts as resource person for training, informs date, time, place of outreach session, takes their help in updating eligible couples, utilize ASHA in motivating pregnant women and married couples for utilizing services at sub-centre. AWW guides ASHA in organizing health day once a month.

JOB RESPONSIBILITIES OF HEALTH WORKER (MALE)

Health worker (male) is available at sub-centre which covers a population of 5,000 in plain and 3,000 in hilly/tribal/desert area. The health worker (male) will make a visit to each family once a fortnight. He will record his visit on the main entrance to the house according to the instructions of the state/UT. His duties pertaining to different national health programmes are:

- Active case detection (active surveillance for malaria): By visiting each family once a fortnight (100 houses per day), preparing thick and thin blood smears of all fever cases and giving full treatment to clinically suspected/confirmed cases of malaria as per guidelines/policy. Nearly 63% of male health worker posts are vaccant.
- Establish Fever Treatment Depot (FTD) with ASHA or with School Teacher/Health Volunteer, in high risk areas of malaria. Replenish both drugs and glass slides and rapid diagnostic kits (RDK) and get account of consumption of drugs and RDKs from each FTD.
- To dispatch blood smear slides to PHC laboratory twice a week and make results available within 24 hours.
- Administer radical treatment to all malaria positive cases as per drug policy on malaria.
- Assist health supervisor male in supervising spray operations and training of field spray staff.
- Participation in National Filaria Day for Mass Drug Administration (MDA).
- Where kala-azar is endemic: Carry out surveillance for kala-azar in each family and refer and guide the suspected cases to nearest PHC for diagnosis and treatment by Medical Officer. Follow-up all cases of kala-azar and ensure administration of complete treatment besides conducting health education activities.
- He will assist spray operation in his area.
- Where Japanese encephalitis (JE) is endemic: From each family he shall enquire about presence of any fever case with altered sensorium (encephalitis) and guide these *suspected cases* of JE for diagnosis and treatment to Medical Officer. He will follow-up all cases of JE. He will assist health supervisor during the spray activities in his area.
- Where filaria in endemic: He will identify cases of lymphoedema/elephantiasis and hydrocele and their referral to PHC/CHC for appropriate management.
- Training of patients with lymphoedema about care of feet and home-based management remedies.
- He will impart training to drug distributors for Mass Drug administration of DEC on National Filaria Day.
- Identification of cases of leprosy, screening of cataract blindness and tuberculosis (suspect cases) and ensure regular and complete treatment of leprosy and tuberculosis cases and refer suspected cases of Cataract to Medical Officer.
- Environmental sanitation: Chlorinate the public drinking water source including wells at regular interval.
- Educate community—the method of disposal of liquid wastes, solid wastes, home sanitation, construction and use of sanitary latrines and smokeless chullah.
- Coordination with *Village Health and Sanitation Committee* (VHSC).
- Prevention and control of *non-communicable diseases* in the area. (Health promotion and opportunistic screening.)
- Communicable diseases: Recognize and report diseases under Integrated Disease surveillance for rapids response in outbreak situation at local level, with the help and guidance of MO of PHC and district teams. Also educate people on prevention and control of communicable diseases and non-communicable diseases.
- Universal Immunization Programme: Assist health Worker female in organizing *outreach session* on Immunization day at Anganwadi centre 'or' organize himself outreach session in remote and difficult area.
- School health: Assist the health supervisor Male and Female in the school health programme.
- Reproductive and Child Health Programme (RCH): Distribute conventional contraceptives and oral contraceptives to the couples and help prospective

acceptors of sterilization in obtaining the services, if necessary by accompanying them or arranging for the ASHA/DAI to accompany them to PHC/CHC/Hospital. Provide follow-up services to acceptors of family planning, in particular male acceptors.

- Identify male community leaders in each village and assist health supervisor male in training leaders in the community and ensure participation of community.
- Identify women requiring help in medical termination of pregnancy and refer them to nearest approved institution.
- Identify and refer cases of genital sore or urethral discharge or non-itchy rash over the body to MO.
- Primary medical care: Provide treatment for common ailments, first aid and emergencies and refer cases beyond his competence to nearest facility.
- Health education: He is a part of sub-centre team for nutrition and health education activities.
- Vital events: Record births and deaths of his area and share/coordinate this information with ANM and report these events to health assistant male.
- Records and reports: Maintain the records of activities performed and report the activities performed on the prescribed monthly report proforma to health supervisor.
- Functions of ASHAs and AWWs: Explained under ICDS and NRHM respectively.

ACTIVITIES OF DAI (BIRTH ATTENDANT)

Traditional birth attendants (TBA) have been trained to conduct safe home deliveries. From now on they are being retrained as skilled birth attendants which include care of mother and newborn.

TBA is a village level functionary who is helpful in early recognition and registration of all pregnant women, promotion of institutional deliveries and conducting safe home deliveries and provides care after delivery to mothers and newborn as also registration of births and deaths with health worker female. She refers high risk women and difficult deliveries to sub-centre or PHC or CHC. She is depot holder for contraceptives and motivates eligible couples for acceptance of contraceptives. She refers unwanted pregnancies for medical termination of pregnancy to recognized facility.

PLANNING OF HEALTH SERVICES

Planning is one of the major function of management. For any work, planning is essential. Planning essentially means what needs to be done, how and when it has to be done; by whom and with what resources? The planning means a blue print or a written protocol that guides our action (Fig. 15.5). "Good plans shape good decisions".

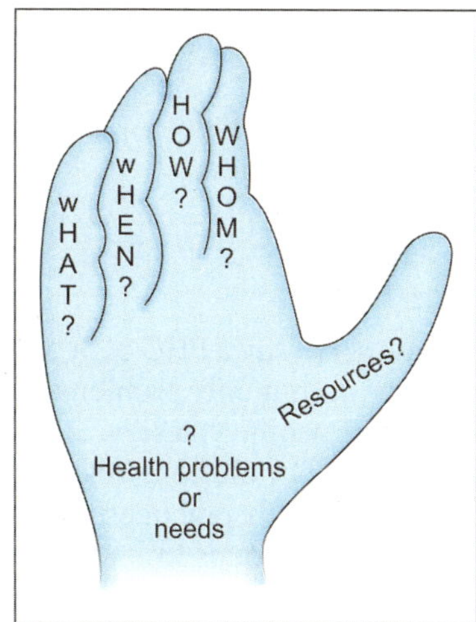

Fig. 15.5: Planning process

DEFINITION

Health Planning

"Health planning is the process of defining community health problems, identifying needs and resources, establishing priority goals, setting out the administrative action needed to reach those goals".

Some of the services/functions which need to be planned at the primary health centre/community health centre level include:

1. Antenatal care and coverage, safe deliveries, postnatal care and contraception services for eligible couples.
2. Newborn care and neonatal care.
3. Immunization services for pregnant women and children, pulse-polio and National Immunization days.
4. Integrated management of neonatal and childhood illness.
5. Management of reproductive tract infection and sexually transmitted infection (RTI/STI).
6. Adolescent health.
7. School health services special campaigns.
8. Health education and community participation.
9. National health programmes implementation (for communicable and non-communicable diseases).
10. Disease surveillance
11. Training and continuing education.
12. Records and reports (information management).

STEPS IN PLANNING OF SUB-CENTRE ACTION PLAN

A. Identification of health problems or needs.
B. Prioritization of problems.
C. What do we want to achieve? or define objectives.
D. Workout resources needed (men, money and material).
E. Programming—arranging the activities in order and with time frame.
F. Implementation of chosen plan or activities.

15

G Monitoring and supervision of activities.

H Coordination of activities.

I Evaluation of activities/plan.

J Replanning after evaluation.

A. Methods of Assessment of Health Problems/Needs

The community you serve say a PHC of 30,000 population, you need to know the community problems. These are best known by knowing the people you serve, the villages, their topographical access, population, resources, drinking water, sanitation and health practices. Meet people and their leaders and women groups to know their felt needs. *Listening* and *observing* the community, and discussing with community leaders, talking with ICDS functionaries, development workers, and the teachers can give you sufficient idea for a health or health-related problems, *besides records, reports* and *direct observation* on people. Similarly, look at the household survey records undertaken by the health workers wherein all members of the family have their names, age, sex and health status in terms of their source of drinking water, excreta disposal, immunization and nutritional status, disability and common diseases. With the help of **household survey registers** which are updated once in a year in the month of January and February you can have lot of information or some information of sub-centre area that helps you to make decision and prepare a "sub-centre action plan" (micro-plan for 5,000 people). You must have the information on number of villages and their population, number of Anganwadi workers and traditional birth attendants (trained and untrained) and other health practitioners in the village. It is better if the health workers have village-wise and anganwadi-wise household survey records for better tracking. If births, deaths, and pregnancy records are updated continuously by surveillance there is no need for annual surveys. Medical officers and supervisors must insist on regular updating (surveillance) of these vital events. Household survey data of health workers (female and male) help the workers to evolve an action plan for sub-centre and work their own workload and work schedule.

In essence, the community health needs/problems can be assessed by rapid methods, such as:

- Contacting people regularly and listening directly from clients their felt health needs or problems.
- Making rapid observations in community/village.
- Household survey data of health worker.
- From health services utilization data of past year available with health workers.
- From available records and reports such as demographic records (age and sex composition of population morbidity and mortality data).
- Health facility survey data contraceptive prevalence from eligible couple surveys.

One Example is Cited

Decentralized Participatory Planning (DPP) Community Need Assessment Approach at Sub-centre Level

Workers have used their own data (Tables 15.8 to 15.11):

1 Sub-centre (Ghironthi) population 4,463

2 Total eligible couples enumerated 746

3 Break up of couples by birth order (Table 15.8)

Workload (What Needs to be Done?)

From sub-centre action plan, workload of year 2004–2005 for a population of 4,463 was assessed as follow:

- 377 eligible couples need contraceptives (Table 15.8).
- 169 antenatals need antenatal care per year, as also safe deliveries and postanatal care (Table 15.9).
- 125 births or infants need newborn and neonatal care and immunization every year (Table 15.10).
- 200 children under-five (grade I and grade II) need to improve their nutritional status (Table 15.11).
- High fertility rate of 28.4/1000 (crude birth rate) was evident.
- 77.6% of deliveries were home deliveries and 22.4% are institutional deliveries. Only 25% deliveries were

Table 15.8: Users of contraceptive at sub-centre Ghironthi year 2003

Birth order	Total number of couples	No. of couples already covered under					Unprotected = Total – (Sterilization + IUD)
		Sterilization					
		Tub	Vas	IUD	CC	Oral pills	
0	73	–	–	–	–	7	73
1	132	1	1	23	3	15	107
2	189	95	–	19	6	13	75
3	216	142	–	24	5	13	50
≥4	136	52	–	12	2	2	72
Total	**746**	**290**	**1**	**78**	**16**	**50**	**377**

15

Table 15.9: Year-wise antenatal cases registered at SC Ghironthi

Year	Brought forward (from previous year)	New ANCs	Total
1999	22	144	166
2000	26	100	126
2001	27	114	141
2002	33	135	168
2003	35	134	169
2004 (till 27th Dec)	39	121	160

Table 15.10: Year-wise births and infant deaths at SC Ghironthi

Year	Live births	Infant deaths	Sub-centre population	Birth rate	IMR
1999	114	04	4292	26.5	35.1
2000	95	07	4310	21.6	73.6
2001	112	09	4360	25.6	80.3
2002	108	06	4390	24.6	55.5
2003	125	05	4458	28.4	40.0
2004 (till 27th Dec.)	121	05	4463	22.6	49.5

Table 15.11: Nutritional status of 0–5 years children SC Ghironthi, 2003

Age	Nutritional status (weight-for-age)					Total
	Normal	Grade I	Grade II	Grade III	Grade IV	
0–6 mth	37	19	1	0	0	57
6 mth–1 yr	22	17	3	0	0	42
1–3 yr	136	65	19	0	0	220
3–5 yr	115	65	11	0	0	191
Total	**310**	**166**	**34**	0	0	**510**

conducted by health worker female and the rest have been conducted by trained birth attendant.

- Postnatal and newborn care by health worker was negligible.
- Immunization and antenatal coverage is good (over 85%). Contraceptive prevalence rate was over 58%.

From the analysis of these data, following needs stand out clearly. In other words, major data based (evidence based) health needs emerging for sub-centre population were:

1 Large number of unprotected eligible couples needing contraceptive services.
2 Needs of pregnant women for antenatal care and safe delivery as also postnatal care.
3 Needs of infants for immunization, vitamin A prophylaxis, control and prevention of acute respiratory infection and diarrhoeal disease.
4 Widespread insanitary conditions—unsafe drinking water and indiscriminate human excreta disposal.

B. Prioritization of Problems

Coverage of pregnant women, infants, eligible couples, may be low in your area. That becomes an urgent need or priority for ensuring high level of coverage of care to antenatals, infants and eligible couples. Coverage norms for immunization is 100% and same is true for antenatal examination (atleast four check-ups). The coverage norms are laid down by state/district/or CHC incharge. Priority clients are: poorest and needy, below poverty line families having infants, under fives, pregnant women, postnatal mothers, sick children and acceptors of contraceptives, adolescents and old people.

From the present report and action plan of sub-centre Ghironthi, it is evident that the worker has:

i Used her own data to make annual sub-centre action plan. The Government has provided them the standard formats for sub-centre action plan.
ii The past year performance has been used as a base line for setting targets for the next year, it is **best practice** (*see* Form-1-SC Action Plan).
iii Worker has not used any formula or rate of district/state/nation to arrive at the number of expected beneficiaries in her area and they themselves have calculated their workload based on local birth rate and actual registered events (pregnancies, and births) by regular surveillance (Tables 15.9 and 15.10): **A best practice.**
iv The community has been consulted and contacted on regular basis, i.e. once a month. The data has been validated by contacting all Anganwadi workers and traditional birth attendants in the area.
v The workers have prepared the records of eligible couples, pregnant women and young children Anganwadi-wise.
vi There is regular tracking of antenatals and young children. Surveillance of antenatals, births and deaths in the area is a regular practice (best practice).
vii Resources available at sub-centre have been identified (the people, their skills, material and money).

Decentralized Participatory Planning

Flexible decentralized participatory planning is the pivot on which the entire concept of the NRHM revolves. The planning process in the health sector is now initiated by the Village Health Sanitation and Nutrition Committee. Composition of this committee is—Sarpanch, ASHA, MPHW (F), School teacher, AWW, and member of self-help group. Rs 10,000 per annum has been sanctioned as untied fund to each village panchayat. Over 5.2 lakh village health sanitation and nutrition committees have been made functional and provided untied grant.

The committee initiates a village health action plan. The aggregation of village health plans will lead to SC; PHC, and Block plan. The Blocks plan would eventually converge to district plans which would thereafter converge into State plans. Funding shall be given for agreed upon performance indicators.

Goal

Goal is purpose towards which effort is directed or the desired destination where you want your institution to be in future.

or

The goal is a broad, direction-setting, positive statement, describing what we want to achieve through our efforts. The goal usually cannot be objectively measured.

Example: To achieve 'health for all', to stabilize population and to improve quality of life.

C. Objectives or What we Want to Achieve?

These are measurable actions to be achieved. An objective is a brief statement specifying the desired impact or effect of a health promotion programme (i.e. how much of what should happen to whom by when) or objective is the aim or the end of an action. Objectives can be measured in terms of accomplishment.

Good objectives are: **SMART**

S: *Specific (clear and precise):* So that everyone involved interpret them in the same way.

M: *Measurable (amenable to evaluation):* To monitor progress or evaluate performance.

A: *Appropriate and relevant:* These should be appropriate and relevant to your organisation's policies, goals and strategies.

R: *Realistic:* The objectives should be realistic in view of limited resources (money, manpower and material).

T: *Time-bound:* The objectives should be achieved within time frame.

Examples of objectives

- To register all pregnant women in sub-centre area.
- To provide minimum four antenatal check-ups to all registered pregnant women in sub-centre area.
- To cover all infants for primary immunization.
- To have 80% of all deliveries in institutions.

These objectives are specific and measurable and feasible or realistic: Every month we get report on coverage of antenatals and infants. In a way, these are *short-term* or "operational objectives" for a programme or service. At the end of the year, we can assess the level of coverage of antenatals and infants for antenatal care and immunization respectively, from regular reports to a reasonable extent or by coverage evaluation surveys. The second set of objectives like:

- Reduction of infant mortality to 25 by the year 2020.
- Reductions of Total Fertility Rate to 2.1 by the year 2020 are *long-term* objectives at national and state levels.

15

These are achievable over a long period of time by effective interventions. These are also known as impact objectives.

Planning of Activities at Sub-centre (How to do it?)

1 Rapid household surveys—built into the programme or updating of household surveys every year or ideally every month by regular surveillance activity for identification of target groups for services, e.g. eligible couples, infants, pregnant women, adolescents, an aged, etc. by regular home visit/contact with families.
2 Segmentation of eligible couples according to parity and age of mother who need your help most for limiting and spacing methods.
3 Register all marriages on continuous basis in your area,
4 Continuous registration of all pregnant women for health check-up and safe pregnancy and delivery.
5 Identification and registration of all births continuously in the area for immunization and growth monitoring.

These activities are to be done by all health workers continuously in their geographical area.

D. Resources at Sub-centre (Men, Material and Money)

The resources at village and sub-centre level include "people" themselves and elected representatives, especially woman members of Panchayat, *Mahila Swasthya Sangh* and *Mahila Mandals* and non-governmental voluntary organizations. Besides these, there are "honorary and voluntary workers" like AWW, ASHA, traditional birth attendants, village chowkidar, health guides and school teachers and private practitioners of various systems. Development functionaries like *Gram Sevikas* are also available in a few villages. At the sub-centre level, "health workers male and female" are available and accountable to medical officer or in some situations to village Panchayats. Besides manpower, the other resources include building—community centre, vocational centre and Anganwadi centres; "medicines (drug kit A and B)" and "equipment" for maternal and child health care are also available. Drug kits are also available at Anganwadi centre.

At sub-centre level, *untied grant* of ₹ 10,000 per year is available for local health actions, such as purchase of emergency medicines, repairs of equipment, and cleanliness. Besides this incentive money to be paid to ASHA (performance-based incentive) is also available.

These resources must be marshalled and used by the sub-centre health teams. The medical officers and supervisors are responsible to ensure proper utilization of available services at sub-centre by the community. The available services must be depicted and made known to the people of the sub-centre area, especially to village Panchayats and women groups (citizen's charter).

Time is also an important resource and hence time management is critical. Time devoted by medical officers

FORM-1 SUB-CENTRE (SC) ACTION PLAN			
General Information **State: Haryana** District: Rohtak P.H.C.: Chiri Sub-centre: Ghironthi No. of villages under the sub-centre:1		**Year 2004** **Population of SC-4463** Birth Rate of Sub-centre-28.4 Eligible Couples-746 (As on 1st April, 2004)	
Sr. No.	**Consultation with**	**No. of consultation**	**When consultation made (month of year)**
1.	Panchayat or health committee of the Panchayat	12	Once a month
2.	Anganwadi worker/TBA	4	Once a week
3.	Women in Mahila Swasthya Sangh	12	Once a month
4.	Families on house-to-house basis		Once in 3 months
Sr. No.	**Services**	**Performance in last year**	**Planned performance in current year**
1.	Antenatal care Total no. of ANC cases registered in the area	169	179
2.	No. of high-risk pregnant women detected and referred	20	25
3.	**No. of TT doses given**		
	(a) TT1	125	150
	(b) TT2	85	90
	(c) Booster	–	–
4.	No. of pregnant women with anaemia treated	72	75
5.	No. of pregnant women given prophylaxis with IFA tablets	69	75
6.	**Natal care** Total no. of deliveries in the area	125	125
7.	**Home** deliveries		–
	(a) by ANM/LHV	31	40
	(b) Trained birth attendant	66	25
	(c) Others	–	
8.	No. of institutional deliveries	28	60
9.	No. of pregnant women referred to PHC/FRU for delivery	28	30
10.	**Neonatal Care**	31	100
	No. of sick newborns referred	5	13
11.	**MTP** No. of women referred for MTP	7	5

Contd...

Contd...

Sr. No.	Services		Performance in last year		Planned performance in current year	
			Male	Female	Male	Female
12.	**RTI/STI** No. of cases detected No. of cases referred		7	134	10	140
			7	106		
13.	No. of infant immunized (0–1 year)	BCG	58	64	60	65
		DPT-1	65	61	67	62
		DPT-2	59	57	60	58
		DPT-3	57	51	58	52
		OPV-0	47	53	48	54
		OPV-1	65	61	66	62
		OPV-2	59	57	60	58
		OPV-3	57	51	58	52
		Measles	55	52	56	53
		Fully immunized				
14.	No. of children immunized (more than 18 months)	DPT Booster	67	44	70	46
		OPV Booster	67	44	70	46
15.	No. of children immunized (more than 5 years)	**DT**	69	73	72	75
16.	No. of children immunized (more than 10 years)	**TT**	28	50	30	52
17.	No. of children immunized (more than 16 years)	**TT**	32	44	35	48
18.	No. of children given IFA small (below 5 years)	**IFA**	234	241	240	240
19.	Vitamin A No. of children administered vitamin A (9 months to 5 years)	Dose 1	55	52	52	54
		Dose 2	67	44	69	46
		Dose 3–9	85	95	88	96
20.	ARI (Acute respiratory infection) no. of cases under 5 with pneumonia	Treated with cotrimoxazole	45	40	47	42
		Referred	15	17	17	19
21.	Acute diarrhoeal diseases no. of cases under 5 years	Treated with ORS	46	43	48	45
		Referred	–	–	–	–
22.	Family planning—number of eligible couples who accepted permanent methods out of couples with:	3 or more children	–	15	–	12
		2 children	–	10	–	14
		1 child	–	2	–	–
23.	No. of eligible couples who accepted temporary methods	(A) IUD	–	35	–	38
		(B) Oral pills	–	16	–	14
		(C) Condoms	100	–	100	–

15

INVENTORY OF DRUGS/CONTRACEPTIVES AND OTHER MATERIALS					
Sr. No.	**Item**	**Requirement assessed last year**	**Actual quantity received last year**	**Surplus or shortage last year**	**Requirement for current year**
1.	ORS packets zinc tablets	300	520	–	400
2.	Tab. Metronidazole	2000	1000	–	2000
3.	Tab. Cotrimoxazole	2000	1000	–	2000
4.	Tab. Paracetamol	2000	2000	500	2500
5.	Tab. Chloroquine	–	–	–	–
6.	Tab. CPM				
7.	Tab. Diclofenac				
8.	Tab. Albendazole				
9.	Inj Methergan				
10.	Inj Syntocinin				
11.	Povidine iodine solution	4	4	–	4
12.	Uristix	50	–	50	50
13.	DD kits (disposable delivery kits)	116	–	150	150
14.	Slides for blood tests or RDT kits	–	–	–	–
15.	Thermometer	–	–	1	1
16.	Gloves	12	12	–	12
17.	IFA large	30000	35000	–	30000
18.	IFA small tablets	26000	39000	–	26000
19.	Vitamin A solution	1200 ml	1500 ml	–	1200 ml
20.	Condoms	18000	12000	–	12000
21.	Oral pills	200	200	–	200
22.	IUDs	40	36	–	40
23.	Syringes and needles	–	–	–	–

CHECKLIST OF FACILITY AT SUB-CENTRE				
Sr. No.	Selected equipment and supplies	Available		Functional status
		Yes	No	
A.	**Facilities**			
1.	ANM/MPW (Male and Female)	✓		
2.	Accommodation (including residence)	✓		
3.	Water	✓		
4.	Electricity	–	✓	✓
B.	**Furniture and equipment**			
1.	Examination table	✓		✓
2.	Benches for clients	✓		✓
3.	Cupboard for drugs	✓		✓
4.	Foot stools	✓		✓
5.	Vessels for water storage	✓		✓
6.	Water disposal containers	✓		✓
7.	Brooms and mops for cleaning	–	✓	✓
8.	Steam sterilizer	✓		✓
9.	Delivery kits	✓		✓
10.	Torch light	✓		✓
11.	Stove	✓		✓
12.	Weighing scale	✓		✓
13.	BP apparatus	✓		✓
14.	Haemoglobinometer	✓		✓
15.	Vaccine carrier	✓		✓
16.	IUD kits Pregnancy test kits	✓		✓
17.	**Newborn Care Corner—Material:**			
	• Radiant warmer			×
	• 200 watt bulb in labour room			
	• Foot operated suction machine			
	• Resuscitator (Ambu-bags)			×
	• Mucus extractor (mucus sucker)			
	• Baby weighing scale			×
	• Oxygen cylinder with flowmeter			
	• Red and black waste bags			
C.	**IEC material**			
1.	Posters	✓		
2.	Models	–	✓	
3.	Flip chart	✓		

15

for management and technical jobs should be balanced to ensure that management functions are not neglected. **Information** is also an important resource.

E. Programming Work Plan

A programme is grouping of continuous and related *activities* designed to achieve the set objective. *Activities* include home visits, immunization, MCH and FP clinic, growth monitoring, communication and counselling and visit to Anganwadi, recording and reporting, group meetings, etc. The activities of sub-centre area will be planned and fixed work plan or schedule of visits will be worked out day-wise and village-wise as exemplified in Table 15.12. It should be flexible enough to adjust to changed conditions and to unusual or unexpected situations like outbreak or intensive activities/campaigns.

Organization of Activities

The antenatal care clinic will be either organized at sub-centre or as an outreach session at Anganwadi centre in non-sub-centre village with the help of traditional birth attendants, Anganwadi workers and ASHAs.

When it will be done: A fixed work plan or schedule of visits will be followed by the health worker female to cover all 5 Anganwadi areas or whole sub-centre areas/villages (Table 15.12). When all the activities are worked out and time-line defined with responsibility, it will give an overview of activities against which monitoring can be undertaken. In other words, this matrix will facilitate in not only providing information on when the activities have to be initiated and completed but can be effectively used for tracking the status of each of the defined activity along with monthly monitoring by health worker female.

- This is just one model programme schedule of sub-centre. This fixed visit schedule can be modified suiting local conditions. Mothers meetings and contact with informants for community-based surveillance and supervision of ORS/chloroquine/condom depot holders will be held as part of AWW visit or home visit at the village level. All efforts would be made to dovetail the activities with Anganwadi workers. Mothers meetings and home visits can be done jointly with AWW and ASHA of the area. That will have more impact and provide security to health worker female.
- *On open days*, the immunization sessions in hamlets or mothers meetings or Health and Nutrition Day or PHC meetings can be held.
- One *home visit* should cover at least 10–15 households and part of that day could be spent at Anganwadi. The events of birth/death/pregnancy and marriage can be collected through home visits or at Anganwadi centre or on Health and Nutrition Day at Anganwadi centre. Home visits are meant for tracking of beneficiaries or follow-up as also identification of new beneficiaries and for counseling and group meetings. The whole of the work schedule should be linked with Anganwadi worker.

F. Implement Plan of Activities and Schedule

A plan is only as good as its implementation. Implementation is the key step in the planning process, which needs special attention. The time table made by workers must be implemented. The implementation of plan of work schedule of health workers must be ensured and the work schedule must be made more efficient. The field workers should spend more time with priority clients especially the poorest and needy. The home visit/contact programme should focus on:

1 Young eligible couples (20–25 years).
2 Pregnant and lactating women of weaker section.
3 Children below one year of age.
4 Register all pregnancies at the earliest with the help of traditional birth attendants, Anganwadi workers, *Mahila Swasthaya Sanghs* and ensure antenatal care, delivery and follow-up of the child regularly till infancy at least. Since large number of pregnant women (169) and infants (125) are to be followed up in homes/clinic, more help from above named functionaries would help increase coverage and facilitate the work of ANMs.
5 Make sure that the workers are mobile—help their mobility. Provide mopeds/bicycles for mobility and arrange loan to purchase mopeds.
6 Additional ANMs should be posted for difficult or remote areas to increase access and to implement the schedule.
7 Male worker should take adequate responsibility of sharing the work with female worker in areas like

Table 15.12: Monthly work plan of health worker, female (MPHW, female)

Week	Monday	Tuesday	Wednesday*	Thursday	Friday	Saturday
First	Home visit village-1	MCH and F.P. clinic	Immunization village-3	MCH and FP clinic	AW visit-1	AW visit-5
Second	Home visit village-2	-do-	Immunization village-4	MCH and FP clinic	AW visit-2	Open day
Third	Home visit village-3	-do-	Immunization village-1	-do-	AW visit-3	Open day
Fourth	Home visit village-4	-do-	Immunization village-2	-do-	AW visit-4	Open day
Fifth	For missed work on any day of above due to leave or holiday or meetings					Open day

*Village health and nutrition day with ASHA and AWW once a month.

immunization and procuring supplies and vaccines and coverage of inaccessible area with the help of traditional birth attendants/ASHA.

8 Provide adequate support and supervision to health worker female to ensure implementation of her work schedule.
9 The work schedule should be known to community, all Anganwadi workers and ASHAs. *Mahila Swasthya Sanghs* and *Mahila Mandals* can help to implement the work schedule of health workers.
10 The whole effort is to enhance coverage of the services through Anganwadi centres and ASHAs.
11 Planning and implementation of outreach session with AWW helps achieve better coverage and better quality of services as also preparation of quality records and reports. It is better if the health worker maintains household survey records/births and antenatal records Anganwadi-wise to ensure better tracking and coverage.
12 ***Logistics and supplies:*** The supplies must reach the sub-centre on regular basis and "stock outs" should be prevented. During rains, the sub-centre access becomes difficult, ensure adequate stocks beforehand. Essential drugs and contraceptives must be made available in sufficient quantities.
13 The schedule is likely to be followed if adequate support of referral services is ensured at the level of PHC and CHC and FRUs. At the moment, this component is quite weak and it needs to be strengthened.

Example of Planning of Antenatal Care in a Sub-centre Area

- *Problem:* Pregnant women do not come to sub-centre and do not get registered for antenatal care.
- *Why:* All pregnant women of the sub-centre area need essential obstetric care at least four antenatal check-ups for safe pregnancy and for timely detection of complications of pregnancy/danger signals and timely referral of antenatals for prompt treatment. Any pregnant woman may develop complication/danger signs any time, i.e. during pregnancy—during delivery or following delivery hence all need to be cared and supervised.
- *The delay:* Most pregnant women report late, i.e. during second and third trimester of pregnancy and thus most valuable time is lost to control and correct anaemia. Therefore, it is most desirable that all pregnancies are identified at the earliest and registered at sub-centre for early action/care.
- *What is to be done?* Ensure 100% registration of all pregnant women at the earliest (before 12 weeks of pregnancy) and ensure 100% coverage of pregnant women for at least four complete health check-ups (full antenatal care). One full antenatal check-up includes past history, general examination for anaemia and swelling over feet, measuring weight and blood pressure, urine and haemoglobin examination, abdominal examination, tetanus toxoid and giving iron and folic acid tablets for one month besides nutrition and health education.
- *How it will be done?* The identification of pregnant women: All married women in reproductive age group who miss their periods are pregnant unless proved otherwise. Such women must report for help and motivated to seek help of health workers. Pregnancy test can be done by the health worker/ASHA.
- *Who will do it?* Health worker female holds primary responsibility for antenatal care. She will seek assistance/help of Anganwadi workers and traditional birth attendants, ASHAs and women groups and also pregnant women who can be helpful in informing other women in their neighbourhood.
- *Which things are needed?* Place for examination, examination table, BP apparatus, weighing machine, register for record and home-based *mother and child protection card*, iron and folic acid tablets and tetanus toxoid, syringes and needles and educational material.

Alternate Strategies and Plan of Action

Different alternatives to ensure near 100% registration and coverage of pregnant women:

1 Should all antenatals come to clinic or workers meet them in their home? It is difficult question. Answer lies in combination of both the approaches. Home visit by health worker female all alone: It will take 3–4 months time to cover the whole area, i.e. 5000 population or 1000 households/families.
2 Joint home visits with Anganwadi worker who works for 150 households—which are intimately known to resident anganwadi workers and their helpers. Taking the help of Anganwadi workers and ASHA can enhance the coverage of antenatal mothers.
3 Using traditional birth attendants (trained and untrained) can also cover more antenatal mothers.
4 Using women groups (*Mahila Swasthya Sanghs* and other women groups or pregnant mothers) for early registration and care at sub-centre.
5 Ensuring regular clinic on fixed days at sub-centre or at village and women report by themselves because of availability of quality services and adequate check-ups and counselling on one-to-one basis.

Implementation of Programme of Antenatal Care

It involves series of activities like:

- Identification or recognition of all pregnant women.
- Registration of pregnant women.
- Health check-ups of all pregnant women and referral of risky mothers.

15

- Immunization and prevention of anaemia.
- Education in groups—explaining danger signals—prepare them for breastfeeding and care of nipples as also limiting the family size and spacing births.
- Deciding place of delivery and ensuring safe delivery.

Mechanisms

- Contact programme in community (home visit schedule) for identification of pregnant women.
- Arranging registers for registration and recording of essential information of all antenatals.
- Arranging examination site—room, table, weighing machine, blood pressure apparatus.
- Conducting clinic on fixed days—areawise preferably Anganwadi-wise.
- Conducting immunization session on fixed dates/days.
- Referrals of high-risk cases and follow-up visits.
- Reporting of progress of work to PHC (new antenatals registered and total antenatals covered).
- Sub-centres to report on their performance to panchayats every month.

G. Monitoring and Supervision of Work Schedule

Monthly monitoring reports (MMR): Monthly monitoring reports provide useful information on monitoring of services of sub-centre. Any deviation detected are brought to the notice of health workers for corrective actions by better planning and implementation of the programme. MMR measures the progress of work each month and serves a useful tool to know the performance level of the worker against the norms or standards.

The purpose of monitoring and supervision is to improve work/service standards. The health supervisors will ensure monitoring of work and spot supervision. Health supervisors ensure supervision and supporting the service in difficult areas and upgrading the skills of workers by on the job training/continued duction.

H. Coordination—"Coming together is a begining, Keeping together is Progress, Working together is Success"

Convergence of work and services with Anganwadi workers and traditional birth attendant can enhance the coverage of antenatal mothers. Supervisory support of medical officers and health supervisors can have a positive influence on coverage and quality of services. Coordinating the work of Anganwadi workers and health workers, traditional birth attendants and *Mahila Swasthya Sangh* is an essential task of all supervisors. All these persons act as one team and understand their common objectives of safe pregnancy and ensuring full utilization of essential obstetrical care services made available at village/ Anganwadi/sub-centre level. Regular meeting of these workers is one of the mechanism to achieve better coordination. Linkage of services and work of these functionaries at village level helps to achieve better results. For example, TBAs and ASHA can be used as link workers, train them together and provide them delivery kits and necessary support; pay her performance-based incentive.

Similarly, health worker female works with and works through anganwadi workers and ASHA, ensure joint visits, joint survey, meeting with antenatals and women groups. Anganwadi centre is a hub or convergence point of all services for women and children.

Further all these health team members must know their assigned role and work schedule of sub-centre and anganwadi as also available services.

Coordinating the work between AWW and health worker female, as also between health workers (female and male), TBAs, ASHAs and NGOs is essential for convergence.

I. Evaluation of Sub-centre Performance

The evaluation means, how far the stated objectives of sub-centre action plan have been met and reasons for not meeting the objectives are identified for replanning of programme/services.

Performance reports (monthly monitoring reports) provide useful information for monitoring and evaluation of services. The purpose of evaluation is to improve the services by mechanism of feedback to the programme and providers. Simple indicators have been evolved for rapid evaluation and medical officer and health supervisors can use these indicators to assess the services at sub-centre. Much of the information is obtained through regular supervisory field visits and by looking into the routine reports. Some of the suggested indicators are mentioned below:

1. Total number of outreach sessions planned and number of sessions actually held in sub-centre area.
2. No. of antenatal mothers provided four check-ups.
3. No. of home deliveries/institutional deliveries and deliveries done/supervised by health worker female.
4. No. of traditional birth attendants trained.
5. No. of infants fully immunized or immunized against measles.
6. No. of antenatals referred.
7. No. of neonates referred.
8. No. of village health and nutrition days organized.

J. Replanning

The evaluation discovers gaps in the planning process. It also pin points shortcomings in the planning process. The replanning takes care of these gaps and shortcomings in the planning cycle.

Other Examples of Planning

See planning implementation and evaluation of communication programme and national health programmes like malaria, filaria, NIDDCP, blindness, cancer, HIV/AIDS and tuberculosis and data of district level household surveys (DLHS) as shown in Boxes 15.1A and B.

Box 15.1A: District level household survey—RCH 2004 key indicators

1	Population of the district (Kaimur in Bihar)	128,9000
2	Percentage of girls married at age less than 18 years	48.6
3	Total fertility rate	3.1
	Birth orders 3 and above	54.4
4	Crude death rate	3.60
5	Knowledge of family planning methods % of women knowing	100.0
6	Percentage of eligible women/husbands	
	• Using any method of contraception	29.2
	• Using modern method of contraception	26.9
	• Female sterilization	20.9
	• Condom users	2.5
	• Male sterilization	0.1
7	Any antenatal-check up received	40.1
	Three or more antenatal check-ups	17.8
	• Tetanus toxoid two or more	53.4
	• Iron and folic acid tablets received	26.1
	• Received full antenatal care (three or more ANC visits + Tetanus toxoid + 100 or more IFA tablets)	2.1
8	Institutional deliveries	33.6
	Home deliveries	66.4
9	Breastfeeding initiated within 2 hours of birth	26.5
	Breastfeeding initiated after 3 days	31.9
10	Children who received full immunization	12.3
11	Children who had diarrhoea in last two weeks	4.5
	• Children who had pneumonia in last two weeks of survey	15.7
	Diarrhoeas treated with ORS	30.4
12	Women having symptoms of RTI/STI	54.4
13	Home visits by health workers in the past 3 months	100.0
14	Utilization of Government health services ANC	8.5
	• Treatment for post-delivery	20.9
	• Treatment for RTI/STI	27.7

Source: IIPS Mumbai. Reproductive and child health project district level household survey-2004. Population Research Centre Dept. of Statistics, Patna University.

Under RCH district household survey data for each district in the country is available on every alternate year. It includes key indicators like: Mean age of marriage, major illnesses, utilization of antenatal care and delivery services and their sources, breastfeeding practices, immunization coverage, ORS use rate, contraceptive prevalence rate, home visits by workers, prevalence of RTIs/STIs, knowledge of HIV/AIDS and incidence of diarrhoea and pneumonia, birth rate and death rate, etc.

- This data base/information is most valuable source for planning and evaluation of reproductive and child health services, behaviour change communication and in-service training of health teams. Data of Kaimur district of Bihar state as presented can be used for these purposes. One can access and use data of the district in which medical college is located. DLHS-4 has been completed and district data cards released.

Box 15.1B: Key findings of district level household survey 2007–08 and CES of 2009 in India

	DLHS-2	DLHS-3	CES 2009
Population	*1129 million*	*1170 m*	
Literacy rate in female	57.6	59	
Households using iodized salt	30	–	
Mean age of marriage for girls	19.4 years	19.9	
Girls married before 18 years	28.5	21.5	
• Total fertility rate	4	4	
• Improvident maternity (Birth orders 3 and above)	42	–	
• Three antenatal check-ups	50.4	51.0	68.7
• Full package of antenatal care	16.5	19.1	26.5
• Institutional deliveries	41	47	73
Private institutions 22%			26
Government institutions 19%		–	47
Initiating breastfeeding within one hour	27.8	40.2	33.5
Fully immunized children	46	54.1	61
ORS use rate	30	33.7	43
Contraceptive prevalence rate	53	54.1	
Use of Government facility by women	29	–	
Women reported symptom of RTI/STI	32	18.3	
Men reported symptom of RTI/STI	8	–	
Unmet need for family planning	21.4	21.5	

Figures in percentages.

SUPERVISION AS MANAGEMENT TOOL

What is Not Supervision?

The supervision is often misused and misunderstood by many. It is not an inspection or fault-finding mission. It is also not a checking or marking only presence or absence of subordinates or just signing the registers.

What is Supportive Supervision?

Supervision is a helping process.

i The supervision means guidance, supporting and facilitating the work.

ii Its objective is to improve the quality of work and health services. It also aims at development of health worker and health teams to improve or upgrade their skills by—on the job training and guidance.

iii The supervisors should make use of management information system and field visits to identify unmet needs of community and help health workers to evolve action plans to meet these needs.

Definition

Supervision is described as: "A process by which a designated individual or a group of individuals, oversee the work of others and establish such controls and procedures as will improve that work through development of worker and working group or through manipulation of the conditions under which the work takes place."[4]

Supervisors must facilitate the work and motivate the workers to perform better and render quality services as per standards. The problems of the workers must be solved by their supervisors and deficiency be rectified by rapid action to sustain the interest of workers.

Methods of Supervision

There are various methods of supervision:

1. ***Observing workers on the job (concurrent supervision):*** When the workers are doing their job the designated supervisor oversees that they are doing the work as per laid down standard. This gives an opportunity to judge the quality aspect of services. There is no other method to judge the quality of services provided to people but for on the job observation.

This is an opportunity to train the worker on the job concurrently. Supervisor also gets a chance to see the relationship of worker with client and community and accessibility and acceptability of services. You can look whether the pieces of equipment are functional and being used. Once the worker is being observed directly they may try to overdo or the situation may be abnormal on that particular day, or the workers may become nervous, these should be guarded and taken care of. No judgment should be passed for an abnormal situation.

2. ***Meeting clients and community leaders (consecutive supervision):*** Consumer or client is a *king* in service delivery system. The supervisors can meet users/ clients and community. A sample of 10 households can be observed to elicit their reactions and satisfaction about services. Their unmet needs can be assessed and reasons of dissatisfaction can be ascertained for rectification. The whole purpose is to improve the system of services. Clients views and consultation always help to improve the system. Action plans should incorporate the view points and suggestions of consumer. Involvement of community and leaders in health system can be worked out by meeting the leaders and organized women groups apart from their demand and satisfaction about services.

3. ***Review of records and reports:*** The records and reports are evidence of work done or work performed by the workers. The accuracy and completeness of records can be assessed by supervisors. Similarly, unmet needs also can be assessed through records and reports. How the workers are using these records for preparing the sub-centre action plans, can also be assessed by supervisors. Whether records are being shared with community and community leaders can be judged. Again, the purpose is to encourage workers to maintain essential records and use that information to improve their work and quality of services and coverage.

4. ***By checklist:*** Health supervisors are required to maintain a 'checklist' for each sub-centre/village to ensure adequate supportive supervision. Use of checklist helps observing performance and identification of deficiencies in standard outputs and procedures and their causes. The supervisors must make a note of deficient skills and rectify these through on the job training. The supervisors must be able to use the management information system to identify the unmet client needs and deficient skills in the workers; client satisfaction and quality of services. Whole machinery of supervision (medical officers and health supervisors and district supervisors) would focus on development of health teams at the sub-centre level. Ensure availability of all supplies for services by regularly supervising these through checklist system. Data on Sub-centre, PHC and CHC facility checklist and survey helps better planning/decision-making.

***Example of checklist*: *See* Sub-centre Action Plan.**

5. ***Staff meetings:*** Staff meetings with health workers provide an opportunity to get information and to give information to health teams. It also helps to coordinate the work between health workers male and female as also Anganwadi workers. It is an occasion to review the deficiencies in work performance and ways and means to improve the work. Some of the pressing problems can be solved in these meetings. It is also a best forum to plan the work for the next month. During review meetings, continuous education session can be organized to improve the skills of health teams.

6. ***Feedback to worker:*** Give feedback to workers about your supervision. Give positive as well as negative feedback about his/her work performance with a view to improve the performance in future. Sector meeting provides an opportunity to provide feedback to the workers on their performance and problems are solved on the spot and joint plan is made, for the next month.

7. ***Solve problem:*** Solving problems related to work and worker or the system are a part of supportive supervision.

Functions of Supervisor

The functions of supervisors include:

1 Facilitation of work, guidance and trdining.
2 Establishing qualitative and quantitative control of the work and improve quality of service.
3 Promoting effectiveness of the individual worker.
4 Promoting effectiveness of the group.

5 Serving a link between field and administrative staff at higher level.
6 Monitoring and evaluation of performance.

Obstacles in Supervision

Lack of training, poor understanding of concept of supervision and its objective, lack of mobility and transport, no fixed schedule of visits, lack of accountability of supervisors are the major obstacles in the supervision.

There is no account of work supervised or assessed. It should be built into the system of monthly reporting. The accountability of the system right now is to the bureaucracy. It should be reversed to the client and community plus health and family welfare staff. Adequate mobility or advance money for supervisory visits should be ensured. Adequate management training to health supervisors, workers during undergraduate and internship period must be strived.

The criteria for measuring the performance of supervisors should focus on their success in using the health management information system and field visits to identify unmet client needs and deficient skills and to rectify these through on the job training.

Present Scenario

The health workers on their job do not get the guidance for improving their deficient skills. Medical officer spend 80% of his time on curative work at the health centre and not available to supervise and support their work with the result the workers are left to themselves to perform and continue to do their job what they know and seldom know whether they are doing things right or as per standard. In the past, the whole focus of supervision was on targets achieved and there was no concern to improve the quality of work, worker and group performance.[11, 12]

The supervisors must have a fixed schedule of visit to sub-centre, it should be known to both people and the health workers of the area.

The supervisors must go well prepared to meet the situation and have all the facts and figures with him/her of that sub-centre. If the supplies were deficient, the supplies must be ensured in that visit. Reaching supplies and material to workers is part of the job of supervisors. Workers should not run all the times to collect supplies.

The best example is sustaining outreach sessions on immunization: The vaccines in vaccine carrier, syringes, needles and necessary cards and reporting formats must be reached to the worker by supervisors and reports and left over vaccines are collected on the same day. Ensure that immunization sessions are held along with Anganwadi workers, preferably at Anganwadi centre or sub-centre as per standard; and high level of coverage and quality is ensured.

Examples: Supervisor observes that planned session of outreach immunization has been missed by the worker. Reason was supplies (vaccines) had not reached to location.

Action by supervisor/manager: To ensure that session is held on subsequent week or on open day of work schedule for the next month.

Similarly, supervisors ensure availability of necessary supplies for quality antenatal care.

- Securing and maintenance of sub-centre buildings.
- Involving people in the health care delivery system.
- Helping workers to prepare and implement efficient work schedule.

These are some examples cited to develop the concept and method of supervision.

All the supervisors must use check list system for supervision and keep a record in their diaries for follow-up action. Supervision without actions is useless exercise.

Training and Continuing Education of Health Teams—a Management Responsibility

Since the workers have been trained at district level and at institutions for their initial training of one year for male and one and a half year for female, they need a system of continuing education to upgrade their skills. These health workers have been imparted some skill training but it is inadequate by all standards. Training schools impart less of community-based training and focus more on theoretical training based in the hospital and in the institutions far away from the community. Basic training faculty is poorly trained and training is a last priority with the state Governments. Basic training of health workers—the syllabus and contents are much more than MBBS or doctorate in community medicine, the implementation of training is faulty in many ways.

In our opinion and experience whole of the basic training of health workers and health team must be based in the community and their teachers should be traditional birth attendants, experienced health workers and Anganwadi workers and senior medical officers of CHC. Given this situation, the medical officer and senior medical officers are responsible to provide on the job training to health workers, continuing education and orientation training.

Of late, quite a transformation of family welfare training system has occurred during the past one decade. A new infrastructure of state institutes of health and family welfare, regional and divisional training centres, and district training centres (DTCs) and district training teams has been created. States are beginning to recognize the critical importance of training for improving service quality. Most staff at the periphery now have received in-service training under CSSM, RCH and NRHM programmes. However, by and large the training and continuing education has been neglected. The skills of trainers and method of training need to be improved. Field staff need more training in; how to plan their work routines and help them preparing an efficient work schedule.[13, 14]

The training, particularly in-service training of health workers can be best carried out at PHC and CHC and at sub-centre level, it gives them an opportunity of hands on training and practice. Major emphasis should be to improve the quality of technical care delivered by auxiliary nurse midwife (female health workers) especially in clinical skills like pelvic examination, IUD insertions, abdominal examination and safe deliveries. Training in work planning and *preparing efficient work schedule* and interpersonal communication can be best provided at block level.

The role of medical officer as manager is to ensure that all the workers and health teams are adequately trained in skills. Deficient skills are to be identified and upgraded during supervisory visits and continuing education sessions at sector meeting or monthly meetings.

Worker to worker training can be arranged by medical officer in PHC or CHC area where better skilled and experienced health workers can impart training to their fellow colleagues. Health supervisors and lady medical officer can ensure skill training at the level of PHC/CHC.

Integrated skill training under RCH leaves much to be desired. The role of medical officer becomes critical in the area of training and continuing education of health teams under his/her charge. Usually this role is not accepted well. Whatever medical officer knows he just lectures on that subject. The training has to be skill-based, need-based, and deficiencies in skills observed during field visits, must be rectified. The training has to be learning by doing and focus on skills of the trainees rather than on the subject. Method should be demonstration; return demonstration and no lectures are needed. Audiovisual methods would be used maximally. *Training needs are assessed* through supervisory visits and if a new technology has come, that becomes the focus of training.

Maternal and child health care (antenatal check-ups, deliveries, postnatal care, neonatal care, immunization, IUD insertion, treatment of diarrhoeal diseases, pneumonia and other common ailments) have been delegated to health workers. Health workers can best discharge this responsibility when trained adequately and supported by supervisors and on the job training. Therefore, team leader and health supervisors are responsible for hands on training of health workers for pelvic and cervical examination by speculum and copper T insertion and conduct of normal delivery as also safe injections. Coverage and quality of maternal and child health services will largely depend on the skills of health workers and their continuous training.

Training and continued education on non-communicable diseases, intersectoral co-ordination and interaction and involvement of people in planning is an imperative need, apart from communication skills.

Controlling

The work done (antenatals examined and care provided) will be reported to primary health centre once a month by fixed date. The sector or monthly meeting day will be used to collect the report and compilation of reports. The supervisors will ensure compiling and collection of reports of each sub-centre area in the sector meeting, where 25–30 Anganwadi workers assemble along with 5–6 health workers female and as also health workers male once every month. The deficiencies are rectified on the spot and performance for the month is assessed. Reasons for short falls are discussed and rectified. The workers and supervisors are assessed on the basis of their annual work performance. The performance of every worker is assessed annually by way of annual confidential reports. Grades of performance are assigned. The objective of this excercise is to improve the performance of workers and health teams as also to establish control.

HEALTH SYSTEM MONITORING

Health system is a set of elements, which function together to accomplish an objective or purpose. The digestive system, e.g. consists of mouth, gullet, stomach, small intestine and large intestine, all of which function together to digest food. The elements in the system are those components, which function, belong together, and work in a synchronized manner, to achieve a common goal, purpose or objective. The health system requires *inputs* to carry out programme activities, which result in *outcome*. These *outcomes* are in the form of *outputs* (immediate products and services produced by the programme), *effects* (the knowledge, attitudes, and behaviour/practice and changes that result from outputs) and *impacts* (changes in health or fertility status due to the effects).[15, 16]

- **Programme inputs** are resources (men, money and materials) that are invested in the health programme.
- **Processes (activities):** Inputs are processed in several ways, which include discrete actions such as weighing, counselling, diagnosis, treatment, referral, immunization, home visit, educating, antenatal check up, delivery, training and laboratory tests as also surveillance, screening, chlorination, and preparation of reports.
- **Outcomes:** The processes (activities and tasks) lead to results which are called outcomes. The outcomes are of three types: (i) outputs, (ii) effects and (iii) impacts.
  - *Outputs (results):* The activities lead to some results. The immediate results are called "outputs" and these are products and the services, growth monitoring and immunization cards (mother and child protection card) and iron folic acid tablets distributed are: products and children weighed and pregnant women contacted and examined are: services. Other examples of services are number of deliveries conducted; number or postnatal mothers and neonates provided required services.
  - *Effects*: The outputs produce effects on client's knowledge, attitude, skills and behaviour and individual gets motivated to use service, e.g. use of

15

ORT, contraceptive, use of antenatal clinic, immunizations, and quit smoking.

- ***Impact***: Ultimate result is impact of outputs, which is reduction in morbidity, mortality, fertility or disability or malnutrition.

The system framework and planning evaluation cycle are shown in Fig. 15.6.

Thus, the system approach converts men, money and material resources into activities, which lead on to outcomes such as outputs in the form of services or products and which produce effects on person and ultimately results into improved health status in the form of reduced disease, fertility, death and disability rates (like reduction in diarrhoea, malaria, decreased infant mortality, decreased birth rate, etc.).

Indicator

An indicator is a variable that helps to measure change.

Indicator is an indirect/direct measure of an event or condition. An indicator is constructed from a set of measurements but is more than the measurement itself.

Example: A child's weight is a measurement. If this weight is compared to a "standard" or reference weight, it indicates the child's nutritional status.

Weight-for-age is a measurement and if it is expressed in terms of percentage of children above or below –2SD of reference value it becomes an "indicator". Weight-for-age is an indirect measure of nutritional status of a child.

Target: Reduce prevalence of underweight in children below 5 years of age to the level of 25% by 2020.

Indicator

$$\frac{\text{Children aged } 0-59 \text{ months who are below minus two standard deviations from median weight for age of WHO child growth standards}}{\text{Total number of children } 0-59 \text{ months of age}} \times 100$$

Uses

Indicators can be used to measure achievement of targets, assess changes/trends in health status and compare the level of achievement between sub-centres, PHCs and CHCs.

Monitoring

Definition

Monitoring is the periodic continuous collection and analysis of selected indicators to enable managers to determine whether key activities are being carried out as planned and are having the expected effects on the target population.

Monitoring provides feedback to project management in order to improve operational plans and to take corrective actions.

The monitoring involves collection and analysis of information of actual operation to detect deviation from planned operation, to ensure mid course corrections.

Purpose

The purpose of monitoring is to detect changes or deviations soon after they occur and action taken at the earliest to correct the root causes of deviations. The whole purpose is to detect deviations at the earliest and ensure corrective action (Table 15.13).

How?

Monitoring information is gene rated from

i Routine reports: are used for monitoring of the programme or health services. Monthly monitoring reports of Sub-centre, PHC, CHC are used as good tools for monitoring of progress of activities and to observe any deviation or changes or alterations from the accepted levels or path or direction and corrective actions are ensured at the earliest.

ii Field visits—observations made by supervisors.

iii By Gnatt chart.

iv Community monitoring.

Types of Indicators for Monitoring[15,17–19]

Health system consists of model of inputs, processes, outputs, effects and impacts. Accordingly, the indicators of monitoring are (Fig. 15.6):

- Input indicators
- Process indicators
- Output indicators
- Effect indicators
- Impact indicators

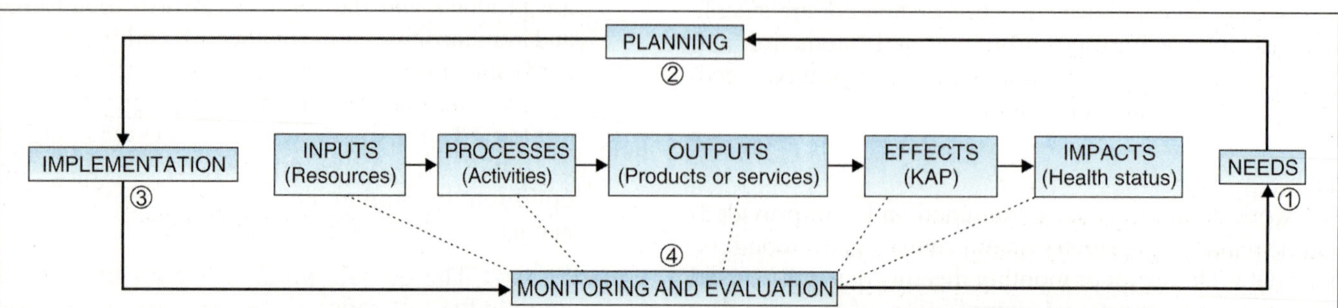

Fig. 15.6: Health system analysis to identify service delivery problems and their causes[15]

15

Table 15.13: Monitoring and surveillance

	Monitoring	Surveillance
NATURE	It is a management tool	It is an epidemiological tool
DEFINITION	Continuous collection and analysis of indicators/indicator	Continuous collection and analysis of disease event mainly, can be extended to collection and analysis of health events as well
PURPOSE	To track the programme implementation To detect deviation from established practice for early and prompt action	To monitor trends To monitor incidence To monitor prevalence To monitor geographical spread and high risk groups To predict outbreaks and control outbreaks
SCOPE/FOCUS	Wide-scope To monitor health programmes or health care delivery system	Limited to a specific, disease of national significance when we intend to eradicate or eliminate disease or control the specific disease
ESSENTIALS	To identify the desired indicators	To set out standard case definitions
METHODS	Periodical routine reports and field visits	Routine reports Sentinel surveillance Surveys and special studies or annual surveys Case or outbreak investigations Vital registration system Census
SIMILARITIES	Data collection for action and fixed periodicity	Data collection for action and fixed periodicity

Input Indicators

Inputs are resources needed to carry out activities or programme. The common input indicators would monitor the availability of:

i *Personnel* (available number of doctors, health supervisors, workers, traditional birth attendants) against the sanctioned posts or against the population norms or against Indian public health standards.

ii *Supplies* are sufficient or insufficient, e.g. ORS packets, essential drugs, equipment and other material for activities, e.g. percentage of sub-centres without drug kit A and B or weighing machines.

iii *Equipment:* Number or percentage of sub-centres without weighing machines and BP appratus and, copper T insertion equipment.

iv *Money:* Budget—Untied money, maintenance grant, JSY money, etc. money spent against sanctioned budget.

The manager must monitor all these to ensure supplies wherever these are deficient before you expect the results or service or performance. Adequate inputs should be ensured and should be in place. Whether SC, PHC, CHC is accessible, population covered by each of these set-up against the norms (Indian Public Health Standards).

Process Indicators

These are activity indicators, how often an activity happens against the planned, e.g. no. of outreach sessions planned and actual numbers held. Number of antenatal clinic days/ sessions held against planned and how often the workers make home visits and contact the Panchayati Raj Institutions against the planned schedule.

Output Indicators

Service output data can be collected through routine reports and it can be used for planning, monitoring, and evaluation purposes at local level. However, the reports are generally incorrect, and coverage is incomplete, not timely available, but nevertheless it provides good information for actions.

Number of beneficiaries covered for immunization, antenatal care, deliveries, postnatal care, and neonatal care in the last one year are output indicators. More specific outputs are:

- Percentage of infant covered for immunization.
- Percentage of antenatal registered and covered for minimum four antenatal check ups.
- Proportion of deliveries performed by health workers and skilled birth attendants.
- Percentage of eligible couples covered by different methods of contraception.
- Number of newborn weighed at birth.
- Quality of care: Percentage of antenatals registered in the first trimester.
- Percentage of antenatals provided care as per norms or standards.

Effect Indicators

Effect indicators include change in knowledge attitude and behaviour or practices observed as a result of activity. Health services utilization may increase after change in behaviour as also coverage, access and quality.

Impact Indicators

i Decline in incidence of diarrhoea, acute respiratory infection and other diseases of national significance.

ii Decline in malnutrition in young children (0–3 years)
iii Decline in birth rate.
iv Decline in death rate.
v Decline in infant and child mortality rate.
vi Initiation of breastfeeding within an hour after birth (percentage of newborn).
vii Exclusive breastfeeding rate.
viii Complementary feeding rate (complementary feeding at right age).

The impact indicators such as improvement of nutritional status, birth rates, death rates, and infant mortality rates are available through routine records/ reports, but these reports are incomplete most of the times. The system generates lot of data and impact indicators can become available through routine reports if the quality of data is improved by regular monitoring. In the absence of good routine reports, these data are collected by special surveys, or through national data of Sample Registration System, National Family Health Surveys Data, and District Level Household Survey Data or Annual Health Surveys.

EVALUATION OF HEALTH PROGRAMME OR HEALTH SERVICES

Evaluation may be defined as the process of assessing the results of the programme to determine whether the stated goals and objectives have been achieved.[19]

Evaluation also answers some critical questions:

- To what extent the stated objectives have been achieved?
- At what cost the objectives have been achieved?
- Should the programme be continued as such?
- Should the programme be modified in view of results/ observations of evaluation?
- Should the programme be abandoned?
- Should the programme and objectives be modified?

Purpose

The whole purpose of the evaluation is to improve the health system/programmes and the health infrastructure development and to guide the allocation of resources in current and future programmes.

Components of Evaluation

The evaluation of programme has the following components:

1 ***What:*** Be clear as to what is to be evaluated? Is it a programme, service or health centre or hospital, which is being evaluated.

2 ***Information:*** What information support is available on the subject. These could be monitoring reports, i.e. data on service outputs and field observations on client satisfaction/reactions, work diaries or some official published reports.

3 ***Verify relevance:*** Are the health policies relevant to country's overall social and economic policies? Is it directed towards defined national health goals? Does it contribute in improving health of population concerned?

Frequency of Evaluation

While monitoring is a continuous process the evaluation is a terminal activity or final step in the programme implementation. It is better to assess the progress and efficiency once a year at least and to assess the impact of programme longer time is required and evaluation should be done at least 5 years from the start of programme.

Indicators and Criteria for Evaluation

Indicators are variables that help to measure changes. They are evaluation tools, which can measure the change directly or indirectly. Keep it short and specific (KISS), i.e. list of indicators should be short and specific.

The indicator should be "valid", i.e. indicator actually measures what it is supposed to measure.

It should be "reliable", it means that even if the indicator is used by different people at different times and under different circumstances the result should be the same or consistent.

It should be "sensitive", it means it should measure the changes as soon as these occur. It should be "specific" it means that the indicator reflects changes only in a situation or phenomenon concerned. It should be "feasible" it means it should be simple to collect and analyse the data for it and lastly it should be "precise", i.e. it should have sufficient details (e.g. age, sex and geographical area). Various indicators for evaluation have been explained in National Health Programmes Evaluation.

Design of Evaluation

There are 57 research designs to conduct evaluation however, most practical, simple and basic designs are given below:

1 *The one time study:* This is expressed as **EXO**, where **'E'** is the experimental group, **'X'** is the programme intervention and **'O'** is the observation.

It is the most common, fast, and inexpensive design, but there is no baseline data, nor is there any control group. Therefore, it is **weakest design.**

2 *One group: Before and after* study or baseline/repeat observation. It may be expressed as **EOXO** where:

E is the experimental group (beneficiaries)

O is the baseline observations (before programme intervention)

X is programme intervention

O is repeat survey observation (after programme intervention).

15

This design is also fast and inexpensive but there is no control group and there is no random selection.

3 *Time series study:* It may be expressed as:

E O O O X O O O

E is experimental group (beneficiaries)

O O O are observations or surveys in time series.

X is programme intervention

O O O—before and after programme intervention.

This design is time consuming, but it determines the impact of the programme over a period of time. However, there is no control group to eliminate extraneous variables, and there is no random selection in the design.

4 *Non-equivalent baseline/repeat observation study (with and without study).* It may be expressed as:

E O X O

C O O

where:

E is experimental group

C is control group

O is baseline observation in experimental group.

O is baseline information in control group

(**O** and **O** are conducted simultaneously)

X is programme intervention

O is repeat observation in experimental group after programme intervention and **O** is repeat observation in control group at the time **O** is conducted.

This is quasi-experimental design, where baseline and repeat observations are conducted on experimental group as well as on the control group. There is no random selection.

5 *Post-programme observations—control group study:* It may be expressed as:

E R X O

C R O

where:

E is experimental group

C is control group

R stands for random selection

X is programme intervention

O is post-programme observation in experimental group.

O is observation on control group at the time O is conducted.

This is true experimental design; it has control group as well as random selection. But there is no baseline data for comparing the impact of the programme.

6 *Baseline/repeat observation control group study:* It may be expressed as:

E R O X O

C R O O

where:

E is experimental group

C is control group

R stands for random selection

O is baseline observation in experimental group

O is baseline observation in control group

(**O** and **O** are conducted simultaneously)

X is programme intervention

O is repeat observation in experimental group after programme intervention, and

O is repeat observation in control group at the time **O** is conducted.

This is true experimental design. It has control group, it involves random selection; and baseline as well as repeat observation are available.

(Adapted from Manual on Integrated Management Information System for ICDS-1986 Ist Ed. MOHRD, New Delhi).

Examples of evaluation: Coverage evaluation survey for immunization in children of 12–23 months of age. Improvement of nutritional status of under 5 years by weight-for-age at one year interval. Using data of sample registration survey to collect birth rate, death rate, and infant mortality rate to know the impact of interventions.

Other examples: HIV sentinel surveillance surveys, surveillance of AFP, Goitre surveys.

PROGRAMME EVALUATION AND REVIEW TECHNIQUE (PERT)

One technique of control in the planning process highly applicable is PERT (programme evaluation and review technique), sometimes called critical path method (CPM), which means to:

1 Identify key activities in a project.
2 Devise the sequence of activities and arrange them in a flow diagram;
3 Assign duration of time for performance of each phase of the work to be done.
4 ***Develop PERT network:*** List the activities horizontally on paper. To make this look like a formal PERT chart put circles at the beginning and end of each activity. Draw lines between beginning and ending circles. These circles are events representing the beginning and completion of each activity. The line represents the activity. Add other circles for other events not related to activities.
5 ***Identify the critical path:*** Begin at the right side where the large task has been completed. Choose the last task that has taken the most time. Now connect that activity with the precedent activity that required the most time, continue this process across the page from right to left. Review this carefully by reading left to right. The objective is to identify a sequence of activities which will accomplish the larger task in the shortest amount of time.

6 ***Perform network time calculations:*** Add up the time allotments along the critical path. The sum will indicate the total time required to complete the project.

7 ***Re-plan:*** Try other routes through the activities always ensuring that no activity commences before the precedents are completed, e.g. training of Anganwadi workers cannot occur unless they are recruited and appointed.

The point of this exercise is to identify the activity/activities which need manager's keenest interest.

The biggest disadvantage of PERT is overemphasis on time and almost no attention to cost (Fig. 15.7).

Critical Path Analysis is Effective and Powerful Method of Assessing

- What tasks must be carried out?
- Where parallel activity can be performed.
- The shortest time in which you can complete a project
- Resources needed to execute a project.
- The sequence of activities, scheduling and timings involved
- Task priorities.
- The most efficient way of shortening time on urgent projects.

Planning Programming Budgeting System (PPBS)

PPBS which combines the best of programme budgeting and performance budgeting has following steps:

A Identify the objectives.

B Present alternative ways to achieve those objectives with cost-benefit ratio for each.

C Identify activities necessary for each programme;

D Evaluate the results so that corrective actions can be taken.

HEALTH CARE FINANCING

The financing of health care in India is based on two basic tenets. **First**, the provision of health care service to people is the responsibility of the state government and **secondly**, comprehensive health care should be available to entire population irrespective of their ability to pay. Health investments bring benefit to economic development.

Since independence health care has been recognized as an essential social sector investment, it was therefore initially envisaged that health services in Government institutions will be provided free of cost to all. During 1990s, it was recognized that given the increasing awareness and expectations of the people, and the escalating cost of health care, this policy could not continue. The 9th plan envisaged that major public health priorities such as essential primary health care, emergency life saving services, services under the disease control and family welfare programme will be provided free of cost to all. The Ninth plan advocated that the centre and state Government should work out appropriate norms for levying user charges on people above the poverty line for other services and hospitalization and evolve mechanisms for collection and utilization of funds. Kerala experimented the user charges model at district level and under European Commission assistance several states introduced users charges for select services and most of the states were allowed to retain user charges for effecting improvement in quality of services.

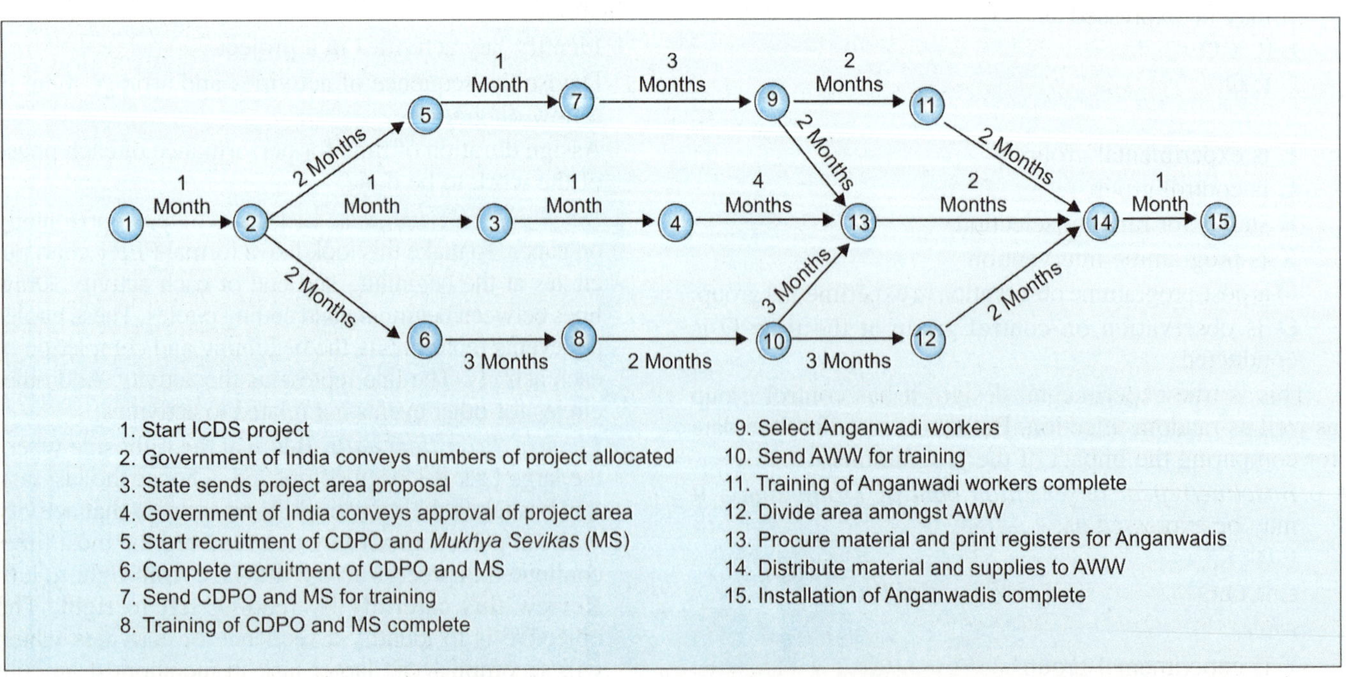

Fig. 15.7: PERT chart for installation of ICDS project in a block

The WHO has estimated that India at present is spending 5.2% of gross domestic product (GDP) on health of which 0.9% is public expenditure and the rest of three-fourths is *out of pocket spending*. India ranks 13th from the bottom in terms of public spending on health (World Health Report 2000), being lowest in the world.

Based on the need and broad goals of National Health Policy 2002, a national health accounts and health statistics was established.[20] Emphasis should shift from *financial* allocation to *outcomes*.

HEALTH FINANCING AT A GLANCE

There are four major *sources* of health financing in India, i. the *out of pocket*, ii. *private insurance* (private sector share 84%), iii. *public sector,* and iv. *social insurance* (government sector share 16%).

Private Health Sector

i It is dominant provider of curative care and caters to 80% of ambulatory (outdoor) care and 60% of indoor hospital care in India. Services provided are of variable quality without any regulation. This sector is financed primarily by out of pocket resources. Nearly 83% of health expenditure is ***out of pocket expenditure*** and major burden falls on poor people. About 63 million people getting impoverished every year on account of OOP health expenditure. Results from National Health Accounts (2004–05) show households expenditure amount to 71.13% of total health expenditure. An important achievement of NRHM has been a considerable reduction in out of pocket expenditure from 72 to 60% by 2012.

ii **Private insurance** coverage and access is limited, confined to mainly urban set up. Private health insurance expenditure is barely 0.6% in India. Health insurance will be promoted especially social insurance for the poor. To promote healthy lifestyles, "no claim bonus"/adjustment of premium could be made on the basis of previous year's hospitalization cost reimbursed by the insurance scheme. According to National Health Accounts social insurance funds contribution in India is only 1.13%.

iii **Public sector—Government revenues (financed from general taxation):** Government health expenditure is only 1% of GDP which caters to 22% of the outdoor (ambulatory) care and 40% of indoor hospital care. Public spending on health in India has increased from 0.22% of GDP in 1950–51 to 1.05% of GDP during the mid 1980s and stagnated at around 0.9% of GDP during the later years. Of late core public health spending has risen to 1.45% of GDP (Economic Survey 2009–10) is given in Table 15.14.

Table 15.14: Trends in public health expenditure in India 1950–51 to 2009–10

Years	*Health expenditure as % of GDP*
1950–51	0.22
1955–56	0.49
1960–61	0.63
1965–66	0.61
1970–71	0.74
1975–76	0.81
1980–81	0.91
1985–86	1.05
1990–91	0.96
1995–96	0.88
2000–01	0.90
2001–02	0.83
2002–03	0.86
2003–04	0.91
2006–07	0.98
2007–08	1.03
2008–09	1.10
2009–10	1.45
2011–12	1.04
2012–17 (Proposed)	1.87

Source: National Commission on Macroeconomics and Health (2005) and NRHM

Government spending on health in India is amongst the lowest in the world, whereas the proportion of private spending on health is one of the highest. More than 1,00,000 crore is being spent annually as household expenditure on health which is more than three times the public (government) expenditure on health. Most of it was out of pocket and was incurred during health distress in unregulated private facilities, leading to vicious **cycle of indebtedness and poverty**. There is therefore imperative need for setting up effective risk pool system of social insurance or community based insurance system. NRHM advocates and promotes such a system.

The allocation for health in the revenue budget of almost all the states has been much less than what is required to maintain the health delivery system in respective states. To make the health system functional at all the levels NRHM commits raising of public spending on health from 0.9% of GDP to 2% of GDP by the end of year 2012. NRHM has initiated several interventions, such as district health action plans, national health accounting system, management capacity at all levels and improved financial management with greater flexibility.[21]

iv **Compulsory social insurance:** Coverage of health insurance in India is pathetically limited. Current health insurance in government and private sector covers around 11% of the population. Besides ESIS, CGHS and Ex-serviceman Contributory Health Scheme, National Health Insurance Scheme (RSBY) has been launched now to cover unorganized sector with focus on below poverty line families. This has increased the pool of public insurance. The Government is further encouraging risk pooling approach besides Community-based Health Insurance. The compulsory social insurance schemes include the Central Government Health Scheme (CGHS) and the Employees State Insurance Scheme (ESIS).

a *CGHS:* This covers 4.5 million beneficiaries at ₹ 450 per beneficiary.

b *ESIS:* Meant for organized sector employees, covers 32 million ESI beneficiaries at ₹ 365 per beneficiary.

c *Other public sector employees:*

- Cess based welfare funds (mines, beedi, plantation, cinema). This covers 5.16 million persons with ₹ 302 million on medical benefits.
- Post and telecom ₹ 1500 million.
- Railways for 8 million population at ₹ 812 per beneficiary.
- Defence services ₹ 8000 million for 5 million beneficiaries at ₹ 1600 per beneficiary.
- Other employees in organized public sector units (PSUs) 8 million beneficaries at ₹ 3000 per employee.
- Schemes for unorganized sector with direct and indirect health protection through various ministries and public insurance corporations (*Rashtriya Swasthya Bima Yojna* and Ex-servicemen contributory health services).[20]

Encourage Community Risk Pooling

Local governments can identify population at risk and provide a revolving fund to be managed by a consortium of self-help groups to give needy households a cash support of ₹ 5,000 to 10,000 for hospitalization, catastrophic illness, and death. This would save household from immediate financial debt at the point of crisis. They would repay this money at a modest interest rate within an appropriate timeframe so that the Village/Ward health risk pool does not fall below ₹ 1 lakh.

Health Spending

The health care system in India predominantly is catered to by the *private sector* and a miniscule contribution through external flows. Expenditure in the private sector contributes to 78.05% of total health expenditure, public sector accounts for 19.67% and external flows 2.28%. In totality, health expenditure formed 4.13% of Gross Domestic Product (GDP) during the year 2008–09. The distribution of total health expenditure and its share in GDP is reflected in Table 15.15.

By source households contributed significant proportion at 71.13% followed by state government 11.97%, central government 6.78%, firms 5.73%, external flow 2.28% and social insurance accounted for 1.13% of total financing for health in India (Fig. 15.8)

NHP-2002 AND NHM POLICY PRESCRIPTION

The paucity of public health investment is a stark reality. Given the extremely difficult fiscal position of the state Governments, the central Government will have to play a key role in augmenting public health investment. Taking into account the gap in health care facilities, it is planned under the policy to increase total health expenditure to 6% of GDP, with 2% of GDP being contributed as public health investment by 2010. The central Government

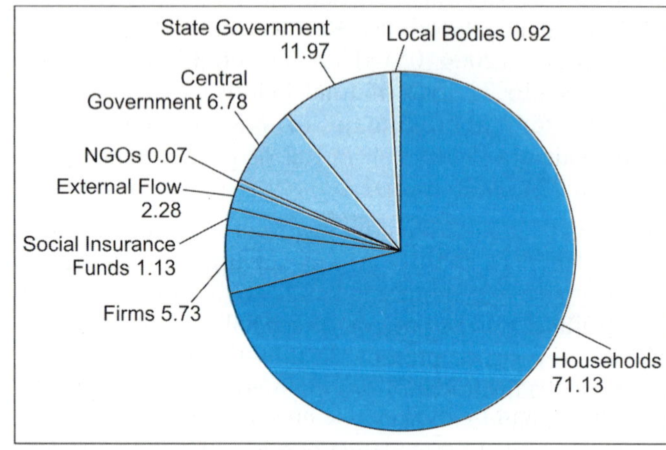

Fig. 15.8: Sources of health financing in India, 2009

Table 15.15: Levels of expenditure on health in India, 2004–05 to 2008–09[22]

	Selected National Health Accounts Indicators	*2004–05*	*2005–06*	*2006–07*	*2007–08*	*2008–09*
1.	Total expenditure on health as % of GDP	4.25	4.23	4.12	4.11	4.13
2.	Public expenditure on health as % of GDP	0.84	0.96	0.98	1.03	1.10
3.	General Government expenditure on health as % of total expenditure on health	19.67	22	24	25	27
4.	Private expenditure on health as % of total expenditure on health	78.05	76	75	73	72
5.	Per capita public expenditure on health	Rs. 242				1904
6.	Per capita private expenditure on health	Rs. 959				

Source: World Health Report 2007, NCMH-2005 and National Health Accounts (2009).

contribution would rise to 25% from the existing 15% by 2010.[21]

In order to achieve equity, NHP-2002 sets out an increased allocation of 55% of total public health investment for the primary health sector; the secondary and tertiary health sector being targeted to 35% and 10% respectively. High level expert group on UHC recommended 70% all health expenditure on primary health care. The policy projects that increased aggregate outlays for the primary health sector will be utilized for strengthening existing facilities and opening additional public health service outlets, consistent with the norms for such facilities.

Under-funding

The investment by the public sector for health care has been inadequate to meet the demands of the people. The State has over the years committed not more than 3.5% of its resources to the health sector. The existing level of government expenditure on health in India is about 1.2% of GDP, which is unacceptably low and woefully short of the World Health Organization (WHO) recommendation of 5%.

The per capita health expenditure for India in 2004–05 was no more than ₹ 1201 of which share of *public* expenditure was ₹ 242 (20.18%) and that of *private* was ₹ 959 (79.82%). Public expenditure as a share of State Domestic Product (SDP) was less than 1% for all major states. Further as a share of total state expenditure, public expenditure varied within 3–4% for all major states. The draft National Health Policy 2015 suggests tax based financing as the predominant source of financing health care costs of at least 70% of the population who are poor.

Catastrophic Health Expenditure

Health care cost exceeding 10% of its total monthly consumption expenditure or 40% of its non food consumption expenditure is designated as catastrophic health expenditure and is declared as an unacceptable level of health care cost. Impoverishment due to health care cost is of course even more unacceptable (63 million people per year in India get impoverished).

Zero-based Budgeting (ZBB)

This newer technique is not concerned with what happened previously but with what is required in the future. It emphasizes planning, fosters understanding of the total organization, identifies priorities, and then states it in terms of cost. Each unit of the budget is justified and placed in a hierarchy. Two important steps are:

A **Identify** "decision packages" which should be the lowest unit for which a budget can be prepared.

B **Rank** "decision packages" by setting priorities within each unit of the organization to force decision making as to the most important activities within that unit.

Management by Objectives (MBO)

What one wants to accomplish, means setting an objective (a goal, a purpose, a target).

The objective should state clearly

What is to be accomplished? .... (purpose)

How much of it? .... (quantification)

Where it is to be done? .... (place)

When it is to be completed? .... (time frame)

Example: As a leader of health team PHC doctor sets his objectives as follow:

- By December, 2014 in PHC "A"
  - There will be no case of neonatal tetanus
  - 90% of pregnant women will receive tetanus toxoid.
  - All the deliveries will be aseptic
- And by August, 2014 the team objectives may be:
  - To hold antenatal clinic regularly once a week.
  - To train one skilled birth attendant per village.

Achieving these objectives by management technique is known as management by objectives (MBO).

The whole MBO process rests upon several premises:

1 Clearly stated objectives;
2 A succession of specific objectives;
3 Delegation of specific objectives;
4 Freedom to act;
5 Verifiable results;
6 Clear communication;
7 Shared responsibilities.
8 Personal accountability;
9 Improving management ability.

MANAGEMENT PROBLEMS AND THEIR CAUSES

Analysis of management problem is essential to find the root causes of the problem so that the action taken is true solution.

***Methods of analysis of problem*:** There are 3 methods to analyse a problem. I Ask *"Why?"* five times, II *Process flow* chart and III *Fishbone diagram.*[23]

i. The why tree: The stakeholders identify chains of causes of a **performance gap,** for example, in low coverage of immunization with the why tree technique, also known as why, why, why, why, why technique. This simple technique for understanding the search for root causes is—by asking "why" five times (Fig. 15.9). Too often we focus

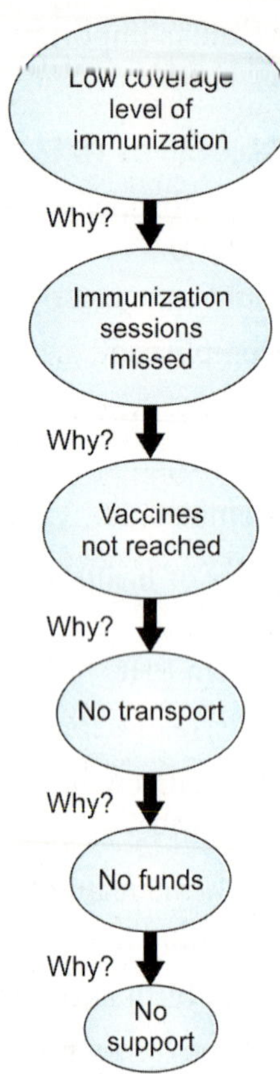

Fig. 15.9: The why tree root cause analysis

on the first cause of a problem, trying to solve it before asking about other causes. Thus, deeper problems go undetected. While there is nothing magic about the number five, repeatedly asking why will lead us to find a number of causes, some that can be addressed, others that cannot. When stakeholder can think no more answer to the question "why"—the facilitator asks if there are any other causes of the gap and begins another chain. Recorded on paper, the **performance gap** appears at the top of the page with a root system of causes. Each root of the why tree describes a cause of performance gap, and the lowest item in the root indicates how to address the cause, in this case, supportive supervision, i.e. supervisor to arrange alternate methods to deliver vaccine to the site of outreach session. This process requires an open mind of manager as also participation of health teams, and looking at the familiar problem as if it was new.

ii. Process flow chart: A process flow chart is another analytical tool that can provide a great deal of insight into the management process. The flow chart can be used to map out how a process is actually functioning. This helps the team to understand the process better and to find ways to streamline to improve it (*see* referral system).

iii. Fishbone diagram (Kaoru Ishikawa diagram)**:** It is one of the tool for analysis of causes and the identification of root causes of management problem by cause and effect diagram, commonly called fishbone diagram. This method *organises* the *information graphically* from sources. The spine of the fishbone diagram extends from the performance gap in a box on the right. The long bones extending from the spine stand for the performance factors (root causes). Generally, the major categories of causes (such as human resources, budget equipment, facility and supplies) are listed on the major branches or *bones* and all the possible causes related to that category are listed there. The objective of the excercise is to look for the most likely root causes of the problem for necessary action/actions. An example of fishbone diagram dealing with low level of coverage of immunization is shown in Fig. 15.10.

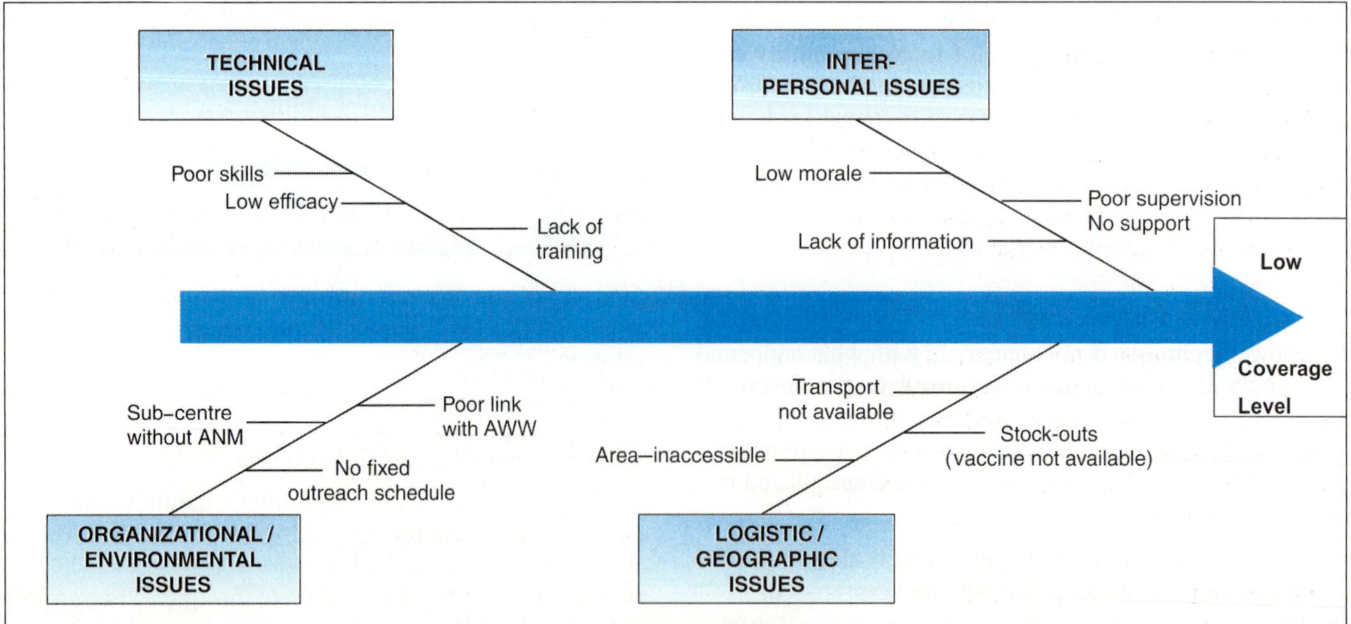

Fig. 15.10: Causes of low level of coverage of immunization cause and effect diagram

SWOT Analysis of National Rural Health Mission for DHAP (District Health Action Plan) for Idenification of Performance Gaps

SWOT stands for strengths, weaknesses, opportunities and threats.

Strengths of NRHM

- Increased access to health care through 8.9 lakhs ASHAs.
- Decentralized management of health facilities and programmes—increased participation and ownership by the PRIs and the community, decentralized village, SC, PHC, block and district health action plans with programme implementation plan (PIP) by each state.
- **Indian public health standards** for assured services and norms for manpower, buildings, equipment, drugs and materials at SC, PHC, CHC, sub-district and district hospital to enhance quality of health services.
- Improved programme management—building up management and public health skills in the existing workforce, supplemented by programme management units at state, district and block level.
- Flexible financing—untied money at SC, PHC, CHC and district level for local health action.
- Innovations in human resource management—contractual appointment route to immediately fill the human resource gap, multi-skilling, and public–private partnership.
- 5.12 lakhs VHSCs constituted to increase demand for health services.

Weaknesses

Lack of integration/convergence with nutrition, sanitation and safe drinking water and education sector (determinants of health and development).

- Village Health Action Plan not initiated.
- Weak community monitoring system.
- Inadequate community participation due to inadequate transfer of administrative and financial powers to PRIs.
- Inaequate capacity of district CHC, PHC and SC to prepare health action plans at local level.
- CHCs not developed to the level of FRUs because of deficiency of specialists (80% shortages of specialists), resulting in poor referral services, such as emergency obstetric and neonatal care.
- Weak logistic and supply chain management system.

Opportunities

The launch of NRHM and NUHM and NHM has provided the Central and State governments with a unique opportunity for carrying out necessary reforms in the health sector. The reforms are necessary for restructuring the health care delivery systems as well as for developing better health financing mechanisms. The strengthening and effectiveness of health institution like SCs/PHCs/CHCs/Taluk/district hospitals have positive influence on all national health programmes (TB, malaria, HIV/AIDS, filaria, family welfare, leprosy, disease surveillance, etc.) as all programmes are based on the assumption that a functional public health system actually exists.

Threats

Lack of workforce management policies for contractual staff of programme management units, data entry and account staff resulting into high attrition rate of these human resources. Stagnation of training programmes due to lack of institutional capacity at State Institute of Health and Family Welfare, District Training Centre, and Training Centres for Health Workers (males) and Nursing Personnels.

State and District Level Bureaucratic Control and administration over SC, PHC, CHCs and district get diminished as PRI's takeover management, administrative and financial control over these institutions.

Conclusion of SWOT Analysis

SWOT analysis helps to identify the weaknesses in the programme and helps to fill the gaps so discovered in the analysis to improve the system of health care delivery. The "weaknesses" identified in SWOT analysis should be, converted into "strengths" and similarly the "threats" be converted into "opportunities" of the health programme and organization.

This analysis leads to identification of issues in terms of **access, quality, demand** and **utilization** of health services.

REFERENCES

1 WHO. On being in charge—a guide for middle level management in primary health care. Geneva: WHO; 1980.

2 NIHFW. Management training modules for medical officers primary health centre. New Delhi: NIHFW; 1987.

3 Arole RS, Rhode JE. Organization of health services and training of physicians for child health services. A consultant report to USAID. New York: USAID; 1983.

4 GOI. National Population Policy 2000. New Delhi: MOH and FW, GOI; 2000.

5 GOI. National health policy (revised) 2002. New Delhi: MOH and FW, GOI; 2002.

6 GOI. Bulletin on rural health statistics in India. New Delhi: MOH and FW, GOI; 2006.

7 Planning Commission. Eleventh five-year plan, volume II. New Delhi: Planning Commission GOI; 2007–12.

8 GOI. Manual on target free approach in family welfare programme. New Delhi: MOH and FW, GOI; 1996.

9 GOI. Manual on community needs assessment approach (formerly target free approach) in family welfare. New Delhi: MOH and FW, GOI; 1998.

10 GOI. IPHS for Sub-centre, Primary Health Centre and Community Health Centre, NRHM, MOH and FW. GOI; New Delhi, 2007.

11 Public health services. 1st edn; United States of America: WB Sounders Company; 1960.
12 Morley D. Paediatric priorities in the developing world – Postgraduate paediatric series, 1st edn; London (U.K.): Butterworth Co. Ltd.; 1973.
13 Measham AR, Heaver RA. India's Family Welfare Programme moving to reproductive and child health approach. Washington DC: World Bank; 1996.
14 NIHFW. Management training for primary health care—Assessment of management training needs. New Delhi: NIHFW; 1986.
15 GOI. Management of integrated management information system for ICDS. New Delhi: Ministry of human resource development; 1986.
16 Aga Khan Foundation. Primary health care management advancement programme modules (1,4,5). Washington (USA): Aga Khan Foundation; 1993.
17 WHO. The health aspects of food and nutrition—a manual for developing countries in Western Pacific Region of WHO. 3rd edn. Regional office for the Western Pacific Manila: WHO; 1979.
18 GOI. National child survival and safe motherhood programme—Plan and implement MCH services. New Delhi: MOH and FW, GOI; 1992.
19 WHO. Health programme evaluation guiding principles. Geneva: WHO; 1981.
20 Ranbaxy Science Foundation. Improving Access to Health Care. Reaching the unreached. Proceedings of 16th Round Table Conference held on Nov. 11th, 2005, New Delhi, pp. 9–19.
21 GOI. National Rural Health Mission, 2005.
22 GOI. National Health Accounts India, 2004–05, MOH and FW, Government of India.
23 AKF. PHC MAP Modules Assessing the quality of management users guide module 7. AKF, USA, 1993.

HOSPITAL STATISTICS

Hospital statistics are used as a measure of evaluation of quality of medical care. It also helps in planning and allocation of resources in different areas.

The major uses of hospital statistics are to

- evaluate quality of medical care rendered,
- identify the deficiencies at various levels, i.e. input process and outcome of the services, and
- evaluate the effectiveness and efficiency of the administration.

The generation of hospital statistics should be purely on the basis of administrative requirement of the hospital. Hence, these vary with the type of hospital. It may be generated daily, weekly, monthly, quarterly and annually depending upon the requirement. Still broadly it can be divided into following types:[1,2]

15

1. ***Patient movement statistics:*** Number of admissions/discharges/deaths, OPD patients.
2. ***Morbidity statistics:*** Number of patients under various diagnosis.
3. ***Administrative statistics:*** Manpower, material, money finances, etc.
4. ***Hospital services statistics:*** Number of operation theatres (OTs), number of surgeries (major/minor), number of specialities and their utilization indicators, etc.

Patient Movement Statistics

Average Daily Census

Average daily census is the average number of patients in the hospital at a given time per day; and is expressed as:

$$\frac{\text{Sum of daily census for a given period}}{\text{Number of calendar days in the period}}$$

TURNOVER INTERVAL OR T INTERVAL

T interval is the mean number of days a bed remains vacant between two admissions, and is expressed as:

$$T = \frac{\text{Number of vacant bed days in a defined period}}{\text{Total number of discharges, deaths and transfers during that period}}$$

The value of T may be negative or positive.

i. A negative T is indicative of scarcity of beds and over-utilization.
ii. A long positive T is indicative of under-utilization because of either defective admission procedures or poor quality medical care.
iii. A short positive T is indicative of optimum utilization.

T interval is a very sensitive index of hospital utilization. It can also be used to measure the demand for or pressure on beds.

Bed Turnover Rate

It is an important measure of hospital utilization indices. It gives the net effect of changes in occupancy rate and AVLS (average length of stay):

$$\frac{\text{Number of discharges for a given period of time}}{\text{Average bed count for that period of time}} \times 100$$

Percentage of Occupancy or Bed Occupancy Rate

This is the ratio of occupied bed days to the available bed days as determined by bed capacity, during any given period of time.

Calculation

$$\frac{\text{Actual number of occupied bed days}}{\text{Available bed days}} \times 100$$

Bed occupancy ratio is used to measure the utilization of health facility beds. 80–85% occupancy is considered ideal for good quality of patient care. A hospital has always some beds vacant for emergency, maternity, isolation, intensive care units, etc. This space is called "dead bed space". This accounts for 15–20% of beds in a hospital. That is why 80–85% occupancy indicates full utilization of hospital beds. 100% occupancy means over-utilization which leads to fall in the quality of care. Occupancy of more than 100 means patients on floors, overtaxed hospital, physical facilities and over worked staff. All this adds up to substandard medical care.

The bed occupancy rate for different units can be monitored to plan hospital services and evaluate the efficiency/ utilization.

An occupancy of less than 80% is uneconomical and indicates lack of response from the public. Too rigid compartmentation of hospital wards does not afford flexibility and may result in under-utilization of one department while another department may be short of beds. Built in flexibility is desirable for proper and optimum utilization of hospital beds.

Average Length of Stay

Average length of stay is the average number of days of service rendered to each discharged patient (including deaths and transfers) during a given period of time (exclusive of newborn babies). Inpatient days are compiled from the discharge summary of discharged patients. In computing the length of stay, the day of admission is counted but the day of discharge is not counted. Admission and discharge on the same day is counted as one day.

Calculation

$$\frac{\text{Total inpatient days during a given period}}{\text{Total discharges (including deaths and transfers) during the same period}}$$

In teaching hospital (PGIMS, Rohtak) during the year 2007, the average length of stay was 6.02 days. If the admission procedures are streamlined, time is not wasted in investigations, early diagnosis and treatment will help bring down the average length of stay of inpatients. On one bed 36 patients can be taken care of in a year if the average length of stay is 10 days. If it is 20 days then only 18 patients can be admitted on this bed. Projecting this principle to a 1000 beds indicates the importance of reduction in the average length of stay. At the same time, care should be taken against too early discharge of patients. For this purpose readmission rate should also be calculated and watched. This index may be used to plan a waiting list.

Average daily OPD attendance

$$\frac{\text{Total number of outpatient attended}}{\text{Number of working days during that period}}$$

Average OPD attendance per patient, i.e. the number of time on an average a patient attends OPD.

$$\frac{\text{Total number of OPD attendance during a given period}}{\text{Total number of new OPD cases during that period}}$$

Autopsy rate

$$\frac{\text{Number of pathological autopsies performed}}{\text{Number of deaths during a period}} \times 100$$

Autopsy rate of more than 15–20% indicates enquiry type of medical staff, progressive in outlook.

Caesarean Section (CS) Rate

Calculation

$$\frac{\text{Total CS performed}}{\text{Total number of deliveries}} \times 100$$

The normal value of this rate is 3–4%. A higher CS rate should be enquired into.

Consultation Rate

Calculation

$$\frac{\text{Total written consultations during a period}}{\text{Total discharges (including deaths) during that period}} \times 100$$

A consultation rate of more than 15–20% is indicative of high quality of medical care.

Hospital Infection Rate (Postoperative Infection Rate)

$$\frac{\text{All infections in clean surgical cases in a year}}{\text{Total number of surgeries in that year}} \times 100$$

Death Rates

Gross Death Rate

$$\frac{\text{Total number of hospital deaths during a given period}}{\text{Total discharges (including deaths and transfers) during the same period}} \times 100$$

Net Death Rate

$$\frac{\text{Total deaths of inpatients after 48 hours or more after admission}}{\text{Total discharges (minus deaths occurring within 48 hours after admission)}} \times 100$$

15

Specific Death Rate

$$\frac{\text{Number of net deaths in a ward or department during a given period}}{\text{Total discharges (including deaths) in that department during the same period}} \times 100$$

Net death rate is used as an indicator of quality of patient care in an institution. In advanced countries, the value of this rate is about 4%. Excessive death rates of hospital should be investigated.

Anaesthesia Death Rate

Calculation

$$\frac{\text{Number of deaths due to anaesthesia}}{\text{Number of patients anaesthetized during a period}} \times 5{,}000$$

An anaesthesia death rate of more than 1 in 5,000 calls for scrutiny of the staff, equipment and procedures in this department.

Postoperative Death Rate (POP Death Rate)

Calculation

$$\frac{\text{POP deaths (within 10 days after surgery)}}{\text{Total operations during a given period}} \times 100$$

The usual value of this rate is 1–2%. But it varies greatly with the type of surgery being undertaken in an institution.

Maternal Death Rate

Calculation

$$\frac{\text{Total deaths of obstetric patients}}{\text{Total discharges (including deaths) of the obstetric patients}} \times 100$$

The usual value is less than 0.25%. Excessive rate should be enquired into.

Neonatal Death Rate

Calculation

$$\frac{\text{Total deaths of neonates during a given period}}{\text{Total viable newborns discharged (including deaths) during the same period}} \times 100$$

A neonatal death rate of more than 2% should be investigated.

Beds and Death Rate

An extensive study of vital statistics and hospital data of different areas has revealed that a close relationship exists between the deaths in a population and number of hospital beds needed. It has been found that 0.5 general beds are needed per annual death in a population of 100.

In a population having 10 deaths per 1000, 5 beds per 1000 are needed in the acute general hospitals for optimum medical care.

If total number of annual deaths in a region are 200, then this population needs 100 general beds. This formula is used extensively for planning medical care facilities in a region. In India, current death rate is 8 per 1000, hence we need 4 beds per 1000 population but we have only 0.96 bed per 1000 population. In Government sector, we have 6,75,779 beds and estimated beds in private sector are 6,69,022 which makes total bed strength of 13,44,801 for population of 1295 million.[3] Only 31.9% all governmental hospital beds are available in rural areas as compared to 68.1% for urban populationd—a paradox.[4]

National Health Policy goal is to have 1 bed per 1000 population. There has been steady decline in utilization of public health facilities for inpatient care (42%).

PREVENTIVE AND PROMOTIVE HEALTH SERVICES IN HOSPITALS

Promotive and preventive health services in hospital set up, such as eduction on health for general public and waiting patients and their attendants in OPD/Indoor, counseling on health and disease through various speciality clinics, ICTC, PPTCT, Comprehensive immunization clinic, trauma centre (prevention of injuries and accidents), contraceptive services, family planning sterilization, adolescent friendly health clinics, clinics for non-communicable diseases and reproductive and child health services can be linked with referral stations (District, sub-district, CHC, PHC and sub-centre), homes and community for continuum of health services.

Hospital data on morbidity and mortality (causes of death) can be most useful for planning of health services. Sentinel surveillance of diseases in hospital (malaria, dengue and chikungunya, STI, RTI, HIV, Acute flaccid paralysis, vaccine preventable diseases, and epidemic prone and notifiable diseases can provide warning signal for early response and action. Geographical pathology can be mapped based on hospital morbidity. Hospitals can take responsibility for a defined geographical area for community based services. Teaching hospitals produce human resources for health and provide referral support for specialist services/national health programme besides continuing education of human resources and support of laboratory services for validating surveillance data.

REFERENCES

1 NIHFW. Training Module for Medical Officers (PHC). New Delhi: NIHFW; 1987.
2 GOI. RCH II family planning programme implementation plan (PIP). New Delhi: Dept. of Family Welfare, MOH and FW; 2004.
3 GOI. National Health Profile 2015. CBHI, DGHS, MOH and FW—Nirman Bhavan, New Delhi.
4 Yadav K, Jarhyan P, Gupta V, Pandav. CS. Revitalizing Rural Health Care Delivery: Can rural health practitioners be the answer? IJCM 2009, 34, 1 view point.

CHAPTER

16

Occupational Safety and Health

Occupational safety and health is essential in preventing workplace ailments and promoting health and welfare of workers. Occupational health is a comprehensive subject comprising the health, safety and welfare of the workers at the "workplace" and "off work" environments. In the country like India, large workforce has been employed in diverse settings. Today we have about 360 million workforce of which about 120 million are in the industrial sector.[1] The organized sector of industries employs less than 30 million workers and this small segment of workforce is generally assured of legally regulated working conditions. Notably, there is no substantive account of the unrecognized small industrial units (estimated to be over 3.5 million units) that employ workforce several times larger than the registered enterprises. Also the occurrence of injury and fatalities has been recorded highest in small enterprises. 225 million workforce spread over in 6,40,000 villages dependent on farming, for them occupational health safety almost is non-existent; thus rural farming sector and unorganized workforce in small industries is a big challenge to assure occupational health and safety.[1]

Now the unorganized sector workers are covered under *Rashtriya Swasthya Bima Yojna (RSBY).*

Occupational health can be defined as—"aiming at health protection and health promotion for gainfully employed and adaptation of work to man and of each man to his job".

Joint committee of WHO and ILO in 1950 defined occupational health as "promotion and maintenance of the highest degree of physical, mental and social well-being of workers in all occupations". Modern concern of "occupational health" is "Environmental health".

Occupational Hazards

Common hazards to which an industrial worker is exposed are as under:

1 Physical hazards (heat, noise, vibration, inadequate light, radiation, pressure, and injuries).
2 Chemical hazards (lead and other heavy metals, dusts-fumes and gases).
3 Biological hazards (anthrax, leptospirosis, brucellosis have association with occupation).
4 Social and psychological hazards (problems of adjustment and interaction with fellow colleagues, and unhealthy lifestyles).

These hazards have been controlled to a large extent under the Factories Act, 1948 (by Legislation) but still the control and preventive measures tend to be ineffective and consequently the workers are exposed to these hazards. These hazards have been discussed in this chapter and some have been discussed in Chapters 7, 8, 12 and 13.

Social and Psychological Hazards

These are not essentially due to occupation, but may be related to family circumstances, interaction with fellow colleagues and lifestyles. The symptoms and signs which are not related to any organic cause fall in this category of hazards.

Mostly single male migrate to industrial towns/cities in search of job leave their families behind in the village or city. They lead life in urban slums and create urban slums and live in precarious sub-human conditions and may not be able to adjust in new environment. Therefore, industrial workforce leads a typical lifestyle of loneliness and indulge into extramarital sexual intercourse or get into the cycle of substance abuse and acquire STD and HIV infection. The psychological signs include tiredness, fatigue, headache, backache, absenteeism and other vague symptoms for which no organic cause can be established. Feeling of isolation, loneliness, depression, unable to cope with stressful situation, frequent change over of jobs, loss of interest in work are some of the other manifestations.

Industrial Hazards to Population

Industries are essential for economic development of the nation. Industrialization leads to many inherent problems as well and these are to be managed effectively. Apart from affecting the health of industrial workers, industry may pose problems to population around the zone of industry. The major problems and hazards are:

- Unplanned development and increase in urban slums because workers migrate to these areas to get jobs and start a new life in deplorable slum conditions apart from social problems like STDs, HIV and drugs.
- The atmospheric air pollution by smoke and poisonous gases fumes and dusts.
- Soil pollution by industrial effluents and wastes.
- Noise pollution.
- Water pollution with toxic material—like arsenic and fluorides which leads to arsenic toxicity and fluorosis and produce crippling effects in human beings.

These have been regulated under the factory Act, 1948 but still the implementation is a problem. Environmental degradation is a growing problem due to uncontrolled and unplanned industrial activity. The problem of environmental pollution has been partially addressed through Water (Prevention and control of pollution) Act, 1974 and Environmental Protection Act, 1986.

PNEUMOCONIOSES

Pneumoconioses means group of occupational lung diseases caused by inhalation of insoluble dusts.

Common pneumoconioses associated with occupational health are as under:

- Pneumoconioses caused by sclerogenous mineral dust include silicosis, asbestosis and anthracosilicosis.
- Due to inhalation of vegetable dusts: Byssinosis, Bagassosis, Tobaccossis, and Farmer's lung on account of inhalation of cotton dust, sugarcane dust, tobacco dust and hay and grain dust respectively.
- Silicosis is the commonest pneumoconioses.[2]

SILICOSIS

Silicosis is a pneumoconioses caused by inhalation of crystalline particles of free silica (silicon dioxide or SiO_2). Silicon contributes to about 28% of earth's crust. Silicon being very reactive combines with oxygen and forms free silica (SiO_2).

Occurrence and uses

16

Earth crust contains about 12% free silica mostly in the form of quartz, mining and tunnelling are the occupations most closely related to the hazard of silica exposure. Most rocks contain silica. Air-borne particles of free silica are produced by blasting, grinding, drilling, and milling of rocks (Sandstones and Granite).

Occupations

Workers engaged in hard rock mining and extraction, stone cutters, crushing, polishing of stone, quarries, sandblasting in foundries, ceramic potteries, etc. are exposed to the risk of silicosis. Around 3 million workers are exposed to the risk in these occupations. Exposure to large amount of free silica can pass unnoticed because silica is colorless, non-irritant, and does not cause any immediate noticeable effect.

Silicosis is an age-old occupational disease and remains a major occupational health problem in India. It is responsible for high morbidity and mortality in industrial workers. There is no specific treatment for this progressive and irreversible disease.

There are many cross-sectional studies on silicosis in India. Prevalence of silicosis ranges from low of 3.5% in ordnance factory to 54.6% in slate pencil industry (Table 16.1).

Mechanism of Action

The dust particles of 5–15 μm diameter are deposited in airway and cleared by mucociliary movement but particles of 0.5–5 μm diameter leading in terminal airway or beyond are retained. The dust particles retained in the lung are taken up by macrophages (mononuclear phagocytes) and transported to lung parenchyma when the dust containing cell die, other cells take up the released particles but these are also killed; creating a continuous low grade reaction leading to formation of localized scars (nodules) which mostly occur around terminal airways. It produces fibrogenesis. The silicotic nodules are 2–5 μm in diameter, homo-

Table 16.1: Industry-wise prevalence of silicosis in India

Industry	*Prevalence* (%)
Gold mines	8.84–13.90
Mica mines and mica processing industries in Bihar	34.0
Manganese mines	4.1
Lead and zinc mines	30.4
Stone cutters	20.0–35.2
Foundries	27.2
Ordnance factory	3.5
Agate workers	38.0
Glass bangle workers	7.3
Slate pencil workers	54.6
Mica mines and mica processing	5.2
Quartz crushing	12.0
Stone quarry	22.0
Sand grinding	27.8
Ceramic and potteries	15.1

Source: ICMR Bulletin 29(9): Sep 1999.

genous in density and usually bilaterally symmetrical can be detected on X-ray of chest.

The radiographs are typical and should be interpreted using the ILO International classification of radiographs of pneumoconioses (1980).

On continued dust exposure, the nodules increase in size and number and eventually cover most parts of the lung. Sometimes the nodules unite and form conglomerate shadows; which are described as progressive massive fibrosis (PMF).

Symptoms: Dyspnoea on exertion is considered to be most frequent and directly related to symptoms of silicosis. Silicosis may develop within a few months to 2 years of massive exposure. Exposure to 1–2 mg quartz/m^3 may cause detectable disease in 5–15 years, the X-ray changes starting first, followed by lung function abnormalities and appearance of symptoms.

Silicosis is irreversible and progressive disease with no specific treatment.

Risk of tuberculosis: Persons who develop silicosis are more prone to develop pulmonary tuberculosis. Silicotics are high-risk group for tuberculosis and hence sputum for AFB test is essential along with X-ray chest. Recently crystalline silica has been classified as a human carcinogen.

Environmental Assessment

The best means of assessment of exposure to crystalline silica in a workplace is by size selective dust sampling in the breathing zone preferably by using personal sampler. Exposure may also be assessed by analyzing respirable dust for crystalline silica content by X-ray or infrared radiation. Environmental control of silica dust is the best prevention of silicosis. Periodical health examination of worker by chest X-ray, lung function tests and sputum examination is advisable.

Control Measures

The suppression of dust by technical control measures (pre-wetting, wet drilling) should be rigidly enforced and any residual dust should be controlled by proper ventilation. National Institute of Occupational Health (NIOH) at Ahmedabad has developed exhaust system for grinding machines which effectively collects the dust in filter bag and thereby it cuts down the level of dust by 93% in work environments. Dust collected in bag filter can be reused for polishing. Respirable dust levels and free silica content of dust should be monitored regularly. Whenever explosives are used, workers should be prevented from entering the dusty area until the dust is cleared by ventilation. Dust should be filtered out of exhaust air.

Personal protective measures include wearing of mask, pressure hoods, etc. Air-conditioned cabs for truck drivers and operators of excavators and cranes should be provided.

ASBESTOSIS

Asbestosis is a progressive, irreversible silicatosis caused by inhalation of asbestos fibres.

These are silicates of magnesium, iron, calcium and sodium and occur in fine fibre forms.

Asbestos is a generic term for a group of naturally occurring fibrous mineral silicates. They are crystalline in form and are capable of splitting longitudinally into single fibrils or fibre bundles.

Uses

Asbestos is used in making cement products such as pipes and roofing sheets, other roofing materials, papers, electrical insulator, floor tiles, paints and coatings, plastics, brake lining, etc.

Workers engaged in mining, milling and processing of asbestos, transport of mined or milled asbestos, manufacture of asbestos products and disposal of waste material from asbestos mining, milling, etc. are exposed to the risk of inhaling asbestos dust.

Mechanism of Action

Inhaled air-borne fibres of asbestos of less than 3 mm diameter penetrate the airways and retained in the lungs. After a long heavy exposure of 5–10 years there is substantial retention of asbestos fibres. This gradually leads to progressive, diffuse, interstitial pulmonary fibrosis. Persons exposed to air-borne dust swallow asbestos fibres with saliva or sputum. Sometimes water drinks and food may also contain small quantities of fibres. Some of the swallowed fibres may penetrate gut wall and migrate to other parts.

After a latent period, rarely less than 20 years and up to 40 years or more after first occupational exposure, lung cancer, malignant mesothelioma of the pleura or gastrointestinal cancer may develop. The mechanism of carcinogenesis are unknown.

Assessment of exposure may be assessed by sampling static air at fixed locations by membrane filters, impingers and thermal precipitators. Most favoured method is personal air sampling by a membrane filter.

Biological assessment includes radiography by using the ILO International classification of radiographs of pneumoconioses. This can be an indicator for monitoring of exposure. Respiratory function tests are less specific compared to radiography. Sputum test: **Asbestos bodies** in the sputum may be counted to give a rough estimate of relatively recent asbestos exposure.

ANTHRACOSILICOSIS

It is also called coal workers pneumoconioses. It is caused by exposure to mixed dust in which the free silica is not the dominant fibrogenic component.

Coal contains mostly carbon and some hydrogen, sulfur and phosphorus and a variety of rocks, some containing free silica.

Occupations: Mixed dust formed during coal mining is most liable to accumulate in deep mines, especially where mechanical cutting is involved and ventilation is ineffective or poor. All workers in deep mines, workers in loading operations of those industries using coal are at greatest risk of exposure.

Reactions: Fine particles of 0.5–5.0 µm may be retained in the lung tissue and low grade tissue reaction leads to disturbance of lung function.

There are no signs or symptoms in early stages. Clinical disease is preceded by many years of X-ray signs of simple pneumoconioses. Complicated pneumoconioses develop only when the dust burden is very high. If dust exposure is stopped at an early stage of simple pneumoconioses, little disabling disease occurs unless the miners develop rheumatoid disease with synergistic lung changes (*Caplan syndrome*). In anthracosilicosis, serious disability occurs after exposure to much higher dust levels than in the case in silicosis. Furthermore disease is less likely to progress.

There is no specific treatment. Control measures recommended for silicosis also are applicable for anthracosilicosis.

Bronchopulmonary Diseases Caused by Hard Metal Dusts

Hard metal dust is derived from carbides of tungsten, iron, nickel, etc.

Hard or sintered metals are used in the manufacture of tools, drills and metal parts of particular hardness.

Occupations

Workers who are engaged in the production of sintered carbides (mixing, pulverising, forming, furnace, heating, machining, precision grinding) and in the manufacture of tools and machine parts as well as those responsible for sharpening of tools produced.

Mechanism of Action

Absorption of hard metal dust takes place exclusively via the lungs. The absorbed dust is distributed to other parts of the body in the same way as other dust particles. Insoluble dust particles are retained in the lung tissue, while the soluble components are carried by blood to other parts of the body. Only cobalt in small amount is excreted in the urine.

Effects

In majority of those, exposed variety of irritative symptoms are seen, including cough, allergic rhinitis, asthma like dyspnoea and dyspnoea on exertion. The symptoms improve after the cessation of exposure. Diffuse interstitial fibrosis is far less common and affects about 1–4% of workers.

Signs tend to appear after 3 years of exposure. Mostly there is progressive aggravation, with respiratory insufficiency and right ventricular failure and some regression of the signs of disease may be noted following withdrawal from exposure, at least at an early stage.

Control Measures

The exposure of workers must be controlled by appropriate technical measures (enclosing machines, applying local exhaust ventilation, etc.) in order to reduce dust concentration below the recommended exposure limits apart from personal protective measures.

BAGASSOSIS

It is an allergic condition due to inhalation of dust from the fibres left after the sugar has been extracted from the cane. These fibres are known as bagasse and are used for the manufacture of fibre board and similar boards. Moist and hot conditions lead to growth of moulds or fungus on the bagasse, called *Thermoactinomyces vulgaris*. Exposure of 2–4 years is usually enough to produce symptoms like breathlessness and low grade fever. Fibre board which is sterilized in the process of manufacture does not produce symptoms of bagassosis.

Preventive measures consist of suppression of dust, use of personal protection measures apart from periodical health examination and engineering methods of control.

FARMER'S LUNG

Thresher's disease, "broken wind" in horses are allergic phenomenon due to moulds occurring in damp hay and straw. Farmer's lung has a seasonal distribution related to harvesting of crops. Since India is agriculture economy most farmers are exposed to the risk of hay-dust or grain dust. On mouldy hay, the fungus growth of *Micropolyspora feeni* and *Thermoactinomyces vulgaris* act as antigen for allergic pneumonitis due to hypersensitive reactions. Similar symptoms may occur after exposure to wood dust or furniture dust.

BYSSINOSIS

Byssinosis is caused by exposure to air-borne dusts of cotton, flax and soft hemp. Cotton dust is composed of four fractions: Cellulose fibre, plant debris, earthy matter and saprophytic microorganisms (usually Gram-negative bacteria and fungi that grow on the cotton during storage).

Occupations

Workers in textile industry carrying out dusty operations are at great risk. Flax breaking and spinning are performed at home causing dust exposure to the workers and their families. Smokers seem to be more susceptible to byssinosis than non-smokers. They are also more likely to suffer from advanced form of disease.

Mechanism of Action

The pathogenesis is not yet fully clear. There is an evidence that a toxic histamine releasing substance may be responsible for the typical symptoms of byssinosis, namely respiratory tightness, on the first day of work after the weekend holiday. It is widely believed that this histamine releasing action of cotton dust is caused by a water soluble, heat stable, small molecular compound derived from the bracts of the cotton plant.

Byssinosis is characterized by symptoms of chest tightness (towards the end of workshift). There is often a decline in forced expiratory volume (FEV), which may be symptomless in some workers. Within one or two days most of the symptoms tend to disappear. As disease progresses, chest tightness is accompanied by breathlessness followed by chronic bronchitis and emphysema.

At early stage, the disease is reversible. With long history of dust exposure FEV declines to a great extent.

Control Measures

This mainly involves dust suppression, by enclosing dusty operations and improved ventilation (exhaust ventilation), personal protective measures such as masks and monitoring of dust level as also examination for lung function tests.

Prevention of Pneumoconioses

This can be achieved by prevention of dust formation, prevention of escape of dusts and by removal of harmful dust besides other measures.

1 ***Prevention of dust formation:*** This prevents or minimizes dust formation by appropriate technology in the industry. Wet drilling or steam drilling or wet process in stone crushing minimizes dust formation. "Wet method" is extremely useful in pottery and lead industry.
2 ***Prevention of escape of dust in the air:*** When the first level of prevention fails attempt is made to isolate the dust forming areas or zone by use of special enclosures or cabinet for machinery and use of localized exhaust ventilation. Reclamation of dust is a practice in some industries for its recycling. Electrostatic precipitators are used in modern industrial plants to control dust and its escape to the environments. The thermal power plant which use coal as fuel deploy most modern procedures to prevent the escape of dust to atmosphere.
3 ***Removal of dust:*** When the dust formation and prevention of escape of dust fails it is attempted to remove the dust by safe procedures such as vacuum suction and special ventilating arrangements.
4 ***Other measures—personal protective measures***
   a Use of masks and special respirators prevents the entry of dusts in respiratory system. The masks and respirators are most difficult to use as these get blocked and cause lot of uneasiness and hence not used.
   b Personal hygiene and strict cleanliness is helpful. Do not allow the dust to accumulate. Vacuum cleaning or wet cleaning should be resorted for cleaning the premises.
   c Training and education of workers and supervisors on harmful effects of dust should be organized regularly.
   d Early detection of impairments in workers by periodical health examination to prevent the disability.

EXTRINSIC ALLERGIC PNEUMONITIS

These are group of disorders caused by a hypersensitivity reaction to inhaled dust especially dust containing material of fungal origin.

Dust containing organic antigens (particularly thermophilic microorganisms and moulds) or animal protein are the main causes of this disease. The most common dust responsible antigens and disease conditions are as under:

Causative agents of extrinsic allergic pneumonitis

Type of dust	*Responsible antigen*	*Disease*
Mouldy hay	*Micropolyspora feeni Thermoactinomyces vulgaris*	Allergic pneumonitis
Mouldy bagasse	*Thermoactinomyces vulgaris*	Bagasse pneumonitis
Mushroom compost	*Micropolyspora feeni Thermoactinomyces vulgaris*	Allergic pneumonitis
Cork dust	Cork dust	Allergic pneumonitis due to cork dust
Redwood saw dust	*Graphium pullaria*	Allergic pneumonitis due to graphium
Wood pulp	Alternaria	Allergic pneumonitis due to wood dust
Mouldy barley	*Aspergillus clavatus Aspergillus fumigatus*	Allergic aspergillosis
Mouldy straw	*Aspergillus versicolor*	Allergic aspergillosis
Wheat flour	*Sitophilus granarius*	Allergic pneumonitis
Pigeon-parrot and other birds dropping	Sera-protein and dropping	Allergic pneumonitis
Animal hair	–	Allergic pneumonitis

Source: WHO, 1986

Occupations

Workers in agriculture, beverage industries, wood and furniture industries and animal keepers are at risk.

Mechanism of Action

Inhaled dust particles that are small enough to be retained in the alveoli and small airways, that contain antigenic materials which are responsible for the disease. In acute stage, there is formation of sarcoid—type granulomata and in chronic stage diffuse interstitial fibrosis occurs.

Symptoms and Signs

Symptoms develop 4–8 hours after heavy exposure to dust containing antigen. Common symptoms are vomiting, chest tightness, breathlessness and cough, there may be cyanosis and crepitations. X-ray may show small opacities in lung. Acute stage and subacute stage may progress to chronic stage.

Prognosis

Acute disease is usually reversible within several weeks. However, it may progress into chronic form if the exposure continues. Chronic disease may worsen steadily and result in congestive heart failure.

Prevention and Control

Immediate removal from exposure should be the first step. Acute stage requires management with corticosteroids. Changes should be made in work practices in order to avoid the multiplication of fungi and bacteria. Technical measures to be applied to control the dust in the air at workplaces apart from personal protective measures.

OCCUPATIONAL ASTHMA

Occupational asthma is caused by inhalation of sensitizing agents or irritants present in the working environments, such as dusts, droplets and gases. This may be material of plant origin or chemical irritants.

Workers who handle grains and cereals, grain storage workers, farmers, saw mill workers are at risk.

They manifest reversible obstruction of airway, like bronchospasm, airway oedema and inflammation. Most individuals feel better if there is no further exposure, and therefore, person should be withdrawn from exposure. In some subjects the condition may persist.

Pre-placement and periodical examination helps. Technical measures should be applied to control the concentration of air pollutants in the working environment.

DISEASES CAUSED BY LEAD AND ITS TOXIC COMPOUNDS

Properties

16

Lead is bluish grey heavy metal with melting and boiling points of 327°C and 1620°C, respectively. At a temperature of 550–600°C, lead evaporates and combines with oxygen to form lead oxide. Its most common oxidation state is lead (II) and the most important organometallic compounds are lead tetraethyl, lead tetramethyl and lead stearate.

Uses

Metallic lead is used in shielding, electrical cables, production of pipes, cisterns, roof coverings, sealing joints, coating metals exposed to weather/sea water (red lead), paints.

Occupations

Workers in smelting and storage battery manufacturing plants, scrap workers, painters, workers in ceramic industry, foundry workers, welders and petrol blenders are among those at greatest risk of exposure.

Lead Absorption

Lead is absorbed into body by inhalation and ingestion. Lead tetraethyl is absorbed through skin. The health hazard from air-borne lead is related to its particle size. Particle smaller than 10 µm can be retained in the lungs.

Distribution

The absorbed lead is transported to other organs. About 95% of blood lead is bound to red blood cells. A fraction of plasma lead is in the diffusible form, which can be deposited into hard tissues (bones, hair, nails, teeth) and soft tissues (bone marrow, nervous system, kidneys, liver). It is thought that only lead in soft tissues is directly toxic. Lead in hard tissues remains tightly bound to the tissues and toxic only when the pool serves as a source to soft tissues.

Excretion: Lead is excreted via both urine (75–80%) and faeces (about 15%).

Toxic Effects

Lead may exert toxic effects on the gastrointestinal, haematopoietic, nervous (peripheral and central) and renal systems.

Gastrointestinal System

Intestinal colic (spasms of the small intestines) is the commonest clinical manifestation of lead poisoning. It is usually preceded by constipation. Greyish pigmentation of the gums ("lead line") is also sign of lead exposure.

Haematopoietic System

Lead inhibits the activity of enzyme delta aminolevulinate dehydratase (ALAD) in erythroblasts in the bone marrow and in the erythrocytes. This leads to increased concentration of delta ALA in the serum and urine. Clustered ribosomes are visible in the basophilic stippled cells as punctate basophilia even in the absence of anaemia. Lead toxicity thus causes progressive anaemia. High level of ALAD may have neurotoxic effect.

Nervous System

The most serious manifestations of acute encephalopathy are, convulsions, comatose and deliriousness. These effects of lead may not be completely reversible and the risk of permanent complications increases with repeated exposure. The most prominent abnormalities in chronic and subclinical encephalopathy include slowness of performance, psychomotor disturbances, slight intelligence defects and personality changes.

Renal System

During acute phase of lead poisoning, there is often functional renal involvement but permanent renal damage is not certain. Renal failure has been postulated but not confirmed. Chronic renal failure and lead encephalopathy may be fatal.

Assessment

Environmental assessment of lead and regular fixed station air lead monitoring is considered essential.

Biological Assessment

i Measurement of ALAD in blood.
ii Amount of delta ALA in urine.
iii The amount of coproporphyrin in urine.
iv Concentration of zinc protoporphyrin IX (ZnPP) in red blood cells.
v Decreased content of haemoglobin.
vi Decreased number of erythrocytes and their short lifespan.
vii Increased number of reticulocytes (young erythrocytes).
viii Increased number of basophilic stippled erythrocytes.

Independently, none of the above test can be regarded as diagnostic. However, two or more of them may be used together to assess exposure (past or present) and to determine the form of clinical poisoning (acute or chronic).

Control measures: Strict attention should be paid to any source of lead dust or fumes and technical control measures should be applied wherever necessary.

- Industrial and personal hygiene are of great importance. Food and drink must not be brought into workrooms and smoking at work must not be allowed.
- Exposure limit should be maintained.
- Pre-placement and periodic examination of workers and screening test should be done at regular interval.
- If toxicity is detected worker should be removed from exposure and placed on some other job.

EFFECTS OF HEAT

In certain occupational conditions and ambient environments, the workers/persons are exposed to high heat conditions: Mine workers, tea plantation workers, furnace workers and desert climate. In hot summer, the workers are exposed to adverse heat conditions.

Heat Exhaustion

The heat exhaustion is a condition where there is excessive loss of water and salt from the body through excessive sweating in hot environments or atmospheric temperature. It is essentially water and salt depletion due to excessive sweating, it leads to development of tachycardia, pulse becomes weak, blood pressure falls and urine output decreases. Excessive water and salt excretion in sweat beyond a critical level thus causes dehydration, haemostatic exhaustion, metabolic disruption and failure to the general adaptation mechanism. Thus, sweating which is so essential for maintaining thermal balance becomes a threat to the body.

Management

Removal of person to cool place and drinking salt and water and saltish tea is recommended. Best drink is ORS (oral rehydration salt) if a person can drink orally. Recovery is very fast and some cases may need appropriate intravenous fluids.

Heat Stroke

This condition is also called, heat hyperpyrexia and typically occurs when the environmental temperature is very high. The outstanding features are:

- Absence of sweating, and
- High body temperature.

Heat stroke is due to failure of the heat regulating mechanism in the hypothalamus. Temperature usually rises above 40°C and individual may become unconscious. The cardinal signs consist of lack of sweating, hot-dry-skin, which may be red and mottled, hyperthermia with rectal temperature more than 40°C with central nervous system disturbances. Breathing is rapid and may become acidotic or Cheyne-Stokes type later.

Case management is symptomatic. Temperature should be rapidly reduced by spraying cool water and fanning; quenching thirst by giving enough cool water and referring the patient to nearby health facility.

Control

By effective monitoring of temperature and rest pauses with adequate ventilation and adequate cool water.

Heat Cramps

This is also due to excessive heat conditions in the environments. This occurs due to intracellular overhydration and diminished chloride in the tissues. Cramps occur in legs and arms.

Prickly Heat

This occurs due to hyperactivity of acrine sweat glands, blocking of the sweat ducts by epithelial debris due to excessive heat and sweating and poor personal hygiene. Secondary infection may lead to furunculosis.

RADIATION

A. Ultraviolet Radiation

It is mainly from sun energy. These radiations form only small part of the whole spectrum of electromagnetic radiations. Ultraviolet visible light infrared region: More than 90% of ultraviolet radiation, which is incident on earth atmosphere is absorbed by the ozone layer surrounding the earth. Exposure to infrared rays and ultraviolet rays (UV) occurs to farmers, blast furnace workers, sailors, blacksmiths, welders and metal moulders. These may be injurious to eye lens, conjunctiva, and skin. Squamous cell carcinoma is associated with UV rays and effect on eye include keratitis and cataract.[3,4]

B. Ionizing Radiation

Ionizing radiation (both natural and artificial) is of two types:

i Electromagnetic

ii Corpuscular

- ***Electromagnetic ionizing*** radiation consists of X-rays and gamma rays. Frequency range of more than 3.0 $\times 10^{15}$ Hz and energy per photon range.
- ***Corpuscular*** radiation consists of alpha and beta particles, electrons, protons, deuterons and neutrons, etc.

Mechanism of Action

The absorption of radiant energy by the tissues leads to adverse biological effects. The amount of radiant energy absorbed by the tissues depends upon the wavelength of the radiation and the energy, size and charge of the particles.

X-rays and gamma rays of short wavelength and neutron particles travel a long distance in the air and penetrate deep into the tissues before being absorbed.

On the other hand, X-rays of long wavelength and alpha particles travel only a few millimeters in the air, and are absorbed by thin layers of matter (tissues of less than a few millimeters' thickness). Alpha particles have little power of penetration. The unit of absorbed dose of radiation is the gray (Gy) (1 Gy = 1J/kg = 100 rad).

Alpha particles: They have little power of penetration passing into soft tissues or only a few millimeter and hence irradiation of body from outside with alpha particles is of little significance.

Beta particles: These are fast moving energy carrying particles (electrons) of very small mass with negative charge. In general, beta particles are more penetrating than alpha particles and can traverse distances up to a centimeter or more in soft tissues. For this reason, they are valuable therapeutically and radioactive substances emitting beta radiations are used for destruction of superficial tumours. It damages superficial tissues.

Gamma rays: These are electromagnetic radiation of high energy emitted by atomic nuclei. Gamma rays have great penetrating power in comparison to alpha and beta particles. Gamma rays can traverse the whole body with relatively little absorption. Gamma rays have more energy and penetrating power than X-rays.

Exposures: This occurs in two ways—external and internal.

External exposure to radiation occurs from sources localized outside the body. The effect depends upon penetrating power of the radiation. Radiation of low penetrating power is confined to outer integuments while highly penetrating radiation reaches deep seated organs and tissues.

Internal exposure is caused by radioactive substances that have entered the body by inhalation of radioactive dusts, vapours and gases, by ingestion of contaminated water and food and through skin penetration.

Assessment of Exposure

Environmental exposure assessment is by Geiger Muller counters and scintillation counters. Dosimeters used for measurement of ionizing radiation include ionizing chambers, film strips or thermoluminescent devices.

Effects

The harmful effects of irradiation may be somatic or genetic. Somatic effects develop directly in the irradiated individual, while the genetic effects appear in his or her progeny.

Radiation effect may be either stochastic or non-stochastic. Stochastic effects are those whose probability of occurrence, though not necessarily their severity, is considered to be function of dose received. The dose in such cases is assumed to be without threshold. Thus, with increasing dose, the incidence of stochastic effects increase in the exposed population. Genetic and carcinogenic effects are stochastic. The risk of increased incidence of malignant tumours induced by radiation is the main stochastic somatic risk. Non-stochastic is applied to the somatic effects for which the severity of the effect varies with the dose and for which there is a threshold value, e.g. include cataract, nonmalignant skin damage, suppression of haematopoiesis, and damage to gametes leading to loss of fertility.

Acute Effects

Whole body irradiation: Irradiation to whole body with over 1 Gy of penetrating radiation in a single exposure or over 1–2 days results in the so-called acute radiation syndrome which is characterized by cell damage and death in the exposed tissues. Under current occupational conditions, such exposures are extremely rare and are only seen in cases of accidents. Radiation dose of 0.05 and 0.25 Gy may not produce any symptoms.

Doses of 1–2.5 Gy produce prodromal symptoms of nausea, vomiting and fatigue and early haematological changes and suppression of bone marrow after latent phase.

Local irradiation to hands or body parts is more frequent and it leads to skin reactions.

Chronic Effects

- Chronic radiation sickness occurs to individuals who have been repeatedly exposed to ionizing radiation.
- Chronic radio-dermatitis: It occurs when radiation dose to skin reaches at least 20–30 Gy.
- **Eye cataract** by X-rays and gamma rays and neutrons. It occurs after long-term exposure.

Delayed Effects

A variety of cancers have been observed following ionizing radiation. The following types of cancers are related to occupational exposures:

Skin cancer, bone tumours, leukaemias, lung cancer.

The period between exposure to ionizing radiation and the development of cancer may vary from a few years to several decades. It is not known whether a threshold dose exists below which cancers do not occur.

Control Measures

Exposure to radiation from both sealed sources (X-ray equipment, nuclear power plants) and unsealed sources (e.g. radioactive chemicals in medical and industrial laboratories) can be controlled by:

- Reducing the duration of exposure.
- Maintaining a safe distance between the worker and the source of radiation.
- Shielding the source of radiation.

Personal protection devices such as lead rubber gloves and lead aprons should always be used during work involving radiation exposure. In the case of unsealed sources of ionizing radiation, good personal hygiene should be strictly enforced.

Exposure limits for ionizing radiation have been recommended jointly by ILO, WHO, IAEA and NEA. For the control of stochastic effects, the annual effective dose equivalent limit is 50 mSv (5 rem). For non-stochastic effects, the annual dose equivalent limit for individual organ and tissue is 500 mSv (50 rem); except for the eye lens, for which the limit is 150 mSv (15 rem).

Pregnant women should not be subjected to annual exposures exceeding 30% of the dose equivalent limits.

DISEASES CAUSED BY COMPRESSED AIR

Compressed air is air at pressures higher than that at sea level (normal atmospheric pressure). It causes **caissons disease.**

Caissons filled with compressed air are used for underwater construction and repairs of tunnels and bridge piers. Compressed air in caissons is limited to a maximum pressure of 330 kPa.

Mechanism of Action

Compressed air may cause either mechanical effects (barotrauma) or physiological effects. The **decompression sickness** is due to formation of nitrogen bubbles in the blood. Under normal pressure, 12 ml of nitrogen are dissolved in 1 litre of blood. At a pressure of 196 kPa, the nitrogen concentration in blood is 22 ml/litre and at 390 kPa the concentration is about 39 ml/litre. When a diver suddenly comes to surface the compressed or dissolved nitrogen tries to come out of blood rapidly and it forms the air bubbles in the blood vessels and may stop circulation to body parts including vital organs. Effect occurring due to bubbles of nitrogen is called decompression sickness.

Now with advanced technology, the decompression is slow and regulated, hence the bad effect of nitrogen bubbles is not seen.

Effects of Decompression Sickness

Sudden decompression leads to middle ear and sinus trauma leading to rupture of eardrum. It may lead to burst lung and cerebral air embolism.

Most workers complain joint pains (bends) and in serious decompression sickness, it causes spinal cord and brain injuries due to air embolism. Aseptic necrosis is also observed.

With modern advancement in decompression, the ill effects are rare.

HEARING IMPAIRMENT CAUSED BY NOISE

Noise is unwanted sound: The sound frequency audible to human ear lies between 16 Hz and 20,000 Hz (Hertz). The intensity of sound is measured in decibels (dB). The adverse effect of noise is proportional to duration of exposure. Sound of 90 dB and above at 1000 Hz is harmful. In industries, increased mechanization results in increased noise levels. The occupations that cause high-risk of hearing loss include mining, tunnelling, quarrying (detonations drilling) heavy engineering, etc. Hearing loss can be either temporary or permanent. Noise induced temporary threshold shift (NITTS) is temporary loss of hearing acuity. Hearing recovers fairly rapidly after cessation of the noise. Noise induced permanent threshold shift (NIPTS) is an irreversible loss of hearing that is caused by prolonged exposure to a noise.

Control Measures

Pre-placement and periodical health examination is helpful to detect early impairment and prompt action.

Sound levels should be controlled by technical means, either as corrective measures (sound absorbing, anti-reflection panels, baffle plating, hooding, etc.) or preferably by designing less noisy machinery. Individual protections such as plastic ear plugs, muff type ear defenders and headphones are effective.

DISEASES CAUSED BY VIBRATION

Vibration tools are widely used in industry. The most commonly used tools are pneumatic drills, vibratory chisels, grinding appliances, motor saws, polishing machines and pneumatic hammers.

Effects

The continuous and long vibration exposure leads to disturbance of vascular system, peripheral nerves and musculoskeletal system.

Angioneurosis of the fingers or **Raynaud's phenomenon** (white finger) leads to feeling of numbness in the fingers during work and shortly afterwards. The advanced stage of disease is characterized by paroxysmal pallor, which not only affects the tips but spreads over most of the fingers but rarely affects thumbs. The paroxysm is provoked by cold.

Osteoarticular pathology is mostly localized to carpal bones and there are minor subjective symptoms of pain. The X-ray changes show arthrosis of carpal bones.

***Neuropathy*:** Peripheral neuritis due to compressive neuropathy or due to angioneurosis.

Control and Prevention

By improving the design of the vibrating tools and by using the protective "antivibration" gloves.

OCCUPATIONAL DERMATOSIS

Dermatosis in industrial workers is a common problem and cause of absence from work.

Causes

These include physical, chemical and biological agents.

Physical agents include—pressure or friction, excessive heat and sweating and radiations.

Chemical agents: These include:

- Primary irritants like acid and alkalies, lipid solvents and detergents
- Sensitizers metals and their salts
- Acnegenic conditions and
- Photosensitizers.

Biological agents include fungi, bacteria and skin parasites.

Occupations

Agriculture workers, and in most of the industries, chemical agents are used and these may occur as undesirable contaminants. Dyers, painters and chemical production workers as also animal handlers are exposed to the risk of dermatosis.

Signs/Effects

Common effects are erythema, oedema, papules, vesicles or bullae localized on hands, forearms or face, lichenification and fissuring, acne, etc.

Control Measures

Whenever possible strong allergens, sensitizers and carcinogens should be replaced by less dangerous substances, elimination of skin contact with harmful substances by wearing protective clothing, aprons, gloves, boots, face masks, using barrier creams. Personal hygiene and cleanliness help to ward off skin diseases.

CARBON MONOXIDE (CO) POISONING

It is a colourless, odourless, tasteless, combustible and explosive gas. It is produced whenever there is incomplete burning of organic material. Petrol and diesel powered internal combustion engines, boilers and furnaces and blasting operations and fires generate lot of CO in some industries. Motor vehicles generate lot of CO in the atmosphere due to burning of petrol and diesel in internal combustion engine.

Occupations

Workers in the manufacture and distribution of gas (coal gas) made from solid fuel, garage mechanics, engine operators, traffic personnel's, miners, fire fighters and boiler room workers are most at risk. Accidental deaths from CO are not uncommon in private houses during cold weather when people sleep with all doors and windows closed and keep an oil lamp or charcoal fire burning within the room.

Distribution

CO has great affinity with haemoglobin and it forms a stable compound with haemoglobin called as *carboxy-*

haemoglobin and it also binds with myoglobin and cytochrome oxidases. The red blood cells which carry oxygen to different parts of body are unable to carry oxygen as haemoglobin is not available for this function.

Assessment

- Assessment of levels of CO in environments to know hazardous concentration.
- By measuring carboxyhaemoglobin in blood—normal level is 0.5 g/100 g of haemoglobin.
- By measuring CO concentration in expired air.

Effects

The effects are due to oxygen deprivation which deranges the normal metabolism of body cells. It can cause acute or chronic poisoning. Common signs and symptoms include headache, dizziness, drowsiness, nausea and vomiting. If the level or concentration of CO is more, collapse, coma and death may occur. The central nervous system and heart are most sensitive to CO poisoning. Mostly the effects are acute and seldom the chronic effects are observed.

In acute poisoning, patient is removed from the exposure and administered oxygen until carboxyhaemoglobin concentration in blood falls below 5 g/100 g of haemoglobin. As a first aid measure, mouth-to-mouth breathing and extra-thoracic heart massage may save life.

Control Measures

Technical control measures should be applied to reduce CO concentration in the air and possibility of its accidental exposure. Personal protective measures should be used whenever necessary (clean air ventilation hood or apparatus with closed circuit of air in emergency situation).

CO concentration may be high when traffic is held up or during traffic jams. Regulating traffic and efficient public system of transport can reduce the level of CO in atmosphere.

COAL MINES AND OTHER MINES—HEALTH PROBLEMS

The miners have to work underground and in unnatural conditions. It involves special hazards of inadequate illumination, high temperature and humidity, inadequate ventilation, which makes the occupation more risky and more prone to accidents. Because of peculiar posture during the work, they may suffer from musculoskeletal problems, "beat elbow" and "beat knee" followed by bursitis. Visual problems related to darkness may lead to miner's nystagmus. Because of lack of sanitation in mines, they may contract diseases related to insanitary conditions.

Accidents

In the past, accidents of serious nature have occurred in mines like flooding, explosion of fire damp, fall of roof. "Fire damp" consists of methane (CH_4), or ethane (C_2H_6), and "after damp" (carbon monoxide) and "white damp" (carbon dioxide and H_2S). Methane is combustible and it can accumulate in mines and can cause serious explosion as it gets ignited by short circuits of faulty wiring and when it gets mixed with oxygen of the air.

Prevention

Mines need effective ventilation by modern techniques. Effective ventilation prevents accumulation of harmful gases in mines and prevents explosion apart from maintaining comfortable temperature. Most mines have been modernized and adequate safeguards have been provided against flooding, bad illumination. Mines operations have been mechanized. Mines Act, 1952 regulates the health, safety and welfare of the mining population.

INDUSTRIAL ACCIDENTS

Occupational accidents still constitute a major health problem for the working population. It has been estimated that over 15 million occupational accidents occur the world over everyday.

Industrial accidents lead to loss of man hours, loss of production, injuries, deaths and disability. Accidents in mines and quarries are most fatal. Industrial accidents and injuries are notifiable under the factory Act, 1948. In occurrence of industrial accidents, interaction between worker, machine and environments plays significant role. Some determinants of accidents may also exist for long period before the accident occurs. These may be in man himself, in the environments or with the machine and in combination of all these. Safe worker, safe environments and safe machine prevents accident.

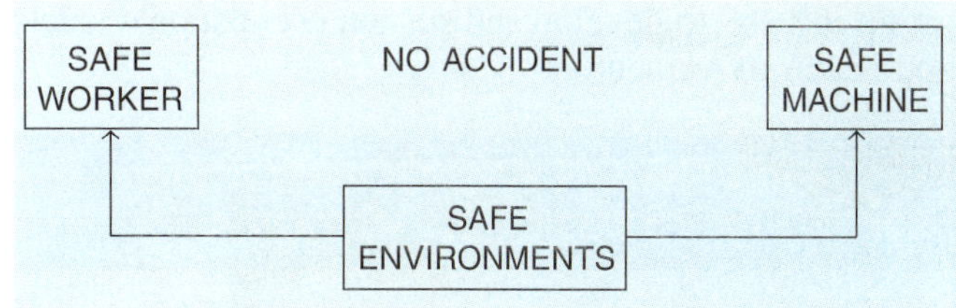

Human Factor

Industrial worker or human factor is responsible for over 90% of the accidents. Human failure is predominant factor in causation of accidents. The human factors include poor visual acuity, impaired hearing, physical defect, negligence, non-use of personal protective measures, industrial fatigue, emotional instability, psychosocial problems, addiction and abuse of substance, age and sex, literacy status, experience and training status of the worker.

ILO (International labour organization) has standardized the following ratio of frequency and severity of accidents in industry.

Frequency rate = E/C × 1,00,000

Severity rate = F/C × 1,00,000

E = Number of accidents causing loss of working time in a given period

C = Total man hours worked in a given period.

F = Total hours lost through accidents occurring in given period.

For death and permanent disabilities, the ILO has prepared standard time losses (death and permanent disability is equivalent to 48,000 hours loss) and these times should be included in the calculation of severity rate less time already lost and accounted as the rate before the permanent nature of the disability became known.

Environmental Factors

The environmental factors which are responsible for occurrence of accidents are overcrowding, less of physical space, slippery floor, inadequate light, uncomfortable temperature, excessive humidity, noise, vibrations, uncovered drains, bad housekeeping, and poor ventilation.

Machine

Machine fault is minimal. Faulty design, lack of guard and fencing, bad maintenance and poor monitoring are some of the faults which can be attributed to machine.

Prevention of Accidents

This includes selection of right man for the right job through pre-placement examination and periodical health examination, adequate on the job training and supervision, ensuring use of personal protective measures, good housekeeping, monitoring of environmental hazards (temperature, humidity, noise, radiation, ventilation, illumination, etc.), safety performance and maintenance of machines. National Safety Council of India (NSCI) was set up in 1966 to develop and sustain occupational safety and health movement.

PREVENTION AND CONTROL OF OCCUPATIONAL HAZARDS

ERGONOMICS

Ergonomics is derived from Greek word 'ergon' means work and 'nomos' meaning law. It primarily aims at "adjusting the job to the worker's characteristic."

Definition

16

According to International Ergonomics Association (IEA): Ergonomics, "Integrates knowledge derived from human sciences to match jobs, systems, products and environments to the physical and mental abilities and limitations of people."

According to Clerk and Corlett (Clerk and Corlett, 1984): Ergonomics is the study of human abilities and characteristics which affect the design of equipment, systems and jobs and its aims are to improve efficiency, safety and well-being. Ergonomics is preventive in action and it prevents fatigue, ill health and accidents. It is more satisfying to the worker, safer and productive.[5,6]

Objectives

i It reduces the physical and mental stress as also fatigue on the job

ii Increases work efficiency

iii Reduces ill health

iv Accelerates response to emergency situation.

Human Characteristics to Ergonomics

Anatomical

The anatomy of human being in terms of height, sitting height, length of arm and body size varies considerably. The design of the good workstation, tools, machines, tables and chairs must be adjustable to individual differences in body size and individual should not be forced to make body adjustment according to what is designed. The workstations should take into consideration the anthropometric characteristic of human beings in terms of sitting height, standing height, eye level, shoulder height, elbow height and knee height. It will reduce the postural defects, apart from this it will increase work efficiency and production and reduce accidents. Most sitting chairs are ill-designed and lumbar support is inappropriate and consequently the sign of fatigue appear faster and *musculoskeletal disorders* appear in large number of persons. Industrial workstations must be workers-friendly. The individual should be able to reach, bend and stretch and adopt natural posture and movements to perform the task.

Working tools and equipment should be 'designed' in such a way that it does not produce pressure signs or vibrations.

Physical Work Capacity

The physical work capacity of human beings varies in children, young and old people. The physical work capacity is at its peak between 20 and 30 years age group and thereafter it gradually decreases. Women capacity is lower. Therefore, the work task must be designed to fit the capacities of range of people. The human system (cardiovascular, aerobic and muscular) should not be taxed to 100%. The norms of weight to be lifted by men and women and children have been fixed in industry.

There should not be undue stress on the cardiovascular, aerobic and muscular system otherwise *musculoskeletal problem* are likely to develop. This can be taken care of by training of workers to adopt correct methods of lifting of weight to reduce the musculoskeletal trauma and wear and tears among those performing physical heavy work. Increased mechanization has led to reduction of these problems.

Sensory Capability

Human beings perceive the happening around through sensory system of vision, hearing, touch, smell and taste. The vision, hearing and touch are important factors in our perception of the environment for quick response to signals from machines, displays, warning signs and other signs and information from fellow workers or supervisors. Taste and smell though less important for ergonomics but may be life-saving in toxic environments.

In ergonomics, the response by senses is quick if we adopt the principle of "contrast" the "alarm bell" must produce high level of sound not to be masked by the usual industry noise. Aged people may require even higher level of sound. For easy perception, alarm buttons are of red colour and easily accessible. Alarm systems have been developed and to be perceived through senses. The senses must have high acuity and the perception can be further enhanced by having colour coded switches, knobs, adequate illumination, sound-based warning system and training of workers. Warning signs must be symbols and icons familiar to the workers.

Planning of Building, Equipment and Machinery

Planning of building, ensuring adequate workspace, illumination ventilation, control of temperature. Similarly, redesign the workstation to avoid unnecessary bending or repetitive bending, excessive stretching to minimize ergonomic hazard. Adjust the machine process and environments to the physical and psychological abilities and limitation of the workers is key to production and increase efficiency and reduce accidents. Control of noise and vibration should be done by designs and proofing.

PRE-PLACEMENT EXAMINATION

The primary purpose of pre-placement examination is to assess the fitness for work. The objective is to choose a right person for right job. In industrial set-up, it protects employee and employer.

All workers should undergo a medical examination before entering industrial employment for the first time (engagement or pre-placement examination) within 15 days of employment.

The examination also enables the management to place workers in jobs suited to their capacities and limitation. The medical information needed is recorded on pre-employment examination form, the design of which varies with different occupations.

Pre-placement examination should consist of general, physical and clinical examinations and special investigations where indicated. If the person shows accident-proneness he should not be employed. The general clinical examination covers visual acuity, hearing, locomotor function, physical capacity, mental capacity, X-ray chest, haemoglobin and urine examination and if history of exposure is present some special investigations are also undertaken, e.g. audiometry. The pre-placement health examination should take account of individual risk factors such as age, sex and individual susceptibility.

Persons having anaemia are unfit to be employed where lead exposure is there. Similarly, person with cough and bronchitis and healed tuberculosis should not be employed in silica industry (mining and stone cutting, etc.). Proper job analysis would be done for all the jobs and each person should be placed in such a way that he fits in the job and the job fits him.

Early Detection of Health Impairment on Occupational Exposure to Health Hazards by 'Periodical Health Examination'

This is secondary level of prevention in occupational health. When the exposure has already set, the efforts are directed to minimize the impact of the exposure and delay the development of disease in exposed individual by periodical health check-up at regular interval.

The objective of periodical examination is to detect the impairment at the earliest.

Early Detection of Occupational Impairment and Diseases/Exposures

Aim

1. To detect susceptible workers and remove them from exposure before they suffer any permanent incapacitation.
2. To provide knowledge on natural history of respiratory disease that is essential for its management in early stage.
3. To identify the nature of hazardous exposure.

Examples are

- i In exposure to dusts and organic fibres:
  - Use of lung function test: Determination of forced expiratory volume (FEV) and forced vital capacity (FVC). Vital capacity and peak flow rate are useful for early detection of respiratory impairment.
  - These tests may be supplemented by a standard questionnaire and an X-ray examination.
- ii For exposure to organophosphorus insecticides, a number of field kits for measurement of total cholinesterase activity in blood are available.
- iii For evaluating, the hazards of lead exposure, simple practical tests include the semiquantitative test for coproporphyrin in the urine and simplified kits for determining ALA in the urine.

iv For exposure to volatile agents; some field kits are available for measuring the agents in exhaled air (especially alcohol and carbon monoxide), however, there is need to develop more practical tests for exhaled air.
v For exposure that affect the blood and haematopoiesis, one can measure haemoglobin, sedimentation rate, and total and differential leucocyte counts, all of which may be nonspecific for an agent but may indicate early impairment.
vi Analysis of urine for protein may be of value for certain exposures such as cadmium and trichlorethylene.
vii Audiometry for noise exposures.
viii Basophilic stippling of red blood cells can be detected at periodical health examination.

Periodic medical examination means medical inspection of worker at specified intervals (monthly, quarterly and yearly) to prevent risk either to worker or fellow employees and to detect an impairment at the earliest.

Risk to fellow workers: The workers employed as railway engine drivers, pilots, lorry drivers pose risk to passengers. They are subjected to periodical examination under the regulation. They are subjected to visual acuity, colour blindness, hearing tests. The norms or standards are fixed for these tests. These workers should not have any disease such as epilepsy or locomotor abnormality.

Risk to the workers: Many of the processes involved in industry are dangerous or potentially dangerous to the workers such as exposure to lead, radiation, silica, heavy metals and mineral oils, etc. Apart from general physical examination, special tests are indicated for specific exposures at specified intervals with the aim of early detection of an impairment.

Environments

Environments such as poor illumination, noise, vibrations, slippery floors, thermal conditions, excessive humidity adversely affect the work capacity and productivity apart from health. The standards of these have been laid down under the factory Act, 1948 and its enforcement helps to improve the environments.

Hazard Elimination

The substances which are hazardous and proven carcinogenic should be eliminated from the processes, e.g. asbestos free products, benzene free solvents and unleaded petrol.

Substitution of Hazard

A process which is hazardous can be substituted by non-hazardous process such as sandblasting may be substituted by shot blasting. Acetone may be used in place of benzol as solvent. Use of yellow phosphorus in match industry leads to characteristic necrosis of bone "phossy jaw" yellow phosphorus has been substituted by sesquisulphide in match industry.

Suppression of Hazard (Engineering Measures)

Suppressing the substances or hazard by process such as "wet process" in drilling of rocks or stone cutting, it suppresses silica dust and similarly exhaust method is another example of *engineering control* of dust at the source.

Other engineering measures to control the hazard are improving ventilation, illumination, enclosing and isolation of hazardous process, local exhaust ventilation, and good housekeeping.

Environment Monitoring of Hazard

Monitoring of toxic substances in the work environments and keeping their level below the permissible limits so that the worker does not suffer any health impairment.

Permissible exposure limit (PEL): It is defined as exposure to a minimum time weighted average (TWA) of concentration of a toxicant for an 8-hour-work. The PEL of some important substances by Factories Act, 1948 (modified in 1987) are given as under:[7, 8]

Permissible exposure limits of gases and Vapours Factory Act, 1948 (Amended, 1987)

Substance	*Parts per million of air by volume*
Acetone	750
Ammonia	0.25
Arsenic	0.2 mg/m^3
Bromine	0.7
Benzene	10
Carbon disulphide (skin)	10
Carbon monoxide	50
Formic acid	5
Hydrogen cyanide (skin)	10
Phenol (skin)	3
Phosgene	5
Pyridine	0.1
Sulphur dioxide	5
Toluene	100
Trichloroethylene	50
Vinylchloride	5
Xylene	100

Permissible levels have their limitations, all efforts must be made to keep the exposure levels as low as possible.

Personal Protective Measures

Lead aprons to protect radiations, gloves, masks, helmets, goggles, earmuffs, ear plugs, use of respirators, footwear and barrier creams, helps and ensures safety against hazard. These appliances must be kept clean and tidy to enhance their acceptability and use. It is, however, not to be used as substitute to other engineering methods to control hazards as elaborated above. Personal protection should be used in conjunction with engineering methods of control of hazard.

Personal Hygiene

Adequate personal hygiene like washing hands, feet and bathing should be observed by all workers to prevent the entry of hazardous substances in the body (lead, chrome and radioactive substances). Industry should provide facilities for hand washing and bathing. Prohibition of preparation and taking meals and smoking in workrooms should be observed.

Health Education

Worker needs to be educated on the hazards reduction, personal hygiene and use of safety measures to protect their own health as also the health of the fellow colleagues. Do's and Don'ts should be displayed on all the work-stations. Workers cooperation is extremely important and this can come through regular information to workers on all aspects of health promotion and prevention of injuries.

Notifiable Disease

Disease notification helps to plan prevention and control programme and learn lessons. The ultimate objective of disease notification is to reduce the incidence of ill health and diseases by controlling the toxic exposure. Disease notification also provides evidence-based information on the effectiveness of engineering control measures and other measures. In essence, notification provides direction for future action. Following diseases are notifiable under Factory Act, 1948 (Amended in 1987).

1. ***Lead poisoning:*** Poisoning by any preparation or compound of lead or its sequelae.
2. Lead tetraethyl poisoning.
3. Phosphorus poisoning or its sequelae.
4. Mercury poisoning or its sequelae.
5. Manganese poisoning or its sequelae.
6. Arsenic poisoning or its sequelae.
7. Poisoning of nitrous fumes.
8. Carbon bisulphate poisoning.
9. Benzene poisoning including poisoning by any of its analogue their nitro- or amino-derivatives or its sequelae.
10. Chrome ulceration or its sequelae.
11. Anthrax.
12. Silicosis.
13. Poisoning by halogens or halogen derivatives of the hydrocarbons of aliphatic series.
14. Pathological manifestation due to radium or other radioactive substances and X-rays.
15. Primary epithelioma of the skin.
16. Toxic anaemia.
17. Jaundice due to hepatotoxic substances.
18. Oil acne or dermatitis due to mineral oils and compounds containing mineral oil base.
19. Byssinosis.
20. Asbestosis.
21. Occupational or contact dermatitis caused by direct contact with chemicals and paints. These are of two types, that is, primary irritants and allergic sensitizers.
22. Noise induced hearing loss (exposure to high noise levels).
23. Berylium poisoning.
24. Carbon monoxide poisoning.
25. Coal mines pneumoconioses.
26. Phosgene poisoning.
27. Occupational cancer.
28. Isocyanide poisoning.
29. Toxic nephritis.

LEGISLATIVE MEASURES: UNDER FACTORIES ACT, 1948

This Act was enacted by Parliament in 1948 and amended from time to time and last amendment was done in 1987. The Act applies to whole of India except Jammu & Kashmir.

Factory: The Act defined "factory" as an establishment employing 10 or more workers where power is used, and 20 or more workers where power is not used. The state Governments are authorized to appoint besides the chief inspector of factories as many additional chief inspectors of factories, joint chief inspectors, deputy chief inspectors as they think fit to enforce the provisions of the law.

Employment of Young Persons and Women

The Act prohibits employment of children below 14 years of age, persons between 15 and 18 years are to be dully certified as adolescents by "certifying surgeon" and also deemed thus fit to work. Adolescent employees and women are restricted from employment in certain dangerous occupations and hazardous processes and are allowed to work between 6 am and 7 pm.

Hours of Work

The Act has prescribed a maximum of 56 hours of work (60 hours including overtime) per week with maximum spread over of work up to 12 hours per day (including rest interval of ½ hour after every 5 hours of work. For adolescents, the maximum hours of work per day have been restricted to 4½ hours.

Leaves and Wages

The Act lays down that besides weekly holidays, every worker will be entitled to leave with wage after 12 months of continuous work at the rate of one day after every 20 days of work for adults and one day for every 15 days of work for adolescents.

No woman or young person unaided by another person can lift, carry, or move by hand or on the head, any material, article, tool appliance exceeding the following limits:

Adult female 29.5 kg, adolescent male 29.5 kg, adolescent female 20 kg, male child 16 kg and female child 13.5 kg.

The state government is empowered to prescribe maximum weights which may be lifted or carried by men, women and children.

If an accident occurs in any factory causing death or bodily injury or prevents a worker from working for more than 48 hours, the manager must immediately send notice to the prescribed authority (labour commissioner).

Similarly, all notifiable diseases shall be notified on occurrence to the appropriate authority.

Work Environments

Design of Building

All buildings, permanent or temporary should be structurally safe and sound to withstand the stress and strain of machinery. Single storey construction is the usual rule as it allows flexibility of layout. Any intensity of natural light can be obtained in it by a combination of wall and roof lighting and it is easier to manage natural ventilation. By careful orientation, direct exposure to the tropical sun can be avoided. Protection from conducted heat can be achieved by a choice of suitable material. Asbestos lining of the walls and ceilings will reduce the noise of machines by controlling the reverberation, resonance and sympathetic vibrations. This will also make the building fireproof.

Space

A floor area of 3.8 m^2 and 14.2 m^3 of space per worker should be provided. The height of the workroom should not be less than 3 meters and height above 4.2 meters should be excluded.

Lighting

Workrooms should be adequately provided with natural and/or artificial lighting. Any special type of work should have special, extra or spot lighting suitable for the operations. In all places, where persons work or pass through, enough diffuse background lighting should be ensured. Natural lighting is ensured by provision of skylights and windows located and spaced with devices to avoid glare. Artificial lighting should be provided where day lighting is insufficient. It should be uniform and free from sharp and contrast shadows and direct or reflected glare. Fluorescent tube in strip light is being increasingly used to have uniform illumination.

Ventilation

Modern concept of ventilation requires replacement of vitiated air by supply of fresh outdoor air. The quality of incoming air should be such that its temperature, humidity and purity are conducive for healthful working. Clean fresh air should be supplied to enclosed workplaces and it is recommended that in workrooms and assemblies there should be 4–6 air changes in one hour. If the air is changed more frequently, i.e. more than 6 times in one hour, it is likely to produce drought which should be avoided. Where the adequate supply of fresh air cannot be obtained by natural ventilation, mechanical ventilation should be provided. All dust, fumes, gases, vapours or mists generated and released in industrial processes should be removed by local exhaust ventilation at their point of origin.

Thermal Comfort

Temperature and humidity should be maintained in enclosed workplaces suitable to the kind of work performed. In localities subject to high or low seasonal temperature appropriate means such as heat insulation of roofs, walls and floors and even of doors and windows should be adopted. All employees should be protected against radiation heat and excessive temperature from heated machines or hot processes by heat insulation of the equipment and/or low temperature. "Transition rooms" should be provided so that the workers can gradually adjust themselves to the external climatic environments. Roof shelters and window breakers should be provided for yard workers where necessary. Measurement and indices of thermal comfort have been specified.

Working Comforts

Seats and workbenches of suitable shape and height should be provided for workers. The seat should be so placed that working material can be reached easily without strain or having to bend forward unduly. Seats should also be provided for all workers, who have to work in standing position, for rest during occasional short interruptions in their work.

Housekeeping

It implies general cleanliness and orderliness of the plants, the tools and the products. Cleaning and sweeping should be done during non-working hours; vacuum cleaning or wet mopping should be adopted. Effective drainage should be maintained where wet processing is carried out. False floors, platforms, mats or other dry standing places along with suitable footwear should be provided in oily and greasy places. However, 'housekeeping' means much more than merely keeping the working places clean. That there is a place for everything and everything in its right place, is a tried and true axiom of industrial safety. Stumbling and tripping due to improper housekeeping is another potential cause of accidents.

Miscellaneous Requirements

Infestation with rodents, insects and vermin should be eliminated by suitable measures. Workrooms and workplaces should not be used as living or sleeping quarters.

No food, drink, betel nut or leaves or tobacco should be consumed or brought by any worker into any workroom in which dangerous and obnoxious materials, particularly lead and radioactive substances, are in use. Anyone suffering from communicable diseases should be at once isolated and preventive and control measures instituted.

Machinery

Accident

The most important industrial hazard due to machinery is the accidental injury. Accidents in industrial environments are due to various causes. Bad housekeeping, faulty and unguarded machinery, faulty work methods, carelessness, ignorance, physical and mental illness, accident-proneness, and slackness in the maintenance of machinery, are the important factors. The components of machinery are the main causes of accidents. Though the loss of productive capacity due to accidental disabilities—major and minor, and even deaths cannot be measured definitely, it is obviously of same magnitude, as judged by the man-days or working time lost. Practical preventive measures are therefore essential to safeguard the workers against accidents. The safety officer must investigate all accidents with a view to ascertaining the cause, adopt safety measures against recurrence and to train personnel in accident prevention. Most of the accidents are preventable by the close collaboration of the factory engineer, safety officer, welfare officer, chemist, industrial hygienist and the medical officer. The worker plays an important role in the prevention of accidents. Some particular industries, occupations and processes cause particular types of injuries on particular parts of the body.

Welfare

Chapter 5 of the Act relates to welfare measures for the worker. The Act specifies that wherein more than 250 workers are ordinarily employed, a canteen shall be provided. In every factory, wherein 30 or more women workers are ordinarily employed, a crèche should be provided. Provisions have been made under the Act to ensure adequate washing facilities, facilities for storing and drying clothes, sitting, first aid appliances, shelters, rest rooms and lunchrooms. There should be a welfare officer for every factory employing more than 500 workers.

Employment in Hazardous Processes

Chapter 4 A, incorporated by the Factories (Amendment) Act, 1987 relates to hazardous processes. A Site Appraisal Committee consisting of chief inspector and other members, not more than 14 in number, is to be constituted to submit recommendations on the siting of factories using hazardous processes. Provisions have been made for workers participation in safety management in industries involving hazardous processes.

Sanitary Conveniences

These should be conveniently located:

- ***Latrines:*** Scale of latrine accommodation is 4 for the first 100 workers and 2 for subsequent 100 workers or part thereof.
- ***Urinals:*** Two urinals for every 100 workers up to 500 and thereafter one for 100 workers are to be provided. For female workers, separate sanitary conveniences are to be provided.
- ***Wash basins:*** Adequate hand washing facilities should be provided. For persons whose work involves contact with any injurious substances, there should be at least one tap for every 15 workers.
- ***Bathrooms:*** Adequate number of bathrooms for bathing and washing of clothes should be provided.

REFERENCES

1 ICMR. A National Priority on occupational health and safety management system. ICMR Bulletin. Nov-Dec 2003; 33 (11–12).

2 ICMR. Silicosis—An uncommonly diagnosed common occupational disease. ICMR Bulletin Sept 1999; 29(9).

3 World Health Organization. Early Detection of Occupational Diseases. Geneva: World Health Organization; 1986.

4 ICMR. Nuclear Medicine—Practice and radiation doses to patient in India. Status of Nuclear Medicine in India. New Delhi: ICMR, 2005.

5 World Health Organization. Psychosocial Factors at work and their relation to health. Geneva: World Health Organization; 1987.

6 WHO. Early detection of health impairment in occupational exposure to health hazards. Technical report series. Geneva: WHO; 1975 Report No. 571.

7 Health Dialogue: Health and safety at work No. 34 July–September 2003, CMAI, New Delhi.

8 Factory Act, 1948 (Amended upto 1987).

EMPLOYEES STATE INSURANCE SCHEME (ESIS) OF INDIA

The social security is as old a concept as the society itself. Though the workmen's compensation Act was promulgated in India in 1923 to safeguard the interests of industrial workers in the event of death and disability, there was no provision to take care of other happenings, more pressing and more frequent such as sickness, temporary disablement and maternity, etc. and even medical care facilities. The ESI Act, 1948 was the first major landmark legislation on social security that covered a variety of risks that the workers in the organized sector were exposed to:[1]

The ESI Act, 1948

The ESI Act was passed in 1948, which was the largest social insurance scheme in India that protects the interests of workers employed in industrial sector/establishment in the event of sickness, maternity, temporary and physical disablement resulting in loss of wages, or earning capacity and death due to employment injury. The Act also guarantees reasonable good medical care to workers and their immediate dependents.

The ESI scheme was first implemented in 1952 at Kanpur and Delhi in Feb., 1952 covering just 1.2 lakh employees. Over the last 63 years, ESI corporation has emerged as the country's leading "multidimensional health insurance" organization. Today, it has a vast network of ESI hospitals, dispensaries, and panel clinics providing, primary, specialist and inpatient services to about 32 million ESI beneficiaries all over the country. ESI corporation has also decided to set-up atleast one model hospital in each state. ESI has also set-up medical colleges.

Coverage of Factories

The ESI Act applies to all non-seasonal factories, using power and employing 10 or more persons, and to non-power using factories employing 20 or more persons for wages on any day in implemented areas. There is enabling provision in the Act to extend coverage to other classes of establishment—industrial, commercial, agricultural or otherwise. Most of the state Governments have extended the provisions of the Act to shops, hotels restaurants, cinemas, road motor transport agencies, newspaper establishment, etc. The Act does not apply to mining operations and railways which are covered under separate Acts similar to ESI Act.

Coverage of Employees

An employee under the Act means any person employed for wages or in connection with the work of a factory or establishment to which this Act applies. The wage ceiling in 1997 was ₹ 6500 per month, raised to ₹ 10,000 in 2008 and further raised to ₹ 15,000 per month in 2010.

Contribution

ESI scheme is contributory in nature; all the employees in the factories or establishment to which the Act applies shall be insured in a manner provided by the Act. Currently, the employee's contribution rate is 1.75% of the wages and that of the employer's 4.75% of the wages paid/payable in respect of the employees in every wage period. Employees in receipt of daily average wage up to ₹ 70 per day are exempted from payment of contribution but entitled for benefits. The state government contribution is 12.5%, while the ESI corporation share is 87.5% towards the medical care of employees.

Infrastructure

The ESI scheme over the last 64 years has come of age in terms of coverage, growth and development. By the end of March, 2014, the scheme has been implemented at 642 industrial centres across the country covering about 19.5 million employees. The total number of beneficiaries were touching 75 million whereas the number of establishments and factories brought within the purview of Act had risen to over 2.20 lakh.

The corporation has already set up. 151 ESI hospitals, 1418 service dispensaries, 42 annexes, 37 specialist centres and has also empanelled about 7763 medical insurance officers. The corporation has set-up 61 regional offices/ subregional offices and 812 local offices and cash offices for the administration of scheme including disbursement of cash benefits to ESI beneficiaries.

Organization and Administration

The ESI scheme is administered by a corporate body called the ESI Corporation (ESIC). This is the apex body constituted and notified by the Central Government for 4 years term, it has representative of employees, employers, the central and state Governments besides, Parliament and medical profession (Fig. 16.1).

MEDICAL BENEFITS UNDER THE ESI SCHEME

The Act provides reasonable medical care in the form of medical treatment and attendance to insured person (IP) and their families in respect of medical, surgical and obstetric treatment.

System of Treatment

Generally, the allopathic system of medicine is used for providing benefits, however, where substantial number of workers demand treatment by Indian system of medicine and homeopathy, treatment facilities may be provided under the scheme.

Scale of Benefits

- To insured persons (IPs): IPs are entitled to avail treatment at ESI dispensary/hospital/diagnostic centre and recognized institutions to which he is attached. The scale of treatment consist of:
  - Outpatient treatment.
  - Inpatient treatment (hospitalization).
  - Domiciliary treatment by visits at their residences.
  - Specialist consultations.
  - Free supply of drugs/dressings/artificial limbs/ hearing aids and appliances.
  - Imaging and laboratory services.
  - Integrated family welfare immunization and MCH programme and other national health programmes, etc.
  - Ambulance service or reimbursement of conveyance charges for going to hospitals, diagnostic centres, etc.
  - Medical certification.

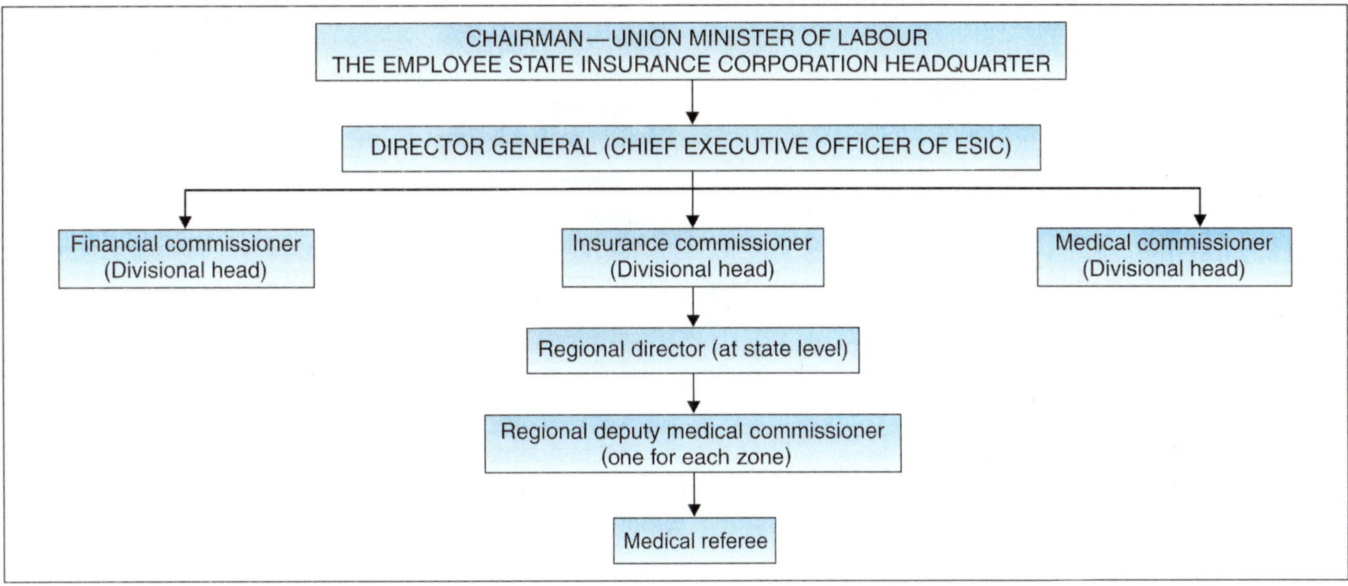

Fig. 16.1: Administrative set-up of ESIS

Special Provision

Family Members of Insured Persons (IPs)

While in all implemented areas, IPs are entitled to medical care as detailed above, members of the family of an IP are entitled to one of the following scales of medical benefits.

- Full medical care, i.e. all facilities as for IPs including hospitalization.
- Expanded medical care, i.e. all facilities as for IPs except hospitalization. A small number of IPs in the state of Gujarat and Bihar fall under this category.

The ESI corporation aims at providing uniform scale of medical care to the family members in all implemented areas, as the rates of contribution by the employees and the employers are the same throughout the country.

Management of Occupational Diseases under ESI

Occupational diseases under ESI are treated as *employment injuries*. Occupational health hazards can be acute or chronic in onset. Acute onset is induced by large doses of toxic substances in an industrial environment (short-term high doses) and chronic onset, which is the result of repeated or continuous exposure of small doses of substance (long-term low doses).

Outpatient Care

The outpatient care is provided through full time insurance medical officers (IMOs) of ESI dispensaries, manned by medical officers of the state Government or by "Panel system", i.e. by private medical practitioners working for ESI scheme, i.e. insurance medical practitioners (IMP) clinic. Generally, a two doctors dispensary should be opened for 3000 IP family units, 3 doctors dispensary for 5000 IP family units and 5 doctors dispensary for 10,000 IP family units. If the number of IPs is less than 3000 IP family units, the services are provided through mobile dispensaries.

Inpatient Treatment

Inpatient facilities are made available by ESI hospitals or by reservation of beds in the hospitals owned by state Government, local fund organization or private bodies. ESI scheme pays for these beds on the basis of occupied bed days.

Domiciliary Treatment

The IP and his family members are entitled free medical attendance by IMO/IMP at their residence when the condition of the patient is such that he/she cannot reasonably be expected to attend the dispensary/clinic.

Specialist Consultation

Under ESI specialist consultation facilities are made available through ESI hospitals or by appointed specialists and super-specialists.

Cash Benefits

Benefits under the ESI Scheme

The following six social security benefits are being provided:

- Medical benefits (in kind)—already discussed.

  Following are the cash benefits admissible under the scheme:
- Sickness benefit (SB) including extended sickness benefit (ESB) and enhanced sickness benefit.

16

- Maternity benefit.
- Disablement benefit:
  - Temporary disablement benefit (TDB)
  - Permanent disablement benefit (PDB)
  - Dependent benefit (DB)
  - Funeral expenses.

An interesting feature of the ESI scheme is that the contributions are related to the paying capacity as a fixed percentage of the worker's wages, whereas, they are provided social security according to individual needs without distinction or discrimination. There are certain additional benefits such as:

i Rehabilitation allowance.

ii Vocational rehabilitation allowance.

Sickness Benefit

Sickness benefit is paid at standard benefit rate which is 50% of the average daily wages and is payable for 91 days during two consecutive benefit period. An employee becomes eligible for sickness benefit if an IP has paid contribution for not less than 78 days during the corresponding contribution period or half the number of days in the first contribution period on initial appointment.

Extended Sickness Benefit (ESB)

IPs suffering from long-term illness face great hardship on expiry of 91 days of sickness benefit. Often, they are not fit for duty, but passes for a final certificate. Hence, a provision for paying sickness benefit for an extended period (extended sickness benefit) of up to 2 years in an ESB period of 3 years was made. IPs suffering from certain long-term diseases are entitled to ESB, only after exhausting sickness benefit to which they may be eligible. The chronic sickness list includes leprosy, tuberculosis, industrial lung disease, malignant diseases, diabetes, monoplegia, hemiplegia, paraplegia, coronary heart disease, chronic obstructive lung diseases, cirrhosis of liver and orthopaedic and psychoses problems as also certain other problems.

Disablement Benefit

Temporary disablement benefit (TDB): TDB is payable to an employee who suffers from employment injury (EI) or occupational disease and is certified to be temporarily incapable to work. "Employment injury" has been defined as a personal injury to an employee caused by an accident or occupational disease arising out of and in the course of his employment, being in insurable employment, whether the accident occurs or the occupational disease is contracted within or outside the territorial limits of India. Examples of occupational sickness include silicosis, asbestosis, bagassosis, byssinosis, farmer's long, pneumoconioses, accidents, etc.

16

TDB rate is 40% over and above the standard benefit rate. This works out to be nearly 70% of the average daily wages. There is no prescribed limit or duration of TDB. This is payable as long as temporary disablement lasts and significant improvement by treatment is possible.

Permanent disability benefit (PDB): The PDB is payable to an IP who suffers permanent residual disablement as a result of EI (employment injury including occupational disease) that results in loss of earning capacity. The permanent disability rate is calculated as percentage of loss of earning capacity as assessed by medical board. The maximum rate of PDB can be equal to the rate of TDB.

Dependents benefit (DB): When an IP dies as a result of EI, the dependent is paid the benefit. The minimum rate of DB is Rs. 14 per day.

Maternity benefit: Maternity benefit is payable to an insured woman in the following cases subject to contributory conditions. Confinement—payable for a period of 12 weeks (84 days) and miscarriage or medical termination of pregnancy (MTP) payable for 6 weeks (42 days) from the date of following miscarriage. Sickness arising out of pregnancy, confinement, premature birth payable for a period not exceeding one month. Maternity benefit rate is double the standard benefit rate or roughly equal to average daily wage.

Funeral benefit: Funeral expenses not exceeding ₹ 1500 is payable towards expenditure on the funeral of a deceased IP and persons in receipt of periodical payments of PDB.

Physical rehabilitation allowance: Disabled insured persons who remain admitted in an artificial limb centre for fixation or repair or replacement of the artificial limb are entitled to a rehabilitation allowance for each day on which they remain admitted at artificial limb centre at double the standard benefit rate. This is not subject to any contribution condition.

Vocational rehabilitation scheme for permanently disabled IPs: This scheme has been designed to provide financial assistance to the IPs who are referred to vocational rehabilitation centre for training. Under the scheme, the insured persons aged not more than 45 years, who are permanently disabled as a result of an employment injury (EI) with loss of earning capacity of not less than 40% and are not in gainful employment subsequent to EI are entitled to receive cash allowance equal to the expenditure charged by the vocational rehabilitation centre or ₹ 45 per day whichever is more during his stay at the vocational rehabilitation centre.

Medical Certification under ESI

The principles of governing the issue of certificates for sickness (including sickness arising out of pregnancy/

confinement and extended sickness benefit (ESB) and temporary disablement) are similar.

'Sickness' means a condition which requires a medical treatment and attendance and necessitates absence from work on medical grounds. Before a certificate is issued, two conditions must be met namely: (1) that a person requires medical treatment and attendance, and (2) that his condition temporarily necessitates abstention from work on medical grounds.

ESI scheme is a good example of health insurance.[2] This achieves the objective of 'increasing productivity, by ensuring good health to working population in factories and establishments. This has national perspective rather than narrow cash benefits scheme. The intention is to keep them fit and make them fittest by curative, preventive and promotive services. Employer should focus on the health status of employee and their families and ensure other important measures such as prevention of injuries and exposure to harmful substances which could be injurious to the health of employees to minimize the loss of man days, finances and to increase the productivity. The doctors working in ESI should ensure prevention of diseases in the IP and their families by providing adequate preventive services.

REFERENCES

1 GOI. ESI Medical Manual (incorporating instructions up to March 2000). 4th edn; New Delhi: DG Employees State Insurance Corporation; 2002, ammended up to 2011.

2 Lal S, Vashisht BM, Reforms in health system in India. Ind J Comm Med 2002; 27(3): 99–105.

CHAPTER

17

Disaster Preparedness and Management

Think globally and act locally holds true to disaster management

Definition

WHO's definition of disaster is: "Any occurrence that causes damage, economic disruption, loss of human life and deterioration in health and the health services on a scale sufficient to warrant an extraordinary response from outside the affected community or area." Under this definition a disaster occurs somewhere in the world, almost everyday. By its very definition, it is clear that response to a disaster must involve all sectors of government.[1,2]

Disaster means a catastrophe, mishap, calamity or grave occurrence, in any area, arising from natural or man-made causes or by accident or negligence which results in substantial loss of life or human suffering or damage to, and destruction of property, or damage to, or degradation of environment, and is of such a nature and magnitude as to beyond the coping capacity of the community of the affected area.

GLOBAL PHENOMENON

Disaster occurrence is a global phenomenon. The greatest number of disasters occur in those countries that are already most adversely affected by ill health and poor-economic conditions. Furthermore, with the continuing deterioration of the environments, including deforestation and misuse of land, we have every reason to believe that frequency of disasters, such as floods, droughts will increase in the coming decades. Japan was hit by devastating earthquake and tsunami on 11th March 2011 which killed more than 19,000 people and crippled three nuclear reactors leading to radiation exposure with a threat of nuclear disaster.

The report from UN agency for disaster risk reduction (UNISDR) in 2015, said: "Floods, storms and other extreme weather events have killed 606000 people since 1995, with an addition 4.1 billion people injured, left homeless or in need of emergency assistance. Floods alone account for 47% of all weather disasters over the post 20 years.

The International Decade for Natural Disaster Reduction (IDNDR) 1990–99 was proclaimed in 1989 by UN General Assembly.[2] The purpose of the decade was to promote activities, which lessen the impact of natural disaster on human environment. The health sector has a particular interest in supporting activities, which will reduce mortality and morbidity resulting from disaster.

Unfortunately, it is virtually impossible to prevent most disasters. Nevertheless, we can forestall or alleviate many of their worst effects by anticipating them and by being prepared. WHO's concern is—reducing the adverse impact of disasters on human health, through preparedness and by bringing the right technology to bear in a timely, coordinated and effective manner, for each phase of operation, i.e. relief, rehabilitation and reconstruction (RRR).

DISASTER PREPAREDNESS

Part of the preparedness for disasters, as for many other conditions of ill health, is to have a sound understanding of the epidemiological situation and the ability to anticipate disaster events. WHO in cooperation with governmental and non-governmental organizations, with organizations and bodies of United Nation System, is engaged in tracking the history of major disasters, in time and place and in magnitude of effects. By better monitoring of weather and climatic pattern overtime, we can anticipate some types of disasters. We can reduce the impact of such events when they occur, e.g. by planning and designing building correctly, starting with health facilities, which could also serve as a model of construction. We also know that certain sequelae of specific types of disaster occur repeatedly including epidemics of diarrhoeal diseases with floods; malnutrition, if not downright famine, with prolonged drought and burns from volcanic eruption or forest fires. This has allowed us to prepare for and respond in the most efficacious way to a specific type of disaster.

Response

Unless response is properly coordinated, the well-intentioned donor community may end up by supplying excessive amounts of some types of supplies, while ignoring others that may be needed more. Standard list of supplies can be useful in responding to defined emergency situations, as important as immediate response to emergency is the long-term rehabilitation and reconstruction of the affected area and this should be considered part of the emergency preparedness. International solidarity and cooperation are essential in reducing the adverse effects of disasters. For this reason, the United Nations declared the 1990s to be International Decade for Natural Disaster Reduction. Countries in WHOs South East Asia region are prone to various types of natural disasters like floods, cyclones, drought, earthquakes, volcano eruption, and because of high density of population in this region the effects are felt by largest number of people.

NATURAL DISASTERS IN INDIA

Impact of over 191 disaster events in India, from 1960 to 1989 and 258 events from 1975 to 2000 are given in Tables 17.1 and 17.2 respectively. India is large country and we have silent disaster of population explosion and HIV/AIDS bomb ticking in with heavy burden of diseases, like tuberculosis for which a global emergency has been proclaimed. India with a wide range of topographic and climatic conditions is prone to a number of natural disasters and hazards. It is a major disaster prone country in the Asia Pacific region. Among all the disasters that country faces, river floods are the most frequent and often devastating. The shortfall in the rainfall causes droughts or drought-like situation in various parts of the country. The country has faced some severe earthquakes causing widespread damage to life and property. India has coastline of about 8,000 km, which is prone to severe cyclonic formation in Arabian Sea and Bay of Bengal. Another major problem faced by the country is in the form of landslide and avalanches.

Man-made chemical disaster struck in Bhopal in 1984 wherein methyl isocyanate (MIC) leaked and killed about 3000 people. While droughts and floods in many states are perpetual and occurrence is witnessed almost every year in states like Bihar, Odisha and northeastern states. Severe and supercyclone hit Odisha in 1999, killing 10,000

Table 17.1: Disaster events from 1960 to 1989 in India (past)[1]

Type	*Frequency*	*Killed*	*Injured*	*Affected*
Accidents	40	5512	101359	351010
Avalanche	1	250	0	0
Civil strife	2	5660	0	10400000
Cold wave	7	1555	0	0
Cyclone	26	31730	1700	33474172
Drought	9	0	0	710666000
Epidemic	19	16150	0	35723
Earthquake	8	595	2424	50000
Fire	7	60857	103059	754926905
Floods	38	24988	1000	223296610
Heat wave	7	1235	0	0
Storm	27	2647	1993	9672267
Total	**191**	**151179**	**211535**	**1742872687**

Table 17.2: Natural disaster impacts in India, 1975–2000

Hazards	*Frequency*	*Population affected (millions)*
Drought	08	701
Floods	83	511
Cyclones	76	68.5
Earthquakes	17	20.1
Landslide	22	3.8
Industrial hazards	52	0.5
Total	**258**	**1.3 Billions**

Source: Reference 11

persons and severe cyclone (Phailin) revisited Odisha and Andhra Pradesh in October 2013, this time because of adequate preparedness lives were saved as 8 lakhs people were evacuated to safer places. Gujarat was affected with severe earthquake in January 2001 which left over 16,000 people dead and many disabled besides loss of property and homes. One keeps on reading occurrence of epidemics, fire accidents and stampede on festivals in many parts of the country every now and then. It appears that in coming years the threat will persist and losses are likely to be more because of dense population and population growth.

Present Scenario 2001 to 2015

During the year 2001–2002, over 16 states were affected with heavy rains, landslides and floods. This affected 115 districts involving more than 17,000 villages. About 379 districts in 18 states were affected by drought due to sluggish monsoon.[3]

During 2003, 16 states were affected by heavy rains landslides and floods. This affected 236 districts involving more than 41,408 villages. About 158 districts in the other states were affected by drought.[4]

On December 26, 2004 a massive undersea earthquake originating in Indonesia, followed by killer sea waves (tsunami) affected many countries in the region including India. This natural disaster affected Indonesia, Sri Lanka, India, Thailand, Malaysia, Mynamar, Bangladesh, Maldives, Somalia, Tanzania and Kenya. Over 1,30,000 people lost their lives by January 2, 2005 and many were missing. In India over 13,000 people lost their lives with widespread damages to property and homes and it rendered many people homeless. The response was swift and mostly from local area and local organizations. It was unpredictable disaster and consequently took a heavy toll.[5–7] In August 2008 devastating floods caused by river Kosi affected 27 lakh people in Bihar (India). Many lives were lost and it was declared as national calamity. A cyclonic storm struck the state of West Bengal on 25th and 26th May 2009 affecting 39 lakh people from 19 districts. Over six thousands people lost their lives in Uttarakhand Flash Flood disaster in July, 2013. State of J & K was affected by flash floods in September 2014. Cyclone (Hudhud) lashed Andhra and Odisha in 2014. Devastating Earthquake hit Nepal, and Bihar killing over 8250 persons in April 2015.

Types of Disasters in India

1. *Water and climate-related disasters*
   Floods, cyclones, tornadoes and hurricanes, hailstorm, cloud burst, heat wave and cold wave, snow avalanches, drought, sea erosion, and thunder and lightening.
2. *Geologically-related disasters*
   Earthquakes, landslides and mud flow, dam failures/ dam bursts, and mine fires.
3. *Biologically-related disasters*
   Epidemics, pest attacks, cattle epidemics, and food poisoning.
4. *Chemical, industrial and nuclear-related disasters*
   Chemical and industrial disasters, and nuclear disasters.
5. *Accident-related disasters*
   Forest fire, urban fire, mine flooding, oil spill, major building collapse, serial bomb blasts, festival related disaster, electrical disasters and fires, air, road and rail accidents, boat capsizing, and village fire.

Types: Disasters are *natural* as also *man-made*. Natural disasters include earthquakes, heavy rains, cyclones, hurricanes, tidal waves and lightening forest fires.

Man-made Disasters

Biggest disaster is population increase and shortages of resources. Widespread pollution of environments by human and industrial activities has led to many disasters. Soil pollution, water pollution and air pollution occur due to human activities and disasters resulting as a consequence of these activities are called man-made disasters.

Wars and conflicts, leaks from nuclear plants, industrial gases and Bhopal tragedy (methyl isocyanate leak). Serial bomb blasts, oil spills, festival related, building collapse, rail road and air accidents are other examples of man-made disasters.

Deforestation and widespread use of fossil fuels in automobiles has led to **global warming**, air pollution and depletion of ozone layer and is a constant threat for rise of sea levels, tidal waves, etc.

General Effects

- Loss of life.
- Injury.
- Damage of property.
- Damage of cash.
- Loss of livelihood.
- Disruption of lifestyle.
- Disruption of essential services.
- Loss/disruption of infrastructure.
- National/state economic loss.
- Sociological/psychological after effects.

Health Effects of Disaster

1. Accidents and trauma, loss of life and disposal of dead bodies.
2. Outbreaks of diarrhoea, cholera and bloody diarrhoea, hepatitis A and E, meningitis, measles, pneumonia and respiratory infections as a consequence of contamination of drinking water and breakdown of water supply system, and large-scale aggregation of people with poor hygienic and environmental conditions.
3. Vector-borne diseases like malaria, dengue, JE are common aftermath of floods and heavy rains. Plague outbreak occurred after earthquake in Latur and Beed after aggregation of people in temporary shelters which led to increased population of rats due to bad environments and lack of sanitation after disaster.
4. Problem of malnutrition, psychological trauma, problems of orphans and shelter.[8]

Response to Disaster

Local People Come First

People affected by disasters are active actors in rebuilding their lives and livelihood and they are not just helpless victims. People's capacities are used and built on their participation and victims should not be looked on as passive recipients of external aid. Damage, needs and capacity assessment are done with people's participation, considering gender, culture and age. Local assistance includes material aid and organizational/motivational aspects to address root causes of vulnerabilities. The focus should be on community and strengthening its organization. It is the community, who should participate in decision-making to prioritize needs. The goal should remain to reduce long-term vulnerabilities and to increase people's capacities to better cope with disaster.

Since disasters hinder development, it needs management.

Disaster management refers to activities like prevention, mitigation, preparedness, emergency response and recovery, to maintain control over disaster and emergency situation. It also provides a framework for helping people at risk to avoid/recover from the impact of the disaster.

The broad areas of disaster management and response consist of:

1. Defining the nature of disasters and emergencies
2. Pre-disaster activities (assessing vulnerability prevention and mitigation, preparedness and planning).
3. Emergency response based on rapid assessment of problem.
4. Recovery and sustainable development.

Technical aspects consist of food, shelter and emergency settlement, water supply and sanitation, vector and pest control, control of communicable diseases and prevention of outbreaks, community participation and training of staff and volunteers.

Nodal Agency and Organization

It was noted that there was need for building up holistic capabilities for disaster management—so as to be able to handle both natural and man-made disasters. Accordingly, it was decided that from June 2002 that Ministry of Home Affairs will be Nodal Agency for disasters management (except draught and epidemics and those emergencies/disasters which were specifically allotted to other Ministries, Table 17.3).

The National Contingency Action Plan (NCAP) facilitates launching of relief and rescue operations without delay. There are various committees at the national level for disaster managements, such as cabinet committee for effective implementation of relief measures in the wake of natural calamity; National Crisis Management Committee (NCMC) at the national level headed by the cabinet secretary who is incharge of various types of disasters and supporting ministries as members; crisis management group reviews various measures required for dealing with a natural disaster and coordinates activities of the central ministries and the state governments pertaining to disaster preparedness and relief and obtains information from nodal officers on measures relating to the above.

Table 17.3: Ministries responsible for various categories of disasters[9]

Disaster	*Nodal ministry*
• Natural disaster management	Ministry of Home Affairs
• Draught and draught relief	Ministry of Agriculture
• Air accidents	Ministry of Civil Aviation
• Railways accidents	Ministry of Railways
• Chemical disasters	Ministry of Environment and Forests
• Biological disasters	Ministry of Health
• Nuclear disasters	Department of Atomic Energy

The state governments are autonomous in organizing relief operations in the event of natural disaster and long-term preparedness/rehabilitation measures. The state governments efforts are supplemented by central government. There is a state crisis management group (SCMG) under the chairmanship of chief secretary/relief commissioner to take into consideration the infrastructure and guidance received from time to time, from government of India and formulate action plans for dealing with different natural disasters. There is a state level control room set-up whenever a disaster situation develops.

States are further divided into districts, each headed by the district collector (also known as the district magistrate or deputy commissioner), who is the focal point at the district level for directing, supervising and monitoring relief measures for disaster and for preparation of district level plans. The collector exercises coordinating and supervisory powers over functionaries of all the departments at the district level. The relief measures are reviewed by the District Disaster Management Authority consisting of official and non-official members, including local legislators and member of parliament. In the wake of Natural disasters, a control room is set-up in the district for day-to-day monitoring of the rescue and relief operations on continuing basis.

The collector/deputy commissioner maintains close liaison with the central government authorities, namely Army, Air Force and Navy, Ministry of Water Resources, etc., who supplement the efforts of district administration in the rescue and relief operation. They all coordinate voluntary efforts by mobilising the non-governmental organisations capable of working in such situations.

The armed forces of the country have played a vital role during disaster emergencies providing prompt relief to the victims even in the most inaccessible and remote areas of the country. The organizational strength of the armed forces with their disciplined and systematised approach, and with their skills in technical and human resource management make them indispensable for such emergency situations. India having a federal structure the integrated disaster management mechanism exists within the government framework.

Response of Health Sector

Disaster management is a multi-sector and proactive approach. Health sector has special and specific responsibility to manage large-scale epidemics of communicable diseases besides emergency services to tackle trauma, saving life and limbs. It calls for rapid response and rapid assessment of the situation. It is an emergency epidemiology and application of principles of epidemiology on massive scale. The other sectors will help in evacuation of causalities and establishing temporary shelters and camps, which the health sector will organize.[2]

1 ***Emergency medical relief (EMR) measures for trauma or diseases:*** This was organized by Gujarat government on massive and rapid scale to save lives and limbs of people affected by the earthquake in the year 2001. Local health authorities were first to respond to the needs on massive scale.

   Israel flew its advance trauma and life support system and reached Bhuj on 31st January, i.e. 5 days after the occurrence of disaster (earthquake) and established hospital under tents and performed 53 major surgeries. It was the fastest international help with tremendous speed and it was self-contained hospital, which supported the local efforts magnificently.

2 ***Chlorination of water supplies for safe water:*** Whatever sources of water supply are left over the health department is responsible for chlorination and monitoring of water supply to people in camps or in their homes after disaster. This was done on war footing when flood struck Rohtak town in September 1995. Home chlorination was ensured through massive efforts deploying all the paramedical workers, Anganwadi workers, medical interns and medical officers besides nursing students and national service scheme volunteers. The occurrence of diarrhoeal diseases, cholera and hepatitis was kept in control.

   - Medical relief measures were extensively organized to respond to occurrence of common morbidities like diarrhoea, fever, multiple boils, eye problem and minor injuries, etc. mobile teams were set-up. Drugs were purchased and arranged by special budget allocation. These teams also monitored the occurrence of diseases and thus acted as rapid response and surveillance teams to monitor epidemic prone diseases at the village level.
   - The laboratory services like examination of blood slides and microscopy centres were established right in the affected villages itself to diagnose malaria and treatment of malaria. Surveillance of fever cases by health teams as also mass fever therapy was done by the mobile teams by home-to-home visit. This was the rapid response to tackle falciparum malaria and fever menace following floods.
   - 1995 floods in Haryana resulted in widespread occurrence of falciparum malaria in many villages as consequence of vector density and poor surveillance operation. Health sector had to tackle it on massive scale even after 4 months of occurrence of flood in the area.
   - ***Insecticide spray and fogging:*** This was stepped up, on massive scale following floods to reduce the vector density and transmission of malaria and other vector-borne diseases. The success was partial. Control of vectors and rodents after floods or other natural disasters becomes an important public health activity.
   - ***Immunization:*** In the floods of 1995 in district Rohtak no vaccination against cholera or typhoid was done. On the other hand, time was spent to educate people on observing personal hygiene measures, washing hands and eating clean food and use of chlorinated water. However, routine immunization against measles; polio, diphtheria, whooping cough and tetanus was stepped up in subsequent months.

CASE STUDY

In an outbreak of cholera in National Capital of Delhi slums (Nand Nagri), there was an over enthusiasm and thousands of people were vaccinated against cholera. Following cholera mass vaccination, many cases of Hepatitis B were reported due to unsafe injections. Thus, iatrogenic outbreak of hepatitis had to be dealt with as an aftermath of mass cholera vaccination. WHO guidelines do not recommend cholera vaccination and travel and trade restrictions for control of an outbreak of cholera or for its prevention and spread to other area.

The occurrence of cholera (outbreak) in National capital of Delhi Urban slums (Nand Nagri) was a boon as Prime Minister of India himself visited the area and thereafter the life of locality and slum of this part of Delhi was totally transformed. Safe water supply for 24 hours was in place, sanitary latrines were constructed, sewer facilities got upgraded besides sanitation of area and housing conditions improved. Today Nand Nagri, owes for all modern developments to the late Prime Minister Rajiv Gandhi. This is a living example of area development and real rehabilitation, which altogether changed and transformed the quality of life following man-made disaster, i.e. outbreak of cholera.[10] Plague epidemic in Surat in 1994 transformed the life of people, as sanitation measures were organized on war footing and sustained thereafter.

Setting up of Shelter, Food and Health Facilities in Camps

The occurrence of natural disaster like flood in 1995 in district Rohtak, forced people to leave their homes and these people had to stay in camps in the vicinity of their locality, or town. These residential camps were organized in school buildings, college buildings and other community places (Dharamshalas) besides temporary shelters of tents, the sanitary arrangements and adequate supply of safe water and mobile teams to manage the sickness were made available. Monitoring the occurrence of unusual events (diseases and outbreaks) and their management is the responsibility of health sector. Hospitals provided referral support besides arranging mobile teams for these camps, and sanitary latrines were arranged by public health department for safe disposal of human excreta.

Education

Education of people during the occurrence of disaster helps building a favourable climate to prevent outbreaks. Educational material on epidemic prone diseases and also adopting healthy practices for eating clean food, drinking safe water and reporting of illness like diarrhoea and taking prompt treatment formed an important plank of disaster management.

Training of People/Students/Volunteers

Training and utilizing people and students for chlorination of pots and sources of water was undertaken by the health sector during the floods of 1995. It paid us rich dividends as trained women and students undertook chlorination themselves in their homes or at source (tube well or hand pump). ORS and chloroquine depots and bleaching powder depots were established in the community and trained volunteers manned these depots themselves. It had a positive impact and people to people services and help was widely accepted. There was tremendous zeal and enthusiasm amongst students and philanthropists to help the affected people. Drug distribution centres (DDCs) were operated by volunteers to prevent mortality due to malaria.

National Disaster Management Authority and Disaster Preparedness (Prevention and Planning)

"Should disaster strike be prepared", holds true for disaster preparedness. Emergency preparedness is a "Programme of long-term development activities whose goals are to strengthen, the overall capacity and capability of a country to manage efficiently all types of emergencies and bring about a transition from relief through recovery and back to sustained development" (WHO 1995).

Following tsunami, it has been decided that the government will soon constitute a national disaster management authority and install an early warning system to tackle calamities like tsunami. Disaster Management Act, 2005 has been passed and the National Disaster Management Authority (NDMA) has been constituted headed by the Prime Minister as ex-officio-chairperson and national plan for disaster management has been drawn up. NDMA has released series of guidelines (15 guidelines) on formulating policies, plans, capacity building, ensuring prevention, mitigation and preparedness for various disasters. The guidelines have been released in the areas of—earthquakes, chemical (industrial) disasters, and floods, preparation of state disaster management plans, medical preparedness and mass casualty management (based on triage approach consisting of colour coding of victims to determine priority. Red colour tag means critically ill, yellow means moderately ill, green means ambulatory and black means dead or moribund). Guidelines on pandemic preparedness beyond health, floods, cyclones, guidelines for training regimens for disaster response, biological disasters, nuclear and radiological emergencies (Part 1), landslides and avalanches, chemical (terrorism disasters), psychological support and mental health services in disasters have been prepared. The 15th guideline on **Incident Response System** (IRS) in disaster was released on 21st July 2010. The **Incident Response Teams** are pre-designated at state, district, subdivision and Tehsil/block level. Now there is a paradigm shift from erstwhile post event relief—centric response to one of proactive prevention, mitigation and preparedness driven approach. Key feature of IRS are—management by objectives, unity of command and chain of command, transfer command, organization, flexibility, span of control, area command, unified command, common terminology, accountability, integrated communications, resources management and incident action plan. National institute of disaster management has been set-up. Similarly, state disaster management and district disaster management authorities have been constituted for rapid response.[10, 11] Disaster preparedness means—a pre-disaster plan in the form of an epidemiological surveillance and support. In India, as has been discussed, we have national, state, and district level plans and committees on disaster management to meet the challenge of disaster. All big hospitals have evolved a disaster management plans. Periodically these committees meet and review the preparedness to deal with any contingency.[11, 12]

The epidemiological surveillance data helps to predict the occurrence of biological disaster and similarly data of National Nutrition Monitoring Bureau helps to predict the occurrence of nutritional deficiency and drought. National Geographical Information System (GIS) and internet and remote sensing facilities forecast on rainfall, floods and landslides and seismic hazards. Similarly, Indian Meteorological Department (IMD) provides cyclone warning from Advance cyclone warning centres (ACWCs) in coastal areas.[13]

Emergency Medical Relief Division (EMR) of Directorate General Health Services, MOH and FW, Government of India coordinates health relief activities and plays a supportive role in terms of physical and logistics support to the states to counter the effects of disaster in the state by health sector. Besides this the existing contingency plan for drought and floods are circulated every year in the pre-monsoon period to all states to keep them at the highest level of preparedness so as to improve their response and capacity to mitigate the health consequences of disaster. Similarly, all state governments send a contingency plan before monsoon to all the districts. Drug supplies are sent in advance to meet any emergency due to disaster.

17

Central medical stores at Karnal, Mumbai, Chennai, Hyderabad, Kolkata and Guwahati are kept in readiness to provide essential drugs and other medical supplies to states as and when demanded. Emergency medicines were given to Odisha on credit payment in the year 2003 to tide over the crisis. Central Research Institute, Kasauli is also kept on alert to provide necessary vaccines.

The National Institute of Communicable Diseases (NICD) Delhi, All India Institute of Hygiene and Public Health, Kolkata and National Environmental Engineering Research Institute (NEERI) at Nagpur are national collaborating centres for disaster preparedness to provide technical support to states and districts in the event of any disaster. Similarly, states have developed their own epidemiological units to monitor and ensure the state of preparedness to meet any health challenge in future. State and district is the most appropriate level to ensure adequate state of preparedness.

Preparedness and Response for Disasters

Crisis management plan for biological disasters and Emergency Support Function Plan were reviewed in 2013 and circulated to all concerned. Now the centre of gravity stands visibly shifted to preparedness, prevention and planning from earlier response and relief centric approach.

Training and continuing education of paramedicals and medical officers is a critical input in disaster preparedness.[2] Regular training and continuing education on disaster management and its prediction is key element. Getting ready before the situation or proactive than reactive is essential lesson of preparedness. National Scouts, St. John Ambulance, National Cadet Corps, Homeguards, National Service Scheme volunteers and students are potential trained resource in first aid. They have been trained in first aid, fire-fighting and casuality evacuation. Regular training of this force helps to ensure state of preparedness. Indian Red Cross Society (IRS) offers postgraduate diploma course in disaster preparedness and rehabilitation at its national headquarter. Preparedness at most levels tends to be weak in the chain of disaster management. We only react and manage a crisis whenever it arises and then forget and wait for the next crisis to occur.[14, 15]

Bioterrorism (Biological Warfare)

Some 82 pathogens and biological toxins like anthrax, plague, and smallpox have been identified by the United States as posing a great risk to public which can be used for mass killing. Disease pathogens can now be manufactured using DNA synthesis. Significantly, defence scientists were able to recreate SARS virus in 2008 using DNA technology. Earlier, the 1918 flu virus was reconstituted, the worldwide pandemic it had caused and killed an estimated 50 million people. Elaborate safeguards are in place to prevent bioterrorism.

REFERENCES

1. WHO. "Should disaster strike be prepared". World Health Day 7th April, 1991. Emergency Preparedness and response. Geneva: WHO, 1991.
2. National Teachers Training Centre. Proceedings of the task force meeting of the collaborating centres for disaster preparedness and response; 1993 July 19–22; JIPMER, Pondicherry, India.
3. GOI/MOH and FW. Annual Report 2002–03. New Delhi: Ministry of Health and Family Welfare Government of India, 2003.
4. GOI/MOH and FW. Annual Report 2003–04. New Delhi: Ministry of Health and Family Welfare, Government of India, 2004.
5. Tsunami Smashes Asia. Hindustan Times, 2004 Dec. 27.
6. Hindustan Times, 2005 January 2; page 1.
7. Disaster control body to be set-up. Hindustan Times, 2005 January 10.
8. GOI/NICD. Management of health problems on account of natural disaster with special reference to earthquakes. CD Alert 2000 Dec; 4(12).
9. GOI (August 2004). Disaster Management in India A—Status Report. NDM Division Ministry of Home Affairs, GOI; New Delhi.
10. GOI/NICD: Cholera—Need for a constant and continuing vigil. CD Alert 2000 January; 4(1).
11. Government of India. The Disaster Management Act, 2005, No 53 of 2005 (23rd December 2005).
12. Disaster Management. An IAF Perspective 10 May 2006.
13. Gupta A. Information Technology and Natural Disaster Management in India. New Delhi: National Centre for Disaster Management (NCDM). Indian Institute of Public Administration, 1991.
14. WHO/International federation of Red Cross and Red Crescent Societies. Environmental health in emergencies and disaster a practical guide. International strategy for disaster reduction. Geneva: WHO/International federation of Red Cross and Red Crescent Societies; 2002.
15. Sharma VK, Kaushik AD. National Disaster Management in India 'Yojana' March 2012. Indian Institute of Public Administration and NIDM, New Delhi.

CHAPTER

18

Infection Management and Environment Plan—Biomedical Waste Management

PURPOSE OF INFECTION MANAGEMENT AND ENVIRONMENT PLAN (IMEP)

IMEP is an approach or framework for managing, avoiding, reducing and controlling health and environmental risks arising from health care facilities. Health and environmental risk arise out of poor infection control practices and unsound environmental management systems such as (i) inappropriate disinfection, (ii) poor sterilization, (iii) inadequate use to protective gears, (iv) poor biomedical waste handling, treatment and disposal practices, (v) unhygienic conditions and inadequate potable water within the health care facilities.

Biomedical waste is a universal phenomenon. Waste management is one of the important public health measure. Biomedical waste if not handled properly may pose hazards to human health and environment in the form of fatal infections, genotoxicity and cytotoxicity, physical injuries and public sensitivity.[1]

Waste: Everything is made for a defined purpose. "Anything which is not intended for further use is termed waste." With industrialization and increasing urbanization, the quantum of urban solid waste is increasing and health care is also one of the industry.

Hospital: It is a residential establishment which provides a short-term and long-term medical care consisting of observational, diagnostic, therapeutic and rehabilitative services for a person suffering or suspected to be suffering from disease or injury and for parturient. It may also provide services for ambulatory patients on an outpatient basis.

Biomedical Waste Generation

Waste generated in health care facilities include different kinds of **infectious** and **non-infectious** waste. The former tends to be of smaller volume than non-infectious waste, but once mixed the total *"unseggregated"* waste is deemed as infectious. Table 18.1 gives the break down of the type and quantity of waste generated in a typical 30 bedded Community Health Centre[2]. For this reason WHO recommends that the daily amount of biomedical wastes in health care facilities without a proper waste management system be calculated using the estimate of 1 kg/bed/day.

Table 18.1: Type and quantity of waste in a 30-bedded CHC

Waste type	*Quantity kg/day*	*Percentage of each type of waste*
A Infectious waste		
A1 Pathological and anatomical	1.5	6
A2 Sharps including syringes	1.0	4
A3 Non-sharp waste	7.5	30
B General waste	15.0	60
Total	**25.0**	**100**

General

The hospital waste like body parts, organs, tissues, blood and body fluids along with soiled linen, cotton bandages and plaster casts from infected and contaminated areas are very essential to be properly collected, segregated, stored, transported, treated and disposed off in a safe manner to prevent nosocomial and hospital acquired infections. Various communicable diseases that spread through water, sweat, blood, body fluids and contaminated organs are important to be prevented. The biomedical waste scattered in and around hospitals invites flies, insects, rodents, cats and dogs that are responsible for the spread of communicable diseases. Rag pickers in the hospital, sorting out the garbage, are at risk of infections. The recycling of disposable syringes, needles, IV sets and article like glass bottles without proper sterilization are responsible for spread of dangerous infection. With the proliferation of blood-borne diseases, more attention is being focused on the issues of infectious medical waste and its disposal.

Hazards of Biomedical/Health Care Waste

Hospital waste/health care waste includes all the waste generated by health care establishments, research facilities, and laboratories including minor or scattered source—such as health care taken at home (insulin injection).

About 75 to 90% of the waste produced by health care providers is non-hazardous "general waste" comparable to domestic waste.

Classification of Hazardous Waste

WHO has classified hazardous waste into following categories:

1 ***Infectious waste*** (suspected to contain pathogens): For example, laboratory culture, waste from isolation wards, tissue-swabs, material in contact with infected patient and excreta.
2 ***Pathological waste*** (containing human tissues or fluids): For example, body parts, blood and other body fluids, fetuses.
3 ***Sharps*** (sharp material): For example, needles, infusion sets, scalpels, knives, blades, broken glass.
4 ***Pharmaceutical waste*** (containing pharmaceuticals): For example, expired drugs; contaminated bottles; boxes.
5 ***Genotoxic waste:*** For example, waste containing cytostatic drugs; genotoxic chemicals.
6 ***Chemical waste:*** For example, laboratory reagents; film developer expired disinfectants, solvents.
7 ***Waste with heavy metals:*** For example, batteries; broken thermometers.
8 ***Pressurized containers:*** For example, gas cylinders, gas cartridges; aerosol cans.
9 ***Radioactive material:*** For example, unused liquid from radiotherapy; contaminated glassware; urine, excreta from patient treated with unsealed radio nucleotides.

Types of Hazards

The exposure to hazardous health care waste can result into:

1 Infection
2 Genotoxicity and cytotoxicity
3 Chemical toxicity
4 Radioactivity hazards
5 Physical injuries
6 Public sensitivity

1. Infection

18

The infectious agents can enter in the body through a puncture, abrasion, or cut in the skin; through mucous membranes; by inhalation and ingestion. Commonest infections, which can result from mishandling of hospital/health care waste, are gastroenteric through faeces and/or vomit (*Salmonella*, *Shigella* spp., *Vibrio cholerae*, Helminths; Hepatitis A), respiratory through inhaled secretions; saliva (*Mycobacterium tuberculosis*; measles virus; *Streptococcus pneumoniae*), ocular infections through eye secretions (herpes virus), genital infections (*Neisseria gonorrhoeae*; herpes virus), skin infection through pus (*Streptococcus* spp.), meningitis through cerebrospinal fluid (*Neisseria meningitidis*), AIDS/HIV through blood and sexual secretions (HIV), haemorrhagic fevers through body fluids (Junin, Lassa, Ebola and Marburg viruses), septicaemia and bacteraemia through blood (*Staphylococcus aureus*, *Enterococcus*, *Enterobacter*, *Klebsiella* and *Streptococcus*) and viral hepatitis B and C through blood and body fluids.

Infection Control

Infection control is the responsibility of all health care professionals. *Preventing nosocomial infections* requires a hygienic and sanitized environment and maintenance of good practices and use of protective gears. Routine cleaning of the health facility is absolutely essential, as that will keep the environment free from dust and dirt. Running water, soap or antiseptic and facilities for drying without contamination are required for health care workers to maintain cleanliness at all times.

2. Genotoxicity and Cytotoxicity

Many cytotoxic drugs are extremely irritant and have harmful local effects after direct contact with skin and eyes (alkylating agents; intercalating agents; vinca alkaloids and derivatives and epipodophyllotoxins). Many neoplastic drugs are carcinogenic and mutagenic; secondary neoplasia is known to be associated with chemotherapy.

3. Chemical Toxicity

Many of chemicals and pharmaceutical drugs used in health care establishments are hazardous (e.g. toxic, genotoxic, corrosive, flammable, reactive, explosive and shock-sensitive). They may cause intoxication by acute or chronic exposure, injuries including burns, and poisoning.

4. Radioactivity Hazards

The radioactive waste exposure may cause headache, dizziness, vomiting, genotoxicity and tissue damage.

5. Physical Injuries

May result from sharps, chemicals and explosive agents.

6. Public Sensitivity

The general public is very sensitive about visual impact of the anatomical waste, recognizable body parts including fetuses if handled improperly.

NATIONAL GUIDELINES FOR HOSPITAL WASTE MANAGEMENT

Objectives are to prevent hazards to human health and prevent environmental pollution.

Government of India has prepared the National Guidelines on the Biomedical Waste (Management and Handling) Rules, 1998; (Amended in 2000 and 2003 and 2016) which were notified under the Environment Protection Act, 1986 (29 of 1986) by the Ministry of Environment and Forest, Government of India on 28th July, 1998. Each hospital should implement the said rules by developing comprehensive plan for hospital waste management smoothly in terms of segregation, collection, transporta-tion, treatment and disposal of waste.[3]

1. Policy on Hospital Waste Management

The policy statement aims "to provide for a system for management of all potentially infectious and hazardous waste in accordance with the Biomedical Waste (Management and Handling) Rules, 2016 (BMW, 1016).

2. Definition of Biomedical Waste

Biomedical waste means any waste which is generated during the diagnosis, treatment or immunization of human beings or animal or in research activities pertaining thereto or in the production or testing of biologicals, including categories mentioned in the Schedule I of the Biomedical waste (Management and Handling) Rules, 1016.

3. Categories of Biomedical Waste

Hazardous, toxic and biomedical waste should be segregated into following categories for the purpose of its safe transportation to a specific site for specific treatment (Tables 18.2). Certain specific categories of toxic and hazardous waste require specific treatment (disinfection/ decontamination) before transportation for treatment, which can also be done under the categorization as mentioned.

4. Segregation of Waste

It should be done at the source of generation of biomedical waste, e.g. all patient care activity areas, diagnostic services areas, operation theatres, labour rooms, treatment rooms, etc.

The responsibility of segregation should be with generator of biomedical waste, i.e. doctors, nurses, technicians, etc. The biomedical waste should be segregated as per categories applicable (Table 18.2).

5. Collection of Biomedical Waste

Collection of biomedical waste should be done as per Biomedical Waste (Management and Handling) Rules, 2016.

All the items sent to incinerator/deep burial should be placed in yellow coloured bags.

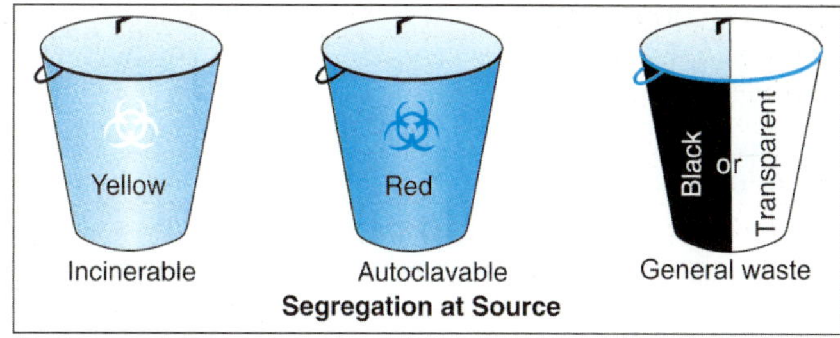

Segregation at Source

All the biomedical waste sent for microwave/autoclave/ chemical treatment should be placed in red coloured bags.

Any waste which is sent to shredder after autoclaving/ microwaving/chemical treatment is to be packed in blue/ white translucent bag.

Location of containers: All containers having different coloured plastic bags should be located at the point of generation of waste, i.e. near OT tables, injection rooms, diagnostic service areas. The colour of container/plastic bags used for collection of segregated biomedical waste should be identifiable.

Labelling: All the bags/containers must be labelled according to the rules (Schedule III of Biomedical Waste Rules, 2016).

Bags: It should be ensured that waste bags are filled up to only three-fourths—capacity, tied securely and removed from the site of the generation regularly and timely.

Certain categories of waste, which may need pre-treatment (decontamination/disinfection) at the site of generation such as plastic, sharp materials, etc. should be removed from the site of generation only after treatment.

The process of collection should be documented in a register, the colour plastic bags should be replaced and the garbage bin should be cleaned with disinfectant regularly.

6. Storage of Waste

Storage refers to the holding of biomedical waste for a certain period of time, after which it is sent for treatment and disposal. In other words, it means the duration of time wastes are kept at the site of generation and transit till the point of treatment and final disposal.

SCHEDULE III
LABEL FOR BIOMEDICAL WASTE CONTAINERS/BAGS

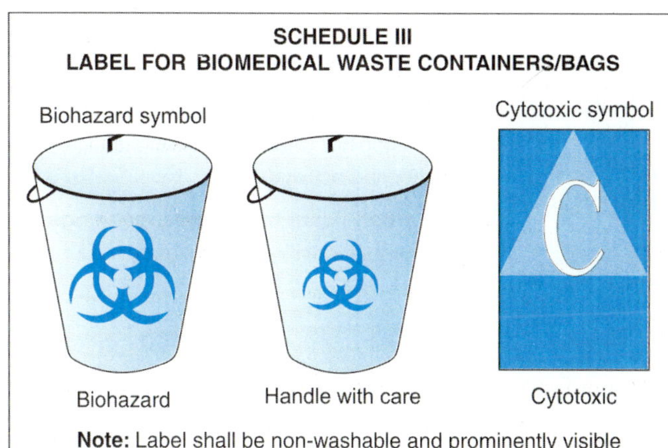

Note: Label shall be non-washable and prominently visible

Table 18.2: Biomedical wastes categories and their segregation, collection, treatment, processing and disposal options[4,5]

Category	*Type of waste*	*Type of bag or container to be used*	*Treatment and disposal options*
1	2	3	4
Yellow	a. **Human anatomical waste** Human tissues, organs, body parts and fetus below the viability period (as per the medical termination of pregnancy Act 1971, amended from time to time)	Yellow coloured non-chlorinated plastic bags	Incineration or plasma pyrolysis or deep burial
	b. **Animal anatomical waste** Experimental animal carcasses, body parts, organs, tissues, including the waste generated from animals used in experiments or testing in veterinary hospitals or colleges or animal houses		
	c. **Soiled waste** Items contaminated with blood, body fluids like dressings, plaster casts, cotton swabs and bags contining residual or discarded blood and blood components	Do	Incineration or plasma pyrolysis or deep burial* In absence of above facilities, autoclaving or micro-waving/hydroclaving followed by shredding or mutilation or combination of steriliza tion and shredding. Treated waste to be sent for energy recovery
	d. **Expired or discarded medicines** Pharmaceutical waste like antibiotics, cytotoxic drugs including all items contaminated with cytotoxic drugs along with glass or plastic ampoules, vials, etc.	Yellow coloured non-chlorinated plastic bags or containers	Expired cytotoxic drugs and items contaminated with cytotoxic drugs to be returned back to the manufacturer or supplier for incineration at temperature >1200°C or to common bio-medical waste treatment facility or hazardous waste treatment, storage and disposal facility for incineration at >1200°C or encapsulation or plasma pyrolysis at >1200°C All other discarded medicines shall be either sent back to manufacturer or disposed by incineration
	e. **Chemical waste** Chemicals used in production of biological and used or discarded disinfectants.	Yellow coloured containers or non-chlorinated plastic bags	Disposed of by incineration or plasma pyrolysis or encapsulation in hazardous waste • Treatment, storage and disposal facility
	f. **Chemical liquid waste** Liquid waste generated due to use of chemicals in production of biological and used or discarded disinfectants, silver X-ray film developing liquid, discarded formalin, infected secretions, aspirated body fluids, liquid from laboratories and floor washing, cleaning, housekeeping, disinfecting activities, etc.	Separate collection system leading to effluent treatment system	After resource recovery, the chemical liquid waste shall be pre-treated before mixing with other waste water. The combined discharge shall conform to the discharge norms given in Schedule III
	g. **Discarded linen, mattresses, beddings** Contaminated with blood or body fluid	Non-chlorinated yellow plastic bags or suitable packing material	Non-chlorinated chemical disinfection followed by incineration of plazma pyrolysis or for energy recovery In absence of above facilities, shredding or mutilation or combination of sterilization and shredding. Treated waste to be sent for energy recovery or incineration or plazma pyrolysis

(Contd...)

Table 18.2: Biomedical wastes categories and their segregation, collection, treatment, processing and disposal options[4,5] *(Contd...)*

Category	*Type of waste*	*Type of bag or Container to be used*	*Treatment and disposal options*
1	**2**	**3**	**4**
	h. Microbiology, biotechnology and other clinical laboratory waste Blood bags, laboratory cultures, stocks or specimens of microorganisms, live or attenuated vaccines, human and animal cell cultures used in research, industrial laboratories, production of biological, residual toxins, dishes and devices used for cultures	Autoclave safe plastic bags or containers	Pre-treat to sterilize with non-chlorinated chemicals on-site as per national AIDS Control Organisation or World Health Organisation guidelines thereafter for incineration
Red	**Contaminated waste (recyclable)** Wastes generated from disposable items such as tubing, bottles, intravenous tubes and sets, catheters, urine bags, syringes (without needles and fixed needle syringes and vaccutainers with their needles cut) and gloves	Puncture proff, leak proof, tamper proff containers	Autoclaving or micro-waving/hydroclaving followed by shredding or mutilation or combination of sterilization and shredding. Treated waste to be sent to registered or authorized recyclers or for energy recovery or plastics to diesel or fuel oil or for road making, whichever is possible Plastic waste should not be sent to landfill sites
White (translucent)	**Waste sharps including metals** Needles, syringes with fixed needles, needles from needle tip cutter or burner, scalpels, blades, or any other contaminated sharp object that may cause puncture and cuts. This includes both used, discarded and contaminated metal sharps	Puncture proof, leak proff, tamper proof containers	Autoclaving or dry heat sterilization followed by shredding or mutilation or encapsulation in metal container or cement concrete; combination of shredding cum autoclaving; and sent for final disposal to iron foundries (having consent to operate from the sate pollution control boards or polution control committees) or sanitary landfill or designated concrete waste sharp pit
Blue	**a. Glassware** Broken or discarded and contaminated glass including medicine vials and ampoules except those contaminated with cytotoxic wastes.	Cardboard boxes with blue colored marking	Disinfection (by soaking the washed glass waste after cleaning with detergent and sodium hypochlorite treatment) or through autoclaving or microwaving or hydroclaving and then sent for recycling
	b. Metallic body implants	Cardboard boxes with blue colored marking	

*Disposal by deep burial is permitted only in rural or remote areas where there is no access to common biomedical waste treatment facility. This will be carried out with prior approval from the prescribed authority and as per the standards specified in schedule III. The deep burial facility shall be located as per the provisions and guidelines issued by central pollution control board from time to time.

No untreated biomedical waste shall be kept, stored beyond a period of 48 hours.

The authorized person must take the permission of the prescribed authority, if for any reason; it becomes necessary to store the waste beyond 48 hours.

The authorized person should take measures to ensure that the waste does not adversely affect human health and the environment, in case; it is kept beyond the prescribed limit.

7. Transportation

Transportation within the hospital.

Within hospital, waste routes must be designated to avoid the passage of waste through patient care areas as far as possible.

Separate time should be earmarked for transportation of biomedical waste to reduce chances of its mixing with general waste as far as possible.

Designated wheeled containers, trolleys or carts should be used to transport the waste bins/plastic bags to the site of storage/treatment.

Trolleys or carts should be thoroughly cleaned and disinfected in the event of any spillage.

The wheeled containers should be designated that the waste can be easily loaded, remains secure during transportation, does not have any sharp edges and easy to clean and disinfection.

Transportation of clinical waste to treatment/disposal outside the hospital: Untreated biomedical waste will be transported only in such vehicles as may be authorized for the purpose by the competent authority as specified by the Government under the Motor Vehicle Act, 1988.

The containers for transportation must be labelled as given in of BMW Rules, 2016.

8. Treatment of Hospital Waste (Methods)[4,5]

General waste (non-hazardous, nontoxic, noninfectious): The safe disposal of this waste should be ensured through local municipal authority by sanitary landfill, composting, etc.

Biomedical waste: Incineration is the process of burning the solids at very high temperature in a furnace. This technology is widely practiced for hospital waste disposal which is hazardous. The old days incinerators designs were closed beehive incinerator, open brick incinerator and drum incinerator. However, the modern technology deploys modern methods and the process of incineration has been regulated and centralized. This costs lot of money to install and operate. Fuel cost is quite heavy. But it is a necessity. Under the Act, 1998, the designs and working efficiency have been prescribed and we should stick to these specifications.

Incineration: The incinerator should be installed and made operational as per specifications under the BMW Rules, 2016 and a certificate may be taken from SPCB (State Pollution Control Board). Specific requirement regarding the incinerator and norms of combustion efficiency and emission levels, etc. have been defined in the Biomedical Waste (Management and Handling) Rules, 2016. In case of small hospitals, joint facilities for incineration can be developed depending upon the local policies of the hospital and feasibility. The plastic bags made of chlorinated plastic should not be incinerated.

Deep burial: Standard for deep burial is also laid down in Biomedical Waste (Management and Handling) Rules, 2016. Disposal by deep burial is permitted only in rural and remote areas.

Autoclave and microwave treatment: Standards for the autoclaving and microwaving are also laid down in the Biomedical Waste (Management and Handling) Rules, 2016. All equipment installed/shared should meet these standards.

Shredding: The plastic (IV bottle, IV sets, syringes, catheters, etc.), sharps (needles, blades, glass, etc.) should be shredded but only after chemical treatment/microwaving/autoclaving ensuring disinfection.

Needles destroyers can be used for disposal of needles directly without chemical treatment.

Secured landfill: The incinerator ash, discarded medicines, cytotoxic substances and solid chemical waste should be treated by this option.

18

It may be noted that there are multiple options available for disposal of certain category of waste. The individual hospital can choose the best option depending upon treatment facilities available.

Radioactive waste: The management of the radioactive waste should be undertaken as per the guidelines of BARC (Bhabha Atomic Research Centre).

Liquid and chemical waste should be disinfected, neutralized and then put into the sewer system.

Chemical disinfection: This is widely practiced in hospitals and clinics. Sodium hypochlorite solution with 10% available chlorine can be used or 100 g of bleach in 1 litre of water has been prescribed concentration. After chemical treatment the hazardous material should be disposed off. This process renders the material safe for disposal.

Needles, disposable syringes and gloves can be treated with sodium hypochlorite solution 20 ml/litre if the condition of material is clean or 100 ml/litre if the condition of the material is unclean, is recommended. Similarly, calcium hypochlorite solution (70% available chlorine) is also available.

Non-chlorine releasing compounds such as Savlon 1%, Dettol 5% and cresol 2.5–5%, formaldehyde 3–4% and ethanol 70% can be used if chlorine releasing agents are not suitable.

9. Safety Measures

Personal protection: Hospitals and health care facilities have to ensure that the following personal protective equipment are provided.

- Gloves
  - Disposable vinyl gloves
  - Latex surgical gloves for invasive procedures
  - Heavy-duty rubber gloves uptil elbow for cleaners.
- *Masks:* Simple and cheap deflector mask to prevent health care workers against aerosols and splashes. Incinerator staff should wear dust masks.
- Protective glasses
- Plastic aprons.
- Special footwear, e.g. gum boots for hospital waste handlers.

Immunization: Hepatitis B and tetanus for health staff.

Reporting accident and spillages: There should be a procedure for reporting accident or incident and records should be kept. The report should include the nature of accident when and where it occurred and which staff were directly involved.

All the generators of biomedical waste should adopt *universal precautions* and appropriate safety measures while doing therapeutic and diagnostic activities and also while handling the biomedical waste.

All the sanitation workers engaged in the handling and transporting should be made aware of the risks involved in handling the biomedical waste.

10. Training

The entire medical profession must be made aware of Biomedical Waste (Management and Handling) Rules, 2016.

Each and every hospital must have well-planned awareness and training programmes for all categories of personnel including administrators.

To make aware the staff about safe hospital waste management practices.

Training should be conducted categorywise and more emphasis should be given in training modules as per category of personnel.

Training should be conducted in appropriate language/medium and in an acceptable manner.

Wherever possible audiovisual material and experienced trainers should be used.

Training should be interactive and should include awareness sessions, demonstration sessions. Behavioural science approach should be adopted with emphasis on establishing proper practices. It is a continuous process and will need constant reinforcement.

11. Management and Administration

The head of the hospital shall form a waste management committee under his chairmanship. The waste management committee shall meet regularly to review the performance of waste disposal. This committee should be responsible for making hospital specific action plan for hospital waste management and its supervision, monitoring and implementation.

The head of each hospital will have to take authorization for generation of waste from appropriate authorities as notified by the concerned State/UT Government well in time and get it renewed as per time schedule laid in the rules. The application is to be made as per format given in form 1 of BMW rules.

The annual reports, accident reporting as required under BMW rules should be submitted to the concerned authorities as per BMW rules format (form II and form III respectively).

12. Coordination between Hospital and Outside Agencies

Municipal authorities: As quite a large percentage of waste (in India up to 90%) generated in Indian hospital belongs to general category (nontoxic and non-hazardous), hospital should have constant interaction with municipal authorities so that this category of waste is regularly taken out of the hospital premises for further disposal.

Coordinated efforts should be made by health authorities and municipal authorities to involve private sector/NGOs for creation of common facilities for treatment.

Health authorities in coordination with municipal authorities should facilitate optimal utilization of waste treatment facility in the area.

Coordination with NGOs and environmental groups for public awareness and education is essential.

Sharing of facility: Hospitals which are not in possession of their own facility for treatment may get their waste treated in a shared facility. The hospitals having excess for treatment should extend the facility to nearby smaller hospital or health care units.

There should be coordinated agencies to take care of exigencies/disruption of waste treatment equipment in a unit.

Biodegradable Plastic and Medical Waste

Plastics are primarily synthetic polymers combined with ingredients such as curative, fillers, reinforcing agents and plasticizers, etc. which can attain desired shape, very easy to store, economical and long-lasting. Chemically, it is chain of macromolecules formed by combination of repeated group of monomers linked together, e.g. polyethylene ($H_2C: CH_2$)

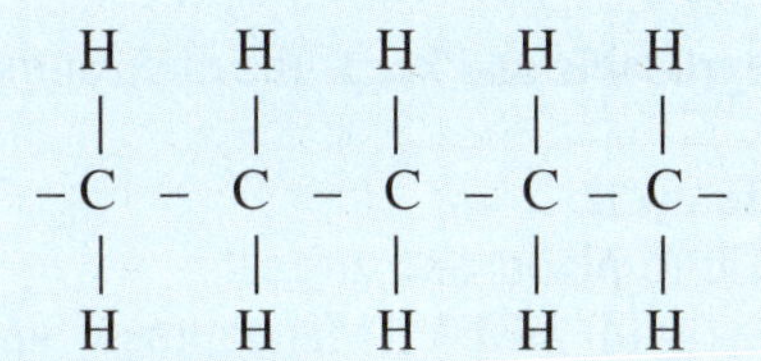

Global Consumption

The global consumption of various types of plastic was estimated to the tune of 70 million tonnes in the year 1990 which has further grown to 145 million tonnes (year 2001) in the beginning of 21st century and its usage is increasing manifold. India generates 15000 tonnes of plastic waste daily, 60% of which is recycled resulting in inferior product. The rest is tossed around to choke the environments.[7] As much as 30 kg of plastic can be found in the stomach of every dead cow or buffalo.

Plastic—A Significant Contribution of Twentieth Century

Plastic is one of the significant contribution of chemistry to mankind which has replaced the most conventional material, being light weight, durable aesthetically appealing preserving nature and in general improving the quality of life for mankind. Plastic has invaded almost every facet of human life and over the last few decades it has brought revolution in variety of application areas such as commodity items, electronics, packaging biomedical waste, sports, entertainment, agriculture, horticulture and so on.

Today we Cannot Visualise Life without Plastic

Conventional plastic has raised eyebrow of many and a big "No." has come in existence.

Hazards of Plastic

- Causing infertility to soil.
- Depleting underground water resource.
- Burning of plastics emits toxic gases causing serious damage to environment.
- A serious threat to life of all living creatures like man, mammals and marine life.
- Creator of unhygienic conditions when left unattended in the atmosphere.
- Food in polybags gets contaminated with toxic dyes that leak.
- Plastic toxicity results in drop in sperm counts, genital abnormality and breast cancer.
- Dioxin, a carcinogenic by-product is passed on through breast to infants.

Merit of Biodegradable Plastics in Service of Nature and Mankind

- Fully degradable and keeps the environment clean and green.
- Short life cycle.
- Non-toxic to plants and animals.
- Complies with BMW (Management and Handling) Rules, 1998 and its amendments 2000, 2003, and 2016.
- Burns like paper without emitting toxic gases
- Increase the soil fertility
- Prevents underground water depletion.

ADVICE

Use of biodegradable plastic should be encouraged replacing regular plastic to reduce hazards to human health and environment specially in context of biomedical waste. "Plastic carry bag free India" with people participation campaign is an urgency in India.

Conclusion

- Thus the biomedical waste must be treated effectively as per Biomedical Waste (BMW) Management and Handling Rules, 2016 which are applicable to all health care establishments in order to achieve objectives of healthy environments and healthy human life.
- All biomedical waste should be segregated at the source of generation in colour coded bags/containers.
- State health authorities to control and regulate the health care establishments for pollution control.
- Dead foetus, placenta and amputated body parts also form biomedical waste.
- Defaulters are liable to be prosecuted/fined up to Rs. 1,00,000 and 5 years of imprisonment.

REFERENCES

1 GOI. Infection Management and Environment Plan (IMEP). Policy Framework March 2007. MOH and FW, Government of India, DFID and the World Bank.

2 Government of NCT Delhi. Biomedical Waste Management Status in National Capital of Delhi. New Delhi: Waste Management Cell DHS; 2003.

3 GOI. Biomedical Waste (Management and Handling) Rules 1998 amended 2000 and 2003. New Delhi: GOI; 2003.

4 Ministry of environment, forest and climate change notification—Biomedical waste management rules, 2016 new delhi.

5 Kishore J, Ingle GK. Biomedical waste management in India. 1st edn. New Delhi: Century Publications; 2004.

6 Shah HK, Ganguli SK, Hospital waste management—A review. Ind J Comm Med July 2000; 25(3):136–7.

7 How best to beat plastic boom? Bharati Chaturvedi. Hindustan Times, September 6, 2005. 'Nation' Hindustan Times, Chandigarh, p. 11.

CHAPTER

19

Medical Ethics and Research in Public Health

Ethics in Medicine

Ethics is the branch of philosophy dealing with the distinction between right and wrong with the moral consequences of our actions (last 1989); it also refers to moral issues involved in statistical investigations in medicine, the scientific integrity of the investigator and the obligations implicit in the doctor–patient relationship. Doctor is at the central stage bound by medical ethics of Hippocrates oath.[1]

Doctor is responsible for care of sick individuals, health care of community and training of health teams. The ethical responsibilities extend to very large domain and in particular the area of medical ethics has become much more important *in view* of recent advances in medicine like:

- ***Genome project:*** Genetic counselling in hereditary diseases, *in vitro* fertilization, growing foetus in the womb of surrogate mothers are important areas.
- Termination of pregnancy on medical grounds.
- Ethics in contraceptives and family planning practices.
- HIV/AIDS.
- Vaccine and drug trials and medical research.
- Distribution and allocation of resources according to health needs of masses and urban and rural areas.
- Doctor–patient relationship.
- Health policies.
- Policies of care of terminal ill patients and voluntary passive euthanasia.
- It is mandatory that every medical institution should have an ethical committee to approve the plan of research work in relation to human beings and animals.
- Besides this the doctors must practice medicine ethically in terms of doctor–patient relationship, avoid unnecessary investigations and consultation and avoid negligence in care. *Consumer Protection Act* (CPA) safeguards the rights of client and it improves the quality of medical care. Under CPA, the negligence in medical care is an offence. Negligence means that a person who holds himself ready to give medical advice and treatment implied, undertakes that he is possessing skill and knowledge for the purpose. Such a person, who is consulted by a patient, owes him certain duties, namely a duty of care in deciding what treatment to give or a duty of care in the administration of that treatment. A breach of any of these duties gives a right of action for negligence to the patient. Doctors in private practice, hospitals, clinics who charge for patient care/hospital paid by an insurance firm for treatment/hospitals having free as well as paying patients come under the purview of this Act.

Hippocratic Oath

Modern Version

- I swear to fulfil, to the best of my ability and judgement, this covenant (solemn agreement):
- I will respect the hard-won scientific gains of those physicians in whose steps I walk and gladly share such knowledge as is mine with those who are to follow.
- I will apply, for the benefit of the sick, all measures which are required, avoiding those twin traps of over treatment and therapeutic nihilism.
- I will remember that there is art to medicine as well as science, and that warmth, sympathy and understanding may outweigh the surgeon's knife or the chemist's drug.
- I will not be ashamed to say "I know not", nor will I fail to call in my colleagues when the skills of another are needed for a patient's recovery.
- I will respect the privacy of my patients, for their problems are not disclosed to me that the world may know. Most especially must I treat with care in matters of life and death. If it is given me to save a life, all

thanks. But it may also be within my power to take a life; this awesome responsibility must be faced with great humbleness and awareness of my own frailty. Above all, I must not play at God.

- I will remember that I do not treat a fever chart, a cancerous growth, but a sick human being, whose illness may affect the person's family and economic stability. My responsibility includes these related problems, if I am to care adequately for the sick.
- I will prevent disease whenever I can, for prevention is preferable to cure.
- I will remember that I remain a member of society, with special obligations to all my fellow human beings, those sound of mind and body as well as the infirm.
- If I do not violate this oath, may I enjoy life and art, respected while I live and remembered with affection thereafter. May, I always act so as to preserve the finest traditions of my calling and may I long experience the joy of healing those who seek my help.

Fifth Century, BC

- I swear by Apollo the physician, by Aesculapius, and health and all-heal, and all the gods and goddesses, that according to my ability and my judgement, I will keep this oath and this stipulation to reckon him who taught me this art equally dear to me as my parents, to share my substance with him, and relieve his necessities if required; to look upon his offspring in the same footing as my own brothers, and to teach them this art, if they wish to learn it, without fee or stipulation; and that by precept, lecture, and every mode of instruction, I will impart a knowledge of the art to my own sons, and of my teachers, and to disciples bound by a stipulation and oath according to the law of medicine, but to none others.
- I will follow that system or regimen which, according to my ability and judgment, I consider for the benefit of my patients, and abstain from whatever is deleterious and mischievous.
- I will give no deadly medicine to any one if asked, nor suggest any such counsel; and in like manner I will not give to a woman a pessary to produce abortion.
- With purity and with holiness, I will pass my life and practice my art. I will not cut persons labouring under the stone, but will leave this to be done by men who are practitioners of this work. Into whatever houses I enter, I will go into them for the benefit of the sick, and will abstain from every voluntary act of mischief and corruption; and further, from the seduction of females or males, of freemen and slaves.
- Whatever, in connection with my professional service, or not in connection with it, I see or hear, in the life of men, which ought not to be spoken of abroad, I will not divulge, as reckoning that all such should be kept secret.
- While I continue to keep this oath inviolated, may it be granted to me to enjoy life and the practice of the art, respected by all men, in all times. But should I trespass and violate this oath, may the reverse be my lot.

Declaration of Geneva

(Written in 1948 and amended to the current form in 1983 by the World Medical Association)

- I solemnly pledge myself to consecrate my life to the service of humanity;
- I will give to my teachers the respect and gratitude which is their due;
- I will practice my profession with conscience and dignity;
- The health of my patient will be my first consideration;
- I will respect the secrets which are confided in me, even after the patient has died;
- I will maintain by all means in my power the honour and the noble traditions of the medical profession;
- My colleagues will be my brothers;
- I will not permit considerations of religion, nationality, race, party politics or social standing to intervene between my duty and my patient;
- I will maintain the utmost respect for human life from its beginning even under threat and I will not use my medical knowledge contrary to the laws of humanity;
- I make these promises solemnly, freely, and upon my honour.

Nuremberg Code of Ethics in Medical Research[2]

1 The voluntary consent of the human subject is absolutely essential. This means that the consent should be free and without force, fraud, deceit duress or any other ulterior motive. The person giving consent should have the legal capacity to do so. It should be intelligent and given only after understanding the nature of experiment, its purpose, duration, methods, its hazards and after effects that may arise out of the experiment.

2 The experiment should be such as to yield fruitful results for the good of society, unprocurably by other methods or means of study, and not random and unnecessary in nature.

3 The experiment should be so designed and based on the results of animal experimentation and a knowledge of the natural history of the disease or other problems under study that the anticipated results will justify the performance of the experiment.

4 The experiment should be conducted to avoid all unnecessary physical and mental suffering and injury.

5 The experiment should be conducted where there is a prior reason to believe that death or disabling injury will occur; except, perhaps in those experiments where the experimental physicians also serve as subjects.

6 The degree of risk to be taken should never exceed that determined by the humanitarian importance of the problem to be solved by the experiment.
7 Proper preparations should be made and adequate facilities provided to protect the experimental subject against even remote possibilities of injury, disability or death.
8 The experiment should be conducted only by scientifically qualified persons. The highest degree of skill and care should be required through all stages of the experiment of those who conduct or engage in the experiment.
9 During the course of the experiment, the human subject should be at liberty to bring the experiment to an end if he has reached the physical and mental state where continuation of the experiment seems to him to be impossible.
10 During the course of the experiment, the scientist in charge must be prepared to terminate the experiment at any stage, if he had probable cause to believe, in the exercise of good faith, superior skill and careful judgement required of him, that a continuation of the experiment is likely to result in injury, disability, or death to the experimental subject.

This code got to the subjects of consent the voluntariness of consent, the right of a patient to withdraw if he wished, and the basic question of doing things in accordance with proper medical standards and safeguards. However, among other limitations, it did not explicitly deal with the subject of children. Probably nobody at that time, thought it would be necessary.

Declaration of Helsinki[2]

World Health Association has prepared the following recommendations as a guide to every doctor in biomedical research involving human subjects. They should be kept under review in future. It must be remembered that these are only a guide to physicians all over the world. Doctors are not relieved from criminal, civil and ethical responsibilities under the laws of their own countries.

I. Basic Principles

1 Biomedical research involving human subjects must conform to generally accepted scientific principles and should be based on adequately performed laboratory and animal experimentation and on a thorough knowledge of the scientific tradition.
2 The design and performance of each experimental procedure involving human subjects should be clearly formulated in an experiment protocol which should be transmitted to specially appointed independent committee for consideration, comment and guidance.
3 Biomedical research involving human subject should be conducted only by scientifically qualified persons and under the supervision of a clinically competent medical person. The responsibility for the human subject must always rest with a medically qualified person and never rest on the subject of the research, even though the subject has given his or her consent.
4 Biomedical research involving humans subjects cannot legitimately be carried out unless the importance of the objective is in proportion to the inherent risk to the subject.
5 Every biomedical research project involving human subjects should be proceeded by careful assessment of predictable risks in comparison with foreseeable benefits to the subject or to others. Concern for the interests of the subjects must always prevail over the interest of science and society.
6 The right of the research subject to safeguard his or her integrity must always be respected. Every precaution should be taken to respect the privacy of the subject and to minimize the impact of the study on the subject's physical mental integrity and on the personality of the subject.
7 Doctors should abstain from engaging in research projects involving human subjects unless they are satisfied that the hazards involved are believed to be predictable. Doctors should cease any investigation if the hazards are found to outweigh the potential benefits.
8 In publication of the results of his or her research, the doctor is obliged to preserve the accuracy of the results. Reports of experimentation not in accordance with the principles laid down in this declaration should not be accepted for publication.
9 In any research on human beings, each potential subject must be adequately informed of the aims, methods, anticipated benefits and potential hazards of the study and the discomfort it may entail. He or she should be informed that he or she is at liberty to abstain from participation in the study and that he or she is free to withdraw his or her consent to participation at any time. The doctor should then obtain the subject's freely given informed consent, preferably in writing.
10 When obtaining informed consent for the research project the doctor should be particularly cautious if the subject is in a dependent relationship to him or her or may consent under duress. In that case, the informed consent should be obtained by a doctor who is not engaged in the investigation and who is completely independent of the official relationship.
11 In case of legal incompetence informed consent should be obtained from the legal guardian in accordance with national legislation. Where physical or mental incapacity makes it impossible to obtain informed consent, or when the subject is a minor, permission from the responsible relative replaces that of the subject in accordance with national legislation.
12 The research protocol should always contain a statement of the ethical considerations involved and should indicate that the principles enunciated in the present declaration are complied with.

II. Medical Research Combined with Professional Care (Clinical Research)

1 In the treatment of the sick person, the doctor must be free to use a new diagnostic and therapeutic measure, if in his or her judgement it offers hope of saving life, re-establishing health or alleviating suffering.

2 The potential benefits, hazards and discomfort of the new method should be weighed against the advantages of the best current diagnostic and therapeutic methods.

3 In any medical study, every patient including those of a control group, if any should be assured of the best proven diagnostic and therapeutic methods.

4 The refusal of the patient to participate in a study must never interfere with the doctor–patient relationship.

5 If the doctor considers, it essential not to obtain informed consent, the specific reasons for this proposal should be stated in the experimental protocol for transmission to the independent committee.

6 The doctor can combine medical research with professional care, the objective being the acquisition of new medical knowledge, only to the extent that medical research is justified by its potential diagnostic or therapeutic value for the patient.

III. Non-therapeutic Biomedical Research Involving Human Subjects (Non-clinical Biomedical Research)

1 In the purely scientific application of medical research carried out on human beings, it is the duty of the doctor to remain the protector of the life and health of that person on whom biomedical research is being carried out.

2 The subjects should be volunteers—either healthy persons or patient for whom the experimental design is not related to the patient's illness.

3 The investigator or the investigating team should discontinue the research if in his/her or their judgement it may, if continued, be harmful to the individual.

4 In research to man, the interest of science and society should never take precedence over consideration related to the well-being of the subject.

EUTHANASIA

Euthanasia has its origin from Greek word, the term 'Eu' means well and Thanatos means death and it literally means an easy death.[2] It is a form of peaceful or dignified death which is specially advocated when life becomes a punishment and dying comes as pleasure to patient, suffering from some incurable disease like cancer with severe intolerable and uncontrollable pain.

The constitution of India provides "Right to life" and it does not provide "Right to die or take away life" by the individual himself. "Suicide is an offence."

19

The individual is forbidden even from taking his own life, one who does is guilty of suicide. A person who can be declared dead under law in USA and UK, is considered to be alive in India. Though this may appear illogical, it is true because brain death is not legally recognized as death of a person and our law is silent on the issue of brain death. The main problem arises in road traffic accident victims who are being maintained on continuous artificial respiration by means of mechanical ventilators after sustaining permanent structural brain damage. In such patients, doctors are not lawfully authorized to switch off the respirator.

The right to life is conferred good and no amount of autonomy can give one a right to take it away. Another approach in legislation is the projected danger facing physicians who wish to withdraw life sustaining treatment lest they be accused to neglect. In India, the law demands reasonable and competent care.

Normally a doctor is not lawfully authorized to switch off a respirator in a patient who suffers irreversible structural brain damage. The recognition of brain death legally as death of a person will save the doctor from responsibility in such cases of terminal injury.

Advantages of legal recognition of brain death in terminal injury:

- It will facilitate organ transplantation.
- It will ensure economy of intensive care resources.
- It will have maximum impact in the matter of property rights, negligence claims, insurance and workers compassionate.

Duties of Physicians to their Patients (Medical Council of India)[3]

Obligations to Sick

2.1.1 Though a physician is not bound to treat each and every person asking his services, he should not only be ever ready to respond to the calls of the sick and the injured, but should be mindful of the high/character of his mission and the responsibility he discharges in the course of his professional duties. In his treatment, he should never forget that the health and the lives of those entrusted to his care depend on his skill and attention. A physician should endeavour to add to the comfort of the sick by making his visits at the hour indicated to the patients. A physician advising a patient to seek service of another physician is acceptable, however, in case of emergency a physician must treat the patient. No physician shall arbitrarily refuse treatment to a patient. However, for good reason, when a patient is suffering from an ailment which is not within the range of experience of the treating physician, the physician may refuse treatment and refer the patient to another physician.

2.1.2 Medical practitioner having any incapacity detrimental to the patient or which can affect his performance vis-à-vis the patient is not permitted to practice his profession.

2.2 ***Patience, delicacy and secrecy:*** Patience and delicacy should characterize the physician. Confidences concerning individual or domestic life entrusted by patients to a physician and defects in the disposition or character of patients observed during medical attendance should never be revealed unless their revelation is required by the laws of the state. Sometimes, however, a physician must determine whether his duty to society requires him to employ knowledge, obtained through confidence as a physician to protect a healthy person against a communicable disease to which he is about to be exposed. In such instance, the physician should act as he would wish another to act toward one of his own family in like circumstances.

2.3 ***Prognosis:*** The physician should neither exaggerate not minimize the gravity of patient's condition. He should ensure himself that the patient, his relatives or his responsible friends have such knowledge of the patient's condition as will serve the best interests of the patient and the family.

2.4 ***The patient must not be neglected:*** A physician is free to choose whom he will serve. He should however, respond to any request for his assistance in an emergency. Once having undertaken a case, the physician should not neglect the patient, nor should he withdraw from the case without giving adequate notice to the patient and his family. Provisionally or fully registered medical practitioner shall not wilfully commit an act of negligence that may deprive his patient or patients from necessary medical care.

2.5 ***Engagement for an obstetric case:*** When a physician who has been engaged to attend an obstetric case is absent and another is sent for and delivery accomplished, the acting physician is entitled to his professional fees, but should secure the patient's consent to resign on the arrival of the physician engaged.

Duties of Physician in Consultation

Unnecessary Consultations should be Avoided

3.1.1 However in case of serious illness and in doubtful or difficult conditions, the physician should request consultation, but under any circumstances such consultation should be justifiable and in the interest of the patient only and not for any other consideration.

3.1.2 Consulting pathologists/radiologists or asking for any other diagnostic laboratory investigation should be done judiciously and not in a routine manner.

3.2 ***Consultation for patient's benefit:*** In every consultation, the benefit to the patient is of foremost importance. All physician as engaged in the case should be frank with the patient and his attendants.

3.3 ***Punctuality in consultation:*** Utmost punctuality should be observed by physicians in making themselves available for consultations.

3.4 ***Statement to patient after consultation***

3.4.1 All statements to the patient or his representatives should take place in the presence of the consulting physicians, except as otherwise agreed. The disclosure of the opinion to the patient or his relatives or friends shall rest with the medical attendant.

3.4.2 Differences of opinion should not be divulged unnecessarily but when there is irreconcilable difference of opinion the circumstances should be frankly and impartially explained to the patient or his relatives or friends. It would be open to them to seek further advise as they so desire.

3.5 ***Treatment after consultation:*** No decision should restrain the attending physician from making such subsequent variations in the treatment if any unexpected change occurs, but at the next consultation, reasons for the variations should be discussed/explained. The same privilege, with its obligations, belongs to the consultant when sent for in an emergency during the absence of attending physician. The attending physician may prescribe medicine at any time for the patient, whereas the consultant may prescribe only in case of emergency or as an expert when called for.

3.6 ***Patients referred to specialists:*** When a patient is referred to a specialist by the attending physician, a case summary of the patient should be given to the specialist, who should communicate his opinion in writing to the attending physician.

3.7 ***Fees and other charges***

3.7.1 A physician will clearly display his fees and other charges on the board of his chamber and/or the hospitals he is visiting. Prescription should also make clear if the physician himself dispensed any medicine.

3.7.2 A physician will write his name and designation in full along with registration particulars in his prescription letter head.

Note: In government hospital where the patient load is heavy, the name of the prescribing doctor must be written below his/her signature.

Unethical Acts

A physician will not aid or abet or commit any of the following acts which shall be construed as unethical:

6.1 ***Advertising:***

6.1.1 Soliciting of patients directly or indirectly by a physician, by a group of physicians or by institutions or organizations is unethical. A physician will not make use of his/her (or his/her name) as subject of any form or manner of advertising or publicity through any mode either alone or in conjunction with others which is of such a character as to invite attention to him or to his professional position, skill, qualifications, achievements, attainments, specialities, appointment, associations, affiliations or honours and/ or of such character as would ordinarily result in his self-aggrandizement. A physician will not give to any person, whether for compensation or otherwise, any approval, recommendation, endorsement, certificate report or statement with respect of any drug, medicine, nostrum remedy, surgical, or therapeutic article, apparatus or appliance or any commercial product or article with respect of any propriety, quality or use thereof or any test, demonstration or trial thereof, for use in connection with his name, signature, or photograph in any form or manner of advertising through any mode nor shall he boast of cases, operations, cures or remedies or permit the publication of report thereof through any mode. A medical practitioner is, however, permitted to make a formal announcement in press regarding the following:

- On starting practice.
- On change of type practice
- On changing address
- On temporary absence from duty
- On resumption of another practice
- On succeeding to another practice
- Public declaration of charges.

6.1.2 Printing of self-photograph or any such material of publicity in the letter head or on sign board of the consulting room or any such clinical establishment will be regarded as acts of self-advertisement and unethical conduct on the part of the physician. However, printing of sketches, diagrams, picture of human system shall not be treated as unethical.

6.2 ***Patent and copyright:*** A physician may patent surgical instruments, appliances and medicine or copyright applications, methods and procedures. However, it will be unethical if the benefits of such patents or copyrights are not made available in situations where the interest of large population is involved.

6.3 ***Running an open shop (dispensing of drugs and appliances by physicians):*** A physician should not run an open shop for sale of medicine for dispensing prescriptions prescribed by doctors other than himself or for sale of medical or surgical appliances. It is not unethical for a physician to prescribe or supply drugs, remedies or appliances as long as there is no exploitation of the patient. Drugs prescribed by a physician or brought from the market for a patient should explicitly state the proprietary formulae as well as generic name of the drug.

Rebates and Commission

6.4.1 A physician will not give, solicit or receive nor will he offer to given solicit or receive, any gift, gratuity, commission or bonus in consideration of or return for the referring, recommending or procuring of any patient for medical, surgical or other treatment. A physician will not directly or indirectly, participate in or be a party to act of division, transference, assignment, subordination, rebating, splitting or refunding of any fee for medical, surgical or other treatment.

6.4.2 Provisions of para 6.4.1 shall apply with equal force to the referring, recommending or procuring by a physician or any person, specimen or material for diagnostic purposes or other study/ work. Nothing in this section, however, will prohibit payment of salaries by a qualified physician to other duly qualified person rendering medical care under his supervision.

6.5 ***Secret remedies:*** The prescribing or dispensing by a physician of secret remedial agents of which he does not know the composition, or the manufacture or promotion of their use is unethical and as such prohibited. All the drugs prescribed by a physician should always carry a proprietary formula and clear name.

6.6 ***Human rights:*** The physician will not aid or abet torture nor will he be a party to either infliction of mental or physical trauma or concealment of torture inflicted by some other person or agency in clear violation of human rights.

6.7 ***Euthanasia:*** Practising euthanasia will constitute unethical conduct. However on specific occasion, the question of withdrawing supporting devices to sustain cardiopulmonary function even after brain death, shall be decided only by a team of doctors and not merely by the treating physician alone. A team of doctors shall declare withdrawal of support system. Such team shall consist of the doctor in change of the patient, CMO/MO incharge of the hospital and a doctor nominated by the incharge of the hospital from the hospital staff or in accordance with the provisions of the Transplantation of Human Organ Act, 1994.

Misconduct

The following acts of commission or omission on the part of a physician will constitute professional misconduct rendering him/her liable for disciplinary action:

7.1 Violation of the regulations: If he/she commits any violation of these regulations.

7.2 If he/she does not maintain the medical records of his/her indoor patients for a period of 3 years as per regulation 1.3 and refuses to provide the same within 72 hours when the patient or his/her authorized representative makes a request for it as per the regulation 1.3.2.

7.3 If he/she does not display the registration number accorded to him/her by the State Medical Council or the Medical Council of India in his clinic, prescriptions, certificates, etc. issued by him/her or violates the provisions of regulation.

7.4 **Adultery or improper conduct:** Abuse of professional position by committing adultery or improper conduct with a patient or by maintaining an improper association with a patient will render a physician liable for disciplinary action as provided under the Indian Medical Council Act, 1956 or the concerned State Medical Council Act.

7.5 **Conviction by Court of Law:** Conviction by a court of law for offences involving moral turpitude/criminal acts.

7.6 **Sex determination tests:** On no account sex determination test shall be undertaken with the intent to terminate the life of a female foetus developing in her mother's womb, unless there are other absolute indications for termination of pregnancy as specified in the Medical Termination of Pregnancy Act, 1971. Any Act of termination of pregnancy of normal female foetus amounting to female foeticide shall be regarded as professional misconduct on the part of the physician leading to erasing from panel, besides rendering him liable to criminal proceedings as per the provisions of this Act.

7.7 **Signing professional certificates reports and other documents:** Registered medical practitioners are in certain cases bound by law to give, or may from time to time be called upon or requested to give certificates, notification, reports and other documents of similar character signed by them in their professional capacity for subsequent use in the courts or for administrative purposes, etc.

7.8 A registered medical practitioner will not contravene the provisions of the drugs and cosmetics Act and regulations made thereunder. Accordingly, prescribing steroids/psychotropic drugs when there is no absolute medical indication; selling schedule 'H' and 'L' drugs and poisons to the public except to his patient; in contravention of the above provisions shall constitute gross professional misconduct on the part of the physician.

7.9 Performing or enabling unqualified person to perform an abortion or any illegal operation for which there is no medical, surgical or psychological indication.

7.10 A registered medical practitioner will not issue certificates of efficiency in modern medicine to unqualified or non-medical person.

Note: The foregoing does not restrict the proper training and instruction of bonafide students, midwives, dispensers, surgical attendants, or skilled mechanical and technical assistant and therapy assistants under the personal supervision of physicians.

7.11 A physician should not contribute to the lay press articles and give interviews regarding diseases and treatments which may have the effect of advertising himself or soliciting practices; but is open to write to the lay press under his own name on matters of public health, hygienic living or to deliver public lectures, give talks on the radio/TV/internet chat for the same purpose and send announcement of the same to lay press.

7.12 An institution run by a physician for a particular purpose such as a maternity home, nursing home, private hospital, rehabilitation centre or any type of training institution, etc. may be advertised in the lay press, but such advertisements should not contain anything more than the name of the institution, type of patients admitted, type of training and other facilities offered and the fees.

7.13 It is improper for a physician to use an unusually large sign board and write on it anything other than his name, qualifications obtained from a university or a statutory body, titles and name of his speciality, registration number including the name of the State Medical Council under which registered. The same should be the contents of his prescription papers. It is improper to affix a sign board on a chemist's shop or in places where he does not reside or work.

7.14. The registered medical practitioner will not disclose the secrets of a patient that have been learnt in the exercise of his/her profession except:

- In a court of law under order of the presiding judge;
- In circumstances where there is a serious and identified risk to a specific person and/or community; and
- Notifiable diseases.

In case of communicable/notifiable diseases, concerned public health authorities should be informed immediately.

7.15 The registered medical practitioner will not refuse on religious grounds alone to give assistance in or conduct of sterility, birth control, circumcision and medical termination of pregnancy when there is medical indication, unless the medical practitioner feels himself/herself incompetent to do so.

7.16 Before performing an operation the physician should obtain in writing the consent from the husband or wife, parent or guardian in the case of minor, or the patient himself as the case may be. In an operation which may result in sterility the consent of both husband and wife is needed.

7.17 A registered medical practitioner will not publish photographs or case reports of his/her patients without their permission, in any medical or other journal in a manner by which their identity could be made out. If the identity is not to be disclosed, the consent is not needed.

7.18 In the case of running of a nursing home by a physician and employing assistants to help him/her, the ultimate responsibility rests on the physician.

7.19 A physician will not use touts or agents for procuring patients.

7.20 A physician will not claim to be specialist unless he has a special qualification in that branch.

7.21 No act of *in vitro* fertilization or artificial insemination will be undertaken without the informed consent of the female patient and her spouse as well as the donor. Such consent will be obtained in writing only after the patient is provided, at her own level of comprehension, with sufficient information about the purpose, methods, risks, inconveniences, disappointments of the procedure and possible risks and hazards.

7.22 *Research:* Clinical drug trials or other research involving patients or volunteers as per the guidelines of ICMR can be undertaken, provided ethical considerations are borne in mind. Violation of existing ICMR guidelines in this regard will constitute misconduct. Consent taken from the patient for trial of drug or therapy which is not as per the guidelines will also be construed as misconduct.

7.23 If a physician posted in rural area is found absent on more than two occasions during inspection by the head of the district health authority or the chairman, Zila Parishad, the same will be construed as a misconduct if it is recommended to the Medical Council of India/State Medical Council by the state Government for action under these regulations.

7.24. If a physician posted in a medical college/institution both as teaching faculty or otherwise will remain in hospital/college during the assigned duty hours. If he is found absent on more than two occasions during this period, the same will be construed as a misconduct if it is certified by the principal/medical superintendent and forwarded through the state Government to Medical Council of India/State Medical Council for action under these regulations.

Punishment and Disciplinary Action

8.1–8.6 If the medical practitioner is found to be guilty of committing professional misconduct, the appropriate Medical Council may award such punishment as deemed necessary or may direct the removal altogether or for a specified period, from the register of the name of the delinquent registered practitioner. Deletion from the register will be widely publicized in local press as well as in the publications of different medical association/societies/bodies.

REFERENCES

1 J. Kishore. Dictionary of public health. First (edn), Century Publication, Okhla, New Delhi, 2002.

2 ICMR (1986). Proceedings of International Conference on Health Policy, ethics and human values, ICMR, New Delhi.

3 Medical Council of India. Regulations of Professional Conduct etiquette and ethics published in Health Action; Bombay, May 2005.

RESEARCH

Research simply means, either application of the known scientific advances/evidence to improve the quality of life and to prevent diseases and promote positive health or it could mean gain in new knowledge/evidence for the development of mankind. Both are essential. Putting today's essential health knowledge into practice is a real challenge. Putting health knowledge at the disposal of families and communities for appropriate action is most essential for our country where resources are limited. The department of health research (DHR) was created on 5th October 2007 with the merger of ICMR.

Research can be put into the broad categories:

- ***Fundamental and basic research:*** It is basic research conducted in laboratories to establish a theory which can subsequently be applied in the field. It could be a stepping stone for applied research.
- ***Applied research*** is essentially from laboratory to land/field or community. It means application of essential scientific knowledge for the development of health of community, to promote health, prevent disease, treat

diseases and eradication of diseases of public health significance.

- ***Action-oriented research (AOR)*** is also an applied research wherein the data are collected, analyzed rapidly to ensure an action. Actions are concurrent with the stage of investigation and actions are modified in the existing environments and suiting to the needs of the consumer and moreover actions are user-friendly and flexible to respect the local cultural practices beliefs and faith.
- ***Operational research (OR):*** It means using a strategy or tactic to make the operation successful. Alternate strategies of health care are designed to achieve the results or goals. India is very large country and has lot of diverse culture and no uniform or single strategy or tactic works.

Definition: OR is defined as "Scientific method for providing executive department a quantitative basis for decision-making regarding the operation under control." It is also defined as "the application of scientific methods, techniques and tools to operations of systems with optimum solution to the problem".[1]

Its purpose is to improve the efficiency of health system or working of the system or health teams. The technique of operational research includes network analysis, programme evaluation and review techniques (PERT), critical path analysis, linear programming, computer simulation procedures and application of queuing theory, cost-effective analysis and work study.

Priority Areas in Research in India

The frontiers of medical science are expanding at a phenomenal pace. Priority attention would require to contain and eradicate the existing widely prevalent disease as well as to deal with emerging health problems. The basic objective of medical research and ultimate test of its utility would involve the translation of available know how (translational research) into simple, low cost, easily applicable low cost technologies, devices and interventions thus placing within the reach of health personnel and to the front line health workers and to the community in the remotest corners of the country. Therefore, besides devotion to basic, fundamental, high priority should be given to applied, operational research including action research for continuously improving cost-effective delivery health services.[2–4] Priority helps in correcting 10/90 gap, which relates to the fact that only 10% of funding for global health research is allocated to health problems that affect 90% of the world's population (Global Forum for Research 2009).

Priority Areas

1. Health system research (policy and systems analysis and programme development) should have high priority which includes primary health care, and its different aspects such as information support, manpower development, appropriate technology, management needs assessment, training needs assessment besides communication needs assessment, and community involvement. This essentially includes operation and action oriented research components. The system framework includes: Inputs → Processes → Outputs → Effects → Impacts.
2. Epidemiology is another area of significance. It is necessary to build up an adequate data base for the proper development of the health programmes.
3. Basic science and fundamental research.

Basic research efforts should devote high priority to the discovery and development of more effective treatment and preventive procedures (vaccines for prevention of diseases) in respect of communicable and tropical diseases. Priority areas include HIV/AIDS, blindness, leprosy, tuberculosis, and malaria. Very high priority should be given to contraception research to improve their effectiveness and acceptance and discover new devices. Nutrition is another area of priority. The fast emerging non-communicable diseases (NCDs), coronary heart disease, strokes, diabetes, hypertension, cancer and accidents need a behaviour change or adopting healthy lifestyle. Protection of environments and ensuring safe water and sanitation remain a challenging area for research.

Department of Health Research would aim to increase share of extramural funding from the current 33 to 50% by the end of 12th plan.

Operational Research (OR)[5]

Directly observed treatment and short-course (DOTS) has evolved through years of research—much of it was done in India. Operational research provides programme managers the data and tools they need to analyze and continuously improve the services/system they offer. The goal is to improve the diagnosis and treatment of tuberculosis by translating the results of research into policy and practice. But world class research is not enough. Researchers must make every efforts to ensure that their findings are promptly translated into more rapid and accurate diagnosis and more reliable and effective treatment of TB patient.

DOTS has become the accepted standard for diagnosis, treatment and monitoring of tuberculosis worldwide. The Director General of the World Health Organization declared "The DOTS strategy represent the most important public health breakthrough of the decade in terms of lives which will be saved." But DOTS is not new. In fact, the essential principles of DOTS are a product of India's long and distinguished tradition of tuberculosis operational research.

- National Tuberculosis Institute (NTI) at Bangalore demonstrated the efficacy and feasibility of case detection by *sputum microscopy* and not by X-ray as tool for diagnosis.

- Studies at Tuberculosis Research Centre in Chennai demonstrated the efficiency and safety of *home treatment* of tuberculosis, the effectiveness of *intermittent chemotherapy* (medications were given two or three times a week) and necessity and feasibility of direct observation in the community.
- Thus, use of supervised treatment—now known as directly observed treatment and short-course (DOTS) in which patients are observed taking their anti-tuberculosis treatment, was shown to be essentially in India. Thus, these 3 cardinal principles of DOTS were developed in India after adequate operational research studies and these were adopted the world over and in India by launching Revised National Tuberculosis Control Programme. Cure rate of TB has increased to 86–90% with DOTS strategy.

Other examples of operational researches are:

1 Enhancing coverage and quality of routine immunization, antenatal care, postnatal and neonatal care by integration of health and ICDS system.
2 Joint home visits of AWW and ANM to recognize community needs and effective response.
3 Promotion of institutional deliveries by setting up of delivery rooms (huts) in subcentre and PHCs.
4 Public–private partnership in health care delivery.
5 Devolution of powers to Village Panchayats to manage subcentres.
6 Alternate methods of delivery of ORS packets, vaccines diagnosis and treatment of malaria and contraceptives at village level. Operational research studies have clearly demonstrated that about 50% cases of diarrhoea in the community can be managed by mothers with home-available fluids and the rest can be treated by health guides with ORS and only a few may be required to be referred to the health facility. With the education of mothers for use of HAF and availability of ORS packets with health guides, it is expected that diarrhoea-related mortality in children will be reduced considerably.
7 People's participation in primary health care.
8 Alternate model of adolescent health (teachers to adolescent, adolescent to adolescent).

Action-oriented Research/Action Research[6,7]

It is research for action:

- Promoting use of home-available fluids as a first response by family or mother when acute watery diarrhoea strikes in young children.
  - Continue breastfeeding and feeding during diarrhoea and promotion of use of ORS packets.
  - Avoiding unnecessary antibiotics for treatment of diarrhoea.

  These are examples of action-oriented research. When women groups and mother groups are empowered and well trained by local health workers they themselves effectively respond to first of all to prevent dehydration and deaths due to diarrhoea and early recovery. Most mothers succeeded in preventing diarrhoea. They kept away drugs and doctors and themselves managed the diarrhoea episodes.
- Promotion of sanitary latrines in rural areas: Only 33% of families in rural areas use sanitary latrines and the rest 67% resort to open field defecation. The programme for sanitary latrines in rural areas has not much succeeded. Action-oriented research undertaken in rural setting by non-governmental organizations and UNICEF supported projects has resulted into acceptance and use of sanitary latrines in rural areas.[8,9] Major steps involved in action-oriented research included:
  - Behavioural research to promote the behaviour to use sanitary latrine to avoid excreta-borne diseases.
  - To promote low cost acceptable and affordable latrines requiring least amount of water to flush.
  - To generate demand for sanitary latrines.
  - To involve community and community leaders for popularization of sanitary latrines.

A comprehensive baseline survey on knowledge, attitudes and practices in rural water supply and sanitation was conducted during 1996–1997 by the Indian Institute of Mass Communication, which showed that 55% of those with private latrines were self-motivated. Only 2% of the respondents claimed the existence of subsidy as the major motivating factor, while 54% claimed to have gone in for sanitary latrines due to convenience and privacy. The study also revealed that 51% of the beneficiaries were willing to spend up to ₹ 1000/- to acquire sanitary toilets.

- Keeping in view the above facts, the Central Rural Sanitation Programme which was launched in 1986 moved towards a "demand driven approach". The revised approach in the programme titled "total sanitation campaign (TSC)" now emphasizes more on information, education and communication (IEC), human resource development, capacity development activities to increase awareness and demand generation for sanitary facilities in houses, schools and villages. This approach has enhanced people's capacity to choose appropriate options with beneficiary participation to meet their demands. Subsidy for individual household latrine units has been reduced.[10]

Research-cum-Action (RCA) Project of ICMR

Number of action-oriented research/action research studies were undertaken to develop suitable rural latrines acceptable to people. Action research was directed towards developing suitable designs of latrine—type of latrine, suitable pan and trap, slab or squating plate, pit, cost, quantity of water required for flushing, life of latrine, utilization of contents as manure, sociological factors like existing beliefs, habits and reactions of people of using the latrine and chances of ground water pollution.

The institutes which participated in action research consisted of: The Planning Research and Action Institute (PRAI) Lucknow, Research-cum-Action (RCA) Project in 1956 by Union Ministry of Health with the assistance of Ford Foundation, Central Public Health Engineering Research Institute (Nagpur), WHO Project at Ramanagram (Mysore), and Sanitation wing at Gandhigram (Chennai). RCA did great deal of useful action research on latrines at three centres—Poonamalee (Chennai), Singur (West-Bengal) and Najafgarh (Delhi). One of the outstanding contributions of the RCA Project was the development of suitable engineering design for the rural latrine.[11]

1. As a first step efforts were made to collect all the available latrine designs in the country including PRAI designs and observe the efficiency of performance in the field.
2. On the basis of field observations on their performance, composite and best design was developed towards the end of 1958 and all the observed defects were corrected.
3. Thus, on the basis of critical studies of earlier designs; a new type of latrine was finally developed known as the RCA (Research-cum-Action) type.
4. This design was further tested in all centres of RCA and other field stations in the country and found to be very satisfactory.

RCA latrine is dug well latrine which can be constructed with local resources and technology. It could be a single pit or two pits hand flushed latrine at affordable cost.

Research Methodology

The research methodologies have been discussed under epidemiological studies. Broadly these are:

1. Observational Studies

a. ***Descriptive studies:*** The scientist or investigator observes the occurrence of disease or an event and orients it to time, place and person distribution. The observations made on occurrence could be the first step towards scientific investigation. Observations generate hypothesis. We call this as descriptive method of epidemiology of research study.

b. ***Analytical methods:*** While descriptive method describes the health status or situation (prevalence and incidence) the analytical method focuses on causes and reasons for such situations or status in the population. Analytical methods could be ecological studies, cross-sectional studies (surveys), cohort study and case control studies.

2. Experimental or Intervention Studies

Here results of intervention are evaluated, e.g. drug trial and efficacy of vaccine or other interventions like iodized salt, supplementary nutrition, safe disposal of human excreta. Details of experimental studies have been discussed under epidemiological methods.

Methods of Data Collection

Data on research purposes can be collected by following methods:

1. Observation
2. Interview
3. Examination
4. Investigations (epidemic, surveillance and laboratory)

1. Observations

The investigator makes observations and collects the facts. Observation could lead to community diagnosis. *Examples:* Observation of health practices such as child feeding and rearing practices, excreta disposal practices, safe water storage practices, etc. Similarly, observations on resources available in the community for health work, can be carried out. Quality of services can be judged by observation mostly, one can observe the technique of immunization, antenatal check up, etc. supervisors can observe the work by way of checklist system (structured observations) and can give feedback to managers. Observation is thus a powerful tool to collect evidence or data on research.

Participant Observations

Here the researcher/observer lives with the community for some period and becomes part of that community to understand the behavior/practice and perception of the community members.

2. Interviews

Here the investigator collects data by asking set of questions or by conversation in a friendly manner. Data on client satisfaction and their reactions towards hospitals, primary health centre and doctors or paramedical workers can be obtained by interview technique. Exit interviews, opinion polls and groups interviews are rapid methods of collection of data from users of services or prospective users of services. 24 hours recall method of dietary survey is quite popular to obtain information by interview on the qualitative and quantitative consumption of dietary items/foods. Drawbacks of an interview are recall lapse (memory) and sensitivity level of a question.

Delphi method is also an interview technique where we get opinion or experiences of key informants and experts on the subject. This is the rapid method of collecting data on disease and high risk individuals and risk factors of a disease.

In clinical practice, interview is the most commonly used method. The first and foremost step in diagnosis of disease is asking the chief complaints of the patients and their duration and sequence of events. This is known as history taking. Apart from chief complaints or presenting complaints, we also obtain past history of illness, family history of illness, dietary intakes, dietary habits, food avoided during illness or food preferred during illness. Experienced doctors and experts can conduct interview easily but for a beginner it may be difficult and hence it requires training—retraining or practice.

The quality of information generated by interview depends upon interviewer and interviewee and the sensitivity level of the information. Essential requirements for successful interview are repeated contacts building the confidence and trust of the client, and keeping the information confidential. Health workers and Anganwadi workers are able to obtain information on health/disease events and other relevant information on households and family members by interview technique, because of their intimate contact with the families. Interview information depends upon memory (recall lapse), literacy level of the respondent as also on the sensitivity level of the information. Interview method is least costlier method of data collection and even paramedical health workers or trained investigators can conduct interview. WHO step-wise approach for surveillance of risk factors of non-communicable diseases makes use of interview technique to collect data on socio-demogrphic and behavioural aspects.

3. Health Examination

a. Clinical examination of patient can collect valuable data from patient. Clinical examination is a standard practice to obtain information on physical signs such as enlargement of liver, spleen, heart sounds, murmurs, abnormal breathing, etc.
b. Apart from clinical examination of patient, one can examine the health records maintained at subcentre. Primary health centre or community health centre or hospital to get an information on common diseases, trends of illness, information on fertility and mortality, availability of drug kits A and B as also equipment. This helps to assess the health needs of the community or community diagnosis.

4. Investigations

Apart from epidemic investigation and surveillance data, laboratory data, imaging and other tests provide quantitative data which can be processed to draw valuable information. The laboratory investigations help to confirm the diagnosis or disease condition in the individual or in the community.

Various epidemiological research methods described above are mostly *Quantitative Methods* of research, which collects specific information and facts that can be expressed as numbers, e.g. number of children, number of household with safe water and latrines.

19

Qualitative Methods of Research

The qualitative methods of research are also useful and complementary to quantitative methods of research.

Qualitative methods of research focus on:

a. Attitudes, beliefs and behaviour of persons, e.g. health seeking behaviour in relation to an illness, utilization of health services, dietary preferences, child rearing practices, use of sanitary latrines.
b. Subjects or persons—mainly to understand human behaviour.
c. These methods explore and analyse the "top of mind of a person" or perceptions.
d. These methods use purposive sampling and analyse the perceptions and personality of a person.

There are various methods adopted for data collection in qualitative research. These methods include: Interviewing, conversations, unstructured, semistructured and structured interviews, narratives, participant observation, non-participant observation, projective techniques, focus group discussion, rapid assessment procedures, rapid rural appraisal, sorting and ranking methods, transit walk and case studies. Some of these methods are being discussed below.

Participatory research: Involving local communities themselves in planning the survey and doing the interview to collect information is known as participatory research.

Interview method: The interview can be conducted by asking series of questions, or by group discussion or by focus group discussion with 'key informants'.

a. ***Questionnaire:*** Here the investigator prepares a questionnaire (a set of questions) and arranges these questions in sequential order to elicit the responses from the subjects. The questionnaire can be structured or open ended. Questionnaire method can be quite useful to collect and record information on knowledge, attitudes, beliefs and practices of respondents.

To literate persons, the questionnaire can be mailed or they themselves can fill-up their responses. From illiterate respondents, the responses have to be collected by asking questions in the language and dialect they understand. The responses can be coded for quick analysis by computer.

Likert scale: A scale measuring the degree to which people agree or disagree with a statement; usually on a 3–, 5–, or 7–, point scale. This is most commonly used to assess the attitudes of respondents.

b. ***Group discussion:*** This is a rapid method of collection of information, e.g. *Mahila Swasthya Sangh* group members can choose and discuss a problem and express their views and opinions and can come to consensus for solution of the problem. Group discussion method can be used to assess the community health needs as also Behaviour Change Communication (BCC) needs or needs of specific groups, e.g. needs of pregnant women, lactating mother and young children. AWWs and ANMs commonly conduct mothers meeting and group discussion to elicit community participation and to improve the service delivery.

Focus Group Discussions (FGDs)

Focus group discussions are thematic discussions among small homogenous group of potential programme beneficiaries. It is a method of learning directly from the "clients" in the clients own words, what they think of certain products or why they uphold certain practices and what benefits they hope to experience from both. FGD is a technique adapted from applied psychology to obtain "top of the mind" responses from clients or beneficiaries of the programme. A theme is chosen on the basis of observations made by the workers during their home visits or contact with the clients during mother and child protection sessions or contacts at subcentre or Anganwadi. The theme could be use of ORS to prevent dehydration and deaths in children having diarrhoea or use of home available fluids to prevent dehydration.

Participants in FGD: Their number should be 6–8. They could be young mothers with child under 36 months, whose child has had diarrhoea at sometime in the past. The FGDs are conducted by a moderator and someone takes the notes and analyses the results of discussion. Recruiters recruit the participants. This way consultation of consumers is obtained and right message for right client, at right place and right time is delivered, suited to their need and cultural practices.

FGD method is commonly used in social marketing to popularize a product or service such as contraceptives, ORS, immunizations, etc. Thus, FGD is an extremely valuable research technique and can be used along with other research techniques to collect information directly from the clients on Behaviour Change Communication (BCC) needs.

Projective Methods

Like FGD, projective techniques are also adapted from applied psychology to collect data on perception of individuals or more complex emotional information. The projective tests have been standardized to know the personality of a person. Standard set of pictorials are used and inferences drawn based on established criteria. We can analyse the make-up of a person by these research methods.

Case Study

This method conducts in-depth analysis of a social unit and is widely used for learning purposes and assessing management needs (Management Needs Assessment). Case could be an institution such as functioning of sub-centre or primary health centre or it could be a person such as work schedule or home visit of health worker or it could be a disease event or beneficiary of a programme.[12]

REFERENCES

1 Kishore J. A Dictionary of Public Health 2002. Century Publication, Okhla, New Delhi.
2 GOI. National Health Policy 1983.
3 GOI. Revised National Health Policy. New Delhi: GOI; 2002.
4 ICSSR and ICMR. Health for All—An alternative strategy 1981. Pune: Indian Institute of Education; 1981.
5 WHO. Research for action. Understanding and controlling tuberculosis in India. New Delhi: WHO Regional Office for South-East Asia; 2000.
6 Anand D. Action oriented research for Primary Health care and use of PHC MAP Modules. 1st edn. New Delhi: Sakshi; 1998.
7 AKF. Assessing information needs user's guide. PHC MAP Modules, Washington DC: AKF; 1993.
8 UNICEF, WATSAN India. Rural water supply and environmental sanitation programme. New Delhi: UNICEF, WATSAN India; 2000.
9 GOI. Training of Doctors on Treatment of Diarrhoeal Diseases and Programme Management. National Diarrhoeal Disease Control Programmes, DGHS, MOH and FW, New Delhi. Prepared by NIC and ED (ICMR), Calcutta; GOI.
10 GOI, Central Rural Sanitation Programme (Total Sanitation Campaign) Department of Drinking water supply, Ministry of Rural Development. Government of India, May 2002.
11 ICMR. Review of work done on Rural latrines in India special Report Series No. 54 by TR Bhaskaran, MA Sampath Kumaran (AIIH and PH, Calcutta), ICMR. New Delhi 1966.
12 Lal S. ASHA's Work Plan. Case studies in Health Management. First Edition, June 1987; pp 21–27. NIHFW, New Delhi.

CHAPTER

20

International Health and International Health Regulations

Before the conclusion of the Second World War, some of the important powers decided to set-up an organization for the purpose of more effectively consolidating the forces for order and for the prevention of any likely recrudescence of the unfortunate trends that led to the Second World War. As a result of an appeal by the four great powers Britain, France, USA and the Union of Soviet Socialist Republic, a conference was held in 1945 at San Francisco and an organization called the United Nations emerged therefrom.

It is significant that one of the first acts of the United Nations Organization through its Economic and Social Council was resolution adopted for the constitution of a World Health Organization as one of the specialised agencies of the United Nations. The activities of this organization are now well-known throughout the world and the influence it has exercised on many problems of health in different countries has materially helped in the tackling of some of the major and urgent problems on a global scale.

WORLD HEALTH ORGANIZATION (WHO)

The WHO is one of the specialized agencies of the United Nations and came into being in 1948. This organization has more than 199 member states, which collaborates in the task of achieving the highest possible level of health throughout the world. The WHO deals with problems of health like malaria, cholera, plague, yellow-fever and other communicable and non-communicable diseases which have an international as well as a national impact. Advice and assistance are given to countries requesting for such help in the fields of maternal and child health, nutrition, environmental sanitation, professional education, nursing, health, education of the public, mental health, etc.

The WHO was established on 7th April 1948 and since then 7th April of every year is observed as "World Health Day". The WHO is a non-political, international health organization of United Nations committed to promotion of attainment of highest standard of health by all citizens of the world. Over the years, its membership has grown and it has 199 countries as its members.

The Constitution of the WHO defines "health" as a "state of complete physical, mental and social well-being and not merely the absence of disease or infirmity" and goes on to say that one of the fundamental right of every human being without distinction of race, religion, political belief, etc. is the enjoyment of the highest attainable standard of health. The objective of the WHO being the "attainment by all people, the highest possible level of health", its functions are described interalias as:

Functions of WHO

- It coordinates international health through international health regulations of 1969 which are amended from time to time. New regulations are in place since 2005.
- It collects and disseminates the information on an international notifiable diseases through weekly epidemiological reports; thereby serves as a warning centre for epidemics, and pandemics.
- Helps in establishment of national surveillance system of diseases of public health significance.
- It strives for "Health for All" through primary health care systems.
- It publishes weekly epidemiological reports, world health statistics quarterly, world health statistic annually, world health reports on public health problems.
- For the purpose of uniformity and comparison, WHO has brought out international classification of diseases and gives standard definition of various morbid conditions and events. This system helps to achieve comparison and uniformity in reporting and recording. The latest international classification of diseases (ICD) is ICD-10 which is due for revision.

- It promotes and supports biomedical research at national, regional and international levels. Notably MONICA research on cardiovascular diseases is an example worth citing.
- WHO helps certifies eradication of diseases/disease from a territory-based on established international criteria. It certified eradication of smallpox way back in 1978 and it also certified eradication of guinea worm disease from India in the year 2000. Polio free India Certified by WHO on 27th March, 2014.
- It establishes international reference laboratories for research and identification of emerging diseases.
- It supports the Nations by providing health experts in different fields.
- Supports fellowship programmes.
- Helps/supports eradication of diseases and national health programmes to control diseases of public health significance (communicable and non-communicable).

WHO has established 6 regional offices:

1 South-East Asia with HQ at New Delhi (India).
2 Africa with HQ at Harare (Zimbabwe).
3 The American HQ at Washington DC (USA).
4 Europe HQ at Copenhagen (Denmark).
5 Eastern Mediterranean HQ at Alexandria (Egypt).
6 Western Pacific HQ at Manila (Philippines).

UNITED NATIONS INTERNATIONAL CHILDREN'S EMERGENCY FUND (UNICEF)

The UNICEF is one of the specialized agencies of the United Nations created for the purpose of providing aid, primarily in the fields of health welfare and nutrition of the mothers and children. It works in close cooperation with other specialized agencies of the United Nations like the WHO, FAO and UNESCO. The UNICEF provides and supplies equipment not available within the country when asked for such help. It gives material help for the training of national personnel and technical advice is provided by the WHO and the FAO. Every type of UNICEF assistance has, as its basic purpose—the improvement of maternal and child health.

United Nations International Children's Emergency Fund (UNICEF) was born in 1946 to deal with the problems of children after Second World War; many of them left as orphans and suffered increased morbidity and mortality after war. Though the emergency functions are over it continues to retain its old name UNICEF and the new name is "United Nations Children's Fund".

Functions

It plays the role of advocacy for mother and child and supports the programmes and services for mother and child development all over the world. Initially, it focused its attention on children only and mothers were forgotten. Its concern for mother developed subsequently. Major functions and supports provided in all the areas of women and child development covers the areas of feeding and nutrition, immunization, water and sanitation, education, integrated child development services, programme for adolescent, literacy, integrated management of childhood illness and many welfare programmes. UNICEF supports training, research and service programmes in the area of mother and child.

It provides equipment, machinery and other materials to support the health and development of mothers and children. Salt iodation plants have been set-up with the assistance of UNICEF. The assistance given falls into the following major categories:

1 Basic maternal and child health services including health centres and training of national personnel.
2 Disease control including control and eradication of diseases such as malaria, TB, leprosy, etc. which affect large number of children.
3 Nutrition including supply of milk for child feeding.
4 Social services for children.
5 Emergency aid to mothers in time of disasters—earthquakes, famine, etc.

India, which has undertaken intensive rural health development work by the establishment of primary health centres in collaboration with the community development centres, has received aid from the UNICEF in the shape of technical equipment, midwives and nurses kit, drugs, milk, vitamins, motor vehicles, bicycles, etc.

The major underlying cause of infant and child mortality being malnutrition, the UNICEF has been donating powdered skimmed milk for distribution to infants and children through the maternal and child welfare centres, schools, clinics, etc. They have gone one step forward and have set-up milk conservation plants for the production and distribution of safe milk in larger quantities. Aid for nine dairy plants have also been executed. This has increased production, processing and distribution of pure milk, as *cheaply* as possible. They train the national staff to plan, supervise and carry-out the nutrition programmes. In collaboration with the FAO, the UNICEF is helping to increase the production and consumption of protective foods (applied nutrition programme) besides iodation of salt to control iodine deficiency disorders.

COLOMBO PLAN

The Colombo Plan is cooperative enterprise of member governments of the commonwealth countries in order to further economic and social progress and to make these countries self-reliant. The Colombo Plan has contributed to the higher training of a large number of medical and auxiliary personnel in all fields. The All India Institute of Medical Sciences at Delhi was established with the financial assistance from one of the Colombo Plan countries, viz. New Zealand. The plan provides for visits to countries by experts who can offer advice on local problems and train the local people, and supply of equipment, especially to teaching institutions. Mention may also be made of the contribution by the New Zealand Government of a Dairy Plant to Delhi under the Colombo Plan. The contribution of Canada in supplying cobalt therapy units to medical institutions in India is another important item of aid under the Colombo Plan.

TECHNICAL COOPERATION MISSION (TCM)

The programme commenced in the first year of the first 5-year plan and is based on an agreement signed between the Governments of US and India on the 5th January, 1952, with the view of promoting and accelerating integrated economic development of India. Under this agreement, projects of technical cooperation mutually agreed upon between the two countries are executed. A separate agreement is again signed for each of the projects in question. The schemes are jointly financed by both the governments. The contribution of the TCM is for meeting overseas' costs of equipment and materials, freight exports and training facilities. The US International Cooperation Administration provides the financial assistance for the TCM programmes.

The following projects under the TCM are included in the field of health:

- i Malaria control and malaria eradication.
- ii National water supply and sanitation.
- iii Assistance of medical colleges and allied institutions.
- iv Health institutions training centres.
- v Control of filaria.
- vi Medical education.
- vii General nursing.
- viii Vector-borne disease control.

ROCKEFELLER FOUNDATION

The Rockefeller Foundation has been operating in India from 1920. It began with a scheme for the prevention and control of Hookworm disease in the Madras Presidency. Later the foundation was associated with several health and medical programmes in India. In the beginning the foundation had treated fields of public health and medical education as two separate issues. Since 1951, however, the two have been combined under a single programme with wide objectives.

The establishment of the All India Institute of Hygiene and Public Health at Calcutta was in a large measure due to the cooperation of the Rockefeller Foundation. The foundation's programme included the training of competent teachers and research workers in a certain number of selected medical colleges, training abroad of candidates from India through fellowships and travel grants, research on fundamental health problems and the adoption of research as an integral part of the medical course and the sponsoring of visits of a large number of medical specialists from the USA. Mention should also be made of the establishment of the Virus Research Centre in Pune by the ICMR in collaboration with the Rockefeller Foundation. The foundation has not only provided equipment and supplies, but also provided some of the staff members and facilities for the training of research work on insect-borne viral diseases. The ICMR has been receiving financial aid from the Foundation for the implementation of their fellowship programme for training junior medical teachers in Indian institutions. The Christian Medical College and Hospital at Vellore, The Seth GS Medical College, Bombay, The Christian Medical College, Ludhiana, The K.G. Medical College, Lucknow, are some of the institutions which have been constantly helped by the Rockefeller Foundation over a period of years. Mention should also be made of the contribution of the Rockefeller Foundation to the All India Institute of Medical Sciences, New Delhi, for the purchase of equipment and for construction work. Fellowships and travel grants in the fields of public health, medical education, research, and nursing have been awarded by the Rockefeller Foundation. International Clinical Epidemiology Network (INCLEN) was started by the Rockefeller Foundation to build-up critical mass of researchers in clinical epidemiology.

FORD FOUNDATION

This is another agency from which India has received aid for the implementation of some of its national health programmes. Their contribution has been mainly in the public health field. For instance, the Foundation has helped in the establishment of public health orientation training centres, research-cum-action projects in environmental sanitation, pilot projects in rural services at Gandhigram and the Rural Latrine Programme. The orientation Training Centres at Singur, Poonamallee and Najafgarh provide training courses in public health for doctors, nurses, health visitors, sanitary inspectors, midwives and other public health personnel all over India. The basic public health principles and health education techniques are emphasized in the training of such personnel. The Ford Foundation has also made available a large sum of money to support programmes of education and family planning for the action-cum-research centres.

FOOD AND AGRICULTURE ORGANIZATION (FAO)

The FAO is mostly concerned with the problem of increased food production and banishment of hunger from the face of the earth. Herein comes the nutritional aspect of the people of India and the impairment of health through undernutrition and malnutrition. In this respect, the FAO has been working in close collaboration with other international organizations and with the Ministries of Food and Agriculture and Health through Government of India. The FAO had recommended at its conference in Rome in

1957 that due attention should be paid to the nutritional status of the people while formulating policies of food production in all countries.

COOPERATIVE FOR AMERICAN RELIEF EVERYWHERE (CARE)

The CARE is a non-profit, non-sectarian and non-governmental organization of the United States created in 1946 with the primary objective of sending food from American donors to people of war-devastated Europe. Today this organization serves many countries and supplies food packages and kits for use in vocational training, agriculture, health and education programmes. Mid-day school meal programme in India was supported by CARE.

WORLD BANK

World Bank assists the developing countries to improve the quality of life by advancing loans. The areas/domain where World Bank has provided assistance include: education, control of communicable diseases, water supply and sanitation, communication, population control, malaria, and HIV/AIDS. Notably in India roll back malaria kala-azar, IDSP, RCH programme, blindness control and construction of roads have been supported by World Bank apart from state health systems development projects to improve secondary health care.

DEPARTMENT FOR INTERNATIONAL DEVELOPMENT (DFID)

This is the bilateral agency of United Kingdom (UK). In India, this organization has supported the programme on reproductive and child health, financing of National Family Health Survey-3 as also Revised National Tuberculosis Control Programme phase-2, besides HIV/AIDS, and polio eradication. Globally, it works for elimination of world poverty, illiteracy and gender inequality.

UNITED NATIONS POPULATION FUNDS (UNFPA)

The UNFPA assisted 6th Country Programme (CP-6). It supports the programme activities on reproductive health, population and development strategies and advocacy in India. The four complementary interventions included in CP-6 were: HIV/AIDS, adolescent health, gender issues and monitoring through result based programming.

UNITED STATES AGENCY FOR INTERNATIONAL DEVELOPMENT (USAID)

This agency supports the innovations in family-planning services (IFPS) project in Uttar Pradesh and now extended to Uttarakhand and Jharkhand. The project includes reproductive health, child survival and HIV/AIDS with emphasis on increasing public/private partnership, catalytic role for technical assistance, integrated client centred services and sustainability.

INTERNATIONAL RED CROSS SOCIETY (IRCS)

It works on the principle of "Peace through humanity". The primary activities of IRCS are, evacuation of war casualities, disaster relief, promotion of voluntary blood donation and collection of blood for transfusion, maternity and child welfare, medical relief and rehabilitation, community services, ambulance and nursing services, and training courses in first aid/rescue operations, promotion of junior/youth red cross, establishment of working women hostels, homes for aged and mentally retarded, and destitutes apart from HIV/AIDS prevention programme. This is the largest humanitarian organization which strives towards the creation of better society.

DANISH INTERNATIONAL DEVELOPMENT AGENCY (DANIDA)

This agency has supported the National Blindness Control Programme in India in terms of development and training of manpower, funding equipment and material apart from establishment of district blindness societies. Another thrust area of DANIDA is poverty reduction in developing nations.

INTERNATIONAL HEALTH REGULATIONS (IHR)

The purpose of the International Health Regulations, adopted by the World Health Assembly in 1969, is to help prevent the international spread of diseases, and in the context of international travel, to do so with the minimum of inconvenience to the passenger. This requires international collaboration in the detection, reduction and elimination of the sources from which infection spreads rather than attempts to prevent the introduction of disease by legalistic barriers that over the years have proved to be ineffective. Ultimately, however, the risk of an infective agent becoming established in a country is determined by the quality of the **national epidemiological services**, and in particular, by the day-to-day national health and disease surveillance activities and the ability to implement prompt and effective control measures.[1]

No regulations can be expected to foresee every disease eventuality, and in certain situations, diseases and conditions other than those covered by the International Health Regulations may be of concern to national health authorities and the travelling public. The International Health Regulations obviously cannot refer specifically to diseases that were not known at the time they were last revised; this is the case with acquired immunodeficiency syndrome (AIDS) and SARS (severe acute respiratory syndrome). Nevertheless, any requirement of an HIV antibody test certificate (AIDS-free certificate) is contrary to the regulations.

International Vaccination Requirements

Smallpox

The eradication of smallpox was confirmed by WHO nearly 38 years ago (1978). Smallpox vaccination is no longer indicated, and may be dangerous to those who are vaccinated and those in close contact with them.

Plague

- Vaccination against plague shall not be required as a condition of admission of any person to a territory.
- For the purposes of these regulations, the incubation period of plague is 6 days for quantine purpose.

Cholera

Vaccination against cholera cannot prevent the introduction of the infection into a country. The World Health Assembly therefore, amended the International Health Regulations in 1973 so that cholera vaccination should no longer be required of any traveller.

The traditional parenteral cholera vaccine conveys incomplete, unreliable protection of short duration and its use is, therefore, not recommended (WHO-official record no. 209, 1973). For the purpose of these regulations, the incubation period for cholera is 5 days.

Yellow-fever Vaccination Certificate

Urban and jungle yellow-fever occurs only in parts of Africa and South America. Urban yellow-fever is an epidemic viral disease of humans transmitted from infected to susceptible persons by the *Aedes aegypti* mosquito. Jungle yellow-fever is an enzootic viral disease transmitted among non-human primate hosts, and occasionally to humans, by a variety of mosquito vectors.

For the purpose of these regulations, the incubation period of yellow fever is 6 days.

A yellow-fever vaccination certificate is now the only certificate that should be required in international travel, and that only for a limited number of travellers.

Many countries require a valid international certificate of vaccination from travellers arriving from infected areas or from countries with infected areas, or who have been in transit. Although there is no epidemiological justification for this latter requirement, which is clearly in excess of the International Health Regulations, travellers may find that it is strictly enforced, particularly for people arriving in Asia from Africa or South America.

On the other hand, vaccination is strongly recommended for travel outside the urban areas of countries in the yellow-fever endemic zone, even if these countries have not officially reported the disease and do not require evidence of vaccination on entry.

The vaccination has almost total efficacy, while the case-fatality rate for the disease is more than 60% in adults who are not immune. Tolerance of the present vaccine is excellent. The only contraindication to its use, apart from true allergy to egg protein, is cellular immunodeficiency (congenital or acquired, the latter sometimes being only temporary).

The period of validity of an international certificate of vaccination against yellow-fever is 10 years, beginning 10 days after vaccination. If a person is revaccinated before the end of this period, the validity is extended for a further 10 years from the date of revaccination. If the revaccination is recorded on a new certificate, travellers are advised to retain the old certificate for 10 days until the new certificate becomes valid.

20

Meningococcal vaccine—for Haj pilgrims.

GLOBAL HEALTH SECURITY

International Health Regulations (IHR) May, 2005

The purpose of the revision of IHR is to develop regulations that are adapted to the present volume of international traffic and trade and take account of current trends in the epidemiology of communicable diseases, including emerging disease threats.

IHR have been revised in May 2005 and have come into effect from June 2007. The revision and updating of IHR on global health security, epidemic alert and global public health response to natural occurrence, accidental release or deliberate use of biological and chemical agents or radionuclear material that affect health, has enlarged the scope of public health emergencies to be notified to the WHO for rapid response (*see* Flowchart 20.1). Major uses of IHR are:

- IHR is the key global instrument for protection against the international spread of diseases.[2]
- IHR encourages the nations to establish effective surveillance system and build capacity at various levels.
- Ensures prompt notification of events that may constitute public health emergency of international concern, to WHO within 24 hours.
- Provides appropriate public health emergency response.

In each country, the national focal point has been established. In India, National Centre for Disease Control (NCDC) has been identified as national focal Point for IHR. Toll free telephone no. 1075 is set-up to encourage lay reporting to health authorities for recognition and response to an unusual event or outbreak. Rapid response teams (RRTs) have since been constituted at national level and checklist for Central Rapid Response Teams for disease outbreak investigations have been prepared.[3]

Core Capacity Requirements for Surveillance and Response

1. At the Local Community Level and/or Primary Public Health Response Level

Capacities

a To detect events involving disease or deaths above expected levels for the particular time and place in all areas within the territory of the state.

b To report all available information to appropriate level of health care response.

c To implement preliminary control measures.

2. At the Intermediate Public Health Response Levels

Capacities

a To confirm the status of reported events and to support or implement additional control measures.

Flowchart 20.1: Decision instrument for the assessment and notification of events that may constitute a public health emergency of international concern

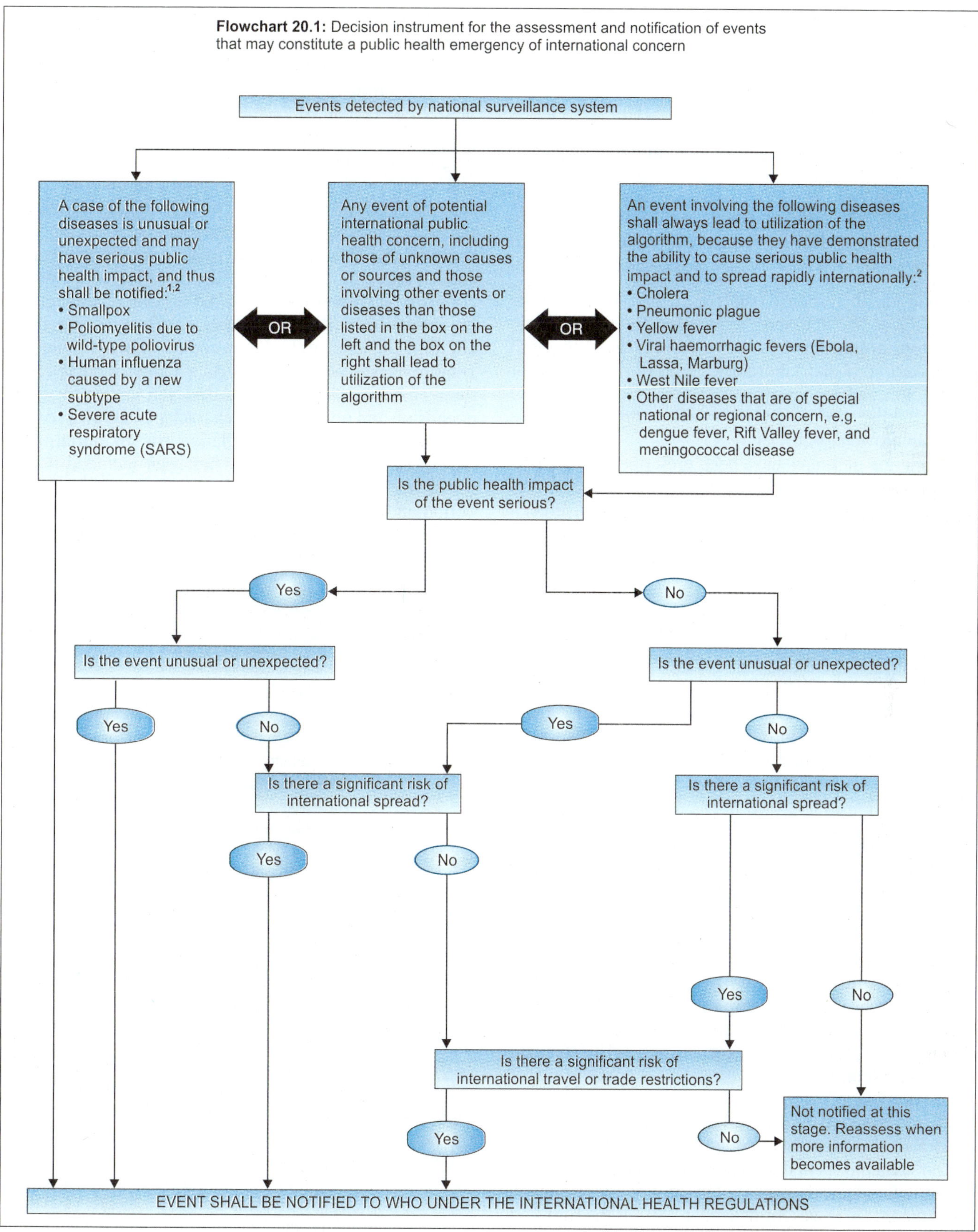

[1] As per WHO case definitions.

[2] The disease list shall be used only for the purposes of these regulations.

b To assess reported events immediately and, if found urgent, to report all essential information to national level. The criteria for urgent events include serious public health impact and/or unusual or unexpected nature with high potential for spread.

3. At National Level—Assessment and Notification

Capacities

a To assess all reports of urgent events within 48 hours.
b To notify to WHO immediately through the national focal point for IHR.

Public health response, **the capacities:** To determine rapidly the control measures required to prevent domestic and international spread, to provide support through specialized staff and laboratory, rapid dissemination of information and recommendations received from WHO and to establish, operate and maintain emergency response plan (*see* Flowchart 20.1).

Quarantine measures have been prescribed under IHR. Specific measures for vector-borne diseases like disinsecting, derating, disinfection of aircraft and ship have been specified and similarly core capacity requirements for airports, ports and ground crossing have been laid out.

REFERENCES

1. WHO. International Health Regulations. 3rd annotated ed. Geneva: WHO; 1969.
2. WHO. International Health Regulations (2005) Second Edition.
3. GOI. NICD, DGHS, MOH and FW—Checklist for Central Rapid. Response Team for disease outbreak investigation including Avian Influenza, 2005.

INTERNATIONAL STATISTICAL CLASSIFICATION OF DISEASES AND RELATED HEALTH PROBLEMS (ICD-10)

A classification of diseases may be defined as a system of categories to which morbid entities are assigned according to some established criteria. ICD is used to translate diagnoses of disease and cause of death from words into an alphanumeric code which permits easy storage, retrieval and analysis of data. ICD-10 accepted as a WHO standard came into effect from 1993.

The purpose of international classification of diseases (ICD) is to compare the disease burden with different areas, states and countries and to compare the disease burden over different time period within the same country. This helps to plan and evaluate the impact of health services and health programmes.[1] ICD was formalized in 1893 as the Bertillon classification or international list of causes of death.

The 10th revision of international statistical classification of diseases and related health problem is the latest in the series (ICD-10).

ICD-10 contains XXI chapters or major groups of diseases, which are shown in Table 20.1.

Each chapter has categories and subcategories and blocks. **The main innovations of ICD 10th revision:** It replaces *numerical system* of coding frame with *alphanumeric* coding frame. Chapters have been assigned a unique letter or group of letters, each capable of providing 100 three character categories. It uses an alphanumeric coding scheme of one letter followed by two or three numbers at the three character categories and four character categories respectively. This has resulted in large coding frame and a stable coding frame (doubling the size of coding frame in comparison with 9th revision). Of 26 available letters, 25 have been used, the letter U being left vacant for future addition and changes and to accommodate new emerging conditions between revisions. As a matter of policy, some three character categories had been left vacant for future expansion and revision. Four character categories (A00.0) are optional. Four special tabulation lists for mortality and one special list for morbidity has been included in 10th revision.[2] The ICD is revised at an interval of 10 years period and accordingly ICD-10 which came into force in Jan 1993 was due for its revision in 2003. International form of medical certificate of cause of death is mandatory.

Table 20.1: XXI chapters of ICD-10

Chapter no.	*Nomenclature of chapters*
I	Certain infectious and parasitic diseases
II	Neoplasms
III	Diseases of blood and blood forming organs and certain disorders involving the immune mechanism
IV	Endocrine, nutritional and metabolic diseases
V	Mental and behavioral disorders
VI	Diseases of nervous system
VII	Diseases of eye and adnexa
VIII	Diseases of the ear and mastoid process
IX	Diseases of the circulatory system
X	Diseases of the respiratory system
XI	Diseases of the digestive system
XII	Diseases of the skin and subcutaneous tissues
XIII	Diseases of the musculoskeletal system and connective tissue
XIV	Diseases of the genitourinary system
XV	Pregnancy, childbirth and puerperium
XVI	Certain conditions originating in perinatal period
XVII	Congenital malformations, deformities and chromosomal abnormalities
XVIII	Symptoms, signs and abnormal clinical and laboratory findings, not elsewhere classified
XIX	Injury, poisoning and certain other consequences of external causes
XX	External causes of morbidity and mortality
XXI	Factors influencing health status and contact with health services

Serial No. of chapter	Nomenclature of chapter	Letter/letters assigned
Chapter I	Certain infectious and parasitic diseases	(A00–B99)
Block	Intestinal infectious diseases	A00–A09
	A00	Cholera
	A01	Typhoid and paratyphoid fevers
	:	
	:	
	:	
	A09	Diarrhoea and gastro-enteritis of presumed infectious origin
	A10-A11-A12-A13-A14-left vaccant for future expansion	
Block	Tuberculosis	(A15–A19)

INTERNATIONAL FORM OF MEDICAL CERTIFICATE OF CAUSE OF DEATH

Cause of death		Approximate interval between onset and death
I		
Disease or condition directly leading to death*	(a) .... due to (or as a consequence of)	....
Antecedent causes		
Morbid conditions, if any, giving rise to the above cause, stating the underlying condition last	(b) .... due to (or as a consequence of)	....
	(c) .... due to (or as a consequence of)	....
	(d) .... due to (or as a consequence of)	
II		
Other significant conditions contributing to the death, but not related to the disease or condition causing it	....	....

* This does not mean the mode of dying, e.g. heart failure, respiratory failure. It means the disease, injury, or complication that caused death.

Causes of Death

The causes of death to be entered on the medical certificate of cause of death are all those diseases, morbid conditions or injuries, which either resulted in or contributed to death and the circumstances of the accident or violence, which produced any such injuries. Death certificates are the main source of mortality data.

Underlying Cause of Death

The underlying cause of death is defined as:

- a Disease or injury which initiated the train of morbid events leading directly to death.
- b "The circumstances of the accident or violence which produced the fatal injury."

Underlying cause of death is used for tabulation purpose.

Example

A 67-year male admitted with retention of urine died of uraemia in the hospital. The chain of events followed were:

- a Uraemia
- b Hydronephrosis
- c Retention of urine
- d Hypertrophy of prostate
  1. The immediate cause of death in this case is uraemia and underlying cause of death was hypertrophy of prostate.
  2. Other significant conditions contributing to death: Old age.

REFERENCES

1. WHO. International Classification of Diseases 1975 Revision, Volume 1, ICD-9. Geneva: World Health Organization; 1977.
2. WHO. International Statistical Classification of Diseases and Related Health Conditions. Tenth Revision Volume 2, ICD-10. Geneva: WHO.

Index